PROFESSIONAL EDITION

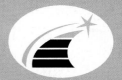

2017
ICD-10-PCS

INCLUDES NETTER'S ANATOMY ART

Carol J. Buck
MS, CPC, CCS-P

Former Program Director
Medical Secretary Programs
Northwest Technical College
East Grand Forks, Minnesota

D1401297

ELSEVIER

ELSEVIER

3251 Riverport Lane
St. Louis, Missouri 63043

2017 ICD-10-PCS PROFESSIONAL EDITION

ISBN: 978-0-323-43118-7

Notice

Knowledge and best practice in this field are constantly changing. As new research and experience broaden our understanding, changes in research methods, professional practices, or medical treatment may become necessary.

Practitioners and researchers must always rely on their own experience and knowledge in evaluating and using any information, methods, compounds, or experiments described herein. In using such information or methods they should be mindful of their own safety and the safety of others, including parties for whom they have a professional responsibility.

With respect to any drug or pharmaceutical products identified, readers are advised to check the most current information provided (i) on procedures featured or (ii) by the manufacturer of each product to be administered, to verify the recommended dose or formula, the method and duration of administration, and contraindications. It is the responsibility of practitioners, relying on their own experience and knowledge of their patients, to make diagnoses, to determine dosages and the best treatment for each individual patient, and to take all appropriate safety precautions.

To the fullest extent of the law, neither the Publisher nor the authors, contributors, or editors, assume any liability for any injury and/or damage to persons or property as a matter of products liability, negligence or otherwise, or from any use or operation of any methods, products, instructions, or ideas contained in the material herein.

Library of Congress Cataloging-in-Publication Data

Names: Buck, Carol J., author.
Title: 2017 ICD-10-PCS / Carol J. Buck.
Other titles: ICD-10-PCS (Professional edition)
Description: Professional edition. | St. Louis, Missouri : Elsevier, [2017]
|
    "Includes Netter's anatomy art." | Includes index. | Preceded by: 2016
    ICD-10-PCS / Carol J. Buck. Professional edition. 2016.
Identifiers: LCCN 2016016065 | ISBN 9780323431187 (pbk.)
Subjects: | MESH: International statistical classification of diseases and
    related health problems. 10th revision. Procedure coding system. |
    Disease--classification | International Classification of Diseases |
    Medical Records | Forms and Records Control--methods
Classification: LCC RB115 | NLM WB 15 | DDC 616.001/2--dc23 LC record available
    at https://lccn.loc.gov/2016016065

Director, Private Sector Education & Professional/References: Jeanne R. Olson
Content Development Manager: Luke Held
Associate Content Development Specialist: Anna Miller
Publishing Services Manager: Jeffrey Patterson
Project Manager: Lisa A. P. Bushey
Design Manager: Julia Dummitt

Printed in United States of America

Last digit is the print number: 9   8   7   6   5   4   3   2

Working together
to grow libraries in
developing countries

www.elsevier.com • www.bookaid.org

DEDICATION

To all the brave medical coders who transitioned the nation into a new coding system.
Decades of waiting finally concluded with the implementation of I-10,
and you have been the pioneers leading the way.

With greatest appreciations for your efforts!

Carol J. Buck, MS, CPC, CCS-P

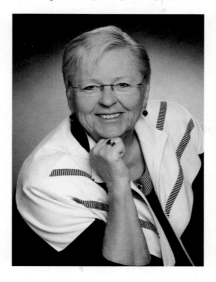

DEVELOPMENT OF THIS EDITION

Query Team

Patricia Cordy Henricksen, MS, CHCA, CPC-I, CPC, CCP-P, ASC-PM
Auditing and Coding Educator
Soterion Medical Services
Lexington, Kentucky

Jackie L. Grass, CPC
Coding and Reimbursement Specialist
Grand Forks, North Dakota

Kathleen Buchda, CPC, CPMA
Revenue Recognition
New Richmond, Wisconsin

Elsevier/MC Strategies Revenue Cycle, Coding and Compliance Staff

"Experts in providing e-learning on revenue cycle, coding and compliance."

Deborah Neville, RHIA, CCS-P
Director

Lynn-Marie D. Wozniak, MS, RHIT
Content Manager

Sandra L. Macica, MS, RHIA, CCS, ROCC
Content Manager

Editorial Consultant

Jenna Price, CPC-A
President
Price Editorial Services, LLC
St. Louis, Missouri

CONTENTS

SYMBOLS AND CONVENTIONS

Annotated

Throughout the manual, revisions, additions, and deleted codes or words are indicated by the following symbols:

New and revised content from the previous edition are indicated by green font.

deleted **Deleted:** Deletions from the previous edition are struck through.

ICD-10-PCS Table Symbols

Throughout the manual information is indicated by the following symbols:

♀♂ **Sex conflict:** *Definitions of Medicare Code Edits* (MCE) detects inconsistencies between a patient's sex and any diagnosis or procedure on the patient's record. For example, a male patient with cervical cancer (diagnosis) or a female patient with a prostatectomy (procedure). In both instances, the indicated diagnosis or the procedure conflicts with the stated sex of the patient. Therefore, either the patient's diagnosis, procedure, or sex is presumed to be incorrect.

 Non-covered: There are some procedures for which Medicare does not provide reimbursement. There are also procedures that would normally not be reimbursed by Medicare but due to the presence of certain diagnoses are reimbursed.

 Limited Coverage: For certain procedures whose medical complexity and serious nature incur extraordinary associated costs, Medicare limits coverage to a portion of the cost.

DRG Non-OR A **non-operating room procedure that does affect MS-DRG assignment** is indicated by a purple highlight.

Non-OR A **non-operating room procedure that does not affect MS-DRG assignment** is indicated by a yellow highlight.

⊡ **Combination:** Certain combinations of procedures are treated differently than their constituent codes.

 Hospital-Acquired Condition: Some procedures are always associated with Hospital Acquired Conditions (HAC) according to the MS-DRG.

Coding Clinic: American Hospital Association's *Coding Clinic®* citations provide reference information to official ICD-10-PCS coding advice.

OGCR The *Official Guidelines for Coding and Reporting* symbol includes the placement of a portion of a guideline as that guideline pertains to the code by which it is located. The complete OGCR are located in the Introduction.

[ ] Brackets below the tables enclose the alphanumeric options for Non-covered, Limited Coverage, DRG Non-OR, Non-OR, and HAC.

Note: The final FY2017 MS-DRG and Medicare Code Edits were unavailable at the time of printing, therefore the proposed FY2017 MS-DRG and Medicare Code Edits were used in this text. Please check codingupdates.com for the final FY2017 MS-DRG and MCE information.

GUIDE TO THE 2017 UPDATES

ICD-10-PCS Tables that have changed this year are shown in table format in the pages below.

SECTION: Ø **MEDICAL AND SURGICAL**
BODY SYSTEM: 2 HEART AND GREAT VESSELS
OPERATION: 1 **BYPASS:** Altering the route of passage of the contents of a tubular body part

	Body Part	Approach	Device	Qualifier
FY2017	Ø Coronary Artery, One Artery 1 Coronary Artery, Two Arteries 2 Coronary Artery, Three Arteries 3 Coronary Artery, Four or More Arteries	Ø Open	8 Zooplastic Tissue 9 Autologous Venous Tissue A Autologous Arterial Tissue J Synthetic Substitute K Nonautologous Tissue Substitute	3 Coronary Artery 8 Internal Mammary, Right 9 Internal Mammary, Left C Thoracic Artery F Abdominal Artery W Aorta
Revise to	Ø Coronary Artery, One Artery 1 Coronary Artery, Two Arteries 2 Coronary Artery, Three Arteries 3 Coronary Artery, Four or More Arteries	Ø Open	Z No Device	3 Coronary Artery 8 Internal Mammary, Right 9 Internal Mammary, Left C Thoracic Artery F Abdominal Artery
Revise to	Ø Coronary Artery, One Artery 1 Coronary Artery, Two Arteries 2 Coronary Artery, Three Arteries 3 Coronary Artery, Four or More Arteries	3 Percutaneous	4 Drug-eluting Intraluminal Device D Intraluminal Device	4 Coronary Vein
Revise to	Ø Coronary Artery, One Artery 1 Coronary Artery, Two Arteries 2 Coronary Artery, Three Arteries 3 Coronary Artery, Four or More Arteries	4 Percutaneous Endoscopic	4 Drug-eluting Intraluminal Device D Intraluminal Device	4 Coronary Vein
FY2017	Ø Coronary Artery, One Artery 1 Coronary Artery, Two Arteries 2 Coronary Artery, Three Arteries 3 Coronary Artery, Four or More Arteries	4 Percutaneous Endoscopic	8 Zooplastic Tissue 9 Autologous Venous Tissue A Autologous Arterial Tissue J Synthetic Substitute K Nonautologous Tissue Substitute	3 Coronary Artery 8 Internal Mammary, Right 9 Internal Mammary, Left C Thoracic Artery F Abdominal Artery W Aorta
Revise to	Ø Coronary Artery, One Artery 1 Coronary Artery, Two Arteries 2 Coronary Artery, Three Arteries 3 Coronary Artery, Four or More Arteries	4 Percutaneous Endoscopic	Z No Device	3 Coronary Artery 8 Internal Mammary, Right 9 Internal Mammary, Left C Thoracic Artery F Abdominal Artery
FY2017	6 Atrium, Right	Ø Open 4 Percutaneous Endoscopic	8 Zooplastic Tissue 9 Autologous Venous Tissue A Autologous Arterial Tissue J Synthetic Substitute K Nonautologous Tissue Substitute	P Pulmonary Trunk Q Pulmonary Artery, Right R Pulmonary Artery, Left

SECTION: Ø MEDICAL AND SURGICAL
BODY SYSTEM: 2 HEART AND GREAT VESSELS
OPERATION: 1 BYPASS: Altering the route of passage of the contents of a tubular body part

Body Part	Approach	Device	Qualifier
7 Atrium, Left V Superior Vena Cava	Ø Open 4 Percutaneous Endoscopic	8 Zooplastic Tissue 9 Autologous Venous Tissue A Autologous Arterial Tissue J Synthetic Substitute K Nonautologous Tissue Substitute Z No Device	P Pulmonary Trunk Q Pulmonary Artery, Right R Pulmonary Artery, Left S Pulmonary Vein, Right T Pulmonary Vein, Left U Pulmonary Vein, Confluence
K Ventricle, Right L Ventricle, Left	Ø Open 4 Percutaneous Endoscopic	8 Zooplastic Tissue 9 Autologous Venous Tissue A Autologous Arterial Tissue J Synthetic Substitute K Nonautologous Tissue Substitute	P Pulmonary Trunk Q Pulmonary Artery, Right R Pulmonary Artery, Left
P Pulmonary Trunk Q Pulmonary Artery, Right R Pulmonary Artery, Left	Ø Open 4 Percutaneous Endoscopic	8 Zooplastic Tissue 9 Autologous Venous Tissue A Autologous Arterial Tissue J Synthetic Substitute K Nonautologous Tissue Substitute Z No Device	A Innominate Artery B Subclavian D Carotid
W Thoracic Aorta, Descending X Thoracic Aorta, Ascending/Arch	Ø Open 4 Percutaneous Endoscopic	8 Zooplastic Tissue 9 Autologous Venous Tissue A Autologous Arterial Tissue J Synthetic Substitute K Nonautologous Tissue Substitute Z No Device	B Subclavian D Carotid P Pulmonary Trunk Q Pulmonary Artery, Right R Pulmonary Artery, Left

FY2017 (marked beside each body part row)

SECTION: Ø MEDICAL AND SURGICAL
BODY SYSTEM: 2 HEART AND GREAT VESSELS
OPERATION: 4 CREATION: Putting in or on biological or synthetic material to form a new body part that to the extent possible replicates the anatomic structure or function of an absent body part

Body Part	Approach	Device	Qualifier
F Aortic Valve	Ø Open	7 Autologous Tissue Substitute 8 Zooplastic Tissue J Synthetic Substitute K Nonautologous Tissue Substitute	J Truncal Valve
G Mitral Valve J Tricuspid Valve	Ø Open	7 Autologous Tissue Substitute 8 Zooplastic Tissue J Synthetic Substitute K Nonautologous Tissue Substitute	2 Common Atrioventricular Valve

FY2017

SECTION: Ø MEDICAL AND SURGICAL

BODY SYSTEM: 2   HEART AND GREAT VESSELS

OPERATION: 5 **DESTRUCTION:** Physical eradication of all or a portion of a body part by the direct use of energy, force, or a destructive agent

FY2Ø17

Body Part	Approach	Device	Qualifier
4 Coronary Vein 5 Atrial Septum 6 Atrium, Right 7 Atrium, Left 8 Conduction Mechanism 9 Chordae Tendineae D Papillary Muscle F Aortic Valve G Mitral Valve H Pulmonary Valve J Tricuspid Valve K Ventricle, Right L Ventricle, Left M Ventricular Septum N Pericardium P Pulmonary Trunk Q Pulmonary Artery, Right R Pulmonary Artery, Left S Pulmonary Vein, Right T Pulmonary Vein, Left V Superior Vena Cava W Thoracic Aorta, Descending X Thoracic Aorta, Ascending/Arch	Ø Open 3 Percutaneous 4 Percutaneous Endoscopic	Z No Device	Z No Qualifier

SECTION: Ø MEDICAL AND SURGICAL

BODY SYSTEM: 2   HEART AND GREAT VESSELS

OPERATION: 7 **DILATION:** *(on multiple pages)*
Expanding an orifice or the lumen of a tubular body part

Body Part	Approach	Device	Qualifier
Ø Coronary Artery, One Artery 1 Coronary Artery, Two Arteries 2 Coronary Artery, Three Arteries 3 Coronary Artery, Four or More Arteries	Ø Open 3 Percutaneous 4 Percutaneous Endoscopic	4 Drug-eluting Intraluminal Device 5 Intraluminal Device, Drug-eluting, Two 6 Intraluminal Device, Drug-eluting, Three 7 Intraluminal Device, Drug-eluting, Four or More D Intraluminal Device E Intraluminal Device, Two F Intraluminal Device, Three G Intraluminal Device, Four or More T Radioactive Intraluminal Device Z No Device	6 Bifurcation Z No Qualifier
F Aortic Valve G Mitral Valve H Pulmonary Valve J Tricuspid Valve K Ventricle, Right P Pulmonary Trunk Q Pulmonary Artery, Right S Pulmonary Vein, Right T Pulmonary Vein, Left V Superior Vena Cava W Thoracic Aorta, Descending X Thoracic Aorta, Ascending/Arch	Ø Open 3 Percutaneous 4 Percutaneous Endoscopic	4 Drug-eluting Intraluminal Device D Intraluminal Device Z No Device	Z No Qualifier

FY2Ø17

FY2Ø17

SECTION: Ø MEDICAL AND SURGICAL
BODY SYSTEM: 2 HEART AND GREAT VESSELS
OPERATION: **B EXCISION:** Cutting out or off, without replacement, a portion of a body part

FY2Ø17

Body Part	Approach	Device	Qualifier
4 Coronary Vein 5 Atrial Septum 6 Atrium, Right 8 Conduction Mechanism 9 Chordae Tendineae D Papillary Muscle F Aortic Valve G Mitral Valve H Pulmonary Valve J Tricuspid Valve K Ventricle, Right L Ventricle, Left M Ventricular Septum N Pericardium P Pulmonary Trunk Q Pulmonary Artery, Right R Pulmonary Artery, Left S Pulmonary Vein, Right T Pulmonary Vein, Left V Superior Vena Cava W Thoracic Aorta, Descending X Thoracic Aorta, Ascending/Arch	Ø Open 3 Percutaneous 4 Percutaneous Endoscopic	Z No Device	X Diagnostic Z No Qualifier

SECTION: Ø MEDICAL AND SURGICAL
BODY SYSTEM: 2 HEART AND GREAT VESSELS
OPERATION: **C EXTIRPATION:** Taking or cutting out solid matter from a body part

FY2Ø17

FY2Ø17

Body Part	Approach	Device	Qualifier
Ø Coronary Artery, One Artery 1 Coronary Artery, Two Arteries 2 Coronary Artery, Three Arteries 3 Coronary Artery, Four or More Arteries	Ø Open 3 Percutaneous 4 Percutaneous Endoscopic	Z No Device	6 Bifurcation Z No Qualifier
4 Coronary Vein 5 Atrial Septum 6 Atrium, Right 7 Atrium, Left 8 Conduction Mechanism 9 Chordae Tendineae D Papillary Muscle F Aortic Valve G Mitral Valve H Pulmonary Valve J Tricuspid Valve K Ventricle, Right L Ventricle, Left M Ventricular Septum N Pericardium P Pulmonary Trunk Q Pulmonary Artery, Right R Pulmonary Artery, Left S Pulmonary Vein, Right T Pulmonary Vein, Left V Superior Vena Cava W Thoracic Aorta, Descending X Thoracic Aorta, Ascending/Arch	Ø Open 3 Percutaneous 4 Percutaneous Endoscopic	Z No Device	Z No Qualifier

SECTION: Ø MEDICAL AND SURGICAL
BODY SYSTEM: 2 HEART AND GREAT VESSELS
OPERATION: H INSERTION: Putting in a nonbiological appliance that monitors, assists, performs, or prevents a physiological function but does not physically take the place of a body part

	Body Part	Approach	Device	Qualifier
FY2Ø17	4 Coronary Vein 6 Atrium, Right 7 Atrium, Left K Ventricle, Right L Ventricle, Left	Ø Open 3 Percutaneous 4 Percutaneous Endoscopic	Ø Monitoring Device, Pressure Sensor 2 Monitoring Device 3 Infusion Device D Intraluminal Device J Cardiac Lead, Pacemaker K Cardiac Lead, Defibrillator M Cardiac Lead N Intracardiac Pacemaker	Z No Qualifier
FY2Ø17	P Pulmonary Trunk Q Pulmonary Artery, Right R Pulmonary Artery, Left S Pulmonary Vein, Right T Pulmonary Vein, Left V Superior Vena Cava W Thoracic Aorta, Descending X Thoracic Aorta, Ascending/Arch	Ø Open 3 Percutaneous 4 Percutaneous Endoscopic	Ø Monitoring Device, Pressure Sensor 2 Monitoring Device 3 Infusion Device D Intraluminal Device	Z No Qualifier

SECTION: Ø MEDICAL AND SURGICAL
BODY SYSTEM: 2 HEART AND GREAT VESSELS
OPERATION: L OCCLUSION: Completely closing an orifice or the lumen of a tubular body part

	Body Part	Approach	Device	Qualifier
FY2Ø17	H Pulmonary Valve S Pulmonary Vein, Right T Pulmonary Vein, Left V Superior Vena Cava	Ø Open 3 Percutaneous 4 Percutaneous Endoscopic	C Extraluminal Device D Intraluminal Device Z No Device	Z No Qualifier

SECTION: Ø MEDICAL AND SURGICAL
BODY SYSTEM: 2 HEART AND GREAT VESSELS
OPERATION: N RELEASE: Freeing a body part from an abnormal physical constraint by cutting or by the use of force

FY2Ø17

Body Part	Approach	Device	Qualifier
4 Coronary Vein 5 Atrial Septum 6 Atrium, Right 7 Atrium, Left 8 Conduction Mechanism 9 Chordae Tendineae D Papillary Muscle F Aortic Valve G Mitral Valve H Pulmonary Valve J Tricuspid Valve K Ventricle, Right L Ventricle, Left M Ventricular Septum N Pericardium P Pulmonary Trunk Q Pulmonary Artery, Right R Pulmonary Artery, Left S Pulmonary Vein, Right T Pulmonary Vein, Left V Superior Vena Cava W Thoracic Aorta, Descending X Thoracic Aorta, Ascending/Arch	Ø Open 3 Percutaneous 4 Percutaneous Endoscopic	Z No Device	Z No Qualifier

SECTION: Ø MEDICAL AND SURGICAL
BODY SYSTEM: 2 HEART AND GREAT VESSELS
OPERATION: P REMOVAL: Taking out or off a device from a body part

FY2Ø17

Body Part	Approach	Device	Qualifier
A Heart	Ø Open 3 Percutaneous 4 Percutaneous Endoscopic	2 Monitoring Device 3 Infusion Device 7 Autologous Tissue Substitute 8 Zooplastic Tissue C Extraluminal Device D Intraluminal Device J Synthetic Substitute K Nonautologous Tissue Substitute M Cardiac Lead N Intracardiac Pacemaker Q Implantable Heart Assist System R External Heart Assist System	Z No Qualifier

SECTION: **Ø MEDICAL AND SURGICAL**
BODY SYSTEM: 2   HEART AND GREAT VESSELS
OPERATION: **Q REPAIR:** Restoring, to the extent possible, a body part to its normal anatomic structure and function

	Body Part	Approach	Device	Qualifier
FY2017	Ø Coronary Artery, One Artery 1 Coronary Artery, Two Arteries 2 Coronary Artery, Three Arteries 3 Coronary Artery, Four or More Arteries 4 Coronary Vein 5 Atrial Septum 6 Atrium, Right 7 Atrium, Left 8 Conduction Mechanism 9 Chordae Tendineae A Heart B Heart, Right C Heart, Left D Papillary Muscle F Aortic Valve G Mitral Valve H Pulmonary Valve J Tricuspid Valve K Ventricle, Right L Ventricle, Left M Ventricular Septum N Pericardium P Pulmonary Trunk Q Pulmonary Artery, Right R Pulmonary Artery, Left S Pulmonary Vein, Right T Pulmonary Vein, Left V Superior Vena Cava W Thoracic Aorta, Descending X Thoracic Aorta, Ascending/Arch	Ø Open 3 Percutaneous 4 Percutaneous Endoscopic	Z No Device	Z No Qualifier
FY2017	F Aortic Valve	Ø Open 3 Percutaneous 4 Percutaneous Endoscopic	Z No Device	J Truncal Valve Z No Qualifier
FY2017	G Mitral Valve	Ø Open 3 Percutaneous 4 Percutaneous Endoscopic	Z No Device	E Atrioventricular Valve, Left Z No Qualifier
FY2017	J Tricuspid Valve	Ø Open 3 Percutaneous 4 Percutaneous Endoscopic	Z No Device	G Atrioventricular Valve, Right Z No Qualifier

SECTION: Ø MEDICAL AND SURGICAL

BODY SYSTEM: 2 HEART AND GREAT VESSELS

OPERATION: R REPLACEMENT: Putting in or on biological or synthetic material that physically takes the place and/or function of all or a portion of a body part

FY2Ø17

Body Part	Approach	Device	Qualifier
5 Atrial Septum	Ø Open	7 Autologous Tissue Substitute	Z No Qualifier
6 Atrium, Right	4 Percutaneous Endoscopic	8 Zooplastic Tissue	
7 Atrium, Left		J Synthetic Substitute	
9 Chordae Tendineae		K Nonautologous Tissue Substitute	
D Papillary Muscle			
J Tricuspid Valve			
K Ventricle, Right			
L Ventricle, Left			
M Ventricular Septum			
N Pericardium			
P Pulmonary Trunk			
Q Pulmonary Artery, Right			
R Pulmonary Artery, Left			
S Pulmonary Vein, Right			
T Pulmonary Vein, Left			
V Superior Vena Cava			
W Thoracic Aorta, Descending			
X Thoracic Aorta, Ascending/Arch			

SECTION: Ø MEDICAL AND SURGICAL

BODY SYSTEM: 2 HEART AND GREAT VESSELS

OPERATION: S REPOSITION: Moving to its normal location, or other suitable location, all or a portion of a body part

FY2Ø17

Body Part	Approach	Device	Qualifier
Ø Coronary Artery, One Artery	Ø Open	Z No Device	Z No Qualifier
1 Coronary Artery, Two Arteries			
P Pulmonary Trunk			
Q Pulmonary Artery, Right			
R Pulmonary Artery, Left			
S Pulmonary Vein, Right			
T Pulmonary Vein, Left			
V Superior Vena Cava			
W Thoracic Aorta, Descending			
X Thoracic Aorta, Ascending/Arch			

SECTION: Ø MEDICAL AND SURGICAL

BODY SYSTEM: 2 HEART AND GREAT VESSELS

OPERATION: **U SUPPLEMENT:** Putting in or on biological or synthetic material that physically reinforces and/or augments the function of a portion of a body part

	Body Part	Approach	Device	Qualifier
FY2Ø17	5 Atrial Septum 6 Atrium, Right 7 Atrium, Left 9 Chordae Tendineae A Heart D Papillary Muscle H Pulmonary Valve K Ventricle, Right L Ventricle, Left M Ventricular Septum N Pericardium P Pulmonary Trunk Q Pulmonary Artery, Right R Pulmonary Artery, Left S Pulmonary Vein, Right T Pulmonary Vein, Left V Superior Vena Cava W Thoracic Aorta, Descending X Thoracic Aorta, Ascending/Arch	Ø Open 3 Percutaneous 4 Percutaneous Endoscopic	7 Autologous Tissue Substitute 8 Zooplastic Tissue J Synthetic Substitute K Nonautologous Tissue Substitute	Z No Qualifier
FY2Ø17	F Aortic Valve	Ø Open 3 Percutaneous 4 Percutaneous Endoscopic	7 Autologous Tissue Substitute 8 Zooplastic Tissue J Synthetic Substitute K Nonautologous Tissue Substitute	J Truncal Valve Z No Qualifier
FY2Ø17	G Mitral Valve	Ø Open 3 Percutaneous 4 Percutaneous Endoscopic	7 Autologous Tissue Substitute 8 Zooplastic Tissue J Synthetic Substitute K Nonautologous Tissue Substitute	E Atrioventricular Valve, Left Z No Qualifier
FY2Ø17	J Tricuspid Valve	Ø Open 3 Percutaneous 4 Percutaneous Endoscopic	7 Autologous Tissue Substitute 8 Zooplastic Tissue J Synthetic Substitute K Nonautologous Tissue Substitute	G Atrioventricular Valve, Right Z No Qualifier

SECTION: Ø MEDICAL AND SURGICAL
BODY SYSTEM: 2 HEART AND GREAT VESSELS
OPERATION: V RESTRICTION: Partially closing an orifice or the lumen of a tubular body part

	Body Part	Approach	Device	Qualifier
FY2Ø17	P Pulmonary Trunk Q Pulmonary Artery, Right S Pulmonary Vein, Right T Pulmonary Vein, Left V Superior Vena Cava	Ø Open 3 Percutaneous 4 Percutaneous Endoscopic	C Extraluminal Device D Intraluminal Device Z No Device	Z No Qualifier
FY2Ø17	W Thoracic Aorta, Descending X Thoracic Aorta, Ascending/Arch	Ø Open 3 Percutaneous 4 Percutaneous Endoscopic	C Extraluminal Device D Intraluminal Device E Intraluminal Device, Branched or Fenestrated, One or Two Arteries F Intraluminal Device, Branched or Fenestrated, Three or More Arteries Z No Device	Z No Qualifier

SECTION: Ø MEDICAL AND SURGICAL
BODY SYSTEM: 2 HEART AND GREAT VESSELS
OPERATION: W REVISION: Correcting, to the extent possible, a portion of a malfunctioning device or the position of a displaced device

	Body Part	Approach	Device	Qualifier
FY2Ø17	A Heart	Ø Open 3 Percutaneous 4 Percutaneous Endoscopic X External	2 Monitoring Device 3 Infusion Device 7 Autologous Tissue Substitute 8 Zooplastic Tissue C Extraluminal Device D Intraluminal Device J Synthetic Substitute K Nonautologous Tissue Substitute M Cardiac Lead N Intracardiac Pacemaker Q Implantable Heart Assist System R External Heart Assist System	Z No Qualifier

SECTION: Ø MEDICAL AND SURGICAL
BODY SYSTEM: 3 UPPER ARTERIES
OPERATION: 7 **DILATION:** Expanding an orifice or the lumen of a tubular body part

FY2Ø17

Body Part	Approach	Device	Qualifier
Ø Internal Mammary Artery, Right 1 Internal Mammary Artery, Left 2 Innominate Artery 3 Subclavian Artery, Right 4 Subclavian Artery, Left 5 Axillary Artery, Right 6 Axillary Artery, Left 7 Brachial Artery, Right 8 Brachial Artery, Left 9 Ulnar Artery, Right A Ulnar Artery, Left B Radial Artery, Right C Radial Artery, Left D Hand Artery, Right F Hand Artery, Left G Intracranial Artery H Common Carotid Artery, Right J Common Carotid Artery, Left K Internal Carotid Artery, Right L Internal Carotid Artery, Left M External Carotid Artery, Right N External Carotid Artery, Left P Vertebral Artery, Right Q Vertebral Artery, Left R Face Artery S Temporal Artery, Right T Temporal Artery, Left U Thyroid Artery, Right V Thyroid Artery, Left Y Upper Artery	Ø Open 3 Percutaneous 4 Percutaneous Endoscopic	4 Intraluminal Device, Drug-eluting 5 Intraluminal Device, Drug-eluting, Two 6 Intraluminal Device, Drug-eluting, Three 7 Intraluminal Device, Drug-eluting, Four or More D Intraluminal Device E Intraluminal Device, Two F Intraluminal Device, Three G Intraluminal Device, Four or More Z No Device	6 Bifurcation Z No Qualifier

SECTION: Ø MEDICAL AND SURGICAL
BODY SYSTEM: 3 UPPER ARTERIES
OPERATION: C **EXTIRPATION:** Taking or cutting out solid matter from a body part

Body Part	Approach	Device	Qualifier
Ø Internal Mammary Artery, Right 1 Internal Mammary Artery, Left 2 Innominate Artery 3 Subclavian Artery, Right 4 Subclavian Artery, Left 5 Axillary Artery, Right 6 Axillary Artery, Left 7 Brachial Artery, Right 8 Brachial Artery, Left 9 Ulnar Artery, Right A Ulnar Artery, Left B Radial Artery, Right C Radial Artery, Left D Hand Artery, Right F Hand Artery, Left G Intracranial Artery H Common Carotid Artery, Right J Common Carotid Artery, Left K Internal Carotid Artery, Right L Internal Carotid Artery, Left M External Carotid Artery, Right N External Carotid Artery, Left P Vertebral Artery, Right Q Vertebral Artery, Left R Face Artery S Temporal Artery, Right T Temporal Artery, Left U Thyroid Artery, Right V Thyroid Artery, Left Y Upper Artery	Ø Open 3 Percutaneous 4 Percutaneous Endoscopic	Z No Device	6 Bifurcation Z No Qualifier

FY2Ø17

xx GUIDE TO THE 2017 UPDATES

SECTION: Ø MEDICAL AND SURGICAL

BODY SYSTEM: 4 LOWER ARTERIES

OPERATION: 7 DILATION: Expanding an orifice or the lumen of a tubular body part

	Body Part	Approach	Device	Qualifier
FY2Ø17	Ø Abdominal Aorta 1 Celiac Artery 2 Gastric Artery 3 Hepatic Artery 4 Splenic Artery 5 Superior Mesenteric Artery 6 Colic Artery, Right 7 Colic Artery, Left 8 Colic Artery, Middle 9 Renal Artery, Right A Renal Artery, Left B Inferior Mesenteric Artery C Common Iliac Artery, Right D Common Iliac Artery, Left E Internal Iliac Artery, Right F Internal Iliac Artery, Left H External Iliac Artery, Right J External Iliac Artery, Left P Anterior Tibial Artery, Right Q Anterior Tibial Artery, Left R Posterior Tibial Artery, Right S Posterior Tibial Artery, Left T Peroneal Artery, Right U Peroneal Artery, Left V Foot Artery, Right W Foot Artery, Left Y Lower Artery	Ø Open 3 Percutaneous 4 Percutaneous Endoscopic	4 Intraluminal Device, Drug-eluting 5 Intraluminal Device, Drug-eluting, Two 6 Intraluminal Device, Drug-eluting, Three 7 Intraluminal Device, Drug-eluting, Four or More D Intraluminal Device E Intraluminal Device, Two F Intraluminal Device, Three G Intraluminal Device, Four or More Z No Device	6 Bifurcation Z No Qualifier
FY2Ø17	K Femoral Artery, Right L Femoral Artery, Left M Popliteal Artery, Right N Popliteal Artery, Left	Ø Open 3 Percutaneous 4 Percutaneous Endoscopic	4 Intraluminal Device, Drug-eluting D Intraluminal Device Z No Device	1 Drug-Coated Balloon 6 Bifurcation Z No Qualifier
FY2Ø17	K Femoral Artery, Right L Femoral Artery, Left M Popliteal Artery, Right N Popliteal Artery, Left	Ø Open 3 Percutaneous 4 Percutaneous Endoscopic	5 Intraluminal Device, Drug-eluting, Two 6 Intraluminal Device, Drug-eluting, Three 7 Intraluminal Device, Drug-eluting, Four or More E Intraluminal Device, Two F Intraluminal Device, Three G Intraluminal Device, Four or More	6 Bifurcation Z No Qualifier

SECTION: Ø MEDICAL AND SURGICAL
BODY SYSTEM: 4 LOWER ARTERIES
OPERATION: C EXTIRPATION: Taking or cutting out solid matter from a body part

Body Part	Approach	Device	Qualifier
Ø Abdominal Aorta	Ø Open	Z No Device	6 Bifurcation
1 Celiac Artery	3 Percutaneous		Z No Qualifier
2 Gastric Artery	4 Percutaneous Endoscopic		
3 Hepatic Artery			
4 Splenic Artery			
5 Superior Mesenteric Artery			
6 Colic Artery, Right			
7 Colic Artery, Left			
8 Colic Artery, Middle			
9 Renal Artery, Right			
A Renal Artery, Left			
B Inferior Mesenteric Artery			
C Common Iliac Artery, Right			
D Common Iliac Artery, Left			
E Internal Iliac Artery, Right			
F Internal Iliac Artery, Left			
H External Iliac Artery, Right			
J External Iliac Artery, Left			
K Femoral Artery, Right			
L Femoral Artery, Left			
M Popliteal Artery, Right			
N Popliteal Artery, Left			
P Anterior Tibial Artery, Right			
Q Anterior Tibial Artery, Left			
R Posterior Tibial Artery, Right			
S Posterior Tibial Artery, Left			
T Peroneal Artery, Right			
U Peroneal Artery, Left			
V Foot Artery, Right			
W Foot Artery, Left			
Y Lower Artery			

FY2017

SECTION: Ø MEDICAL AND SURGICAL
BODY SYSTEM: 4 LOWER ARTERIES
OPERATION: V RESTRICTION: Partially closing an orifice or the lumen of a tubular body part

	Body Part	Approach	Device	Qualifier
FY2017	Ø Abdominal Aorta	Ø Open 3 Percutaneous 4 Percutaneous Endoscopic	C Extraluminal Device E Intraluminal Device, Branched or Fenestrated, One or Two Arteries F Intraluminal Device, Branched or Fenestrated, Three or More Arteries Z No Device	6 Bifurcation Z No Qualifier
FY2017	Ø Abdominal Aorta	Ø Open 3 Percutaneous 4 Percutaneous Endoscopic	D Intraluminal Device	6 Bifurcation J Temporary Z No Qualifier
FY2017	1 Celiac Artery 2 Gastric Artery 3 Hepatic Artery 4 Splenic Artery 5 Superior Mesenteric Artery 6 Colic Artery, Right 7 Colic Artery, Left 8 Colic Artery, Middle 9 Renal Artery, Right A Renal Artery, Left B Inferior Mesenteric Artery E Internal Iliac Artery, Right F Internal Iliac Artery, Left H External Iliac Artery, Right J External Iliac Artery, Left K Femoral Artery, Right L Femoral Artery, Left M Popliteal Artery, Right N Popliteal Artery, Left P Anterior Tibial Artery, Right Q Anterior Tibial Artery, Left R Posterior Tibial Artery, Right S Posterior Tibial Artery, Left T Peroneal Artery, Right U Peroneal Artery, Left V Foot Artery, Right W Foot Artery, Left Y Lower Artery	Ø Open 3 Percutaneous 4 Percutaneous Endoscopic	C Extraluminal Device D Intraluminal Device Z No Device	Z No Qualifier
FY2017	C Common Iliac Artery, Right D Common Iliac Artery, Left	Ø Open 3 Percutaneous 4 Percutaneous Endoscopic	C Extraluminal Device D Intraluminal Device E Intraluminal Device, Branched or Fenestrated, One or Two Arteries F Intraluminal Device, Branched or Fenestrated, Three or More Arteries Z No Device	Z No Qualifier

SECTION: Ø MEDICAL AND SURGICAL
BODY SYSTEM: 5 UPPER VEINS

OPERATION: **H INSERTION:** Putting in a nonbiological appliance that monitors, assists, performs, or prevents a physiological function but does not physically take the place of a body part

Body Part	Approach	Device	Qualifier
Ø Azygos Vein	Ø Open 3 Percutaneous 4 Percutaneous Endoscopic	2 Monitoring Device 3 Infusion Device D Intraluminal Device M Neurostimulator Lead	Z No Qualifier
1 Hemiazygos Vein 5 Subclavian Vein, Right 6 Subclavian Vein, Left 7 Axillary Vein, Right 8 Axillary Vein, Left 9 Brachial Vein, Right A Brachial Vein, Left B Basilic Vein, Right C Basilic Vein, Left D Cephalic Vein, Right F Cephalic Vein, Left G Hand Vein, Right H Hand Vein, Left L Intracranial Vein M Internal Jugular Vein, Right N Internal Jugular Vein, Left P External Jugular Vein, Right Q External Jugular Vein, Left R Vertebral Vein, Right S Vertebral Vein, Left T Face Vein, Right V Face Vein, Left	Ø Open 3 Percutaneous 4 Percutaneous Endoscopic	3 Infusion Device D Intraluminal Device	Z No Qualifier
3 Innominate Vein, Right 4 Innominate Vein, Left	Ø Open 3 Percutaneous 4 Percutaneous Endoscopic	3 Infusion Device D Intraluminal Device M Neurostimulator Lead	Z No Qualifier

FY2Ø17 (Azygos Vein row)

FY2Ø17 (Hemiazygos Vein block)

FY2Ø17 (Innominate Vein row)

SECTION: Ø MEDICAL AND SURGICAL

BODY SYSTEM: 5 UPPER VEINS

OPERATION: P REMOVAL: Taking out or off a device from a body part

	Body Part	Approach	Device	Qualifier
FY2017	Ø Azygos Vein	Ø Open 3 Percutaneous 4 Percutaneous Endoscopic X External	2 Monitoring Device M Neurostimulator Lead	Z No Qualifier
FY2017	3 Innominate Vein, Right 4 Innominate Vein, Left	Ø Open 3 Percutaneous 4 Percutaneous Endoscopic X External	M Neurostimulator Lead	Z No Qualifier

SECTION: Ø MEDICAL AND SURGICAL

BODY SYSTEM: 5 UPPER VEINS

OPERATION: W REVISION: Correcting, to the extent possible, a portion of a malfunctioning device or the position of a displaced device

	Body Part	Approach	Device	Qualifier
FY2017	Ø Azygos Vein	Ø Open 3 Percutaneous 4 Percutaneous Endoscopic X External	2 Monitoring Device M Neurostimulator Lead	Z No Qualifier
FY2017	3 Innominate Vein, Right 4 Innominate Vein, Left	Ø Open 3 Percutaneous 4 Percutaneous Endoscopic X External	M Neurostimulator Lead	Z No Qualifier

SECTION: Ø MEDICAL AND SURGICAL
BODY SYSTEM: S LOWER JOINTS
OPERATION: P REMOVAL: Taking out or off a device from a body part

	Body Part	Approach	Device	Qualifier
FY2Ø17	A Hip Joint, Acetabular Surface, Right E Hip Joint, Acetabular Surface, Left R Hip Joint, Femoral Surface, Right S Hip Joint, Femoral Surface, Left T Knee Joint, Femoral Surface, Right U Knee Joint, Femoral Surface, Left V Knee Joint, Tibial Surface, Right W Knee Joint, Tibial Surface, Left	Ø Open 3 Percutaneous 4 Percutaneous Endoscopic	J Synthetic Substitute	Z No Qualifier
FY2Ø17	C Knee Joint, Right D Knee Joint, Left	Ø Open	Ø Drainage Device 3 Infusion Device 4 Internal Fixation Device 5 External Fixation Device 7 Autologous Tissue Substitute 8 Spacer 9 Liner K Nonautologous Tissue Substitute	Z No Qualifier
FY2Ø17	C Knee Joint, Right D Knee Joint, Left	Ø Open	J Synthetic Substitute	C Patellar Surface Z No Qualifier
FY2Ø17	C Knee Joint, Right D Knee Joint, Left	3 Percutaneous 4 Percutaneous Endoscopic	Ø Drainage Device 3 Infusion Device 4 Internal Fixation Device 5 External Fixation Device 7 Autologous Tissue Substitute 8 Spacer K Nonautologous Tissue Substitute	Z No Qualifier
FY2Ø17	C Knee Joint, Right D Knee Joint, Left	3 Percutaneous 4 Percutaneous Endoscopic	J Synthetic Substitute	C Patellar Surface Z No Qualifier

SECTION: Ø MEDICAL AND SURGICAL
BODY SYSTEM: S LOWER JOINTS
OPERATION: R REPLACEMENT: Putting in or on biological or synthetic material that physically takes the place and/or function of all or a portion of a body part

	Body Part	Approach	Device	Qualifier
FY2Ø17	C Knee Joint, Right D Knee Joint, Left	Ø Open	7 Autologous Tissue Substitute K Nonautologous Tissue Substitute	Z No Qualifier
FY2Ø17	C Knee Joint, Right D Knee Joint, Left	Ø Open	J Synthetic Substitute L Synthetic Substitute, Unicondylar	9 Cemented A Uncemented Z No Qualifier
FY2Ø17	F Ankle Joint, Right G Ankle Joint, Left T Knee Joint, Femoral Surface, Right U Knee Joint, Femoral Surface, Left V Knee Joint, Tibial Surface, Right W Knee Joint, Tibial Surface, Left	Ø Open	7 Autologous Tissue Substitute K Nonautologous Tissue Substitute	Z No Qualifier
FY2Ø17	F Ankle Joint, Right G Ankle Joint, Left T Knee Joint, Femoral Surface, Right U Knee Joint, Femoral Surface, Left V Knee Joint, Tibial Surface, Right W Knee Joint, Tibial Surface, Left	Ø Open	J Synthetic Substitute	9 Cemented A Uncemented Z No Qualifier

SECTION: Ø MEDICAL AND SURGICAL

BODY SYSTEM: S LOWER JOINTS

OPERATION: W REVISION: Correcting, to the extent possible, a portion of a malfunctioning device or the position of a displaced device

	Body Part	Approach	Device	Qualifier
FY2017	A Hip Joint, Acetabular Surface, Right E Hip Joint, Acetabular Surface, Left R Hip Joint, Femoral Surface, Right S Hip Joint, Femoral Surface, Left T Knee Joint, Femoral Surface, Right U Knee Joint, Femoral Surface, Left V Knee Joint, Tibial Surface, Right W Knee Joint, Tibial Surface, Left	Ø Open 3 Percutaneous 4 Percutaneous Endoscopic X External	J Synthetic Substitute	Z No Qualifier
FY2017	C Knee Joint, Right D Knee Joint, Left	Ø Open	Ø Drainage Device 3 Infusion Device 4 Internal Fixation Device 5 External Fixation Device 7 Autologous Tissue Substitute 8 Spacer 9 Liner K Nonautologous Tissue Substitute	Z No Qualifier
FY2017	C Knee Joint, Right D Knee Joint, Left	Ø Open	J Synthetic Substitute	C Patellar Surface Z No Qualifier
FY2017	C Knee Joint, Right D Knee Joint, Left	3 Percutaneous 4 Percutaneous Endoscopic X External	Ø Drainage Device 3 Infusion Device 4 Internal Fixation Device 5 External Fixation Device 7 Autologous Tissue Substitute 8 Spacer K Nonautologous Tissue Substitute	Z No Qualifier
FY2017	C Knee Joint, Right D Knee Joint, Left	3 Percutaneous 4 Percutaneous Endoscopic X External	J Synthetic Substitute	C Patellar Surface Z No Qualifier

Revise to

SECTION: Ø **MEDICAL AND SURGICAL**
BODY SYSTEM: W ANATOMICAL REGIONS, GENERAL
OPERATION: **3 CONTROL:** Stopping, or attempting to stop, postprocedure or other acute bleeding

Revise to

SECTION: Ø **MEDICAL AND SURGICAL**
BODY SYSTEM: W ANATOMICAL REGIONS, GENERAL
OPERATION: **4 CREATION:** Putting in or on biological or synthetic material to form a new body part that to the extent possible replicates the anatomic structure or function of an absent body part

FY2Ø17

SECTION: Ø **MEDICAL AND SURGICAL**
BODY SYSTEM: W ANATOMICAL REGIONS, GENERAL
OPERATION: **Y TRANSPLANTATION:** Putting in or on all or a portion of a living body part taken from another individual or animal to physically take the place and/or function of all or a portion of a similar body part

FY2Ø17

Body Part	Approach	Device	Qualifier
2 Face	Ø Open	Z No Device	Ø Allogeneic 1 Syngeneic

Revise to

SECTION: Ø **MEDICAL AND SURGICAL**
BODY SYSTEM: X ANATOMICAL REGIONS, UPPER EXTREMITIES
OPERATION: **3 CONTROL:** Stopping, or attempting to stop, postprocedure or other acute bleeding

FY2Ø17

SECTION: Ø **MEDICAL AND SURGICAL**
BODY SYSTEM: X ANATOMICAL REGIONS, UPPER EXTREMITIES
OPERATION: **Y TRANSPLANTATION:** Putting in or on all or a portion of a living body part taken from another individual or animal to physically take the place and/or function of all or a portion of a similar body part

FY2Ø17

Body Part	Approach	Device	Qualifier
J Hand, Right K Hand, Left	Ø Open	Z No Device	Ø Allogeneic 1 Syngeneic

Revise to

SECTION: Ø **MEDICAL AND SURGICAL**
BODY SYSTEM: Y ANATOMICAL REGIONS, LOWER EXTREMITIES
OPERATION: **3 CONTROL:** Stopping, or attempting to stop, postprocedure or other acute bleeding

SECTION: 3 ADMINISTRATION
BODY SYSTEM: Ø CIRCULATORY
OPERATION: 2 TRANSFUSION: Putting in blood or blood products

	Body System / Region	Approach	Substance	Qualifier
FY2017	3 Peripheral Vein 4 Central Vein	Ø Open 3 Percutaneous	G Bone Marrow X Stem Cells, Cord Blood Y Stem Cells, Hematopoietic	Ø Autologous 2 Allogeneic, Related 3 Allogeneic, Unrelated 4 Allogeneic, Unspecified
FY2017	3 Peripheral Vein 4 Central Vein	Ø Open 3 Percutaneous	H Whole Blood J Serum Albumin K Frozen Plasma L Fresh Plasma M Plasma Cryoprecipitate N Red Blood Cells P Frozen Red Cells Q White Cells R Platelets S Globulin T Fibrinogen V Antihemophilic Factors W Factor IX	Ø Autologous 1 Nonautologous

SECTION: 3 ADMINISTRATION
BODY SYSTEM: E PHYSIOLOGICAL SYSTEMS AND ANATOMICAL REGIONS
OPERATION: Ø INTRODUCTION: Putting in or on a therapeutic, diagnostic, nutritional, physiological, or prophylactic substance except blood or blood products

	Body System / Region	Approach	Substance	Qualifier
FY2017	Q Cranial Cavity and Brain	Ø Open 3 Percutaneous	Ø Antineoplastic	4 Liquid Brachytherapy Radioisotope 5 Other Antineoplastic M Monoclonal Antibody
FY2017	Q Cranial Cavity and Brain	Ø Open 3 Percutaneous	2 Anti-infective	8 Oxazolidinones 9 Other Anti-infective
FY2017	Q Cranial Cavity and Brain	Ø Open 3 Percutaneous	3 Anti-inflammatory 6 Nutritional Substance 7 Electrolytic and Water Balance Substance A Stem Cells, Embryonic B Local Anesthetic H Radioactive Substance K Other Diagnostic Substance N Analgesics, Hypnotics, Sedatives T Destructive Agent	Z No Qualifier
FY2017	Q Cranial Cavity and Brain	Ø Open 3 Percutaneous	E Stem Cells, Somatic	Ø Autologous 1 Nonautologous
FY2017	Q Cranial Cavity and Brain	Ø Open 3 Percutaneous	G Other Therapeutic Substance	C Other Substance
FY2017	Q Cranial Cavity and Brain	Ø Open 3 Percutaneous	S Gas	F Other Gas

SECTION: 4 MEASUREMENT AND MONITORING
BODY SYSTEM: A PHYSIOLOGICAL SYSTEMS
OPERATION: 1 MONITORING: Determining the level of a physiological or physical function repetitively over a period of time

	Body System	Approach	Function / Device	Qualifier
FY2017	2 Cardiac	X External	S Vascular Perfusion	H Indocyanine Green Dye
FY2017	B Gastrointestinal	X External	S Vascular Perfusion	H Indocyanine Green Dye
FY2017	G Skin and Breast	X External	S Vascular Perfusion	H Indocyanine Green Dye

SECTION: 6 EXTRACORPOREAL THERAPIES
FY2017   *BODY SYSTEM:* A PHYSIOLOGICAL SYSTEMS
OPERATION: B PERFUSION: Extracorporeal treatment by diffusion of therapeutic fluid

	Body System	Duration	Qualifier	Qualifier
FY2017	5 Circulatory B Respiratory System F Hepatobiliary System and Pancreas T Urinary System	Ø Single	B Donor Organ	Z No Qualifier

SECTION: X NEW TECHNOLOGY
FY2017   *BODY SYSTEM:* 2 CARDIOVASCULAR SYSTEM
OPERATION: A ASSISTANCE: Taking over a portion of a physiological function by extracorporeal means

	Body Part	Approach	Device / Substance / Technology	Qualifier
FY2017	5 Innominate Artery and Left Common Carotid Artery	3 Percutaneous	1 Cerebral Embolic Filtration, Dual Filter	2 New Technology Group 2

SECTION: X NEW TECHNOLOGY
BODY SYSTEM: 2 CARDIOVASCULAR SYSTEM
OPERATION: C EXTIRPATION: Taking or cutting out solid matter from a body part

	Body Part	Approach	Device / Substance / Technology	Qualifier
Revise to	Ø Coronary Artery, One Artery 1 Coronary Artery, Two Arteries 2 Coronary Artery, Three Arteries 3 Coronary Artery, Four or More Arteries	3 Percutaneous	6 Orbital Atherectomy Technology	1 New Technology Group 1

SECTION: X NEW TECHNOLOGY

FY2017 **BODY SYSTEM: 2 CARDIOVASCULAR SYSTEM**

OPERATION: R REPLACEMENT: Putting in or on biological or synthetic material that physically takes the place and/or function of all or a portion of a body part

Body Part	Approach	Device / Substance / Technology	Qualifier
F Aortic Valve	Ø Open 3 Percutaneous 4 Percutaneous Endoscopic	3 Zooplastic Tissue, Rapid Deployment Technique	2 New Technology Group 2

SECTION: X NEW TECHNOLOGY

FY2017 **BODY SYSTEM: H SKIN, SUBCUTANEOUS TISSUE, FASCIA AND BREAST**

OPERATION: R REPLACEMENT: Putting in or on biological or synthetic material that physically takes the place and/or function of all or a portion of a body part

Body Part	Approach	Device / Substance / Technology	Qualifier
P Skin	X External	L Skin Substitute, Porcine Liver Derived	2 New Technology Group 2

SECTION: X NEW TECHNOLOGY

FY2017 **BODY SYSTEM: N BONES**

OPERATION: S REPLACEMENT: Moving to its normal location, or other suitable location, all or a portion of a body part

Body Part	Approach	Device / Substance / Technology	Qualifier
Ø Lumbar Vertebra 3 Cervical Vertebra 4 Thoracic Vertebra	Ø Open 4 Percutaneous Endoscopic	3 Magnetically Controlled Growth Rod(s)	2 New Technology Group 2

SECTION: X NEW TECHNOLOGY

FY2017 **BODY SYSTEM:** R JOINTS

OPERATION: G **FUSION:** Joining together portions of an articular body part rendering the articular body part immobile

Body Part	Approach	Device / Substance / Technology	Qualifier
Ø Occipital-cervical Joint 1 Cervical Vertebral Joint 2 Cervical Vertebral Joints, 2 or more 4 Cervicothoracic Vertebral Joint 6 Thoracic Vertebral Joint 7 Thoracic Vertebral Joints, 2 to 7 8 Thoracic Vertebral Joints, 8 or more A Thoracolumbar Vertebral Joint B Lumbar Vertebral Joint C Lumbar Vertebral Joints, 2 or more D Lumbosacral Joint	Ø Open	9 Interbody Fusion Device, Nanotextured Surface	2 New Technology Group 2

FY2017

SECTION: X NEW TECHNOLOGY

BODY SYSTEM: W ANATOMICAL REGIONS

OPERATION: Ø **INTRODUCTION:** Putting in or on a therapeutic, diagnostic, nutritional, physiological, or prophylactic substance except blood or blood products

	Body Part	Approach	Device / Substance / Technology	Qualifier
FY2017	3 Peripheral Vein	3 Percutaneous	2 Ceftazidime-Avibactam Anti-infective 3 Idarucizumab, Dabigatran Reversal Agent 4 Isavuconazole Anti-infective 5 Blinatumomab Antineoplastic Immunotherapy	1 New Technology Group 1
FY2017	3 Peripheral Vein	3 Percutaneous	7 Andexanet Alfa, Factor Xa Inhibitor Reversal Agent 9 Defibrotide Sodium Anticoagulant	2 New Technology Group 2
FY2017	4 Central Vein	3 Percutaneous	2 Ceftazidime-Avibactam Anti-infective 3 Idarucizumab, Dabigatran Reversal Agent 4 Isavuconazole Antiinfective 5 Blinatumomab Antineoplastic Immunotherapy	1 New Technology Group 1
FY2017	4 Central Vein	3 Percutaneous	7 Andexanet Alfa, Factor Xa Inhibitor Reversal Agent 9 Defibrotide Sodium Anticoagulant	2 New Technology Group 2
FY2017	D Mouth and Pharynx	X External	8 Uridine Triacetate	2 New Technology Group 2

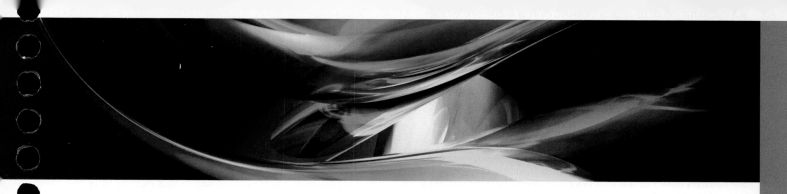

Introduction

ICD-10-PCS Official Guidelines for Coding and Reporting

2017

The Centers for Medicare and Medicaid Services (CMS) and the National Center for Health Statistics (NCHS), two departments within the U.S. Federal Government's Department of Health and Human Services (DHHS) provide the following guidelines for coding and reporting using the International Classification of Diseases, 10th Revision, Procedure Coding System (ICD-10-PCS). These guidelines should be used as a companion document to the official version of the ICD-10-PCS as published on the CMS website. The ICD-10-PCS is a procedure classification published by the United States for classifying procedures performed in hospital inpatient health care settings.

These guidelines have been approved by the four organizations that make up the Cooperating Parties for the ICD-10-PCS: the American Hospital Association (AHA), the American Health Information Management Association (AHIMA), CMS, and NCHS.

These guidelines are a set of rules that have been developed to accompany and complement the official conventions and instructions provided within the ICD-10-PCS itself. The instructions and conventions of the classification take precedence over guidelines. These guidelines are based on the coding and sequencing instructions in the Tables, Index and Definitions of ICD-10-PCS, but provide additional instruction. Adherence to these guidelines when assigning ICD-10-PCS procedure codes is required under the Health Insurance Portability and Accountability Act (HIPAA). The procedure codes have been adopted under HIPAA for hospital inpatient healthcare settings. A joint effort between the healthcare provider and the coder is essential to achieve complete and accurate documentation, code assignment, and reporting of diagnoses and procedures. These guidelines have been developed to assist both the healthcare provider and the coder in identifying those procedures that are to be reported. The importance of consistent, complete documentation in the medical record cannot be overemphasized. Without such documentation accurate coding cannot be achieved.

Table of Contents

Conventions

A1
ICD-10-PCS codes are composed of seven characters. Each character is an axis of classification that specifies information about the procedure performed. Within a defined code range, a character specifies the same type of information in that axis of classification.
Example: The fifth axis of classification specifies the approach in sections 0 through 4 and 7 through 9 of the system.

A2
One of 34 possible values can be assigned to each axis of classification in the seven-character code: they are the numbers 0 through 9 and the alphabet (except I and O because they are easily confused with the numbers 1 and 0). The number of unique values used in an axis of classification differs as needed.
Example: Where the fifth axis of classification specifies the approach, seven different approach values are currently used to specify the approach.

A3
The valid values for an axis of classification can be added to as needed.
Example: If a significantly distinct type of device is used in a new procedure, a new device value can be added to the system.

A4

As with words in their context, the meaning of any single value is a combination of its axis of classification and any preceding values on which it may be dependent.

Example: The meaning of a body part value in the Medical and Surgical section is always dependent on the body system value. The body part value Ø in the Central Nervous body system specifies Brain and the body part value Ø in the Peripheral Nervous body system specifies Cervical Plexus.

A5

As the system is expanded to become increasingly detailed, over time more values will depend on preceding values for their meaning.

Example: In the Lower Joints body system, the device value 3 in the root operation Insertion specifies Infusion Device and the device value 3 in the root operation Replacement specifies Ceramic Synthetic Substitute.

A6

The purpose of the alphabetic index is to locate the appropriate table that contains all information necessary to construct a procedure code. The PCS Tables should always be consulted to find the most appropriate valid code.

A7

It is not required to consult the index first before proceeding to the tables to complete the code. A valid code may be chosen directly from the tables.

A8

All seven characters must be specified to be a valid code. If the documentation is incomplete for coding purposes, the physician should be queried for the necessary information.

A9

Within a PCS table, valid codes include all combinations of choices in characters 4 through 7 contained in the same row of the table. In the example below, ØJHT3VZ is a valid code, and ØJHW3VZ is *not* a valid code.

A1Ø

"And," when used in a code description, means "and/or."

Example: Lower Arm and Wrist Muscle means lower arm and/or wrist muscle.

A11

Many of the terms used to construct PCS codes are defined within the system. It is the coder's responsibility to determine what the documentation in the medical record equates to in the PCS definitions. The physician is not expected to use the terms used in PCS code descriptions, nor is the coder required to query the physician when the correlation between the documentation and the defined PCS terms is clear.

Example: When the physician documents "partial resection" the coder can independently correlate "partial resection" to

the root operation Excision without querying the physician for clarification.

Medical and Surgical Section Guidelines (section Ø)

B2. Body System

General guidelines

B2.1a

The procedure codes in the general anatomical regions body systems can be used when the procedure is performed on an anatomical region rather than a specific body part (e.g., root operations Control and Detachment, Drainage of a body cavity) or on the rare occasion when no information is available to support assignment of a code to a specific body part.

Examples: Control of postoperative hemorrhage is coded to the root operation Control found in the general anatomical regions body systems.

Chest tube drainage of the pleural cavity is coded to the root operation Drainage found in the general anatomical regions body systems. Suture repair of the abdominal wall is coded to the root operation Repair in the general anatomical regions body system.

B2.1b

Where the general body part values "upper" and "lower" are provided as an option in the Upper Arteries, Lower Arteries, Upper Veins, Lower Veins, Muscles and Tendons body systems, "upper" or "lower" specifies body parts located above or below the diaphragm respectively.

Example: Vein body parts above the diaphragm are found in the Upper Veins body system; vein body parts below the diaphragm are found in the Lower Veins body system.

B3. Root Operation

General guidelines

B3.1a

In order to determine the appropriate root operation, the full definition of the root operation as contained in the PCS Tables must be applied.

B3.1b

Components of a procedure specified in the root operation definition and explanation are not coded separately. Procedural steps necessary to reach the operative site and close the operative site, including anastomosis of a tubular body part, are also not coded separately.

Examples: Resection of a joint as part of a joint replacement procedure is included in the root operation definition of Replacement and is not coded separately. Laparotomy performed to reach the site of an open liver biopsy is not coded separately. In a resection of sigmoid colon with anastomosis of descending colon to rectum, the anastomosis is not coded separately.

SECTION: Ø   MEDICAL AND SURGICAL

BODY SYSTEM: J   SUBCUTANEOUS TISSUE AND FASCIA

OPERATION: H   **INSERTION:** Putting in a nonbiological appliance that monitors, assists, performs, or prevents a physiological function but does not physically take the place of a body part

Body Part	Approach	Device	Qualifier
S Subcutaneous Tissue and Fascia, Head and Neck V Subcutaneous Tissue and Fascia, Upper Extremity W Subcutaneous Tissue and Fascia, Lower Extremity	Ø Open 3 Percutaneous	1 Radioactive Element 3 Infusion Device	Z No Qualifier
T Subcutaneous Tissue and Fascia, Trunk	Ø Open 3 Percutaneous	1 Radioactive Element 3 Infusion Device V Infusion Pump	Z No Qualifier

Multiple procedures
B3.2
During the same operative episode, multiple procedures are coded if:
  a. The same root operation is performed on different body parts as defined by distinct values of the body part character.
  Examples: Diagnostic excision of liver and pancreas are coded separately.
  b. The same root operation is repeated in multiple body parts, and those body parts are separate and distinct body parts classified to a single ICD-10-PCS body part value.
  Examples: Excision of the sartorius muscle and excision of the gracilis muscle are both included in the upper leg muscle body part value, and multiple procedures are coded.
  Extraction of multiple toenails are coded separately.
  c. Multiple root operations with distinct objectives are performed on the same body part.
  Example: Destruction of sigmoid lesion and bypass of sigmoid colon are coded separately.
  d. The intended root operation is attempted using one approach, but is converted to a different approach.
  Example: Laparoscopic cholecystectomy converted to an open cholecystectomy is coded as percutaneous endoscopic Inspection and open Resection.

Discontinued procedures
B3.3
If the intended procedure is discontinued, code the procedure to the root operation performed. If a procedure is discontinued before any other root operation is performed, code the root operation Inspection of the body part or anatomical region inspected.
Example: A planned aortic valve replacement procedure is discontinued after the initial thoracotomy and before any incision is made in the heart muscle, when the patient becomes hemodynamically unstable. This procedure is coded as an open Inspection of the mediastinum.

Biopsy procedures
B3.4a
Biopsy procedures are coded using the root operations Excision, Extraction, or Drainage and the qualifier Diagnostic.
Examples: Fine needle aspiration biopsy of fluid in the lung is coded to the root operation Drainage with the qualifier Diagnostic. Biopsy of bone marrow is coded to the root operation Extraction with the qualifier Diagnostic. Lymph node sampling for biopsy is coded to the root operation Excision with the qualifier Diagnostic.

Biopsy followed by more definitive treatment
B3.4b
If a diagnostic Excision, Extraction, or Drainage procedure (biopsy) is followed by a more definitive procedure, such as Destruction, Excision or Resection at the same procedure site, both the biopsy and the more definitive treatment are coded.
Example: Biopsy of breast followed by partial mastectomy at the same procedure site, both the biopsy and the partial mastectomy procedure are coded.

Overlapping body layers
B3.5
If the root operations Excision, Repair or Inspection are performed on overlapping layers of the musculoskeletal system, the body part specifying the deepest layer is coded.
Example: Excisional debridement that includes skin and subcutaneous tissue and muscle is coded to the muscle body part.

Bypass procedures
B3.6a
Bypass procedures are coded by identifying the body part bypassed "from" and the body part bypassed "to." The fourth character body part specifies the body part bypassed from, and the qualifier specifies the body part bypassed to.
Example: Bypass from stomach to jejunum, stomach is the body part and jejunum is the qualifier.
B3.6b
Coronary artery bypass procedures are coded differently than other bypass procedures as described in the previous guideline. Rather than identifying the body part bypassed from, the body part identifies the number of coronary artery sites bypassed to, and the qualifier specifies the vessel bypassed from.
Example: Aortocoronary artery bypass of the left anterior descending coronary artery and the obtuse marginal coronary artery is classified in the body part axis of classification as two coronary arteries, and the qualifier specifies the aorta as the body part bypassed from.
B3.6c
If multiple coronary arteries are bypassed, a separate procedure is coded for each coronary artery that uses a different device and/or qualifier.
Example: Aortocoronary artery bypass and internal mammary coronary artery bypass are coded separately.

Control vs. more definitive root operations
B3.7
The root operation Control is defined as, "Stopping, or attempting to stop, postprocedural or other acute bleeding." If an attempt to stop postprocedural or other acute bleeding is initially unsuccessful, and to stop the bleeding requires performing any of the definitive root operations Bypass, Detachment, Excision, Extraction, Reposition, Replacement, or Resection, then that root operation is coded instead of Control.
Example: Resection of spleen to stop bleeding is coded to Resection instead of Control.

Excision vs. Resection
B3.8
PCS contains specific body parts for anatomical subdivisions of a body part, such as lobes of the lungs or liver and regions of the intestine. Resection of the specific body part is coded whenever all of the body part is cut out or off, rather than coding Excision of a less specific body part.
Example: Left upper lung lobectomy is coded to Resection of Upper Lung Lobe, Left rather than Excision of Lung, Left.

Excision for graft
B3.9
If an autograft is obtained from a different procedure site in order to complete the objective of the procedure, a separate procedure is coded.
Example: Coronary bypass with excision of saphenous vein graft, excision of saphenous vein is coded separately.

Fusion procedures of the spine
B3.10a
The body part coded for a spinal vertebral joint(s) rendered immobile by a spinal fusion procedure is classified by the level of the spine (e.g. thoracic). There are distinct body part values for a single vertebral joint and for multiple vertebral joints at each spinal level.
Example: Body part values specify Lumbar Vertebral Joint, Lumbar Vertebral Joints, 2 or More and Lumbosacral Vertebral Joint.

B3.10b

If multiple vertebral joints are fused, a separate procedure is coded for each vertebral joint that uses a different device and/or qualifier.

Example: Fusion of lumbar vertebral joint, posterior approach, anterior column and fusion of lumbar vertebral joint, posterior approach, posterior column are coded separately.

B3.10c

Combinations of devices and materials are often used on a vertebral joint to render the joint immobile. When combinations of devices are used on the same vertebral joint, the device value coded for the procedure is as follows:

- If an interbody fusion device is used to render the joint immobile (alone or containing other material like bone graft), the procedure is coded with the device value Interbody Fusion Device
- If bone graft is the *only* device used to render the joint immobile, the procedure is coded with the device value Nonautologous Tissue Substitute or Autologous Tissue Substitute
- If a mixture of autologous and nonautologous bone graft (with or without biological or synthetic extenders or binders) is used to render the joint immobile, code the procedure with the device value Autologous Tissue Substitute

Examples: Fusion of a vertebral joint using a cage style interbody fusion device containing morsellized bone graft is coded to the device Interbody Fusion Device. Fusion of a vertebral joint using a bone dowel interbody fusion device made of cadaver bone and packed with a mixture of local morsellized bone and demineralized bone matrix is coded to the device Interbody Fusion Device.

Fusion of a vertebral joint using both autologous bone graft and bone bank bone graft is coded to the device Autologous Tissue Substitute.

Inspection procedures

B3.11a

Inspection of a body part(s) performed in order to achieve the objective of a procedure is not coded separately.

Example: Fiberoptic bronchoscopy performed for irrigation of bronchus, only the irrigation procedure is coded.

B3.11b

If multiple tubular body parts are inspected, the most distal body part (the body part furthest from the starting point of the inspection) is coded. If multiple non-tubular body parts in a region are inspected, the body part that specifies the entire area inspected is coded.

Examples: Cystoureteroscopy with inspection of bladder and ureters is coded to the ureter body part value. Exploratory laparotomy with general inspection of abdominal contents is coded to the peritoneal cavity body part value.

B3.11c

When both an Inspection procedure and another procedure are performed on the same body part during the same episode, if the Inspection procedure is performed using a different approach than the other procedure, the Inspection procedure is coded separately.

Example: Endoscopic Inspection of the duodenum is coded separately when open

Excision of the duodenum is performed during the same procedural episode.

Occlusion vs. Restriction for vessel embolization procedures

B3.12

If the objective of an embolization procedure is to completely close a vessel, the root operation Occlusion is coded. If the objective of an embolization procedure is to narrow the lumen of a vessel, the root operation Restriction is coded.

Examples: Tumor embolization is coded to the root operation Occlusion, because the objective of the procedure is to cut off the blood supply to the vessel.

Embolization of a cerebral aneurysm is coded to the root operation Restriction, because the objective of the procedure is not to close off the vessel entirely, but to narrow the lumen of the vessel at the site of the aneurysm where it is abnormally wide.

Release procedures

B3.13

In the root operation Release, the body part value coded is the body part being freed and not the tissue being manipulated or cut to free the body part.

Example: Lysis of intestinal adhesions is coded to the specific intestine body part value.

Release vs. Division

B3.14

If the sole objective of the procedure is freeing a body part without cutting the body part, the root operation is Release. If the sole objective of the procedure is separating or transecting a body part, the root operation is Division.

Examples: Freeing a nerve root from surrounding scar tissue to relieve pain is coded to the root operation Release. Severing a nerve root to relieve pain is coded to the root operation Division.

Reposition for fracture treatment

B3.15

Reduction of a displaced fracture is coded to the root operation Reposition and the application of a cast or splint in conjunction with the Reposition procedure is not coded separately. Treatment of a nondisplaced fracture is coded to the procedure performed.

Examples: Casting of a nondisplaced fracture is coded to the root operation Immobilization in the Placement section. Putting a pin in a nondisplaced fracture is coded to the root operation Insertion.

Transplantation vs. Administration

B3.16

Putting in a mature and functioning living body part taken from another individual or animal is coded to the root operation Transplantation. Putting in autologous or nonautologous cells is coded to the Administration section.

Example: Putting in autologous or nonautologous bone marrow, pancreatic islet cells or stem cells is coded to the Administration section.

B4. Body Part

General guidelines

B4.1a

If a procedure is performed on a portion of a body part that does not have a separate body part value, code the body part value corresponding to the whole body part.

Example: A procedure performed on the alveolar process of the mandible is coded to the mandible body part.

B4.1b

If the prefix "peri" is combined with a body part to identify the site of the procedure, and the site of the procedure is not further specified, then the procedure is coded to the body part named. This guideline applies only when a more specific body part value is not available.

Examples: A procedure site identified as perirenal is coded to the kidney body part when the site of the procedure is not further specified. A procedure site described in the documentation as peri-urethral, and the documentation also indicates that it is the vulvar tissue and not the urethral tissue that is the site of the procedure, then the procedure is coded to the vulva body part.

Branches of body parts
B4.2
Where a specific branch of a body part does not have its own body part value in PCS, the body part is typically coded to the closest proximal branch that has a specific body part value. In the cardiovascular body systems, if a general body part is available in the correct root operation table, and coding to a proximal branch would require assigning a code in a different body system, the procedure is coded using the general body part value.
Example: A procedure performed on the mandibular branch of the trigeminal nerve is coded to the trigeminal nerve body part value.

Bilateral body part values
B4.3
Bilateral body part values are available for a limited number of body parts. If the identical procedure is performed on contralateral body parts, and a bilateral body part value exists for that body part, a single procedure is coded using the bilateral body part value. If no bilateral body part value exists, each procedure is coded separately using the appropriate body part value.
Examples: The identical procedure performed on both fallopian tubes is coded once using the body part value Fallopian Tube, Bilateral. The identical procedure performed on both knee joints is coded twice using the body part values Knee Joint, Right and Knee Joint, Left.

Coronary arteries
B4.4
The coronary arteries are classified as a single body part that is further specified by number of arteries treated. One procedure code specifying multiple arteries is used when the same procedure is performed, including the same device and qualifier values. Separate body part values are used to specify the number of sites treated when the same procedure is performed on multiple sites in the coronary arteries.
Examples: Angioplasty of two distinct arteries in the left anterior descending coronary artery with placement of two stents is coded as Dilation of Coronary Arteries, Two Arteries, with Intraluminal Device.
Angioplasty of two distinct arteries in the left anterior descending coronary artery, one with stent placed and one without, is coded separately as Dilation of Coronary Artery, One Artery with Intraluminal Device, and Dilation of Coronary Artery, One Artery with no device.

Tendons, ligaments, bursae and fascia near a joint
B4.5
Procedures performed on tendons, ligaments, bursae and fascia supporting a joint are coded to the body part in the respective body system that is the focus of the procedure. Procedures performed on joint structures themselves are coded to the body part in the joint body systems.
Examples: Repair of the anterior cruciate ligament of the knee is coded to the knee bursae and ligament body part in the bursae and ligaments body system. Knee arthroscopy with shaving of articular cartilage is coded to the knee joint body part in the Lower Joints body system.

Skin, subcutaneous tissue and fascia overlying a joint
B4.6
If a procedure is performed on the skin, subcutaneous tissue or fascia overlying a joint, the procedure is coded to the following body part:
- Shoulder is coded to Upper Arm
- Elbow is coded to Lower Arm
- Wrist is coded to Lower Arm

- Hip is coded to Upper Leg
- Knee is coded to Lower Leg
- Ankle is coded to Foot

Fingers and toes
B4.7
If a body system does not contain a separate body part value for fingers, procedures performed on the fingers are coded to the body part value for the hand. If a body system does not contain a separate body part value for toes, procedures performed on the toes are coded to the body part value for the foot.
Example: Excision of finger muscle is coded to one of the hand muscle body part values in the Muscles body system.

Upper and lower intestinal tract
B4.8
In the Gastrointestinal body system, the general body part values Upper Intestinal Tract and Lower Intestinal Tract are provided as an option for the root operations Change, Inspection, Removal and Revision. Upper Intestinal Tract includes the portion of the gastrointestinal tract from the esophagus down to and including the duodenum, and Lower Intestinal Tract includes the portion of the gastrointestinal tract from the jejunum down to and including the rectum and anus.
Example: In the root operation Change table, change of a device in the jejunum is coded using the body part Lower Intestinal Tract.

B5. Approach
Open approach with percutaneous endoscopic assistance
B5.2
Procedures performed using the open approach with percutaneous endoscopic assistance are coded to the approach Open.
Example: Laparoscopic-assisted sigmoidectomy is coded to the approach Open.

External approach
B5.3a
Procedures performed within an orifice on structures that are visible without the aid of any instrumentation are coded to the approach External.
Example: Resection of tonsils is coded to the approach External.
B5.3b
Procedures performed indirectly by the application of external force through the intervening body layers are coded to the approach External.
Example: Closed reduction of fracture is coded to the approach External.

Percutaneous procedure via device
B5.4
Procedures performed percutaneously via a device placed for the procedure are coded to the approach Percutaneous.
Example: Fragmentation of kidney stone performed via percutaneous nephrostomy is coded to the approach Percutaneous.

B6. Device
General guidelines
B6.1a
A device is coded only if a device remains after the procedure is completed. If no device remains, the device value No Device is coded.

B6.1b

Materials such as sutures, ligatures, radiological markers and temporary post-operative wound drains are considered integral to the performance of a procedure and are not coded as devices.

B6.1c

Procedures performed on a device only and not on a body part are specified in the root operations Change, Irrigation, Removal and Revision, and are coded to the procedure performed.

Example: Irrigation of percutaneous nephrostomy tube is coded to the root operation Irrigation of indwelling device in the Administration section.

Drainage device

B6.2

A separate procedure to put in a drainage device is coded to the root operation Drainage with the device value Drainage Device.

Obstetric Section Guidelines (section 1)

C. Obstetrics Section

Products of conception

C1

Procedures performed on the products of conception are coded to the Obstetrics section. Procedures performed on the pregnant female other than the products of conception are coded to the appropriate root operation in the Medical and Surgical section.

Example: Amniocentesis is coded to the products of conception body part in the Obstetrics section. Repair of obstetric urethral laceration is coded to the urethra body part in the Medical and Surgical section.

Procedures following delivery or abortion

C2

Procedures performed following a delivery or abortion for curettage of the endometrium or evacuation of retained products of conception are all coded in the Obstetrics section, to the root operation Extraction and the body part Products of Conception, Retained. Diagnostic or therapeutic dilation and curettage performed during times other than the postpartum or post-abortion period are all coded in the Medical and Surgical section, to the root operation Extraction and the body part Endometrium.

New Technology Section Guidelines (section X)

D. New Technology Section

General guidelines

D1

Section X codes are standalone codes. They are not supplemental codes. Section X codes fully represent the specific procedure described in the code title, and do not require any additional codes from other sections of ICD-10-PCS. When section X contains a code title which describes a specific new technology procedure, only that X code is reported for the procedure. There is no need to report a broader, non-specific code in another section of ICD-10-PCS.

Example: XW04321 Introduction of Ceftazidime-Avibactam Anti-infective into Central Vein, Percutaneous Approach, New Technology Group 1, can be coded to indicate that Ceftazidime-Avibactam Anti-infective was administered via a central vein. A separate code from table 3E0 in the Administration section of ICD-10-PCS is not coded in addition to this code.

Selection of Principal Procedure

The following instructions should be applied in the selection of principal procedure and clarification on the importance of the relation to the principal diagnosis when more than one procedure is performed:

1. Procedure performed for definitive treatment of both principal diagnosis and secondary diagnosis
   a. Sequence procedure performed for definitive treatment most related to principal diagnosis as principal procedure.
2. Procedure performed for definitive treatment and diagnostic procedures performed for both principal diagnosis and secondary diagnosis
   a. Sequence procedure performed for definitive treatment most related to principal diagnosis as principal procedure
3. A diagnostic procedure was performed for the principal diagnosis and a procedure is performed for definitive treatment of a secondary diagnosis.
   a. Sequence diagnostic procedure as principal procedure, since the procedure most related to the principal diagnosis takes precedence.
4. No procedures performed that are related to principal diagnosis; procedures performed for definitive treatment and diagnostic procedures were performed for secondary diagnosis
   a. Sequence procedure performed for definitive treatment of secondary diagnosis as principal procedure, since there are no procedures (definitive or nondefinitive treatment) related to principal diagnosis.

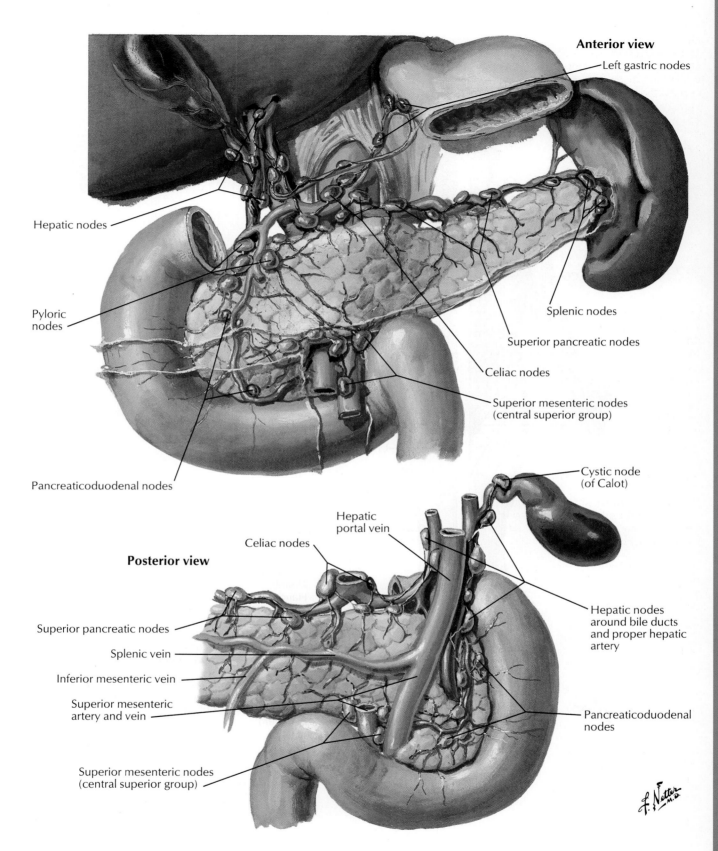

Anterior view

Left gastric nodes

Hepatic nodes

Pyloric nodes

Pancreaticoduodenal nodes

Splenic nodes

Superior pancreatic nodes

Celiac nodes

Superior mesenteric nodes (central superior group)

Posterior view

Cystic node (of Calot)

Hepatic portal vein

Celiac nodes

Hepatic nodes around bile ducts and proper hepatic artery

Superior pancreatic nodes

Splenic vein

Inferior mesenteric vein

Superior mesenteric artery and vein

Pancreaticoduodenal nodes

Superior mesenteric nodes (central superior group)

Plate 315   Lymph Vessels and Nodes of Pancreas. (Netter: Atlas of Human Anatomy, 4 ed, 2006, Saunders.)

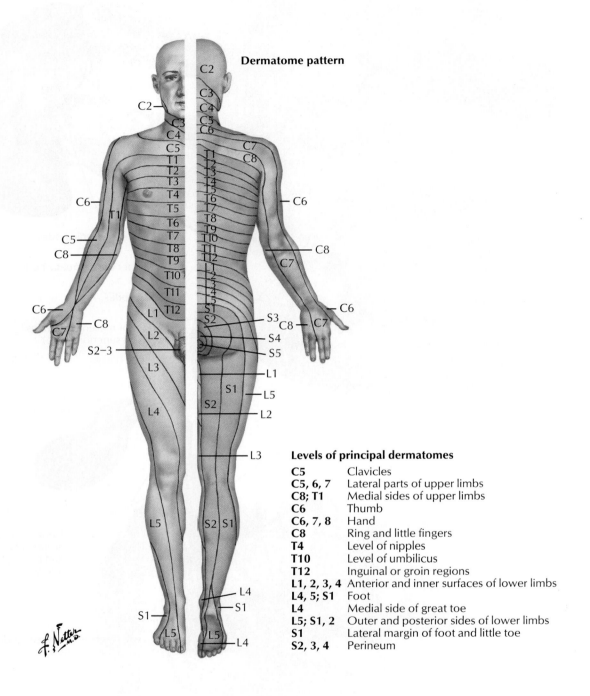

Dermatome pattern

Levels of principal dermatomes

C5	Clavicles
C5, 6, 7	Lateral parts of upper limbs
C8; T1	Medial sides of upper limbs
C6	Thumb
C6, 7, 8	Hand
C8	Ring and little fingers
T4	Level of nipples
T10	Level of umbilicus
T12	Inguinal or groin regions
L1, 2, 3, 4	Anterior and inner surfaces of lower limbs
L4, 5; S1	Foot
L4	Medial side of great toe
L5; S1, 2	Outer and posterior sides of lower limbs
S1	Lateral margin of foot and little toe
S2, 3, 4	Perineum

Plate 164 Dermatomes. (Netter: Atlas of Human Anatomy, 4 ed, 2006, Saunders.)

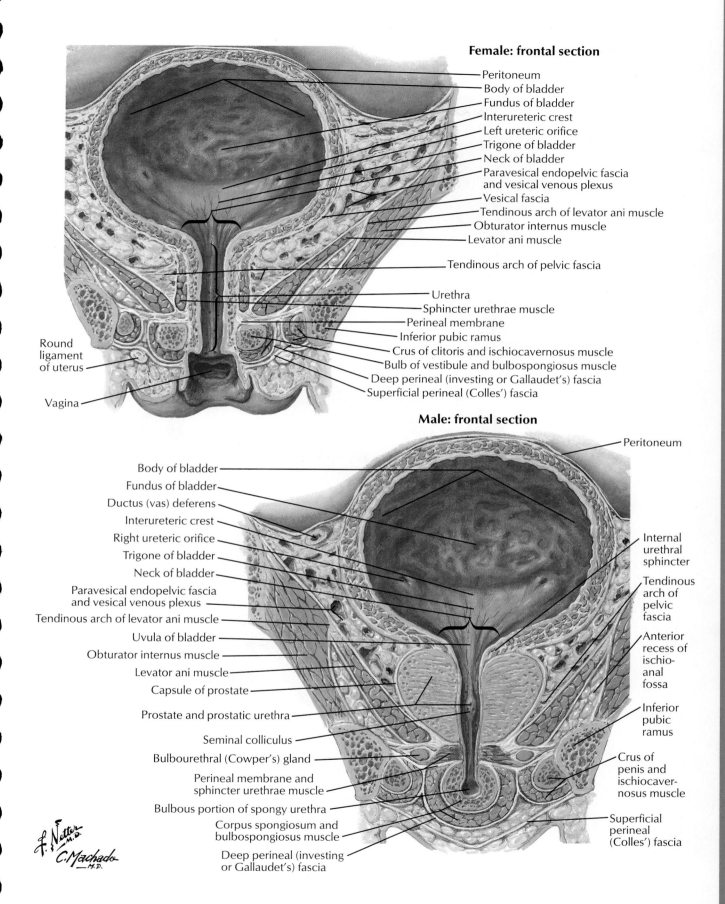

Female: frontal section

- Peritoneum
- Body of bladder
- Fundus of bladder
- Interureteric crest
- Left ureteric orifice
- Trigone of bladder
- Neck of bladder
- Paravesical endopelvic fascia and vesical venous plexus
- Vesical fascia
- Tendinous arch of levator ani muscle
- Obturator internus muscle
- Levator ani muscle
- Tendinous arch of pelvic fascia
- Urethra
- Sphincter urethrae muscle
- Perineal membrane
- Inferior pubic ramus
- Crus of clitoris and ischiocavernosus muscle
- Bulb of vestibule and bulbospongiosus muscle
- Deep perineal (investing or Gallaudet's) fascia
- Superficial perineal (Colles') fascia

Round ligament of uterus

Vagina

Male: frontal section

- Body of bladder
- Fundus of bladder
- Ductus (vas) deferens
- Interureteric crest
- Right ureteric orifice
- Trigone of bladder
- Neck of bladder
- Paravesical endopelvic fascia and vesical venous plexus
- Tendinous arch of levator ani muscle
- Uvula of bladder
- Obturator internus muscle
- Levator ani muscle
- Capsule of prostate
- Prostate and prostatic urethra
- Seminal colliculus
- Bulbourethral (Cowper's) gland
- Perineal membrane and sphincter urethrae muscle
- Bulbous portion of spongy urethra
- Corpus spongiosum and bulbospongiosus muscle
- Deep perineal (investing or Gallaudet's) fascia

- Peritoneum
- Internal urethral sphincter
- Tendinous arch of pelvic fascia
- Anterior recess of ischio-anal fossa
- Inferior pubic ramus
- Crus of penis and ischiocavernosus muscle
- Superficial perineal (Colles') fascia

Plate 366 Urinary Bladder: Female and Male. (Netter: Atlas of Human Anatomy, 4 ed, 2006, Saunders.)

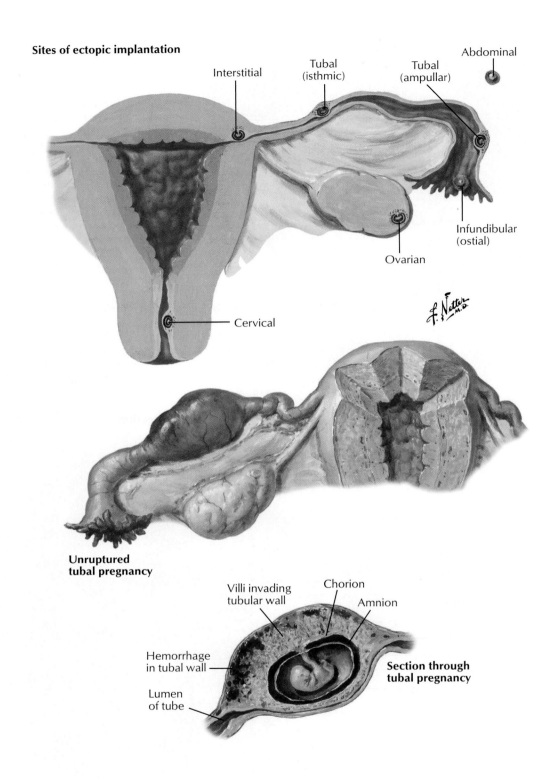

Sites of ectopic implantation

Interstitial

Tubal (isthmic)

Tubal (ampullar)

Abdominal

Infundibular (ostial)

Ovarian

Cervical

Unruptured tubal pregnancy

Villi invading tubular wall

Chorion

Amnion

Hemorrhage in tubal wall

Lumen of tube

Section through tubal pregnancy

Plate 375 Ectopic Pregnancy. (Netter: Atlas of Human Anatomy, 4 ed, 2006, Saunders.)

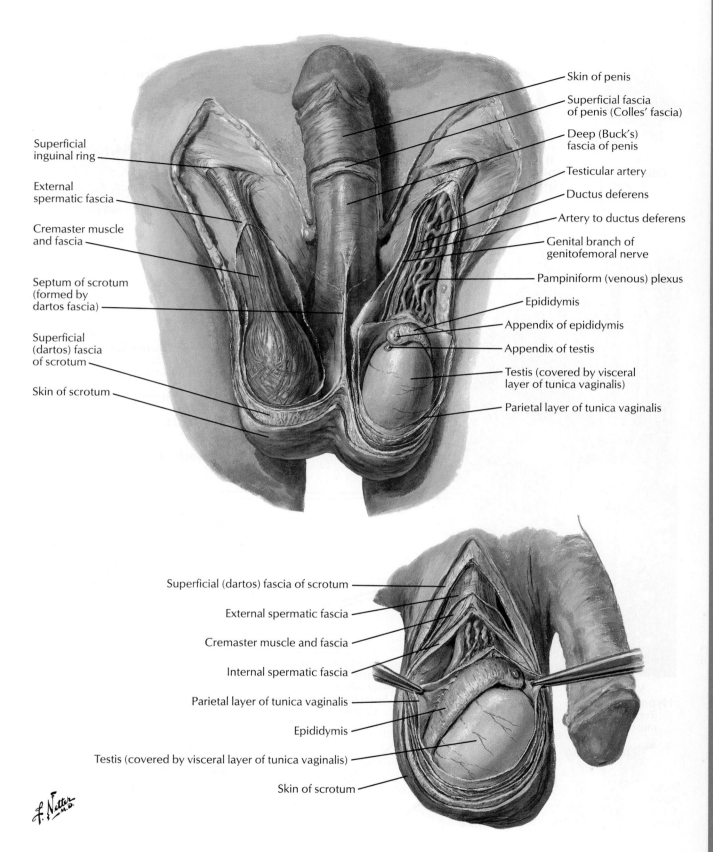

Superficial inguinal ring

External spermatic fascia

Cremaster muscle and fascia

Septum of scrotum (formed by dartos fascia)

Superficial (dartos) fascia of scrotum

Skin of scrotum

Skin of penis

Superficial fascia of penis (Colles' fascia)

Deep (Buck's) fascia of penis

Testicular artery

Ductus deferens

Artery to ductus deferens

Genital branch of genitofemoral nerve

Pampiniform (venous) plexus

Epididymis

Appendix of epididymis

Appendix of testis

Testis (covered by visceral layer of tunica vaginalis)

Parietal layer of tunica vaginalis

Superficial (dartos) fascia of scrotum

External spermatic fascia

Cremaster muscle and fascia

Internal spermatic fascia

Parietal layer of tunica vaginalis

Epididymis

Testis (covered by visceral layer of tunica vaginalis)

Skin of scrotum

Plate 387   Scrotum and Contents. (Netter: Atlas of Human Anatomy, 4 ed, 2006, Saunders.)

NETTER'S ANATOMY ILLUSTRATIONS

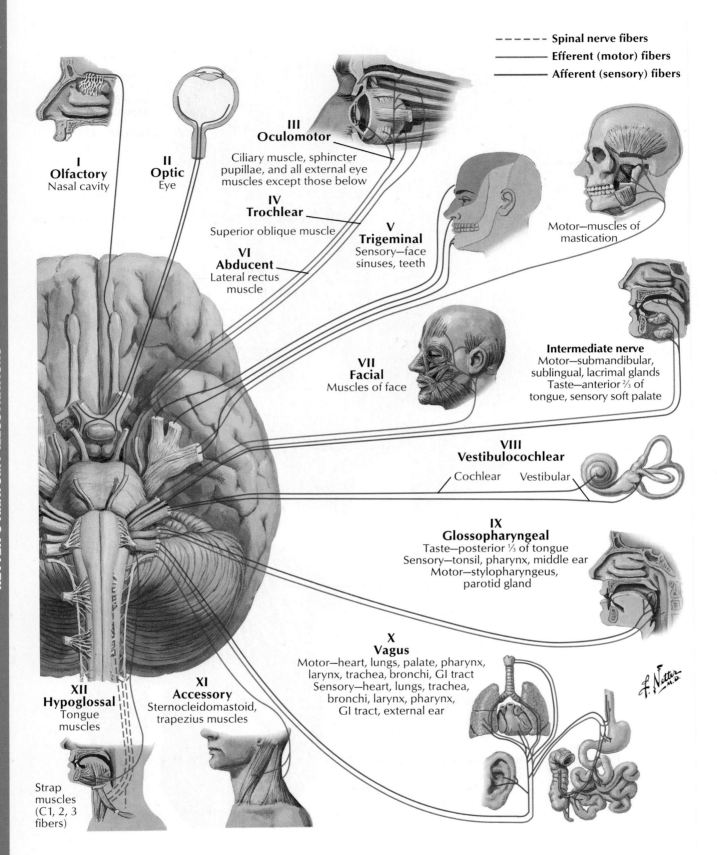

----- Spinal nerve fibers
——— Efferent (motor) fibers
——— Afferent (sensory) fibers

I
Olfactory
Nasal cavity

II
Optic
Eye

III
Oculomotor
Ciliary muscle, sphincter pupillae, and all external eye muscles except those below

IV
Trochlear
Superior oblique muscle

V
Trigeminal
Sensory—face sinuses, teeth

VI
Abducent
Lateral rectus muscle

Motor—muscles of mastication

VII
Facial
Muscles of face

Intermediate nerve
Motor—submandibular, sublingual, lacrimal glands
Taste—anterior ⅔ of tongue, sensory soft palate

VIII
Vestibulocochlear
Cochlear   Vestibular

IX
Glossopharyngeal
Taste—posterior ⅓ of tongue
Sensory—tonsil, pharynx, middle ear
Motor—stylopharyngeus, parotid gland

X
Vagus
Motor—heart, lungs, palate, pharynx, larynx, trachea, bronchi, GI tract
Sensory—heart, lungs, trachea, bronchi, larynx, pharynx, GI tract, external ear

XII
Hypoglossal
Tongue muscles

XI
Accessory
Sternocleidomastoid, trapezius muscles

Strap muscles (C1, 2, 3 fibers)

Plate 118   Cranial Nerves (Motor and Sensory Distribution): Schema. (Netter: Atlas of Human Anatomy, 4 ed, 2006, Saunders.)

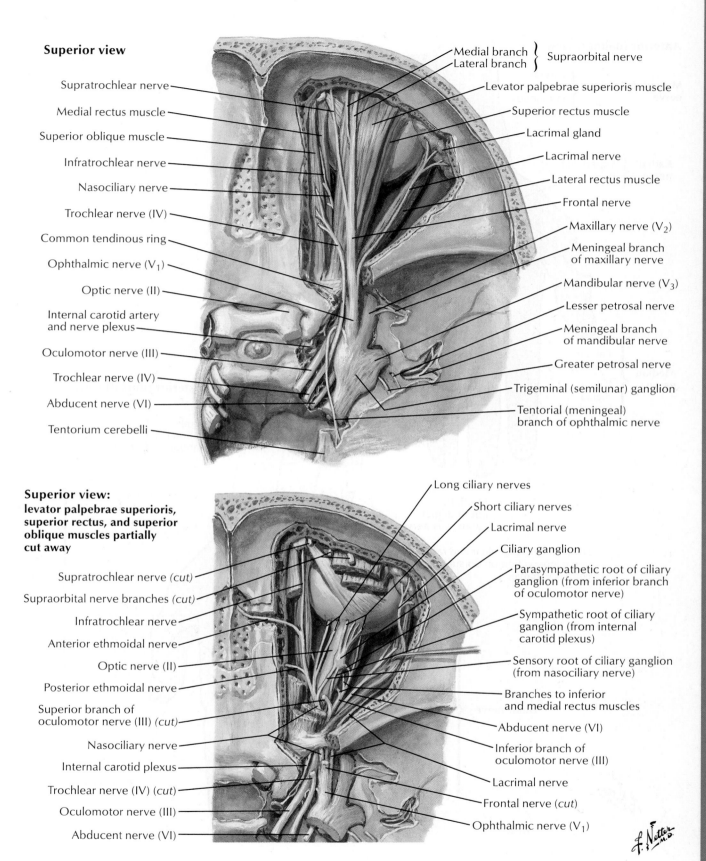

Superior view

Supratrochlear nerve

Medial rectus muscle

Superior oblique muscle

Infratrochlear nerve

Nasociliary nerve

Trochlear nerve (IV)

Common tendinous ring

Ophthalmic nerve (V₁)

Optic nerve (II)

Internal carotid artery and nerve plexus

Oculomotor nerve (III)

Trochlear nerve (IV)

Abducent nerve (VI)

Tentorium cerebelli

Medial branch } Supraorbital nerve
Lateral branch }

Levator palpebrae superioris muscle

Superior rectus muscle

Lacrimal gland

Lacrimal nerve

Lateral rectus muscle

Frontal nerve

Maxillary nerve (V₂)

Meningeal branch of maxillary nerve

Mandibular nerve (V₃)

Lesser petrosal nerve

Meningeal branch of mandibular nerve

Greater petrosal nerve

Trigeminal (semilunar) ganglion

Tentorial (meningeal) branch of ophthalmic nerve

Superior view:
levator palpebrae superioris, superior rectus, and superior oblique muscles partially cut away

Supratrochlear nerve *(cut)*

Supraorbital nerve branches *(cut)*

Infratrochlear nerve

Anterior ethmoidal nerve

Optic nerve (II)

Posterior ethmoidal nerve

Superior branch of oculomotor nerve (III) *(cut)*

Nasociliary nerve

Internal carotid plexus

Trochlear nerve (IV) *(cut)*

Oculomotor nerve (III)

Abducent nerve (VI)

Long ciliary nerves

Short ciliary nerves

Lacrimal nerve

Ciliary ganglion

Parasympathetic root of ciliary ganglion (from inferior branch of oculomotor nerve)

Sympathetic root of ciliary ganglion (from internal carotid plexus)

Sensory root of ciliary ganglion (from nasociliary nerve)

Branches to inferior and medial rectus muscles

Abducent nerve (VI)

Inferior branch of oculomotor nerve (III)

Lacrimal nerve

Frontal nerve *(cut)*

Ophthalmic nerve (V₁)

Plate 86 Nerves of Orbit. (Netter: Atlas of Human Anatomy, 4 ed, 2006, Saunders.)

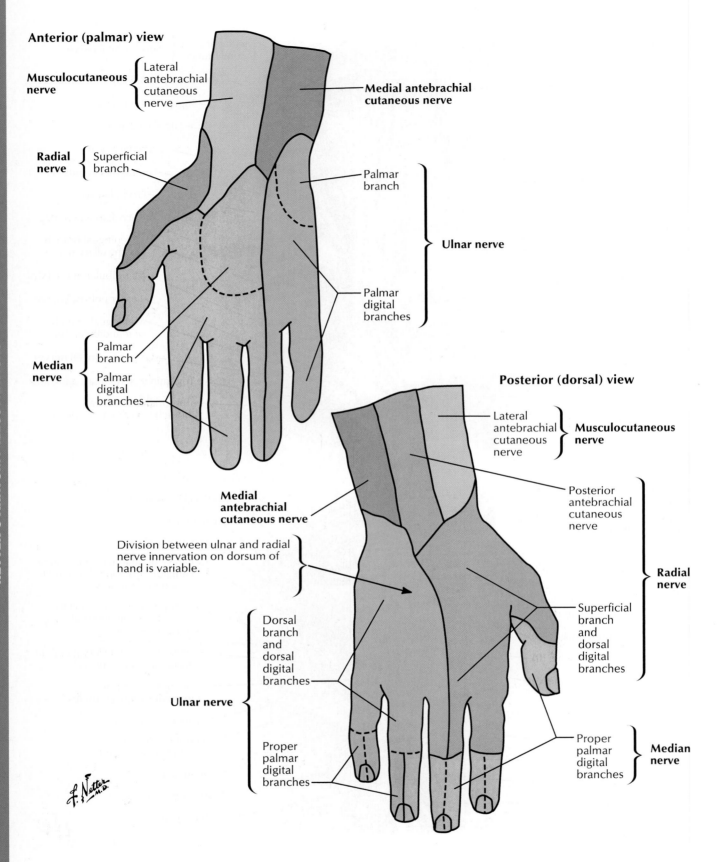

Anterior (palmar) view

Musculocutaneous nerve { Lateral antebrachial cutaneous nerve

Medial antebrachial cutaneous nerve

Radial nerve { Superficial branch

Palmar branch

Ulnar nerve

Palmar digital branches

Median nerve { Palmar branch / Palmar digital branches

Posterior (dorsal) view

Lateral antebrachial cutaneous nerve **Musculocutaneous nerve**

Posterior antebrachial cutaneous nerve

Medial antebrachial cutaneous nerve

Division between ulnar and radial nerve innervation on dorsum of hand is variable.

Radial nerve

Superficial branch and dorsal digital branches

Dorsal branch and dorsal digital branches

Ulnar nerve

Proper palmar digital branches

Proper palmar digital branches **Median nerve**

Plate 472 Cutaneous Innervation of Wrist and Hand. (Netter: Atlas of Human Anatomy, 4 ed, 2006, Saunders.)

Anterior view

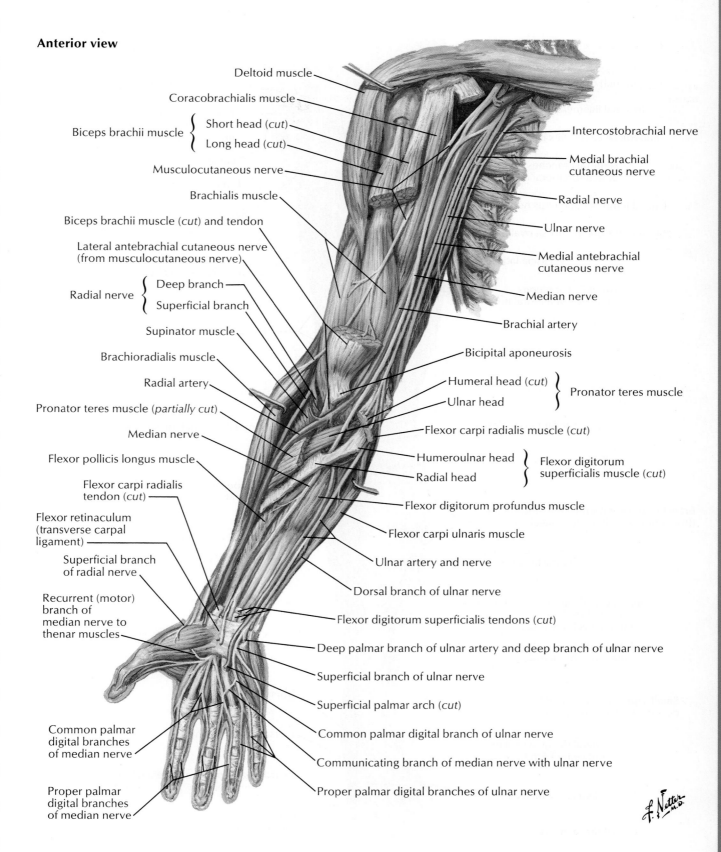

Deltoid muscle

Coracobrachialis muscle

Biceps brachii muscle { Short head (*cut*)

Long head (*cut*)

Musculocutaneous nerve

Brachialis muscle

Biceps brachii muscle (*cut*) and tendon

Lateral antebrachial cutaneous nerve (from musculocutaneous nerve)

Radial nerve { Deep branch

Superficial branch

Supinator muscle

Brachioradialis muscle

Radial artery

Pronator teres muscle (*partially cut*)

Median nerve

Flexor pollicis longus muscle

Flexor carpi radialis tendon (*cut*)

Flexor retinaculum (transverse carpal ligament)

Superficial branch of radial nerve

Recurrent (motor) branch of median nerve to thenar muscles

Common palmar digital branches of median nerve

Proper palmar digital branches of median nerve

Intercostobrachial nerve

Medial brachial cutaneous nerve

Radial nerve

Ulnar nerve

Medial antebrachial cutaneous nerve

Median nerve

Brachial artery

Bicipital aponeurosis

Humeral head (*cut*) } Pronator teres muscle

Ulnar head

Flexor carpi radialis muscle (*cut*)

Humeroulnar head } Flexor digitorum superficialis muscle (*cut*)

Radial head

Flexor digitorum profundus muscle

Flexor carpi ulnaris muscle

Ulnar artery and nerve

Dorsal branch of ulnar nerve

Flexor digitorum superficialis tendons (*cut*)

Deep palmar branch of ulnar artery and deep branch of ulnar nerve

Superficial branch of ulnar nerve

Superficial palmar arch (*cut*)

Common palmar digital branch of ulnar nerve

Communicating branch of median nerve with ulnar nerve

Proper palmar digital branches of ulnar nerve

Plate 473   Arteries and Nerves of Upper Limb. (Netter: Atlas of Human Anatomy, 4 ed, 2006, Saunders.)

NETTER'S ANATOMY ILLUSTRATIONS

15

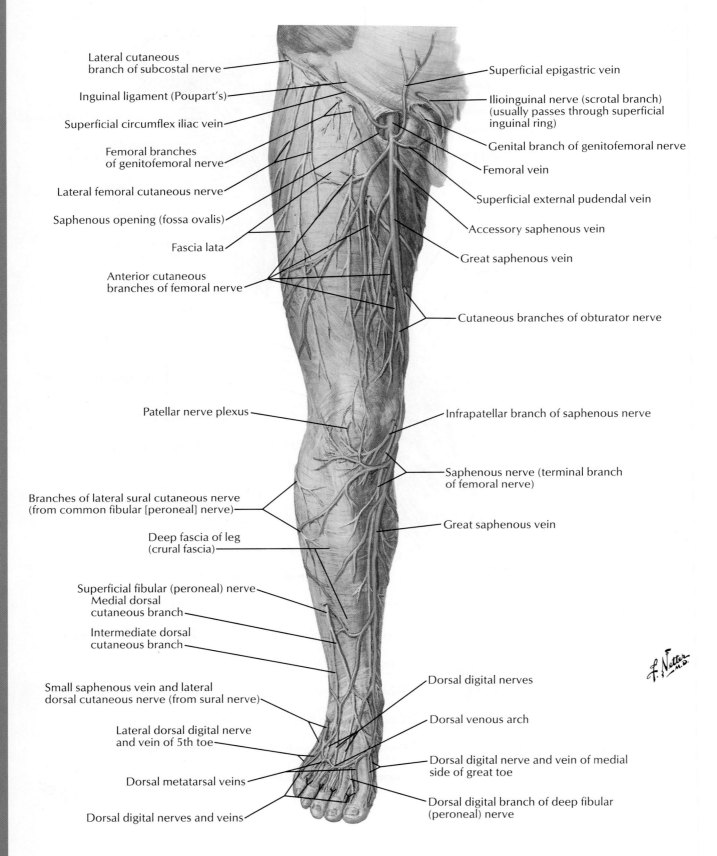

Lateral cutaneous
branch of subcostal nerve

Inguinal ligament (Poupart's)

Superficial circumflex iliac vein

Femoral branches
of genitofemoral nerve

Lateral femoral cutaneous nerve

Saphenous opening (fossa ovalis)

Fascia lata

Anterior cutaneous
branches of femoral nerve

Patellar nerve plexus

Branches of lateral sural cutaneous nerve
(from common fibular [peroneal] nerve)

Deep fascia of leg
(crural fascia)

Superficial fibular (peroneal) nerve
Medial dorsal
cutaneous branch

Intermediate dorsal
cutaneous branch

Small saphenous vein and lateral
dorsal cutaneous nerve (from sural nerve)

Lateral dorsal digital nerve
and vein of 5th toe

Dorsal metatarsal veins

Dorsal digital nerves and veins

Superficial epigastric vein

Ilioinguinal nerve (scrotal branch)
(usually passes through superficial
inguinal ring)

Genital branch of genitofemoral nerve

Femoral vein

Superficial external pudendal vein

Accessory saphenous vein

Great saphenous vein

Cutaneous branches of obturator nerve

Infrapatellar branch of saphenous nerve

Saphenous nerve (terminal branch
of femoral nerve)

Great saphenous vein

Dorsal digital nerves

Dorsal venous arch

Dorsal digital nerve and vein of medial
side of great toe

Dorsal digital branch of deep fibular
(peroneal) nerve

Plate 544 Superficial Nerves and Veins of Lower Limb: Anterior View. (Netter: Atlas of Human Anatomy, 4 ed, 2006, Saunders.)

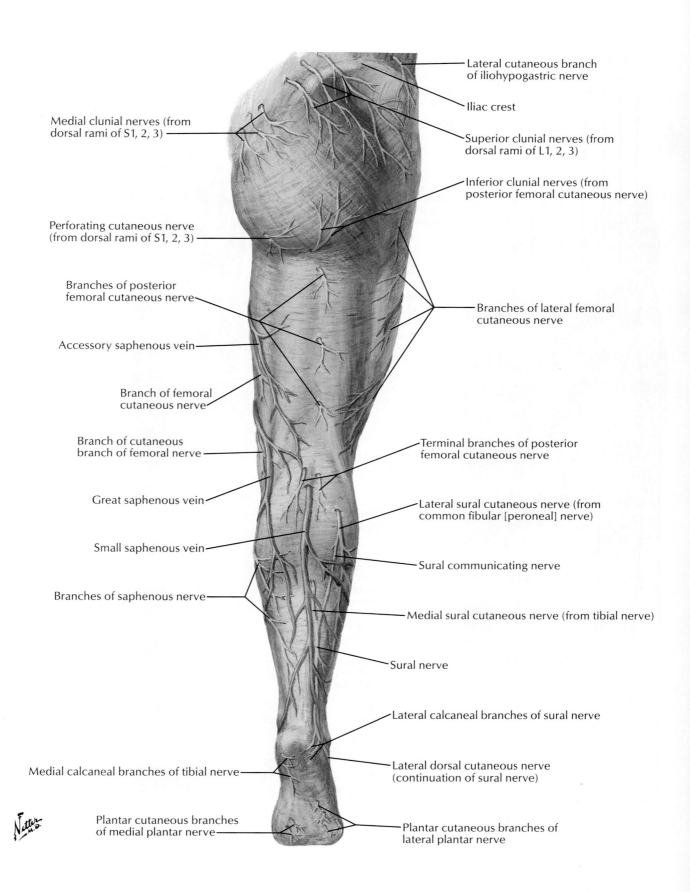

Lateral cutaneous branch of iliohypogastric nerve

Iliac crest

Superior clunial nerves (from dorsal rami of L1, 2, 3)

Inferior clunial nerves (from posterior femoral cutaneous nerve)

Medial clunial nerves (from dorsal rami of S1, 2, 3)

Perforating cutaneous nerve (from dorsal rami of S1, 2, 3)

Branches of posterior femoral cutaneous nerve

Branches of lateral femoral cutaneous nerve

Accessory saphenous vein

Branch of femoral cutaneous nerve

Branch of cutaneous branch of femoral nerve

Terminal branches of posterior femoral cutaneous nerve

Great saphenous vein

Lateral sural cutaneous nerve (from common fibular [peroneal] nerve)

Small saphenous vein

Sural communicating nerve

Branches of saphenous nerve

Medial sural cutaneous nerve (from tibial nerve)

Sural nerve

Lateral calcaneal branches of sural nerve

Medial calcaneal branches of tibial nerve

Lateral dorsal cutaneous nerve (continuation of sural nerve)

Plantar cutaneous branches of medial plantar nerve

Plantar cutaneous branches of lateral plantar nerve

Plate 545 Superficial Nerves and Veins of Lower Limb: Posterior View. (Netter: Atlas of Human Anatomy, 4 ed, 2006, Saunders.)

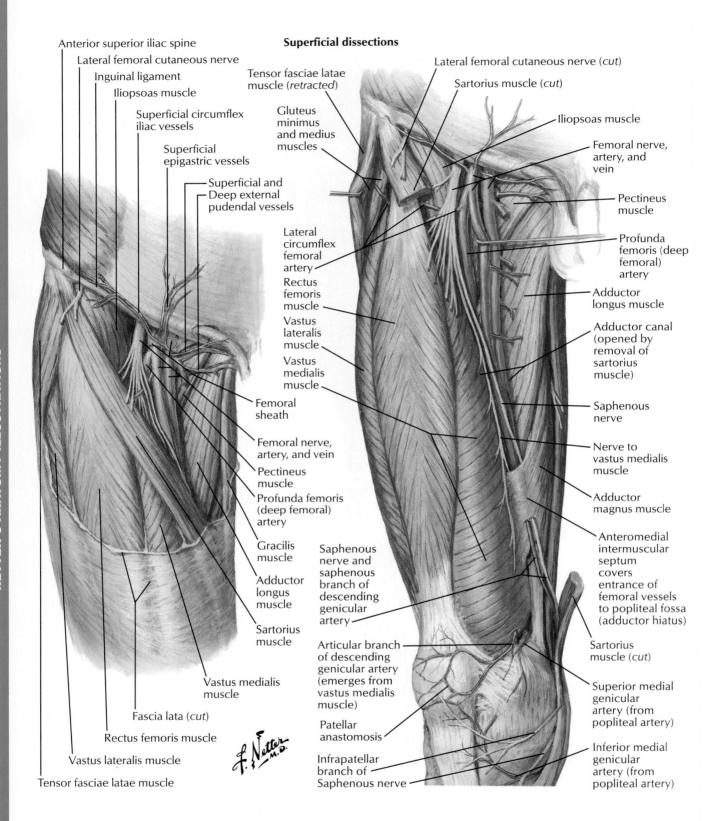

Superficial dissections

Anterior superior iliac spine
Lateral femoral cutaneous nerve
Inguinal ligament
Iliopsoas muscle
Superficial circumflex iliac vessels
Superficial epigastric vessels
Superficial and Deep external pudendal vessels

Tensor fasciae latae muscle (*retracted*)
Gluteus minimus and medius muscles
Lateral circumflex femoral artery
Rectus femoris muscle
Vastus lateralis muscle
Vastus medialis muscle
Femoral sheath
Femoral nerve, artery, and vein
Pectineus muscle
Profunda femoris (deep femoral) artery
Gracilis muscle
Adductor longus muscle
Sartorius muscle

Saphenous nerve and saphenous branch of descending genicular artery

Articular branch of descending genicular artery (emerges from vastus medialis muscle)

Patellar anastomosis

Infrapatellar branch of Saphenous nerve

Lateral femoral cutaneous nerve (*cut*)
Sartorius muscle (*cut*)
Iliopsoas muscle
Femoral nerve, artery, and vein
Pectineus muscle
Profunda femoris (deep femoral) artery
Adductor longus muscle
Adductor canal (opened by removal of sartorius muscle)
Saphenous nerve
Nerve to vastus medialis muscle
Adductor magnus muscle
Anteromedial intermuscular septum covers entrance of femoral vessels to popliteal fossa (adductor hiatus)
Sartorius muscle (*cut*)
Superior medial genicular artery (from popliteal artery)
Inferior medial genicular artery (from popliteal artery)

Vastus medialis muscle
Fascia lata (*cut*)
Rectus femoris muscle
Vastus lateralis muscle
Tensor fasciae latae muscle

Plate 500 Arteries and Nerves of Thigh: Anterior Views. (Netter: Atlas of Human Anatomy, 4 ed, 2006, Saunders.)

Deep dissection

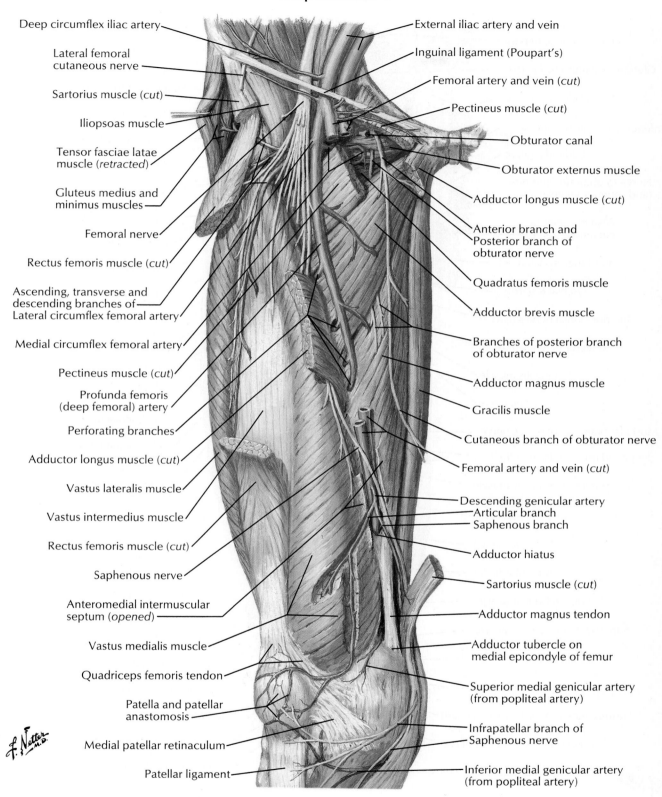

Deep circumflex iliac artery

Lateral femoral cutaneous nerve

Sartorius muscle (*cut*)

Iliopsoas muscle

Tensor fasciae latae muscle (*retracted*)

Gluteus medius and minimus muscles

Femoral nerve

Rectus femoris muscle (*cut*)

Ascending, transverse and descending branches of Lateral circumflex femoral artery

Medial circumflex femoral artery

Pectineus muscle (*cut*)

Profunda femoris (deep femoral) artery

Perforating branches

Adductor longus muscle (*cut*)

Vastus lateralis muscle

Vastus intermedius muscle

Rectus femoris muscle (*cut*)

Saphenous nerve

Anteromedial intermuscular septum (*opened*)

Vastus medialis muscle

Quadriceps femoris tendon

Patella and patellar anastomosis

Medial patellar retinaculum

Patellar ligament

External iliac artery and vein

Inguinal ligament (Poupart's)

Femoral artery and vein (*cut*)

Pectineus muscle (*cut*)

Obturator canal

Obturator externus muscle

Adductor longus muscle (*cut*)

Anterior branch and Posterior branch of obturator nerve

Quadratus femoris muscle

Adductor brevis muscle

Branches of posterior branch of obturator nerve

Adductor magnus muscle

Gracilis muscle

Cutaneous branch of obturator nerve

Femoral artery and vein (*cut*)

Descending genicular artery
Articular branch
Saphenous branch

Adductor hiatus

Sartorius muscle (*cut*)

Adductor magnus tendon

Adductor tubercle on medial epicondyle of femur

Superior medial genicular artery (from popliteal artery)

Infrapatellar branch of Saphenous nerve

Inferior medial genicular artery (from popliteal artery)

Plate 501   Arteries and Nerves of Thigh: Posterior View. (Netter: Atlas of Human Anatomy, 4 ed, 2006, Saunders.)

Deep dissection

Superior clunial nerves

Gluteus maximus muscle (*cut*)

Medial clunial nerves

Inferior gluteal artery and nerve

Pudendal nerve

Nerve to obturator internus
(and superior gemellus)

Posterior femoral
cutaneous nerve

Sacrotuberous ligament

Ischial tuberosity

Inferior clunial nerves (*cut*)

Adductor magnus muscle

Gracilis muscle

Sciatic nerve

Muscular branches of sciatic nerve

Semitendinosus muscle (*retracted*)

Semimembranosus muscle

Sciatic nerve

Articular branch

Adductor hiatus

Popliteal vein and artery

Superior medial genicular artery

Medial epicondyle of femur

Tibial nerve

Gastrocnemius muscle (medial head)

Medial sural cutaneous nerve

Small saphenous vein

Iliac crest

Gluteal aponeurosis and
gluteus medius muscle (*cut*)

Superior gluteal artery and nerve

Gluteus minimus muscle

Tensor fasciae latae muscle

Piriformis muscle

Gluteus medius muscle (*cut*)

Superior gemellus muscle

Greater trochanter of femur

Obturator internus muscle

Inferior gemellus muscle

Gluteus maximus muscle (*cut*)

Quadratus femoris muscle

Medial circumflex femoral
artery

Vastus lateralis muscle
and iliotibial tract

Adductor minimus part of
adductor magnus muscle

1st perforating artery (from
profunda femoris artery)

Adductor magnus muscle

2nd and 3rd perforating arteries
(from profunda femoris artery)

4th perforating artery (from
profunda femoris artery)

Long head (*retracted*) ⎫ Biceps femoris
Short head ⎬ muscle
⎭

Superior lateral genicular artery

Common fibular (peroneal) nerve

Plantaris muscle

Gastrocnemius muscle (lateral head)

Lateral sural cutaneous nerve

F. Netter
M.D.

Plate 5Ø2 Arteries and Nerves of Thigh: Posterior View. (Netter: Atlas of Human Anatomy, 4 ed, 2006, Saunders.)

Horizontal section

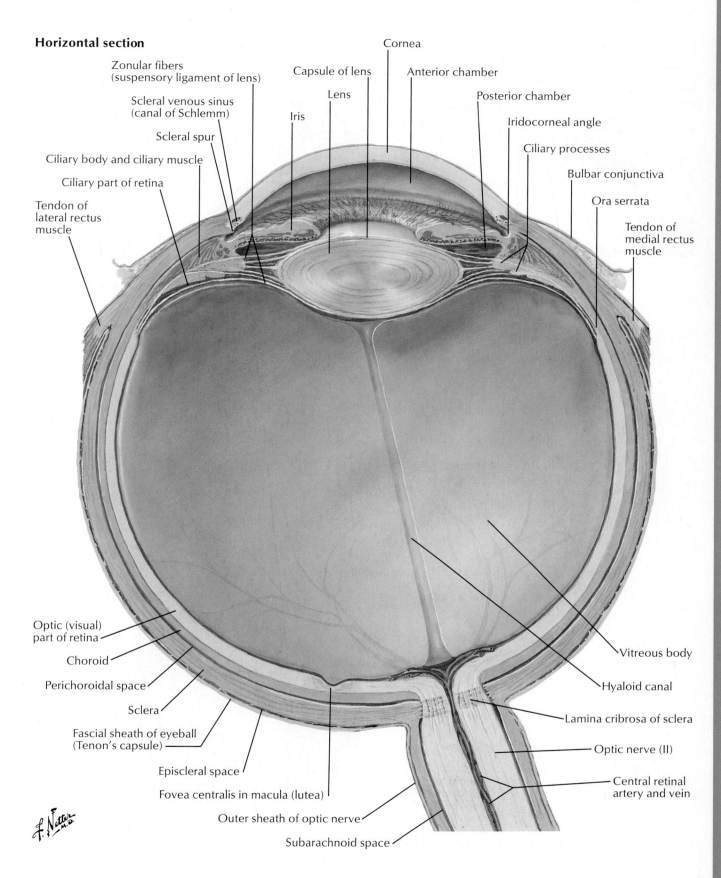

Zonular fibers
(suspensory ligament of lens)

Scleral venous sinus
(canal of Schlemm)

Scleral spur

Ciliary body and ciliary muscle

Ciliary part of retina

Tendon of
lateral rectus
muscle

Iris

Capsule of lens

Lens

Cornea

Anterior chamber

Posterior chamber

Iridocorneal angle

Ciliary processes

Bulbar conjunctiva

Ora serrata

Tendon of
medial rectus
muscle

Optic (visual)
part of retina

Choroid

Perichoroidal space

Sclera

Fascial sheath of eyeball
(Tenon's capsule)

Episcleral space

Fovea centralis in macula (lutea)

Outer sheath of optic nerve

Subarachnoid space

Vitreous body

Hyaloid canal

Lamina cribrosa of sclera

Optic nerve (II)

Central retinal
artery and vein

Plate 87   Eyeball. (Netter: Atlas of Human Anatomy, 4 ed, 2006, Saunders.)

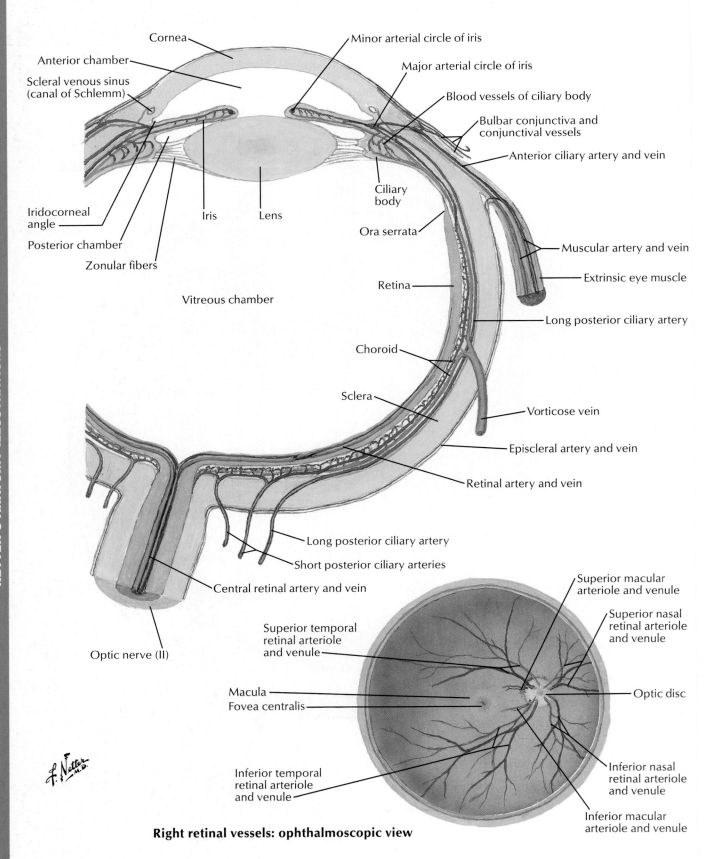

Cornea

Minor arterial circle of iris

Anterior chamber

Major arterial circle of iris

Scleral venous sinus
(canal of Schlemm)

Blood vessels of ciliary body

Bulbar conjunctiva and
conjunctival vessels

Anterior ciliary artery and vein

Ciliary
body

Iridocorneal
angle

Iris

Lens

Ora serrata

Muscular artery and vein

Posterior chamber

Extrinsic eye muscle

Zonular fibers

Retina

Long posterior ciliary artery

Vitreous chamber

Choroid

Sclera

Vorticose vein

Episcleral artery and vein

Retinal artery and vein

Long posterior ciliary artery

Short posterior ciliary arteries

Central retinal artery and vein

Optic nerve (II)

Superior macular
arteriole and venule

Superior temporal
retinal arteriole
and venule

Superior nasal
retinal arteriole
and venule

Macula

Fovea centralis

Optic disc

Inferior nasal
retinal arteriole
and venule

Inferior temporal
retinal arteriole
and venule

Inferior macular
arteriole and venule

Right retinal vessels: ophthalmoscopic view

Plate 90   Intrinsic Arteries and Veins of Eye. (Netter: Atlas of Human Anatomy, 4 ed, 2006, Saunders.)

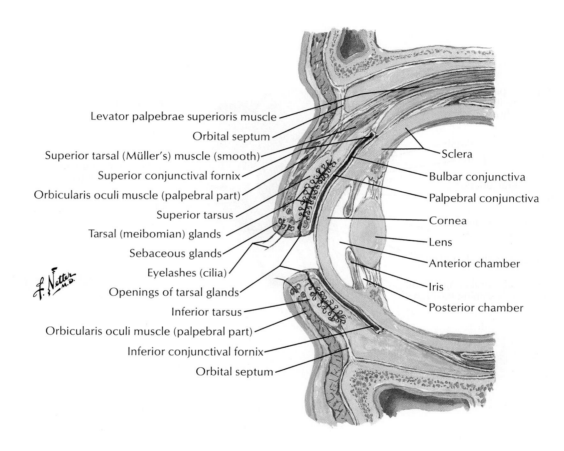

Levator palpebrae superioris muscle

Orbital septum

Superior tarsal (Müller's) muscle (smooth)

Superior conjunctival fornix

Orbicularis oculi muscle (palpebral part)

Superior tarsus

Tarsal (meibomian) glands

Sebaceous glands

Eyelashes (cilia)

Openings of tarsal glands

Inferior tarsus

Orbicularis oculi muscle (palpebral part)

Inferior conjunctival fornix

Orbital septum

Sclera

Bulbar conjunctiva

Palpebral conjunctiva

Cornea

Lens

Anterior chamber

Iris

Posterior chamber

Plate 81, Middle   Eyelids. (Netter: Atlas of Human Anatomy, 4 ed, 2006, Saunders.)

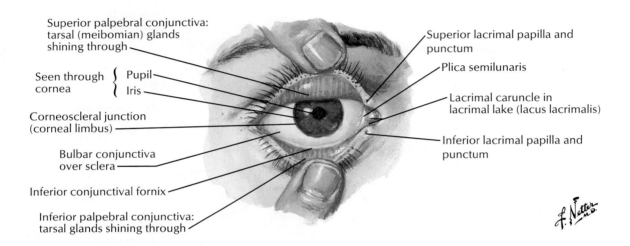

Superior palpebral conjunctiva: tarsal (meibomian) glands shining through

Seen through cornea { Pupil / Iris

Corneoscleral junction (corneal limbus)

Bulbar conjunctiva over sclera

Inferior conjunctival fornix

Inferior palpebral conjunctiva: tarsal glands shining through

Superior lacrimal papilla and punctum

Plica semilunaris

Lacrimal caruncle in lacrimal lake (lacus lacrimalis)

Inferior lacrimal papilla and punctum

Plate 81, Upper Eyelid. (Netter: Atlas of Human Anatomy, 4 ed, 2006, Saunders.)

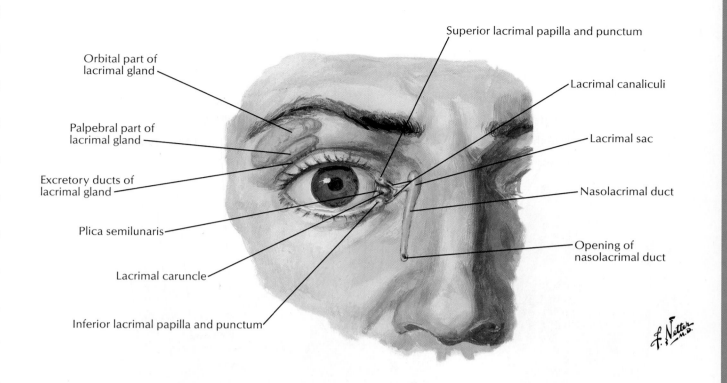

Orbital part of lacrimal gland

Palpebral part of lacrimal gland

Excretory ducts of lacrimal gland

Plica semilunaris

Lacrimal caruncle

Inferior lacrimal papilla and punctum

Superior lacrimal papilla and punctum

Lacrimal canaliculi

Lacrimal sac

Nasolacrimal duct

Opening of nasolacrimal duct

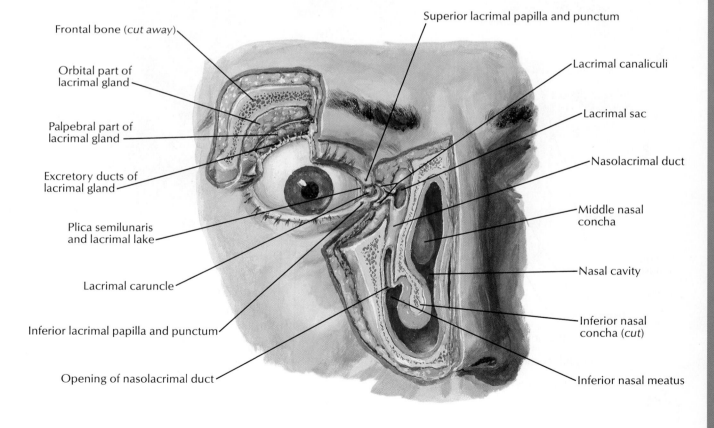

Frontal bone (*cut away*)

Orbital part of lacrimal gland

Palpebral part of lacrimal gland

Excretory ducts of lacrimal gland

Plica semilunaris and lacrimal lake

Lacrimal caruncle

Inferior lacrimal papilla and punctum

Opening of nasolacrimal duct

Superior lacrimal papilla and punctum

Lacrimal canaliculi

Lacrimal sac

Nasolacrimal duct

Middle nasal concha

Nasal cavity

Inferior nasal concha (*cut*)

Inferior nasal meatus

Plate 82   Lacrimal Apparatus. (Netter: Atlas of Human Anatomy, 4 ed, 2006, Saunders.)

Frontal section

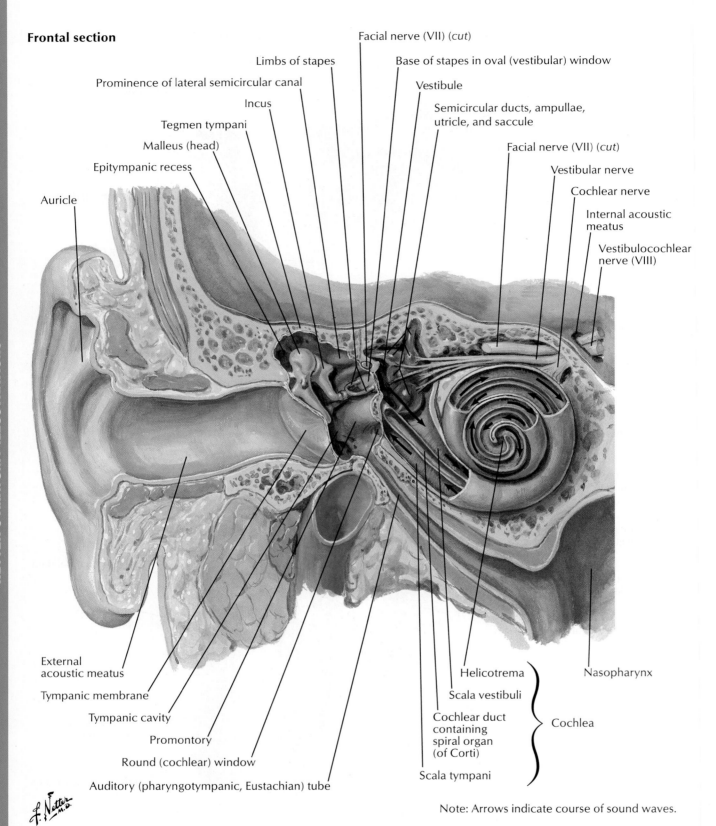

Facial nerve (VII) (*cut*)

Limbs of stapes

Base of stapes in oval (vestibular) window

Prominence of lateral semicircular canal

Vestibule

Incus

Semicircular ducts, ampullae, utricle, and saccule

Tegmen tympani

Malleus (head)

Facial nerve (VII) (*cut*)

Epitympanic recess

Vestibular nerve

Auricle

Cochlear nerve

Internal acoustic meatus

Vestibulocochlear nerve (VIII)

External acoustic meatus

Helicotrema

Nasopharynx

Tympanic membrane

Scala vestibuli

Tympanic cavity

Cochlear duct containing spiral organ (of Corti)

Promontory

Cochlea

Round (cochlear) window

Scala tympani

Auditory (pharyngotympanic, Eustachian) tube

Note: Arrows indicate course of sound waves.

Plate 92 Pathway of Sound Reception. (Netter: Atlas of Human Anatomy, 4 ed, 2006, Saunders.)

Medial wall of tympanic cavity: lateral view

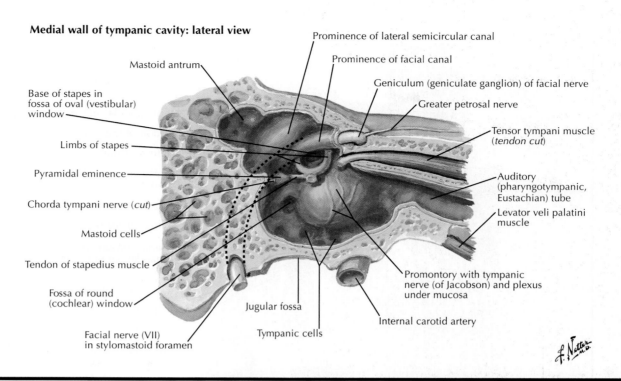

Mastoid antrum

Prominence of lateral semicircular canal

Prominence of facial canal

Geniculum (geniculate ganglion) of facial nerve

Greater petrosal nerve

Base of stapes in fossa of oval (vestibular) window

Limbs of stapes

Pyramidal eminence

Chorda tympani nerve (*cut*)

Mastoid cells

Tendon of stapedius muscle

Fossa of round (cochlear) window

Facial nerve (VII) in stylomastoid foramen

Jugular fossa

Tympanic cells

Tensor tympani muscle (*tendon cut*)

Auditory (pharyngotympanic, Eustachian) tube

Levator veli palatini muscle

Promontory with tympanic nerve (of Jacobson) and plexus under mucosa

Internal carotid artery

Plate 94 Tympanic Cavity. (Netter: Atlas of Human Anatomy, 4 ed, 2006, Saunders.)

Otoscopic view of right tympanic membrane

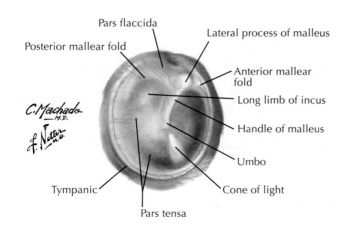

Pars flaccida

Posterior mallear fold

Lateral process of malleus

Anterior mallear fold

Long limb of incus

Handle of malleus

Umbo

Tympanic

Cone of light

Pars tensa

Plate 93 Tympanic Cavity. (Netter: Atlas of Human Anatomy, 4 ed, 2006, Saunders.)

Dissected right bony labyrinth (otic capsule): membranous labyrinth removed

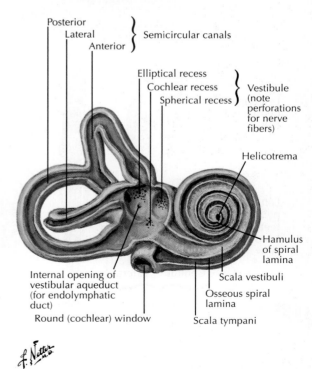

Posterior

Lateral

Anterior

Semicircular canals

Elliptical recess

Cochlear recess

Spherical recess

Vestibule (note perforations for nerve fibers)

Helicotrema

Hamulus of spiral lamina

Internal opening of vestibular aqueduct (for endolymphatic duct)

Round (cochlear) window

Scala vestibuli

Osseous spiral lamina

Scala tympani

Plate 95 Bony Membranous Labyrinth. (Netter: Atlas of Human Anatomy, 4 ed, 2006, Saunders.)

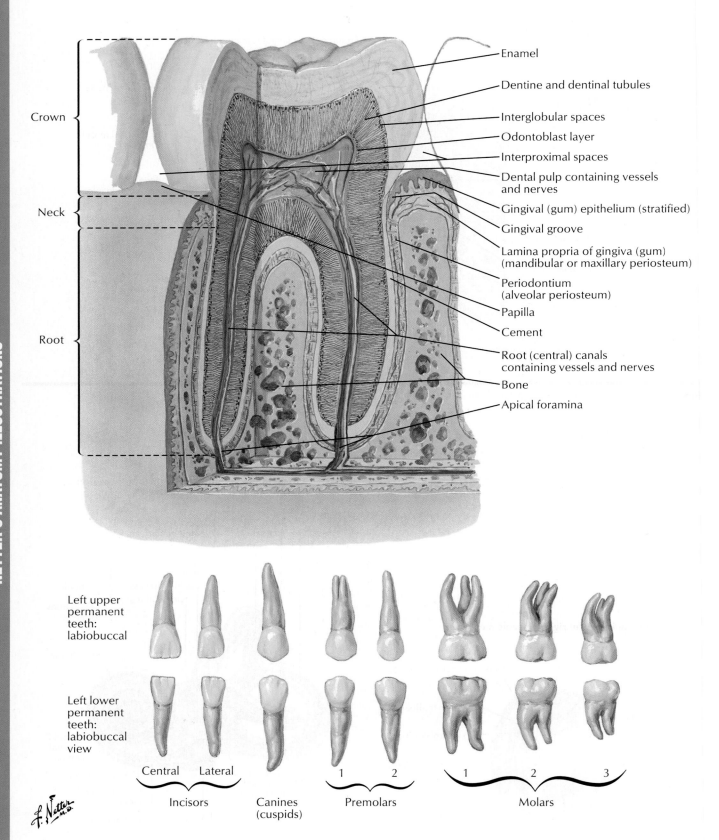

Crown

Neck

Root

Enamel

Dentine and dentinal tubules

Interglobular spaces

Odontoblast layer

Interproximal spaces

Dental pulp containing vessels and nerves

Gingival (gum) epithelium (stratified)

Gingival groove

Lamina propria of gingiva (gum) (mandibular or maxillary periosteum)

Periodontium (alveolar periosteum)

Papilla

Cement

Root (central) canals containing vessels and nerves

Bone

Apical foramina

Left upper permanent teeth: labiobuccal

Left lower permanent teeth: labiobuccal view

Central   Lateral

1   2

1   2   3

Incisors

Canines (cuspids)

Premolars

Molars

Plate 57 Teeth. (Netter: Atlas of Human Anatomy, 4 ed, 2006, Saunders.)

Tongue

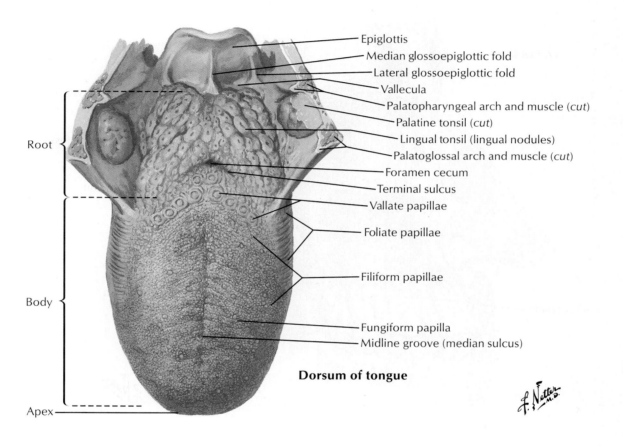

Epiglottis
Median glossoepiglottic fold
Lateral glossoepiglottic fold
Vallecula
Palatopharyngeal arch and muscle (*cut*)
Palatine tonsil (*cut*)
Lingual tonsil (lingual nodules)
Palatoglossal arch and muscle (*cut*)
Foramen cecum
Terminal sulcus
Vallate papillae
Foliate papillae
Filiform papillae
Fungiform papilla
Midline groove (median sulcus)

Root

Body

Apex

Dorsum of tongue

Plate 58   Tongue. (Netter: Atlas of Human Anatomy, 4 ed, 2006, Saunders.)

29

NETTER'S ANATOMY ILLUSTRATIONS

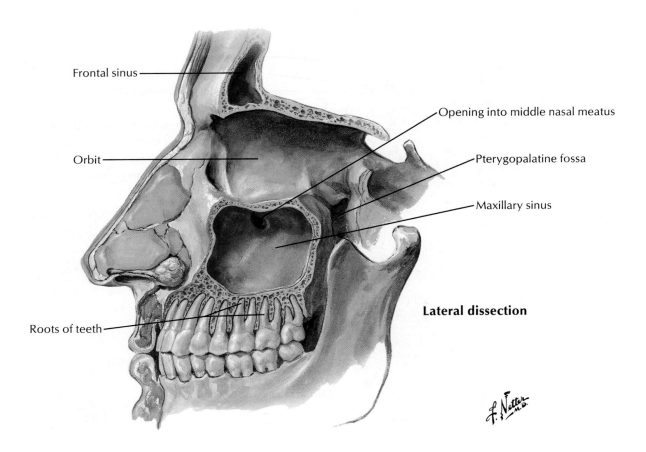

Frontal sinus

Opening into middle nasal meatus

Orbit

Pterygopalatine fossa

Maxillary sinus

Lateral dissection

Roots of teeth

f. Netter m.d.

Plate 49   Paranasal Sinuses. (Netter: Atlas of Human Anatomy, 4 ed, 2006, Saunders.)

30

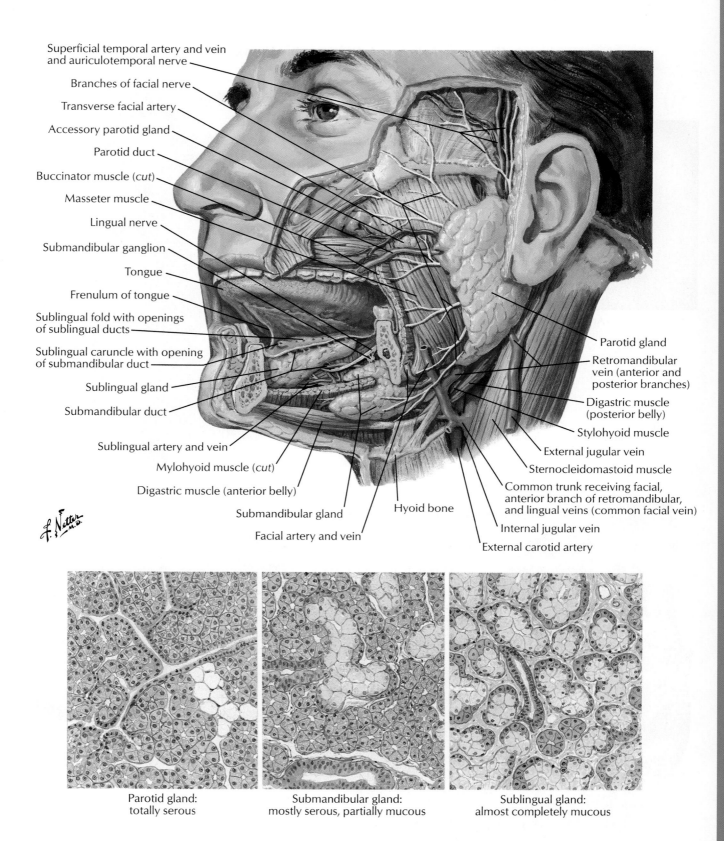

Superficial temporal artery and vein and auriculotemporal nerve

Branches of facial nerve

Transverse facial artery

Accessory parotid gland

Parotid duct

Buccinator muscle (*cut*)

Masseter muscle

Lingual nerve

Submandibular ganglion

Tongue

Frenulum of tongue

Sublingual fold with openings of sublingual ducts

Sublingual caruncle with opening of submandibular duct

Sublingual gland

Submandibular duct

Sublingual artery and vein

Mylohyoid muscle (*cut*)

Digastric muscle (anterior belly)

Submandibular gland

Facial artery and vein

Hyoid bone

Parotid gland

Retromandibular vein (anterior and posterior branches)

Digastric muscle (posterior belly)

Stylohyoid muscle

External jugular vein

Sternocleidomastoid muscle

Common trunk receiving facial, anterior branch of retromandibular, and lingual veins (common facial vein)

Internal jugular vein

External carotid artery

Parotid gland: totally serous

Submandibular gland: mostly serous, partially mucous

Sublingual gland: almost completely mucous

Plate 61 Salivary Glands. (Netter: Atlas of Human Anatomy, 4 ed, 2006, Saunders.)

Coronary Arteries: Arteriographic Views

Right coronary artery: left anterior oblique view

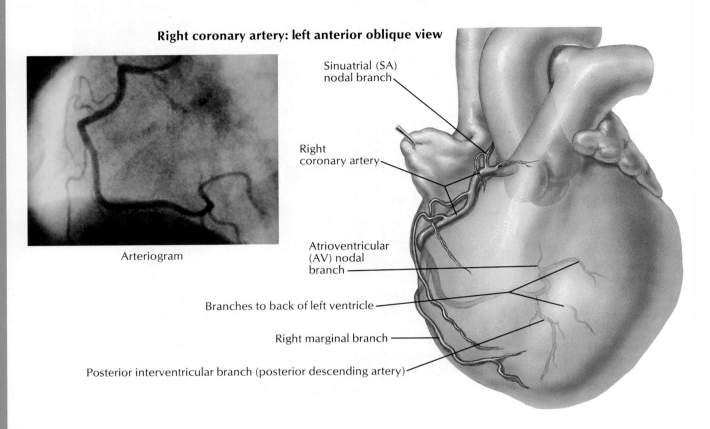

Sinuatrial (SA) nodal branch

Right coronary artery

Atrioventricular (AV) nodal branch

Branches to back of left ventricle

Right marginal branch

Posterior interventricular branch (posterior descending artery)

Arteriogram

Right coronary artery: right anterior oblique view

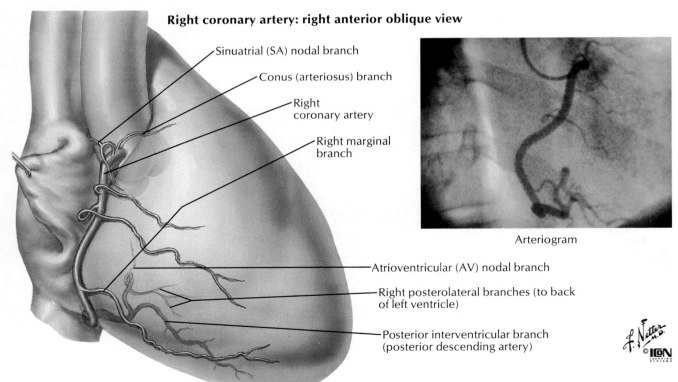

Sinuatrial (SA) nodal branch

Conus (arteriosus) branch

Right coronary artery

Right marginal branch

Atrioventricular (AV) nodal branch

Right posterolateral branches (to back of left ventricle)

Posterior interventricular branch (posterior descending artery)

Arteriogram

Plate 218 Coronary Arteries: Arteriographic Views. (Netter: Atlas of Human Anatomy, 4 ed, 2006, Saunders.)

Left coronary artery: left anterior oblique view

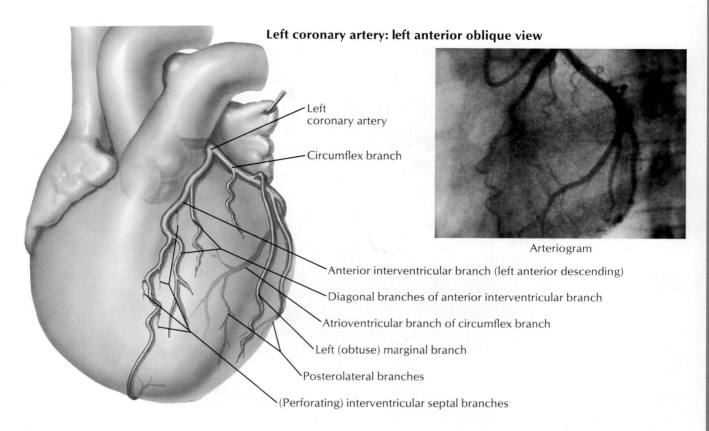

Left coronary artery

Circumflex branch

Arteriogram

Anterior interventricular branch (left anterior descending)

Diagonal branches of anterior interventricular branch

Atrioventricular branch of circumflex branch

Left (obtuse) marginal branch

Posterolateral branches

(Perforating) interventricular septal branches

Left coronary artery: right anterior oblique view

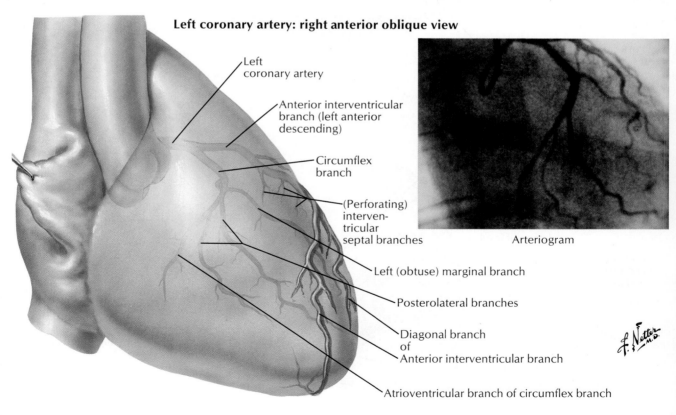

Left coronary artery

Anterior interventricular branch (left anterior descending)

Circumflex branch

(Perforating) interventricular septal branches

Arteriogram

Left (obtuse) marginal branch

Posterolateral branches

Diagonal branch of Anterior interventricular branch

Atrioventricular branch of circumflex branch

Plate 219 Coronary Arteries: Arteriographic Views. (Netter: Atlas of Human Anatomy, 4 ed, 2006, Saunders.)

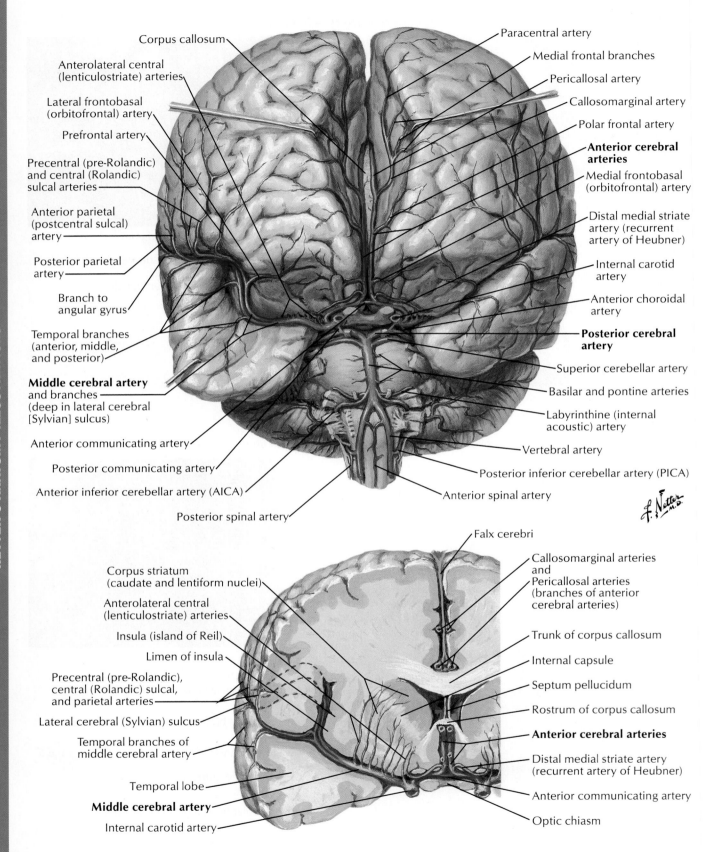

Corpus callosum

Anterolateral central (lenticulostriate) arteries

Lateral frontobasal (orbitofrontal) artery

Prefrontal artery

Precentral (pre-Rolandic) and central (Rolandic) sulcal arteries

Anterior parietal (postcentral sulcal) artery

Posterior parietal artery

Branch to angular gyrus

Temporal branches (anterior, middle, and posterior)

Middle cerebral artery and branches (deep in lateral cerebral [Sylvian] sulcus)

Anterior communicating artery

Posterior communicating artery

Anterior inferior cerebellar artery (AICA)

Posterior spinal artery

Paracentral artery

Medial frontal branches

Pericallosal artery

Callosomarginal artery

Polar frontal artery

Anterior cerebral arteries

Medial frontobasal (orbitofrontal) artery

Distal medial striate artery (recurrent artery of Heubner)

Internal carotid artery

Anterior choroidal artery

Posterior cerebral artery

Superior cerebellar artery

Basilar and pontine arteries

Labyrinthine (internal acoustic) artery

Vertebral artery

Posterior inferior cerebellar artery (PICA)

Anterior spinal artery

Corpus striatum (caudate and lentiform nuclei)

Anterolateral central (lenticulostriate) arteries

Insula (island of Reil)

Limen of insula

Precentral (pre-Rolandic), central (Rolandic) sulcal, and parietal arteries

Lateral cerebral (Sylvian) sulcus

Temporal branches of middle cerebral artery

Temporal lobe

Middle cerebral artery

Internal carotid artery

Falx cerebri

Callosomarginal arteries and Pericallosal arteries (branches of anterior cerebral arteries)

Trunk of corpus callosum

Internal capsule

Septum pellucidum

Rostrum of corpus callosum

Anterior cerebral arteries

Distal medial striate artery (recurrent artery of Heubner)

Anterior communicating artery

Optic chiasm

Plate 141 Arteries of Brain: Frontal View and Section. (Netter: Atlas of Human Anatomy, 4 ed, 2006, Saunders.)

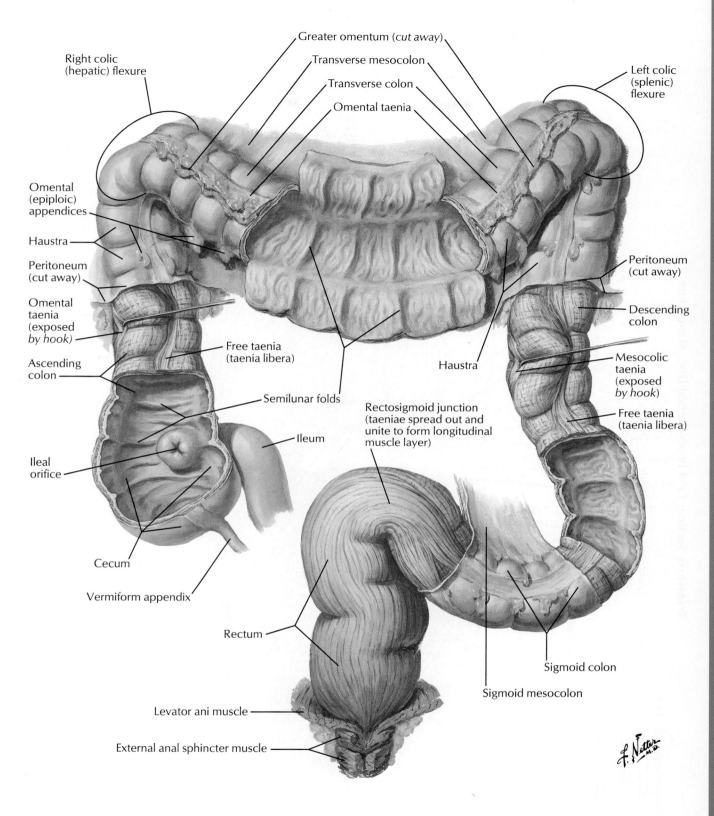

Greater omentum (*cut away*)

Transverse mesocolon

Transverse colon

Omental taenia

Right colic (hepatic) flexure

Left colic (splenic) flexure

Omental (epiploic) appendices

Haustra

Peritoneum (cut away)

Omental taenia (exposed *by hook*)

Ascending colon

Free taenia (taenia libera)

Semilunar folds

Ileal orifice

Cecum

Vermiform appendix

Ileum

Rectosigmoid junction (taeniae spread out and unite to form longitudinal muscle layer)

Haustra

Peritoneum (cut away)

Descending colon

Mesocolic taenia (exposed *by hook*)

Free taenia (taenia libera)

Sigmoid colon

Sigmoid mesocolon

Rectum

Levator ani muscle

External anal sphincter muscle

Plate 284 Mucosa and Musculature of Large Intestine. (Netter: Atlas of Human Anatomy, 4 ed, 2006, Saunders.)

Transverse Section: T3–4 Intervertebral Disc, Manubrium

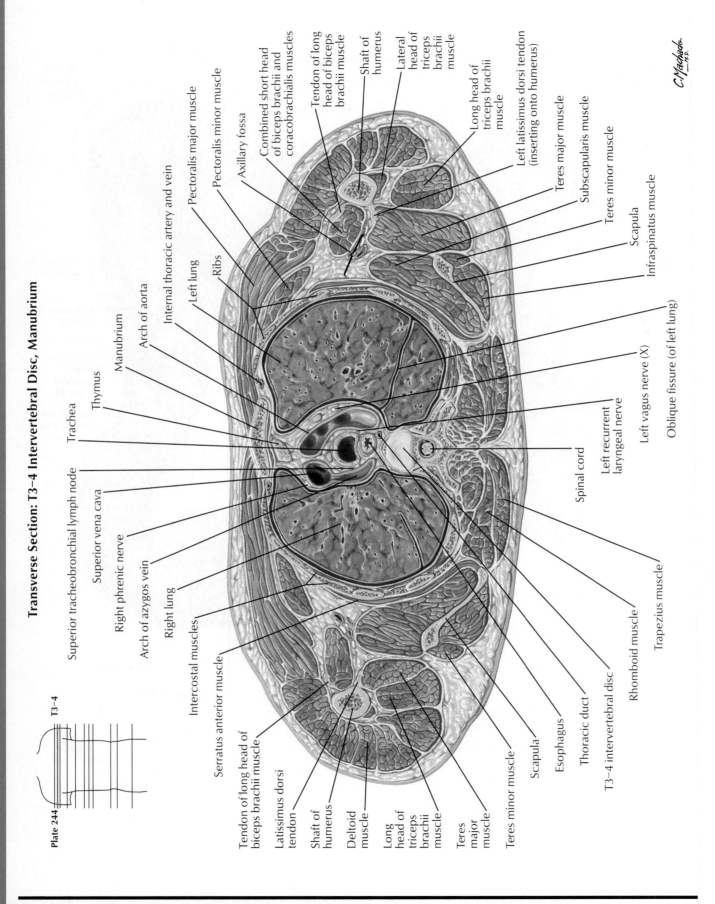

Superior tracheobronchial lymph node

Trachea

Thymus

Manubrium

Arch of aorta

Internal thoracic artery and vein

Pectoralis major muscle

Left lung

Ribs

Pectoralis minor muscle

Axillary fossa

Combined short head of biceps brachii and coracobrachialis muscles

Tendon of long head of biceps brachii muscle

Shaft of humerus

Lateral head of triceps brachii muscle

Long head of triceps brachii muscle

Left latissimus dorsi tendon (inserting onto humerus)

Teres major muscle

Subscapularis muscle

Teres minor muscle

Scapula

Infraspinatus muscle

Oblique fissure (of left lung)

Left vagus nerve (X)

Left recurrent laryngeal nerve

Spinal cord

Trapezius muscle

Rhomboid muscle

T3–4 intervertebral disc

Thoracic duct

Esophagus

Scapula

Teres minor muscle

Teres major muscle

Long head of triceps brachii muscle

Deltoid muscle

Shaft of humerus

Latissimus dorsi tendon

Tendon of long head of biceps brachii muscle

Serratus anterior muscle

Intercostal muscles

Right lung

Arch of azygos vein

Right phrenic nerve

Superior vena cava

Plate 244

T3–4

Plate 244   Cross Section of Thorax at T3-4 Disc Level. (Netter: Atlas of Human Anatomy, 4 ed, 2006, Saunders.)

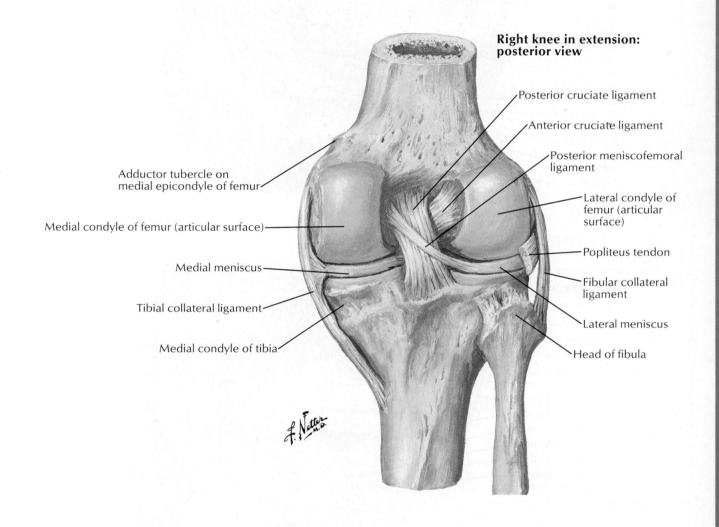

Right knee in extension: posterior view

Adductor tubercle on medial epicondyle of femur

Medial condyle of femur (articular surface)

Medial meniscus

Tibial collateral ligament

Medial condyle of tibia

Posterior cruciate ligament

Anterior cruciate ligament

Posterior meniscofemoral ligament

Lateral condyle of femur (articular surface)

Popliteus tendon

Fibular collateral ligament

Lateral meniscus

Head of fibula

Plate 5Ø9 Knee: Cruciate and Collateral Ligaments. (Netter: Atlas of Human Anatomy, 4 ed, 2006, Saunders.)

NETTER'S ANATOMY ILLUSTRATIONS

Paramedian (sagittal) dissection

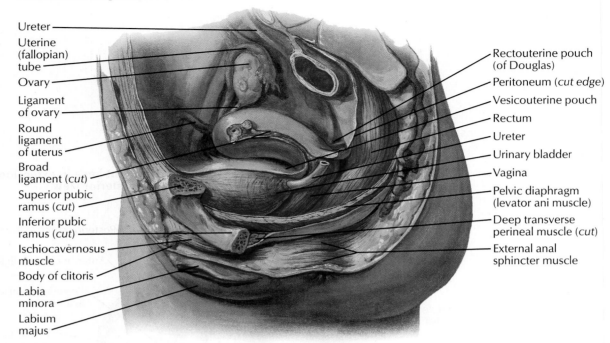

Ureter

Uterine (fallopian) tube

Ovary

Ligament of ovary

Round ligament of uterus

Broad ligament (*cut*)

Superior pubic ramus (*cut*)

Inferior pubic ramus (*cut*)

Ischiocavernosus muscle

Body of clitoris

Labia minora

Labium majus

Rectouterine pouch (of Douglas)

Peritoneum (*cut edge*)

Vesicouterine pouch

Rectum

Ureter

Urinary bladder

Vagina

Pelvic diaphragm (levator ani muscle)

Deep transverse perineal muscle (*cut*)

External anal sphincter muscle

Median (sagittal) section

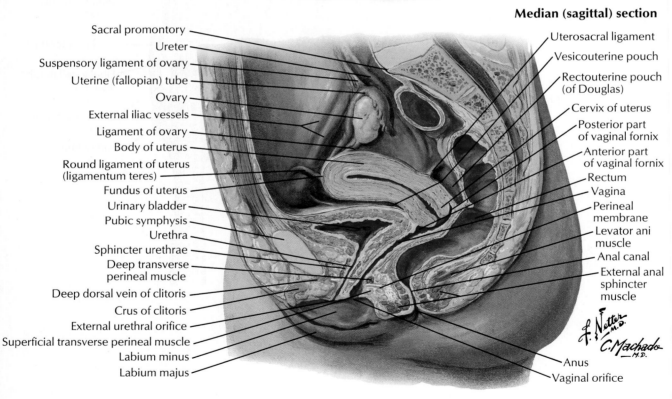

Sacral promontory

Ureter

Suspensory ligament of ovary

Uterine (fallopian) tube

Ovary

External iliac vessels

Ligament of ovary

Body of uterus

Round ligament of uterus (ligamentum teres)

Fundus of uterus

Urinary bladder

Pubic symphysis

Urethra

Sphincter urethrae

Deep transverse perineal muscle

Deep dorsal vein of clitoris

Crus of clitoris

External urethral orifice

Superficial transverse perineal muscle

Labium minus

Labium majus

Uterosacral ligament

Vesicouterine pouch

Rectouterine pouch (of Douglas)

Cervix of uterus

Posterior part of vaginal fornix

Anterior part of vaginal fornix

Rectum

Vagina

Perineal membrane

Levator ani muscle

Anal canal

External anal sphincter muscle

Anus

Vaginal orifice

Plate 360   Pelvic Viscera and Perineum: Female. (Netter: Atlas of Human Anatomy, 4 ed, 2006, Saunders.)

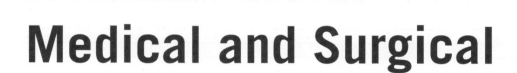

TABLES

Medical and Surgical

New/Revised Text in Green   ~~deleted~~ Deleted   ♀ Females Only   ♂ Males Only   **Coding Clinic**

Non-covered   Limited Coverage   ⊞ Combination (See Appendix E)   DRG Non-OR   Non-OR   Hospital-Acquired Condition

SECTION: Ø MEDICAL AND SURGICAL

BODY SYSTEM: Ø CENTRAL NERVOUS SYSTEM

OPERATION: 1 **BYPASS:** Altering the route of passage of the contents of a tubular body part

Body Part	Approach	Device	Qualifier
6 Cerebral Ventricle	Ø Open 3 Percutaneous	7 Autologous Tissue Substitute J Synthetic Substitute K Nonautologous Tissue Substitute	Ø Nasopharynx 1 Mastoid Sinus 2 Atrium 3 Blood Vessel 4 Pleural Cavity 5 Intestine 6 Peritoneal Cavity 7 Urinary Tract 8 Bone Marrow B Cerebral Cisterns
U Spinal Canal	Ø Open 3 Percutaneous	7 Autologous Tissue Substitute J Synthetic Substitute K Nonautologous Tissue Substitute	4 Pleural Cavity 6 Peritoneal Cavity 7 Urinary Tract 9 Fallopian Tube

Coding Clinic: 2013, Q2, P37 – 00163J6

SECTION: Ø MEDICAL AND SURGICAL

BODY SYSTEM: Ø CENTRAL NERVOUS SYSTEM

OPERATION: 2 **CHANGE:** Taking out or off a device from a body part and putting back an identical or similar device in or on the same body part without cutting or puncturing the skin or a mucous membrane

Body Part	Approach	Device	Qualifier
Ø Brain E Cranial Nerve U Spinal Canal	X External	Ø Drainage Device Y Other Device	Z No Qualifier

Non-OR All Values

SECTION: Ø MEDICAL AND SURGICAL

BODY SYSTEM: Ø CENTRAL NERVOUS SYSTEM

OPERATION: 5 DESTRUCTION: Physical eradication of all or a portion of a body part by the direct use of energy, force, or a destructive agent

Body Part	Approach	Device	Qualifier
Ø Brain	Ø Open	Z No Device	Z No Qualifier
1 Cerebral Meninges	3 Percutaneous		
2 Dura Mater	4 Percutaneous Endoscopic		
6 Cerebral Ventricle			
7 Cerebral Hemisphere			
8 Basal Ganglia			
9 Thalamus			
A Hypothalamus			
B Pons			
C Cerebellum			
D Medulla Oblongata			
F Olfactory Nerve			
G Optic Nerve			
H Oculomotor Nerve			
J Trochlear Nerve			
K Trigeminal Nerve			
L Abducens Nerve			
M Facial Nerve			
N Acoustic Nerve			
P Glossopharyngeal Nerve			
Q Vagus Nerve			
R Accessory Nerve			
S Hypoglossal Nerve			
T Spinal Meninges			
W Cervical Spinal Cord			
X Thoracic Spinal Cord			
Y Lumbar Spinal Cord			

Non-OR ØØ5[FGHJKLMNPQRS][Ø34]ZZ

SECTION: Ø MEDICAL AND SURGICAL

BODY SYSTEM: Ø CENTRAL NERVOUS SYSTEM

OPERATION: 8 DIVISION: Cutting into a body part, without draining fluids and/or gases from the body part, in order to separate or transect a body part

Body Part	Approach	Device	Qualifier
Ø Brain	Ø Open	Z No Device	Z No Qualifier
7 Cerebral Hemisphere	3 Percutaneous		
8 Basal Ganglia	4 Percutaneous Endoscopic		
F Olfactory Nerve			
G Optic Nerve			
H Oculomotor Nerve			
J Trochlear Nerve			
K Trigeminal Nerve			
L Abducens Nerve			
M Facial Nerve			
N Acoustic Nerve			
P Glossopharyngeal Nerve			
Q Vagus Nerve			
R Accessory Nerve			
S Hypoglossal Nerve			
W Cervical Spinal Cord			
X Thoracic Spinal Cord			
Y Lumbar Spinal Cord			

Ø: CENTRAL NERVOUS SYSTEM   5: DESTRUCTION   8: DIVISION   Ø: M/S

SECTION: Ø MEDICAL AND SURGICAL
BODY SYSTEM: Ø CENTRAL NERVOUS SYSTEM
OPERATION: 9 **DRAINAGE:** *(on multiple pages)*
Taking or letting out fluids and/or gases from a body part

Body Part	Approach	Device	Qualifier
Ø Brain 1 Cerebral Meninges 2 Dura Mater 3 Epidural Space 4 Subdural Space 5 Subarachnoid Space 6 Cerebral Ventricle 7 Cerebral Hemisphere 8 Basal Ganglia 9 Thalamus A Hypothalamus B Pons C Cerebellum D Medulla Oblongata F Olfactory Nerve G Optic Nerve H Oculomotor Nerve J Trochlear Nerve K Trigeminal Nerve L Abducens Nerve M Facial Nerve N Acoustic Nerve P Glossopharyngeal Nerve Q Vagus Nerve R Accessory Nerve S Hypoglossal Nerve T Spinal Meninges U Spinal Canal W Cervical Spinal Cord X Thoracic Spinal Cord Y Lumbar Spinal Cord	Ø Open 3 Percutaneous 4 Percutaneous Endoscopic	Ø Drainage Device	Z No Qualifier

Non-OR   ØØ9U[34]ØZ

Coding Clinic: 2Ø15, Q2, P3Ø – ØØ9WØØZ

SECTION: Ø MEDICAL AND SURGICAL

BODY SYSTEM: Ø CENTRAL NERVOUS SYSTEM

OPERATION: 9 DRAINAGE: *(continued)*

Taking or letting out fluids and/or gases from a body part

Body Part	Approach	Device	Qualifier
Ø Brain	Ø Open	Z No Device	X Diagnostic
1 Cerebral Meninges	3 Percutaneous		Z No Qualifier
2 Dura Mater	4 Percutaneous Endoscopic		
3 Epidural Space			
4 Subdural Space			
5 Subarachnoid Space			
6 Cerebral Ventricle			
7 Cerebral Hemisphere			
8 Basal Ganglia			
9 Thalamus			
A Hypothalamus			
B Pons			
C Cerebellum			
D Medulla Oblongata			
F Olfactory Nerve			
G Optic Nerve			
H Oculomotor Nerve			
J Trochlear Nerve			
K Trigeminal Nerve			
L Abducens Nerve			
M Facial Nerve			
N Acoustic Nerve			
P Glossopharyngeal Nerve			
Q Vagus Nerve			
R Accessory Nerve			
S Hypoglossal Nerve			
T Spinal Meninges			
U Spinal Canal			
W Cervical Spinal Cord			
X Thoracic Spinal Cord			
Y Lumbar Spinal Cord			

Non-OR   ØØ9[Ø123456789ABCDFGHJKLMNPQRSU][34]ZX
Non-OR   ØØ9U[34]ZZ

Coding Clinic: 2015, Q3, P12-13 – ØØ9[46]3ØZ

New/Revised Text in Green   ~~deleted~~ Deleted   ♀ Females Only   ♂ Males Only   **Coding Clinic**
Non-covered   Limited Coverage   ⊞ Combination (See Appendix E)   DRG Non-OR   Non-OR   Hospital-Acquired Condition

SECTION: 0 MEDICAL AND SURGICAL

BODY SYSTEM: 0 CENTRAL NERVOUS SYSTEM

OPERATION: B EXCISION: Cutting out or off, without replacement, a portion of a body part

Body Part	Approach	Device	Qualifier
0 Brain	0 Open	Z No Device	X Diagnostic
1 Cerebral Meninges	3 Percutaneous		Z No Qualifier
2 Dura Mater	4 Percutaneous Endoscopic		
6 Cerebral Ventricle			
7 Cerebral Hemisphere			
8 Basal Ganglia			
9 Thalamus			
A Hypothalamus			
B Pons			
C Cerebellum			
D Medulla Oblongata			
F Olfactory Nerve			
G Optic Nerve			
H Oculomotor Nerve			
J Trochlear Nerve			
K Trigeminal Nerve			
L Abducens Nerve			
M Facial Nerve			
N Acoustic Nerve			
P Glossopharyngeal Nerve			
Q Vagus Nerve			
R Accessory Nerve			
S Hypoglossal Nerve			
T Spinal Meninges			
W Cervical Spinal Cord			
X Thoracic Spinal Cord			
Y Lumbar Spinal Cord			

Non-OR 00B[0126789ABCDFGHJKLMNPQRS][34]ZX

Coding Clinic: 2015, Q1, P13 – 00B00ZZ
Coding Clinic: 2016, Q2, P13 – 00B[MRS]0ZZ
Coding Clinic: 2016, Q2, P18 – 00B70ZZ

SECTION: Ø MEDICAL AND SURGICAL
BODY SYSTEM: Ø CENTRAL NERVOUS SYSTEM
OPERATION: C EXTIRPATION: Taking or cutting out solid matter from a body part

Body Part	Approach	Device	Qualifier
Ø Brain	Ø Open	Z No Device	Z No Qualifier
1 Cerebral Meninges	3 Percutaneous		
2 Dura Mater	4 Percutaneous Endoscopic		
3 Epidural Space			
4 Subdural Space			
5 Subarachnoid Space			
6 Cerebral Ventricle			
7 Cerebral Hemisphere			
8 Basal Ganglia			
9 Thalamus			
A Hypothalamus			
B Pons			
C Cerebellum			
D Medulla Oblongata			
F Olfactory Nerve			
G Optic Nerve			
H Oculomotor Nerve			
J Trochlear Nerve			
K Trigeminal Nerve			
L Abducens Nerve			
M Facial Nerve			
N Acoustic Nerve			
P Glossopharyngeal Nerve			
Q Vagus Nerve			
R Accessory Nerve			
S Hypoglossal Nerve			
T Spinal Meninges			
W Cervical Spinal Cord			
X Thoracic Spinal Cord			
Y Lumbar Spinal Cord			

Coding Clinic: 2015, Q1, P12 – 00C00ZZ
Coding Clinic: 2016, Q2, P29; 2015, Q3, P11 – 00C40ZZ
Coding Clinic: 2015, Q3, P13 – 00C74ZZ

C: EXTIRPATION

Ø: CENTRAL NERVOUS SYSTEM

Ø: M/S

New/Revised Text in Green   ~~deleted~~ Deleted   ♀ Females Only   ♂ Males Only   **Coding Clinic**
🚫 Non-covered   🚫 Limited Coverage   ⊡ Combination (See Appendix E)   DRG Non-OR   Non-OR   🚫 Hospital-Acquired Condition

SECTION: Ø MEDICAL AND SURGICAL

BODY SYSTEM: Ø CENTRAL NERVOUS SYSTEM

OPERATION: D EXTRACTION: Pulling or stripping out or off all or a portion of a body part by the use of force

Body Part	Approach	Device	Qualifier
1 Cerebral Meninges 2 Dura Mater F Olfactory Nerve G Optic Nerve H Oculomotor Nerve J Trochlear Nerve K Trigeminal Nerve L Abducens Nerve M Facial Nerve N Acoustic Nerve P Glossopharyngeal Nerve Q Vagus Nerve R Accessory Nerve S Hypoglossal Nerve T Spinal Meninges	Ø Open 3 Percutaneous 4 Percutaneous Endoscopic	Z No Device	Z No Qualifier

Coding Clinic: 2015, Q3, P14 – ØØD2ØZZ

SECTION: Ø MEDICAL AND SURGICAL

BODY SYSTEM: Ø CENTRAL NERVOUS SYSTEM

OPERATION: F FRAGMENTATION: Breaking solid matter in a body part into pieces

Body Part	Approach	Device	Qualifier
3 Epidural Space 🐾 4 Subdural Space 🐾 5 Subarachnoid Space 🐾 6 Cerebral Ventricle 🐾 U Spinal Canal	Ø Open 3 Percutaneous 4 Percutaneous Endoscopic X External	Z No Device	Z No Qualifier

🐾 ØØF[3456]XZZ
Non-OR ØØF[3456]XZZ

SECTION: Ø MEDICAL AND SURGICAL

BODY SYSTEM: Ø CENTRAL NERVOUS SYSTEM

OPERATION: H INSERTION: Putting in a nonbiological appliance that monitors, assists, performs, or prevents a physiological function but does not physically take the place of a body part

Body Part	Approach	Device	Qualifier
Ø Brain ⊞ 6 Cerebral Ventricle ⊞ E Cranial Nerve ⊞ U Spinal Canal ⊞ V Spinal Cord ⊞	Ø Open 3 Percutaneous 4 Percutaneous Endoscopic	2 Monitoring Device 3 Infusion Device M Neurostimulator Lead	Z No Qualifier

⊞ ØØH[Ø6EUV][Ø34]MZ
Non-OR ØØH[UV][Ø34]3Z

New/Revised Text in Green   deleted Deleted   ♀ Females Only   ♂ Males Only   **Coding Clinic**
🐾 Non-covered   🐾 Limited Coverage   ⊞ Combination (See Appendix E)   DRG Non-OR   Non-OR   🐾 Hospital-Acquired Condition

47

J: INSPECTION   K: MAP

Ø: CENTRAL NERVOUS SYSTEM

Ø: M/S

SECTION: Ø MEDICAL AND SURGICAL
BODY SYSTEM: Ø CENTRAL NERVOUS SYSTEM
OPERATION: J **INSPECTION:** Visually and/or manually exploring a body part

Body Part	Approach	Device	Qualifier
Ø Brain E Cranial Nerve U Spinal Canal V Spinal Cord	Ø Open 3 Percutaneous 4 Percutaneous Endoscopic	Z No Device	Z No Qualifier

DRG Non-OR ØØJ[ØEUV]3ZZ

SECTION: Ø MEDICAL AND SURGICAL
BODY SYSTEM: Ø CENTRAL NERVOUS SYSTEM
OPERATION: K **MAP:** Locating the route of passage of electrical impulses and/or locating functional areas in a body part

Body Part	Approach	Device	Qualifier
Ø Brain 7 Cerebral Hemisphere 8 Basal Ganglia 9 Thalamus A Hypothalamus B Pons C Cerebellum D Medulla Oblongata	Ø Open 3 Percutaneous 4 Percutaneous Endoscopic	Z No Device	Z No Qualifier

SECTION: Ø MEDICAL AND SURGICAL

BODY SYSTEM: Ø CENTRAL NERVOUS SYSTEM

OPERATION: N RELEASE: Freeing a body part from an abnormal physical constraint by cutting or by the use of force

Body Part	Approach	Device	Qualifier
Ø Brain 1 Cerebral Meninges 2 Dura Mater 6 Cerebral Ventricle 7 Cerebral Hemisphere 8 Basal Ganglia 9 Thalamus A Hypothalamus B Pons C Cerebellum D Medulla Oblongata F Olfactory Nerve G Optic Nerve H Oculomotor Nerve J Trochlear Nerve K Trigeminal Nerve L Abducens Nerve M Facial Nerve N Acoustic Nerve P Glossopharyngeal Nerve Q Vagus Nerve R Accessory Nerve S Hypoglossal Nerve T Spinal Meninges W Cervical Spinal Cord X Thoracic Spinal Cord Y Lumbar Spinal Cord	Ø Open 3 Percutaneous 4 Percutaneous Endoscopic	Z No Device	Z No Qualifier

Coding Clinic: 2015, Q2, P22 – ØØNWØZZ
Coding Clinic: 2016, Q2, P29 – ØØNØØZZ

SECTION: Ø MEDICAL AND SURGICAL
BODY SYSTEM: Ø CENTRAL NERVOUS SYSTEM
OPERATION: P REMOVAL: Taking out or off a device from a body part

Body Part	Approach	Device	Qualifier
Ø Brain V Spinal Cord	Ø Open 3 Percutaneous 4 Percutaneous Endoscopic	Ø Drainage Device 2 Monitoring Device 3 Infusion Device 7 Autologous Tissue Substitute J Synthetic Substitute K Nonautologous Tissue Substitute M Neurostimulator Lead	Z No Qualifier
Ø Brain V Spinal Cord	X External	Ø Drainage Device 2 Monitoring Device 3 Infusion Device M Neurostimulator Lead	Z No Qualifier
6 Cerebral Ventricle U Spinal Canal	Ø Open 3 Percutaneous 4 Percutaneous Endoscopic	Ø Drainage Device 2 Monitoring Device 3 Infusion Device J Synthetic Substitute M Neurostimulator Lead	Z No Qualifier
6 Cerebral Ventricle U Spinal Canal	X External	Ø Drainage Device 2 Monitoring Device 3 Infusion Device M Neurostimulator Lead	Z No Qualifier
E Cranial Nerve	Ø Open 3 Percutaneous 4 Percutaneous Endoscopic	Ø Drainage Device 2 Monitoring Device 3 Infusion Device 7 Autologous Tissue Substitute M Neurostimulator Lead	Z No Qualifier
E Cranial Nerve	X External	Ø Drainage Device 2 Monitoring Device 3 Infusion Device M Neurostimulator Lead	Z No Qualifier

Non-OR ØØP[ØV]X[Ø23M]Z
Non-OR ØØP6X[Ø3]Z
Non-OR ØØPEX[Ø23]Z
Non-OR ØØPUX[Ø23M]Z

New/Revised Text in Green   deleted Deleted   ♀ Females Only   ♂ Males Only   **Coding Clinic**
🌑 Non-covered   🌑 Limited Coverage   ⊟ Combination (See Appendix E)   DRG Non-OR   Non-OR   🌑 Hospital-Acquired Condition

SECTION: Ø MEDICAL AND SURGICAL
BODY SYSTEM: Ø CENTRAL NERVOUS SYSTEM
OPERATION: Q REPAIR: Restoring, to the extent possible, a body part to its normal anatomic structure and function

Body Part	Approach	Device	Qualifier
Ø Brain 1 Cerebral Meninges 2 Dura Mater 6 Cerebral Ventricle 7 Cerebral Hemisphere 8 Basal Ganglia 9 Thalamus A Hypothalamus B Pons C Cerebellum D Medulla Oblongata F Olfactory Nerve G Optic Nerve H Oculomotor Nerve J Trochlear Nerve K Trigeminal Nerve L Abducens Nerve M Facial Nerve N Acoustic Nerve P Glossopharyngeal Nerve Q Vagus Nerve R Accessory Nerve S Hypoglossal Nerve T Spinal Meninges W Cervical Spinal Cord X Thoracic Spinal Cord Y Lumbar Spinal Cord	Ø Open 3 Percutaneous 4 Percutaneous Endoscopic	Z No Device	Z No Qualifier

Coding Clinic: 2013, Q3, P25 – 00Q20ZZ

SECTION: Ø MEDICAL AND SURGICAL
BODY SYSTEM: Ø CENTRAL NERVOUS SYSTEM
OPERATION: S REPOSITION: Moving to its normal location, or other suitable location, all or a portion of a body part

Body Part	Approach	Device	Qualifier
F Olfactory Nerve G Optic Nerve H Oculomotor Nerve J Trochlear Nerve K Trigeminal Nerve L Abducens Nerve M Facial Nerve N Acoustic Nerve P Glossopharyngeal Nerve Q Vagus Nerve R Accessory Nerve S Hypoglossal Nerve W Cervical Spinal Cord X Thoracic Spinal Cord Y Lumbar Spinal Cord	Ø Open 3 Percutaneous 4 Percutaneous Endoscopic	Z No Device	Z No Qualifier

SECTION: Ø MEDICAL AND SURGICAL
BODY SYSTEM: Ø CENTRAL NERVOUS SYSTEM
OPERATION: T RESECTION: Cutting out or off, without replacement, all of a body part

Body Part	Approach	Device	Qualifier
7 Cerebral Hemisphere	Ø Open 3 Percutaneous 4 Percutaneous Endoscopic	Z No Device	Z No Qualifier

SECTION: Ø MEDICAL AND SURGICAL
BODY SYSTEM: Ø CENTRAL NERVOUS SYSTEM
OPERATION: U SUPPLEMENT: Putting in or on biological or synthetic material that physically reinforces and/or augments the function of a portion of a body part

Body Part	Approach	Device	Qualifier
1 Cerebral Meninges 2 Dura Mater T Spinal Meninges	Ø Open 3 Percutaneous 4 Percutaneous Endoscopic	7 Autologous Tissue Substitute J Synthetic Substitute K Nonautologous Tissue Substitute	Z No Qualifier
F Olfactory Nerve G Optic Nerve H Oculomotor Nerve J Trochlear Nerve K Trigeminal Nerve L Abducens Nerve M Facial Nerve N Acoustic Nerve P Glossopharyngeal Nerve Q Vagus Nerve R Accessory Nerve S Hypoglossal Nerve	Ø Open 3 Percutaneous 4 Percutaneous Endoscopic	7 Autologous Tissue Substitute	Z No Qualifier

New/Revised Text in Green   ~~deleted~~ Deleted   ♀ Females Only   ♂ Males Only   **Coding Clinic**
Non-covered   Limited Coverage   ⊞ Combination (See Appendix E)   DRG Non-OR   Non-OR   Hospital-Acquired Condition

SECTION: Ø MEDICAL AND SURGICAL

BODY SYSTEM: Ø CENTRAL NERVOUS SYSTEM

OPERATION: W REVISION: Correcting, to the extent possible, a portion of a malfunctioning device or the position of a displaced device

Body Part	Approach	Device	Qualifier
Ø Brain V Spinal Cord	Ø Open 3 Percutaneous 4 Percutaneous Endoscopic X External	Ø Drainage Device 2 Monitoring Device 3 Infusion Device 7 Autologous Tissue Substitute J Synthetic Substitute K Nonautologous Tissue Substitute M Neurostimulator Lead	Z No Qualifier
6 Cerebral Ventricle U Spinal Canal	Ø Open 3 Percutaneous 4 Percutaneous Endoscopic X External	Ø Drainage Device 2 Monitoring Device 3 Infusion Device J Synthetic Substitute M Neurostimulator Lead	Z No Qualifier
E Cranial Nerve	Ø Open 3 Percutaneous 4 Percutaneous Endoscopic X External	Ø Drainage Device 2 Monitoring Device 3 Infusion Device 7 Autologous Tissue Substitute M Neurostimulator Lead	Z No Qualifier

Non-OR ØØW[ØV]X[Ø237JKM]Z
Non-OR ØØW[6U]X[Ø23JM]Z
Non-OR ØØWEX[Ø237M]Z

SECTION: Ø MEDICAL AND SURGICAL

BODY SYSTEM: Ø CENTRAL NERVOUS SYSTEM

OPERATION: X TRANSFER: Moving, without taking out, all or a portion of a body part to another location to take over the function of all or a portion of a body part

Body Part	Approach	Device	Qualifier
F Olfactory Nerve G Optic Nerve H Oculomotor Nerve J Trochlear Nerve K Trigeminal Nerve L Abducens Nerve M Facial Nerve N Acoustic Nerve P Glossopharyngeal Nerve Q Vagus Nerve R Accessory Nerve S Hypoglossal Nerve	Ø Open 4 Percutaneous Endoscopic	Z No Device	F Olfactory Nerve G Optic Nerve H Oculomotor Nerve J Trochlear Nerve K Trigeminal Nerve L Abducens Nerve M Facial Nerve N Acoustic Nerve P Glossopharyngeal Nerve Q Vagus Nerve R Accessory Nerve S Hypoglossal Nerve

New/Revised Text in Green ~~deleted~~ Deleted ♀ Females Only ♂ Males Only **Coding Clinic**

Non-covered Limited Coverage ⊞ Combination (See Appendix E) DRG Non-OR Non-OR Hospital-Acquired Condition

SECTION: Ø MEDICAL AND SURGICAL

BODY SYSTEM: 1 PERIPHERAL NERVOUS SYSTEM

OPERATION: 2 **CHANGE:** Taking out or off a device from a body part and putting back an identical or similar device in or on the same body part without cutting or puncturing the skin or a mucous membrane

Body Part	Approach	Device	Qualifier
Y Peripheral Nerve	X External	Ø Drainage Device Y Other Device	Z No Qualifier

Non-OR Ø12YX[ØY]Z

SECTION: Ø MEDICAL AND SURGICAL

BODY SYSTEM: 1 PERIPHERAL NERVOUS SYSTEM

OPERATION: 5 **DESTRUCTION:** Physical eradication of all or a portion of a body part by the direct use of energy, force, or a destructive agent

Body Part	Approach	Device	Qualifier
Ø Cervical Plexus 1 Cervical Nerve 2 Phrenic Nerve 3 Brachial Plexus 4 Ulnar Nerve 5 Median Nerve 6 Radial Nerve 8 Thoracic Nerve 9 Lumbar Plexus A Lumbosacral Plexus B Lumbar Nerve C Pudendal Nerve D Femoral Nerve F Sciatic Nerve G Tibial Nerve H Peroneal Nerve K Head and Neck Sympathetic Nerve L Thoracic Sympathetic Nerve M Abdominal Sympathetic Nerve N Lumbar Sympathetic Nerve P Sacral Sympathetic Nerve Q Sacral Plexus R Sacral Nerve	Ø Open 3 Percutaneous 4 Percutaneous Endoscopic	Z No Device	Z No Qualifier

Non-OR Ø15[Ø234569ACDFGHQ][Ø34]ZZ
Non-OR Ø15[18BR]3ZZ

SECTION: Ø MEDICAL AND SURGICAL
BODY SYSTEM: 1 **PERIPHERAL NERVOUS SYSTEM**
OPERATION: 8 **DIVISION:** Cutting into a body part, without draining fluids and/or gases from the body part, in order to separate or transect a body part

Body Part	Approach	Device	Qualifier
Ø Cervical Plexus	Ø Open	Z No Device	Z No Qualifier
1 Cervical Nerve	3 Percutaneous		
2 Phrenic Nerve	4 Percutaneous Endoscopic		
3 Brachial Plexus			
4 Ulnar Nerve			
5 Median Nerve			
6 Radial Nerve			
8 Thoracic Nerve			
9 Lumbar Plexus			
A Lumbosacral Plexus			
B Lumbar Nerve			
C Pudendal Nerve			
D Femoral Nerve			
F Sciatic Nerve			
G Tibial Nerve			
H Peroneal Nerve			
K Head and Neck Sympathetic Nerve			
L Thoracic Sympathetic Nerve			
M Abdominal Sympathetic Nerve			
N Lumbar Sympathetic Nerve			
P Sacral Sympathetic Nerve			
Q Sacral Plexus			
R Sacral Nerve			

SECTION: Ø MEDICAL AND SURGICAL
BODY SYSTEM: 1 PERIPHERAL NERVOUS SYSTEM
OPERATION: 9 DRAINAGE: Taking or letting out fluids and/or gases from a body part

Body Part	Approach	Device	Qualifier
Ø Cervical Plexus 1 Cervical Nerve 2 Phrenic Nerve 3 Brachial Plexus 4 Ulnar Nerve 5 Median Nerve 6 Radial Nerve 8 Thoracic Nerve 9 Lumbar Plexus A Lumbosacral Plexus B Lumbar Nerve C Pudendal Nerve D Femoral Nerve F Sciatic Nerve G Tibial Nerve H Peroneal Nerve K Head and Neck Sympathetic Nerve L Thoracic Sympathetic Nerve M Abdominal Sympathetic Nerve N Lumbar Sympathetic Nerve P Sacral Sympathetic Nerve Q Sacral Plexus R Sacral Nerve	Ø Open 3 Percutaneous 4 Percutaneous Endoscopic	Ø Drainage Device	Z No Qualifier
Ø Cervical Plexus 1 Cervical Nerve 2 Phrenic Nerve 3 Brachial Plexus 4 Ulnar Nerve 5 Median Nerve 6 Radial Nerve 8 Thoracic Nerve 9 Lumbar Plexus A Lumbosacral Plexus B Lumbar Nerve C Pudendal Nerve D Femoral Nerve F Sciatic Nerve G Tibial Nerve H Peroneal Nerve K Head and Neck Sympathetic Nerve L Thoracic Sympathetic Nerve M Abdominal Sympathetic Nerve N Lumbar Sympathetic Nerve P Sacral Sympathetic Nerve Q Sacral Plexus R Sacral Nerve	Ø Open 3 Percutaneous 4 Percutaneous Endoscopic	Z No Device	X Diagnostic Z No Qualifier

DRG Non-OR Ø19[Ø12345689ABCDFGHKLMNPQR]3ØZ
DRG Non-OR Ø19[Ø12345689ABCDFGHKLMNPQR]3ZZ
Non-OR Ø19[Ø12345689ABCDFGHQR][34]ZX

New/Revised Text in Green   deleted Deleted   ♀ Females Only   ♂ Males Only   **Coding Clinic**
🅠 Non-covered   🅠 Limited Coverage   ⊞ Combination (See Appendix E)   DRG Non-OR   Non-OR   🅠 Hospital-Acquired Condition

SECTION: Ø MEDICAL AND SURGICAL
BODY SYSTEM: 1 PERIPHERAL NERVOUS SYSTEM
OPERATION: **B EXCISION:** Cutting out or off, without replacement, a portion of a body part

Body Part	Approach	Device	Qualifier
Ø Cervical Plexus 1 Cervical Nerve 2 Phrenic Nerve 3 Brachial Plexus ⊞ 4 Ulnar Nerve 5 Median Nerve 6 Radial Nerve 8 Thoracic Nerve 9 Lumbar Plexus A Lumbosacral Plexus B Lumbar Nerve C Pudendal Nerve D Femoral Nerve F Sciatic Nerve G Tibial Nerve H Peroneal Nerve K Head and Neck Sympathetic Nerve L Thoracic Sympathetic Nerve ⊞ M Abdominal Sympathetic Nerve N Lumbar Sympathetic Nerve P Sacral Sympathetic Nerve Q Sacral Plexus R Sacral Nerve	Ø Open 3 Percutaneous 4 Percutaneous Endoscopic	Z No Device	X Diagnostic Z No Qualifier

⊞ Ø1B[3L]ØZZ
Non-OR Ø1B[Ø12345689ABCDFGHQR][34]ZX

SECTION: Ø MEDICAL AND SURGICAL
BODY SYSTEM: 1 PERIPHERAL NERVOUS SYSTEM
OPERATION: **C EXTIRPATION:** Taking or cutting out solid matter from a body part

Body Part	Approach	Device	Qualifier
Ø Cervical Plexus 1 Cervical Nerve 2 Phrenic Nerve 3 Brachial Plexus 4 Ulnar Nerve 5 Median Nerve 6 Radial Nerve 8 Thoracic Nerve 9 Lumbar Plexus A Lumbosacral Plexus B Lumbar Nerve C Pudendal Nerve D Femoral Nerve F Sciatic Nerve G Tibial Nerve H Peroneal Nerve K Head and Neck Sympathetic Nerve L Thoracic Sympathetic Nerve M Abdominal Sympathetic Nerve N Lumbar Sympathetic Nerve P Sacral Sympathetic Nerve Q Sacral Plexus R Sacral Nerve	Ø Open 3 Percutaneous 4 Percutaneous Endoscopic	Z No Device	Z No Qualifier

New/Revised Text in Green   ~~deleted~~ Deleted   ♀ Females Only   ♂ Males Only   **Coding Clinic**
🜢 Non-covered   🜢 Limited Coverage   ⊞ Combination (See Appendix E)   DRG Non-OR   Non-OR   🜢 Hospital-Acquired Condition

SECTION: Ø MEDICAL AND SURGICAL

BODY SYSTEM: 1 PERIPHERAL NERVOUS SYSTEM

OPERATION: D **EXTRACTION:** Pulling or stripping out or off all or a portion of a body part by the use of force

Body Part	Approach	Device	Qualifier
Ø Cervical Plexus	Ø Open	Z No Device	Z No Qualifier
1 Cervical Nerve	3 Percutaneous		
2 Phrenic Nerve	4 Percutaneous Endoscopic		
3 Brachial Plexus			
4 Ulnar Nerve			
5 Median Nerve			
6 Radial Nerve			
8 Thoracic Nerve			
9 Lumbar Plexus			
A Lumbosacral Plexus			
B Lumbar Nerve			
C Pudendal Nerve			
D Femoral Nerve			
F Sciatic Nerve			
G Tibial Nerve			
H Peroneal Nerve			
K Head and Neck Sympathetic Nerve			
L Thoracic Sympathetic Nerve			
M Abdominal Sympathetic Nerve			
N Lumbar Sympathetic Nerve			
P Sacral Sympathetic Nerve			
Q Sacral Plexus			
R Sacral Nerve			

SECTION: Ø MEDICAL AND SURGICAL

BODY SYSTEM: 1 PERIPHERAL NERVOUS SYSTEM

OPERATION: H **INSERTION:** Putting in a nonbiological appliance that monitors, assists, performs, or prevents a physiological function but does not physically take the place of a body part

Body Part	Approach	Device	Qualifier
Y Peripheral Nerve ⊞	Ø Open	2 Monitoring Device	Z No Qualifier
	3 Percutaneous	M Neurostimulator Lead	
	4 Percutaneous Endoscopic		

⊞ 01HY[034]MZ

SECTION: Ø MEDICAL AND SURGICAL

BODY SYSTEM: 1 PERIPHERAL NERVOUS SYSTEM

OPERATION: J **INSPECTION:** Visually and/or manually exploring a body part

Body Part	Approach	Device	Qualifier
Y Peripheral Nerve	Ø Open	Z No Device	Z No Qualifier
	3 Percutaneous		
	4 Percutaneous Endoscopic		

DRG Non-OR   01JY3ZZ

SECTION: Ø MEDICAL AND SURGICAL

BODY SYSTEM: 1 PERIPHERAL NERVOUS SYSTEM

OPERATION: N **RELEASE:** Freeing a body part from an abnormal physical constraint by cutting or by the use of force

Body Part	Approach	Device	Qualifier
Ø Cervical Plexus 1 Cervical Nerve 2 Phrenic Nerve 3 Brachial Plexus 4 Ulnar Nerve 5 Median Nerve 6 Radial Nerve 8 Thoracic Nerve 9 Lumbar Plexus A Lumbosacral Plexus B Lumbar Nerve C Pudendal Nerve D Femoral Nerve F Sciatic Nerve G Tibial Nerve H Peroneal Nerve K Head and Neck Sympathetic Nerve L Thoracic Sympathetic Nerve M Abdominal Sympathetic Nerve N Lumbar Sympathetic Nerve P Sacral Sympathetic Nerve Q Sacral Plexus R Sacral Nerve	Ø Open 3 Percutaneous 4 Percutaneous Endoscopic	Z No Device	Z No Qualifier

Coding Clinic: 2Ø16, Q2, P16; 2Ø15, Q2, P34 – Ø1NBØZZ
Coding Clinic: 2Ø16, Q2, P17 – Ø1N1ØZZ
Coding Clinic: 2Ø16, Q2, P23 – Ø1N3ØZZ

SECTION: Ø MEDICAL AND SURGICAL

BODY SYSTEM: 1 PERIPHERAL NERVOUS SYSTEM

OPERATION: P **REMOVAL:** Taking out or off a device from a body part

Body Part	Approach	Device	Qualifier
Y Peripheral Nerve	Ø Open 3 Percutaneous 4 Percutaneous Endoscopic	Ø Drainage Device 2 Monitoring Device 7 Autologous Tissue Substitute M Neurostimulator Lead	Z No Qualifier
Y Peripheral Nerve	X External	Ø Drainage Device 2 Monitoring Device M Neurostimulator Lead	Z No Qualifier

Non-OR Ø1PYX[Ø2]Z

New/Revised Text in Green   ~~deleted~~ Deleted   ♀ Females Only   ♂ Males Only   **Coding Clinic**
🚱 Non-covered   🚱 Limited Coverage   ⊞ Combination (See Appendix E)   DRG Non-OR   Non-OR   🚱 Hospital-Acquired Condition

Sidebar: N: RELEASE   P: REMOVAL
1: PERIPHERAL NERVOUS SYSTEM
Ø: M/S

SECTION: Ø MEDICAL AND SURGICAL
BODY SYSTEM: 1 PERIPHERAL NERVOUS SYSTEM
OPERATION: Q REPAIR: Restoring, to the extent possible, a body part to its normal anatomic structure and function

Body Part	Approach	Device	Qualifier
Ø Cervical Plexus	Ø Open	Z No Device	Z No Qualifier
1 Cervical Nerve	3 Percutaneous		
2 Phrenic Nerve	4 Percutaneous Endoscopic		
3 Brachial Plexus			
4 Ulnar Nerve			
5 Median Nerve			
6 Radial Nerve			
8 Thoracic Nerve			
9 Lumbar Plexus			
A Lumbosacral Plexus			
B Lumbar Nerve			
C Pudendal Nerve			
D Femoral Nerve			
F Sciatic Nerve			
G Tibial Nerve			
H Peroneal Nerve			
K Head and Neck Sympathetic Nerve			
L Thoracic Sympathetic Nerve			
M Abdominal Sympathetic Nerve			
N Lumbar Sympathetic Nerve			
P Sacral Sympathetic Nerve			
Q Sacral Plexus			
R Sacral Nerve			

SECTION: Ø MEDICAL AND SURGICAL
BODY SYSTEM: 1 PERIPHERAL NERVOUS SYSTEM
OPERATION: S REPOSITION: Moving to its normal location, or other suitable location, all or a portion of a body part

Body Part	Approach	Device	Qualifier
Ø Cervical Plexus	Ø Open	Z No Device	Z No Qualifier
1 Cervical Nerve	3 Percutaneous		
2 Phrenic Nerve	4 Percutaneous Endoscopic		
3 Brachial Plexus			
4 Ulnar Nerve			
5 Median Nerve			
6 Radial Nerve			
8 Thoracic Nerve			
9 Lumbar Plexus			
A Lumbosacral Plexus			
B Lumbar Nerve			
C Pudendal Nerve			
D Femoral Nerve			
F Sciatic Nerve			
G Tibial Nerve			
H Peroneal Nerve			
Q Sacral Plexus			
R Sacral Nerve			

New/Revised Text in Green   ~~deleted~~ Deleted   ♀ Females Only   ♂ Males Only   **Coding Clinic**
Non-covered   Limited Coverage   ⊞ Combination (See Appendix E)   DRG Non-OR   Non-OR   Hospital-Acquired Condition

61

SECTION: Ø MEDICAL AND SURGICAL

BODY SYSTEM: 1 PERIPHERAL NERVOUS SYSTEM

OPERATION: U SUPPLEMENT: Putting in or on biological or synthetic material that physically reinforces and/or augments the function of a portion of a body part

Body Part	Approach	Device	Qualifier
1 Cervical Nerve 2 Phrenic Nerve 4 Ulnar Nerve 5 Median Nerve 6 Radial Nerve 8 Thoracic Nerve B Lumbar Nerve C Pudendal Nerve D Femoral Nerve F Sciatic Nerve G Tibial Nerve H Peroneal Nerve R Sacral Nerve	Ø Open 3 Percutaneous 4 Percutaneous Endoscopic	7 Autologous Tissue Substitute	Z No Qualifier

SECTION: Ø MEDICAL AND SURGICAL

BODY SYSTEM: 1 PERIPHERAL NERVOUS SYSTEM

OPERATION: W REVISION: Correcting, to the extent possible, a portion of a malfunctioning device or the position of a displaced device

Body Part	Approach	Device	Qualifier
Y Peripheral Nerve	Ø Open 3 Percutaneous 4 Percutaneous Endoscopic X External	Ø Drainage Device 2 Monitoring Device 7 Autologous Tissue Substitute M Neurostimulator Lead	Z No Qualifier

Non-OR Ø1WYX[Ø27M]Z

SECTION: Ø MEDICAL AND SURGICAL
BODY SYSTEM: 1 PERIPHERAL NERVOUS SYSTEM
OPERATION: X TRANSFER: Moving, without taking out, all or a portion of a body part to another location to take over the function of all or a portion of a body part

Body Part	Approach	Device	Qualifier
1 Cervical Nerve 2 Phrenic Nerve	Ø Open 4 Percutaneous Endoscopic	Z No Device	1 Cervical Nerve 2 Phrenic Nerve
4 Ulnar Nerve 5 Median Nerve 6 Radial Nerve	Ø Open 4 Percutaneous Endoscopic	Z No Device	4 Ulnar Nerve 5 Median Nerve 6 Radial Nerve
8 Thoracic Nerve	Ø Open 4 Percutaneous Endoscopic	Z No Device	8 Thoracic Nerve
B Lumbar Nerve C Pudendal Nerve	Ø Open 4 Percutaneous Endoscopic	Z No Device	B Lumbar Nerve C Pudendal Nerve
D Femoral Nerve F Sciatic Nerve G Tibial Nerve H Peroneal Nerve	Ø Open 4 Percutaneous Endoscopic	Z No Device	D Femoral Nerve F Sciatic Nerve G Tibial Nerve H Peroneal Nerve

Ø: M/S

1: PERIPHERAL NERVOUS SYSTEM

X: TRANSFER

02. Heart and Great Vessels

SECTION: 0 MEDICAL AND SURGICAL

BODY SYSTEM: 2 HEART AND GREAT VESSELS

OPERATION: 1 BYPASS: *(on multiple pages)*

Altering the route of passage of the contents of a tubular body part

Body Part	Approach	Device	Qualifier
0 Coronary Artery, One Artery 🦠 1 Coronary Artery, Two Arteries 🦠 2 Coronary Artery, Three Arteries 🦠 3 Coronary Artery, Four or More Arteries 🦠	0 Open	8 Zooplastic Tissue 9 Autologous Venous Tissue A Autologous Arterial Tissue J Synthetic Substitute K Nonautologous Tissue Substitute	3 Coronary Artery 8 Internal Mammary, Right 9 Internal Mammary, Left C Thoracic Artery F Abdominal Artery W Aorta
0 Coronary Artery, One Artery 🦠 1 Coronary Artery, Two Arteries 🦠 2 Coronary Artery, Three Arteries 🦠 3 Coronary Artery, Four or More Arteries 🦠	0 Open	Z No Device	3 Coronary Artery 8 Internal Mammary, Right 9 Internal Mammary, Left C Thoracic Artery F Abdominal Artery
0 Coronary Artery, One Artery 1 Coronary Artery, Two Arteries 2 Coronary Artery, Three Arteries 3 Coronary Artery, Four or More Arteries	3 Percutaneous	4 Drug-eluting Intraluminal Device D Intraluminal Device	4 Coronary Vein
0 Coronary Artery, One Artery 1 Coronary Artery, Two Arteries 2 Coronary Artery, Three Arteries 3 Coronary Artery, Four or More Arteries	4 Percutaneous Endoscopic	4 Drug-eluting Intraluminal Device D Intraluminal Device	4 Coronary Vein
0 Coronary Artery, One Artery 🦠 1 Coronary Artery, Two Arteries 🦠 2 Coronary Artery, Three Arteries 🦠 3 Coronary Artery, Four or More Arteries 🦠	4 Percutaneous Endoscopic	8 Zooplastic Tissue 9 Autologous Venous Tissue A Autologous Arterial Tissue J Synthetic Substitute K Nonautologous Tissue Substitute	3 Coronary Artery 8 Internal Mammary, Right 9 Internal Mammary, Left C Thoracic Artery F Abdominal Artery W Aorta
0 Coronary Artery, One Artery 🦠 1 Coronary Artery, Two Arteries 🦠 2 Coronary Artery, Three Arteries 🦠 3 Coronary Artery, Four or More Arteries 🦠	4 Percutaneous Endoscopic	Z No Device	3 Coronary Artery 8 Internal Mammary, Right 9 Internal Mammary, Left C Thoracic Artery F Abdominal Artery
6 Atrium, Right	0 Open 4 Percutaneous Endoscopic	8 Zooplastic Tissue 9 Autologous Venous Tissue A Autologous Arterial Tissue J Synthetic Substitute K Nonautologous Tissue Substitute	P Pulmonary Trunk Q Pulmonary Artery, Right R Pulmonary Artery, Left
6 Atrium, Right	0 Open 4 Percutaneous Endoscopic	Z No Device	7 Atrium, Left P Pulmonary Trunk Q Pulmonary Artery, Right R Pulmonary Artery, Left
7 Atrium, Left ⊞ V Superior Vena Cava	0 Open 4 Percutaneous Endoscopic	8 Zooplastic Tissue 9 Autologous Venous Tissue A Autologous Arterial Tissue J Synthetic Substitute K Nonautologous Tissue Substitute Z No Device	P Pulmonary Trunk Q Pulmonary Artery, Right R Pulmonary Artery, Left S Pulmonary Vein, Right T Pulmonary Vein, Left U Pulmonary Vein, Confluence

🦠 02170Z[PQR]

Non-OR 021[0123]3[4D]4

Non-OR 021[0123]4[4F]4

🦠 021[0123]0[9AJK][389CFW] when reported with Secondary Diagnosis J98.5

🦠 021[0123]0Z[389CF] when reported with Secondary Diagnosis J98.5

🦠 021[0123]4[9AJK][389CFW] when reported with Secondary Diagnosis J98.5

🦠 021[0123]4Z[389CF] when reported with Secondary Diagnosis J98.5

Coding Clinic: 2015, Q4, P23 P25, Q3, P17 – 021K0KP

Coding Clinic: 2016, Q1, P28 – 02100Z9, 021209W

0: M/S

2: HEART AND GREAT VESSELS

1: BYPASS

SECTION: Ø MEDICAL AND SURGICAL
BODY SYSTEM: 2 HEART AND GREAT VESSELS
OPERATION: 1 BYPASS: *(continued)*
Altering the route of passage of the contents of a tubular body part

Body Part	Approach	Device	Qualifier
K Ventricle, Right L Ventricle, Left	Ø Open 4 Percutaneous Endoscopic	8 Zooplastic Tissue 9 Autologous Venous Tissue A Autologous Arterial Tissue J Synthetic Substitute K Nonautologous Tissue Substitute	P Pulmonary Trunk Q Pulmonary Artery, Right R Pulmonary Artery, Left
K Ventricle, Right L Ventricle, Left	Ø Open 4 Percutaneous Endoscopic	Z No Device	5 Coronary Circulation 8 Internal Mammary, Right 9 Internal Mammary, Left C Thoracic Artery F Abdominal Artery P Pulmonary Trunk Q Pulmonary Artery, Right R Pulmonary Artery, Left W Aorta
P Pulmonary Trunk Q Pulmonary Artery, Right R Pulmonary Artery, Left	Ø Open 4 Percutaneous Endoscopic	8 Zooplastic Tissue 9 Autologous Venous Tissue A Autologous Arterial Tissue J Synthetic Substitute K Nonautologous Tissue Substitute Z No Device	A Innominate Artery B Subclavian D Carotid
W Thoracic Aorta, Descending X Thoracic Aorta, Ascending/Arch	Ø Open 4 Percutaneous Endoscopic	8 Zooplastic Tissue 9 Autologous Venous Tissue A Autologous Arterial Tissue J Synthetic Substitute K Nonautologous Tissue Substitute Z No Device	B Subclavian D Carotid P Pulmonary Trunk Q Pulmonary Artery, Right R Pulmonary Artery, Left

SECTION: Ø MEDICAL AND SURGICAL
BODY SYSTEM: 2 HEART AND GREAT VESSELS
OPERATION: 4 CREATION: Putting in or on biological or synthetic material to form a new body part that to the extent possible replicates the anatomic structure or function of an absent body part

Body Part	Approach	Device	Qualifier
F Aortic Valve	Ø Open	7 Autologous Tissue Substitute 8 Zooplastic Tissue J Synthetic Substitute K Nonautologous Tissue Substitute	J Truncal Valve
G Mitral Valve J Tricuspid Valve	Ø Open	7 Autologous Tissue Substitute 8 Zooplastic Tissue J Synthetic Substitute K Nonautologous Tissue Substitute	2 Common Atrioventricular Valve

Side tab (vertical): 1: BYPASS 4: CREATION | 2: HEART AND GREAT VESSELS | Ø: M/S

New/Revised Text in Green ~~deleted~~ Deleted ♀ Females Only ♂ Males Only **Coding Clinic**
🕭 Non-covered 🕭 Limited Coverage ⊡ Combination (See Appendix E) DRG Non-OR Non-OR 🕭 Hospital-Acquired Condition

SECTION: Ø MEDICAL AND SURGICAL

BODY SYSTEM: 2 HEART AND GREAT VESSELS

OPERATION: 5 DESTRUCTION: Physical eradication of all or a portion of a body part by the direct use of energy, force, or a destructive agent

Body Part	Approach	Device	Qualifier
4 Coronary Vein 5 Atrial Septum 6 Atrium, Right 7 Atrium, Left 8 Conduction Mechanism 9 Chordae Tendineae D Papillary Muscle F Aortic Valve G Mitral Valve H Pulmonary Valve J Tricuspid Valve K Ventricle, Right L Ventricle, Left M Ventricular Septum N Pericardium P Pulmonary Trunk Q Pulmonary Artery, Right R Pulmonary Artery, Left S Pulmonary Vein, Right T Pulmonary Vein, Left V Superior Vena Cava W Thoracic Aorta, Descending X Thoracic Aorta, Ascending/Arch	Ø Open 3 Percutaneous 4 Percutaneous Endoscopic	Z No Device	Z No Qualifier
7 Atrium, Left	Ø Open 3 Percutaneous 4 Percutaneous Endoscopic	Z No Device	K Left Atrial Appendage Z No Qualifier

DRG Non-OR   Ø257[Ø34]ZK

Coding Clinic: 2Ø13, Q2, P39 – Ø25S3ZZ, Ø25T3ZZ
Coding Clinic: 2Ø16, Q2, P18 – Ø25NØZZ

SECTION: Ø MEDICAL AND SURGICAL
BODY SYSTEM: 2 HEART AND GREAT VESSELS

OPERATION: **7 DILATION:** Expanding an orifice or the lumen of a tubular body part

Body Part	Approach	Device	Qualifier
Ø Coronary Artery, One Artery 1 Coronary Artery, Two Arteries 2 Coronary Artery, Three Arteries 3 Coronary Artery, Four or More Arteries	Ø Open 3 Percutaneous 4 Percutaneous Endoscopic	4 Drug-eluting Intraluminal Device 5 Intraluminal Device, Drug-eluting, Two 6 Intraluminal Device, Drug-eluting, Three 7 Intraluminal Device, Drug-eluting, Four or More D Intraluminal Device E Intraluminal Device, Two F Intraluminal Device, Three G Intraluminal Device, Four or More T Radioactive Intraluminal Device Z No Device	6 Bifurcation Z No Qualifier
F Aortic Valve G Mitral Valve H Pulmonary Valve J Tricuspid Valve K Ventricle, Right P Pulmonary Trunk Q Pulmonary Artery, Right S Pulmonary Vein, Right T Pulmonary Vein, Left V Superior Vena Cava W Thoracic Aorta, Descending X Thoracic Aorta, Ascending/Arch	Ø Open 3 Percutaneous 4 Percutaneous Endoscopic	4 Drug-eluting Intraluminal Device D Intraluminal Device Z No Device	Z No Qualifier
R Pulmonary Artery, Left	Ø Open 3 Percutaneous 4 Percutaneous Endoscopic	4 Drug-eluting Intraluminal Device D Intraluminal Device Z No Device	T Ductus Arteriosus Z No Qualifier

Coding Clinic: 2Ø15, Q2, P3-5 – Ø27234Z, Ø27Ø3[4D]Z, Ø27Ø346, Ø27134Z
Coding Clinic: 2Ø15, Q3, P1Ø, P17 – Ø27Ø3ZZ, Ø27QØDZ
Coding Clinic: 2Ø15, Q4, P14 – Ø27Ø34Z
Coding Clinic: 2Ø16, Q1, P17 – Ø27HØZZ

7: DILATION

2: HEART AND GREAT VESSELS

Ø: M/S

New/Revised Text in Green ~~deleted~~ Deleted ♀ Females Only ♂ Males Only **Coding Clinic**
Non-covered Limited Coverage ⊕ Combination (See Appendix E) DRG Non-OR Non-OR Hospital-Acquired Condition

SECTION: Ø MEDICAL AND SURGICAL

BODY SYSTEM: 2 HEART AND GREAT VESSELS

OPERATION: 8 DIVISION: Cutting into a body part, without draining fluids and/or gases from the body part, in order to separate or transect a body part

Body Part	Approach	Device	Qualifier
8 Conduction Mechanism 9 Chordae Tendineae D Papillary Muscle	Ø Open 3 Percutaneous 4 Percutaneous Endoscopic	Z No Device	Z No Qualifier

SECTION: Ø MEDICAL AND SURGICAL

BODY SYSTEM: 2 HEART AND GREAT VESSELS

OPERATION: B EXCISION: Cutting out or off, without replacement, a portion of a body part

Body Part	Approach	Device	Qualifier
4 Coronary Vein 5 Atrial Septum 6 Atrium, Right 8 Conduction Mechanism 9 Chordae Tendineae D Papillary Muscle F Aortic Valve G Mitral Valve H Pulmonary Valve J Tricuspid Valve K Ventricle, Right ⚕ ⊞ L Ventricle, Left ⚕ M Ventricular Septum N Pericardium P Pulmonary Trunk Q Pulmonary Artery, Right R Pulmonary Artery, Left S Pulmonary Vein, Right T Pulmonary Vein, Left V Superior Vena Cava W Thoracic Aorta, Descending X Thoracic Aorta, Ascending/Arch	Ø Open 3 Percutaneous 4 Percutaneous Endoscopic	Z No Device	X Diagnostic Z No Qualifier
7 Atrium, Left	Ø Open 3 Percutaneous 4 Percutaneous Endoscopic	Z No Device	K Left Atrial Appendage X Diagnostic Z No Qualifier

⚕ 02B[KL][034]ZZ
⊞ 02BKØZZ
`DRG Non-OR` 02B7[034]ZK
`Non-OR` 02B[45689DFGHJKLM][034]ZX
`Non-OR` 02B7[034]ZX

Coding Clinic: 2015, Q2, P24 – 02BGØZZ

New/Revised Text in Green ~~deleted~~ Deleted ♀ Females Only ♂ Males Only **Coding Clinic**
⚕ Non-covered ⚕ Limited Coverage ⊞ Combination (See Appendix E) `DRG Non-OR` `Non-OR` ⚕ Hospital-Acquired Condition

69

C: EXTIRPATION   F: FRAGMENTATION

2: HEART AND GREAT VESSELS

0: M/S

SECTION: Ø MEDICAL AND SURGICAL
BODY SYSTEM: 2 HEART AND GREAT VESSELS
OPERATION: C EXTIRPATION: Taking or cutting out solid matter from a body part

Body Part	Approach	Device	Qualifier
Ø Coronary Artery, One Artery 1 Coronary Artery, Two Arteries 2 Coronary Artery, Three Arteries 3 Coronary Artery, Four or More Arteries	Ø Open 3 Percutaneous 4 Percutaneous Endoscopic	Z No Device	6 Bifurcation Z No Qualifier
4 Coronary Vein 5 Atrial Septum 6 Atrium, Right 7 Atrium, Left 8 Conduction Mechanism 9 Chordae Tendineae D Papillary Muscle F Aortic Valve G Mitral Valve H Pulmonary Valve J Tricuspid Valve K Ventricle, Right L Ventricle, Left M Ventricular Septum N Pericardium P Pulmonary Trunk Q Pulmonary Artery, Right R Pulmonary Artery, Left S Pulmonary Vein, Right T Pulmonary Vein, Left V Superior Vena Cava W Thoracic Aorta, Descending X Thoracic Aorta, Ascending/Arch	Ø Open 3 Percutaneous 4 Percutaneous Endoscopic	Z No Device	Z No Qualifier

Coding Clinic: 2Ø16, Q2, P25 – Ø2CGØZZ

SECTION: Ø MEDICAL AND SURGICAL
BODY SYSTEM: 2 HEART AND GREAT VESSELS
OPERATION: F FRAGMENTATION: Breaking solid matter in a body part into pieces

Body Part	Approach	Device	Qualifier
N Pericardium 🇶	Ø Open 3 Percutaneous 4 Percutaneous Endoscopic X External	Z No Device	Z No Qualifier

🇶 Ø2FNXZZ
Non-OR Ø2FNXZZ

New/Revised Text in Green   ~~deleted~~ Deleted   ♀ Females Only   ♂ Males Only   **Coding Clinic**
🇶 Non-covered   🇶 Limited Coverage   ⊟ Combination (See Appendix E)   DRG Non-OR   Non-OR   🇶 Hospital-Acquired Condition

SECTION: 0 MEDICAL AND SURGICAL

BODY SYSTEM: 2 HEART AND GREAT VESSELS

OPERATION: H INSERTION: Putting in a nonbiological appliance that monitors, assists, performs, or prevents a physiological function but does not physically take the place of a body part

Body Part	Approach	Device	Qualifier
4 Coronary Vein ⊞ ◌ 6 Atrium, Right ⊞ ◌ 7 Atrium, Left ⊞ ◌ K Ventricle, Right ⊞ ◌ L Ventricle, Left ⊞ ◌	0 Open 3 Percutaneous 4 Percutaneous Endoscopic	0 Monitoring Device, Pressure Sensor 2 Monitoring Device 3 Infusion Device D Intraluminal Device J Cardiac Lead, Pacemaker K Cardiac Lead, Defibrillator M Cardiac Lead N Intracardiac Pacemaker	Z No Qualifier
A Heart ◌ ◌	0 Open 3 Percutaneous 4 Percutaneous Endoscopic	Q Implantable Heart Assist System	Z No Qualifier
A Heart ⊞	0 Open 3 Percutaneous 4 Percutaneous Endoscopic	R External Heart Assist System	S Biventricular Z No Qualifier
N Pericardium ⊞ ◌	0 Open 3 Percutaneous 4 Percutaneous Endoscopic	0 Monitoring Device, Pressure Sensor 2 Monitoring Device J Cardiac Lead, Pacemaker K Cardiac Lead, Defibrillator M Cardiac Lead	Z No Qualifier
P Pulmonary Trunk Q Pulmonary Artery, Right R Pulmonary Artery, Left S Pulmonary Vein, Right T Pulmonary Vein, Left V Superior Vena Cava W Thoracic Aorta, Descending X Thoracic Aorta, Ascending/Arch	0 Open 3 Percutaneous 4 Percutaneous Endoscopic	0 Monitoring Device, Pressure Sensor 2 Monitoring Device 3 Infusion Device D Intraluminal Device	Z No Qualifier

◌ 02HA[34]QZ
◌ 02HA0QZ
⊞ 02H[467LN][034][JKM]Z
⊞ 02HK[034][02JKM]Z
⊞ 02HA[04]R[SZ]
⊞ 02HA3RS
DRG Non-OR 02H[467][04][JM]Z
DRG Non-OR 02H[67]3JZ
DRG Non-OR 02H[KL][034][JM]Z
DRG Non-OR 02H[47L]3[23]Z
DRG Non-OR 02H[6K]32Z
DRG Non-OR 02HN32Z
DRG Non-OR 02H[STVW]32Z
Non-OR 02H[6K]33Z
Non-OR 02HP[034][023]Z
Non-OR 02H[QR][034][23]Z
Non-OR 02H[STV][034]3Z
Non-OR 02HW[034][03]Z

◌ 02H43[JKM]Z when reported with Secondary Diagnosis K68.11, T81.4XXA, T82.6XXA, or T82.7XXA
◌ 02H[67]3[JM]Z when reported with Secondary Diagnosis K68.11, T81.4XXA, T82.6XXA, or T82.7XXA
◌ 02H[KL]3JZ when reported with Secondary Diagnosis K68.11, T81.4XXA, T82.6XXA, or T82.7XXA
◌ 02HN[034][JM]Z when reported with Secondary Diagnosis K68.11, T81.4XXA, T82.6XXA, or T82.7XXA

Coding Clinic: 2013, Q3, P18 – 02HV33Z
Coding Clinic: 2015, Q2, P32-33 – 02HK3DZ, 02HV33Z
Coding Clinic: 2015, Q3, P35 – 02HP32Z
Coding Clinic: 2015, Q4, P14, P28-32 – 02HV33Z
Coding Clinic: 2016, Q2, P15 – 02H633Z

New/Revised Text in Green   ~~deleted~~ Deleted   ♀ Females Only   ♂ Males Only   **Coding Clinic**
◌ Non-covered   ◌ Limited Coverage   ⊞ Combination (See Appendix E)   DRG Non-OR   Non-OR   ◌ Hospital-Acquired Condition

SECTION: Ø MEDICAL AND SURGICAL
BODY SYSTEM: 2 HEART AND GREAT VESSELS
OPERATION: **J INSPECTION:** Visually and/or manually exploring a body part

Body Part	Approach	Device	Qualifier
A Heart Y Great Vessel	Ø Open 3 Percutaneous 4 Percutaneous Endoscopic	Z No Device	Z No Qualifier

Non-OR 02J[AY]3ZZ

Coding Clinic: 2015, Q3, P9 – 02JA3ZZ

SECTION: Ø MEDICAL AND SURGICAL
BODY SYSTEM: 2 HEART AND GREAT VESSELS
OPERATION: **K MAP:** Locating the route of passage of electrical impulses and/or locating functional areas in a body part

Body Part	Approach	Device	Qualifier
8 Conduction Mechanism	Ø Open 3 Percutaneous 4 Percutaneous Endoscopic	Z No Device	Z No Qualifier

DRG Non-OR 02K8[034]ZZ

SECTION: Ø MEDICAL AND SURGICAL
BODY SYSTEM: 2 HEART AND GREAT VESSELS
OPERATION: **L OCCLUSION:** Completely closing an orifice or the lumen of a tubular body part

Body Part	Approach	Device	Qualifier
7 Atrium, Left	Ø Open 3 Percutaneous 4 Percutaneous Endoscopic	C Extraluminal Device D Intraluminal Device Z No Device	K Left Atrial Appendage
H Pulmonary Valve S Pulmonary Vein, Right ⊞ T Pulmonary Vein, Left ⊞ V Superior Vena Cava	Ø Open 3 Percutaneous 4 Percutaneous Endoscopic	C Extraluminal Device D Intraluminal Device Z No Device	Z No Qualifier
R Pulmonary Artery, Left ⊞	Ø Open 3 Percutaneous 4 Percutaneous Endoscopic	C Extraluminal Device D Intraluminal Device Z No Device	T Ductus Arteriosus

⊞ 02LRØZT
⊞ 02L[ST]ØZZ
DRG Non-OR 02L7[034][CDZ]K

Coding Clinic: 2015, Q4, P24 – 02LRØZT
Coding Clinic: 2016, Q2, P26 – 02LS3DZ

SECTION: Ø MEDICAL AND SURGICAL

BODY SYSTEM: 2 HEART AND GREAT VESSELS

OPERATION: N RELEASE: Freeing a body part from an abnormal physical constraint by cutting or by the use of force

Body Part	Approach	Device	Qualifier
4 Coronary Vein 5 Atrial Septum 6 Atrium, Right 7 Atrium, Left 8 Conduction Mechanism 9 Chordae Tendineae D Papillary Muscle F Aortic Valve G Mitral Valve H Pulmonary Valve ⊞ J Tricuspid Valve K Ventricle, Right L Ventricle, Left M Ventricular Septum N Pericardium P Pulmonary Trunk Q Pulmonary Artery, Right R Pulmonary Artery, Left S Pulmonary Vein, Right T Pulmonary Vein, Left V Superior Vena Cava W Thoracic Aorta, Descending X Thoracic Aorta, Ascending/Arch	Ø Open 3 Percutaneous 4 Percutaneous Endoscopic	Z No Device	Z No Qualifier

⊞ Ø2NHØZZ

New/Revised Text in Green   ~~deleted~~ Deleted   ♀ Females Only   ♂ Males Only   **Coding Clinic**

🖑 Non-covered   🖑 Limited Coverage   ⊞ Combination (See Appendix E)   DRG Non-OR   Non-OR   🖑 Hospital-Acquired Condition

SECTION: 0 MEDICAL AND SURGICAL

BODY SYSTEM: 2 HEART AND GREAT VESSELS

OPERATION: **P REMOVAL:** Taking out or off a device from a body part

Body Part	Approach	Device	Qualifier
A Heart ⊞ ⚕	0 Open 3 Percutaneous 4 Percutaneous Endoscopic	2 Monitoring Device 3 Infusion Device 7 Autologous Tissue Substitute 8 Zooplastic Tissue C Extraluminal Device D Intraluminal Device J Synthetic Substitute K Nonautologous Tissue Substitute M Cardiac Lead N Intracardiac Pacemaker Q Implantable Heart Assist System R External Heart Assist System	Z No Qualifier
A Heart ⊞ ⚕	X External	2 Monitoring Device 3 Infusion Device D Intraluminal Device M Cardiac Lead	Z No Qualifier
Y Great Vessel	0 Open 3 Percutaneous 4 Percutaneous Endoscopic	2 Monitoring Device 3 Infusion Device 7 Autologous Tissue Substitute 8 Zooplastic Tissue C Extraluminal Device D Intraluminal Device J Synthetic Substitute K Nonautologous Tissue Substitute	Z No Qualifier
Y Great Vessel	X External	2 Monitoring Device 3 Infusion Device D Intraluminal Device	Z No Qualifier

⊞ 02PA[034][MR]Z

⊞ 02PAXMZ

DRG Non-OR 02PA3[23]Z

DRG Non-OR 02PY3[23]Z

Non-OR 02PAX[23D]Z

Non-OR 02PYX[23D]Z

⚕ 02PA[034]MZ when reported with Secondary Diagnosis K68.11, T81.4XXA, T82.6XXA, or T82.7XXA

⚕ 02PAXMZ when reported with Secondary Diagnosis K68.11, T81.4XXA, T82.6XXA, or T82.7XXA

Coding Clinic: 2015, Q3, P33 – 02PA3MZ
Coding Clinic: 2016, Q2, P15; 2015, Q4, P32 – 02PY33Z

SECTION: Ø MEDICAL AND SURGICAL

BODY SYSTEM: 2 HEART AND GREAT VESSELS

OPERATION: Q REPAIR: Restoring, to the extent possible, a body part to its normal anatomic structure and function

Body Part	Approach	Device	Qualifier
Ø Coronary Artery, One Artery 1 Coronary Artery, Two Arteries 2 Coronary Artery, Three Arteries 3 Coronary Artery, Four or More Arteries 4 Coronary Vein 5 Atrial Septum 6 Atrium, Right 7 Atrium, Left 8 Conduction Mechanism 9 Chordae Tendineae A Heart B Heart, Right C Heart, Left D Papillary Muscle F Aortic Valve G Mitral Valve H Pulmonary Valve J Tricuspid Valve K Ventricle, Right L Ventricle, Left M Ventricular Septum N Pericardium P Pulmonary Trunk Q Pulmonary Artery, Right R Pulmonary Artery, Left S Pulmonary Vein, Right T Pulmonary Vein, Left V Superior Vena Cava W Thoracic Aorta, Descending X Thoracic Aorta, Ascending/Arch	Ø Open 3 Percutaneous 4 Percutaneous Endoscopic	Z No Device	Z No Qualifier
F Aortic Valve	Ø Open 3 Percutaneous 4 Percutaneous Endoscopic	Z No Device	J Truncal Valve Z No Qualifier
G Mitral Valve	Ø Open 3 Percutaneous 4 Percutaneous Endoscopic	Z No Device	E Atrioventricular Valve, Left Z No Qualifier
J Tricuspid Valve	Ø Open 3 Percutaneous 4 Percutaneous Endoscopic	Z No Device	G Atrioventricular Valve, Right Z No Qualifier

Coding Clinic: 2015, Q3, P16 – 02QWØZZ
Coding Clinic: 2015, Q4, P24 – 02Q5ØZZ

Ø: M/S

2: HEART AND GREAT VESSELS

Q: REPAIR

New/Revised Text in Green   ~~deleted~~ Deleted   ♀ Females Only   ♂ Males Only   **Coding Clinic**
🜚 Non-covered   🜚 Limited Coverage   ⊕ Combination (See Appendix E)   DRG Non-OR   Non-OR   🜚 Hospital-Acquired Condition

75

SECTION: Ø MEDICAL AND SURGICAL

BODY SYSTEM: 2 HEART AND GREAT VESSELS

OPERATION: R REPLACEMENT: Putting in or on biological or synthetic material that physically takes the place and/or function of all or a portion of a body part

Body Part	Approach	Device	Qualifier
5 Atrial Septum 6 Atrium, Right 7 Atrium, Left 9 Chordae Tendineae D Papillary Muscle J Tricuspid Valve K Ventricle, Right 🔒 🔒 L Ventricle, Left 🔒 🔒 M Ventricular Septum ⊞ N Pericardium P Pulmonary Trunk ⊞ Q Pulmonary Artery, Right ⊞ R Pulmonary Artery, Left ⊞ S Pulmonary Vein, Right T Pulmonary Vein, Left V Superior Vena Cava W Thoracic Aorta, Descending X Thoracic Aorta, Ascending/Arch	Ø Open 4 Percutaneous Endoscopic	7 Autologous Tissue Substitute 8 Zooplastic Tissue J Synthetic Substitute K Nonautologous Tissue Substitute	Z No Qualifier
F Aortic Valve G Mitral Valve H Pulmonary Valve	Ø Open 4 Percutaneous Endoscopic	7 Autologous Tissue Substitute 8 Zooplastic Tissue J Synthetic Substitute K Nonautologous Tissue Substitute	Z No Qualifier
F Aortic Valve G Mitral Valve H Pulmonary Valve	3 Percutaneous	7 Autologous Tissue Substitute 8 Zooplastic Tissue J Synthetic Substitute K Nonautologous Tissue Substitute	H Transapical Z No Qualifier

🔒 02R[KL]ØJZ except when combined with diagnosis code Z00.6
🔒 02R[KL]ØJZ when combined with Z00.6
⊞ 02R[MP]ØJZ
⊞ 02R[QR]Ø[7J]Z

New/Revised Text in Green   ~~deleted~~ Deleted   ♀ Females Only   ♂ Males Only   **Coding Clinic**
🔒 Non-covered   🔒 Limited Coverage   ⊞ Combination (See Appendix E)   DRG Non-OR   Non-OR   🔒 Hospital-Acquired Condition

SECTION: ∅ MEDICAL AND SURGICAL

BODY SYSTEM: 2 HEART AND GREAT VESSELS

OPERATION: S REPOSITION: Moving to its normal location, or other suitable location, all or a portion of a body part

Body Part	Approach	Device	Qualifier
∅ Coronary Artery, One Artery	∅ Open	Z No Device	Z No Qualifier
1 Coronary Artery, Two Arteries			
P Pulmonary Trunk ⊞			
Q Pulmonary Artery, Right			
R Pulmonary Artery, Left			
S Pulmonary Vein, Right			
T Pulmonary Vein, Left			
V Superior Vena Cava			
W Thoracic Aorta, Descending ⊞			
X Thoracic Aorta, Ascending/Arch			

⊞ ∅2S[PW]∅ZZ

Coding Clinic: 2∅15, Q4, P24 – ∅2S[PW]∅ZZ

SECTION: ∅ MEDICAL AND SURGICAL

BODY SYSTEM: 2 HEART AND GREAT VESSELS

OPERATION: T RESECTION: Cutting out or off, without replacement, all of a body part

Body Part	Approach	Device	Qualifier
5 Atrial Septum	∅ Open	Z No Device	Z No Qualifier
8 Conduction Mechanism	3 Percutaneous		
9 Chordae Tendineae	4 Percutaneous Endoscopic		
D Papillary Muscle			
H Pulmonary Valve			
M Ventricular Septum			
N Pericardium			

SECTION: 0 MEDICAL AND SURGICAL

BODY SYSTEM: 2 HEART AND GREAT VESSELS

OPERATION: U SUPPLEMENT: Putting in or on biological or synthetic material that physically reinforces and/or augments the function of a portion of a body part

Body Part	Approach	Device	Qualifier
5 Atrial Septum 6 Atrium, Right 7 Atrium, Left ⊞ 9 Chordae Tendineae A Heart D Papillary Muscle F ~~Aortic Valve~~ G ~~Mitral Valve~~ H Pulmonary Valve J ~~Tricuspid Valve~~ K Ventricle, Right L Ventricle, Left M Ventricular Septum N Pericardium P Pulmonary Trunk Q Pulmonary Artery, Right R Pulmonary Artery, Left S Pulmonary Vein, Right T Pulmonary Vein, Left V Superior Vena Cava W Thoracic Aorta, Descending X Thoracic Aorta, Ascending/Arch	0 Open 3 Percutaneous 4 Percutaneous Endoscopic	7 Autologous Tissue Substitute 8 Zooplastic Tissue J Synthetic Substitute K Nonautologous Tissue Substitute	Z No Qualifier
F Aortic Valve	0 Open 3 Percutaneous 4 Percutaneous Endoscopic	7 Autologous Tissue Substitute 8 Zooplastic Tissue J Synthetic Substitute K Nonautologous Tissue Substitute	J Truncal Valve Z No Qualifier
G Mitral Valve	0 Open 3 Percutaneous 4 Percutaneous Endoscopic	7 Autologous Tissue Substitute 8 Zooplastic Tissue J Synthetic Substitute K Nonautologous Tissue Substitute	E Atrioventricular Valve, Left Z No Qualifier
J Tricuspid Valve	0 Open 3 Percutaneous 4 Percutaneous Endoscopic	7 Autologous Tissue Substitute 8 Zooplastic Tissue J Synthetic Substitute K Nonautologous Tissue Substitute	G Atrioventricular Valve, Right Z No Qualifier

⊞ 02U70JZ

DRG Non-OR 02U7[34]JZ

Coding Clinic: 2015, Q2, P24 – 02UG0JZ
Coding Clinic: 2015, Q3, P17 – 02U[QR]0KZ
Coding Clinic: 2015, Q4, P23-25 – 02UF08Z, 02UM0JZ, 02UM08Z, 02UW07Z
Coding Clinic: 2016, Q2, P24 – 02U[PR]07Z
Coding Clinic: 2016, Q2, P27 – 02UW0JZ

U: SUPPLEMENT

2: HEART AND GREAT VESSELS

0: M/S

New/Revised Text in Green   ~~deleted~~ Deleted   ♀ Females Only   ♂ Males Only   Coding Clinic
🚫 Non-covered   🚫 Limited Coverage   ⊞ Combination (See Appendix E)   DRG Non-OR   Non-OR   🚫 Hospital-Acquired Condition

SECTION: Ø MEDICAL AND SURGICAL

BODY SYSTEM: 2 HEART AND GREAT VESSELS

OPERATION: V RESTRICTION: Partially closing an orifice or the lumen of a tubular body part

Body Part	Approach	Device	Qualifier
A Heart	Ø Open 3 Percutaneous 4 Percutaneous Endoscopic	C Extraluminal Device Z No Device	Z No Qualifier
P Pulmonary Trunk Q Pulmonary Artery, Right S Pulmonary Vein, Right T Pulmonary Vein, Left V Superior Vena Cava W ~~Thoracic Aorta~~	Ø Open 3 Percutaneous 4 Percutaneous Endoscopic	C Extraluminal Device D Intraluminal Device Z No Device	Z No Qualifier
R Pulmonary Artery, Left ⊟	Ø Open 3 Percutaneous 4 Percutaneous Endoscopic	C Extraluminal Device D Intraluminal Device Z No Device	T Ductus Arteriosus Z No Qualifier
W Thoracic Aorta, Descending X Thoracic Aorta, Ascending/Arch	Ø Open 3 Percutaneous 4 Percutaneous Endoscopic	C Extraluminal Device D Intraluminal Device E Intraluminal Device, Branched or Fenestrated, One or Two Arteries F Intraluminal Device, Branched or Fenestrated, Three or More Arteries Z No Device	Z No Qualifier

⊟ 02VRØZT

Ø: M/S

2: HEART AND GREAT VESSELS

V: RESTRICTION

SECTION: 0 MEDICAL AND SURGICAL
BODY SYSTEM: 2 HEART AND GREAT VESSELS
OPERATION: W REVISION: Correcting, to the extent possible, a portion of a malfunctioning device or the position of a displaced device

Body Part	Approach	Device	Qualifier
5 Atrial Septum M Ventricular Septum	0 Open 4 Percutaneous Endoscopic	J Synthetic Substitute	Z No Qualifier
A Heart 🔖 🔖 ⊞ 🔖	0 Open 3 Percutaneous 4 Percutaneous Endoscopic X External	2 Monitoring Device 3 Infusion Device 7 Autologous Tissue Substitute 8 Zooplastic Tissue C Extraluminal Device D Intraluminal Device J Synthetic Substitute K Nonautologous Tissue Substitute M Cardiac Lead N Intracardiac Pacemaker Q Implantable Heart Assist System R External Heart Assist System	Z No Qualifier
F Aortic Valve G Mitral Valve H Pulmonary Valve J Tricuspid Valve	0 Open 4 Percutaneous Endoscopic	7 Autologous Tissue Substitute 8 Zooplastic Tissue J Synthetic Substitute K Nonautologous Tissue Substitute	Z No Qualifier
Y Great Vessel	0 Open 3 Percutaneous 4 Percutaneous Endoscopic X External	2 Monitoring Device 3 Infusion Device 7 Autologous Tissue Substitute 8 Zooplastic Tissue C Extraluminal Device D Intraluminal Device J Synthetic Substitute K Nonautologous Tissue Substitute	Z No Qualifier

🔖 02WA[34]QZ
🔖 02WA0[JQ]Z
⊞ 02WA[034][QR]Z
Non-OR 02WAX[2378CDJKMQR]Z
Non-OR 025WYX[2378CDJK]Z
🔖 02WA[034]MZ when reported with Secondary Diagnosis K68.11, T81.4XXA, T82.6XXA, or T82.7XXA

Coding Clinic: 2015, Q3, P32 – 02WA3MZ

New/Revised Text in Green ~~deleted~~ Deleted ♀ Females Only ♂ Males Only **Coding Clinic**
🔖 Non-covered 🔖 Limited Coverage ⊞ Combination (See Appendix E) DRG Non-OR Non-OR 🔖 Hospital-Acquired Condition

W: REVISION

2: HEART AND GREAT VESSELS

0: M/S

SECTION: 0 MEDICAL AND SURGICAL

BODY SYSTEM: 2 HEART AND GREAT VESSELS

OPERATION: Y TRANSPLANTATION: Putting in or on all or a portion of a living body part taken from another individual or animal to physically take the place and/or function of all or a portion of a similar body part

Body Part	Approach	Device	Qualifier
A Heart 🔖	0 Open	Z No Device	0 Allogeneic 1 Syngeneic 2 Zooplastic

🔖 02YA0Z[012]

Coding Clinic: 2013, Q3, P19 – 02YA0Z0

SECTION: Ø MEDICAL AND SURGICAL
BODY SYSTEM: 3 UPPER ARTERIES
OPERATION: 1 BYPASS: *(on multiple pages)*
Altering the route of passage of the contents of a tubular body part

Body Part	Approach	Device	Qualifier
2 Innominate Artery 5 Axillary Artery, Right 6 Axillary Artery, Left	Ø Open	9 Autologous Venous Tissue A Autologous Arterial Tissue J Synthetic Substitute K Nonautologous Tissue Substitute Z No Device	Ø Upper Arm Artery, Right 1 Upper Arm Artery, Left 2 Upper Arm Artery, Bilateral 3 Lower Arm Artery, Right 4 Lower Arm Artery, Left 5 Lower Arm Artery, Bilateral 6 Upper Leg Artery, Right 7 Upper Leg Artery, Left 8 Upper Leg Artery, Bilateral 9 Lower Leg Artery, Right B Lower Leg Artery, Left C Lower Leg Artery, Bilateral D Upper Arm Vein F Lower Arm Vein J Extracranial Artery, Right K Extracranial Artery, Left
3 Subclavian Artery, Right 4 Subclavian Artery, Left	Ø Open	9 Autologous Venous Tissue A Autologous Arterial Tissue J Synthetic Substitute K Nonautologous Tissue Substitute Z No Device	Ø Upper Arm Artery, Right 1 Upper Arm Artery, Left 2 Upper Arm Artery, Bilateral 3 Lower Arm Artery, Right 4 Lower Arm Artery, Left 5 Lower Arm Artery, Bilateral 6 Upper Leg Artery, Right 7 Upper Leg Artery, Left 8 Upper Leg Artery, Bilateral 9 Lower Leg Artery, Right B Lower Leg Artery, Left C Lower Leg Artery, Bilateral D Upper Arm Vein F Lower Arm Vein J Extracranial Artery, Right K Extracranial Artery, Left M Pulmonary Artery, Right N Pulmonary Artery, Left
7 Brachial Artery, Right	Ø Open	9 Autologous Venous Tissue A Autologous Arterial Tissue J Synthetic Substitute K Nonautologous Tissue Substitute Z No Device	Ø Upper Arm Artery, Right 3 Lower Arm Artery, Right D Upper Arm Vein F Lower Arm Vein
8 Brachial Artery, Left	Ø Open	9 Autologous Venous Tissue A Autologous Arterial Tissue J Synthetic Substitute K Nonautologous Tissue Substitute Z No Device	1 Upper Arm Artery, Left 4 Lower Arm Artery, Left D Upper Arm Vein F Lower Arm Vein

Ø: M/S

3: UPPER ARTERIES

1: BYPASS

SECTION: Ø MEDICAL AND SURGICAL
BODY SYSTEM: 3 **UPPER ARTERIES**
OPERATION: 1 **BYPASS:** *(continued)*
Altering the route of passage of the contents of a tubular body part

Body Part	Approach	Device	Qualifier
9 Ulnar Artery, Right B Radial Artery, Right ⊞	Ø Open	9 Autologous Venous Tissue A Autologous Arterial Tissue J Synthetic Substitute K Nonautologous Tissue Substitute Z No Device	3 Lower Arm Artery, Right F Lower Arm Vein
A Ulnar Artery, Left C Radial Artery, Left ⊞	Ø Open	9 Autologous Venous Tissue A Autologous Arterial Tissue J Synthetic Substitute K Nonautologous Tissue Substitute Z No Device	4 Lower Arm Artery, Left F Lower Arm Vein
G Intracranial Artery S Temporal Artery, Right ⊘ T Temporal Artery, Left ⊘	Ø Open	9 Autologous Venous Tissue A Autologous Arterial Tissue J Synthetic Substitute K Nonautologous Tissue Substitute Z No Device	G Intracranial Artery
H Common Carotid Artery, Right ⊘	Ø Open	9 Autologous Venous Tissue A Autologous Arterial Tissue J Synthetic Substitute K Nonautologous Tissue Substitute Z No Device	G Intracranial Artery J Extracranial Artery, Right
J Common Carotid Artery, Left ⊘	Ø Open	9 Autologous Venous Tissue A Autologous Arterial Tissue J Synthetic Substitute K Nonautologous Tissue Substitute Z No Device	G Intracranial Artery K Extracranial Artery, Left
K Internal Carotid Artery, Right M External Carotid Artery, Right	Ø Open	9 Autologous Venous Tissue A Autologous Arterial Tissue J Synthetic Substitute K Nonautologous Tissue Substitute Z No Device	J Extracranial Artery, Right
L Internal Carotid Artery, Left N External Carotid Artery, Left	Ø Open	9 Autologous Venous Tissue A Autologous Arterial Tissue J Synthetic Substitute K Nonautologous Tissue Substitute Z No Device	K Extracranial Artery, Left

⊘ Ø31[ST]Ø[9AJKZ]G
⊘ Ø31HØ[9AJKZ]G
⊘ Ø31JØ[9AJKZ]G
⊞ Ø31BØJF
⊞ Ø31CØJF

Coding Clinic: 2Ø13, Q1, P228 – Ø31CØZF

Sidebar: 1: BYPASS 3: UPPER ARTERIES Ø: M/S

New/Revised Text in Green ~~deleted~~ Deleted ♀ Females Only ♂ Males Only **Coding Clinic**
⊘ Non-covered ⊘ Limited Coverage ⊞ Combination (See Appendix E) DRG Non-OR Non-OR ⊘ Hospital-Acquired Condition

SECTION: Ø MEDICAL AND SURGICAL

BODY SYSTEM: 3 UPPER ARTERIES

OPERATION: 5 DESTRUCTION: Physical eradication of all or a portion of a body part by the direct use of energy, force, or a destructive agent

Body Part	Approach	Device	Qualifier
Ø Internal Mammary Artery, Right	Ø Open	Z No Device	Z No Qualifier
1 Internal Mammary Artery, Left	3 Percutaneous		
2 Innominate Artery	4 Percutaneous Endoscopic		
3 Subclavian Artery, Right			
4 Subclavian Artery, Left			
5 Axillary Artery, Right			
6 Axillary Artery, Left			
7 Brachial Artery, Right			
8 Brachial Artery, Left			
9 Ulnar Artery, Right			
A Ulnar Artery, Left			
B Radial Artery, Right			
C Radial Artery, Left			
D Hand Artery, Right			
F Hand Artery, Left			
G Intracranial Artery			
H Common Carotid Artery, Right			
J Common Carotid Artery, Left			
K Internal Carotid Artery, Right			
L Internal Carotid Artery, Left			
M External Carotid Artery, Right			
N External Carotid Artery, Left			
P Vertebral Artery, Right			
Q Vertebral Artery, Left			
R Face Artery			
S Temporal Artery, Right			
T Temporal Artery, Left			
U Thyroid Artery, Right			
V Thyroid Artery, Left			
Y Upper Artery			

Ø: M/S

3: UPPER ARTERIES

5: DESTRUCTION

SECTION: Ø MEDICAL AND SURGICAL
BODY SYSTEM: 3 UPPER ARTERIES
OPERATION: 7 **DILATION:** Expanding an orifice or the lumen of a tubular body part

Body Part	Approach	Device	Qualifier
Ø Internal Mammary Artery, Right 1 Internal Mammary Artery, Left 2 Innominate Artery 3 Subclavian Artery, Right 4 Subclavian Artery, Left 5 Axillary Artery, Right 6 Axillary Artery, Left 7 Brachial Artery, Right 8 Brachial Artery, Left 9 Ulnar Artery, Right A Ulnar Artery, Left B Radial Artery, Right C Radial Artery, Left D Hand Artery, Right F Hand Artery, Left G Intracranial Artery ⚕ H Common Carotid Artery, Right J Common Carotid Artery, Left K Internal Carotid Artery, Right L Internal Carotid Artery, Left M External Carotid Artery, Right N External Carotid Artery, Left P Vertebral Artery, Right Q Vertebral Artery, Left R Face Artery S Temporal Artery, Right T Temporal Artery, Left U Thyroid Artery, Right V Thyroid Artery, Left Y Upper Artery	Ø Open 3 Percutaneous 4 Percutaneous Endoscopic	4 Intraluminal Device, Drug-eluting 5 Intraluminal Device, Drug-eluting, Two 6 Intraluminal Device, Drug-eluting, Three 7 Intraluminal Device, Drug-eluting, Four or More D Intraluminal Device E Intraluminal Device, Two F Intraluminal Device, Three G Intraluminal Device, Four or More Z No Device	6 Bifurcation Z No Qualifier

⚕ Ø37G[34]ZZ

7: DILATION

3: UPPER ARTERIES

Ø: M/S

SECTION: Ø MEDICAL AND SURGICAL
BODY SYSTEM: 3 UPPER ARTERIES
OPERATION: 9 DRAINAGE: *(on multiple pages)*
Taking or letting out fluids and/or gases from a body part

Body Part	Approach	Device	Qualifier
Ø Internal Mammary Artery, Right 1 Internal Mammary Artery, Left 2 Innominate Artery 3 Subclavian Artery, Right 4 Subclavian Artery, Left 5 Axillary Artery, Right 6 Axillary Artery, Left 7 Brachial Artery, Right 8 Brachial Artery, Left 9 Ulnar Artery, Right A Ulnar Artery, Left B Radial Artery, Right C Radial Artery, Left D Hand Artery, Right F Hand Artery, Left G Intracranial Artery H Common Carotid Artery, Right J Common Carotid Artery, Left K Internal Carotid Artery, Right L Internal Carotid Artery, Left M External Carotid Artery, Right N External Carotid Artery, Left P Vertebral Artery, Right Q Vertebral Artery, Left R Face Artery S Temporal Artery, Right T Temporal Artery, Left U Thyroid Artery, Right V Thyroid Artery, Left Y Upper Artery	Ø Open 3 Percutaneous 4 Percutaneous Endoscopic	Ø Drainage Device	Z No Qualifier

Non-OR 039[0123456789ABCDFGHJKLMNPQRSTUVY][034]0Z

SECTION: Ø MEDICAL AND SURGICAL
BODY SYSTEM: 3 **UPPER ARTERIES**
OPERATION: 9 **DRAINAGE:** *(continued)*
Taking or letting out fluids and/or gases from a body part

Body Part	Approach	Device	Qualifier
Ø Internal Mammary Artery, Right	Ø Open	Z No Device	X Diagnostic
1 Internal Mammary Artery, Left	3 Percutaneous		Z No Qualifier
2 Innominate Artery	4 Percutaneous Endoscopic		
3 Subclavian Artery, Right			
4 Subclavian Artery, Left			
5 Axillary Artery, Right			
6 Axillary Artery, Left			
7 Brachial Artery, Right			
8 Brachial Artery, Left			
9 Ulnar Artery, Right			
A Ulnar Artery, Left			
B Radial Artery, Right			
C Radial Artery, Left			
D Hand Artery, Right			
F Hand Artery, Left			
G Intracranial Artery			
H Common Carotid Artery, Right			
J Common Carotid Artery, Left			
K Internal Carotid Artery, Right			
L Internal Carotid Artery, Left			
M External Carotid Artery, Right			
N External Carotid Artery, Left			
P Vertebral Artery, Right			
Q Vertebral Artery, Left			
R Face Artery			
S Temporal Artery, Right			
T Temporal Artery, Left			
U Thyroid Artery, Right			
V Thyroid Artery, Left			
Y Upper Artery			

Non-OR Ø39[Ø123456789ABCDFGHJKLMNPQRSTUVY][Ø34]ZZ

SECTION: 0 MEDICAL AND SURGICAL
BODY SYSTEM: 3 UPPER ARTERIES
OPERATION: B EXCISION: Cutting out or off, without replacement, a portion of a body part

Body Part	Approach	Device	Qualifier
0 Internal Mammary Artery, Right	0 Open	Z No Device	X Diagnostic
1 Internal Mammary Artery, Left	3 Percutaneous		Z No Qualifier
2 Innominate Artery	4 Percutaneous Endoscopic		
3 Subclavian Artery, Right			
4 Subclavian Artery, Left			
5 Axillary Artery, Right			
6 Axillary Artery, Left			
7 Brachial Artery, Right			
8 Brachial Artery, Left			
9 Ulnar Artery, Right			
A Ulnar Artery, Left			
B Radial Artery, Right			
C Radial Artery, Left			
D Hand Artery, Right			
F Hand Artery, Left			
G Intracranial Artery			
H Common Carotid Artery, Right			
J Common Carotid Artery, Left			
K Internal Carotid Artery, Right			
L Internal Carotid Artery, Left			
M External Carotid Artery, Right			
N External Carotid Artery, Left			
P Vertebral Artery, Right			
Q Vertebral Artery, Left			
R Face Artery			
S Temporal Artery, Right			
T Temporal Artery, Left			
U Thyroid Artery, Right			
V Thyroid Artery, Left			
Y Upper Artery			

Coding Clinic: 2016, Q2, P13 – 03BN0ZZ

SECTION: Ø MEDICAL AND SURGICAL
BODY SYSTEM: 3 UPPER ARTERIES
OPERATION: C EXTIRPATION: Taking or cutting out solid matter from a body part

Body Part	Approach	Device	Qualifier
Ø Internal Mammary Artery, Right	Ø Open	Z No Device	6 Bifurcation
1 Internal Mammary Artery, Left	3 Percutaneous		Z No Qualifier
2 Innominate Artery	4 Percutaneous Endoscopic		
3 Subclavian Artery, Right			
4 Subclavian Artery, Left			
5 Axillary Artery, Right			
6 Axillary Artery, Left			
7 Brachial Artery, Right			
8 Brachial Artery, Left			
9 Ulnar Artery, Right			
A Ulnar Artery, Left			
B Radial Artery, Right			
C Radial Artery, Left			
D Hand Artery, Right			
F Hand Artery, Left			
G Intracranial Artery			
H Common Carotid Artery, Right			
J Common Carotid Artery, Left			
K Internal Carotid Artery, Right			
L Internal Carotid Artery, Left			
M External Carotid Artery, Right			
N External Carotid Artery, Left			
P Vertebral Artery, Right			
Q Vertebral Artery, Left			
R Face Artery			
S Temporal Artery, Right			
T Temporal Artery, Left			
U Thyroid Artery, Right			
V Thyroid Artery, Left			
Y Upper Artery			

Coding Clinic: 2Ø16, Q2, P12 – Ø3CKØZZ

SECTION: Ø MEDICAL AND SURGICAL
BODY SYSTEM: 3 UPPER ARTERIES
OPERATION: H **INSERTION:** Putting in a nonbiological appliance that monitors, assists, performs, or prevents a physiological function but does not physically take the place of a body part

Body Part	Approach	Device	Qualifier
Ø Internal Mammary Artery, Right 1 Internal Mammary Artery, Left 2 Innominate Artery 3 Subclavian Artery, Right 4 Subclavian Artery, Left 5 Axillary Artery, Right 6 Axillary Artery, Left 7 Brachial Artery, Right 8 Brachial Artery, Left 9 Ulnar Artery, Right A Ulnar Artery, Left B Radial Artery, Right C Radial Artery, Left D Hand Artery, Right F Hand Artery, Left G Intracranial Artery H Common Carotid Artery, Right J Common Carotid Artery, Left M External Carotid Artery, Right N External Carotid Artery, Left P Vertebral Artery, Right Q Vertebral Artery, Left R Face Artery S Temporal Artery, Right T Temporal Artery, Left U Thyroid Artery, Right V Thyroid Artery, Left	Ø Open 3 Percutaneous 4 Percutaneous Endoscopic	3 Infusion Device D Intraluminal Device	Z No Qualifier
K Internal Carotid Artery, Right ⊞ L Internal Carotid Artery, Left ⊞	Ø Open 3 Percutaneous 4 Percutaneous Endoscopic	3 Infusion Device D Intraluminal Device M Stimulator Lead	Z No Qualifier
Y Upper Artery	Ø Open 3 Percutaneous 4 Percutaneous Endoscopic	2 Monitoring Device 3 Infusion Device D Intraluminal Device	Z No Qualifier

⊞ 03H[KL][034]MZ
DRG Non-OR 03HY32Z
Non-OR 03H[Ø123456789ABCDFGHJMNPQRSTUV][034]3Z
Non-OR 03H[KL][034]3Z
Non-OR 03HY[034]3Z

Coding Clinic: 2016, Q2, P32 – 03HY32Z

L: OCCLUSION   J: INSPECTION   3: UPPER ARTERIES   0: M/S

SECTION: 0 MEDICAL AND SURGICAL
BODY SYSTEM: 3 UPPER ARTERIES
OPERATION: J INSPECTION: Visually and/or manually exploring a body part

Body Part	Approach	Device	Qualifier
Y Upper Artery	0 Open 3 Percutaneous 4 Percutaneous Endoscopic X External	Z No Device	Z No Qualifier

DRG Non-OR 03JY3ZZ
Non-OR 03JY[4X]ZZ

Coding Clinic: 2015, Q1, P29 – 03JY0ZZ

SECTION: 0 MEDICAL AND SURGICAL
BODY SYSTEM: 3 UPPER ARTERIES
OPERATION: L OCCLUSION: Completely closing an orifice or the lumen of a tubular body part

Body Part	Approach	Device	Qualifier
0 Internal Mammary Artery, Right 1 Internal Mammary Artery, Left 2 Innominate Artery 3 Subclavian Artery, Right 4 Subclavian Artery, Left 5 Axillary Artery, Right 6 Axillary Artery, Left 7 Brachial Artery, Right 8 Brachial Artery, Left 9 Ulnar Artery, Right A Ulnar Artery, Left B Radial Artery, Right C Radial Artery, Left D Hand Artery, Right F Hand Artery, Left R Face Artery S Temporal Artery, Right T Temporal Artery, Left U Thyroid Artery, Right V Thyroid Artery, Left Y Upper Artery	0 Open 3 Percutaneous 4 Percutaneous Endoscopic	C Extraluminal Device D Intraluminal Device Z No Device	Z No Qualifier
G Intracranial Artery H Common Carotid Artery, Right J Common Carotid Artery, Left K Internal Carotid Artery, Right L Internal Carotid Artery, Left M External Carotid Artery, Right N External Carotid Artery, Left P Vertebral Artery, Right Q Vertebral Artery, Left	0 Open 3 Percutaneous 4 Percutaneous Endoscopic	B Intraluminal Device, Bioactive C Extraluminal Device D Intraluminal Device Z No Device	Z No Qualifier

Coding Clinic: 2016, Q2, P30 – 03LG0CZ

New/Revised Text in Green   ~~deleted~~ Deleted   ♀ Females Only   ♂ Males Only   **Coding Clinic**
Non-covered   Limited Coverage   Combination (See Appendix E)   DRG Non-OR   Non-OR   Hospital-Acquired Condition

SECTION: 0 MEDICAL AND SURGICAL

BODY SYSTEM: 3 UPPER ARTERIES

OPERATION: N RELEASE: Freeing a body part from an abnormal physical constraint by cutting or by the use of force

Body Part	Approach	Device	Qualifier
0 Internal Mammary Artery, Right	0 Open	Z No Device	Z No Qualifier
1 Internal Mammary Artery, Left	3 Percutaneous		
2 Innominate Artery	4 Percutaneous Endoscopic		
3 Subclavian Artery, Right			
4 Subclavian Artery, Left			
5 Axillary Artery, Right			
6 Axillary Artery, Left			
7 Brachial Artery, Right			
8 Brachial Artery, Left			
9 Ulnar Artery, Right			
A Ulnar Artery, Left			
B Radial Artery, Right			
C Radial Artery, Left			
D Hand Artery, Right			
F Hand Artery, Left			
G Intracranial Artery			
H Common Carotid Artery, Right			
J Common Carotid Artery, Left			
K Internal Carotid Artery, Right			
L Internal Carotid Artery, Left			
M External Carotid Artery, Right			
N External Carotid Artery, Left			
P Vertebral Artery, Right			
Q Vertebral Artery, Left			
R Face Artery			
S Temporal Artery, Right			
T Temporal Artery, Left			
U Thyroid Artery, Right			
V Thyroid Artery, Left			
Y Upper Artery			

P: REMOVAL

3: UPPER ARTERIES

0: M/S

SECTION: 0 MEDICAL AND SURGICAL
BODY SYSTEM: 3 UPPER ARTERIES
OPERATION: P REMOVAL: Taking out or off a device from a body part

Body Part	Approach	Device	Qualifier
Y Upper Artery ⊕	0 Open 3 Percutaneous 4 Percutaneous Endoscopic	0 Drainage Device 2 Monitoring Device 3 Infusion Device 7 Autologous Tissue Substitute C Extraluminal Device D Intraluminal Device J Synthetic Substitute K Nonautologous Tissue Substitute M Stimulator Lead	Z No Qualifier
Y Upper Artery	X External	0 Drainage Device 2 Monitoring Device 3 Infusion Device D Intraluminal Device M Stimulator Lead	Z No Qualifier

⊕ 03PY[034][JM]Z
DRG Non-OR 03PY3[023]Z
Non-OR 03PYX[023DM]Z

New/Revised Text in Green ~~deleted~~ Deleted ♀ Females Only ♂ Males Only **Coding Clinic**
🔖 Non-covered 🔖 Limited Coverage ⊕ Combination (See Appendix E) DRG Non-OR Non-OR 🔖 Hospital-Acquired Condition

SECTION: Ø MEDICAL AND SURGICAL

BODY SYSTEM: 3 UPPER ARTERIES

OPERATION: **Q REPAIR:** Restoring, to the extent possible, a body part to its normal anatomic structure and function

Body Part	Approach	Device	Qualifier
Ø Internal Mammary Artery, Right 1 Internal Mammary Artery, Left 2 Innominate Artery 3 Subclavian Artery, Right 4 Subclavian Artery, Left 5 Axillary Artery, Right 6 Axillary Artery, Left 7 Brachial Artery, Right 8 Brachial Artery, Left 9 Ulnar Artery, Right A Ulnar Artery, Left B Radial Artery, Right C Radial Artery, Left D Hand Artery, Right F Hand Artery, Left G Intracranial Artery H Common Carotid Artery, Right J Common Carotid Artery, Left K Internal Carotid Artery, Right L Internal Carotid Artery, Left M External Carotid Artery, Right N External Carotid Artery, Left P Vertebral Artery, Right Q Vertebral Artery, Left R Face Artery S Temporal Artery, Right T Temporal Artery, Left U Thyroid Artery, Right V Thyroid Artery, Left Y Upper Artery	Ø Open 3 Percutaneous 4 Percutaneous Endoscopic	Z No Device	Z No Qualifier

SECTION:　Ø　MEDICAL AND SURGICAL

BODY SYSTEM: 3　UPPER ARTERIES

OPERATION:　R　**REPLACEMENT:** Putting in or on biological or synthetic material that physically takes the place and/or function of all or a portion of a body part

Body Part	Approach	Device	Qualifier
Ø Internal Mammary Artery, Right 1 Internal Mammary Artery, Left 2 Innominate Artery 3 Subclavian Artery, Right 4 Subclavian Artery, Left 5 Axillary Artery, Right 6 Axillary Artery, Left 7 Brachial Artery, Right 8 Brachial Artery, Left 9 Ulnar Artery, Right A Ulnar Artery, Left B Radial Artery, Right C Radial Artery, Left D Hand Artery, Right F Hand Artery, Left G Intracranial Artery H Common Carotid Artery, Right J Common Carotid Artery, Left K Internal Carotid Artery, Right L Internal Carotid Artery, Left M External Carotid Artery, Right N External Carotid Artery, Left P Vertebral Artery, Right Q Vertebral Artery, Left R Face Artery S Temporal Artery, Right T Temporal Artery, Left U Thyroid Artery, Right V Thyroid Artery, Left Y Upper Artery	Ø Open 4 Percutaneous Endoscopic	7 Autologous Tissue Substitute J Synthetic Substitute K Nonautologous Tissue Substitute	Z No Qualifier

SECTION: Ø MEDICAL AND SURGICAL
BODY SYSTEM: 3 UPPER ARTERIES
OPERATION: S REPOSITION: Moving to its normal location, or other suitable location, all or a portion of a body part

Body Part	Approach	Device	Qualifier
Ø Internal Mammary Artery, Right	Ø Open	Z No Device	Z No Qualifier
1 Internal Mammary Artery, Left	3 Percutaneous		
2 Innominate Artery	4 Percutaneous Endoscopic		
3 Subclavian Artery, Right			
4 Subclavian Artery, Left			
5 Axillary Artery, Right			
6 Axillary Artery, Left			
7 Brachial Artery, Right			
8 Brachial Artery, Left			
9 Ulnar Artery, Right			
A Ulnar Artery, Left			
B Radial Artery, Right			
C Radial Artery, Left			
D Hand Artery, Right			
F Hand Artery, Left			
G Intracranial Artery			
H Common Carotid Artery, Right			
J Common Carotid Artery, Left			
K Internal Carotid Artery, Right			
L Internal Carotid Artery, Left			
M External Carotid Artery, Right			
N External Carotid Artery, Left			
P Vertebral Artery, Right			
Q Vertebral Artery, Left			
R Face Artery			
S Temporal Artery, Right			
T Temporal Artery, Left			
U Thyroid Artery, Right			
V Thyroid Artery, Left			
Y Upper Artery			

Coding Clinic: 2Ø15, Q3, P28 – Ø3SSØZZ

SECTION: Ø MEDICAL AND SURGICAL
BODY SYSTEM: 3 UPPER ARTERIES
OPERATION: U SUPPLEMENT: Putting in or on biological or synthetic material that physically reinforces and/or augments the function of a portion of a body part

Body Part	Approach	Device	Qualifier
Ø Internal Mammary Artery, Right	Ø Open	7 Autologous Tissue Substitute	Z No Qualifier
1 Internal Mammary Artery, Left	3 Percutaneous	J Synthetic Substitute	
2 Innominate Artery	4 Percutaneous Endoscopic	K Nonautologous Tissue Substitute	
3 Subclavian Artery, Right			
4 Subclavian Artery, Left			
5 Axillary Artery, Right			
6 Axillary Artery, Left			
7 Brachial Artery, Right			
8 Brachial Artery, Left			
9 Ulnar Artery, Right			
A Ulnar Artery, Left			
B Radial Artery, Right			
C Radial Artery, Left			
D Hand Artery, Right			
F Hand Artery, Left			
G Intracranial Artery			
H Common Carotid Artery, Right			
J Common Carotid Artery, Left			
K Internal Carotid Artery, Right			
L Internal Carotid Artery, Left			
M External Carotid Artery, Right			
N External Carotid Artery, Left			
P Vertebral Artery, Right			
Q Vertebral Artery, Left			
R Face Artery			
S Temporal Artery, Right			
T Temporal Artery, Left			
U Thyroid Artery, Right			
V Thyroid Artery, Left			
Y Upper Artery			

Coding Clinic: 2Ø16, Q2, P12 – Ø3UKØJZ

U: SUPPLEMENT

3: UPPER ARTERIES

Ø: M/S

New/Revised Text in Green   ~~deleted~~ Deleted   ♀ Females Only   ♂ Males Only   **Coding Clinic**
Non-covered   Limited Coverage   ⊞ Combination (See Appendix E)   DRG Non-OR   Non-OR   Hospital-Acquired Condition

SECTION: Ø MEDICAL AND SURGICAL

BODY SYSTEM: 3 UPPER ARTERIES

OPERATION: V RESTRICTION: Partially closing an orifice or the lumen of a tubular body part

Body Part	Approach	Device	Qualifier
Ø Internal Mammary Artery, Right 1 Internal Mammary Artery, Left 2 Innominate Artery 3 Subclavian Artery, Right 4 Subclavian Artery, Left 5 Axillary Artery, Right 6 Axillary Artery, Left 7 Brachial Artery, Right 8 Brachial Artery, Left 9 Ulnar Artery, Right A Ulnar Artery, Left B Radial Artery, Right C Radial Artery, Left D Hand Artery, Right F Hand Artery, Left R Face Artery S Temporal Artery, Right T Temporal Artery, Left U Thyroid Artery, Right V Thyroid Artery, Left Y Upper Artery	Ø Open 3 Percutaneous 4 Percutaneous Endoscopic	C Extraluminal Device D Intraluminal Device Z No Device	Z No Qualifier
G Intracranial Artery H Common Carotid Artery, Right J Common Carotid Artery, Left K Internal Carotid Artery, Right L Internal Carotid Artery, Left M External Carotid Artery, Right N External Carotid Artery, Left P Vertebral Artery, Right Q Vertebral Artery, Left	Ø Open 3 Percutaneous 4 Percutaneous Endoscopic	B Intraluminal Device, Bioactive C Extraluminal Device D Intraluminal Device Z No Device	Z No Qualifier

Coding Clinic: 2Ø16, Q1, P2Ø – Ø3VG3DZ

SECTION: Ø MEDICAL AND SURGICAL

BODY SYSTEM: 3 UPPER ARTERIES

OPERATION: W REVISION: Correcting, to the extent possible, a portion of a malfunctioning device or the position of a displaced device

Body Part	Approach	Device	Qualifier
Y Upper Artery	Ø Open 3 Percutaneous 4 Percutaneous Endoscopic X External	Ø Drainage Device 2 Monitoring Device 3 Infusion Device 7 Autologous Tissue Substitute C Extraluminal Device D Intraluminal Device J Synthetic Substitute K Nonautologous Tissue Substitute M Stimulator Lead	Z No Qualifier

Non-OR Ø3WYX[Ø237CDJKM]Z

Coding Clinic: 2Ø15, Q1, P33 – ØØWY3DZ

Ø: M/S · 3: UPPER ARTERIES · V: RESTRICTION · W: REVISION

SECTION: Ø MEDICAL AND SURGICAL
BODY SYSTEM: 4 LOWER ARTERIES
OPERATION: 1 **BYPASS:** Altering the route of passage of the contents of a tubular body part

Body Part	Approach	Device	Qualifier
Ø Abdominal Aorta C Common Iliac Artery, Right D Common Iliac Artery, Left	Ø Open 4 Percutaneous Endoscopic	9 Autologous Venous Tissue A Autologous Arterial Tissue J Synthetic Substitute K Nonautologous Tissue Substitute Z No Device	Ø Abdominal Aorta 1 Celiac Artery 2 Mesenteric Artery 3 Renal Artery, Right 4 Renal Artery, Left 5 Renal Artery, Bilateral 6 Common Iliac Artery, Right 7 Common Iliac Artery, Left 8 Common Iliac Arteries, Bilateral 9 Internal Iliac Artery, Right B Internal Iliac Artery, Left C Internal Iliac Arteries, Bilateral D External Iliac Artery, Right F External Iliac Artery, Left G External Iliac Arteries, Bilateral H Femoral Artery, Right J Femoral Artery, Left K Femoral Arteries, Bilateral Q Lower Extremity Artery R Lower Artery
4 Splenic Artery	Ø Open 4 Percutaneous Endoscopic	9 Autologous Venous Tissue A Autologous Arterial Tissue J Synthetic Substitute K Nonautologous Tissue Substitute Z No Device	3 Renal Artery, Right 4 Renal Artery, Left 5 Renal Artery, Bilateral
E Internal Iliac Artery, Right F Internal Iliac Artery, Left H External Iliac Artery, Right J External Iliac Artery, Left	Ø Open 4 Percutaneous Endoscopic	9 Autologous Venous Tissue A Autologous Arterial Tissue J Synthetic Substitute K Nonautologous Tissue Substitute Z No Device	9 Internal Iliac Artery, Right B Internal Iliac Artery, Left C Internal Iliac Arteries, Bilateral D External Iliac Artery, Right F External Iliac Artery, Left G External Iliac Arteries, Bilateral H Femoral Artery, Right J Femoral Artery, Left K Femoral Arteries, Bilateral P Foot Artery Q Lower Extremity Artery
K Femoral Artery, Right L Femoral Artery, Left	Ø Open 4 Percutaneous Endoscopic	9 Autologous Venous Tissue A Autologous Arterial Tissue J Synthetic Substitute K Nonautologous Tissue Substitute Z No Device	H Femoral Artery, Right J Femoral Artery, Left K Femoral Arteries, Bilateral L Popliteal Artery M Peroneal Artery N Posterior Tibial Artery P Foot Artery Q Lower Extremity Artery S Lower Extremity Vein
M Popliteal Artery, Right N Popliteal Artery, Left	Ø Open 4 Percutaneous Endoscopic	9 Autologous Venous Tissue A Autologous Arterial Tissue J Synthetic Substitute K Nonautologous Tissue Substitute Z No Device	L Popliteal Artery M Peroneal Artery P Foot Artery Q Lower Extremity Artery S Lower Extremity Vein

Coding Clinic: 2Ø15, Q3, P28 – Ø41ØØZ3, Ø414ØZ4
Coding Clinic: 2Ø16, Q2, P19 – Ø41KØJN

Ø: M/S   4: LOWER ARTERIES   1: BYPASS

New/Revised Text in Green   ~~deleted~~ Deleted   ♀ Females Only   ♂ Males Only   **Coding Clinic**
Non-covered   Limited Coverage   ⊞ Combination (See Appendix E)   DRG Non-OR   Non-OR   Hospital-Acquired Condition

1Ø1

SECTION: Ø MEDICAL AND SURGICAL

BODY SYSTEM: 4 LOWER ARTERIES

OPERATION: 5 **DESTRUCTION:** Physical eradication of all or a portion of a body part by the direct use of energy, force, or a destructive agent

Body Part	Approach	Device	Qualifier
Ø Abdominal Aorta	Ø Open	Z No Device	Z No Qualifier
1 Celiac Artery	3 Percutaneous		
2 Gastric Artery	4 Percutaneous Endoscopic		
3 Hepatic Artery			
4 Splenic Artery			
5 Superior Mesenteric Artery			
6 Colic Artery, Right			
7 Colic Artery, Left			
8 Colic Artery, Middle			
9 Renal Artery, Right			
A Renal Artery, Left			
B Inferior Mesenteric Artery			
C Common Iliac Artery, Right			
D Common Iliac Artery, Left			
E Internal Iliac Artery, Right			
F Internal Iliac Artery, Left			
H External Iliac Artery, Right			
J External Iliac Artery, Left			
K Femoral Artery, Right			
L Femoral Artery, Left			
M Popliteal Artery, Right			
N Popliteal Artery, Left			
P Anterior Tibial Artery, Right			
Q Anterior Tibial Artery, Left			
R Posterior Tibial Artery, Right			
S Posterior Tibial Artery, Left			
T Peroneal Artery, Right			
U Peroneal Artery, Left			
V Foot Artery, Right			
W Foot Artery, Left			
Y Lower Artery			

5: DESTRUCTION

4: LOWER ARTERIES

Ø: M/S

New/Revised Text in Green   ~~deleted~~ Deleted   ♀ Females Only   ♂ Males Only   **Coding Clinic**
🔖 Non-covered   🔖 Limited Coverage   ⊞ Combination (See Appendix E)   DRG Non-OR   Non-OR   🔖 Hospital-Acquired Condition

SECTION: Ø MEDICAL AND SURGICAL

BODY SYSTEM: 4 LOWER ARTERIES
OPERATION: 7 DILATION: Expanding an orifice or the lumen of a tubular body part

Body Part	Approach	Device	Qualifier
Ø Abdominal Aorta 1 Celiac Artery 2 Gastric Artery 3 Hepatic Artery 4 Splenic Artery 5 Superior Mesenteric Artery 6 Colic Artery, Right 7 Colic Artery, Left 8 Colic Artery, Middle 9 Renal Artery, Right A Renal Artery, Left B Inferior Mesenteric Artery C Common Iliac Artery, Right D Common Iliac Artery, Left E Internal Iliac Artery, Right F Internal Iliac Artery, Left H External Iliac Artery, Right J External Iliac Artery, Left P Anterior Tibial Artery, Right Q Anterior Tibial Artery, Left R Posterior Tibial Artery, Right S Posterior Tibial Artery, Left T Peroneal Artery, Right U Peroneal Artery, Left V Foot Artery, Right W Foot Artery, Left Y Lower Artery	Ø Open 3 Percutaneous 4 Percutaneous Endoscopic	4 Intraluminal Device, Drug-eluting 5 Intraluminal Device, Drug-eluting, Two 6 Intraluminal Device, Drug-eluting, Three 7 Intraluminal Device, Drug-eluting, Four or More D Intraluminal Device E Intraluminal Device, Two F Intraluminal Device, Three G Intraluminal Device, Four or More Z No Device	6 Bifurcation Z No Qualifier
K Femoral Artery, Right L Femoral Artery, Left M Popliteal Artery, Right N Popliteal Artery, Left	Ø Open 3 Percutaneous 4 Percutaneous Endoscopic	4 Intraluminal Device, Drug-eluting D Intraluminal Device Z No Device	1 Drug-Coated Balloon 6 Bifurcation Z No Qualifier
K Femoral Artery, Right L Femoral Artery, Left M Popliteal Artery, Right N Popliteal Artery, Left	Ø Open 3 Percutaneous 4 Percutaneous Endoscopic	5 Intraluminal Device, Drug-eluting, Two 6 Intraluminal Device, Drug-eluting, Three 7 Intraluminal Device, Drug-eluting, Four or More E Intraluminal Device, Two F Intraluminal Device, Three G Intraluminal Device, Four or More	6 Bifurcation Z No Qualifier

Non-OR Ø47[59A]4DZ

Coding Clinic: 2Ø15, Q4, P7 – Ø47K3D1
Coding Clinic: 2Ø15, Q4, P15 – Ø47K3D1, Ø47L3Z1

Ø: M/S

4: LOWER ARTERIES

7: DILATION

New/Revised Text in Green   ~~deleted~~ Deleted   ♀ Females Only   ♂ Males Only   **Coding Clinic**
🔾 Non-covered   🔾 Limited Coverage   ⊞ Combination (See Appendix E)   DRG Non-OR   Non-OR   🔾 Hospital-Acquired Condition

1Ø3

SECTION: Ø MEDICAL AND SURGICAL
BODY SYSTEM: 4 LOWER ARTERIES
OPERATION: 9 DRAINAGE: *(on multiple pages)*
Taking or letting out fluids and/or gases from a body part

Body Part	Approach	Device	Qualifier
Ø Abdominal Aorta	Ø Open	Ø Drainage Device	Z No Qualifier
1 Celiac Artery	3 Percutaneous		
2 Gastric Artery	4 Percutaneous Endoscopic		
3 Hepatic Artery			
4 Splenic Artery			
5 Superior Mesenteric Artery			
6 Colic Artery, Right			
7 Colic Artery, Left			
8 Colic Artery, Middle			
9 Renal Artery, Right			
A Renal Artery, Left			
B Inferior Mesenteric Artery			
C Common Iliac Artery, Right			
D Common Iliac Artery, Left			
E Internal Iliac Artery, Right			
F Internal Iliac Artery, Left			
H External Iliac Artery, Right			
J External Iliac Artery, Left			
K Femoral Artery, Right			
L Femoral Artery, Left			
M Popliteal Artery, Right			
N Popliteal Artery, Left			
P Anterior Tibial Artery, Right			
Q Anterior Tibial Artery, Left			
R Posterior Tibial Artery, Right			
S Posterior Tibial Artery, Left			
T Peroneal Artery, Right			
U Peroneal Artery, Left			
V Foot Artery, Right			
W Foot Artery, Left			
Y Lower Artery			

Non-OR 049[0123456789ABCDEFHJKLMNPQRSTUVWY][034]0Z

New/Revised Text in Green   ~~deleted~~ Deleted   ♀ Females Only   ♂ Males Only   **Coding Clinic**
Non-covered   Limited Coverage   ⊞ Combination (See Appendix E)   DRG Non-OR   Non-OR   Hospital-Acquired Condition

SECTION: Ø MEDICAL AND SURGICAL

BODY SYSTEM: 4 LOWER ARTERIES

OPERATION: 9 DRAINAGE: *(continued)*

Taking or letting out fluids and/or gases from a body part

Body Part	Approach	Device	Qualifier
Ø Abdominal Aorta	Ø Open	Z No Device	X Diagnostic
1 Celiac Artery	3 Percutaneous		Z No Qualifier
2 Gastric Artery	4 Percutaneous Endoscopic		
3 Hepatic Artery			
4 Splenic Artery			
5 Superior Mesenteric Artery			
6 Colic Artery, Right			
7 Colic Artery, Left			
8 Colic Artery, Middle			
9 Renal Artery, Right			
A Renal Artery, Left			
B Inferior Mesenteric Artery			
C Common Iliac Artery, Right			
D Common Iliac Artery, Left			
E Internal Iliac Artery, Right			
F Internal Iliac Artery, Left			
H External Iliac Artery, Right			
J External Iliac Artery, Left			
K Femoral Artery, Right			
L Femoral Artery, Left			
M Popliteal Artery, Right			
N Popliteal Artery, Left			
P Anterior Tibial Artery, Right			
Q Anterior Tibial Artery, Left			
R Posterior Tibial Artery, Right			
S Posterior Tibial Artery, Left			
T Peroneal Artery, Right			
U Peroneal Artery, Left			
V Foot Artery, Right			
W Foot Artery, Left			
Y Lower Artery			

Non-OR Ø49[Ø123456789ABCDEFHJKLMNPQRSTUVWY][Ø34]ZZ

New/Revised Text in Green · ~~deleted~~ Deleted · ♀ Females Only · ♂ Males Only · **Coding Clinic**

🖢 Non-covered · 🖢 Limited Coverage · ⊞ Combination (See Appendix E) · DRG Non-OR · Non-OR · 🖢 Hospital-Acquired Condition

105

SECTION: Ø MEDICAL AND SURGICAL
BODY SYSTEM: 4 LOWER ARTERIES
OPERATION: B EXCISION: Cutting out or off, without replacement, a portion of a body part

Body Part	Approach	Device	Qualifier
Ø Abdominal Aorta	Ø Open	Z No Device	X Diagnostic
1 Celiac Artery	3 Percutaneous		Z No Qualifier
2 Gastric Artery	4 Percutaneous Endoscopic		
3 Hepatic Artery			
4 Splenic Artery			
5 Superior Mesenteric Artery			
6 Colic Artery, Right			
7 Colic Artery, Left			
8 Colic Artery, Middle			
9 Renal Artery, Right			
A Renal Artery, Left			
B Inferior Mesenteric Artery			
C Common Iliac Artery, Right			
D Common Iliac Artery, Left			
E Internal Iliac Artery, Right			
F Internal Iliac Artery, Left			
H External Iliac Artery, Right			
J External Iliac Artery, Left			
K Femoral Artery, Right			
L Femoral Artery, Left			
M Popliteal Artery, Right			
N Popliteal Artery, Left			
P Anterior Tibial Artery, Right			
Q Anterior Tibial Artery, Left			
R Posterior Tibial Artery, Right			
S Posterior Tibial Artery, Left			
T Peroneal Artery, Right			
U Peroneal Artery, Left			
V Foot Artery, Right			
W Foot Artery, Left			
Y Lower Artery			

B: EXCISION

4: LOWER ARTERIES

Ø: M/S

New/Revised Text in Green ~~deleted~~ Deleted ♀ Females Only ♂ Males Only **Coding Clinic**
Non-covered Limited Coverage ⊞ Combination (See Appendix E) DRG Non-OR Non-OR Hospital-Acquired Condition

SECTION: Ø MEDICAL AND SURGICAL
BODY SYSTEM: 4 LOWER ARTERIES
OPERATION: C EXTIRPATION: Taking or cutting out solid matter from a body part

Body Part	Approach	Device	Qualifier
Ø Abdominal Aorta	Ø Open	Z No Device	6 Bifurcation
1 Celiac Artery	3 Percutaneous		Z No Qualifier
2 Gastric Artery	4 Percutaneous Endoscopic		
3 Hepatic Artery			
4 Splenic Artery			
5 Superior Mesenteric Artery			
6 Colic Artery, Right			
7 Colic Artery, Left			
8 Colic Artery, Middle			
9 Renal Artery, Right			
A Renal Artery, Left			
B Inferior Mesenteric Artery			
C Common Iliac Artery, Right			
D Common Iliac Artery, Left			
E Internal Iliac Artery, Right			
F Internal Iliac Artery, Left			
H External Iliac Artery, Right			
J External Iliac Artery, Left			
K Femoral Artery, Right			
L Femoral Artery, Left			
M Popliteal Artery, Right			
N Popliteal Artery, Left			
P Anterior Tibial Artery, Right			
Q Anterior Tibial Artery, Left			
R Posterior Tibial Artery, Right			
S Posterior Tibial Artery, Left			
T Peroneal Artery, Right			
U Peroneal Artery, Left			
V Foot Artery, Right			
W Foot Artery, Left			
Y Lower Artery			

Coding Clinic: 2Ø15, Q1, P36 – Ø4CL3ZZ
Coding Clinic: 2Ø16, Q1, P31 – Ø4CJØZZ

New/Revised Text in Green   deleted Deleted   ♀ Females Only   ♂ Males Only   **Coding Clinic**
⊘ Non-covered   ⊘ Limited Coverage   ⊞ Combination (See Appendix E)   DRG Non-OR   Non-OR   ⊘ Hospital-Acquired Condition

SECTION: Ø MEDICAL AND SURGICAL

BODY SYSTEM: 4 LOWER ARTERIES

OPERATION: H INSERTION: Putting in a nonbiological appliance that monitors, assists, performs, or prevents a physiological function but does not physically take the place of a body part

Body Part	Approach	Device	Qualifier
Ø Abdominal Aorta Y Lower Artery	Ø Open 3 Percutaneous 4 Percutaneous Endoscopic	2 Monitoring Device 3 Infusion Device D Intraluminal Device	Z No Qualifier
1 Celiac Artery 2 Gastric Artery 3 Hepatic Artery 4 Splenic Artery 5 Superior Mesenteric Artery 6 Colic Artery, Right 7 Colic Artery, Left 8 Colic Artery, Middle 9 Renal Artery, Right A Renal Artery, Left B Inferior Mesenteric Artery C Common Iliac Artery, Right D Common Iliac Artery, Left E Internal Iliac Artery, Right F Internal Iliac Artery, Left H External Iliac Artery, Right J External Iliac Artery, Left K Femoral Artery, Right L Femoral Artery, Left M Popliteal Artery, Right N Popliteal Artery, Left P Anterior Tibial Artery, Right Q Anterior Tibial Artery, Left R Posterior Tibial Artery, Right S Posterior Tibial Artery, Left T Peroneal Artery, Right U Peroneal Artery, Left V Foot Artery, Right W Foot Artery, Left	Ø Open 3 Percutaneous 4 Percutaneous Endoscopic	3 Infusion Device D Intraluminal Device	Z No Qualifier

DRG Non-OR Ø4HY32Z
Non-OR Ø4HØ[Ø34][23]Z
Non-OR Ø4HY[Ø34]3Z
Non-OR Ø4H[123456789ABCDEFHJKLMNPQRSTUVW][Ø34]3Z

SECTION: Ø MEDICAL AND SURGICAL

BODY SYSTEM: 4 LOWER ARTERIES

OPERATION: J INSPECTION: Visually and/or manually exploring a body part

Body Part	Approach	Device	Qualifier
Y Lower Artery	Ø Open 3 Percutaneous 4 Percutaneous Endoscopic X External	Z No Device	Z No Qualifier

DRG Non-OR Ø4JY3ZZ
Non-OR Ø4JY[4X]ZZ

New/Revised Text in Green   deleted Deleted   ♀ Females Only   ♂ Males Only   Coding Clinic
Non-covered   Limited Coverage   ⊞ Combination (See Appendix E)   DRG Non-OR   Non-OR   Hospital-Acquired Condition

SECTION: 0 MEDICAL AND SURGICAL
BODY SYSTEM: 4 LOWER ARTERIES
OPERATION: L OCCLUSION: Completely closing an orifice or the lumen of a tubular body part

Body Part	Approach	Device	Qualifier
0 Abdominal Aorta 1 Celiac Artery 2 Gastric Artery 3 Hepatic Artery 4 Splenic Artery 5 Superior Mesenteric Artery 6 Colic Artery, Right 7 Colic Artery, Left 8 Colic Artery, Middle 9 Renal Artery, Right A Renal Artery, Left B Inferior Mesenteric Artery C Common Iliac Artery, Right D Common Iliac Artery, Left H External Iliac Artery, Right J External Iliac Artery, Left K Femoral Artery, Right L Femoral Artery, Left M Popliteal Artery, Right N Popliteal Artery, Left P Anterior Tibial Artery, Right Q Anterior Tibial Artery, Left R Posterior Tibial Artery, Right S Posterior Tibial Artery, Left T Peroneal Artery, Right U Peroneal Artery, Left V Foot Artery, Right W Foot Artery, Left Y Lower Artery	0 Open 3 Percutaneous 4 Percutaneous Endoscopic	C Extraluminal Device D Intraluminal Device Z No Device	Z No Qualifier
E Internal Iliac Artery, Right	0 Open 3 Percutaneous 4 Percutaneous Endoscopic	C Extraluminal Device D Intraluminal Device Z No Device	T Uterine Artery, Right ♀ Z No Qualifier
F Internal Iliac Artery, Left	0 Open 3 Percutaneous 4 Percutaneous Endoscopic	C Extraluminal Device D Intraluminal Device Z No Device	U Uterine Artery, Left ♀ Z No Qualifier

Non-OR 04L23DZ

Coding Clinic: 2015, Q2, P27 – 04LE3DT

0: M/S

4: LOWER ARTERIES

L: OCCLUSION

New/Revised Text in Green deleted Deleted ♀ Females Only ♂ Males Only **Coding Clinic**
 Non-covered   Limited Coverage   Combination (See Appendix E) DRG Non-OR Non-OR Hospital-Acquired Condition

109

SECTION: Ø MEDICAL AND SURGICAL

BODY SYSTEM: 4 LOWER ARTERIES

OPERATION: N RELEASE: Freeing a body part from an abnormal physical constraint by cutting or by the use of force

Body Part	Approach	Device	Qualifier
Ø Abdominal Aorta	Ø Open	Z No Device	Z No Qualifier
1 Celiac Artery	3 Percutaneous		
2 Gastric Artery	4 Percutaneous Endoscopic		
3 Hepatic Artery			
4 Splenic Artery			
5 Superior Mesenteric Artery			
6 Colic Artery, Right			
7 Colic Artery, Left			
8 Colic Artery, Middle			
9 Renal Artery, Right			
A Renal Artery, Left			
B Inferior Mesenteric Artery			
C Common Iliac Artery, Right			
D Common Iliac Artery, Left			
E Internal Iliac Artery, Right			
F Internal Iliac Artery, Left			
H External Iliac Artery, Right			
J External Iliac Artery, Left			
K Femoral Artery, Right			
L Femoral Artery, Left			
M Popliteal Artery, Right			
N Popliteal Artery, Left			
P Anterior Tibial Artery, Right			
Q Anterior Tibial Artery, Left			
R Posterior Tibial Artery, Right			
S Posterior Tibial Artery, Left			
T Peroneal Artery, Right			
U Peroneal Artery, Left			
V Foot Artery, Right			
W Foot Artery, Left			
Y Lower Artery			

Coding Clinic: 2Ø15, Q2, P28 – Ø4N1ØZZ

SECTION: Ø MEDICAL AND SURGICAL
BODY SYSTEM: 4 LOWER ARTERIES
OPERATION: P REMOVAL: Taking out or off a device from a body part

Body Part	Approach	Device	Qualifier
Y Lower Artery	Ø Open 3 Percutaneous 4 Percutaneous Endoscopic	Ø Drainage Device 2 Monitoring Device 3 Infusion Device 7 Autologous Tissue Substitute C Extraluminal Device D Intraluminal Device J Synthetic Substitute K Nonautologous Tissue Substitute	Z No Qualifier
Y Lower Artery	X External	Ø Drainage Device 1 Radioactive Element 2 Monitoring Device 3 Infusion Device D Intraluminal Device	Z No Qualifier

DRG Non-OR 04PY3[Ø23]Z
Non-OR 04PYX[Ø123D]Z

New/Revised Text in Green   deleted Deleted   ♀ Females Only   ♂ Males Only   **Coding Clinic**
Non-covered   Limited Coverage   ⊞ Combination (See Appendix E)   DRG Non-OR   Non-OR   Hospital-Acquired Condition

SECTION: Ø MEDICAL AND SURGICAL

BODY SYSTEM: 4 LOWER ARTERIES

OPERATION: Q REPAIR: Restoring, to the extent possible, a body part to its normal anatomic structure and function

Body Part	Approach	Device	Qualifier
Ø Abdominal Aorta	Ø Open	Z No Device	Z No Qualifier
1 Celiac Artery	3 Percutaneous		
2 Gastric Artery	4 Percutaneous Endoscopic		
3 Hepatic Artery			
4 Splenic Artery			
5 Superior Mesenteric Artery			
6 Colic Artery, Right			
7 Colic Artery, Left			
8 Colic Artery, Middle			
9 Renal Artery, Right			
A Renal Artery, Left			
B Inferior Mesenteric Artery			
C Common Iliac Artery, Right			
D Common Iliac Artery, Left			
E Internal Iliac Artery, Right			
F Internal Iliac Artery, Left			
H External Iliac Artery, Right			
J External Iliac Artery, Left			
K Femoral Artery, Right			
L Femoral Artery, Left			
M Popliteal Artery, Right			
N Popliteal Artery, Left			
P Anterior Tibial Artery, Right			
Q Anterior Tibial Artery, Left			
R Posterior Tibial Artery, Right			
S Posterior Tibial Artery, Left			
T Peroneal Artery, Right			
U Peroneal Artery, Left			
V Foot Artery, Right			
W Foot Artery, Left			
Y Lower Artery			

Q: REPAIR

4: LOWER ARTERIES

Ø: M/S

SECTION: 0 MEDICAL AND SURGICAL

BODY SYSTEM: 4 LOWER ARTERIES

OPERATION: R REPLACEMENT: Putting in or on biological or synthetic material that physically takes the place and/or function of all or a portion of a body part

Body Part	Approach	Device	Qualifier
0 Abdominal Aorta 1 Celiac Artery 2 Gastric Artery 3 Hepatic Artery 4 Splenic Artery 5 Superior Mesenteric Artery 6 Colic Artery, Right 7 Colic Artery, Left 8 Colic Artery, Middle 9 Renal Artery, Right A Renal Artery, Left B Inferior Mesenteric Artery C Common Iliac Artery, Right D Common Iliac Artery, Left E Internal Iliac Artery, Right F Internal Iliac Artery, Left H External Iliac Artery, Right J External Iliac Artery, Left K Femoral Artery, Right L Femoral Artery, Left M Popliteal Artery, Right N Popliteal Artery, Left P Anterior Tibial Artery, Right Q Anterior Tibial Artery, Left R Posterior Tibial Artery, Right S Posterior Tibial Artery, Left T Peroneal Artery, Right U Peroneal Artery, Left V Foot Artery, Right W Foot Artery, Left Y Lower Artery	0 Open 4 Percutaneous Endoscopic	7 Autologous Tissue Substitute J Synthetic Substitute K Nonautologous Tissue Substitute	Z No Qualifier

Coding Clinic: 2015, Q2, P28 – 04R10JZ

0: M/S

4: LOWER ARTERIES

R: REPLACEMENT

SECTION: Ø MEDICAL AND SURGICAL
BODY SYSTEM: 4 LOWER ARTERIES
OPERATION: S REPOSITION: Moving to its normal location, or other suitable location, all or a portion of a body part

Body Part	Approach	Device	Qualifier
Ø Abdominal Aorta	Ø Open	Z No Device	Z No Qualifier
1 Celiac Artery	3 Percutaneous		
2 Gastric Artery	4 Percutaneous Endoscopic		
3 Hepatic Artery			
4 Splenic Artery			
5 Superior Mesenteric Artery			
6 Colic Artery, Right			
7 Colic Artery, Left			
8 Colic Artery, Middle			
9 Renal Artery, Right			
A Renal Artery, Left			
B Inferior Mesenteric Artery			
C Common Iliac Artery, Right			
D Common Iliac Artery, Left			
E Internal Iliac Artery, Right			
F Internal Iliac Artery, Left			
H External Iliac Artery, Right			
J External Iliac Artery, Left			
K Femoral Artery, Right			
L Femoral Artery, Left			
M Popliteal Artery, Right			
N Popliteal Artery, Left			
P Anterior Tibial Artery, Right			
Q Anterior Tibial Artery, Left			
R Posterior Tibial Artery, Right			
S Posterior Tibial Artery, Left			
T Peroneal Artery, Right			
U Peroneal Artery, Left			
V Foot Artery, Right			
W Foot Artery, Left			
Y Lower Artery			

S: REPOSITION

4: LOWER ARTERIES

Ø: M/S

New/Revised Text in Green   ~~deleted~~ Deleted   ♀ Females Only   ♂ Males Only   **Coding Clinic**
🚫 Non-covered   🚫 Limited Coverage   ⊞ Combination (See Appendix E)   DRG Non-OR   Non-OR   🚫 Hospital-Acquired Condition

SECTION: Ø MEDICAL AND SURGICAL

BODY SYSTEM: 4 LOWER ARTERIES

OPERATION: U SUPPLEMENT: Putting in or on biological or synthetic material that physically reinforces and/or augments the function of a portion of a body part

Body Part	Approach	Device	Qualifier
Ø Abdominal Aorta	Ø Open	7 Autologous Tissue Substitute	Z No Qualifier
1 Celiac Artery	3 Percutaneous	J Synthetic Substitute	
2 Gastric Artery	4 Percutaneous Endoscopic	K Nonautologous Tissue Substitute	
3 Hepatic Artery			
4 Splenic Artery			
5 Superior Mesenteric Artery			
6 Colic Artery, Right			
7 Colic Artery, Left			
8 Colic Artery, Middle			
9 Renal Artery, Right			
A Renal Artery, Left			
B Inferior Mesenteric Artery			
C Common Iliac Artery, Right			
D Common Iliac Artery, Left			
E Internal Iliac Artery, Right			
F Internal Iliac Artery, Left			
H External Iliac Artery, Right			
J External Iliac Artery, Left			
K Femoral Artery, Right			
L Femoral Artery, Left			
M Popliteal Artery, Right			
N Popliteal Artery, Left			
P Anterior Tibial Artery, Right			
Q Anterior Tibial Artery, Left			
R Posterior Tibial Artery, Right			
S Posterior Tibial Artery, Left			
T Peroneal Artery, Right			
U Peroneal Artery, Left			
V Foot Artery, Right			
W Foot Artery, Left			
Y Lower Artery			

Coding Clinic: 2016, Q1, P31 – 04UJ0KZ
Coding Clinic: 2016, Q2, P19 – 04UR07Z

SECTION: Ø   MEDICAL AND SURGICAL

BODY SYSTEM: 4   **LOWER ARTERIES**

OPERATION: **V**   **RESTRICTION:** Partially closing an orifice or the lumen of a tubular body part

Body Part	Approach	Device	Qualifier
Ø Abdominal Aorta	Ø Open 3 Percutaneous 4 Percutaneous Endoscopic	C Extraluminal Device E Intraluminal Device, Branched or Fenestrated, One or Two Arteries F Intraluminal Device, Branched or Fenestrated, Three or More Arteries Z No Device	6 Bifurcation Z No Qualifier
Ø Abdominal Aorta	Ø Open 3 Percutaneous 4 Percutaneous Endoscopic	D Intraluminal Device	6 Bifurcation J Temporary Z No Qualifier
1 Celiac Artery 2 Gastric Artery 3 Hepatic Artery 4 Splenic Artery 5 Superior Mesenteric Artery 6 Colic Artery, Right 7 Colic Artery, Left 8 Colic Artery, Middle 9 Renal Artery, Right A Renal Artery, Left B Inferior Mesenteric Artery C ~~Common Iliac Artery, Right~~ D ~~Common Iliac Artery, Left~~ E Internal Iliac Artery, Right F Internal Iliac Artery, Left H External Iliac Artery, Right J External Iliac Artery, Left K Femoral Artery, Right L Femoral Artery, Left M Popliteal Artery, Right N Popliteal Artery, Left P Anterior Tibial Artery, Right Q Anterior Tibial Artery, Left R Posterior Tibial Artery, Right S Posterior Tibial Artery, Left T Peroneal Artery, Right U Peroneal Artery, Left V Foot Artery, Right W Foot Artery, Left Y Lower Artery	Ø Open 3 Percutaneous 4 Percutaneous Endoscopic	C Extraluminal Device D Intraluminal Device Z No Device	Z No Qualifier
C Common Iliac Artery, Right D Common Iliac Artery, Left	Ø Open 3 Percutaneous 4 Percutaneous Endoscopic	C Extraluminal Device D Intraluminal Device E Intraluminal Device, Branched or Fenestrated, One or Two Arteries F Intraluminal Device, Branched or Fenestrated, Three or More Arteries Z No Device	Z No Qualifier

V: RESTRICTION

4: LOWER ARTERIES

Ø: M/S

SECTION: Ø MEDICAL AND SURGICAL
BODY SYSTEM: 4 LOWER ARTERIES
OPERATION: W REVISION: Correcting, to the extent possible, a portion of a malfunctioning device or the position of a displaced device

Body Part	Approach	Device	Qualifier
Y Lower Artery	Ø Open 3 Percutaneous 4 Percutaneous Endoscopic X External	Ø Drainage Device 2 Monitoring Device 3 Infusion Device 7 Autologous Tissue Substitute C Extraluminal Device D Intraluminal Device J Synthetic Substitute K Nonautologous Tissue Substitute	Z No Qualifier

Non-OR   04WYX[0237CDJK]Z

Coding Clinic: 2015, Q1, P37 – 04WY07Z

New/Revised Text in Green   deleted Deleted   ♀ Females Only   ♂ Males Only   **Coding Clinic**
Non-covered   Limited Coverage   Combination (See Appendix E)   DRG Non-OR   Non-OR   Hospital-Acquired Condition

117

SECTION: Ø MEDICAL AND SURGICAL

BODY SYSTEM: 5 UPPER VEINS

OPERATION: 1 **BYPASS:** Altering the route of passage of the contents of a tubular body part

Body Part	Approach	Device	Qualifier
Ø Azygos Vein	Ø Open	7 Autologous Tissue Substitute	Y Upper Vein
1 Hemiazygos Vein	4 Percutaneous Endoscopic	9 Autologous Venous Tissue	
3 Innominate Vein, Right		A Autologous Arterial Tissue	
4 Innominate Vein, Left		J Synthetic Substitute	
5 Subclavian Vein, Right		K Nonautologous Tissue	
6 Subclavian Vein, Left		Substitute	
7 Axillary Vein, Right		Z No Device	
8 Axillary Vein, Left			
9 Brachial Vein, Right			
A Brachial Vein, Left			
B Basilic Vein, Right			
C Basilic Vein, Left			
D Cephalic Vein, Right			
F Cephalic Vein, Left			
G Hand Vein, Right			
H Hand Vein, Left			
L Intracranial Vein			
M Internal Jugular Vein, Right			
N Internal Jugular Vein, Left			
P External Jugular Vein, Right			
Q External Jugular Vein, Left			
R Vertebral Vein, Right			
S Vertebral Vein, Left			
T Face Vein, Right			
V Face Vein, Left			

SECTION: Ø MEDICAL AND SURGICAL
BODY SYSTEM: 5 **UPPER VEINS**
OPERATION: 5 **DESTRUCTION:** Physical eradication of all or a portion of a body part by the direct use of energy, force, or a destructive agent

Body Part	Approach	Device	Qualifier
Ø Azygos Vein 1 Hemiazygos Vein 3 Innominate Vein, Right 4 Innominate Vein, Left 5 Subclavian Vein, Right 6 Subclavian Vein, Left 7 Axillary Vein, Right 8 Axillary Vein, Left 9 Brachial Vein, Right A Brachial Vein, Left B Basilic Vein, Right C Basilic Vein, Left D Cephalic Vein, Right F Cephalic Vein, Left G Hand Vein, Right H Hand Vein, Left L Intracranial Vein M Internal Jugular Vein, Right N Internal Jugular Vein, Left P External Jugular Vein, Right Q External Jugular Vein, Left R Vertebral Vein, Right S Vertebral Vein, Left T Face Vein, Right V Face Vein, Left Y Upper Vein	Ø Open 3 Percutaneous 4 Percutaneous Endoscopic	Z No Device	Z No Qualifier

5: DESTRUCTION

5: UPPER VEINS

Ø: M/S

SECTION: Ø MEDICAL AND SURGICAL
BODY SYSTEM: 5 UPPER VEINS
OPERATION: 7 **DILATION:** Expanding an orifice or the lumen of a tubular body part

Body Part	Approach	Device	Qualifier
Ø Azygos Vein	Ø Open	D Intraluminal Device	Z No Qualifier
1 Hemiazygos Vein	3 Percutaneous	Z No Device	
3 Innominate Vein, Right	4 Percutaneous Endoscopic		
4 Innominate Vein, Left			
5 Subclavian Vein, Right			
6 Subclavian Vein, Left			
7 Axillary Vein, Right			
8 Axillary Vein, Left			
9 Brachial Vein, Right			
A Brachial Vein, Left			
B Basilic Vein, Right			
C Basilic Vein, Left			
D Cephalic Vein, Right			
F Cephalic Vein, Left			
G Hand Vein, Right			
H Hand Vein, Left			
L Intracranial Vein			
M Internal Jugular Vein, Right			
N Internal Jugular Vein, Left			
P External Jugular Vein, Right			
Q External Jugular Vein, Left			
R Vertebral Vein, Right			
S Vertebral Vein, Left			
T Face Vein, Right			
V Face Vein, Left			
Y Upper Vein			

Ø57L[34]ZZ

Ø: M/S

5: UPPER VEINS

7: DILATION

SECTION: Ø MEDICAL AND SURGICAL

BODY SYSTEM: 5 UPPER VEINS

OPERATION: 9 DRAINAGE: Taking or letting out fluids and/or gases from a body part

Body Part	Approach	Device	Qualifier
Ø Azygos Vein 1 Hemiazygos Vein 3 Innominate Vein, Right 4 Innominate Vein, Left 5 Subclavian Vein, Right 6 Subclavian Vein, Left 7 Axillary Vein, Right 8 Axillary Vein, Left 9 Brachial Vein, Right A Brachial Vein, Left B Basilic Vein, Right C Basilic Vein, Left D Cephalic Vein, Right F Cephalic Vein, Left G Hand Vein, Right H Hand Vein, Left L Intracranial Vein M Internal Jugular Vein, Right N Internal Jugular Vein, Left P External Jugular Vein, Right Q External Jugular Vein, Left R Vertebral Vein, Right S Vertebral Vein, Left T Face Vein, Right V Face Vein, Left Y Upper Vein	Ø Open 3 Percutaneous 4 Percutaneous Endoscopic	Ø Drainage Device	Z No Qualifier
Ø Azygos Vein 1 Hemiazygos Vein 3 Innominate Vein, Right 4 Innominate Vein, Left 5 Subclavian Vein, Right 6 Subclavian Vein, Left 7 Axillary Vein, Right 8 Axillary Vein, Left 9 Brachial Vein, Right A Brachial Vein, Left B Basilic Vein, Right C Basilic Vein, Left D Cephalic Vein, Right F Cephalic Vein, Left G Hand Vein, Right H Hand Vein, Left L Intracranial Vein M Internal Jugular Vein, Right N Internal Jugular Vein, Left P External Jugular Vein, Right Q External Jugular Vein, Left R Vertebral Vein, Right S Vertebral Vein, Left T Face Vein, Right V Face Vein, Left Y Upper Vein	Ø Open 3 Percutaneous 4 Percutaneous Endoscopic	Z No Device	X Diagnostic Z No Qualifier

Non-OR   Ø59[Ø13456789ABCDFGHLMNPQRSTVY][Ø34]ØZ
Non-OR   Ø59[Ø13456789ABCDFGHLMNPQRSTVY][Ø34]ZZ

New/Revised Text in Green   ~~deleted~~ Deleted   ♀ Females Only   ♂ Males Only   **Coding Clinic**

🔾 Non-covered   🔾 Limited Coverage   ⊞ Combination (See Appendix E)   DRG Non-OR   Non-OR   🔾 Hospital-Acquired Condition

9: DRAINAGE   **5: UPPER VEINS**   **Ø: M/S**

SECTION: Ø MEDICAL AND SURGICAL

BODY SYSTEM: 5 UPPER VEINS

OPERATION: B EXCISION: Cutting out or off, without replacement, a portion of a body part

Body Part	Approach	Device	Qualifier
Ø Azygos Vein	Ø Open	Z No Device	X Diagnostic
1 Hemiazygos Vein	3 Percutaneous		Z No Qualifier
3 Innominate Vein, Right	4 Percutaneous Endoscopic		
4 Innominate Vein, Left			
5 Subclavian Vein, Right			
6 Subclavian Vein, Left			
7 Axillary Vein, Right			
8 Axillary Vein, Left			
9 Brachial Vein, Right			
A Brachial Vein, Left			
B Basilic Vein, Right			
C Basilic Vein, Left			
D Cephalic Vein, Right			
F Cephalic Vein, Left			
G Hand Vein, Right			
H Hand Vein, Left			
L Intracranial Vein			
M Internal Jugular Vein, Right			
N Internal Jugular Vein, Left			
P External Jugular Vein, Right			
Q External Jugular Vein, Left			
R Vertebral Vein, Right			
S Vertebral Vein, Left			
T Face Vein, Right			
V Face Vein, Left			
Y Upper Vein			

Coding Clinic: 2Ø16, Q2, P13-14 – Ø5B[NQ]ØZZ

Ø: M/S

5: UPPER VEINS

B: EXCISION

SECTION: **Ø MEDICAL AND SURGICAL**

BODY SYSTEM: 5 **UPPER VEINS**

OPERATION: **C EXTIRPATION:** Taking or cutting out solid matter from a body part

Body Part	Approach	Device	Qualifier
Ø Azygos Vein 1 Hemiazygos Vein 3 Innominate Vein, Right 4 Innominate Vein, Left 5 Subclavian Vein, Right 6 Subclavian Vein, Left 7 Axillary Vein, Right 8 Axillary Vein, Left 9 Brachial Vein, Right A Brachial Vein, Left B Basilic Vein, Right C Basilic Vein, Left D Cephalic Vein, Right F Cephalic Vein, Left G Hand Vein, Right H Hand Vein, Left L Intracranial Vein M Internal Jugular Vein, Right N Internal Jugular Vein, Left P External Jugular Vein, Right Q External Jugular Vein, Left R Vertebral Vein, Right S Vertebral Vein, Left T Face Vein, Right V Face Vein, Left Y Upper Vein	Ø Open 3 Percutaneous 4 Percutaneous Endoscopic	Z No Device	Z No Qualifier

SECTION: **Ø MEDICAL AND SURGICAL**

BODY SYSTEM: 5 **UPPER VEINS**

OPERATION: **D EXTRACTION:** Pulling or stripping out or off all or a portion of a body part by the use of force

Body Part	Approach	Device	Qualifier
9 Brachial Vein, Right A Brachial Vein, Left B Basilic Vein, Right C Basilic Vein, Left D Cephalic Vein, Right F Cephalic Vein, Left G Hand Vein, Right H Hand Vein, Left Y Upper Vein	Ø Open 3 Percutaneous	Z No Device	Z No Qualifier

C: EXTIRPATION   D: EXTRACTION

5: UPPER VEINS

Ø: M/S

New/Revised Text in Green   ~~deleted~~ Deleted   ♀ Females Only   ♂ Males Only   **Coding Clinic**

⊘ Non-covered   ⊘ Limited Coverage   ⊞ Combination (See Appendix E)   DRG Non-OR   Non-OR   ⊘ Hospital-Acquired Condition

SECTION: Ø MEDICAL AND SURGICAL

BODY SYSTEM: 5 UPPER VEINS

OPERATION: H INSERTION: Putting in a nonbiological appliance that monitors, assists, performs, or prevents a physiological function but does not physically take the place of a body part

Body Part	Approach	Device	Qualifier
Ø Azygos Vein	Ø Open 3 Percutaneous 4 Percutaneous Endoscopic	2 Monitoring Device 3 Infusion Device D Intraluminal Device M Neurostimulator Lead	Z No Qualifier
Ø Azygos Vein 1 Hemiazygos Vein 3 Innominate Vein, Right 4 Innominate Vein, Left 5 Subclavian Vein, Right ⊞ 6 Subclavian Vein, Left ⊞ 7 Axillary Vein, Right 8 Axillary Vein, Left 9 Brachial Vein, Right A Brachial Vein, Left B Basilic Vein, Right C Basilic Vein, Left D Cephalic Vein, Right F Cephalic Vein, Left G Hand Vein, Right H Hand Vein, Left L Intracranial Vein M Internal Jugular Vein, Right ⊞ ⬤ N Internal Jugular Vein, Left ⊞ ⬤ P External Jugular Vein, Right ⊞ ⬤ Q External Jugular Vein, Left ⊞ ⬤ R Vertebral Vein, Right S Vertebral Vein, Left T Face Vein, Right V Face Vein, Left	Ø Open 3 Percutaneous 4 Percutaneous Endoscopic	3 Infusion Device D Intraluminal Device	Z No Qualifier
3 Innominate Vein, Right 4 Innominate Vein, Left	Ø Open 3 Percutaneous 4 Percutaneous Endoscopic	3 Infusion Device D Intraluminal Device M Neurostimulator Lead	Z No Qualifier
Y Upper Vein	Ø Open 3 Percutaneous 4 Percutaneous Endoscopic	2 Monitoring Device 3 Infusion Device D Intraluminal Device	Z No Qualifier

⊞ Ø5H[56MNPQ]33Z

DRG Non-OR Ø5H[56MNPQ]33Z

DRG Non-OR Ø5HY32Z

Non-OR Ø5HØ[Ø34]3Z

Non-OR Ø5H[13789ABCDFGHLRSTV][Ø34]3Z

Non-OR Ø5H[56MNPQ][Ø4]3Z

Non-OR Ø5H[34][Ø34]3Z

Non-OR Ø5HY[Ø34]3Z

⬤ Ø5H[MNPQ]33Z when reported with Secondary Diagnosis J95.811

Ø: M/S

5: UPPER VEINS

H: INSERTION

SECTION: Ø MEDICAL AND SURGICAL

BODY SYSTEM: 5 UPPER VEINS

OPERATION: J INSPECTION: Visually and/or manually exploring a body part

Body Part	Approach	Device	Qualifier
Y Upper Vein	Ø Open 3 Percutaneous 4 Percutaneous Endoscopic X External	Z No Device	Z No Qualifier

DRG Non-OR Ø5JY3ZZ
Non-OR Ø5JYXZZ

SECTION: Ø MEDICAL AND SURGICAL

BODY SYSTEM: 5 UPPER VEINS

OPERATION: L OCCLUSION: Completely closing an orifice or the lumen of a tubular body part

Body Part	Approach	Device	Qualifier
Ø Azygos Vein 1 Hemiazygos Vein 3 Innominate Vein, Right 4 Innominate Vein, Left 5 Subclavian Vein, Right 6 Subclavian Vein, Left 7 Axillary Vein, Right 8 Axillary Vein, Left 9 Brachial Vein, Right A Brachial Vein, Left B Basilic Vein, Right C Basilic Vein, Left D Cephalic Vein, Right F Cephalic Vein, Left G Hand Vein, Right H Hand Vein, Left L Intracranial Vein M Internal Jugular Vein, Right N Internal Jugular Vein, Left P External Jugular Vein, Right Q External Jugular Vein, Left R Vertebral Vein, Right S Vertebral Vein, Left T Face Vein, Right V Face Vein, Left Y Upper Vein	Ø Open 3 Percutaneous 4 Percutaneous Endoscopic	C Extraluminal Device D Intraluminal Device Z No Device	Z No Qualifier

Side margin: L: OCCLUSION J: INSPECTION 5: UPPER VEINS Ø: M/S

New/Revised Text in Green   ~~deleted~~ Deleted   ♀ Females Only   ♂ Males Only   **Coding Clinic**
🐾 Non-covered   🐾 Limited Coverage   ⊕ Combination (See Appendix E)   DRG Non-OR   Non-OR   🐾 Hospital-Acquired Condition

SECTION: Ø MEDICAL AND SURGICAL
BODY SYSTEM: 5 UPPER VEINS
OPERATION: N RELEASE: Freeing a body part from an abnormal physical constraint

Body Part	Approach	Device	Qualifier
Ø Azygos Vein 1 Hemiazygos Vein 3 Innominate Vein, Right 4 Innominate Vein, Left 5 Subclavian Vein, Right 6 Subclavian Vein, Left 7 Axillary Vein, Right 8 Axillary Vein, Left 9 Brachial Vein, Right A Brachial Vein, Left B Basilic Vein, Right C Basilic Vein, Left D Cephalic Vein, Right F Cephalic Vein, Left G Hand Vein, Right H Hand Vein, Left L Intracranial Vein M Internal Jugular Vein, Right N Internal Jugular Vein, Left P External Jugular Vein, Right Q External Jugular Vein, Left R Vertebral Vein, Right S Vertebral Vein, Left T Face Vein, Right V Face Vein, Left Y Upper Vein	Ø Open 3 Percutaneous 4 Percutaneous Endoscopic	Z No Device	Z No Qualifier

SECTION:　Ø　MEDICAL AND SURGICAL

BODY SYSTEM: 5　UPPER VEINS

OPERATION:　P　REMOVAL: Taking out or off a device from a body part

Body Part	Approach	Device	Qualifier
Ø　Azygos Vein	Ø　Open 3　Percutaneous 4　Percutaneous Endoscopic X　External	2　Monitoring Device M　Neurostimulator Lead	Z　No Qualifier
3　Innominate Vein, Right 4　Innominate Vein, Left	Ø　Open 3　Percutaneous 4　Percutaneous Endoscopic X　External	M　Neurostimulator Lead	Z　No Qualifier
Y　Upper Vein	Ø　Open 3　Percutaneous 4　Percutaneous Endoscopic	Ø　Drainage Device 2　Monitoring Device 3　Infusion Device 7　Autologous Tissue Substitute C　Extraluminal Device D　Intraluminal Device J　Synthetic Substitute K　Nonautologous Tissue Substitute	Z　No Qualifier
Y　Upper Vein	X　External	Ø　Drainage Device 2　Monitoring Device 3　Infusion Device D　Intraluminal Device	Z　No Qualifier

DRG Non-OR　Ø5PY3[Ø23]Z
Non-OR　Ø5PYX[Ø23D]Z

New/Revised Text in Green　~~deleted~~ Deleted　♀ Females Only　♂ Males Only　**Coding Clinic**

Non-covered　Limited Coverage　⊕ Combination (See Appendix E)　DRG Non-OR　Non-OR　Hospital-Acquired Condition

P: REMOVAL

5: UPPER VEINS

Ø: M/S

SECTION: 0 MEDICAL AND SURGICAL

BODY SYSTEM: 5 UPPER VEINS

OPERATION: Q REPAIR: Restoring, to the extent possible, a body part to its normal anatomic structure and function

Body Part	Approach	Device	Qualifier
0 Azygos Vein 1 Hemiazygos Vein 3 Innominate Vein, Right 4 Innominate Vein, Left 5 Subclavian Vein, Right 6 Subclavian Vein, Left 7 Axillary Vein, Right 8 Axillary Vein, Left 9 Brachial Vein, Right A Brachial Vein, Left B Basilic Vein, Right C Basilic Vein, Left D Cephalic Vein, Right F Cephalic Vein, Left G Hand Vein, Right H Hand Vein, Left L Intracranial Vein M Internal Jugular Vein, Right N Internal Jugular Vein, Left P External Jugular Vein, Right Q External Jugular Vein, Left R Vertebral Vein, Right S Vertebral Vein, Left T Face Vein, Right V Face Vein, Left Y Upper Vein	0 Open 3 Percutaneous 4 Percutaneous Endoscopic	Z No Device	Z No Qualifier

SECTION: Ø MEDICAL AND SURGICAL

BODY SYSTEM: 5 UPPER VEINS

OPERATION: R REPLACEMENT: Putting in or on biological or synthetic material that physically takes the place and/or function of all or a portion of a body part

Body Part	Approach	Device	Qualifier
Ø Azygos Vein	Ø Open	7 Autologous Tissue Substitute	Z No Qualifier
1 Hemiazygos Vein	4 Percutaneous Endoscopic	J Synthetic Substitute	
3 Innominate Vein, Right		K Nonautologous Tissue Substitute	
4 Innominate Vein, Left			
5 Subclavian Vein, Right			
6 Subclavian Vein, Left			
7 Axillary Vein, Right			
8 Axillary Vein, Left			
9 Brachial Vein, Right			
A Brachial Vein, Left			
B Basilic Vein, Right			
C Basilic Vein, Left			
D Cephalic Vein, Right			
F Cephalic Vein, Left			
G Hand Vein, Right			
H Hand Vein, Left			
L Intracranial Vein			
M Internal Jugular Vein, Right			
N Internal Jugular Vein, Left			
P External Jugular Vein, Right			
Q External Jugular Vein, Left			
R Vertebral Vein, Right			
S Vertebral Vein, Left			
T Face Vein, Right			
V Face Vein, Left			
Y Upper Vein			

R: REPLACEMENT

5: UPPER VEINS

Ø: M/S

New/Revised Text in Green ~~deleted~~ Deleted ♀ Females Only ♂ Males Only **Coding Clinic**

Non-covered Limited Coverage Combination (See Appendix E) DRG Non-OR Non-OR Hospital-Acquired Condition

SECTION: Ø MEDICAL AND SURGICAL

BODY SYSTEM: 5 UPPER VEINS

OPERATION: S REPOSITION: Moving to its normal location, or other suitable location, all or a portion of a body part

Body Part	Approach	Device	Qualifier
Ø Azygos Vein 1 Hemiazygos Vein 3 Innominate Vein, Right 4 Innominate Vein, Left 5 Subclavian Vein, Right 6 Subclavian Vein, Left 7 Axillary Vein, Right 8 Axillary Vein, Left 9 Brachial Vein, Right A Brachial Vein, Left B Basilic Vein, Right C Basilic Vein, Left D Cephalic Vein, Right F Cephalic Vein, Left G Hand Vein, Right H Hand Vein, Left L Intracranial Vein M Internal Jugular Vein, Right N Internal Jugular Vein, Left P External Jugular Vein, Right Q External Jugular Vein, Left R Vertebral Vein, Right S Vertebral Vein, Left T Face Vein, Right V Face Vein, Left Y Upper Vein	Ø Open 3 Percutaneous 4 Percutaneous Endoscopic	Z No Device	Z No Qualifier

Ø: M/S

5: UPPER VEINS

S: REPOSITION

SECTION: Ø MEDICAL AND SURGICAL

BODY SYSTEM: 5 UPPER VEINS

OPERATION: **U SUPPLEMENT:** Putting in or on biological or synthetic material that physically reinforces and/or augments the function of a portion of a body part

Body Part	Approach	Device	Qualifier
Ø Azygos Vein 1 Hemiazygos Vein 3 Innominate Vein, Right 4 Innominate Vein, Left 5 Subclavian Vein, Right 6 Subclavian Vein, Left 7 Axillary Vein, Right 8 Axillary Vein, Left 9 Brachial Vein, Right A Brachial Vein, Left B Basilic Vein, Right C Basilic Vein, Left D Cephalic Vein, Right F Cephalic Vein, Left G Hand Vein, Right H Hand Vein, Left L Intracranial Vein M Internal Jugular Vein, Right N Internal Jugular Vein, Left P External Jugular Vein, Right Q External Jugular Vein, Left R Vertebral Vein, Right S Vertebral Vein, Left T Face Vein, Right V Face Vein, Left Y Upper Vein	Ø Open 3 Percutaneous 4 Percutaneous Endoscopic	7 Autologous Tissue Substitute J Synthetic Substitute K Nonautologous Tissue Substitute	Z No Qualifier

U: SUPPLEMENT

5: UPPER VEINS

Ø: M/S

SECTION: Ø MEDICAL AND SURGICAL
BODY SYSTEM: 5 UPPER VEINS
OPERATION: V RESTRICTION: Partially closing an orifice or the lumen of a tubular body part

Body Part	Approach	Device	Qualifier
Ø Azygos Vein 1 Hemiazygos Vein 3 Innominate Vein, Right 4 Innominate Vein, Left 5 Subclavian Vein, Right 6 Subclavian Vein, Left 7 Axillary Vein, Right 8 Axillary Vein, Left 9 Brachial Vein, Right A Brachial Vein, Left B Basilic Vein, Right C Basilic Vein, Left D Cephalic Vein, Right F Cephalic Vein, Left G Hand Vein, Right H Hand Vein, Left L Intracranial Vein M Internal Jugular Vein, Right N Internal Jugular Vein, Left P External Jugular Vein, Right Q External Jugular Vein, Left R Vertebral Vein, Right S Vertebral Vein, Left T Face Vein, Right V Face Vein, Left Y Upper Vein	Ø Open 3 Percutaneous 4 Percutaneous Endoscopic	C Extraluminal Device D Intraluminal Device Z No Device	Z No Qualifier

SECTION: Ø MEDICAL AND SURGICAL
BODY SYSTEM: 5 UPPER VEINS
OPERATION: W REVISION: Correcting, to the extent possible, a portion of a malfunctioning device or the position of a displaced device

Body Part	Approach	Device	Qualifier
Ø Azygos Vein	Ø Open 3 Percutaneous 4 Percutaneous Endoscopic X External	2 Monitoring Device M Neurostimulator Lead	Z No Qualifier
3 Innominate Vein, Right 4 Innominate Vein, Left	Ø Open 3 Percutaneous 4 Percutaneous Endoscopic X External	M Neurostimulator Lead	Z No Qualifier
Y Upper Vein	Ø Open 3 Percutaneous 4 Percutaneous Endoscopic X External	Ø Drainage Device 2 Monitoring Device 3 Infusion Device 7 Autologous Tissue Substitute C Extraluminal Device D Intraluminal Device J Synthetic Substitute K Nonautologous Tissue Substitute	Z No Qualifier

Non-OR   Ø5WYX[Ø237CDJK]Z

New/Revised Text in Green ~~deleted~~ Deleted ♀ Females Only ♂ Males Only **Coding Clinic**
Non-covered Limited Coverage Combination (See Appendix E) DRG Non-OR Non-OR Hospital-Acquired Condition

SECTION: Ø MEDICAL AND SURGICAL

BODY SYSTEM: 6 LOWER VEINS

OPERATION: 1 BYPASS: Altering the route of passage of the contents of a tubular body part

Body Part	Approach	Device	Qualifier
Ø Inferior Vena Cava	Ø Open 4 Percutaneous Endoscopic	7 Autologous Tissue Substitute 9 Autologous Venous Tissue A Autologous Arterial Tissue J Synthetic Substitute K Nonautologous Tissue Substitute Z No Device	5 Superior Mesenteric Vein 6 Inferior Mesenteric Vein Y Lower Vein
1 Splenic Vein	Ø Open 4 Percutaneous Endoscopic	7 Autologous Tissue Substitute 9 Autologous Venous Tissue A Autologous Arterial Tissue J Synthetic Substitute K Nonautologous Tissue Substitute Z No Device	9 Renal Vein, Right B Renal Vein, Left Y Lower Vein
2 Gastric Vein 3 Esophageal Vein 4 Hepatic Vein 5 Superior Mesenteric Vein 6 Inferior Mesenteric Vein 7 Colic Vein 9 Renal Vein, Right B Renal Vein, Left C Common Iliac Vein, Right D Common Iliac Vein, Left F External Iliac Vein, Right G External Iliac Vein, Left H Hypogastric Vein, Right J Hypogastric Vein, Left M Femoral Vein, Right N Femoral Vein, Left P Greater Saphenous Vein, Right Q Greater Saphenous Vein, Left R Lesser Saphenous Vein, Right S Lesser Saphenous Vein, Left T Foot Vein, Right V Foot Vein, Left	Ø Open 4 Percutaneous Endoscopic	7 Autologous Tissue Substitute 9 Autologous Venous Tissue A Autologous Arterial Tissue J Synthetic Substitute K Nonautologous Tissue Substitute Z No Device	Y Lower Vein
8 Portal Vein	Ø Open	7 Autologous Tissue Substitute 9 Autologous Venous Tissue A Autologous Arterial Tissue J Synthetic Substitute K Nonautologous Tissue Substitute Z No Device	9 Renal Vein, Right B Renal Vein, Left Y Lower Vein
8 Portal Vein	3 Percutaneous	D Intraluminal Device	Y Lower Vein
8 Portal Vein	4 Percutaneous Endoscopic	7 Autologous Tissue Substitute 9 Autologous Venous Tissue A Autologous Arterial Tissue J Synthetic Substitute K Nonautologous Tissue Substitute Z No Device	9 Renal Vein, Right B Renal Vein, Left Y Lower Vein
8 Portal Vein	4 Percutaneous Endoscopic	D Intraluminal Device	Y Lower Vein

Ø: M/S

6: LOWER VEINS

1: BYPASS

SECTION: Ø MEDICAL AND SURGICAL
BODY SYSTEM: 6 LOWER VEINS

OPERATION: 5 **DESTRUCTION:** Physical eradication of all or a portion of a body part by the direct use of energy, force, or a destructive agent

Body Part	Approach	Device	Qualifier
Ø Inferior Vena Cava 1 Splenic Vein 2 Gastric Vein 3 Esophageal Vein 4 Hepatic Vein 5 Superior Mesenteric Vein 6 Inferior Mesenteric Vein 7 Colic Vein 8 Portal Vein 9 Renal Vein, Right B Renal Vein, Left C Common Iliac Vein, Right D Common Iliac Vein, Left F External Iliac Vein, Right G External Iliac Vein, Left H Hypogastric Vein, Right J Hypogastric Vein, Left M Femoral Vein, Right N Femoral Vein, Left P Greater Saphenous Vein, Right Q Greater Saphenous Vein, Left R Lesser Saphenous Vein, Right S Lesser Saphenous Vein, Left T Foot Vein, Right V Foot Vein, Left	Ø Open 3 Percutaneous 4 Percutaneous Endoscopic	Z No Device	Z No Qualifier
Y Lower Vein	Ø Open 3 Percutaneous 4 Percutaneous Endoscopic	Z No Device	C Hemorrhoidal Plexus Z No Qualifier

New/Revised Text in Green   ~~deleted~~ Deleted   ♀ Females Only   ♂ Males Only   **Coding Clinic**

℞ Non-covered   ℞ Limited Coverage   ⊞ Combination (See Appendix E)   DRG Non-OR   Non-OR   ℞ Hospital-Acquired Condition

SECTION: Ø MEDICAL AND SURGICAL
BODY SYSTEM: 6 LOWER VEINS
OPERATION: 7 DILATION: Expanding an orifice or the lumen of a tubular body part

Body Part	Approach	Device	Qualifier
Ø Inferior Vena Cava 1 Splenic Vein 2 Gastric Vein 3 Esophageal Vein 4 Hepatic Vein 5 Superior Mesenteric Vein 6 Inferior Mesenteric Vein 7 Colic Vein 8 Portal Vein 9 Renal Vein, Right B Renal Vein, Left C Common Iliac Vein, Right D Common Iliac Vein, Left F External Iliac Vein, Right G External Iliac Vein, Left H Hypogastric Vein, Right J Hypogastric Vein, Left M Femoral Vein, Right N Femoral Vein, Left P Greater Saphenous Vein, Right Q Greater Saphenous Vein, Left R Lesser Saphenous Vein, Right S Lesser Saphenous Vein, Left T Foot Vein, Right V Foot Vein, Left Y Lower Vein	Ø Open 3 Percutaneous 4 Percutaneous Endoscopic	D Intraluminal Device Z No Device	Z No Qualifier

Ø: M/S

6: LOWER VEINS

7: DILATION

SECTION: Ø MEDICAL AND SURGICAL
BODY SYSTEM: 6 LOWER VEINS
OPERATION: 9 **DRAINAGE:** Taking or letting out fluids and/or gases from a body part

9: DRAINAGE

6: LOWER VEINS

Ø: M/S

Body Part	Approach	Device	Qualifier
Ø Inferior Vena Cava 1 Splenic Vein 2 Gastric Vein 3 Esophageal Vein 4 Hepatic Vein 5 Superior Mesenteric Vein 6 Inferior Mesenteric Vein 7 Colic Vein 8 Portal Vein 9 Renal Vein, Right B Renal Vein, Left C Common Iliac Vein, Right D Common Iliac Vein, Left F External Iliac Vein, Right G External Iliac Vein, Left H Hypogastric Vein, Right J Hypogastric Vein, Left M Femoral Vein, Right N Femoral Vein, Left P Greater Saphenous Vein, Right Q Greater Saphenous Vein, Left R Lesser Saphenous Vein, Right S Lesser Saphenous Vein, Left T Foot Vein, Right V Foot Vein, Left Y Lower Vein	Ø Open 3 Percutaneous 4 Percutaneous Endoscopic	Ø Drainage Device	Z No Qualifier
Ø Inferior Vena Cava 1 Splenic Vein 2 Gastric Vein 3 Esophageal Vein 4 Hepatic Vein 5 Superior Mesenteric Vein 6 Inferior Mesenteric Vein 7 Colic Vein 8 Portal Vein 9 Renal Vein, Right B Renal Vein, Left C Common Iliac Vein, Right D Common Iliac Vein, Left F External Iliac Vein, Right G External Iliac Vein, Left H Hypogastric Vein, Right J Hypogastric Vein, Left M Femoral Vein, Right N Femoral Vein, Left P Greater Saphenous Vein, Right Q Greater Saphenous Vein, Left R Lesser Saphenous Vein, Right S Lesser Saphenous Vein, Left T Foot Vein, Right V Foot Vein, Left Y Lower Vein	Ø Open 3 Percutaneous 4 Percutaneous Endoscopic	Z No Device	X Diagnostic Z No Qualifier

DRG Non-OR   Ø69330Z
DRG Non-OR   Ø6933ZZ
Non-OR   Ø69[Ø12456789BCDFGHJMNPQRSTVY][Ø34]ØZ
Non-OR   Ø69[Ø12456789BCDFGHJMNPQRSTVY][Ø34]ZZ

New/Revised Text in Green   ~~deleted~~ Deleted   ♀ Females Only   ♂ Males Only   **Coding Clinic**
🚫 Non-covered   🚫 Limited Coverage   ⊞ Combination (See Appendix E)   DRG Non-OR   Non-OR   🚫 Hospital-Acquired Condition

SECTION: Ø MEDICAL AND SURGICAL
BODY SYSTEM: 6 LOWER VEINS
OPERATION: B EXCISION: Cutting out or off, without replacement, a portion of a body part

Body Part	Approach	Device	Qualifier
Ø Inferior Vena Cava 1 Splenic Vein 2 Gastric Vein 3 Esophageal Vein 4 Hepatic Vein 5 Superior Mesenteric Vein 6 Inferior Mesenteric Vein 7 Colic Vein 8 Portal Vein 9 Renal Vein, Right B Renal Vein, Left C Common Iliac Vein, Right D Common Iliac Vein, Left F External Iliac Vein, Right G External Iliac Vein, Left H Hypogastric Vein, Right J Hypogastric Vein, Left M Femoral Vein, Right N Femoral Vein, Left P Greater Saphenous Vein, Right Q Greater Saphenous Vein, Left R Lesser Saphenous Vein, Right S Lesser Saphenous Vein, Left T Foot Vein, Right V Foot Vein, Left	Ø Open 3 Percutaneous 4 Percutaneous Endoscopic	Z No Device	X Diagnostic Z No Qualifier
Y Lower Vein	Ø Open 3 Percutaneous 4 Percutaneous Endoscopic	Z No Device	C Hemorrhoidal Plexus X Diagnostic Z No Qualifier

Coding Clinic: 2016, Q1, P28 – 06BQ4ZZ
Coding Clinic: 2016, Q2, P19 – 06B90ZZ

SECTION: Ø MEDICAL AND SURGICAL
BODY SYSTEM: 6 LOWER VEINS
OPERATION: C EXTIRPATION: Taking or cutting out solid matter from a body part

Body Part	Approach	Device	Qualifier
Ø Inferior Vena Cava	Ø Open	Z No Device	Z No Qualifier
1 Splenic Vein	3 Percutaneous		
2 Gastric Vein	4 Percutaneous Endoscopic		
3 Esophageal Vein			
4 Hepatic Vein			
5 Superior Mesenteric Vein			
6 Inferior Mesenteric Vein			
7 Colic Vein			
8 Portal Vein			
9 Renal Vein, Right			
B Renal Vein, Left			
C Common Iliac Vein, Right			
D Common Iliac Vein, Left			
F External Iliac Vein, Right			
G External Iliac Vein, Left			
H Hypogastric Vein, Right			
J Hypogastric Vein, Left			
M Femoral Vein, Right			
N Femoral Vein, Left			
P Greater Saphenous Vein, Right			
Q Greater Saphenous Vein, Left			
R Lesser Saphenous Vein, Right			
S Lesser Saphenous Vein, Left			
T Foot Vein, Right			
V Foot Vein, Left			
Y Lower Vein			

SECTION: Ø MEDICAL AND SURGICAL
BODY SYSTEM: 6 LOWER VEINS
OPERATION: D EXTRACTION: Pulling or stripping out or off all or a portion of a body part by the use of force

Body Part	Approach	Device	Qualifier
M Femoral Vein, Right	Ø Open	Z No Device	Z No Qualifier
N Femoral Vein, Left	3 Percutaneous		
P Greater Saphenous Vein, Right	4 Percutaneous Endoscopic		
Q Greater Saphenous Vein, Left			
R Lesser Saphenous Vein, Right			
S Lesser Saphenous Vein, Left			
T Foot Vein, Right			
V Foot Vein, Left			
Y Lower Vein			

C: EXTIRPATION   D: EXTRACTION

6: LOWER VEINS

Ø: M/S

New/Revised Text in Green ~~deleted~~ Deleted ♀ Females Only ♂ Males Only **Coding Clinic**
Non-covered Limited Coverage Combination (See Appendix E) DRG Non-OR Non-OR Hospital-Acquired Condition

SECTION: Ø MEDICAL AND SURGICAL
BODY SYSTEM: 6 LOWER VEINS
OPERATION: H INSERTION: Putting in a nonbiological appliance that monitors, assists, performs, or prevents a physiological function but does not physically take the place of a body part

Body Part	Approach	Device	Qualifier
Ø Inferior Vena Cava	Ø Open 3 Percutaneous	3 Infusion Device	T Via Unbilical Vein Z No Qualifier
Ø Inferior Vena Cava	Ø Open 3 Percutaneous	D Intraluminal Device	Z No Qualifier
Ø Inferior Vena Cava	4 Percutaneous Endoscopic	3 Infusion Device D Intraluminal Device	Z No Qualifier
1 Splenic Vein 2 Gastric Vein 3 Esophageal Vein 4 Hepatic Vein 5 Superior Mesenteric Vein 6 Inferior Mesenteric Vein 7 Colic Vein 8 Portal Vein 9 Renal Vein, Right B Renal Vein, Left C Common Iliac Vein, Right D Common Iliac Vein, Left F External Iliac Vein, Right G External Iliac Vein, Left H Hypogastric Vein, Right J Hypogastric Vein, Left M Femoral Vein, Right ⊞ N Femoral Vein, Left ⊞ P Greater Saphenous Vein, Right Q Greater Saphenous Vein, Left R Lesser Saphenous Vein, Right S Lesser Saphenous Vein, Left T Foot Vein, Right V Foot Vein, Left	Ø Open 3 Percutaneous 4 Percutaneous Endoscopic	3 Infusion Device D Intraluminal Device	Z No Qualifier
Y Lower Vein	Ø Open 3 Percutaneous 4 Percutaneous Endoscopic	2 Monitoring Device 3 Infusion Device D Intraluminal Device	Z No Qualifier

⊞ 06H[MN]33Z
DRG Non-OR 06H[MN]33Z
DRG Non-OR 06HY32Z
Non-OR 06HØ[Ø3]3[TZ]
Non-OR 06HØ43Z
Non-OR 06H[123456789BCDFGHJPQRSTV][Ø34]3Z
Non-OR 06H[MN][Ø4]3Z
Non-OR 06HY[Ø34]3Z

Coding Clinic: 2013, Q3, P19 – 06HØ33Z

J: INSPECTION   L: OCCLUSION

6: LOWER VEINS

Ø: M/S

SECTION: Ø MEDICAL AND SURGICAL
BODY SYSTEM: 6 LOWER VEINS
OPERATION: J INSPECTION: Visually and/or manually exploring a body part

Body Part	Approach	Device	Qualifier
Y Lower Vein	Ø Open 3 Percutaneous 4 Percutaneous Endoscopic X External	Z No Device	Z No Qualifier

DRG Non-OR Ø6JY3ZZ
Non-OR Ø6JYXZZ

SECTION: Ø MEDICAL AND SURGICAL
BODY SYSTEM: 6 LOWER VEINS
OPERATION: L OCCLUSION: Completely closing an orifice or the lumen of a tubular
body part

Body Part	Approach	Device	Qualifier
Ø Inferior Vena Cava 1 Splenic Vein 2 Gastric Vein 3 Esophageal Vein 4 Hepatic Vein 5 Superior Mesenteric Vein 6 Inferior Mesenteric Vein 7 Colic Vein 8 Portal Vein 9 Renal Vein, Right B Renal Vein, Left C Common Iliac Vein, Right D Common Iliac Vein, Left F External Iliac Vein, Right G External Iliac Vein, Left H Hypogastric Vein, Right J Hypogastric Vein, Left M Femoral Vein, Right N Femoral Vein, Left P Greater Saphenous Vein, Right Q Greater Saphenous Vein, Left R Lesser Saphenous Vein, Right S Lesser Saphenous Vein, Left T Foot Vein, Right V Foot Vein, Left	Ø Open 3 Percutaneous 4 Percutaneous Endoscopic	C Extraluminal Device D Intraluminal Device Z No Device	Z No Qualifier
Y Lower Vein	Ø Open 3 Percutaneous 4 Percutaneous Endoscopic	C Extraluminal Device D Intraluminal Device Z No Device	C Hemorrhoidal Plexus Z No Qualifier

DRG Non-OR Ø6L3[34][CDZ]Z

New/Revised Text in Green   ~~deleted~~ Deleted   ♀ Females Only   ♂ Males Only   **Coding Clinic**
Non-covered   Limited Coverage   ⊕ Combination (See Appendix E)   DRG Non-OR   Non-OR   Hospital-Acquired Condition

SECTION: Ø MEDICAL AND SURGICAL
BODY SYSTEM: 6 LOWER VEINS
OPERATION: N RELEASE: Freeing a body part from an abnormal physical constraint by cutting or by the use of force

Body Part	Approach	Device	Qualifier
Ø Inferior Vena Cava 1 Splenic Vein 2 Gastric Vein 3 Esophageal Vein 4 Hepatic Vein 5 Superior Mesenteric Vein 6 Inferior Mesenteric Vein 7 Colic Vein 8 Portal Vein 9 Renal Vein, Right B Renal Vein, Left C Common Iliac Vein, Right D Common Iliac Vein, Left F External Iliac Vein, Right G External Iliac Vein, Left H Hypogastric Vein, Right J Hypogastric Vein, Left M Femoral Vein, Right N Femoral Vein, Left P Greater Saphenous Vein, Right Q Greater Saphenous Vein, Left R Lesser Saphenous Vein, Right S Lesser Saphenous Vein, Left T Foot Vein, Right V Foot Vein, Left Y Lower Vein	Ø Open 3 Percutaneous 4 Percutaneous Endoscopic	Z No Device	Z No Qualifier

SECTION: Ø MEDICAL AND SURGICAL
BODY SYSTEM: 6 LOWER VEINS
OPERATION: P REMOVAL: Taking out or off a device from a body part

Body Part	Approach	Device	Qualifier
Y Lower Vein	Ø Open 3 Percutaneous 4 Percutaneous Endoscopic	Ø Drainage Device 2 Monitoring Device 3 Infusion Device 7 Autologous Tissue Substitute C Extraluminal Device D Intraluminal Device J Synthetic Substitute K Nonautologous Tissue Substitute	Z No Qualifier
Y Lower Vein	X External	Ø Drainage Device 2 Monitoring Device 3 Infusion Device D Intraluminal Device	Z No Qualifier

DRG Non-OR 06PY3[023]Z
Non-OR 06PYX[023D]Z

SECTION: Ø MEDICAL AND SURGICAL
BODY SYSTEM: 6 LOWER VEINS
OPERATION: Q REPAIR: Restoring, to the extent possible, a body part to its normal anatomic structure and function

Body Part	Approach	Device	Qualifier
Ø Inferior Vena Cava	Ø Open	Z No Device	Z No Qualifier
1 Splenic Vein	3 Percutaneous		
2 Gastric Vein	4 Percutaneous Endoscopic		
3 Esophageal Vein			
4 Hepatic Vein			
5 Superior Mesenteric Vein			
6 Inferior Mesenteric Vein			
7 Colic Vein			
8 Portal Vein			
9 Renal Vein, Right			
B Renal Vein, Left			
C Common Iliac Vein, Right			
D Common Iliac Vein, Left			
F External Iliac Vein, Right			
G External Iliac Vein, Left			
H Hypogastric Vein, Right			
J Hypogastric Vein, Left			
M Femoral Vein, Right			
N Femoral Vein, Left			
P Greater Saphenous Vein, Right			
Q Greater Saphenous Vein, Left			
R Lesser Saphenous Vein, Right			
S Lesser Saphenous Vein, Left			
T Foot Vein, Right			
V Foot Vein, Left			
Y Lower Vein			

Q: REPAIR

6: LOWER VEINS

Ø: M/S

New/Revised Text in Green — deleted Deleted — ♀ Females Only — ♂ Males Only — **Coding Clinic**
Non-covered — Limited Coverage — ⊞ Combination (See Appendix E) — DRG Non-OR — Non-OR — Hospital-Acquired Condition

SECTION: Ø MEDICAL AND SURGICAL
BODY SYSTEM: 6 LOWER VEINS
OPERATION: R REPLACEMENT: Putting in or on biological or synthetic material that physically takes the place and/or function of all or a portion of a body part

Body Part	Approach	Device	Qualifier
Ø Inferior Vena Cava	Ø Open	7 Autologous Tissue Substitute	Z No Qualifier
1 Splenic Vein	4 Percutaneous Endoscopic	J Synthetic Substitute	
2 Gastric Vein		K Nonautologous Tissue Substitute	
3 Esophageal Vein			
4 Hepatic Vein			
5 Superior Mesenteric Vein			
6 Inferior Mesenteric Vein			
7 Colic Vein			
8 Portal Vein			
9 Renal Vein, Right			
B Renal Vein, Left			
C Common Iliac Vein, Right			
D Common Iliac Vein, Left			
F External Iliac Vein, Right			
G External Iliac Vein, Left			
H Hypogastric Vein, Right			
J Hypogastric Vein, Left			
M Femoral Vein, Right			
N Femoral Vein, Left			
P Greater Saphenous Vein, Right			
Q Greater Saphenous Vein, Left			
R Lesser Saphenous Vein, Right			
S Lesser Saphenous Vein, Left			
T Foot Vein, Right			
V Foot Vein, Left			
Y Lower Vein			

Ø: M/S

6: LOWER VEINS

R: REPLACEMENT

SECTION: Ø MEDICAL AND SURGICAL
BODY SYSTEM: 6 LOWER VEINS
OPERATION: S REPOSITION: Moving to its normal location, or other suitable location, all or a portion of a body part

Body Part	Approach	Device	Qualifier
Ø Inferior Vena Cava	Ø Open	Z No Device	Z No Qualifier
1 Splenic Vein	3 Percutaneous		
2 Gastric Vein	4 Percutaneous Endoscopic		
3 Esophageal Vein			
4 Hepatic Vein			
5 Superior Mesenteric Vein			
6 Inferior Mesenteric Vein			
7 Colic Vein			
8 Portal Vein			
9 Renal Vein, Right			
B Renal Vein, Left			
C Common Iliac Vein, Right			
D Common Iliac Vein, Left			
F External Iliac Vein, Right			
G External Iliac Vein, Left			
H Hypogastric Vein, Right			
J Hypogastric Vein, Left			
M Femoral Vein, Right			
N Femoral Vein, Left			
P Greater Saphenous Vein, Right			
Q Greater Saphenous Vein, Left			
R Lesser Saphenous Vein, Right			
S Lesser Saphenous Vein, Left			
T Foot Vein, Right			
V Foot Vein, Left			
Y Lower Vein			

S: REPOSITION

6: LOWER VEINS

Ø: M/S

New/Revised Text in Green   ~~deleted~~ Deleted   ♀ Females Only   ♂ Males Only   **Coding Clinic**

Non-covered   Limited Coverage   ⊞ Combination (See Appendix E)   DRG Non-OR   Non-OR   Hospital-Acquired Condition

SECTION: Ø MEDICAL AND SURGICAL
BODY SYSTEM: 6 LOWER VEINS
OPERATION: U SUPPLEMENT: Putting in or on biological or synthetic material that physically reinforces and/or augments the function of a portion of a body part

Body Part	Approach	Device	Qualifier
Ø Inferior Vena Cava 1 Splenic Vein 2 Gastric Vein 3 Esophageal Vein 4 Hepatic Vein 5 Superior Mesenteric Vein 6 Inferior Mesenteric Vein 7 Colic Vein 8 Portal Vein 9 Renal Vein, Right B Renal Vein, Left C Common Iliac Vein, Right D Common Iliac Vein, Left F External Iliac Vein, Right G External Iliac Vein, Left H Hypogastric Vein, Right J Hypogastric Vein, Left M Femoral Vein, Right N Femoral Vein, Left P Greater Saphenous Vein, Right Q Greater Saphenous Vein, Left R Lesser Saphenous Vein, Right S Lesser Saphenous Vein, Left T Foot Vein, Right V Foot Vein, Left Y Lower Vein	Ø Open 3 Percutaneous 4 Percutaneous Endoscopic	7 Autologous Tissue Substitute J Synthetic Substitute K Nonautologous Tissue Substitute	Z No Qualifier

Ø: M/S

6: LOWER VEINS

U: SUPPLEMENT

SECTION: Ø MEDICAL AND SURGICAL

BODY SYSTEM: 6 LOWER VEINS

OPERATION: V RESTRICTION: Partially closing an orifice or the lumen of a tubular body part

Body Part	Approach	Device	Qualifier
Ø Inferior Vena Cava 1 Splenic Vein 2 Gastric Vein 3 Esophageal Vein 4 Hepatic Vein 5 Superior Mesenteric Vein 6 Inferior Mesenteric Vein 7 Colic Vein 8 Portal Vein 9 Renal Vein, Right B Renal Vein, Left C Common Iliac Vein, Right D Common Iliac Vein, Left F External Iliac Vein, Right G External Iliac Vein, Left H Hypogastric Vein, Right J Hypogastric Vein, Left M Femoral Vein, Right N Femoral Vein, Left P Greater Saphenous Vein, Right Q Greater Saphenous Vein, Left R Lesser Saphenous Vein, Right S Lesser Saphenous Vein, Left T Foot Vein, Right V Foot Vein, Left Y Lower Vein	Ø Open 3 Percutaneous 4 Percutaneous Endoscopic	C Extraluminal Device D Intraluminal Device Z No Device	Z No Qualifier

SECTION: Ø MEDICAL AND SURGICAL

BODY SYSTEM: 6 LOWER VEINS

OPERATION: W REVISION: Correcting, to the extent possible, a portion of a malfunctioning device or the position of a displaced device

Body Part	Approach	Device	Qualifier
Y Lower Vein	Ø Open 3 Percutaneous 4 Percutaneous Endoscopic X External	Ø Drainage Device 2 Monitoring Device 3 Infusion Device 7 Autologous Tissue Substitute C Extraluminal Device D Intraluminal Device J Synthetic Substitute K Nonautologous Tissue Substitute	Z No Qualifier

Non-OR 06WYX[0237CDJK]Z

New/Revised Text in Green · deleted Deleted · ♀ Females Only · ♂ Males Only · Coding Clinic
Non-covered · Limited Coverage · Combination (See Appendix E) · DRG Non-OR · Non-OR · Hospital-Acquired Condition

SECTION: Ø MEDICAL AND SURGICAL
BODY SYSTEM: 7 LYMPHATIC AND HEMIC SYSTEMS
OPERATION: 2 **CHANGE:** Taking out or off a device from a body part and putting back an identical or similar device in or on the same body part without cutting or puncturing the skin or a mucous membrane

Body Part	Approach	Device	Qualifier
K Thoracic Duct L Cisterna Chyli M Thymus N Lymphatic P Spleen T Bone Marrow	X External	Ø Drainage Device Y Other Device	Z No Qualifier

Non-OR All Values

Coding Clinic: 2016, Q1, P30 – 07T50ZZ

SECTION: Ø MEDICAL AND SURGICAL
BODY SYSTEM: 7 LYMPHATIC AND HEMIC SYSTEMS
OPERATION: 5 **DESTRUCTION:** Physical eradication of all or a portion of a body part by the direct use of energy, force, or a destructive agent

Body Part	Approach	Device	Qualifier
Ø Lymphatic, Head 1 Lymphatic, Right Neck 2 Lymphatic, Left Neck 3 Lymphatic, Right Upper Extremity 4 Lymphatic, Left Upper Extremity 5 Lymphatic, Right Axillary 6 Lymphatic, Left Axillary 7 Lymphatic, Thorax 8 Lymphatic, Internal Mammary, Right 9 Lymphatic, Internal Mammary, Left B Lymphatic, Mesenteric C Lymphatic, Pelvis D Lymphatic, Aortic F Lymphatic, Right Lower Extremity G Lymphatic, Left Lower Extremity H Lymphatic, Right Inguinal J Lymphatic, Left Inguinal K Thoracic Duct L Cisterna Chyli M Thymus P Spleen	Ø Open 3 Percutaneous 4 Percutaneous Endoscopic	Z No Device	Z No Qualifier

New/Revised Text in Green   ~~deleted~~ Deleted   ♀ Females Only   ♂ Males Only   **Coding Clinic**
Non-covered   Limited Coverage   ⊞ Combination (See Appendix E)   DRG Non-OR   Non-OR   Hospital-Acquired Condition

SECTION: Ø MEDICAL AND SURGICAL
BODY SYSTEM: 7 LYMPHATIC AND HEMIC SYSTEMS
OPERATION: 9 **DRAINAGE:** Taking or letting out fluids and/or gases from a body part

Body Part	Approach	Device	Qualifier
Ø Lymphatic, Head 1 Lymphatic, Right Neck 2 Lymphatic, Left Neck 3 Lymphatic, Right Upper Extremity 4 Lymphatic, Left Upper Extremity 5 Lymphatic, Right Axillary 6 Lymphatic, Left Axillary 7 Lymphatic, Thorax 8 Lymphatic, Internal Mammary, Right 9 Lymphatic, Internal Mammary, Left B Lymphatic, Mesenteric C Lymphatic, Pelvis D Lymphatic, Aortic F Lymphatic, Right Lower Extremity G Lymphatic, Left Lower Extremity H Lymphatic, Right Inguinal J Lymphatic, Left Inguinal K Thoracic Duct L Cisterna Chyli M Thymus P Spleen T Bone Marrow	Ø Open 3 Percutaneous 4 Percutaneous Endoscopic	Ø Drainage Device	Z No Qualifier
Ø Lymphatic, Head 1 Lymphatic, Right Neck 2 Lymphatic, Left Neck 3 Lymphatic, Right Upper Extremity 4 Lymphatic, Left Upper Extremity 5 Lymphatic, Right Axillary 6 Lymphatic, Left Axillary 7 Lymphatic, Thorax 8 Lymphatic, Internal Mammary, Right 9 Lymphatic, Internal Mammary, Left B Lymphatic, Mesenteric C Lymphatic, Pelvis D Lymphatic, Aortic F Lymphatic, Right Lower Extremity G Lymphatic, Left Lower Extremity H Lymphatic, Right Inguinal J Lymphatic, Left Inguinal K Thoracic Duct L Cisterna Chyli M Thymus P Spleen T Bone Marrow	Ø Open 3 Percutaneous 4 Percutaneous Endoscopic	Z No Device	X Diagnostic Z No Qualifier

DRG Non-OR 079[0123456789BCDFGHJKLM]30Z
DRG Non-OR 079[0123456789BCDFGHJKLM]3ZZ
Non-OR 079P[34]0Z
Non-OR 079T[034]0Z
Non-OR 079P[34]Z[XZ]
Non-OR 079T[034]Z[XZ]

SECTION: Ø MEDICAL AND SURGICAL

BODY SYSTEM: 7 LYMPHATIC AND HEMIC SYSTEMS

OPERATION: B EXCISION: Cutting out or off, without replacement, a portion of a body part

Body Part	Approach	Device	Qualifier
Ø Lymphatic, Head 1 Lymphatic, Right Neck 2 Lymphatic, Left Neck 3 Lymphatic, Right Upper Extremity 4 Lymphatic, Left Upper Extremity 5 Lymphatic, Right Axillary 6 Lymphatic, Left Axillary 7 Lymphatic, Thorax 8 Lymphatic, Internal Mammary, Right 9 Lymphatic, Internal Mammary, Left B Lymphatic, Mesenteric C Lymphatic, Pelvis D Lymphatic, Aortic F Lymphatic, Right Lower Extremity G Lymphatic, Left Lower Extremity H Lymphatic, Right Inguinal ⊞ J Lymphatic, Left Inguinal ⊞ K Thoracic Duct L Cisterna Chyli M Thymus P Spleen	Ø Open 3 Percutaneous 4 Percutaneous Endoscopic	Z No Device	X Diagnostic Z No Qualifier

⊞ Ø7B[HJ][Ø4]ZZ
Non-OR Ø7BP[34]ZX

SECTION: Ø MEDICAL AND SURGICAL

BODY SYSTEM: 7 LYMPHATIC AND HEMIC SYSTEMS

OPERATION: C EXTIRPATION: Taking or cutting out solid matter from a body part

Body Part	Approach	Device	Qualifier
Ø Lymphatic, Head 1 Lymphatic, Right Neck 2 Lymphatic, Left Neck 3 Lymphatic, Right Upper Extremity 4 Lymphatic, Left Upper Extremity 5 Lymphatic, Right Axillary 6 Lymphatic, Left Axillary 7 Lymphatic, Thorax 8 Lymphatic, Internal Mammary, Right 9 Lymphatic, Internal Mammary, Left B Lymphatic, Mesenteric C Lymphatic, Pelvis D Lymphatic, Aortic F Lymphatic, Right Lower Extremity G Lymphatic, Left Lower Extremity H Lymphatic, Right Inguinal J Lymphatic, Left Inguinal K Thoracic Duct L Cisterna Chyli M Thymus P Spleen	Ø Open 3 Percutaneous 4 Percutaneous Endoscopic	Z No Device	Z No Qualifier

Non-OR Ø7CP[34]ZZ

New/Revised Text in Green · ~~deleted~~ Deleted · ♀ Females Only · ♂ Males Only · **Coding Clinic**
🚫 Non-covered · 🚫 Limited Coverage · ⊞ Combination (See Appendix E) · DRG Non-OR · Non-OR · 🚫 Hospital-Acquired Condition

B: EXCISION   C: EXTIRPATION

7: LYMPHATIC AND HEMIC SYSTEMS

Ø: M/S

SECTION: 0 MEDICAL AND SURGICAL

BODY SYSTEM: 7 LYMPHATIC AND HEMIC SYSTEMS

OPERATION: D EXTRACTION: Pulling or stripping out or off all or a portion of a body part by the use of force

Body Part	Approach	Device	Qualifier
Q Bone Marrow, Sternum R Bone Marrow, Iliac S Bone Marrow, Vertebral	0 Open 3 Percutaneous	Z No Device	X Diagnostic Z No Qualifier

Non-OR All Values

SECTION: 0 MEDICAL AND SURGICAL

BODY SYSTEM: 7 LYMPHATIC AND HEMIC SYSTEMS

OPERATION: H INSERTION: Putting in a nonbiological appliance that monitors, assists, performs, or prevents a physiological function but does not physically take the place of a body part

Body Part	Approach	Device	Qualifier
K Thoracic Duct L Cisterna Chyli M Thymus N Lymphatic P Spleen	0 Open 3 Percutaneous 4 Percutaneous Endoscopic	3 Infusion Device	Z No Qualifier

DRG Non-OR All Values

SECTION: 0 MEDICAL AND SURGICAL

BODY SYSTEM: 7 LYMPHATIC AND HEMIC SYSTEMS

OPERATION: J INSPECTION: Visually and/or manually exploring a body part

Body Part	Approach	Device	Qualifier
K Thoracic Duct L Cisterna Chyli M Thymus T Bone Marrow	0 Open 3 Percutaneous 4 Percutaneous Endoscopic	Z No Device	Z No Qualifier
N Lymphatic P Spleen	0 Open 3 Percutaneous 4 Percutaneous Endoscopic X External	Z No Device	Z No Qualifier

DRG Non-OR 07J[KLM]3ZZ
DRG Non-OR 07JN3ZZ
Non-OR 07JNXZZ
Non-OR 07JP[34X]ZZ
Non-OR 07JT[034]ZZ

SECTION: Ø MEDICAL AND SURGICAL

BODY SYSTEM: 7 LYMPHATIC AND HEMIC SYSTEMS

OPERATION: L OCCLUSION: Completely closing an orifice or the lumen of a tubular body part

Body Part	Approach	Device	Qualifier
Ø Lymphatic, Head	Ø Open	C Extraluminal Device	Z No Qualifier
1 Lymphatic, Right Neck	3 Percutaneous	D Intraluminal Device	
2 Lymphatic, Left Neck	4 Percutaneous Endoscopic	Z No Device	
3 Lymphatic, Right Upper Extremity			
4 Lymphatic, Left Upper Extremity			
5 Lymphatic, Right Axillary			
6 Lymphatic, Left Axillary			
7 Lymphatic, Thorax			
8 Lymphatic, Internal Mammary, Right			
9 Lymphatic, Internal Mammary, Left			
B Lymphatic, Mesenteric			
C Lymphatic, Pelvis			
D Lymphatic, Aortic			
F Lymphatic, Right Lower Extremity			
G Lymphatic, Left Lower Extremity			
H Lymphatic, Right Inguinal			
J Lymphatic, Left Inguinal			
K Thoracic Duct			
L Cisterna Chyli			

SECTION: Ø MEDICAL AND SURGICAL

BODY SYSTEM: 7 LYMPHATIC AND HEMIC SYSTEMS

OPERATION: N RELEASE: Freeing a body part from an abnormal physical constraint by cutting or by the use of force

Body Part	Approach	Device	Qualifier
Ø Lymphatic, Head	Ø Open	Z No Device	Z No Qualifier
1 Lymphatic, Right Neck	3 Percutaneous		
2 Lymphatic, Left Neck	4 Percutaneous Endoscopic		
3 Lymphatic, Right Upper Extremity			
4 Lymphatic, Left Upper Extremity			
5 Lymphatic, Right Axillary			
6 Lymphatic, Left Axillary			
7 Lymphatic, Thorax			
8 Lymphatic, Internal Mammary, Right			
9 Lymphatic, Internal Mammary, Left			
B Lymphatic, Mesenteric			
C Lymphatic, Pelvis			
D Lymphatic, Aortic			
F Lymphatic, Right Lower Extremity			
G Lymphatic, Left Lower Extremity			
H Lymphatic, Right Inguinal			
J Lymphatic, Left Inguinal			
K Thoracic Duct			
L Cisterna Chyli			
M Thymus			
P Spleen			

SECTION: Ø MEDICAL AND SURGICAL
BODY SYSTEM: 7 LYMPHATIC AND HEMIC SYSTEMS
OPERATION: P REMOVAL: Taking out or off a device from a body part

Body Part	Approach	Device	Qualifier
K Thoracic Duct L Cisterna Chyli N Lymphatic	Ø Open 3 Percutaneous 4 Percutaneous Endoscopic	Ø Drainage Device 3 Infusion Device 7 Autologous Tissue Substitute C Extraluminal Device D Intraluminal Device J Synthetic Substitute K Nonautologous Tissue Substitute	Z No Qualifier
K Thoracic Duct L Cisterna Chyli N Lymphatic	X External	Ø Drainage Device 3 Infusion Device D Intraluminal Device	Z No Qualifier
M Thymus P Spleen	Ø Open 3 Percutaneous 4 Percutaneous Endoscopic X External	Ø Drainage Device 3 Infusion Device	Z No Qualifier
T Bone Marrow	Ø Open 3 Percutaneous 4 Percutaneous Endoscopic X External	Ø Drainage Device	Z No Qualifier

Non-OR 07P[KLN]X[03D]Z
Non-OR 07P[MP]X[03]Z
Non-OR 07PT[034X]0Z

SECTION: Ø MEDICAL AND SURGICAL
BODY SYSTEM: 7 LYMPHATIC AND HEMIC SYSTEMS
OPERATION: Q REPAIR: Restoring, to the extent possible, a body part to its normal
anatomic structure and function

Body Part	Approach	Device	Qualifier
Ø Lymphatic, Head 1 Lymphatic, Right Neck 2 Lymphatic, Left Neck 3 Lymphatic, Right Upper Extremity 4 Lymphatic, Left Upper Extremity 5 Lymphatic, Right Axillary 6 Lymphatic, Left Axillary 7 Lymphatic, Thorax 8 Lymphatic, Internal Mammary, Right 9 Lymphatic, Internal Mammary, Left B Lymphatic, Mesenteric C Lymphatic, Pelvis D Lymphatic, Aortic F Lymphatic, Right Lower Extremity G Lymphatic, Left Lower Extremity H Lymphatic, Right Inguinal J Lymphatic, Left Inguinal K Thoracic Duct L Cisterna Chyli M Thymus P Spleen	Ø Open 3 Percutaneous 4 Percutaneous Endoscopic	Z No Device	Z No Qualifier

New/Revised Text in Green ~~deleted~~ Deleted ♀ Females Only ♂ Males Only **Coding Clinic**
🔖 Non-covered 🔖 Limited Coverage ⊕ Combination (See Appendix E) [DRG Non-OR] Non-OR 🔖 Hospital-Acquired Condition

SECTION: Ø MEDICAL AND SURGICAL
BODY SYSTEM: 7 LYMPHATIC AND HEMIC SYSTEMS
OPERATION: S REPOSITION: Moving to its normal location, or other suitable location, all or a portion of a body part

Body Part	Approach	Device	Qualifier
M Thymus P Spleen	Ø Open	Z No Device	Z No Qualifier

SECTION: Ø MEDICAL AND SURGICAL
BODY SYSTEM: 7 LYMPHATIC AND HEMIC SYSTEMS
OPERATION: T RESECTION: Cutting out or off, without replacement, all of a body part

Body Part	Approach	Device	Qualifier
Ø Lymphatic, Head 1 Lymphatic, Right Neck 2 Lymphatic, Left Neck 3 Lymphatic, Right Upper Extremity 4 Lymphatic, Left Upper Extremity 5 Lymphatic, Right Axillary ⊞ 6 Lymphatic, Left Axillary ⊞ 7 Lymphatic, Thorax ⊞ 8 Lymphatic, Internal Mammary, Right ⊞ 9 Lymphatic, Internal Mammary, Left ⊞ B Lymphatic, Mesenteric C Lymphatic, Pelvis D Lymphatic, Aortic F Lymphatic, Right Lower Extremity G Lymphatic, Left Lower Extremity H Lymphatic, Right Inguinal J Lymphatic, Left Inguinal K Thoracic Duct L Cisterna Chyli M Thymus P Spleen	Ø Open 4 Percutaneous Endoscopic	Z No Device	Z No Qualifier

⊞ 07T[56789]ØZZ

Coding Clinic: 2015, Q4, P13 – 07TPØZZ
Coding Clinic: 2016, Q2, P13 – 07T20ZZ

New/Revised Text in Green   ~~deleted~~ Deleted   ♀ Females Only   ♂ Males Only   **Coding Clinic**
🚫 Non-covered   🚫 Limited Coverage   ⊞ Combination (See Appendix E)   DRG Non-OR   Non-OR   🚫 Hospital-Acquired Condition

SECTION: 0 MEDICAL AND SURGICAL
BODY SYSTEM: 7 LYMPHATIC AND HEMIC SYSTEMS
OPERATION: U SUPPLEMENT: Putting in or on biological or synthetic material that physically reinforces and/or augments the function of a portion of a body part

Body Part	Approach	Device	Qualifier
0 Lymphatic, Head	0 Open	7 Autologous Tissue Substitute	Z No Qualifier
1 Lymphatic, Right Neck	4 Percutaneous Endoscopic	J Synthetic Substitute	
2 Lymphatic, Left Neck		K Nonautologous Tissue	
3 Lymphatic, Right Upper Extremity		Substitute	
4 Lymphatic, Left Upper Extremity			
5 Lymphatic, Right Axillary			
6 Lymphatic, Left Axillary			
7 Lymphatic, Thorax			
8 Lymphatic, Internal Mammary, Right			
9 Lymphatic, Internal Mammary, Left			
B Lymphatic, Mesenteric			
C Lymphatic, Pelvis			
D Lymphatic, Aortic			
F Lymphatic, Right Lower Extremity			
G Lymphatic, Left Lower Extremity			
H Lymphatic, Right Inguinal			
J Lymphatic, Left Inguinal			
K Thoracic Duct			
L Cisterna Chyli			

SECTION: 0 MEDICAL AND SURGICAL
BODY SYSTEM: 7 LYMPHATIC AND HEMIC SYSTEMS
OPERATION: V RESTRICTION: Partially closing an orifice or the lumen of a tubular body part

Body Part	Approach	Device	Qualifier
0 Lymphatic, Head	0 Open	C Extraluminal Device	Z No Qualifier
1 Lymphatic, Right Neck	3 Percutaneous	D Intraluminal Device	
2 Lymphatic, Left Neck	4 Percutaneous Endoscopic	Z No Device	
3 Lymphatic, Right Upper Extremity			
4 Lymphatic, Left Upper Extremity			
5 Lymphatic, Right Axillary			
6 Lymphatic, Left Axillary			
7 Lymphatic, Thorax			
8 Lymphatic, Internal Mammary, Right			
9 Lymphatic, Internal Mammary, Left			
B Lymphatic, Mesenteric			
C Lymphatic, Pelvis			
D Lymphatic, Aortic			
F Lymphatic, Right Lower Extremity			
G Lymphatic, Left Lower Extremity			
H Lymphatic, Right Inguinal			
J Lymphatic, Left Inguinal			
K Thoracic Duct			
L Cisterna Chyli			

New/Revised Text in Green   deleted Deleted   ♀ Females Only   ♂ Males Only   **Coding Clinic**
🚫 Non-covered   🚫 Limited Coverage   ⊞ Combination (See Appendix E)   DRG Non-OR   Non-OR   🚫 Hospital-Acquired Condition

W: REVISION   Y: TRANSPLANTATION

7: LYMPHATIC AND HEMIC SYSTEMS

0: M/S

SECTION: Ø MEDICAL AND SURGICAL

BODY SYSTEM: 7 LYMPHATIC AND HEMIC SYSTEMS
OPERATION: W REVISION: Correcting, to the extent possible, a portion of a malfunctioning device or the position of a displaced device

Body Part	Approach	Device	Qualifier
K Thoracic Duct L Cisterna Chyli N Lymphatic	Ø Open 3 Percutaneous 4 Percutaneous Endoscopic X External	Ø Drainage Device 3 Infusion Device 7 Autologous Tissue Substitute C Extraluminal Device D Intraluminal Device J Synthetic Substitute K Nonautologous Tissue Substitute	Z No Qualifier
M Thymus P Spleen	Ø Open 3 Percutaneous 4 Percutaneous Endoscopic X External	Ø Drainage Device 3 Infusion Device	Z No Qualifier
T Bone Marrow	Ø Open 3 Percutaneous 4 Percutaneous Endoscopic X External	Ø Drainage Device	Z No Qualifier

Non-OR 07W[KLN]X[037CDJK]Z
Non-OR 07W[MP]X[03]Z
Non-OR 07WT[034X]0Z

SECTION: Ø MEDICAL AND SURGICAL

BODY SYSTEM: 7 LYMPHATIC AND HEMIC SYSTEMS
OPERATION: Y TRANSPLANTATION: Putting in or on all or a portion of a living body part taken from another individual or animal to physically take the place and/or function of all or a portion of a similar body part

Body Part	Approach	Device	Qualifier
M Thymus P Spleen	Ø Open	Z No Device	Ø Allogeneic 1 Syngeneic 2 Zooplastic

SECTION: Ø MEDICAL AND SURGICAL
BODY SYSTEM: 8 EYE
OPERATION: Ø **ALTERATION:** Modifying the anatomic structure of a body part without affecting the function of the body part

Body Part	Approach	Device	Qualifier
N Upper Eyelid, Right P Upper Eyelid, Left Q Lower Eyelid, Right R Lower Eyelid, Left	Ø Open 3 Percutaneous X External	7 Autologous Tissue Substitute J Synthetic Substitute K Nonautologous Tissue Substitute Z No Device	Z No Qualifier

Non-OR   All Values

SECTION: Ø MEDICAL AND SURGICAL
BODY SYSTEM: 8 EYE
OPERATION: 1 **BYPASS:** Altering the route of passage of the contents of a tubular body part

Body Part	Approach	Device	Qualifier
2 Anterior Chamber, Right 3 Anterior Chamber, Left	3 Percutaneous	J Synthetic Substitute K Nonautologous Tissue Substitute Z No Device	4 Sclera
X Lacrimal Duct, Right Y Lacrimal Duct, Left	Ø Open 3 Percutaneous	J Synthetic Substitute K Nonautologous Tissue Substitute Z No Device	3 Nasal Cavity

SECTION: Ø MEDICAL AND SURGICAL
BODY SYSTEM: 8 EYE
OPERATION: 2 **CHANGE:** Taking out or off a device from a body part and putting back an identical or similar device in or on the same body part without cutting or puncturing the skin or a mucous membrane

Body Part	Approach	Device	Qualifier
Ø Eye, Right 1 Eye, Left	X External	Ø Drainage Device Y Other Device	Z No Qualifier

Non-OR   All Values

SECTION: Ø MEDICAL AND SURGICAL

BODY SYSTEM: 8 EYE

OPERATION: 5 DESTRUCTION: Physical eradication of all or a portion of a body part by the direct use of energy, force, or a destructive agent

Body Part	Approach	Device	Qualifier
Ø Eye, Right 1 Eye, Left 6 Sclera, Right 7 Sclera, Left 8 Cornea, Right 9 Cornea, Left S Conjunctiva, Right T Conjunctiva, Left	X External	Z No Device	Z No Qualifier
2 Anterior Chamber, Right 3 Anterior Chamber, Left 4 Vitreous, Right 5 Vitreous, Left C Iris, Right D Iris, Left E Retina, Right F Retina, Left G Retinal Vessel, Right H Retinal Vessel, Left J Lens, Right K Lens, Left	3 Percutaneous	Z No Device	Z No Qualifier
A Choroid, Right B Choroid, Left L Extraocular Muscle, Right M Extraocular Muscle, Left V Lacrimal Gland, Right W Lacrimal Gland, Left	Ø Open 3 Percutaneous	Z No Device	Z No Qualifier
N Upper Eyelid, Right P Upper Eyelid, Left Q Lower Eyelid, Right R Lower Eyelid, Left	Ø Open 3 Percutaneous X External	Z No Device	Z No Qualifier
X Lacrimal Duct, Right Y Lacrimal Duct, Left	Ø Open 3 Percutaneous 7 Via Natural or Artificial Opening 8 Via Natural or Artificial Opening Endoscopic	Z No Device	Z No Qualifier

SECTION: Ø MEDICAL AND SURGICAL

BODY SYSTEM: 8 EYE

OPERATION: 7 DILATION: Expanding an orifice or the lumen of a tubular body part

Body Part	Approach	Device	Qualifier
X Lacrimal Duct, Right Y Lacrimal Duct, Left	Ø Open 3 Percutaneous 7 Via Natural or Artificial Opening 8 Via Natural or Artificial Opening Endoscopic	D Intraluminal Device Z No Device	Z No Qualifier

SECTION: Ø MEDICAL AND SURGICAL

BODY SYSTEM: 8 EYE

OPERATION: 9 DRAINAGE: *(on multiple pages)*
Taking or letting out fluids and/or gases from a body part

Body Part	Approach	Device	Qualifier
Ø Eye, Right 1 Eye, Left 6 Sclera, Right 7 Sclera, Left 8 Cornea, Right 9 Cornea, Left S Conjunctiva, Right T Conjunctiva, Left	X External	Ø Drainage Device	Z No Qualifier
Ø Eye, Right 1 Eye, Left 6 Sclera, Right 7 Sclera, Left 8 Cornea, Right 9 Cornea, Left S Conjunctiva, Right T Conjunctiva, Left	X External	Z No Device	X Diagnostic Z No Qualifier
2 Anterior Chamber, Right 3 Anterior Chamber, Left 4 Vitreous, Right 5 Vitreous, Left C Iris, Right D Iris, Left E Retina, Right F Retina, Left G Retinal Vessel, Right H Retinal Vessel, Left J Lens, Right K Lens, Left	3 Percutaneous	Ø Drainage Device	Z No Qualifier
2 Anterior Chamber, Right 3 Anterior Chamber, Left 4 Vitreous, Right 5 Vitreous, Left C Iris, Right D Iris, Left E Retina, Right F Retina, Left G Retinal Vessel, Right H Retinal Vessel, Left J Lens, Right K Lens, Left	3 Percutaneous	Z No Device	X Diagnostic Z No Qualifier
A Choroid, Right B Choroid, Left L Extraocular Muscle, Right M Extraocular Muscle, Left V Lacrimal Gland, Right W Lacrimal Gland, Left	Ø Open 3 Percutaneous	Ø Drainage Device	Z No Qualifier

Coding Clinic: 2Ø16, Q2, P21 – Ø8923ZZ

9: DRAINAGE   8: EYE   Ø: M/S

SECTION: Ø MEDICAL AND SURGICAL
BODY SYSTEM: 8 EYE
OPERATION: 9 DRAINAGE: *(continued)*

Taking or letting out fluids and/or gases from a body part

Body Part	Approach	Device	Qualifier
A Choroid, Right B Choroid, Left L Extraocular Muscle, Right M Extraocular Muscle, Left V Lacrimal Gland, Right W Lacrimal Gland, Left	Ø Open 3 Percutaneous	Z No Device	X Diagnostic Z No Qualifier
N Upper Eyelid, Right P Upper Eyelid, Left Q Lower Eyelid, Right R Lower Eyelid, Left	Ø Open 3 Percutaneous X External	Ø Drainage Device	Z No Qualifier
N Upper Eyelid, Right P Upper Eyelid, Left Q Lower Eyelid, Right R Lower Eyelid, Left	Ø Open 3 Percutaneous X External	Z No Device	X Diagnostic Z No Qualifier
X Lacrimal Duct, Right Y Lacrimal Duct, Left	Ø Open 3 Percutaneous 7 Via Natural or Artificial Opening 8 Via Natural or Artificial Opening Endoscopic	Ø Drainage Device	Z No Qualifier
X Lacrimal Duct, Right Y Lacrimal Duct, Left	Ø Open 3 Percutaneous 7 Via Natural or Artificial Opening 8 Via Natural or Artificial Opening Endoscopic	Z No Device	X Diagnostic Z No Qualifier

Non-OR Ø89[NPQR][Ø3X]ØZ
Non-OR Ø89[NPQR][Ø3X]ZZ

Ø: M/S

8: EYE

9: DRAINAGE

New/Revised Text in Green ~~deleted~~ Deleted ♀ Females Only ♂ Males Only **Coding Clinic**
⚕ Non-covered ⚕ Limited Coverage ⊞ Combination (See Appendix E) DRG Non-OR Non-OR ⚕ Hospital-Acquired Condition

163

SECTION: Ø MEDICAL AND SURGICAL

BODY SYSTEM: 8 EYE

OPERATION: B EXCISION: Cutting out or off, without replacement, a portion of a body part

Body Part	Approach	Device	Qualifier
Ø Eye, Right 1 Eye, Left N Upper Eyelid, Right P Upper Eyelid, Left Q Lower Eyelid, Right R Lower Eyelid, Left	Ø Open 3 Percutaneous X External	Z No Device	X Diagnostic Z No Qualifier
4 Vitreous, Right 5 Vitreous, Left C Iris, Right ⊞ D Iris, Left ⊞ E Retina, Right F Retina, Left J Lens, Right K Lens, Left	3 Percutaneous	Z No Device	X Diagnostic Z No Qualifier
6 Sclera, Right ⊞ 7 Sclera, Left ⊞ 8 Cornea, Right 9 Cornea, Left S Conjunctiva, Right T Conjunctiva, Left	X External	Z No Device	X Diagnostic Z No Qualifier
A Choroid, Right B Choroid, Left L Extraocular Muscle, Right M Extraocular Muscle, Left V Lacrimal Gland, Right W Lacrimal Gland, Left	Ø Open 3 Percutaneous	Z No Device	X Diagnostic Z No Qualifier
X Lacrimal Duct, Right Y Lacrimal Duct, Left	Ø Open 3 Percutaneous 7 Via Natural or Artificial Opening 8 Via Natural or Artificial Opening Endoscopic	Z No Device	X Diagnostic Z No Qualifier

⊞ Ø8B[67]XZZ
⊞ Ø8B[CD]3ZZ

New/Revised Text in Green   ~~deleted~~ Deleted   ♀ Females Only   ♂ Males Only   **Coding Clinic**
 Non-covered   Limited Coverage   ⊞ Combination (See Appendix E)   DRG Non-OR   Non-OR   Hospital-Acquired Condition

SECTION: Ø MEDICAL AND SURGICAL

BODY SYSTEM: 8 EYE

OPERATION: C EXTIRPATION: Taking or cutting out solid matter from a body part

Body Part	Approach	Device	Qualifier
Ø Eye, Right 1 Eye, Left 6 Sclera, Right 7 Sclera, Left 8 Cornea, Right 9 Cornea, Left S Conjunctiva, Right T Conjunctiva, Left	X External	Z No Device	Z No Qualifier
2 Anterior Chamber, Right 3 Anterior Chamber, Left 4 Vitreous, Right 5 Vitreous, Left C Iris, Right D Iris, Left E Retina, Right F Retina, Left G Retinal Vessel, Right H Retinal Vessel, Left J Lens, Right K Lens, Left	3 Percutaneous X External	Z No Device	Z No Qualifier
A Choroid, Right B Choroid, Left L Extraocular Muscle, Right M Extraocular Muscle, Left N Upper Eyelid, Right P Upper Eyelid, Left Q Lower Eyelid, Right R Lower Eyelid, Left V Lacrimal Gland, Right W Lacrimal Gland, Left	Ø Open 3 Percutaneous X External	Z No Device	Z No Qualifier
X Lacrimal Duct, Right Y Lacrimal Duct, Left	Ø Open 3 Percutaneous 7 Via Natural or Artificial Opening 8 Via Natural or Artificial Opening Endoscopic	Z No Device	Z No Qualifier

Non-OR 08C[23]XZZ
Non-OR 08C[67]XZZ
Non-OR 08C[NPQR][03X]ZZ

SECTION: Ø MEDICAL AND SURGICAL

BODY SYSTEM: 8 EYE

OPERATION: D EXTRACTION: Pulling or stripping out or off all or a portion of a body part by the use of force

Body Part	Approach	Device	Qualifier
8 Cornea, Right 9 Cornea, Left	X External	Z No Device	X Diagnostic Z No Qualifier
J Lens, Right K Lens, Left	3 Percutaneous	Z No Device	Z No Qualifier

SECTION: Ø MEDICAL AND SURGICAL

BODY SYSTEM: 8 EYE

OPERATION: F FRAGMENTATION: Breaking solid matter in a body part into pieces

Body Part	Approach	Device	Qualifier
4 Vitreous, Right 🜲 5 Vitreous, Left 🜲	3 Percutaneous X External	Z No Device	Z No Qualifier

🜲 08F[45]XZZ

Non-OR 08F[45]XZZ

SECTION: Ø MEDICAL AND SURGICAL

BODY SYSTEM: 8 EYE

OPERATION: H INSERTION: Putting in a nonbiological appliance that monitors, assists, performs, or prevents a physiological function but does not physically take the place of a body part

Body Part	Approach	Device	Qualifier
Ø Eye, Right 1 Eye, Left	Ø Open	5 Epiretinal Visual Prosthesis	Z No Qualifier
Ø Eye, Right 1 Eye, Left	3 Percutaneous X External	1 Radioactive Element 3 Infusion Device	Z No Qualifier

SECTION: Ø MEDICAL AND SURGICAL

BODY SYSTEM: 8 EYE

OPERATION: J INSPECTION: Visually and/or manually exploring a body part

Body Part	Approach	Device	Qualifier
Ø Eye, Right 1 Eye, Left J Lens, Right K Lens, Left	X External	Z No Device	Z No Qualifier
L Extraocular Muscle, Right M Extraocular Muscle, Left	Ø Open X External	Z No Device	Z No Qualifier

DRG Non-OR 08J[Ø1JK]XZZ

DRG Non-OR 08J[LM]XZZ

Coding Clinic: 2015, Q1, P36 – 08JØXZZ

SECTION: Ø MEDICAL AND SURGICAL

BODY SYSTEM: 8 EYE

OPERATION: L OCCLUSION: Completely closing an orifice or the lumen of a tubular body part

Body Part	Approach	Device	Qualifier
X Lacrimal Duct, Right Y Lacrimal Duct, Left	Ø Open 3 Percutaneous	C Extraluminal Device D Intraluminal Device Z No Device	Z No Qualifier
X Lacrimal Duct, Right Y Lacrimal Duct, Left	7 Via Natural or Artificial Opening 8 Via Natural or Artificial Opening Endoscopic	D Intraluminal Device Z No Device	Z No Qualifier

Side tab (vertical): L: OCCLUSION J: INSPECTION H: INSERTION F: FRAGMENTATION 8: EYE Ø: M/S

SECTION: Ø MEDICAL AND SURGICAL

BODY SYSTEM: 8 EYE

OPERATION: M REATTACHMENT: Putting back in or on all or a portion of a separated body part to its normal location or other suitable location

Body Part	Approach	Device	Qualifier
N Upper Eyelid, Right P Upper Eyelid, Left Q Lower Eyelid, Right R Lower Eyelid, Left	X External	Z No Device	Z No Qualifier

SECTION: Ø MEDICAL AND SURGICAL

BODY SYSTEM: 8 EYE

OPERATION: N RELEASE: Freeing a body part from an abnormal physical constraint by cutting or by the use of force

Body Part	Approach	Device	Qualifier
Ø Eye, Right 1 Eye, Left 6 Sclera, Right 7 Sclera, Left 8 Cornea, Right 9 Cornea, Left S Conjunctiva, Right T Conjunctiva, Left	X External	Z No Device	Z No Qualifier
2 Anterior Chamber, Right 3 Anterior Chamber, Left 4 Vitreous, Right 5 Vitreous, Left C Iris, Right D Iris, Left E Retina, Right F Retina, Left G Retinal Vessel, Right H Retinal Vessel, Left J Lens, Right K Lens, Left	3 Percutaneous	Z No Device	Z No Qualifier
A Choroid, Right B Choroid, Left L Extraocular Muscle, Right M Extraocular Muscle, Left V Lacrimal Gland, Right W Lacrimal Gland, Left	Ø Open 3 Percutaneous	Z No Device	Z No Qualifier
N Upper Eyelid, Right P Upper Eyelid, Left Q Lower Eyelid, Right R Lower Eyelid, Left	Ø Open 3 Percutaneous X External	Z No Device	Z No Qualifier
X Lacrimal Duct, Right Y Lacrimal Duct, Left	Ø Open 3 Percutaneous 7 Via Natural or Artificial Opening 8 Via Natural or Artificial Opening Endoscopic	Z No Device	Z No Qualifier

Coding Clinic: 2015, Q2, P25 – 08NC3ZZ

New/Revised Text in Green   deleted Deleted   ♀ Females Only   ♂ Males Only   Coding Clinic
Non-covered   Limited Coverage   ⊞ Combination (See Appendix E)   DRG Non-OR   Non-OR   Hospital-Acquired Condition

SECTION: 0 MEDICAL AND SURGICAL

BODY SYSTEM: 8 EYE

OPERATION: P REMOVAL: Taking out or off a device from a body part

Body Part	Approach	Device	Qualifier
0 Eye, Right 1 Eye, Left	0 Open 3 Percutaneous 7 Via Natural or Artificial Opening 8 Via Natural or Artificial Opening Endoscopic X External	0 Drainage Device 1 Radioactive Element 3 Infusion Device 7 Autologous Tissue Substitute C Extraluminal Device D Intraluminal Device J Synthetic Substitute K Nonautologous Tissue Substitute	Z No Qualifier
J Lens, Right K Lens, Left	3 Percutaneous	J Synthetic Substitute	Z No Qualifier
L Extraocular Muscle, Right M Extraocular Muscle, Left	0 Open 3 Percutaneous	0 Drainage Device 7 Autologous Tissue Substitute J Synthetic Substitute K Nonautologous Tissue Substitute	Z No Qualifier

DRG Non-OR 08P[01][78][03D]Z
Non-OR 08P0X[03CD]Z
Non-OR 08P1X[013CD]Z

P: REMOVAL

8: EYE

0: M/S

SECTION: Ø MEDICAL AND SURGICAL
BODY SYSTEM: 8 EYE
OPERATION: Q REPAIR: Restoring, to the extent possible, a body part to its normal anatomic structure and function

Body Part	Approach	Device	Qualifier
Ø Eye, Right 1 Eye, Left 6 Sclera, Right 7 Sclera, Left 8 Cornea, Right 🦠 9 Cornea, Left 🦠 S Conjunctiva, Right T Conjunctiva, Left	X External	Z No Device	Z No Qualifier
2 Anterior Chamber, Right 3 Anterior Chamber, Left 4 Vitreous, Right 5 Vitreous, Left C Iris, Right D Iris, Left E Retina, Right F Retina, Left G Retinal Vessel, Right H Retinal Vessel, Left J Lens, Right K Lens, Left	3 Percutaneous	Z No Device	Z No Qualifier
A Choroid, Right B Choroid, Left L Extraocular Muscle, Right M Extraocular Muscle, Left V Lacrimal Gland, Right W Lacrimal Gland, Left	Ø Open 3 Percutaneous	Z No Device	Z No Qualifier
N Upper Eyelid, Right P Upper Eyelid, Left Q Lower Eyelid, Right R Lower Eyelid, Left	Ø Open 3 Percutaneous X External	Z No Device	Z No Qualifier
X Lacrimal Duct, Right Y Lacrimal Duct, Left	Ø Open 3 Percutaneous 7 Via Natural or Artificial Opening 8 Via Natural or Artificial Opening Endoscopic	Z No Device	Z No Qualifier

🦠 08Q[89]XZZ
Non-OR 08Q[NPQR][03X]ZZ

0: M/S

8: EYE

Q: REPAIR

SECTION: Ø MEDICAL AND SURGICAL

BODY SYSTEM: 8 EYE

OPERATION: R REPLACEMENT: Putting in or on biological or synthetic material that physically takes the place and/or function of all or a portion of a body part

Body Part	Approach	Device	Qualifier
Ø Eye, Right 1 Eye, Left A Choroid, Right B Choroid, Left	Ø Open 3 Percutaneous	7 Autologous Tissue Substitute J Synthetic Substitute K Nonautologous Tissue Substitute	Z No Qualifier
4 Vitreous, Right 5 Vitreous, Left C Iris, Right D Iris, Left G Retinal Vessel, Right H Retinal Vessel, Left	3 Percutaneous	7 Autologous Tissue Substitute J Synthetic Substitute K Nonautologous Tissue Substitute	Z No Qualifier
6 Sclera, Right 7 Sclera, Left S Conjunctiva, Right T Conjunctiva, Left	X External	7 Autologous Tissue Substitute J Synthetic Substitute K Nonautologous Tissue Substitute	Z No Qualifier
8 Cornea, Right 9 Cornea, Left	3 Percutaneous X External	7 Autologous Tissue Substitute J Synthetic Substitute K Nonautologous Tissue Substitute	Z No Qualifier
J Lens, Right K Lens, Left	3 Percutaneous	Ø Synthetic Substitute, Intraocular Telescope 7 Autologous Tissue Substitute J Synthetic Substitute K Nonautologous Tissue Substitute	Z No Qualifier
N Upper Eyelid, Right P Upper Eyelid, Left Q Lower Eyelid, Right R Lower Eyelid, Left	Ø Open 3 Percutaneous X External	7 Autologous Tissue Substitute J Synthetic Substitute K Nonautologous Tissue Substitute	Z No Qualifier
X Lacrimal Duct, Right Y Lacrimal Duct, Left	Ø Open 3 Percutaneous 7 Via Natural or Artificial Opening 8 Via Natural or Artificial Opening Endoscopic	7 Autologous Tissue Substitute J Synthetic Substitute K Nonautologous Tissue Substitute	Z No Qualifier

Coding Clinic: 2Ø15, Q2, P25-26 – Ø8R8XKZ

New/Revised Text in Green ~~deleted~~ Deleted ♀ Females Only ♂ Males Only **Coding Clinic**

🚫 Non-covered   🚫 Limited Coverage   ⊞ Combination (See Appendix E)   DRG Non-OR   Non-OR   🚫 Hospital-Acquired Condition

SECTION: Ø MEDICAL AND SURGICAL

BODY SYSTEM: 8 EYE

OPERATION: **S REPOSITION:** Moving to its normal location, or other suitable location, all or a portion of a body part

Body Part	Approach	Device	Qualifier
C Iris, Right D Iris, Left G Retinal Vessel, Right H Retinal Vessel, Left J Lens, Right K Lens, Left	3 Percutaneous	Z No Device	Z No Qualifier
L Extraocular Muscle, Right M Extraocular Muscle, Left V Lacrimal Gland, Right W Lacrimal Gland, Left	Ø Open 3 Percutaneous	Z No Device	Z No Qualifier
N Upper Eyelid, Right ⊞ P Upper Eyelid, Left ⊞ Q Lower Eyelid, Right ⊞ R Lower Eyelid, Left ⊞	Ø Open 3 Percutaneous X External	Z No Device	Z No Qualifier
X Lacrimal Duct, Right Y Lacrimal Duct, Left	Ø Open 3 Percutaneous 7 Via Natural or Artificial Opening 8 Via Natural or Artificial Opening Endoscopic	Z No Device	Z No Qualifier

⊞ Ø8S[NPQR][Ø3X]ZZ

SECTION: Ø MEDICAL AND SURGICAL
BODY SYSTEM: 8 EYE
OPERATION: **T** **RESECTION:** Cutting out or off, without replacement, all of a body part

Body Part	Approach	Device	Qualifier
Ø Eye, Right ⊞ 1 Eye, Left ⊞ 8 Cornea, Right 9 Cornea, Left	X External	Z No Device	Z No Qualifier
4 Vitreous, Right 5 Vitreous, Left C Iris, Right D Iris, Left J Lens, Right K Lens, Left	3 Percutaneous	Z No Device	Z No Qualifier
L Extraocular Muscle, Right M Extraocular Muscle, Left V Lacrimal Gland, Right W Lacrimal Gland, Left	Ø Open 3 Percutaneous	Z No Device	Z No Qualifier
N Upper Eyelid, Right P Upper Eyelid, Left Q Lower Eyelid, Right R Lower Eyelid, Left	Ø Open X External	Z No Device	Z No Qualifier

X Lacrimal Duct, Right
Y Lacrimal Duct, Left
	Ø Open
	3 Percutaneous
	7 Via Natural or Artificial
	   Opening
	8 Via Natural or Artificial
	   Opening Endoscopic
		Z No Device	Z No Qualifier

⊞ Ø8T[Ø1]XZZ

Coding Clinic: 2Ø15, Q2, P13 – Ø8T1XZZ, Ø8T[MR]ØZZ

SECTION: Ø MEDICAL AND SURGICAL

BODY SYSTEM: 8 EYE

OPERATION: U **SUPPLEMENT:** Putting in or on biological or synthetic material that physically reinforces and/or augments the function of a portion of a body part

Body Part	Approach	Device	Qualifier
Ø Eye, Right 1 Eye, Left C Iris, Right D Iris, Left E Retina, Right F Retina, Left G Retinal Vessel, Right H Retinal Vessel, Left L Extraocular Muscle, Right M Extraocular Muscle, Left	Ø Open 3 Percutaneous	7 Autologous Tissue Substitute J Synthetic Substitute K Nonautologous Tissue Substitute	Z No Qualifier
8 Cornea, Right 🗫 9 Cornea, Left 🗫 N Upper Eyelid, Right P Upper Eyelid, Left Q Lower Eyelid, Right R Lower Eyelid, Left	Ø Open 3 Percutaneous X External	7 Autologous Tissue Substitute J Synthetic Substitute K Nonautologous Tissue Substitute	Z No Qualifier
X Lacrimal Duct, Right Y Lacrimal Duct, Left	Ø Open 3 Percutaneous 7 Via Natural or Artificial Opening 8 Via Natural or Artificial Opening Endoscopic	7 Autologous Tissue Substitute J Synthetic Substitute K Nonautologous Tissue Substitute	Z No Qualifier

🗫 Ø8U[89][Ø3X]KZ

SECTION: Ø MEDICAL AND SURGICAL

BODY SYSTEM: 8 EYE

OPERATION: V **RESTRICTION:** Partially closing an orifice or the lumen of a tubular body part

Body Part	Approach	Device	Qualifier
X Lacrimal Duct, Right Y Lacrimal Duct, Left	Ø Open 3 Percutaneous	C Extraluminal Device D Intraluminal Device Z No Device	Z No Qualifier
X Lacrimal Duct, Right Y Lacrimal Duct, Left	7 Via Natural or Artificial Opening 8 Via Natural or Artificial Opening Endoscopic	D Intraluminal Device Z No Device	Z No Qualifier

SECTION: ø MEDICAL AND SURGICAL

BODY SYSTEM: 8 EYE

OPERATION: W **REVISION:** Correcting, to the extent possible, a portion of a malfunctioning device or the positon of a displaced device

Body Part	Approach	Device	Qualifier
ø Eye, Right 1 Eye, Left	ø Open 3 Percutaneous 7 Via Natural or Artificial Opening 8 Via Natural or Artificial Opening Endoscopic X External	ø Drainage Device 3 Infusion Device 7 Autologous Tissue Substitute C Extraluminal Device D Intraluminal Device J Synthetic Substitute K Nonautologous Tissue Substitute	Z No Qualifier
J Lens, Right K Lens, Left	3 Percutaneous X External	J Synthetic Substitute	Z No Qualifier
L Extraocular Muscle, Right M Extraocular Muscle, Left	ø Open 3 Percutaneous	ø Drainage Device 7 Autologous Tissue Substitute J Synthetic Substitute K Nonautologous Tissue Substitute	Z No Qualifier

Non-OR ø8W[ø1]X[ø37CDJK]Z
Non-OR ø8W[JK]XJZ

SECTION: ø MEDICAL AND SURGICAL

BODY SYSTEM: 8 EYE

OPERATION: X **TRANSFER:** Moving, without taking out, all or a portion of a body part to another location to take over the function of all or a portion of a body part

Body Part	Approach	Device	Qualifier
L Extraocular Muscle, Right M Extraocular Muscle, Left	ø Open 3 Percutaneous	Z No Device	Z No Qualifier

(Left margin: W: REVISION   X: TRANSFER   8: EYE   ø: M/S)

New/Revised Text in Green   ~~deleted~~ Deleted   ♀ Females Only   ♂ Males Only   **Coding Clinic**

🏷 Non-covered   🏷 Limited Coverage   ⊞ Combination (See Appendix E)   DRG Non-OR   Non-OR   🏷 Hospital-Acquired Condition

SECTION: Ø MEDICAL AND SURGICAL

BODY SYSTEM: 9 EAR, NOSE, SINUS

OPERATION: Ø **ALTERATION:** Modifying the anatomic structure of a body part without affecting the function of the body part

Body Part	Approach	Device	Qualifier
Ø External Ear, Right 1 External Ear, Left 2 External Ear, Bilateral K Nose	Ø Open 3 Percutaneous 4 Percutaneous Endoscopic X External	7 Autologous Tissue Substitute J Synthetic Substitute K Nonautologous Tissue Substitute Z No Device	Z No Qualifier

SECTION: Ø MEDICAL AND SURGICAL

BODY SYSTEM: 9 EAR, NOSE, SINUS

OPERATION: 1 **BYPASS:** Altering the route of passage of the contents of a tubular body part

Body Part	Approach	Device	Qualifier
D Inner Ear, Right E Inner Ear, Left	Ø Open	7 Autologous Tissue Substitute J Synthetic Substitute K Nonautologous Tissue Substitute Z No Device	Ø Endolymphatic

SECTION: Ø MEDICAL AND SURGICAL

BODY SYSTEM: 9 EAR, NOSE, SINUS

OPERATION: 2 **CHANGE:** Taking out or off a device from a body part and putting back an identical or similar device in or on the same body part without cutting or puncturing the skin or a mucous membrane

Body Part	Approach	Device	Qualifier
H Ear, Right J Ear, Left K Nose Y Sinus	X External	Ø Drainage Device Y Other Device	Z No Qualifier

Non-OR All Values

Ø: ALTERATION 1: BYPASS 2: CHANGE

9: EAR, NOSE, SINUS

Ø: M/S

New/Revised Text in Green   deleted Deleted   ♀ Females Only   ♂ Males Only   **Coding Clinic**
🔖 Non-covered   🔖 Limited Coverage   ⊞ Combination (See Appendix E)   DRG Non-OR   Non-OR   🔖 Hospital-Acquired Condition

SECTION: 0 MEDICAL AND SURGICAL
BODY SYSTEM: 9 EAR, NOSE, SINUS
OPERATION: 5 DESTRUCTION: Physical eradication of all or a portion of a body part by the direct use of energy, force, or a destructive agent

Body Part	Approach	Device	Qualifier
0 External Ear, Right 1 External Ear, Left K Nose	0 Open 3 Percutaneous 4 Percutaneous Endoscopic X External	Z No Device	Z No Qualifier
3 External Auditory Canal, Right 4 External Auditory Canal, Left	0 Open 3 Percutaneous 4 Percutaneous Endoscopic 7 Via Natural or Artificial Opening 8 Via Natural or Artificial Opening Endoscopic X External	Z No Device	Z No Qualifier
5 Middle Ear, Right 6 Middle Ear, Left 9 Auditory Ossicle, Right A Auditory Ossicle, Left D Inner Ear, Right E Inner Ear, Left	0 Open	Z No Device	Z No Qualifier
7 Tympanic Membrane, Right 8 Tympanic Membrane, Left F Eustachian Tube, Right G Eustachian Tube, Left L Nasal Turbinate N Nasopharynx	0 Open 3 Percutaneous 4 Percutaneous Endoscopic 7 Via Natural or Artificial Opening 8 Via Natural or Artificial Opening Endoscopic	Z No Device	Z No Qualifier
B Mastoid Sinus, Right C Mastoid Sinus, Left M Nasal Septum P Accessory Sinus Q Maxillary Sinus, Right R Maxillary Sinus, Left S Frontal Sinus, Right T Frontal Sinus, Left U Ethmoid Sinus, Right V Ethmoid Sinus, Left W Sphenoid Sinus, Right X Sphenoid Sinus, Left	0 Open 3 Percutaneous 4 Percutaneous Endoscopic	Z No Device	Z No Qualifier

Non-OR 095[01K][034X]ZZ
Non-OR 095[34][03478X]ZZ
Non-OR 095[FG][03478]ZZ
Non-OR 095M[034]ZZ

0: M/S
9: EAR, NOSE, SINUS
5: DESTRUCTION

SECTION: Ø MEDICAL AND SURGICAL

BODY SYSTEM: 9 EAR, NOSE, SINUS

OPERATION: 7 DILATION: Expanding an orifice or the lumen of a tubular body part

Body Part	Approach	Device	Qualifier
F Eustachian Tube, Right G Eustachian Tube, Left	Ø Open 7 Via Natural or Artificial Opening 8 Via Natural or Artificial Opening Endoscopic	D Intraluminal Device Z No Device	Z No Qualifier
F Eustachian Tube, Right G Eustachian Tube, Left	3 Percutaneous 4 Percutaneous Endoscopic	Z No Device	Z No Qualifier

Non-OR All Values

SECTION: Ø MEDICAL AND SURGICAL

BODY SYSTEM: 9 EAR, NOSE, SINUS

OPERATION: 8 DIVISION: Cutting into a body part, without draining fluids and/or gases from the body part, in order to separate or transect a body part

Body Part	Approach	Device	Qualifier
L Nasal Turbinate	Ø Open 3 Percutaneous 4 Percutaneous Endoscopic 7 Via Natural or Artificial Opening 8 Via Natural or Artificial Opening Endoscopic	Z No Device	Z No Qualifier

SECTION: Ø MEDICAL AND SURGICAL
BODY SYSTEM: 9 EAR, NOSE, SINUS
OPERATION: 9 **DRAINAGE:** *(on multiple pages)*
Taking or letting out fluids and/or gases from a body part

Body Part	Approach	Device	Qualifier
Ø External Ear, Right 1 External Ear, Left K Nose	Ø Open 3 Percutaneous 4 Percutaneous Endoscopic X External	Ø Drainage Device	Z No Qualifier
Ø External Ear, Right 1 External Ear, Left K Nose	Ø Open 3 Percutaneous 4 Percutaneous Endoscopic X External	Z No Device	X Diagnostic Z No Qualifier
3 External Auditory Canal, Right 4 External Auditory Canal, Left	Ø Open 3 Percutaneous 4 Percutaneous Endoscopic 7 Via Natural or Artificial Opening 8 Via Natural or Artificial Opening Endoscopic X External	Ø Drainage Device	Z No Qualifier
3 External Auditory Canal, Right 4 External Auditory Canal, Left	Ø Open 3 Percutaneous 4 Percutaneous Endoscopic 7 Via Natural or Artificial Opening 8 Via Natural or Artificial Opening Endoscopic X External	Z No Device	X Diagnostic Z No Qualifier
5 Middle Ear, Right 6 Middle Ear, Left 9 Auditory Ossicle, Right A Auditory Ossicle, Left D Inner Ear, Right E Inner Ear, Left	Ø Open	Ø Drainage Device	Z No Qualifier
5 Middle Ear, Right 6 Middle Ear, Left 9 Auditory Ossicle, Right A Auditory Ossicle, Left D Inner Ear, Right E Inner Ear, Left	Ø Open	Z No Device	X Diagnostic Z No Qualifier
7 Tympanic Membrane, Right 8 Tympanic Membrane, Left F Eustachian Tube, Right G Eustachian Tube, Left L Nasal Turbinate N Nasopharynx	Ø Open 3 Percutaneous 4 Percutaneous Endoscopic 7 Via Natural or Artificial Opening 8 Via Natural or Artificial Opening Endoscopic	Ø Drainage Device	Z No Qualifier

DRG Non-OR   Ø99N3ØZ
Non-OR   Ø99[Ø1K][Ø34X]ØZ
Non-OR   Ø99[Ø1K][Ø34X]Z[XZ]
Non-OR   Ø99[34][Ø3478X]ØZ
Non-OR   Ø99[34][Ø3478X]Z[XZ]
Non-OR   Ø99[56]ØZZ
Non-OR   Ø99[FGL][Ø3478]ØZ

Ø: M/S

9: EAR, NOSE, SINUS

9: DRAINAGE

New/Revised Text in Green   ~~deleted~~ Deleted   ♀ Females Only   ♂ Males Only   **Coding Clinic**
Non-covered   Limited Coverage   ⊞ Combination (See Appendix E)   DRG Non-OR   Non-OR   Hospital-Acquired Condition

179

SECTION: Ø MEDICAL AND SURGICAL
BODY SYSTEM: 9 EAR, NOSE, SINUS
OPERATION: 9 DRAINAGE: *(continued)*
Taking or letting out fluids and/or gases from a body part

Body Part	Approach	Device	Qualifier
7 Tympanic Membrane, Right 8 Tympanic Membrane, Left F Eustachian Tube, Right G Eustachian Tube, Left L Nasal Turbinate N Nasopharynx	Ø Open 3 Percutaneous 4 Percutaneous Endoscopic 7 Via Natural or Artificial Opening 8 Via Natural or Artificial Opening Endoscopic	Z No Device	X Diagnostic Z No Qualifier
B Mastoid Sinus, Right C Mastoid Sinus, Left M Nasal Septum P Accessory Sinus Q Maxillary Sinus, Right R Maxillary Sinus, Left S Frontal Sinus, Right T Frontal Sinus, Left U Ethmoid Sinus, Right V Ethmoid Sinus, Left W Sphenoid Sinus, Right X Sphenoid Sinus, Left	Ø Open 3 Percutaneous 4 Percutaneous Endoscopic	Ø Drainage Device	Z No Qualifier
B Mastoid Sinus, Right C Mastoid Sinus, Left M Nasal Septum P Accessory Sinus Q Maxillary Sinus, Right R Maxillary Sinus, Left S Frontal Sinus, Right T Frontal Sinus, Left U Ethmoid Sinus, Right V Ethmoid Sinus, Left W Sphenoid Sinus, Right X Sphenoid Sinus, Left	Ø Open 3 Percutaneous 4 Percutaneous Endoscopic	Z No Device	X Diagnostic Z No Qualifier

DRG Non-OR   Ø99N3ZZ
DRG Non-OR   Ø99[BC]3ØZ
DRG Non-OR   Ø99[BC]3ZZ
Non-OR   Ø99[78FG][Ø3478]ZZ
Non-OR   Ø99L[Ø3478]Z[XZ]
Non-OR   Ø99N[Ø3478]ZX
Non-OR   Ø99M[Ø34]ØZ
Non-OR   Ø99[PQRSTUVWX][34]ØZ
Non-OR   Ø99M[Ø34]Z[XZ]
Non-OR   Ø99[PQRSTUVWX][34]Z[XZ]

9: DRAINAGE

9: EAR, NOSE, SINUS

Ø: M/S

New/Revised Text in Green   ~~deleted~~ Deleted   ♀ Females Only   ♂ Males Only   **Coding Clinic**
Non-covered   Limited Coverage   ⊕ Combination (See Appendix E)   DRG Non-OR   Non-OR   Hospital-Acquired Condition

SECTION: 0 MEDICAL AND SURGICAL
BODY SYSTEM: 9 EAR, NOSE, SINUS
OPERATION: B EXCISION: Cutting out or off, without replacement, a portion of a body part

Body Part	Approach	Device	Qualifier
0 External Ear, Right 1 External Ear, Left K Nose	0 Open 3 Percutaneous 4 Percutaneous Endoscopic X External	Z No Device	X Diagnostic Z No Qualifier
3 External Auditory Canal, Right 4 External Auditory Canal, Left	0 Open 3 Percutaneous 4 Percutaneous Endoscopic 7 Via Natural or Artificial Opening 8 Via Natural or Artificial Opening Endoscopic X External	Z No Device	X Diagnostic Z No Qualifier
5 Middle Ear, Right 6 Middle Ear, Left 9 Auditory Ossicle, Right A Auditory Ossicle, Left D Inner Ear, Right E Inner Ear, Left	0 Open	Z No Device	X Diagnostic Z No Qualifier
7 Tympanic Membrane, Right 8 Tympanic Membrane, Left F Eustachian Tube, Right G Eustachian Tube, Left L Nasal Turbinate N Nasopharynx	0 Open 3 Percutaneous 4 Percutaneous Endoscopic 7 Via Natural or Artificial Opening 8 Via Natural or Artificial Opening Endoscopic	Z No Device	X Diagnostic Z No Qualifier
B Mastoid Sinus, Right C Mastoid Sinus, Left M Nasal Septum P Accessory Sinus Q Maxillary Sinus, Right R Maxillary Sinus, Left S Frontal Sinus, Right T Frontal Sinus, Left U Ethmoid Sinus, Right V Ethmoid Sinus, Left W Sphenoid Sinus, Right X Sphenoid Sinus, Left	0 Open 3 Percutaneous 4 Percutaneous Endoscopic	Z No Device	X Diagnostic Z No Qualifier

Non-OR 09B[01K][034X]Z[XZ]
Non-OR 09B[34][03478X]Z[XZ]
Non-OR 09B[FG][03478]Z[XZ]
Non-OR 09B[LN][03478]ZX
Non-OR 09BM[034]ZX
Non-OR 09B[PQRSTUVWX][34]ZX

0: M/S

9: EAR, NOSE, SINUS

B: EXCISION

SECTION: Ø MEDICAL AND SURGICAL

BODY SYSTEM: 9 EAR, NOSE, SINUS

OPERATION: C EXTIRPATION: Taking or cutting out solid matter from a body part

Body Part	Approach	Device	Qualifier
Ø External Ear, Right 1 External Ear, Left K Nose	Ø Open 3 Percutaneous 4 Percutaneous Endoscopic X External	Z No Device	Z No Qualifier
3 External Auditory Canal, Right 4 External Auditory Canal, Left	Ø Open 3 Percutaneous 4 Percutaneous Endoscopic 7 Via Natural or Artificial Opening 8 Via Natural or Artificial Opening Endoscopic X External	Z No Device	Z No Qualifier
5 Middle Ear, Right 6 Middle Ear, Left 9 Auditory Ossicle, Right A Auditory Ossicle, Left D Inner Ear, Right E Inner Ear, Left	Ø Open	Z No Device	Z No Qualifier
7 Tympanic Membrane, Right 8 Tympanic Membrane, Left F Eustachian Tube, Right G Eustachian Tube, Left L Nasal Turbinate N Nasopharynx	Ø Open 3 Percutaneous 4 Percutaneous Endoscopic 7 Via Natural or Artificial Opening 8 Via Natural or Artificial Opening Endoscopic	Z No Device	Z No Qualifier
B Mastoid Sinus, Right C Mastoid Sinus, Left M Nasal Septum P Accessory Sinus Q Maxillary Sinus, Right R Maxillary Sinus, Left S Frontal Sinus, Right T Frontal Sinus, Left U Ethmoid Sinus, Right V Ethmoid Sinus, Left W Sphenoid Sinus, Right X Sphenoid Sinus, Left	Ø Open 3 Percutaneous 4 Percutaneous Endoscopic	Z No Device	Z No Qualifier

Non-OR Ø9C[Ø1K][Ø34X]ZZ
Non-OR Ø9C[34][Ø3478X]ZZ
Non-OR Ø9C[78FGL][Ø3478]ZZ
Non-OR Ø9CM[Ø34]ZZ

C: EXTIRPATION

9: EAR, NOSE, SINUS

Ø: M/S

New/Revised Text in Green · ~~deleted~~ Deleted · ♀ Females Only · ♂ Males Only · **Coding Clinic**
Non-covered · Limited Coverage · ⊕ Combination (See Appendix E) · DRG Non-OR · Non-OR · Hospital-Acquired Condition

SECTION: Ø MEDICAL AND SURGICAL

BODY SYSTEM: 9 EAR, NOSE, SINUS

OPERATION: D EXTRACTION: Pulling or stripping out or off all or a portion of a body part by the use of force

Body Part	Approach	Device	Qualifier
7 Tympanic Membrane, Right 8 Tympanic Membrane, Left L Nasal Turbinate	Ø Open 3 Percutaneous 4 Percutaneous Endoscopic 7 Via Natural or Artificial Opening 8 Via Natural or Artificial Opening Endoscopic	Z No Device	Z No Qualifier
9 Auditory Ossicle, Right A Auditory Ossicle, Left	Ø Open	Z No Device	Z No Qualifier
B Mastoid Sinus, Right C Mastoid Sinus, Left M Nasal Septum P Accessory Sinus Q Maxillary Sinus, Right R Maxillary Sinus, Left S Frontal Sinus, Right T Frontal Sinus, Left U Ethmoid Sinus, Right V Ethmoid Sinus, Left W Sphenoid Sinus, Right X Sphenoid Sinus, Left	Ø Open 3 Percutaneous 4 Percutaneous Endoscopic	Z No Device	Z No Qualifier

SECTION: Ø MEDICAL AND SURGICAL

BODY SYSTEM: 9 EAR, NOSE, SINUS

OPERATION: H INSERTION: Putting in a nonbiological appliance that monitors, assists, performs, or prevents a physiological function but does not physically take the place of a body part

Body Part	Approach	Device	Qualifier
D Inner Ear, Right E Inner Ear, Left	Ø Open 3 Percutaneous 4 Percutaneous Endoscopic	4 Hearing Device, Bone Conduction 5 Hearing Device, Single Channel Cochlear Prosthesis 6 Hearing Device, Multiple Channel Cochlear Prosthesis S Hearing Device	Z No Qualifier
N Nasopharynx	7 Via Natural or Artificial Opening 8 Via Natural or Artificial Opening Endoscopic	B Intraluminal Device, Airway	Z No Qualifier

Non-OR Ø9HN[78]BZ

SECTION: Ø MEDICAL AND SURGICAL
BODY SYSTEM: 9 EAR, NOSE, SINUS
OPERATION: J INSPECTION: Visually and/or manually exploring a body part

Body Part	Approach	Device	Qualifier
7 Tympanic Membrane, Right 8 Tympanic Membrane, Left H Ear, Right J Ear, Left	Ø Open 3 Percutaneous 4 Percutaneous Endoscopic 7 Via Natural or Artificial Opening 8 Via Natural or Artificial Opening Endoscopic X External	Z No Device	Z No Qualifier
D Inner Ear, Right E Inner Ear, Left K Nose Y Sinus	Ø Open 3 Percutaneous 4 Percutaneous Endoscopic X External	Z No Device	Z No Qualifier

DRG Non-OR Ø9J[78][37X]ZZ
DRG Non-OR Ø9J[DE][3X]ZZ
Non-OR Ø9J[78]8ZZ
Non-OR Ø9J[HJ][Ø3478X]ZZ
Non-OR Ø9J[KY][Ø34X]ZZ

SECTION: Ø MEDICAL AND SURGICAL
BODY SYSTEM: 9 EAR, NOSE, SINUS
OPERATION: M REATTACHMENT: Putting back in or on all or a portion of a separated body part to its normal location or other suitable location

Body Part	Approach	Device	Qualifier
Ø External Ear, Right 1 External Ear, Left K Nose	X External	Z No Device	Z No Qualifier

SECTION: Ø MEDICAL AND SURGICAL

BODY SYSTEM: 9 EAR, NOSE, SINUS

OPERATION: N RELEASE: Freeing a body part from an abnormal physical constraint

Body Part	Approach	Device	Qualifier
Ø External Ear, Right 1 External Ear, Left K Nose	Ø Open 3 Percutaneous 4 Percutaneous Endoscopic X External	Z No Device	Z No Qualifier
3 External Auditory Canal, Right 4 External Auditory Canal, Left	Ø Open 3 Percutaneous 4 Percutaneous Endoscopic 7 Via Natural or Artificial Opening 8 Via Natural or Artificial Opening Endoscopic X External	Z No Device	Z No Qualifier
5 Middle Ear, Right 6 Middle Ear, Left 9 Auditory Ossicle, Right A Auditory Ossicle, Left D Inner Ear, Right E Inner Ear, Left	Ø Open	Z No Device	Z No Qualifier
7 Tympanic Membrane, Right 8 Tympanic Membrane, Left F Eustachian Tube, Right G Eustachian Tube, Left L Nasal Turbinate N Nasopharynx	Ø Open 3 Percutaneous 4 Percutaneous Endoscopic 7 Via Natural or Artificial Opening 8 Via Natural or Artificial Opening Endoscopic	Z No Device	Z No Qualifier
B Mastoid Sinus, Right C Mastoid Sinus, Left M Nasal Septum P Accessory Sinus Q Maxillary Sinus, Right R Maxillary Sinus, Left S Frontal Sinus, Right T Frontal Sinus, Left U Ethmoid Sinus, Right V Ethmoid Sinus, Left W Sphenoid Sinus, Right X Sphenoid Sinus, Left	Ø Open 3 Percutaneous 4 Percutaneous Endoscopic	Z No Device	Z No Qualifier

Non-OR Ø9NK[Ø34X]ZZ
Non-OR Ø9N[FGL][Ø3478]ZZ
Non-OR Ø9NM[Ø34]ZZ

New/Revised Text in Green   ~~deleted~~ Deleted   ♀ Females Only   ♂ Males Only   **Coding Clinic**
Non-covered   Limited Coverage   ⊕ Combination (See Appendix E)   DRG Non-OR   Non-OR   Hospital-Acquired Condition

185

SECTION: Ø MEDICAL AND SURGICAL
BODY SYSTEM: 9 EAR, NOSE, SINUS
OPERATION: P REMOVAL: Taking out or off a device from a body part

Body Part	Approach	Device	Qualifier
7 Tympanic Membrane, Right 8 Tympanic Membrane, Left	Ø Open 7 Via Natural or Artificial Opening 8 Via Natural or Artificial Opening Endoscopic X External	Ø Drainage Device	Z No Qualifier
D Inner Ear, Right E Inner Ear, Left	Ø Open 7 Via Natural or Artificial Opening 8 Via Natural or Artificial Opening Endoscopic	S Hearing Device	Z No Qualifier
H Ear, Right J Ear, Left K Nose	Ø Open 3 Percutaneous 4 Percutaneous Endoscopic 7 Via Natural or Artificial Opening 8 Via Natural or Artificial Opening Endoscopic X External	Ø Drainage Device 7 Autologous Tissue Substitute D Intraluminal Device J Synthetic Substitute K Nonautologous Tissue Substitute	Z No Qualifier
Y Sinus	Ø Open 3 Percutaneous 4 Percutaneous Endoscopic X External	Ø Drainage Device	Z No Qualifier

Non-OR Ø9P[78][Ø78X]ØZ
Non-OR Ø9P[HJ][34][ØJK]Z
Non-OR Ø9P[HJ][78][ØD]Z
Non-OR Ø9P[HJ]X[Ø7DJK]Z
Non-OR Ø9PK[Ø3478X][Ø7DJK]Z
Non-OR Ø9PYXØZ

SECTION: Ø MEDICAL AND SURGICAL
BODY SYSTEM: 9 EAR, NOSE, SINUS
OPERATION: Q **REPAIR:** Restoring, to the extent possible, a body part to its normal anatomic structure and function

Body Part	Approach	Device	Qualifier
Ø External Ear, Right 1 External Ear, Left 2 External Ear, Bilateral K Nose ⊞	Ø Open 3 Percutaneous 4 Percutaneous Endoscopic X External	Z No Device	Z No Qualifier
3 External Auditory Canal, Right 4 External Auditory Canal, Left F Eustachian Tube, Right G Eustachian Tube, Left	Ø Open 3 Percutaneous 4 Percutaneous Endoscopic 7 Via Natural or Artificial Opening 8 Via Natural or Artificial Opening Endoscopic X External	Z No Device	Z No Qualifier
5 Middle Ear, Right 6 Middle Ear, Left 9 Auditory Ossicle, Right A Auditory Ossicle, Left D Inner Ear, Right E Inner Ear, Left	Ø Open	Z No Device	Z No Qualifier
7 Tympanic Membrane, Right 8 Tympanic Membrane, Left L Nasal Turbinate N Nasopharynx	Ø Open 3 Percutaneous 4 Percutaneous Endoscopic 7 Via Natural or Artificial Opening 8 Via Natural or Artificial Opening Endoscopic	Z No Device	Z No Qualifier
B Mastoid Sinus, Right C Mastoid Sinus, Left M Nasal Septum P Accessory Sinus Q Maxillary Sinus, Right ⊞ R Maxillary Sinus, Left S Frontal Sinus, Right T Frontal Sinus, Left U Ethmoid Sinus, Right V Ethmoid Sinus, Left W Sphenoid Sinus, Right X Sphenoid Sinus, Left	Ø Open 3 Percutaneous 4 Percutaneous Endoscopic	Z No Device	Z No Qualifier

⊞ 09QK[034]ZZ
⊞ 09QQ[034]ZZ
Non-OR 09Q[012]XZZ
Non-OR 09Q[34]XZZ
Non-OR 09Q[FG][03478X]ZZ

SECTION: Ø MEDICAL AND SURGICAL

BODY SYSTEM: 9 EAR, NOSE, SINUS

OPERATION: R **REPLACEMENT:** Putting in or on biological or synthetic material that physically takes the place and/or function of all or a portion of a body part

Body Part	Approach	Device	Qualifier
Ø External Ear, Right 1 External Ear, Left 2 External Ear, Bilateral K Nose	Ø Open X External	7 Autologous Tissue Substitute J Synthetic Substitute K Nonautologous Tissue Substitute	Z No Qualifier
5 Middle Ear, Right 6 Middle Ear, Left 9 Auditory Ossicle, Right A Auditory Ossicle, Left D Inner Ear, Right E Inner Ear, Left	Ø Open	7 Autologous Tissue Substitute J Synthetic Substitute K Nonautologous Tissue Substitute	Z No Qualifier
7 Tympanic Membrane, Right 8 Tympanic Membrane, Left N Nasopharynx	Ø Open 7 Via Natural or Artificial Opening 8 Via Natural or Artificial Opening Endoscopic	7 Autologous Tissue Substitute J Synthetic Substitute K Nonautologous Tissue Substitute	Z No Qualifier
L Nasal Turbinate	Ø Open 3 Percutaneous 4 Percutaneous Endoscopic 7 Via Natural or Artificial Opening 8 Via Natural or Artificial Opening Endoscopic	7 Autologous Tissue Substitute J Synthetic Substitute K Nonautologous Tissue Substitute	Z No Qualifier
M Nasal Septum	Ø Open 3 Percutaneous 4 Percutaneous Endoscopic	7 Autologous Tissue Substitute J Synthetic Substitute K Nonautologous Tissue Substitute	Z No Qualifier

SECTION: Ø MEDICAL AND SURGICAL

BODY SYSTEM: 9 EAR, NOSE, SINUS

OPERATION: S **REPOSITION:** Moving to its normal location, or other suitable location, all or a portion of a body part

Body Part	Approach	Device	Qualifier
Ø External Ear, Right 1 External Ear, Left 2 External Ear, Bilateral K Nose	Ø Open 4 Percutaneous Endoscopic X External	Z No Device	Z No Qualifier
7 Tympanic Membrane, Right 8 Tympanic Membrane, Left F Eustachian Tube, Right G Eustachian Tube, Left L Nasal Turbinate	Ø Open 4 Percutaneous Endoscopic 7 Via Natural or Artificial Opening 8 Via Natural or Artificial Opening Endoscopic	Z No Device	Z No Qualifier
9 Auditory Ossicle, Right A Auditory Ossicle, Left M Nasal Septum	Ø Open 4 Percutaneous Endoscopic	Z No Device	Z No Qualifier

Non-OR 09S[FG][0478]ZZ

New/Revised Text in Green   ~~deleted~~ Deleted   ♀ Females Only   ♂ Males Only   **Coding Clinic**

🔹 Non-covered   🔹 Limited Coverage   ⊞ Combination (See Appendix E)   DRG Non-OR   Non-OR   🔹 Hospital-Acquired Condition

R: REPLACEMENT   S: REPOSITION

9: EAR, NOSE, SINUS

Ø: M/S

SECTION: Ø MEDICAL AND SURGICAL
BODY SYSTEM: 9 EAR, NOSE, SINUS
OPERATION: T RESECTION: Cutting out or off, without replacement, all of a body part

Body Part	Approach	Device	Qualifier
Ø External Ear, Right 1 External Ear, Left K Nose	Ø Open 4 Percutaneous Endoscopic X External	Z No Device	Z No Qualifier
5 Middle Ear, Right 6 Middle Ear, Left 9 Auditory Ossicle, Right A Auditory Ossicle, Left D Inner Ear, Right E Inner Ear, Left	Ø Open	Z No Device	Z No Qualifier
7 Tympanic Membrane, Right 8 Tympanic Membrane, Left F Eustachian Tube, Right G Eustachian Tube, Left L Nasal Turbinate N Nasopharynx	Ø Open 4 Percutaneous Endoscopic 7 Via Natural or Artificial Opening 8 Via Natural or Artificial Opening Endoscopic	Z No Device	Z No Qualifier
B Mastoid Sinus, Right C Mastoid Sinus, Left M Nasal Septum P Accessory Sinus Q Maxillary Sinus, Right R Maxillary Sinus, Left S Frontal Sinus, Right T Frontal Sinus, Left U Ethmoid Sinus, Right V Ethmoid Sinus, Left W Sphenoid Sinus, Right X Sphenoid Sinus, Left	Ø Open 4 Percutaneous Endoscopic	Z No Device	Z No Qualifier

Non-OR 09T[FG][0478]ZZ

SECTION: Ø MEDICAL AND SURGICAL
BODY SYSTEM: 9 EAR, NOSE, SINUS
OPERATION: U SUPPLEMENT: Putting in or on biological or synthetic material that physically reinforces and/or augments the function of a portion of a body part

Body Part	Approach	Device	Qualifier
Ø External Ear, Right 1 External Ear, Left 2 External Ear, Bilateral K Nose	Ø Open X External	7 Autologous Tissue Substitute J Synthetic Substitute K Nonautologous Tissue Substitute	Z No Qualifier
5 Middle Ear, Right 6 Middle Ear, Left 9 Auditory Ossicle, Right A Auditory Ossicle, Left D Inner Ear, Right E Inner Ear, Left	Ø Open	7 Autologous Tissue Substitute J Synthetic Substitute K Nonautologous Tissue Substitute	Z No Qualifier
7 Tympanic Membrane, Right 8 Tympanic Membrane, Left N Nasopharynx	Ø Open 7 Via Natural or Artificial Opening 8 Via Natural or Artificial Opening Endoscopic	7 Autologous Tissue Substitute J Synthetic Substitute K Nonautologous Tissue Substitute	Z No Qualifier
L Nasal Turbinate	Ø Open 3 Percutaneous 4 Percutaneous Endoscopic 7 Via Natural or Artificial Opening 8 Via Natural or Artificial Opening Endoscopic	7 Autologous Tissue Substitute J Synthetic Substitute K Nonautologous Tissue Substitute	Z No Qualifier
M Nasal Septum	Ø Open 3 Percutaneous 4 Percutaneous Endoscopic	7 Autologous Tissue Substitute J Synthetic Substitute K Nonautologous Tissue Substitute	Z No Qualifier

SECTION: Ø MEDICAL AND SURGICAL
BODY SYSTEM: 9 EAR, NOSE, SINUS
OPERATION: W REVISION: Correcting, to the extent possible, a portion of a malfunctioning device or the position of a displaced device

Body Part	Approach	Device	Qualifier
7 Tympanic Membrane, Right 8 Tympanic Membrane, Left 9 Auditory Ossicle, Right A Auditory Ossicle, Left	Ø Open 7 Via Natural or Artificial Opening 8 Via Natural or Artificial Opening Endoscopic	7 Autologous Tissue Substitute J Synthetic Substitute K Nonautologous Tissue Substitute	Z No Qualifier
D Inner Ear, Right E Inner Ear, Left	Ø Open 7 Via Natural or Artificial Opening 8 Via Natural or Artificial Opening Endoscopic	S Hearing Device	Z No Qualifier
H Ear, Right J Ear, Left K Nose	Ø Open 3 Percutaneous 4 Percutaneous Endoscopic 7 Via Natural or Artificial Opening 8 Via Natural or Artificial Opening Endoscopic X External	Ø Drainage Device 7 Autologous Tissue Substitute D Intraluminal Device J Synthetic Substitute K Nonautologous Tissue Substitute	Z No Qualifier
Y Sinus	Ø Open 3 Percutaneous 4 Percutaneous Endoscopic X External	Ø Drainage Device	Z No Qualifier

Non-OR 09W[HJ][34][JK]Z
Non-OR 09W[HJ][78]DZ
Non-OR 09W[HJ]X[07DJK]Z
Non-OR 09WK[03478X][07DJK]Z
Non-OR 09WYX0Z

SECTION: Ø MEDICAL AND SURGICAL
BODY SYSTEM: **B** RESPIRATORY SYSTEM
OPERATION: **1** **BYPASS:** Altering the route of passage of the contents of a tubular body part

Body Part	Approach	Device	Qualifier
1 Trachea	Ø Open	D Intraluminal Device	6 Esophagus
1 Trachea	Ø Open	F Tracheostomy Device Z No Device	4 Cutaneous
1 Trachea	3 Percutaneous 4 Percutaneous Endoscopic	F Tracheostomy Device Z No Device	4 Cutaneous

DRG Non-OR   ØB113[FZ]4
Non-OR   ØB110D6

SECTION: Ø MEDICAL AND SURGICAL
BODY SYSTEM: **B** RESPIRATORY SYSTEM
OPERATION: **2** **CHANGE:** Taking out or off a device from a body part and putting back an identical or similar device in or on the same body part without cutting or puncturing the skin or a mucous membrane

Body Part	Approach	Device	Qualifier
Ø Tracheobronchial Tree K Lung, Right L Lung, Left Q Pleura T Diaphragm	X External	Ø Drainage Device Y Other Device	Z No Qualifier
1 Trachea	X External	Ø Drainage Device E Intraluminal Device, Endotracheal Airway F Tracheostomy Device Y Other Device	Z No Qualifier

Non-OR   All Values

SECTION: Ø MEDICAL AND SURGICAL

BODY SYSTEM: B RESPIRATORY SYSTEM

OPERATION: 5 **DESTRUCTION:** Physical eradication of all or a portion of a body part by the direct use of energy, force, or a destructive agent

Body Part	Approach	Device	Qualifier
1 Trachea 2 Carina 3 Main Bronchus, Right 4 Upper Lobe Bronchus, Right 5 Middle Lobe Bronchus, Right 6 Lower Lobe Bronchus, Right 7 Main Bronchus, Left 8 Upper Lobe Bronchus, Left 9 Lingula Bronchus B Lower Lobe Bronchus, Left C Upper Lung Lobe, Right D Middle Lung Lobe, Right F Lower Lung Lobe, Right G Upper Lung Lobe, Left H Lung Lingula J Lower Lung Lobe, Left K Lung, Right L Lung, Left M Lungs, Bilateral	Ø Open 3 Percutaneous 4 Percutaneous Endoscopic 7 Via Natural or Artificial Opening 8 Via Natural or Artificial Opening Endoscopic	Z No Device	Z No Qualifier
N Pleura, Right P Pleura, Left R Diaphragm, Right S Diaphragm, Left	Ø Open 3 Percutaneous 4 Percutaneous Endoscopic	Z No Device	Z No Qualifier

Non-OR   ØB5[3456789B]4ZZ
Non-OR   ØB5[CDFGHJKLM]8ZZ

Coding Clinic: 2016, Q2, P18 – ØB5[PS]ØZZ

SECTION: Ø MEDICAL AND SURGICAL

BODY SYSTEM: B RESPIRATORY SYSTEM

OPERATION: 7 **DILATION:** Expanding an orifice or the lumen of a tubular body part

Body Part	Approach	Device	Qualifier
1 Trachea 2 Carina 3 Main Bronchus, Right 4 Upper Lobe Bronchus, Right 5 Middle Lobe Bronchus, Right 6 Lower Lobe Bronchus, Right 7 Main Bronchus, Left 8 Upper Lobe Bronchus, Left 9 Lingula Bronchus B Lower Lobe Bronchus, Left	Ø Open 3 Percutaneous 4 Percutaneous Endoscopic 7 Via Natural or Artificial Opening 8 Via Natural or Artificial Opening Endoscopic	D Intraluminal Device Z No Device	Z No Qualifier

Non-OR   ØB5[3456789B][03478][DZ]Z

SECTION: Ø MEDICAL AND SURGICAL

BODY SYSTEM: B RESPIRATORY SYSTEM

OPERATION: 9 DRAINAGE: Taking or letting out fluids and/or gases from a body part

Body Part	Approach	Device	Qualifier
1 Trachea 2 Carina 3 Main Bronchus, Right 4 Upper Lobe Bronchus, Right 5 Middle Lobe Bronchus, Right 6 Lower Lobe Bronchus, Right 7 Main Bronchus, Left 8 Upper Lobe Bronchus, Left 9 Lingula Bronchus B Lower Lobe Bronchus, Left C Upper Lung Lobe, Right D Middle Lung Lobe, Right F Lower Lung Lobe, Right G Upper Lung Lobe, Left H Lung Lingula J Lower Lung Lobe, Left K Lung, Right L Lung, Left M Lungs, Bilateral	Ø Open 3 Percutaneous 4 Percutaneous Endoscopic 7 Via Natural or Artificial Opening 8 Via Natural or Artificial Opening Endoscopic	Ø Drainage Device	Z No Qualifier
1 Trachea 2 Carina 3 Main Bronchus, Right 4 Upper Lobe Bronchus, Right 5 Middle Lobe Bronchus, Right 6 Lower Lobe Bronchus, Right 7 Main Bronchus, Left 8 Upper Lobe Bronchus, Left 9 Lingula Bronchus B Lower Lobe Bronchus, Left C Upper Lung Lobe, Right D Middle Lung Lobe, Right F Lower Lung Lobe, Right G Upper Lung Lobe, Left H Lung Lingula J Lower Lung Lobe, Left K Lung, Right L Lung, Left M Lungs, Bilateral	Ø Open 3 Percutaneous 4 Percutaneous Endoscopic 7 Via Natural or Artificial Opening 8 Via Natural or Artificial Opening Endoscopic	Z No Device	X Diagnostic Z No Qualifier
N Pleura, Right P Pleura, Left R Diaphragm, Right S Diaphragm, Left	Ø Open 3 Percutaneous 4 Percutaneous Endoscopic	Ø Drainage Device	Z No Qualifier
N Pleura, Right P Pleura, Left R Diaphragm, Right S Diaphragm, Left	Ø Open 3 Percutaneous 4 Percutaneous Endoscopic	Z No Device	X Diagnostic Z No Qualifier

DRG Non-OR ØB9[RS]3ØZ
DRG Non-OR ØB9[RS]3ZZ
Non-OR ØB9[123456789B][3478]ZX
Non-OR ØB9[CDFGHJKLM][347]ZX
Non-OR ØB9[NP][Ø3]ØZ
Non-OR ØB9[NP][Ø3]Z[XZ]
Non-OR ØB9[NP]4ZX

Coding Clinic: 2Ø16, Q1, P26 – ØB948ZX, ØB9B8ZX
Coding Clinic: 2Ø16, Q1, P27 – ØB988ZX

New/Revised Text in Green ~~deleted~~ Deleted ♀ Females Only ♂ Males Only **Coding Clinic**
Non-covered Limited Coverage ⊞ Combination (See Appendix E) DRG Non-OR Non-OR Hospital-Acquired Condition

195

SECTION: Ø MEDICAL AND SURGICAL

BODY SYSTEM: B RESPIRATORY SYSTEM

OPERATION: B EXCISION: Cutting out or off, without replacement, a portion of a body part

Body Part	Approach	Device	Qualifier
1 Trachea 2 Carina 3 Main Bronchus, Right 4 Upper Lobe Bronchus, Right 5 Middle Lobe Bronchus, Right 6 Lower Lobe Bronchus, Right 7 Main Bronchus, Left 8 Upper Lobe Bronchus, Left 9 Lingula Bronchus B Lower Lobe Bronchus, Left C Upper Lung Lobe, Right D Middle Lung Lobe, Right F Lower Lung Lobe, Right G Upper Lung Lobe, Left H Lung Lingula J Lower Lung Lobe, Left K Lung, Right L Lung, Left M Lungs, Bilateral	Ø Open 3 Percutaneous 4 Percutaneous Endoscopic 7 Via Natural or Artificial Opening 8 Via Natural or Artificial Opening Endoscopic	Z No Device	X Diagnostic Z No Qualifier
N Pleura, Right P Pleura, Left R Diaphragm, Right S Diaphragm, Left	Ø Open 3 Percutaneous 4 Percutaneous Endoscopic	Z No Device	X Diagnostic Z No Qualifier

Non-OR ØBB[123456789B][3478]ZX

Non-OR ØBB[3456789BM][48]ZZ

Non-OR ØBB[CDFGHJKLM]3ZX

Non-OR ØBB[CDFGHJKL]8ZZ

Non-OR ØBB[NP][Ø3]ZX

Coding Clinic: 2015, Q1, P16 – ØBB1ØZZ
Coding Clinic: 2016, Q1, P26 – ØBB48ZX, ØBBC8ZX
Coding Clinic: 2016, Q1, P27 – ØBB88ZX

SECTION: Ø MEDICAL AND SURGICAL

BODY SYSTEM: B RESPIRATORY SYSTEM

OPERATION: C EXTIRPATION: *(on multiple pages)*
Taking or cutting out solid matter from a body part

Body Part	Approach	Device	Qualifier
1 Trachea 2 Carina 3 Main Bronchus, Right 4 Upper Lobe Bronchus, Right 5 Middle Lobe Bronchus, Right 6 Lower Lobe Bronchus, Right 7 Main Bronchus, Left 8 Upper Lobe Bronchus, Left 9 Lingula Bronchus B Lower Lobe Bronchus, Left C Upper Lung Lobe, Right D Middle Lung Lobe, Right F Lower Lung Lobe, Right G Upper Lung Lobe, Left H Lung Lingula J Lower Lung Lobe, Left K Lung, Right L Lung, Left M Lungs, Bilateral	Ø Open 3 Percutaneous 4 Percutaneous Endoscopic 7 Via Natural or Artificial Opening 8 Via Natural or Artificial Opening Endoscopic	Z No Device	Z No Qualifier

Non-OR ØBC[123456789B][78]ZZ

New/Revised Text in Green — ~~deleted~~ Deleted — ♀ Females Only — ♂ Males Only — **Coding Clinic**

Non-covered — Limited Coverage — ⊞ Combination (See Appendix E) — DRG Non-OR — Non-OR — Hospital-Acquired Condition

SECTION: Ø MEDICAL AND SURGICAL
BODY SYSTEM: B RESPIRATORY SYSTEM
OPERATION: C EXTIRPATION: *(continued)*
Taking or cutting out solid matter from a body part

Body Part	Approach	Device	Qualifier
N Pleura, Right P Pleura, Left R Diaphragm, Right S Diaphragm, Left	Ø Open 3 Percutaneous 4 Percutaneous Endoscopic	Z No Device	Z No Qualifier

Non-OR ØBC[NP][Ø34]ZZ

SECTION: Ø MEDICAL AND SURGICAL
BODY SYSTEM: B RESPIRATORY SYSTEM
OPERATION: D EXTRACTION: Pulling or stripping out or off all or a portion of a body part by the use of force

Body Part	Approach	Device	Qualifier
N Pleura, Right P Pleura, Left	Ø Open 3 Percutaneous 4 Percutaneous Endoscopic	Z No Device	X Diagnostic Z No Qualifier

SECTION: Ø MEDICAL AND SURGICAL
BODY SYSTEM: B RESPIRATORY SYSTEM
OPERATION: F FRAGMENTATION: Breaking solid matter in a body part into pieces

Body Part	Approach	Device	Qualifier
1 Trachea 🜲 2 Carina 🜲 3 Main Bronchus, Right 🜲 4 Upper Lobe Bronchus, Right 🜲 5 Middle Lobe Bronchus, Right 🜲 6 Lower Lobe Bronchus, Right 🜲 7 Main Bronchus, Left 🜲 8 Upper Lobe Bronchus, Left 🜲 9 Lingula Bronchus 🜲 B Lower Lobe Bronchus, Left 🜲	Ø Open 3 Percutaneous 4 Percutaneous Endoscopic 7 Via Natural or Artificial Opening 8 Via Natural or Artificial Opening Endoscopic X External	Z No Device	Z No Qualifier

🜲 ØBF[123456789B]XZZ
Non-OR ØBF[123456789B]XZZ

New/Revised Text in Green ~~deleted~~ Deleted ♀ Females Only ♂ Males Only **Coding Clinic**
🜲 Non-covered 🜲 Limited Coverage ⊞ Combination (See Appendix E) DRG Non-OR Non-OR 🜲 Hospital-Acquired Condition

197

Ø: M/S

B: RESPIRATORY SYSTEM

C: EXTIRPATION   D: EXTRACTION   F: FRAGMENTATION

SECTION: Ø MEDICAL AND SURGICAL
BODY SYSTEM: B RESPIRATORY SYSTEM
OPERATION: H INSERTION: Putting in a nonbiological appliance that monitors, assists, performs, or prevents a physiological function but does not physically take the place of a body part

H: INSERTION

B: RESPIRATORY SYSTEM

Ø: M/S

Body Part	Approach	Device	Qualifier
Ø Tracheobronchial Tree	Ø Open 3 Percutaneous 4 Percutaneous Endoscopic 7 Via Natural or Artificial Opening 8 Via Natural or Artificial Opening Endoscopic	1 Radioactive Element 2 Monitoring Device 3 Infusion Device D Intraluminal Device	Z No Qualifier
1 Trachea	Ø Open	2 Monitoring Device D Intraluminal Device	Z No Qualifier
1 Trachea	3 Percutaneous	D Intraluminal Device E Intraluminal Device, Endotracheal Airway	Z No Qualifier
1 Trachea	4 Percutaneous Endoscopic	D Intraluminal Device	Z No Qualifier
1 Trachea	7 Via Natural or Artificial Opening 8 Via Natural or Artificial Opening Endoscopic	2 Monitoring Device D Intraluminal Device E Intraluminal Device, Endotracheal Airway	Z No Qualifier
3 Main Bronchus, Right 4 Upper Lobe Bronchus, Right 5 Middle Lobe Bronchus, Right 6 Lower Lobe Bronchus, Right 7 Main Bronchus, Left 8 Upper Lobe Bronchus, Left 9 Lingula Bronchus B Lower Lobe Bronchus, Left	Ø Open 3 Percutaneous 4 Percutaneous Endoscopic 7 Via Natural or Artificial Opening 8 Via Natural or Artificial Opening Endoscopic	G Endobronchial Device, Endobronchial Valve	Z No Qualifier
K Lung, Right L Lung, Left	Ø Open 3 Percutaneous 4 Percutaneous Endoscopic 7 Via Natural or Artificial Opening 8 Via Natural or Artificial Opening Endoscopic	1 Radioactive Element 2 Monitoring Device 3 Infusion Device	Z No Qualifier
R Diaphragm, Right S Diaphragm, Left	Ø Open 3 Percutaneous 4 Percutaneous Endoscopic	2 Monitoring Device M Diaphragmatic Pacemaker Lead	Z No Qualifier

DRG Non-OR ØBH1[78]2Z
DRG Non-OR ØBH[KL][78][23]Z
Non-OR ØBHØ[78][23D]Z
Non-OR ØBH13EZ
Non-OR ØBH1[78]EZ
Non-OR ØBH[3456789B]8GZ

New/Revised Text in Green deleted Deleted ♀ Females Only ♂ Males Only **Coding Clinic**
Non-covered Limited Coverage ⊕ Combination (See Appendix E) DRG Non-OR Non-OR Hospital-Acquired Condition

SECTION: Ø MEDICAL AND SURGICAL
BODY SYSTEM: B RESPIRATORY SYSTEM
OPERATION: J INSPECTION: Visually and/or manually exploring a body part

Body Part	Approach	Device	Qualifier
Ø Tracheobronchial Tree 1 Trachea K Lung, Right L Lung, Left Q Pleura T Diaphragm	Ø Open 3 Percutaneous 4 Percutaneous Endoscopic 7 Via Natural or Artificial Opening 8 Via Natural or Artificial Opening Endoscopic X External	Z No Device	Z No Qualifier

DRG Non-OR   ØBJ[ØKL][37X]ZZ
DRG Non-OR   ØBJ[QT][378X]ZZ
Non-OR   ØBJ[ØKL]8ZZ
Non-OR   ØBJ1[3478X]ZZ

Coding Clinic: 2015, Q2, P31 – ØBJQ4ZZ

SECTION: Ø MEDICAL AND SURGICAL
BODY SYSTEM: B RESPIRATORY SYSTEM
OPERATION: L OCCLUSION: Completely closing an orifice or the lumen of a tubular body part

Body Part	Approach	Device	Qualifier
1 Trachea 2 Carina 3 Main Bronchus, Right 4 Upper Lobe Bronchus, Right 5 Middle Lobe Bronchus, Right 6 Lower Lobe Bronchus, Right 7 Main Bronchus, Left 8 Upper Lobe Bronchus, Left 9 Lingula Bronchus B Lower Lobe Bronchus, Left	Ø Open 3 Percutaneous 4 Percutaneous Endoscopic	C Extraluminal Device D Intraluminal Device Z No Device	Z No Qualifier
1 Trachea 2 Carina 3 Main Bronchus, Right 4 Upper Lobe Bronchus, Right 5 Middle Lobe Bronchus, Right 6 Lower Lobe Bronchus, Right 7 Main Bronchus, Left 8 Upper Lobe Bronchus, Left 9 Lingula Bronchus B Lower Lobe Bronchus, Left	7 Via Natural or Artificial Opening 8 Via Natural or Artificial Opening Endoscopic	D Intraluminal Device Z No Device	Z No Qualifier

New/Revised Text in Green   deleted Deleted   ♀ Females Only   ♂ Males Only   Coding Clinic
Non-covered   Limited Coverage   ⊞ Combination (See Appendix E)   DRG Non-OR   Non-OR   Hospital-Acquired Condition
199

SECTION: Ø MEDICAL AND SURGICAL

BODY SYSTEM: B RESPIRATORY SYSTEM

OPERATION: M REATTACHMENT: Putting back in or on all or a portion of a separated body part to its normal location or other suitable location

Body Part	Approach	Device	Qualifier
1 Trachea	Ø Open	Z No Device	Z No Qualifier
2 Carina			
3 Main Bronchus, Right			
4 Upper Lobe Bronchus, Right			
5 Middle Lobe Bronchus, Right			
6 Lower Lobe Bronchus, Right			
7 Main Bronchus, Left			
8 Upper Lobe Bronchus, Left			
9 Lingula Bronchus			
B Lower Lobe Bronchus, Left			
C Upper Lung Lobe, Right			
D Middle Lung Lobe, Right			
F Lower Lung Lobe, Right			
G Upper Lung Lobe, Left			
H Lung Lingula			
J Lower Lung Lobe, Left			
K Lung, Right			
L Lung, Left			
R Diaphragm, Right			
S Diaphragm, Left			

SECTION: Ø MEDICAL AND SURGICAL

BODY SYSTEM: B RESPIRATORY SYSTEM

OPERATION: N RELEASE: Freeing a body part from an abnormal physical constraint by cutting or by the use of force

Body Part	Approach	Device	Qualifier
1 Trachea	Ø Open	Z No Device	Z No Qualifier
2 Carina	3 Percutaneous		
3 Main Bronchus, Right	4 Percutaneous Endoscopic		
4 Upper Lobe Bronchus, Right	7 Via Natural or Artificial Opening		
5 Middle Lobe Bronchus, Right	8 Via Natural or Artificial Opening Endoscopic		
6 Lower Lobe Bronchus, Right			
7 Main Bronchus, Left			
8 Upper Lobe Bronchus, Left			
9 Lingula Bronchus			
B Lower Lobe Bronchus, Left			
C Upper Lung Lobe, Right			
D Middle Lung Lobe, Right			
F Lower Lung Lobe, Right			
G Upper Lung Lobe, Left			
H Lung Lingula			
J Lower Lung Lobe, Left			
K Lung, Right			
L Lung, Left			
M Lungs, Bilateral			
N Pleura, Right	Ø Open	Z No Device	Z No Qualifier
P Pleura, Left	3 Percutaneous		
R Diaphragm, Right	4 Percutaneous Endoscopic		
S Diaphragm, Left			

Coding Clinic: 2Ø15, Q3, P15 – ØBN1ØZZ

New/Revised Text in Green ~~deleted~~ Deleted ♀ Females Only ♂ Males Only **Coding Clinic**

🞕 Non-covered 🞕 Limited Coverage ⊕ Combination (See Appendix E) | DRG Non-OR | Non-OR 🞕 Hospital-Acquired Condition

SECTION: Ø MEDICAL AND SURGICAL
BODY SYSTEM: B RESPIRATORY SYSTEM
OPERATION: P REMOVAL: *(on multiple pages)*
Taking out or off a device from a body part

Body Part	Approach	Device	Qualifier
Ø Tracheobronchial Tree	Ø Open 3 Percutaneous 4 Percutaneous Endoscopic 7 Via Natural or Artificial Opening 8 Via Natural or Artificial Opening Endoscopic	Ø Drainage Device 1 Radioactive Element 2 Monitoring Device 3 Infusion Device 7 Autologous Tissue Substitute C Extraluminal Device D Intraluminal Device J Synthetic Substitute K Nonautologous Tissue Substitute	Z No Qualifier
Ø Tracheobronchial Tree	X External	Ø Drainage Device 1 Radioactive Element 2 Monitoring Device 3 Infusion Device D Intraluminal Device	Z No Qualifier
1 Trachea	Ø Open 3 Percutaneous 4 Percutaneous Endoscopic 7 Via Natural or Artificial Opening 8 Via Natural or Artificial Opening Endoscopic	Ø Drainage Device 2 Monitoring Device 7 Autologous Tissue Substitute C Extraluminal Device D Intraluminal Device F Tracheostomy Device J Synthetic Substitute K Nonautologous Tissue Substitute	Z No Qualifier
1 Trachea	X External	Ø Drainage Device 2 Monitoring Device D Intraluminal Device F Tracheostomy Device	Z No Qualifier
K Lung, Right L Lung, Left	Ø Open 3 Percutaneous 4 Percutaneous Endoscopic 7 Via Natural or Artificial Opening 8 Via Natural or Artificial Opening Endoscopic X External	Ø Drainage Device 1 Radioactive Element 2 Monitoring Device 3 Infusion Device	Z No Qualifier
Q Pleura	Ø Open 3 Percutaneous 4 Percutaneous Endoscopic 7 Via Natural or Artificial Opening 8 Via Natural or Artificial Opening Endoscopic X External	Ø Drainage Device 1 Radioactive Element 2 Monitoring Device	Z No Qualifier

DRG Non-OR ØBPØ[78][Ø23D]Z
DRG Non-OR ØBP1[Ø34]FZ
DRG Non-OR ØBP1[78][Ø2DF]Z
DRG Non-OR ØBP[KL][78][Ø23]Z
Non-OR ØBPØX[Ø123D]Z
Non-OR ØBP1X[Ø2DF]Z
Non-OR ØBP[KL]X[Ø123]Z
Non-OR ØBPQ[Ø3478X][Ø12]Z

New/Revised Text in Green   ~~deleted~~ Deleted   ♀ Females Only   ♂ Males Only   **Coding Clinic**
🚫 Non-covered   🚫 Limited Coverage   ⊞ Combination (See Appendix E)   DRG Non-OR   Non-OR   🚫 Hospital-Acquired Condition

SECTION: Ø MEDICAL AND SURGICAL

BODY SYSTEM: B RESPIRATORY SYSTEM

OPERATION: P REMOVAL: *(continued)*
Taking out or off a device from a body part

Body Part	Approach	Device	Qualifier

T Diaphragm	Ø Open
	3 Percutaneous
	4 Percutaneous Endoscopic
	7 Via Natural or Artificial
	     Opening
	8 Via Natural or Artificial
	     Opening Endoscopic
		Ø Drainage Device
		2 Monitoring Device
		7 Autologous Tissue Substitute
		J Synthetic Substitute
		K Nonautologous Tissue
		     Substitute
		M Diaphragmatic Pacemaker
		     Lead
			Z No Qualifier

T Diaphragm	X External	Ø Drainage Device 2 Monitoring Device M Diaphragmatic Pacemaker Lead	Z No Qualifier

DRG Non-OR   ØBPT[78][Ø2]Z
Non-OR   ØBPTX[Ø2M]Z

SECTION: Ø MEDICAL AND SURGICAL

BODY SYSTEM: B RESPIRATORY SYSTEM

OPERATION: Q REPAIR: Restoring, to the extent possible, a body part to its normal anatomic structure and function

Body Part	Approach	Device	Qualifier

1   Trachea ⊞
2   Carina
3   Main Bronchus, Right ⊞
4   Upper Lobe Bronchus, Right ⊞
5   Middle Lobe Bronchus, Right ⊞
6   Lower Lobe Bronchus, Right ⊞
7   Main Bronchus, Left ⊞
8   Upper Lobe Bronchus, Left ⊞
9   Lingula Bronchus ⊞
B   Lower Lobe Bronchus, Left ⊞
C   Upper Lung Lobe, Right
D   Middle Lung Lobe, Right
F   Lower Lung Lobe, Right
G   Upper Lung Lobe, Left
H   Lung Lingula
J   Lower Lung Lobe, Left
K   Lung, Right ⊞
L   Lung, Left ⊞
M   Lungs, Bilateral ⊞
	Ø Open
	3 Percutaneous
	4 Percutaneous Endoscopic
	7 Via Natural or Artificial
	     Opening
	8 Via Natural or Artificial
	     Opening Endoscopic
		Z No Device	Z No Qualifier

N Pleura, Right ⊞ P Pleura, Left ⊞ R Diaphragm, Right ⊞ S Diaphragm, Left	Ø Open 3 Percutaneous 4 Percutaneous Endoscopic	Z No Device	Z No Qualifier

⊞ ØBQ[13456789BKLM][Ø3478]ZZ
⊞ ØBQ[NP][Ø34]ZZ

Coding Clinic: 2016, Q2, P23 – ØBQ[RS]ØZZ

New/Revised Text in Green   ~~deleted~~ Deleted   ♀ Females Only   ♂ Males Only   **Coding Clinic**
🚫 Non-covered   🚫 Limited Coverage   ⊞ Combination (See Appendix E)   DRG Non-OR   Non-OR   🚫 Hospital-Acquired Condition

SECTION: Ø MEDICAL AND SURGICAL
BODY SYSTEM: B RESPIRATORY SYSTEM
OPERATION: S REPOSITION: Moving to its normal location, or other suitable location, all or a portion of a body part

Body Part	Approach	Device	Qualifier
1 Trachea 2 Carina 3 Main Bronchus, Right 4 Upper Lobe Bronchus, Right 5 Middle Lobe Bronchus, Right 6 Lower Lobe Bronchus, Right 7 Main Bronchus, Left 8 Upper Lobe Bronchus, Left 9 Lingula Bronchus B Lower Lobe Bronchus, Left C Upper Lung Lobe, Right D Middle Lung Lobe, Right F Lower Lung Lobe, Right G Upper Lung Lobe, Left H Lung Lingula J Lower Lung Lobe, Left K Lung, Right L Lung, Left R Diaphragm, Right S Diaphragm, Left	Ø Open	Z No Device	Z No Qualifier

SECTION: Ø MEDICAL AND SURGICAL
BODY SYSTEM: B RESPIRATORY SYSTEM
OPERATION: T RESECTION: Cutting out or off, without replacement, all of a body part

Body Part	Approach	Device	Qualifier
1 Trachea 2 Carina 3 Main Bronchus, Right 4 Upper Lobe Bronchus, Right 5 Middle Lobe Bronchus, Right 6 Lower Lobe Bronchus, Right 7 Main Bronchus, Left 8 Upper Lobe Bronchus, Left 9 Lingula Bronchus B Lower Lobe Bronchus, Left C Upper Lung Lobe, Right D Middle Lung Lobe, Right F Lower Lung Lobe, Right G Upper Lung Lobe, Left H Lung Lingula J Lower Lung Lobe, Left K Lung, Right ⊞ L Lung, Left ⊞ M Lungs, Bilateral ⊞ R Diaphragm, Right S Diaphragm, Left	Ø Open 4 Percutaneous Endoscopic	Z No Device	Z No Qualifier

⊞ ØBT[KLM]ØZZ

SECTION: Ø MEDICAL AND SURGICAL

BODY SYSTEM: B RESPIRATORY SYSTEM

OPERATION: U SUPPLEMENT: Putting in or on biological or synthetic material that physically reinforces and/or augments the function of a portion of a body part

Body Part	Approach	Device	Qualifier
1 Trachea 2 Carina 3 Main Bronchus, Right 4 Upper Lobe Bronchus, Right 5 Middle Lobe Bronchus, Right 6 Lower Lobe Bronchus, Right 7 Main Bronchus, Left 8 Upper Lobe Bronchus, Left 9 Lingula Bronchus B Lower Lobe Bronchus, Left R Diaphragm, Right S Diaphragm, Left	Ø Open 4 Percutaneous Endoscopic	7 Autologous Tissue Substitute J Synthetic Substitute K Nonautologous Tissue Substitute	Z No Qualifier

Coding Clinic: 2Ø15, Q1, P28 – ØBU3Ø7Z

SECTION: Ø MEDICAL AND SURGICAL

BODY SYSTEM: B RESPIRATORY SYSTEM

OPERATION: V RESTRICTION: Partially closing an orifice or the lumen of a tubular body part

Body Part	Approach	Device	Qualifier
1 Trachea 2 Carina 3 Main Bronchus, Right 4 Upper Lobe Bronchus, Right 5 Middle Lobe Bronchus, Right 6 Lower Lobe Bronchus, Right 7 Main Bronchus, Left 8 Upper Lobe Bronchus, Left 9 Lingula Bronchus B Lower Lobe Bronchus, Left	Ø Open 3 Percutaneous 4 Percutaneous Endoscopic	C Extraluminal Device D Intraluminal Device Z No Device	Z No Qualifier
1 Trachea 2 Carina 3 Main Bronchus, Right 4 Upper Lobe Bronchus, Right 5 Middle Lobe Bronchus, Right 6 Lower Lobe Bronchus, Right 7 Main Bronchus, Left 8 Upper Lobe Bronchus, Left 9 Lingula Bronchus B Lower Lobe Bronchus, Left	7 Via Natural or Artificial Opening 8 Via Natural or Artificial Opening Endoscopic	D Intraluminal Device Z No Device	Z No Qualifier

New/Revised Text in Green deleted Deleted ♀ Females Only ♂ Males Only **Coding Clinic**

Non-covered Limited Coverage ⊞ Combination (See Appendix E) DRG Non-OR Non-OR Hospital-Acquired Condition

SECTION: Ø MEDICAL AND SURGICAL

BODY SYSTEM: B RESPIRATORY SYSTEM

OPERATION: W REVISION: Correcting, to the extent possible, a portion of a malfunctioning device or the position of a displaced device

Body Part	Approach	Device	Qualifier
Ø Tracheobronchial Tree	Ø Open 3 Percutaneous 4 Percutaneous Endoscopic 7 Via Natural or Artificial Opening 8 Via Natural or Artificial Opening Endoscopic X External	Ø Drainage Device 2 Monitoring Device 3 Infusion Device 7 Autologous Tissue Substitute C Extraluminal Device D Intraluminal Device J Synthetic Substitute K Nonautologous Tissue Substitute	Z No Qualifier
1 Trachea	Ø Open 3 Percutaneous 4 Percutaneous Endoscopic 7 Via Natural or Artificial Opening 8 Via Natural or Artificial Opening Endoscopic X External	Ø Drainage Device 2 Monitoring Device 7 Autologous Tissue Substitute C Extraluminal Device D Intraluminal Device F Tracheostomy Device J Synthetic Substitute K Nonautologous Tissue Substitute	Z No Qualifier
K Lung, Right L Lung, Left	Ø Open 3 Percutaneous 4 Percutaneous Endoscopic 7 Via Natural or Artificial Opening 8 Via Natural or Artificial Opening Endoscopic X External	Ø Drainage Device 2 Monitoring Device 3 Infusion Device	Z No Qualifier
Q Pleura	Ø Open 3 Percutaneous 4 Percutaneous Endoscopic 7 Via Natural or Artificial Opening 8 Via Natural or Artificial Opening Endoscopic X External	Ø Drainage Device 2 Monitoring Device	Z No Qualifier
T Diaphragm	Ø Open 3 Percutaneous 4 Percutaneous Endoscopic 7 Via Natural or Artificial Opening 8 Via Natural or Artificial Opening Endoscopic X External	Ø Drainage Device 2 Monitoring Device 7 Autologous Tissue Substitute J Synthetic Substitute K Nonautologous Tissue Substitute M Diaphragmatic Pacemaker Lead	Z No Qualifier

Non-OR ØBWØX[Ø237CDJK]Z
Non-OR ØBW1X[Ø27CDFJK]Z
Non-OR ØBW[KL]X[Ø23]Z
Non-OR ØBWQ[Ø3478X][Ø2]Z
Non-OR ØBWTX[Ø27JKM]Z

Ø: M/S

B: RESPIRATORY SYSTEM

W: REVISION

SECTION: Ø MEDICAL AND SURGICAL

BODY SYSTEM: B RESPIRATORY SYSTEM

OPERATION: Y TRANSPLANTATION: Putting in or on all or a portion of a living body part taken from another individual or animal to physically take the place and/or function of all or a portion of a similar body part

Body Part	Approach	Device	Qualifier
C Upper Lung Lobe, Right 🖘 D Middle Lung Lobe, Right 🖘 F Lower Lung Lobe, Right 🖘 G Upper Lung Lobe, Left 🖘 H Lung Lingula 🖘 J Lower Lung Lobe, Left 🖘 K Lung, Right 🖘 L Lung, Left 🖘 M Lungs, Bilateral 🖘	Ø Open	Z No Device	Ø Allogeneic 1 Syngeneic 2 Zooplastic

🖘 All Values

Y: TRANSPLANTATION

B: RESPIRATORY SYSTEM

Ø: M/S

🖘 Non-covered 🖘 Limited Coverage ⊞ Combination (See Appendix E) New/Revised Text in Green ~~deleted~~ Deleted DRG Non-OR ♀ Females Only ♂ Males Only Non-OR **Coding Clinic** 🖘 Hospital-Acquired Condition

SECTION: 0 MEDICAL AND SURGICAL
BODY SYSTEM: C MOUTH AND THROAT
OPERATION: 0 **ALTERATION:** Modifying the anatomic structure of a body part without affecting the function of the body part

Body Part	Approach	Device	Qualifier
0 Upper Lip 1 Lower Lip	X External	7 Autologous Tissue Substitute J Synthetic Substitute K Nonautologous Tissue Substitute Z No Device	Z No Qualifier

SECTION: 0 MEDICAL AND SURGICAL
BODY SYSTEM: C MOUTH AND THROAT
OPERATION: 2 **CHANGE:** Taking out or off a device from a body part and putting back an identical or similar device in or on the same body part without cutting or puncturing the skin or a mucous membrane

Body Part	Approach	Device	Qualifier
A Salivary Gland S Larynx Y Mouth and Throat	X External	0 Drainage Device Y Other Device	Z No Qualifier

Non-OR   All Values

SECTION: 0 MEDICAL AND SURGICAL
BODY SYSTEM: C MOUTH AND THROAT
OPERATION: 5 **DESTRUCTION:** *(on multiple pages)*
Physical eradication of all or a portion of a body part by the use of direct energy, force, or a destructive agent

Body Part	Approach	Device	Qualifier
0 Upper Lip 1 Lower Lip 2 Hard Palate 3 Soft Palate 4 Buccal Mucosa 5 Upper Gingiva 6 Lower Gingiva 7 Tongue N Uvula P Tonsils Q Adenoids	0 Open 3 Percutaneous X External	Z No Device	Z No Qualifier

Non-OR   0C5[56][03X]ZZ

SECTION: Ø MEDICAL AND SURGICAL

BODY SYSTEM: C MOUTH AND THROAT
OPERATION: 5 DESTRUCTION: *(continued)*
Physical eradication of all or a portion of a body part by the use of direct energy, force, or a destructive agent

Body Part	Approach	Device	Qualifier
8 Parotid Gland, Right 9 Parotid Gland, Left B Parotid Duct, Right C Parotid Duct, Left D Sublingual Gland, Right F Sublingual Gland, Left G Submaxillary Gland, Right H Submaxillary Gland, Left J Minor Salivary Gland	Ø Open 3 Percutaneous	Z No Device	Z No Qualifier
M Pharynx R Epiglottis S Larynx T Vocal Cord, Right V Vocal Cord, Left	Ø Open 3 Percutaneous 4 Percutaneous Endoscopic 7 Via Natural or Artificial Opening 8 Via Natural or Artificial Opening Endoscopic	Z No Device	Z No Qualifier
W Upper Tooth X Lower Tooth	Ø Open X External	Z No Device	Ø Single 1 Multiple 2 All

Non-OR 0C5[WX][ØX]Z[Ø12]

SECTION: Ø MEDICAL AND SURGICAL

BODY SYSTEM: C MOUTH AND THROAT
OPERATION: 7 DILATION: Expanding an orifice or the lumen of a tubular body part

Body Part	Approach	Device	Qualifier
B Parotid Duct, Right C Parotid Duct, Left	Ø Open 3 Percutaneous 7 Via Natural or Artificial Opening	D Intraluminal Device Z No Device	Z No Qualifier
M Pharynx	7 Via Natural or Artificial Opening 8 Via Natural or Artificial Opening Endoscopic	D Intraluminal Device Z No Device	Z No Qualifier
S Larynx ⊞	Ø Open 3 Percutaneous 4 Percutaneous Endoscopic 7 Via Natural or Artificial Opening 8 Via Natural or Artificial Opening Endoscopic	D Intraluminal Device Z No Device	Z No Qualifier

⊞ 0C7S[Ø3478]DZ
Non-OR 0C7[BC][Ø37][DZ]Z
Non-OR 0C7M[78][DZ]Z

SECTION: 0 MEDICAL AND SURGICAL

BODY SYSTEM: C MOUTH AND THROAT

OPERATION: 9 DRAINAGE: *(on multiple pages)*
Taking or letting out fluids and/or gases from a body part

Body Part	Approach	Device	Qualifier
0 Upper Lip 1 Lower Lip 2 Hard Palate 3 Soft Palate 4 Buccal Mucosa 5 Upper Gingiva 6 Lower Gingiva 7 Tongue N Uvula P Tonsils Q Adenoids	0 Open 3 Percutaneous X External	0 Drainage Device	Z No Qualifier
0 Upper Lip 1 Lower Lip 2 Hard Palate 3 Soft Palate 4 Buccal Mucosa 5 Upper Gingiva 6 Lower Gingiva 7 Tongue N Uvula P Tonsils Q Adenoids	0 Open 3 Percutaneous X External	Z No Device	X Diagnostic Z No Qualifier
8 Parotid Gland, Right 9 Parotid Gland, Left B Parotid Duct, Right C Parotid Duct, Left D Sublingual Gland, Right F Sublingual Gland, Left G Submaxillary Gland, Right H Submaxillary Gland, Left J Minor Salivary Gland	0 Open 3 Percutaneous	0 Drainage Device	Z No Qualifier
8 Parotid Gland, Right 9 Parotid Gland, Left B Parotid Duct, Right C Parotid Duct, Left D Sublingual Gland, Right F Sublingual Gland, Left G Submaxillary Gland, Right H Submaxillary Gland, Left J Minor Salivary Gland	0 Open 3 Percutaneous	Z No Device	X Diagnostic Z No Qualifier
M Pharynx R Epiglottis S Larynx T Vocal Cord, Right V Vocal Cord, Left	0 Open 3 Percutaneous 4 Percutaneous Endoscopic 7 Via Natural or Artificial Opening 8 Via Natural or Artificial Opening Endoscopic	0 Drainage Device	Z No Qualifier

DRG Non-OR 0C9[012347NPQ]30Z
DRG Non-OR 0C9[012347NPQ]3ZZ
DRG Non-OR 0C9[MRSTV]30Z
Non-OR 0C9[56][03X]0Z
Non-OR 0C9[01456][03X]ZX

Non-OR 0C9[56][03X]ZZ
Non-OR 0C97[3X]ZX
Non-OR 0C9[89BCDFGHJ][03]0Z
Non-OR 0C9[89BCDFGHJ]3ZX
Non-OR 0C9[89BCDFGHJ][03]ZZ

New/Revised Text in Green deleted Deleted ♀ Females Only ♂ Males Only Coding Clinic
Non-covered Limited Coverage Combination (See Appendix E) DRG Non-OR Non-OR Hospital-Acquired Condition

SECTION: 0 MEDICAL AND SURGICAL

BODY SYSTEM: C MOUTH AND THROAT

OPERATION: 9 DRAINAGE: *(continued)*
Taking or letting out fluids and/or gases from a body part

Body Part	Approach	Device	Qualifier
M Pharynx R Epiglottis S Larynx T Vocal Cord, Right V Vocal Cord, Left	0 Open 3 Percutaneous 4 Percutaneous Endoscopic 7 Via Natural or Artificial Opening 8 Via Natural or Artificial Opening Endoscopic	Z No Device	X Diagnostic Z No Qualifier
W Upper Tooth X Lower Tooth	0 Open X External	0 Drainage Device Z No Device	0 Single 1 Multiple 2 All

DRG Non-OR 0C9[MRSTV]3ZZ
Non-OR 0C9M[03478]ZX

Non-OR 0C9[RSTV][3478]ZX
Non-OR 0C9[WX][0X][0Z][012]

SECTION: 0 MEDICAL AND SURGICAL

BODY SYSTEM: C MOUTH AND THROAT

OPERATION: B EXCISION: Cutting out or off, without replacement, a portion of a body part

Body Part	Approach	Device	Qualifier
0 Upper Lip 1 Lower Lip 2 Hard Palate 3 Soft Palate 4 Buccal Mucosa 5 Upper Gingiva 6 Lower Gingiva 7 Tongue N Uvula P Tonsils Q Adenoids	0 Open 3 Percutaneous X External	Z No Device	X Diagnostic Z No Qualifier
8 Parotid Gland, Right 9 Parotid Gland, Left B Parotid Duct, Right C Parotid Duct, Left D Sublingual Gland, Right F Sublingual Gland, Left G Submaxillary Gland, Right H Submaxillary Gland, Left J Minor Salivary Gland	0 Open 3 Percutaneous	Z No Device	X Diagnostic Z No Qualifier
M Pharynx R Epiglottis S Larynx T Vocal Cord, Right V Vocal Cord, Left	0 Open 3 Percutaneous 4 Percutaneous Endoscopic 7 Via Natural or Artificial Opening 8 Via Natural or Artificial Opening Endoscopic	Z No Device	X Diagnostic Z No Qualifier
W Upper Tooth X Lower Tooth	0 Open X External	Z No Device	0 Single 1 Multiple 2 All

Non-OR 0CB[01456][03X]ZX
Non-OR 0CB[56][03X]ZZ
Non-OR 0CB7[3X]ZX
Non-OR 0CB[89BCDFGHJ]3ZX

Non-OR 0CBM[03478]ZX
Non-OR 0CB[RSTV][3478]ZX
Non-OR 0CB[WX][0X]Z[012]

Coding Clinic: 2016, Q2, P20 – 0CBM8ZX

SECTION: 0 MEDICAL AND SURGICAL

BODY SYSTEM: C MOUTH AND THROAT

OPERATION: C EXTIRPATION: Taking or cutting out solid matter from a body part

Body Part	Approach	Device	Qualifier
0 Upper Lip 1 Lower Lip 2 Hard Palate 3 Soft Palate 4 Buccal Mucosa 5 Upper Gingiva 6 Lower Gingiva 7 Tongue N Uvula P Tonsils Q Adenoids	0 Open 3 Percutaneous X External	Z No Device	Z No Qualifier
8 Parotid Gland, Right 9 Parotid Gland, Left B Parotid Duct, Right C Parotid Duct, Left D Sublingual Gland, Right F Sublingual Gland, Left G Submaxillary Gland, Right H Submaxillary Gland, Left J Minor Salivary Gland	0 Open 3 Percutaneous	Z No Device	Z No Qualifier
M Pharynx R Epiglottis S Larynx T Vocal Cord, Right V Vocal Cord, Left	0 Open 3 Percutaneous 4 Percutaneous Endoscopic 7 Via Natural or Artificial Opening 8 Via Natural or Artificial Opening Endoscopic	Z No Device	Z No Qualifier
W aUpper Tooth X Lower Tooth	0 Open X External	Z No Device	0 Single 1 Multiple 2 All

Non-OR 0CC[012347NPQ]XZZ
Non-OR 0CC[56][03X]ZZ
Non-OR 0CC[89BCDFGHJ][03]ZZ

Non-OR 0CC[MS][78]ZZ
Non-OR 0CC[WX][0X]Z[012]

Coding Clinic: 2016, Q2, P20 – 0CCH3ZZ

SECTION: 0 MEDICAL AND SURGICAL

BODY SYSTEM: C MOUTH AND THROAT

OPERATION: D EXTRACTION: Pulling or stripping out or off all or a portion of a body part by the use of force

Body Part	Approach	Device	Qualifier
T Vocal Cord, Right V Vocal Cord, Left	0 Open 3 Percutaneous 4 Percutaneous Endoscopic 7 Via Natural or Artificial Opening 8 Via Natural or Artificial Opening Endoscopic	Z No Device	Z No Qualifier
W Upper Tooth X Lower Tooth	X External	Z No Device	0 Single 1 Multiple 2 All

Non-OR 0CD[WX]XZ[012]

New/Revised Text in Green   deleted Deleted   ♀ Females Only   ♂ Males Only   **Coding Clinic**
Non-covered   Limited Coverage   Combination (See Appendix E)   DRG Non-OR   Non-OR   Hospital-Acquired Condition

SECTION: Ø MEDICAL AND SURGICAL
BODY SYSTEM: C MOUTH AND THROAT
OPERATION: F FRAGMENTATION: Breaking solid matter in a body part into pieces

Body Part	Approach	Device	Qualifier
B Parotid Duct, Right C Parotid Duct, Left	Ø Open 3 Percutaneous 7 Via Natural or Artificial Opening X External	Z No Device	Z No Qualifier

ØCF[BC]XZZ
Non-OR All Values

SECTION: Ø MEDICAL AND SURGICAL
BODY SYSTEM: C MOUTH AND THROAT
OPERATION: H INSERTION: Putting in a nonbiological appliance that monitors, assists, performs, or prevents a physiological function but does not physically take the place of a body part

Body Part	Approach	Device	Qualifier
7 Tongue	Ø Open 3 Percutaneous X External	1 Radioactive Element	Z No Qualifier
Y Mouth and Throat	7 Via Natural or Artificial Opening 8 Via Natural or Artificial Opening Endoscopic	B Intraluminal Device, Airway	Z No Qualifier

Non-OR ØCHY[78]BZ

SECTION: Ø MEDICAL AND SURGICAL
BODY SYSTEM: C MOUTH AND THROAT
OPERATION: J INSPECTION: Visually and/or manually exploring a body part

Body Part	Approach	Device	Qualifier
A Salivary Gland	Ø Open 3 Percutaneous X External	Z No Device	Z No Qualifier
S Larynx Y Mouth and Throat	Ø Open 3 Percutaneous 4 Percutaneous Endoscopic 7 Via Natural or Artificial Opening 8 Via Natural or Artificial Opening Endoscopic X External	Z No Device	Z No Qualifier

Non-OR All Values

SECTION: Ø MEDICAL AND SURGICAL

BODY SYSTEM: C MOUTH AND THROAT

OPERATION: L OCCLUSION: Completely closing an orifice or the lumen of a tubular body part

Body Part	Approach	Device	Qualifier
B Parotid Duct, Right C Parotid Duct, Left	Ø Open 3 Percutaneous 4 Percutaneous Endoscopic	C Extraluminal Device D Intraluminal Device Z No Device	Z No Qualifier
B Parotid Duct, Right C Parotid Duct, Left	7 Via Natural or Artificial Opening 8 Via Natural or Artificial Opening Endoscopic	D Intraluminal Device Z No Device	Z No Qualifier

SECTION: Ø MEDICAL AND SURGICAL

BODY SYSTEM: C MOUTH AND THROAT

OPERATION: M REATTACHMENT: Putting back in or on all or a portion of a separated body part to its normal location or other suitable location

Body Part	Approach	Device	Qualifier
Ø Upper Lip 1 Lower Lip 3 Soft Palate 7 Tongue N Uvula	Ø Open	Z No Device	Z No Qualifier
W Upper Tooth X Lower Tooth	Ø Open X External	Z No Device	Ø Single 1 Multiple 2 All

Non-OR ØCM[WX][ØX]Z[Ø12]

SECTION: Ø MEDICAL AND SURGICAL
BODY SYSTEM: C MOUTH AND THROAT
OPERATION: N RELEASE: Freeing a body part from an abnormal physical constraint by cutting or by the use of force

Body Part	Approach	Device	Qualifier
Ø Upper Lip 1 Lower Lip 2 Hard Palate 3 Soft Palate 4 Buccal Mucosa 5 Upper Gingiva 6 Lower Gingiva 7 Tongue N Uvula P Tonsils Q Adenoids	Ø Open 3 Percutaneous X External	Z No Device	Z No Qualifier
8 Parotid Gland, Right 9 Parotid Gland, Left B Parotid Duct, Right C Parotid Duct, Left D Sublingual Gland, Right F Sublingual Gland, Left G Submaxillary Gland, Right H Submaxillary Gland, Left J Minor Salivary Gland	Ø Open 3 Percutaneous	Z No Device	Z No Qualifier
M Pharynx R Epiglottis S Larynx T Vocal Cord, Right V Vocal Cord, Left	Ø Open 3 Percutaneous 4 Percutaneous Endoscopic 7 Via Natural or Artificial Opening 8 Via Natural or Artificial Opening Endoscopic	Z No Device	Z No Qualifier
W Upper Tooth X Lower Tooth	Ø Open X External	Z No Device	Ø Single 1 Multiple 2 All

Non-OR ØCN[Ø1567][Ø3X]ZZ
Non-OR ØCN[WX][ØX]Z[Ø12]

SECTION: Ø MEDICAL AND SURGICAL
BODY SYSTEM: C MOUTH AND THROAT
OPERATION: P REMOVAL: Taking out or off a device from a body part

Body Part	Approach	Device	Qualifier
A Salivary Gland	Ø Open 3 Percutaneous	Ø Drainage Device C Extraluminal Device	Z No Qualifier
S Larynx ⊞	Ø Open 3 Percutaneous 7 Via Natural or Artificial Opening 8 Via Natural or Artificial Opening Endoscopic X External	Ø Drainage Device 7 Autologous Tissue Substitute D Intraluminal Device J Synthetic Substitute K Nonautologous Tissue Substitute	Z No Qualifier
Y Mouth and Throat	Ø Open 3 Percutaneous 7 Via Natural or Artificial Opening 8 Via Natural or Artificial Opening Endoscopic X External	Ø Drainage Device 1 Radioactive Element 7 Autologous Tissue Substitute D Intraluminal Device J Synthetic Substitute K Nonautologous Tissue Substitute	Z No Qualifier

⊞ ØCPS[Ø378]DZ
DRG Non-OR ØCPS[78][ØD]Z
Non-OR ØCPA[Ø3][ØC]Z
Non-OR ØCPSX[Ø7DJK]Z
Non-OR ØCPY[78][ØD]Z
Non-OR ØCPYX[Ø17DJK]Z

SECTION: 0 MEDICAL AND SURGICAL
BODY SYSTEM: C MOUTH AND THROAT
OPERATION: Q **REPAIR:** Restoring, to the extent possible, a body part to its normal anatomic structure and function

Body Part	Approach	Device	Qualifier
0 Upper Lip ⊞ 1 Lower Lip ⊞ 2 Hard Palate 3 Soft Palate 4 Buccal Mucosa ⊞ 5 Upper Gingiva 6 Lower Gingiva 7 Tongue N Uvula P Tonsils Q Adenoids	0 Open 3 Percutaneous X External	Z No Device	Z No Qualifier
8 Parotid Gland, Right 9 Parotid Gland, Left B Parotid Duct, Right C Parotid Duct, Left D Sublingual Gland, Right F Sublingual Gland, Left G Submaxillary Gland, Right H Submaxillary Gland, Left J Minor Salivary Gland	0 Open 3 Percutaneous	Z No Device	Z No Qualifier
M Pharynx ⊞ R Epiglottis S Larynx T Vocal Cord, Right V Vocal Cord, Left	0 Open 3 Percutaneous 4 Percutaneous Endoscopic 7 Via Natural or Artificial Opening 8 Via Natural or Artificial Opening Endoscopic	Z No Device	Z No Qualifier
W Upper Tooth X Lower Tooth	0 Open X External	Z No Device	0 Single 1 Multiple 2 All

⊞ 0CQ[01][03]ZZ
⊞ 0CQ4[03X]ZZ
⊞ 0CQM[03478]ZZ
Non-OR 0CQ[01]XZZ
Non-OR 0CQ[56][03X]ZZ
Non-OR 0CQ[WX][0X]Z[012]

New/Revised Text in Green ~~deleted~~ Deleted ♀ Females Only ♂ Males Only **Coding Clinic**
🚫 Non-covered 🚫 Limited Coverage ⊞ Combination (See Appendix E) DRG Non-OR Non-OR 🚫 Hospital-Acquired Condition

217

SECTION: Ø MEDICAL AND SURGICAL

BODY SYSTEM: C MOUTH AND THROAT

OPERATION: R REPLACEMENT: Putting in or on biological or synthetic material that physically takes the place and/or function of all or a portion of a body part

Body Part	Approach	Device	Qualifier
Ø Upper Lip 1 Lower Lip 2 Hard Palate 3 Soft Palate 4 Buccal Mucosa 5 Upper Gingiva 6 Lower Gingiva 7 Tongue N Uvula	Ø Open 3 Percutaneous X External	7 Autologous Tissue Substitute J Synthetic Substitute K Nonautologous Tissue Substitute	Z No Qualifier
B Parotid Duct, Right C Parotid Duct, Left	Ø Open 3 Percutaneous	7 Autologous Tissue Substitute J Synthetic Substitute K Nonautologous Tissue Substitute	Z No Qualifier
M Pharynx R Epiglottis S Larynx ⊞ T Vocal Cord, Right V Vocal Cord, Left	Ø Open 7 Via Natural or Artificial Opening 8 Via Natural or Artificial Opening Endoscopic	7 Autologous Tissue Substitute J Synthetic Substitute K Nonautologous Tissue Substitute	Z No Qualifier
W Upper Tooth X Lower Tooth	Ø Open X External	7 Autologous Tissue Substitute J Synthetic Substitute K Nonautologous Tissue Substitute	Ø Single 1 Multiple 2 All

⊞ ØCRS[Ø78]JZ
Non-OR ØCR[WX][ØX][7JK][Ø12]

SECTION: Ø MEDICAL AND SURGICAL

BODY SYSTEM: C MOUTH AND THROAT

OPERATION: S REPOSITION: Moving to its normal location, or other suitable location, all or a portion of a body part

Body Part	Approach	Device	Qualifier
Ø Upper Lip 1 Lower Lip 2 Hard Palate 3 Soft Palate 7 Tongue N Uvula	Ø Open X External	Z No Device	Z No Qualifier
B Parotid Duct, Right C Parotid Duct, Left	Ø Open 3 Percutaneous	Z No Device	Z No Qualifier
R Epiglottis T Vocal Cord, Right V Vocal Cord, Left	Ø Open 7 Via Natural or Artificial Opening 8 Via Natural or Artificial Opening Endoscopic	Z No Device	Z No Qualifier
W Upper Tooth X Lower Tooth	Ø Open X External	5 External Fixation Device Z No Device	Ø Single 1 Multiple 2 All

Non-OR ØCS[WX][ØX][5Z][Ø12]

New/Revised Text in Green   ~~deleted~~ Deleted   ♀ Females Only   ♂ Males Only   **Coding Clinic**
🚫 Non-covered   🚫 Limited Coverage   ⊞ Combination (See Appendix E)   DRG Non-OR   Non-OR   🚫 Hospital-Acquired Condition

SECTION: Ø MEDICAL AND SURGICAL
BODY SYSTEM: C MOUTH AND THROAT
OPERATION: T RESECTION: Cutting out or off, without replacement, all of a body part

Body Part	Approach	Device	Qualifier
Ø Upper Lip 1 Lower Lip 2 Hard Palate 3 Soft Palate 7 Tongue N Uvula P Tonsils ⊞ Q Adenoids ⊞	Ø Open X External	Z No Device	Z No Qualifier
8 Parotid Gland, Right 9 Parotid Gland, Left B Parotid Duct, Right C Parotid Duct, Left D Sublingual Gland, Right F Sublingual Gland, Left G Submaxillary Gland, Right H Submaxillary Gland, Left J Minor Salivary Gland	Ø Open	Z No Device	Z No Qualifier
M Pharynx R Epiglottis S Larynx T Vocal Cord, Right V Vocal Cord, Left	Ø Open 4 Percutaneous Endoscopic 7 Via Natural or Artificial Opening 8 Via Natural or Artificial Opening Endoscopic	Z No Device	Z No Qualifier
W Upper Tooth X Lower Tooth	Ø Open	Z No Device	Ø Single 1 Multiple 2 All

⊞ ØCT[PQ][ØX]ZZ   Non-OR ØCT[WX]ØZ[Ø12]

Coding Clinic: 2016, Q2, P13 – ØCT9ØZZ

SECTION: Ø MEDICAL AND SURGICAL
BODY SYSTEM: C MOUTH AND THROAT
OPERATION: U SUPPLEMENT: Putting in or on biological or synthetic material that physically reinforces and/or augments the function of a portion of a body part

Body Part	Approach	Device	Qualifier
Ø Upper Lip 1 Lower Lip 2 Hard Palate 3 Soft Palate 4 Buccal Mucosa 5 Upper Gingiva 6 Lower Gingiva 7 Tongue N Uvula	Ø Open 3 Percutaneous X External	7 Autologous Tissue Substitute J Synthetic Substitute K Nonautologous Tissue Substitute	Z No Qualifier
M Pharynx R Epiglottis S Larynx ⊞ T Vocal Cord, Right V Vocal Cord, Left	Ø Open 7 Via Natural or Artificial Opening 8 Via Natural or Artificial Opening Endoscopic	7 Autologous Tissue Substitute J Synthetic Substitute K Nonautologous Tissue Substitute	Z No Qualifier

⊞ ØCUS[Ø78]JZ   Non-OR ØCU2[Ø3]JZ

New/Revised Text in Green   ~~deleted~~ Deleted   ♀ Females Only   ♂ Males Only   **Coding Clinic**
🚫 Non-covered   🚫 Limited Coverage   ⊞ Combination (See Appendix E)   DRG Non-OR   Non-OR   🚫 Hospital-Acquired Condition

Ø: M/S   C: MOUTH AND THROAT   T: RESECTION   U: SUPPLEMENT

SECTION: 0 MEDICAL AND SURGICAL
BODY SYSTEM: C MOUTH AND THROAT
OPERATION: V **RESTRICTION:** Partially closing an orifice or the lumen of a tubular body part

Body Part	Approach	Device	Qualifier
B Parotid Duct, Right C Parotid Duct, Left	0 Open 3 Percutaneous	C Extraluminal Device D Intraluminal Device Z No Device	Z No Qualifier
B Parotid Duct, Right C Parotid Duct, Left	7 Via Natural or Artificial Opening 8 Via Natural or Artificial Opening Endoscopic	D Intraluminal Device Z No Device	Z No Qualifier

SECTION: 0 MEDICAL AND SURGICAL
BODY SYSTEM: C MOUTH AND THROAT
OPERATION: W **REVISION:** Correcting, to the extent possible, a portion of a malfunctioning device or the position of a displaced device

Body Part	Approach	Device	Qualifier
A Salivary Gland	0 Open 3 Percutaneous X External	0 Drainage Device C Extraluminal Device	Z No Qualifier
S Larynx	0 Open 3 Percutaneous 7 Via Natural or Artificial Opening 8 Via Natural or Artificial Opening Endoscopic X External	0 Drainage Device 7 Autologous Tissue Substitute D Intraluminal Device J Synthetic Substitute K Nonautologous Tissue Substitute	Z No Qualifier
Y Mouth and Throat	0 Open 3 Percutaneous 7 Via Natural or Artificial Opening 8 Via Natural or Artificial Opening Endoscopic X External	0 Drainage Device 1 Radioactive Element 7 Autologous Tissue Substitute D Intraluminal Device J Synthetic Substitute K Nonautologous Tissue Substitute	Z No Qualifier

Non-OR 0CWA[03X][0C]Z
Non-OR 0CWSX[07DHJ]Z
Non-OR 0CWY07Z
Non-OR 0CWYX[017DJK]Z

New/Revised Text in Green   ~~deleted~~ Deleted   ♀ Females Only   ♂ Males Only   **Coding Clinic**

Non-covered   Limited Coverage   ⊞ Combination (See Appendix E)   DRG Non-OR   Non-OR   Hospital-Acquired Condition

SECTION: Ø MEDICAL AND SURGICAL

BODY SYSTEM: C MOUTH AND THROAT

OPERATION: X **TRANSFER:** Moving, without taking out, all or a portion of a body part to another location to take over the function of all or a portion of a body part

Body Part	Approach	Device	Qualifier
Ø Upper Lip 1 Lower Lip 3 Soft Palate 4 Buccal Mucosa 5 Upper Gingiva 6 Lower Gingiva 7 Tongue	Ø Open X External	Z No Device	Z No Qualifier

SECTION: Ø MEDICAL AND SURGICAL

BODY SYSTEM: D GASTROINTESTINAL SYSTEM
OPERATION: 1 BYPASS: *(on multiple pages)*

Altering the route of passage of the contents of a tubular body part

Body Part	Approach	Device	Qualifier

1 Esophagus, Upper
2 Esophagus, Middle
3 Esophagus, Lower
5 Esophagus
	Ø Open
	4 Percutaneous Endoscopic
	8 Via Natural or Artificial
	   Opening Endoscopic
		7 Autologous Tissue Substitute
		J Synthetic Substitute
		K Nonautologous Tissue
		   Substitute
		Z No Device
			4 Cutaneous
			6 Stomach
			9 Duodenum
			A Jejunum
			B Ileum

1 Esophagus, Upper 2 Esophagus, Middle 3 Esophagus, Lower 5 Esophagus	3 Percutaneous	J Synthetic Substitute	4 Cutaneous

6 Stomach ⊞ ✎
9 Duodenum
	Ø Open
	4 Percutaneous Endoscopic
	8 Via Natural or Artificial
	   Opening Endoscopic
		7 Autologous Tissue Substitute
		J Synthetic Substitute
		K Nonautologous Tissue
		   Substitute
		Z No Device
			4 Cutaneous
			9 Duodenum
			A Jejunum
			B Ileum
			L Transverse Colon

6 Stomach 9 Duodenum	3 Percutaneous	J Synthetic Substitute	4 Cutaneous

A Jejunum	Ø Open
	4 Percutaneous Endoscopic
	8 Via Natural or Artificial
	   Opening Endoscopic
		7 Autologous Tissue Substitute
		J Synthetic Substitute
		K Nonautologous Tissue
		   Substitute
		Z No Device
			4 Cutaneous
			A Jejunum
			B Ileum
			H Cecum
			K Ascending Colon
			L Transverse Colon
			M Descending Colon
			N Sigmoid Colon
			P Rectum
			Q Anus

A Jejunum	3 Percutaneous	J Synthetic Substitute	4 Cutaneous

B Ileum	Ø Open
	4 Percutaneous Endoscopic
	8 Via Natural or Artificial
	   Opening Endoscopic
		7 Autologous Tissue Substitute
		J Synthetic Substitute
		K Nonautologous Tissue
		   Substitute
		Z No Device
			4 Cutaneous
			B Ileum
			H Cecum
			K Ascending Colon
			L Transverse Colon
			M Descending Colon
			N Sigmoid Colon
			P Rectum
			Q Anus

B Ileum	3 Percutaneous	J Synthetic Substitute	4 Cutaneous

H Cecum	Ø Open
	4 Percutaneous Endoscopic
	8 Via Natural or Artificial
	   Opening Endoscopic
		7 Autologous Tissue Substitute
		J Synthetic Substitute
		K Nonautologous Tissue
		   Substitute
		Z No Device
			4 Cutaneous
			H Cecum
			K Ascending Colon
			L Transverse Colon
			M Descending Colon
			N Sigmoid Colon
			P Rectum

H Cecum	3 Percutaneous	J Synthetic Substitute	4 Cutaneous

⊞ ØD16Ø[7JK]A
⊞ ØD16ØZ[AB]
Non-OR ØD16[Ø48][7JKZ]4
Non-OR ØD163J4

✎ ØD16[Ø48][7JKZ][9ABL] when reported with Principal Diagnosis E66.Ø1 and Secondary Diagnosis K68.11, K95.Ø1, K95.81, or T81.4XXA

Coding Clinic: 2Ø16, Q2, P31 – ØD194ZB

New/Revised Text in Green   ~~deleted~~ Deleted   ♀ Females Only   ♂ Males Only   **Coding Clinic**
✎ Non-covered   ✎ Limited Coverage   ⊞ Combination (See Appendix E)   DRG Non-OR   Non-OR   ✎ Hospital-Acquired Condition

SECTION: Ø MEDICAL AND SURGICAL

BODY SYSTEM: D GASTROINTESTINAL SYSTEM
OPERATION: 1 BYPASS: *(continued)*
Altering the route of passage of the contents of a tubular body part

Body Part	Approach	Device	Qualifier
K Ascending Colon	Ø Open 4 Percutaneous Endoscopic 8 Via Natural or Artificial Opening Endoscopic	7 Autologous Tissue Substitute J Synthetic Substitute K Nonautologous Tissue Substitute Z No Device	4 Cutaneous K Ascending Colon L Transverse Colon M Descending Colon N Sigmoid Colon P Rectum
K Ascending Colon	3 Percutaneous	J Synthetic Substitute	4 Cutaneous
L Transverse Colon	Ø Open 4 Percutaneous Endoscopic 8 Via Natural or Artificial Opening Endoscopic	7 Autologous Tissue Substitute J Synthetic Substitute K Nonautologous Tissue Substitute Z No Device	4 Cutaneous L Transverse Colon M Descending Colon N Sigmoid Colon P Rectum
L Transverse Colon	3 Percutaneous	J Synthetic Substitute	4 Cutaneous
M Descending Colon	Ø Open 4 Percutaneous Endoscopic 8 Via Natural or Artificial Opening Endoscopic	7 Autologous Tissue Substitute J Synthetic Substitute K Nonautologous Tissue Substitute Z No Device	4 Cutaneous M Descending Colon N Sigmoid Colon P Rectum
M Descending Colon	3 Percutaneous	J Synthetic Substitute	4 Cutaneous
N Sigmoid Colon ⊞	Ø Open 4 Percutaneous Endoscopic 8 Via Natural or Artificial Opening Endoscopic	7 Autologous Tissue Substitute J Synthetic Substitute K Nonautologous Tissue Substitute Z No Device	4 Cutaneous N Sigmoid Colon P Rectum
N Sigmoid Colon	3 Percutaneous	J Synthetic Substitute	4 Cutaneous

⊞ ØD1N[Ø4]Z4

SECTION: Ø MEDICAL AND SURGICAL

BODY SYSTEM: D GASTROINTESTINAL SYSTEM
OPERATION: 2 CHANGE: Taking out or off a device from a body part and putting back an identical or similar device in or on the same body part without cutting or puncturing the skin or a mucous membrane

Body Part	Approach	Device	Qualifier
Ø Upper Intestinal Tract D Lower Intestinal Tract	X External	Ø Drainage Device U Feeding Device Y Other Device	Z No Qualifier
U Omentum V Mesentery W Peritoneum	X External	Ø Drainage Device Y Other Device	Z No Qualifier

Non-OR All Values

SECTION: Ø MEDICAL AND SURGICAL

BODY SYSTEM: D GASTROINTESTINAL SYSTEM

OPERATION: 5 **DESTRUCTION:** Physical eradication of all or a portion of a body part by the direct use of energy, force, or a destructive agent

Body Part	Approach	Device	Qualifier
1 Esophagus, Upper 2 Esophagus, Middle 3 Esophagus, Lower 4 Esophagogastric Junction 5 Esophagus 6 Stomach 7 Stomach, Pylorus 8 Small Intestine 9 Duodenum A Jejunum B Ileum C Ileocecal Valve E Large Intestine F Large Intestine, Right G Large Intestine, Left H Cecum J Appendix K Ascending Colon L Transverse Colon M Descending Colon N Sigmoid Colon P Rectum	Ø Open 3 Percutaneous 4 Percutaneous Endoscopic 7 Via Natural or Artificial Opening 8 Via Natural or Artificial Opening Endoscopic	Z No Device	Z No Qualifier
Q Anus	Ø Open 3 Percutaneous 4 Percutaneous Endoscopic 7 Via Natural or Artificial Opening 8 Via Natural or Artificial Opening Endoscopic X External	Z No Device	Z No Qualifier
R Anal Sphincter S Greater Omentum T Lesser Omentum V Mesentery W Peritoneum	Ø Open 3 Percutaneous 4 Percutaneous Endoscopic	Z No Device	Z No Qualifier

Non-OR ØD5[12345679EFGHKLMN][48]ZZ
Non-OR ØD5P[03478]ZZ
Non-OR ØD5Q[48]ZZ
Non-OR ØD5R4ZZ

Ø: M/S

D: GASTROINTESTINAL SYSTEM

5: DESTRUCTION

SECTION: Ø MEDICAL AND SURGICAL

BODY SYSTEM: D GASTROINTESTINAL SYSTEM

OPERATION: 7 **DILATION:** Expanding an orifice or the lumen of a tubular body part

Body Part	Approach	Device	Qualifier

1 Esophagus, Upper
2 Esophagus, Middle
3 Esophagus, Lower
4 Esophagogastric Junction
5 Esophagus
6 Stomach
7 Stomach, Pylorus
8 Small Intestine
9 Duodenum
A Jejunum
B Ileum
C Ileocecal Valve
E Large Intestine
F Large Intestine, Right
G Large Intestine, Left
H Cecum
K Ascending Colon
L Transverse Colon
M Descending Colon
N Sigmoid Colon
P Rectum
Q Anus
	Ø Open
	3 Percutaneous
	4 Percutaneous Endoscopic
	7 Via Natural or Artificial
	   Opening
	8 Via Natural or Artificial
	   Opening Endoscopic
		D Intraluminal Device
		Z No Device
			Z No Qualifier

DRG Non-OR   ØD76[78][DZ]Z
DRG Non-OR   ØD777[DZ]Z
Non-OR   ØD7[1234589ABCEFGHKLMNPQ][78][DZ]Z
Non-OR   ØD77[48]DZ
Non-OR   ØD778ZZ
Non-OR   ØD7[89ABCEFGHKLMN][Ø34]DZ

SECTION: Ø MEDICAL AND SURGICAL

BODY SYSTEM: D GASTROINTESTINAL SYSTEM

OPERATION: 8 **DIVISION:** Cutting into a body part, without draining fluids and/or gases from the body part, in order to separate or transect a body part

Body Part	Approach	Device	Qualifier

4 Esophagogastric Junction
7 Stomach, Pylorus
	Ø Open
	3 Percutaneous
	4 Percutaneous Endoscopic
	7 Via Natural or Artificial
	   Opening
	8 Via Natural or Artificial
	   Opening Endoscopic
		Z No Device	Z No Qualifier

R Anal Sphincter	Ø Open 3 Percutaneous	Z No Device	Z No Qualifier

New/Revised Text in Green   ~~deleted~~ Deleted   ♀ Females Only   ♂ Males Only   **Coding Clinic**
Non-covered   Limited Coverage   ⊞ Combination (See Appendix E)   DRG Non-OR   Non-OR   Hospital-Acquired Condition

7: DILATION   8: DIVISION

D: GASTROINTESTINAL SYSTEM

Ø: M/S

SECTION: Ø MEDICAL AND SURGICAL
BODY SYSTEM: D GASTROINTESTINAL SYSTEM
OPERATION: 9 DRAINAGE: *(on multiple pages)*

Taking or letting out fluids and/or gases from a body part

Body Part	Approach	Device	Qualifier
1 Esophagus, Upper 2 Esophagus, Middle 3 Esophagus, Lower 4 Esophagogastric Junction 5 Esophagus 6 Stomach 7 Stomach, Pylorus 8 Small Intestine 9 Duodenum A Jejunum B Ileum C Ileocecal Valve E Large Intestine F Large Intestine, Right G Large Intestine, Left H Cecum J Appendix K Ascending Colon L Transverse Colon M Descending Colon N Sigmoid Colon P Rectum	Ø Open 3 Percutaneous 4 Percutaneous Endoscopic 7 Via Natural or Artificial Opening 8 Via Natural or Artificial Opening Endoscopic	Ø Drainage Device	Z No Qualifier
1 Esophagus, Upper 2 Esophagus, Middle 3 Esophagus, Lower 4 Esophagogastric Junction 5 Esophagus 6 Stomach 7 Stomach, Pylorus 8 Small Intestine 9 Duodenum A Jejunum B Ileum C Ileocecal Valve E Large Intestine F Large Intestine, Right G Large Intestine, Left H Cecum J Appendix K Ascending Colon L Transverse Colon M Descending Colon N Sigmoid Colon P Rectum	Ø Open 3 Percutaneous 4 Percutaneous Endoscopic 7 Via Natural or Artificial Opening 8 Via Natural or Artificial Opening Endoscopic	Z No Device	X Diagnostic Z No Qualifier

DRG Non-OR   ØD9[123456789ABCEFGHJKLMNP]3ØZ
DRG Non-OR   ØD9[123456789ABCEFGHJKLMNP]3ZZ
Non-OR   ØD9[6789ABEFGHKLMNP][78]ØZ
Non-OR   ØD9[123456789ABCEFGHJKLMNP][3478]ZX

Coding Clinic: 2Ø15, Q2, P29 – ØD967ØZ

Ø: M/S

D: GASTROINTESTINAL SYSTEM

9: DRAINAGE

SECTION: Ø MEDICAL AND SURGICAL
BODY SYSTEM: D GASTROINTESTINAL SYSTEM
OPERATION: 9 DRAINAGE: *(continued)*
Taking or letting out fluids and/or gases from a body part

Body Part	Approach	Device	Qualifier
Q Anus	Ø Open 3 Percutaneous 4 Percutaneous Endoscopic 7 Via Natural or Artificial Opening 8 Via Natural or Artificial Opening Endoscopic X External	Ø Drainage Device	Z No Qualifier
Q Anus	Ø Open 3 Percutaneous 4 Percutaneous Endoscopic 7 Via Natural or Artificial Opening 8 Via Natural or Artificial Opening Endoscopic X External	Z No Device	X Diagnostic Z No Qualifier
R Anal Sphincter S Greater Omentum T Lesser Omentum V Mesentery W Peritoneum	Ø Open 3 Percutaneous 4 Percutaneous Endoscopic	Ø Drainage Device	Z No Qualifier
R Anal Sphincter S Greater Omentum T Lesser Omentum V Mesentery W Peritoneum	Ø Open 3 Percutaneous 4 Percutaneous Endoscopic	Z No Device	X Diagnostic Z No Qualifier

DRG Non-OR   ØD9Q3ØZ
DRG Non-OR   ØD9Q3ZZ
DRG Non-OR   ØD9R3ØZ
DRG Non-OR   ØD9R3ZZ
Non-OR   ØD9Q[Ø3478X]ZX
Non-OR   ØD9[STVW][34]ØZ
Non-OR   ØD9R[Ø34]ZX
Non-OR   ØD9[STVW][34]ZZ

SECTION: Ø MEDICAL AND SURGICAL

BODY SYSTEM: D GASTROINTESTINAL SYSTEM

OPERATION: B **EXCISION:** Cutting out or off, without replacement, a portion of a body part

Body Part	Approach	Device	Qualifier
1 Esophagus, Upper 2 Esophagus, Middle 3 Esophagus, Lower 4 Esophagogastric Junction 5 Esophagus 7 Stomach, Pylorus 8 Small Intestine ⊞ 9 Duodenum ⊞ A Jejunum B Ileum ⊞ C Ileocecal Valve E Large Intestine ⊞ F Large Intestine, Right G Large Intestine, Left H Cecum J Appendix K Ascending Colon L Transverse Colon M Descending Colon N Sigmoid Colon ⊞ P Rectum	Ø Open 3 Percutaneous 4 Percutaneous Endoscopic 7 Via Natural or Artificial Opening 8 Via Natural or Artificial Opening Endoscopic	Z No Device	X Diagnostic Z No Qualifier
6 Stomach	Ø Open 3 Percutaneous 4 Percutaneous Endoscopic 7 Via Natural or Artificial Opening 8 Via Natural or Artificial Opening Endoscopic	Z No Device	3 Vertical X Diagnostic Z No Qualifier
Q Anus	Ø Open 3 Percutaneous 4 Percutaneous Endoscopic 7 Via Natural or Artificial Opening 8 Via Natural or Artificial Opening Endoscopic X External	Z No Device	X Diagnostic Z No Qualifier
R Anal Sphincter S Greater Omentum T Lesser Omentum V Mesentery W Peritoneum	Ø Open 3 Percutaneous 4 Percutaneous Endoscopic	Z No Device	X Diagnostic Z No Qualifier

⊞ ØDB[89BEN]ØZZ

Non-OR ØDB[12345789ABCEFGHKLMNP][3478]ZX
Non-OR ØDB[123579][48]ZZ
Non-OR ØDB[4EFGHKLMNP]8ZZ
Non-OR ØDB6[3478]ZX
Non-OR ØDB6[48]ZZ
Non-OR ØDBQ[Ø3478X]ZX
Non-OR ØDBR[Ø34]ZX
Non-OR ØDB[STVW][34]ZX

Coding Clinic: 2Ø16, Q1, P22 – ØDBP7ZZ
Coding Clinic: 2Ø16, Q1, P24 – ØDB28ZX
Coding Clinic: 2Ø16, Q2, P31 – ØDB64Z3

Ø: M/S

D: GASTROINTESTINAL SYSTEM

B: EXCISION

SECTION: Ø MEDICAL AND SURGICAL
BODY SYSTEM: D GASTROINTESTINAL SYSTEM
OPERATION: C EXTIRPATION: Taking or cutting out solid matter from a body part

Body Part	Approach	Device	Qualifier

1 Esophagus, Upper
2 Esophagus, Middle
3 Esophagus, Lower
4 Esophagogastric Junction
5 Esophagus
6 Stomach
7 Stomach, Pylorus
8 Small Intestine
9 Duodenum
A Jejunum
B Ileum
C Ileocecal Valve
E Large Intestine
F Large Intestine, Right
G Large Intestine, Left
H Cecum
J Appendix
K Ascending Colon
L Transverse Colon
M Descending Colon
N Sigmoid Colon
P Rectum
	Ø Open
	3 Percutaneous
	4 Percutaneous Endoscopic
	7 Via Natural or Artificial
	   Opening
	8 Via Natural or Artificial
	   Opening Endoscopic
		Z No Device	Z No Qualifier

Q Anus	Ø Open
	3 Percutaneous
	4 Percutaneous Endoscopic
	7 Via Natural or Artificial
	   Opening
	8 Via Natural or Artificial
	   Opening Endoscopic
	X External
		Z No Device	Z No Qualifier

R Anal Sphincter S Greater Omentum T Lesser Omentum V Mesentery W Peritoneum	Ø Open 3 Percutaneous 4 Percutaneous Endoscopic	Z No Device	Z No Qualifier

Non-OR ØDC[123456789ABCEFGHKLMNP][78]ZZ
Non-OR ØDCQ[78X]ZZ

New/Revised Text in Green   ~~deleted~~ Deleted   ♀ Females Only   ♂ Males Only   **Coding Clinic**
Non-covered   Limited Coverage   ⊞ Combination (See Appendix E)   DRG Non-OR   Non-OR   Hospital-Acquired Condition

C: EXTIRPATION

D: GASTROINTESTINAL SYSTEM

Ø: M/S

SECTION: Ø MEDICAL AND SURGICAL
BODY SYSTEM: D GASTROINTESTINAL SYSTEM
OPERATION: F FRAGMENTATION: Breaking solid matter in a body part into pieces

Body Part	Approach	Device	Qualifier

5 Esophagus %
6 Stomach %
8 Small Intestine %
9 Duodenum %
A Jejunum %
B Ileum %
E Large Intestine %
F Large Intestine, Right %
G Large Intestine, Left %
H Cecum %
J Appendix %
K Ascending Colon %
L Transverse Colon %
M Descending Colon %
N Sigmoid Colon %
P Rectum %
Q Anus %
	Ø Open
	3 Percutaneous
	4 Percutaneous Endoscopic
	7 Via Natural or Artificial
	   Opening
	8 Via Natural or Artificial
	   Opening Endoscopic
	X External
		Z No Device	Z No Qualifier

% ØDF[5689ABEFGHJKLMNPQ]XZZ
Non-OR ØDF[5689ABEFGHJKLMNPQ]XZZ

New/Revised Text in Green   ~~deleted~~ Deleted   ♀ Females Only   ♂ Males Only   **Coding Clinic**
% Non-covered   % Limited Coverage   ⊞ Combination (See Appendix E)   DRG Non-OR   Non-OR   % Hospital-Acquired Condition

SECTION: Ø MEDICAL AND SURGICAL
BODY SYSTEM: **D GASTROINTESTINAL SYSTEM**
OPERATION: **H INSERTION:** *(on multiple pages)*
Putting in a nonbiological appliance that monitors, assists, performs, or prevents a physiological function but does not physically take the place of a body part

H: INSERTION

D: GASTROINTESTINAL SYSTEM

Ø: M/S

Body Part	Approach	Device	Qualifier
5 Esophagus	Ø Open 3 Percutaneous 4 Percutaneous Endoscopic	1 Radioactive Element 2 Monitoring Device 3 Infusion Device D Intraluminal Device U Feeding Device	Z No Qualifier
5 Esophagus	7 Via Natural or Artificial Opening 8 Via Natural or Artificial Opening Endoscopic	1 Radioactive Element 2 Monitoring Device 3 Infusion Device B Airway D Intraluminal Device U Feeding Device	Z No Qualifier
6 Stomach ⊞	Ø Open 3 Percutaneous 4 Percutaneous Endoscopic	2 Monitoring Device 3 Infusion Device D Intraluminal Device M Stimulator Lead U Feeding Device	Z No Qualifier
6 Stomach	7 Via Natural or Artificial Opening 8 Via Natural or Artificial Opening Endoscopic	2 Monitoring Device 3 Infusion Device D Intraluminal Device U Feeding Device	Z No Qualifier
8 Small Intestine 9 Duodenum A Jejunum B Ileum	Ø Open 3 Percutaneous 4 Percutaneous Endoscopic 7 Via Natural or Artificial Opening 8 Via Natural or Artificial Opening Endoscopic	2 Monitoring Device 3 Infusion Device D Intraluminal Device U Feeding Device	Z No Qualifier
E Large Intestine	Ø Open 3 Percutaneous 4 Percutaneous Endoscopic 7 Via Natural or Artificial Opening 8 Via Natural or Artificial Opening Endoscopic	D Intraluminal Device	Z No Qualifier
P Rectum	Ø Open 3 Percutaneous 4 Percutaneous Endoscopic 7 Via Natural or Artificial Opening 8 Via Natural or Artificial Opening Endoscopic	1 Radioactive Element D Intraluminal Device	Z No Qualifier

⊞ ØDH6[Ø34]MZ
DRG Non-OR ØDH5[78][23]Z
DRG Non-OR ØDH6[78][23]Z
DRG Non-OR ØDH[89AB][78][23]Z
Non-OR ØDH5[Ø34][DU]Z
Non-OR ØDH5[78][BDU]Z

Non-OR ØDH6[34]UZ
Non-OR ØDH6[78]UZ
Non-OR ØDH[89AB][Ø3478][DU]Z
Non-OR ØDHE[Ø3478]DZ
Non-OR ØDHP[Ø3478]DZ

New/Revised Text in Green   ~~deleted~~ Deleted   ♀ Females Only   ♂ Males Only   **Coding Clinic**
🖉 Non-covered   🖉 Limited Coverage   ⊞ Combination (See Appendix E)   DRG Non-OR   Non-OR   🖉 Hospital-Acquired Condition

SECTION: Ø MEDICAL AND SURGICAL
BODY SYSTEM: D GASTROINTESTINAL SYSTEM
OPERATION: H INSERTION: *(Continued)*
Putting in a nonbiological appliance that monitors, assists, performs, or prevents a physiological function but does not physically take the place of a body part

Body Part	Approach	Device	Qualifier
Q Anus	Ø Open 3 Percutaneous 4 Percutaneous Endoscopic	D Intraluminal Device L Artificial Sphincter	Z No Qualifier
Q Anus	7 Via Natural or Artificial Opening 8 Via Natural or Artificial Opening Endoscopic	D Intraluminal Device	Z No Qualifier
R Anal Sphincter	Ø Open 3 Percutaneous 4 Percutaneous Endoscopic	M Stimulator Lead	Z No Qualifier

SECTION: Ø MEDICAL AND SURGICAL
BODY SYSTEM: D GASTROINTESTINAL SYSTEM
OPERATION: J INSPECTION: Visually and/or manually exploring a body part

Body Part	Approach	Device	Qualifier
Ø Upper Intestinal Tract 6 Stomach D Lower Intestinal Tract	Ø Open 3 Percutaneous 4 Percutaneous Endoscopic 7 Via Natural or Artificial Opening 8 Via Natural or Artificial Opening Endoscopic X External	Z No Device	Z No Qualifier
U Omentum V Mesentery W Peritoneum	Ø Open 3 Percutaneous 4 Percutaneous Endoscopic X External	Z No Device	Z No Qualifier

DRG Non-OR ØDJ[UVW]3ZZ
Non-OR ØDJ[Ø6D][378X]ZZ
Non-OR ØDJ[UVW]XZZ

Coding Clinic: 2015, Q3, P25 – ØDJØ8ZZ
Coding Clinic: 2016, Q2, P21 – ØDJØ7ZZ

New/Revised Text in Green   deleted Deleted   ♀ Females Only   ♂ Males Only   Coding Clinic
Non-covered   Limited Coverage   Combination (See Appendix E)   DRG Non-OR   Non-OR   Hospital-Acquired Condition

233

SECTION: Ø MEDICAL AND SURGICAL

BODY SYSTEM: D GASTROINTESTINAL SYSTEM

OPERATION: L OCCLUSION: Completely closing an orifice or the lumen of a tubular body part

L: OCCLUSION

D: GASTROINTESTINAL SYSTEM

Ø: M/S

Body Part	Approach	Device	Qualifier
1 Esophagus, Upper 2 Esophagus, Middle 3 Esophagus, Lower 4 Esophagogastric Junction 5 Esophagus 6 Stomach 7 Stomach, Pylorus 8 Small Intestine 9 Duodenum A Jejunum B Ileum C Ileocecal Valve E Large Intestine F Large Intestine, Right G Large Intestine, Left H Cecum K Ascending Colon L Transverse Colon M Descending Colon N Sigmoid Colon P Rectum	Ø Open 3 Percutaneous 4 Percutaneous Endoscopic	C Extraluminal Device D Intraluminal Device Z No Device	Z No Qualifier
1 Esophagus, Upper 2 Esophagus, Middle 3 Esophagus, Lower 4 Esophagogastric Junction 5 Esophagus 6 Stomach 7 Stomach, Pylorus 8 Small Intestine 9 Duodenum A Jejunum B Ileum C Ileocecal Valve E Large Intestine F Large Intestine, Right G Large Intestine, Left H Cecum K Ascending Colon L Transverse Colon M Descending Colon N Sigmoid Colon P Rectum	7 Via Natural or Artificial Opening 8 Via Natural or Artificial Opening Endoscopic	D Intraluminal Device Z No Device	Z No Qualifier
Q Anus	Ø Open 3 Percutaneous 4 Percutaneous Endoscopic X External	C Extraluminal Device D Intraluminal Device Z No Device	Z No Qualifier
Q Anus	7 Via Natural or Artificial Opening 8 Via Natural or Artificial Opening Endoscopic	D Intraluminal Device Z No Device	Z No Qualifier

Non-OR ØDL[12345][Ø34][CDZ]Z
Non-OR ØDL[12345][78][DZ]Z

New/Revised Text in Green ~~deleted~~ Deleted ♀ Females Only ♂ Males Only **Coding Clinic**

🚫 Non-covered 🚫 Limited Coverage ⊞ Combination (See Appendix E) DRG Non-OR Non-OR 🚫 Hospital-Acquired Condition

SECTION: Ø MEDICAL AND SURGICAL
BODY SYSTEM: D GASTROINTESTINAL SYSTEM
OPERATION: M REATTACHMENT: Putting back in or on all or a portion of a separated body part to its normal location or other suitable location

Body Part	Approach	Device	Qualifier
5 Esophagus 6 Stomach 8 Small Intestine 9 Duodenum A Jejunum B Ileum E Large Intestine F Large Intestine, Right G Large Intestine, Left H Cecum K Ascending Colon L Transverse Colon M Descending Colon N Sigmoid Colon P Rectum	Ø Open 4 Percutaneous Endoscopic	Z No Device	Z No Qualifier

Ø: M/S

D: GASTROINTESTINAL SYSTEM

M: REATTACHMENT

SECTION: Ø MEDICAL AND SURGICAL
BODY SYSTEM: D GASTROINTESTINAL SYSTEM
OPERATION: N RELEASE: Freeing a body part from an abnormal physical constraint by cutting or by the use of force

Body Part	Approach	Device	Qualifier
1 Esophagus, Upper 2 Esophagus, Middle 3 Esophagus, Lower 4 Esophagogastric Junction 5 Esophagus 6 Stomach 7 Stomach, Pylorus 8 Small Intestine 9 Duodenum A Jejunum B Ileum C Ileocecal Valve E Large Intestine F Large Intestine, Right G Large Intestine, Left H Cecum J Appendix K Ascending Colon L Transverse Colon M Descending Colon N Sigmoid Colon P Rectum	Ø Open 3 Percutaneous 4 Percutaneous Endoscopic 7 Via Natural or Artificial Opening 8 Via Natural or Artificial Opening Endoscopic	Z No Device	Z No Qualifier
Q Anus	Ø Open 3 Percutaneous 4 Percutaneous Endoscopic 7 Via Natural or Artificial Opening 8 Via Natural or Artificial Opening Endoscopic X External	Z No Device	Z No Qualifier
R Anal Sphincter S Greater Omentum T Lesser Omentum V Mesentery W Peritoneum	Ø Open 3 Percutaneous 4 Percutaneous Endoscopic	Z No Device	Z No Qualifier

Non-OR ØDN[89ABEFGHKLMN][78]ZZ

Coding Clinic: 2015, Q3, P15-16 – ØDN5ØZZ

SECTION: Ø MEDICAL AND SURGICAL
BODY SYSTEM: D GASTROINTESTINAL SYSTEM
OPERATION: P REMOVAL: (on multiple pages)
Taking out or off a device from a body part

Body Part	Approach	Device	Qualifier
Ø Upper Intestinal Tract D Lower Intestinal Tract	Ø Open 3 Percutaneous 4 Percutaneous Endoscopic 7 Via Natural or Artificial Opening 8 Via Natural or Artificial Opening Endoscopic	Ø Drainage Device 2 Monitoring Device 3 Infusion Device 7 Autologous Tissue Substitute C Extraluminal Device D Intraluminal Device J Synthetic Substitute K Nonautologous Tissue Substitute U Feeding Device	Z No Qualifier
Ø Upper Intestinal Tract D Lower Intestinal Tract	X External	Ø Drainage Device 2 Monitoring Device 3 Infusion Device D Intraluminal Device U Feeding Device	Z No Qualifier
5 Esophagus	Ø Open 3 Percutaneous 4 Percutaneous Endoscopic	1 Radioactive Element 2 Monitoring Device 3 Infusion Device U Feeding Device	Z No Qualifier
5 Esophagus	7 Via Natural or Artificial Opening 8 Via Natural or Artificial Opening Endoscopic	1 Radioactive Element D Intraluminal Device	Z No Qualifier
5 Esophagus	X External	1 Radioactive Element 2 Monitoring Device 3 Infusion Device D Intraluminal Device U Feeding Device	Z No Qualifier
6 Stomach	Ø Open 3 Percutaneous 4 Percutaneous Endoscopic	Ø Drainage Device 2 Monitoring Device 3 Infusion Device 7 Autologous Tissue Substitute C Extraluminal Device D Intraluminal Device J Synthetic Substitute K Nonautologous Tissue Substitute M Stimulator Lead U Feeding Device	Z No Qualifier
6 Stomach	7 Via Natural or Artificial Opening 8 Via Natural or Artificial Opening Endoscopic	Ø Drainage Device 2 Monitoring Device 3 Infusion Device 7 Autologous Tissue Substitute C Extraluminal Device D Intraluminal Device J Synthetic Substitute K Nonautologous Tissue Substitute U Feeding Device	Z No Qualifier

DRG Non-OR ØDP[ØD][78][Ø23D]Z
DRG Non-OR ØDP5[78]DZ
DRG Non-OR ØDP6[78][Ø23]Z

Non-OR ØDP[ØD]X[Ø23DU]Z
Non-OR ØDP5[78]1Z
Non-OR ØDP5X[123DU]Z
Non-OR ØDP6[78]DZ

Ø: M/S

D: GASTROINTESTINAL SYSTEM

P: REMOVAL

SECTION: Ø MEDICAL AND SURGICAL
BODY SYSTEM: D GASTROINTESTINAL SYSTEM
OPERATION: P REMOVAL: *(Continued)*
Taking out or off a device from a body part

Body Part	Approach	Device	Qualifier
6 Stomach	X External	Ø Drainage Device 2 Monitoring Device 3 Infusion Device D Intraluminal Device U Feeding Device	Z No Qualifier
P Rectum	Ø Open 3 Percutaneous 4 Percutaneous Endoscopic 7 Via Natural or Artificial Opening 8 Via Natural or Artificial Opening Endoscopic X External	1 Radioactive Element	Z No Qualifier
Q Anus	Ø Open 3 Percutaneous 4 Percutaneous Endoscopic 7 Via Natural or Artificial Opening 8 Via Natural or Artificial Opening Endoscopic	L Artificial Sphincter	Z No Qualifier
R Anal Sphincter	Ø Open 3 Percutaneous 4 Percutaneous Endoscopic	M Stimulator Lead	Z No Qualifier
U Omentum V Mesentery W Peritoneum	Ø Open 3 Percutaneous 4 Percutaneous Endoscopic	Ø Drainage Device 1 Radioactive Element 7 Autologous Tissue Substitute J Synthetic Substitute K Nonautologous Tissue Substitute	Z No Qualifier

Non-OR ØDP6X[Ø23DU]Z
Non-OR ØDPP[78X]1Z

(side tab) P: REMOVAL

(side tab) D: GASTROINTESTINAL SYSTEM

(side tab) Ø: M/S

New/Revised Text in Green   ~~deleted~~ Deleted   ♀ Females Only   ♂ Males Only   **Coding Clinic**
Non-covered   Limited Coverage   ⊡ Combination (See Appendix E)   DRG Non-OR   Non-OR   Hospital-Acquired Condition

SECTION: Ø MEDICAL AND SURGICAL
BODY SYSTEM: D GASTROINTESTINAL SYSTEM
OPERATION: Q REPAIR: Restoring, to the extent possible, a body part to its normal anatomic structure and function

Body Part	Approach	Device	Qualifier
1 Esophagus, Upper 2 Esophagus, Middle 3 Esophagus, Lower 4 Esophagogastric Junction 5 Esophagus ⊞ 6 Stomach ⊞ 7 Stomach, Pylorus 8 Small Intestine ⊞ 9 Duodenum ⊞ A Jejunum ⊞ B Ileum ⊞ C Ileocecal Valve E Large Intestine ⊞ F Large Intestine, Right ⊞ G Large Intestine, Left ⊞ H Cecum ⊞ J Appendix ⊞ K Ascending Colon ⊞ L Transverse Colon ⊞ M Descending Colon ⊞ N Sigmoid Colon ⊞ P Rectum ⊞	Ø Open 3 Percutaneous 4 Percutaneous Endoscopic 7 Via Natural or Artificial Opening 8 Via Natural or Artificial Opening Endoscopic	Z No Device	Z No Qualifier
Q Anus ⊞	Ø Open 3 Percutaneous 4 Percutaneous Endoscopic 7 Via Natural or Artificial Opening 8 Via Natural or Artificial Opening Endoscopic X External	Z No Device	Z No Qualifier
R Anal Sphincter S Greater Omentum T Lesser Omentum V Mesentery W Peritoneum ⊞	Ø Open 3 Percutaneous 4 Percutaneous Endoscopic	Z No Device	Z No Qualifier

⊞ ØDQ[56JNP][Ø3478]ZZ
⊞ ØDQ[89ABEFGHKLM]ØZZ
⊞ ØDQQ[Ø3478]ZZ
⊞ ØDQW[Ø34]ZZ

Coding Clinic: 2016, Q1, P7-8 – ØDQRØZZ, ØDQPØZZ

SECTION: Ø MEDICAL AND SURGICAL

BODY SYSTEM: D GASTROINTESTINAL SYSTEM

OPERATION: R REPLACEMENT: Putting in or on biological or synthetic material that physically takes the place and/or function of all or a portion of a body part

Body Part	Approach	Device	Qualifier
5 Esophagus	Ø Open 4 Percutaneous Endoscopic 7 Via Natural or Artificial Opening 8 Via Natural or Artificial Opening Endoscopic	7 Autologous Tissue Substitute J Synthetic Substitute K Nonautologous Tissue Substitute	Z No Qualifier
R Anal Sphincter S Greater Omentum T Lesser Omentum V Mesentery W Peritoneum	Ø Open 4 Percutaneous Endoscopic	7 Autologous Tissue Substitute J Synthetic Substitute K Nonautologous Tissue Substitute	Z No Qualifier

SECTION: Ø MEDICAL AND SURGICAL

BODY SYSTEM: D GASTROINTESTINAL SYSTEM

OPERATION: S REPOSITION: Moving to its normal location, or other suitable location, all or a portion of a body part

Body Part	Approach	Device	Qualifier
5 Esophagus 6 Stomach 9 Duodenum A Jejunum B Ileum H Cecum K Ascending Colon L Transverse Colon M Descending Colon N Sigmoid Colon P Rectum Q Anus	Ø Open 4 Percutaneous Endoscopic 7 Via Natural or Artificial Opening 8 Via Natural or Artificial Opening Endoscopic X External	Z No Device	Z No Qualifier

Non-OR ØDS[69ABHKLMNP]XZZ

New/Revised Text in Green   deleted Deleted   ♀ Females Only   ♂ Males Only   **Coding Clinic**
Non-covered   Limited Coverage   Combination (See Appendix E)   DRG Non-OR   Non-OR   Hospital-Acquired Condition

Side tab: R: REPLACEMENT   S: REPOSITION   D: GASTROINTESTINAL SYSTEM   Ø: M/S

SECTION: Ø MEDICAL AND SURGICAL

BODY SYSTEM: D GASTROINTESTINAL SYSTEM

OPERATION: T RESECTION: Cutting out or off, without replacement, all of a body part

Body Part	Approach	Device	Qualifier
1 Esophagus, Upper 2 Esophagus, Middle 3 Esophagus, Lower 4 Esophagogastric Junction 5 Esophagus 6 Stomach 7 Stomach, Pylorus 8 Small Intestine 9 Duodenum ⊞ A Jejunum B Ileum C Ileocecal Valve E Large Intestine F Large Intestine, Right G Large Intestine, Left H Cecum J Appendix K Ascending Colon L Transverse Colon M Descending Colon N Sigmoid Colon ⊞ P Rectum ⊞ Q Anus	Ø Open 4 Percutaneous Endoscopic 7 Via Natural or Artificial Opening 8 Via Natural or Artificial Opening Endoscopic	Z No Device	Z No Qualifier
R Anal Sphincter S Greater Omentum T Lesser Omentum	Ø Open 4 Percutaneous Endoscopic	Z No Device	Z No Qualifier

⊞ ØDT9ØZZ
⊞ ØDTN[Ø4]ZZ
⊞ ØDTP[Ø478]ZZ

0: M/S

D: GASTROINTESTINAL SYSTEM

T: RESECTION

SECTION: Ø MEDICAL AND SURGICAL

BODY SYSTEM: D GASTROINTESTINAL SYSTEM

OPERATION: U SUPPLEMENT: Putting in or on biological or synthetic material that physically reinforces and/or augments the function of a portion of a body part

Body Part	Approach	Device	Qualifier
1 Esophagus, Upper 2 Esophagus, Middle 3 Esophagus, Lower 4 Esophagogastric Junction 5 Esophagus 6 Stomach 7 Stomach, Pylorus 8 Small Intestine 9 Duodenum A Jejunum B Ileum C Ileocecal Valve E Large Intestine F Large Intestine, Right G Large Intestine, Left H Cecum K Ascending Colon L Transverse Colon M Descending Colon N Sigmoid Colon P Rectum	Ø Open 4 Percutaneous Endoscopic 7 Via Natural or Artificial Opening 8 Via Natural or Artificial Opening Endoscopic	7 Autologous Tissue Substitute J Synthetic Substitute K Nonautologous Tissue Substitute	Z No Qualifier
Q Anus	Ø Open 4 Percutaneous Endoscopic 7 Via Natural or Artificial Opening 8 Via Natural or Artificial Opening Endoscopic X External	7 Autologous Tissue Substitute J Synthetic Substitute K Nonautologous Tissue Substitute	Z No Qualifier
R Anal Sphincter S Greater Omentum T Lesser Omentum V Mesentery W Peritoneum	Ø Open 4 Percutaneous Endoscopic	7 Autologous Tissue Substitute J Synthetic Substitute K Nonautologous Tissue Substitute	Z No Qualifier

New/Revised Text in Green deleted Deleted ♀ Females Only ♂ Males Only **Coding Clinic** Non-covered Limited Coverage Combination (See Appendix E) DRG Non-OR Non-OR Hospital-Acquired Condition

SECTION: Ø MEDICAL AND SURGICAL
BODY SYSTEM: D GASTROINTESTINAL SYSTEM
OPERATION: V RESTRICTION: Partially closing an orifice or the lumen of a tubular body part

Body Part	Approach	Device	Qualifier
1 Esophagus, Upper 2 Esophagus, Middle 3 Esophagus, Lower 4 Esophagogastric Junction 5 Esophagus 6 Stomach 🦠 7 Stomach, Pylorus 8 Small Intestine 9 Duodenum A Jejunum B Ileum C Ileocecal Valve E Large Intestine F Large Intestine, Right G Large Intestine, Left H Cecum K Ascending Colon L Transverse Colon M Descending Colon N Sigmoid Colon P Rectum	Ø Open 3 Percutaneous 4 Percutaneous Endoscopic	C Extraluminal Device D Intraluminal Device Z No Device	Z No Qualifier
1 Esophagus, Upper 2 Esophagus, Middle 3 Esophagus, Lower 4 Esophagogastric Junction 5 Esophagus 6 Stomach 🦠 7 Stomach, Pylorus 8 Small Intestine 9 Duodenum A Jejunum B Ileum C Ileocecal Valve E Large Intestine F Large Intestine, Right G Large Intestine, Left H Cecum K Ascending Colon L Colon M Descending Colon N Sigmoid Colon P Rectum	7 Via Natural or Artificial Opening 8 Via Natural or Artificial Opening Endoscopic	D Intraluminal Device Z No Device	Z No Qualifier
Q Anus	Ø Open 3 Percutaneous 4 Percutaneous Endoscopic X External	C Extraluminal Device D Intraluminal Device Z No Device	Z No Qualifier
Q Anus	7 Via Natural or Artificial Opening 8 Via Natural or Artificial Opening Endoscopic	D Intraluminal Device Z No Device	Z No Qualifier

🦠 ØDV6[78]DZ
Non-OR ØDV6[78]DZ
🦠 ØDV64CZ when reported with Principal Diagnosis E66.Ø1 and Secondary Diagnosis K68.11, K95.Ø1, K95.81, or T81.4XXA

Coding Clinic: 2Ø16, Q2, P23 – ØDV4ØZZ

New/Revised Text in Green   ~~deleted~~ Deleted   ♀ Females Only   ♂ Males Only   **Coding Clinic**
🦠 Non-covered   🦠 Limited Coverage   ⊞ Combination (See Appendix E)   `DRG Non-OR`   Non-OR   🦠 Hospital-Acquired Condition

SECTION: Ø MEDICAL AND SURGICAL
BODY SYSTEM: D GASTROINTESTINAL SYSTEM
OPERATION: W REVISION: Correcting, to the extent possible, a portion of a malfunctioning device or the position of a displaced device

W: REVISION

D: GASTROINTESTINAL SYSTEM

Ø: M/S

Body Part	Approach	Device	Qualifier
Ø Upper Intestinal Tract D Lower Intestinal Tract	Ø Open 3 Percutaneous 4 Percutaneous Endoscopic 7 Via Natural or Artificial Opening 8 Via Natural or Artificial Opening Endoscopic X External	Ø Drainage Device 2 Monitoring Device 3 Infusion Device 7 Autologous Tissue Substitute C Extraluminal Device D Intraluminal Device J Synthetic Substitute K Nonautologous Tissue Substitute U Feeding Device	Z No Qualifier
5 Esophagus	7 Via Natural or Artificial Opening 8 Via Natural or Artificial Opening Endoscopic X External	D Intraluminal Device	Z No Qualifier
6 Stomach	Ø Open 3 Percutaneous 4 Percutaneous Endoscopic	Ø Drainage Device 2 Monitoring Device 3 Infusion Device 7 Autologous Tissue Substitute C Extraluminal Device D Intraluminal Device J Synthetic Substitute K Nonautologous Tissue Substitute M Stimulator Lead U Feeding Device	Z No Qualifier
6 Stomach	7 Via Natural or Artificial Opening 8 Via Natural or Artificial Opening Endoscopic X External	Ø Drainage Device 2 Monitoring Device 3 Infusion Device 7 Autologous Tissue Substitute C Extraluminal Device D Intraluminal Device J Synthetic Substitute K Nonautologous Tissue Substitute U Feeding Device	Z No Qualifier
8 Small Intestine E Large Intestine	Ø Open 4 Percutaneous Endoscopic 7 Via Natural or Artificial Opening 8 Via Natural or Artificial Opening Endoscopic	7 Autologous Tissue Substitute J Synthetic Substitute K Nonautologous Tissue Substitute	Z No Qualifier
Q Anus	Ø Open 3 Percutaneous 4 Percutaneous Endoscopic 7 Via Natural or Artificial Opening 8 Via Natural or Artificial Opening Endoscopic	L Artificial Sphincter	Z No Qualifier
R Anal Sphincter	Ø Open 3 Percutaneous 4 Percutaneous Endoscopic	M Stimulator Lead	Z No Qualifier
U Omentum V Mesentery W Peritoneum	Ø Open 3 Percutaneous 4 Percutaneous Endoscopic	Ø Drainage Device 7 Autologous Tissue Substitute J Synthetic Substitute K Nonautologous Tissue Substitute	Z No Qualifier

Non-OR ØDW[ØD]X[0237CDJKU]Z
Non-OR ØDW5XDZ

Non-OR ØDW6X[0237CDJKU]Z
Non-OR ØDW[UVW][034]0Z

New/Revised Text in Green ~~deleted~~ Deleted ♀ Females Only ♂ Males Only **Coding Clinic**
🖉 Non-covered 🖉 Limited Coverage ⊞ Combination (See Appendix E) DRG Non-OR Non-OR 🖉 Hospital-Acquired Condition

SECTION: Ø MEDICAL AND SURGICAL
BODY SYSTEM: D GASTROINTESTINAL SYSTEM
OPERATION: X **TRANSFER:** Moving, without taking out, all or a portion of a body part to another location to take over the function of all or a portion of a body part

Body Part	Approach	Device	Qualifier
6 Stomach 8 Small Intestine E Large Intestine	Ø Open 4 Percutaneous Endoscopic	Z No Device	5 Esophagus

Coding Clinic: 2016, Q2, P24 – ØDX6ØZ5

SECTION: Ø MEDICAL AND SURGICAL
BODY SYSTEM: D GASTROINTESTINAL SYSTEM
OPERATION: Y **TRANSPLANTATION:** Putting in or on all or a portion of a living body part taken from another individual or animal to physically take the place and/or function of all or a portion of a similar body part

Body Part	Approach	Device	Qualifier
5 Esophagus 6 Stomach 8 Small Intestine 🐾 E Large Intestine 🐾	Ø Open	Z No Device	0 Allogeneic 1 Syngeneic 2 Zooplastic

🐾 ØDY[8E]ØZ[Ø12]
Non-OR ØDY5ØZ[Ø12]

New/Revised Text in Green   ~~deleted~~ Deleted   ♀ Females Only   ♂ Males Only   **Coding Clinic**

Non-covered   Limited Coverage   Combination (See Appendix E)   DRG Non-OR   Non-OR   Hospital-Acquired Condition

SECTION: Ø MEDICAL AND SURGICAL
BODY SYSTEM: F HEPATOBILIARY SYSTEM AND PANCREAS
OPERATION: 1 BYPASS: Altering the route of passage of the contents of a tubular body part

Body Part	Approach	Device	Qualifier
4 Gallbladder 5 Hepatic Duct, Right 6 Hepatic Duct, Left 8 Cystic Duct 9 Common Bile Duct ⊞	Ø Open 4 Percutaneous Endoscopic	D Intraluminal Device Z No Device	3 Duodenum 4 Stomach 5 Hepatic Duct, Right 6 Hepatic Duct, Left 7 Hepatic Duct, Caudate 8 Cystic Duct 9 Common Bile Duct B Small Intestine
D Pancreatic Duct F Pancreatic Duct, Accessory G Pancreas ⊞	Ø Open 4 Percutaneous Endoscopic	D Intraluminal Device Z No Device	3 Duodenum B Small Intestine C Large Intestine

⊞ ØF19ØZ3
⊞ ØF1GØZC

SECTION: Ø MEDICAL AND SURGICAL
BODY SYSTEM: F HEPATOBILIARY SYSTEM AND PANCREAS
OPERATION: 2 CHANGE: Taking out or off a device from a body part and putting back an identical or similar device in or on the same body part without cutting or puncturing the skin or a mucous membrane

Body Part	Approach	Device	Qualifier
Ø Liver 4 Gallbladder B Hepatobiliary Duct D Pancreatic Duct G Pancreas	X External	Ø Drainage Device Y Other Device	Z No Qualifier

Non-OR All Values

SECTION: Ø MEDICAL AND SURGICAL
BODY SYSTEM: F HEPATOBILIARY SYSTEM AND PANCREAS
OPERATION: 5 DESTRUCTION: Physical eradication of all or a portion of a body part by the direct use of energy, force, or a destructive agent

Body Part	Approach	Device	Qualifier
Ø Liver 1 Liver, Right Lobe 2 Liver, Left Lobe 4 Gallbladder G Pancreas	Ø Open 3 Percutaneous 4 Percutaneous Endoscopic	Z No Device	Z No Qualifier
5 Hepatic Duct, Right 6 Hepatic Duct, Left 8 Cystic Duct 9 Common Bile Duct C Ampulla of Vater D Pancreatic Duct F Pancreatic Duct, Accessory	Ø Open 3 Percutaneous 4 Percutaneous Endoscopic 7 Via Natural or Artificial Opening 8 Via Natural or Artificial Opening Endoscopic	Z No Device	Z No Qualifier

Non-OR ØF5G4ZZ
Non-OR ØF5[5689CDF][48]ZZ

SECTION: Ø MEDICAL AND SURGICAL
BODY SYSTEM: F HEPATOBILIARY SYSTEM AND PANCREAS
OPERATION: 7 DILATION: Expanding an orifice or the lumen of a tubular body part

Body Part	Approach	Device	Qualifier
5 Hepatic Duct, Right ⊞ 6 Hepatic Duct, Left ⊞ 8 Cystic Duct ⊞ 9 Common Bile Duct ⊞ C Ampulla of Vater D Pancreatic Duct ⊞ F Pancreatic Duct, Accessory	Ø Open 3 Percutaneous 4 Percutaneous Endoscopic 7 Via Natural or Artificial Opening 8 Via Natural or Artificial Opening Endoscopic	D Intraluminal Device Z No Device	Z No Qualifier

⊞ ØF7[5689D][78]DZ
DRG Non-OR ØF7[5689D][78]DZ
Non-OR ØF7[5689][34][DZ]Z
Non-OR ØF7[CF]8DZ
Non-OR ØF7[DF]4[DZ]Z
Non-OR ØF7[5689CDF]8ZZ

Coding Clinic: 2016, Q1, P25 – ØF798DZ, ØF7D8DZ

SECTION: Ø MEDICAL AND SURGICAL
BODY SYSTEM: F HEPATOBILIARY SYSTEM AND PANCREAS
OPERATION: 8 DIVISION: Cutting into a body part, without draining fluids and/or gases from the body part, in order to separate or transect a body part

Body Part	Approach	Device	Qualifier
G Pancreas	Ø Open 3 Percutaneous 4 Percutaneous Endoscopic	Z No Device	Z No Qualifier

SECTION: Ø MEDICAL AND SURGICAL
BODY SYSTEM: F HEPATOBILIARY SYSTEM AND PANCREAS
OPERATION: 9 DRAINAGE: Taking or letting out fluids and/or gases from a body part

Body Part	Approach	Device	Qualifier
Ø Liver 1 Liver, Right Lobe 2 Liver, Left Lobe 4 Gallbladder G Pancreas	Ø Open 3 Percutaneous 4 Percutaneous Endoscopic	Ø Drainage Device	Z No Qualifier
Ø Liver 1 Liver, Right Lobe 2 Liver, Left Lobe 4 Gallbladder G Pancreas	Ø Open 3 Percutaneous 4 Percutaneous Endoscopic	Z No Device	X Diagnostic Z No Qualifier
5 Hepatic Duct, Right 6 Hepatic Duct, Left 8 Cystic Duct 9 Common Bile Duct C Ampulla of Vater D Pancreatic Duct F Pancreatic Duct, Accessory	Ø Open 3 Percutaneous 4 Percutaneous Endoscopic 7 Via Natural or Artificial Opening 8 Via Natural or Artificial Opening Endoscopic	Ø Drainage Device	Z No Qualifier
5 Hepatic Duct, Right 6 Hepatic Duct, Left 8 Cystic Duct 9 Common Bile Duct C Ampulla of Vater D Pancreatic Duct F Pancreatic Duct, Accessory	Ø Open 3 Percutaneous 4 Percutaneous Endoscopic 7 Via Natural or Artificial Opening 8 Via Natural or Artificial Opening Endoscopic	Z No Device	X Diagnostic Z No Qualifier

DRG Non-OR ØF9[4G]3ØZ
DRG Non-OR ØF9G3ZZ
DRG Non-OR ØF9[5689CDF]3ØZ
DRG Non-OR ØF9[568CDF]3ZZ
Non-OR ØF9[Ø12][34]ØZ
Non-OR ØF944ØZ

Non-OR ØF9[Ø124][34]Z[XZ]
Non-OR ØF9G[34]ZX
Non-OR ØF9[9DF]8ØZ
Non-OR ØF9C[48]ØZ
Non-OR ØF9[568][3478]ZX
Non-OR ØF99[3478]Z[XZ]

Non-OR ØF9[CDF][347]ZX
Non-OR ØF994ZZ
Non-OR ØF9C8Z[XZ]
Non-OR ØF9[DF]8ZX

Coding Clinic: 2015, Q1, P32 – ØF963ØZ

SECTION: Ø MEDICAL AND SURGICAL
BODY SYSTEM: F HEPATOBILIARY SYSTEM AND PANCREAS
OPERATION: B EXCISION: Cutting out or off, without replacement, a portion of a body part

Body Part	Approach	Device	Qualifier
Ø Liver 1 Liver, Right Lobe 2 Liver, Left Lobe 4 Gallbladder G Pancreas	Ø Open 3 Percutaneous 4 Percutaneous Endoscopic	Z No Device	X Diagnostic Z No Qualifier
5 Hepatic Duct, Right 6 Hepatic Duct, Left 8 Cystic Duct 9 Common Bile Duct C Ampulla of Vater D Pancreatic Duct F Pancreatic Duct, Accessory	Ø Open 3 Percutaneous 4 Percutaneous Endoscopic 7 Via Natural or Artificial Opening 8 Via Natural or Artificial Opening Endoscopic	Z No Device	X Diagnostic Z No Qualifier

Non-OR ØFB[Ø12]3ZX
Non-OR ØFB[4G][34]ZX

Non-OR ØFB[5689CDF][3478]ZX
Non-OR ØFB[5689CDF][48]ZZ

Coding Clinic: 2016, Q1, P23, P25 – ØFB98ZX
Coding Clinic: 2016, Q1, P25 – ØFBD8ZX

New/Revised Text in Green   ~~deleted~~ Deleted   ♀ Females Only   ♂ Males Only   Coding Clinic
🐾 Non-covered   🐾 Limited Coverage   ⊞ Combination (See Appendix E)   DRG Non-OR   Non-OR   🐾 Hospital-Acquired Condition
                                                                      249

SECTION: Ø MEDICAL AND SURGICAL
BODY SYSTEM: F HEPATOBILIARY SYSTEM AND PANCREAS
OPERATION: C EXTIRPATION: Taking or cutting out solid matter from a body part

Body Part	Approach	Device	Qualifier
Ø Liver 1 Liver, Right Lobe 2 Liver, Left Lobe 4 Gallbladder G Pancreas	Ø Open 3 Percutaneous 4 Percutaneous Endoscopic	Z No Device	Z No Qualifier
5 Hepatic Duct, Right 6 Hepatic Duct, Left 8 Cystic Duct 9 Common Bile Duct C Ampulla of Vater D Pancreatic Duct F Pancreatic Duct, Accessory	Ø Open 3 Percutaneous 4 Percutaneous Endoscopic 7 Via Natural or Artificial Opening 8 Via Natural or Artificial Opening Endoscopic	Z No Device	Z No Qualifier

Non-OR ØFC[5689][3478]ZZ   Non-OR ØFCC[48]ZZ   Non-OR ØFC[DF][348]ZZ

SECTION: Ø MEDICAL AND SURGICAL
BODY SYSTEM: F HEPATOBILIARY SYSTEM AND PANCREAS
OPERATION: F FRAGMENTATION: Breaking solid matter in a body part into pieces

Body Part	Approach	Device	Qualifier
4 Gallbladder 🔖 5 Hepatic Duct, Right 🔖 6 Hepatic Duct, Left 🔖 8 Cystic Duct 🔖 9 Common Bile Duct 🔖 C Ampulla of Vater 🔖 D Pancreatic Duct 🔖 F Pancreatic Duct, Acessory 🔖	Ø Open 3 Percutaneous 4 Percutaneous Endoscopic 7 Via Natural or Artificial Opening 8 Via Natural or Artificial Opening Endoscopic X External	Z No Device	Z No Qualifier

🔖 ØFF[45689CDF]XZZ   Non-OR ØFF[45689C][8X]ZZ   Non-OR ØFF[DF]XZZ

SECTION: Ø MEDICAL AND SURGICAL
BODY SYSTEM: F HEPATOBILIARY SYSTEM AND PANCREAS
OPERATION: H INSERTION: Putting in a nonbiological appliance that monitors, assists, performs, or prevents a physiological function but does not physically take the place of a body part

Body Part	Approach	Device	Qualifier
Ø Liver 1 Liver, Right Lobe 2 Liver, Left Lobe 4 Gallbladder G Pancreas	Ø Open 3 Percutaneous 4 Percutaneous Endoscopic	2 Monitoring Device 3 Infusion Device	Z No Qualifier
B Hepatobiliary Duct ⊞ D Pancreatic Duct	Ø Open 3 Percutaneous 4 Percutaneous Endoscopic 7 Via Natural or Artificial Opening 8 Via Natural or Artificial Opening Endoscopic	1 Radioactive Element 2 Monitoring Device 3 Infusion Device D Intraluminal Device	Z No Qualifier

⊞ ØFHB[78]DZ   DRG Non-OR ØFH[BD][78][23]Z   Non-OR ØFH[BD][Ø34]3Z
DRG Non-OR ØFH[Ø124G][Ø34]3Z   DRG Non-OR ØFHB8DZ   Non-OR ØFH[BD]4DZ
DRG Non-OR ØFH[BD][Ø34]3Z   Non-OR ØFH[Ø124G][Ø34]3Z   Non-OR ØFHD8DZ

New/Revised Text in Green   ~~deleted~~ Deleted   ♀ Females Only   ♂ Males Only   **Coding Clinic**
🔖 Non-covered   🔖 Limited Coverage   ⊞ Combination (See Appendix E)   DRG Non-OR   Non-OR   🔖 Hospital-Acquired Condition

Side tabs (left margin): H: INSERTION | F: FRAGMENTATION | C: EXTIRPATION | F: HEPATOBILIARY SYSTEM AND PANCREAS | Ø: M/S

SECTION: Ø MEDICAL AND SURGICAL
BODY SYSTEM: F HEPATOBILIARY SYSTEM AND PANCREAS
OPERATION: J INSPECTION: Visually and/or manually exploring a body part

Body Part	Approach	Device	Qualifier
Ø Liver 4 Gallbladder G Pancreas	Ø Open 3 Percutaneous 4 Percutaneous Endoscopic X External	Z No Device	Z No Qualifier
B Hepatobiliary Duct D Pancreatic Duct	Ø Open 3 Percutaneous 4 Percutaneous Endoscopic 7 Via Natural or Artificial Opening 8 Via Natural or Artificial Opening Endoscopic	Z No Device	Z No Qualifier

DRG Non-OR ØFJ[Ø4G]3ZZ
DRG Non-OR ØFJ[BD][378]ZZ
Non-OR ØFJ[Ø4G]XZZ

SECTION: Ø MEDICAL AND SURGICAL
BODY SYSTEM: F HEPATOBILIARY SYSTEM AND PANCREAS
OPERATION: L OCCLUSION: Completely closing an orifice or the lumen of a tubular body part

Body Part	Approach	Device	Qualifier
5 Hepatic Duct, Right 6 Hepatic Duct, Left 8 Cystic Duct 9 Common Bile Duct C Ampulla of Vater D Pancreatic Duct F Pancreatic Duct, Accessory	Ø Open 3 Percutaneous 4 Percutaneous Endoscopic	C Extraluminal Device D Intraluminal Device Z No Device	Z No Qualifier
5 Hepatic Duct, Right 6 Hepatic Duct, Left 8 Cystic Duct 9 Common Bile Duct C Ampulla of Vater D Pancreatic Duct F Pancreatic Duct, Accessory	7 Via Natural or Artificial Opening 8 Via Natural or Artificial Opening Endoscopic	D Intraluminal Device Z No Device	Z No Qualifier

Non-OR ØFL[5689][34][CDZ]Z
Non-OR ØFL[5689][78][DZ]Z

Ø: M/S

F: HEPATOBILIARY SYSTEM AND PANCREAS

J: INSPECTION   L: OCCLUSION

SECTION: Ø MEDICAL AND SURGICAL
BODY SYSTEM: F HEPATOBILIARY SYSTEM AND PANCREAS
OPERATION: M REATTACHMENT: Putting back in or on all or a portion of a separated body part to its normal location or other suitable location

Body Part	Approach	Device	Qualifier
Ø Liver 1 Liver, Right Lobe 2 Liver, Left Lobe 4 Gallbladder 5 Hepatic Duct, Right 6 Hepatic Duct, Left 8 Cystic Duct 9 Common Bile Duct C Ampulla of Vater D Pancreatic Duct F Pancreatic Duct, Accessory G Pancreas	Ø Open 4 Percutaneous Endoscopic	Z No Device	Z No Qualifier

Non-OR   ØFM[45689]4ZZ

SECTION: Ø MEDICAL AND SURGICAL
BODY SYSTEM: F HEPATOBILIARY SYSTEM AND PANCREAS
OPERATION: N RELEASE: Freeing a body part from an abnormal physical constraint by cutting or by the use of force

Body Part	Approach	Device	Qualifier
Ø Liver 1 Liver, Right Lobe 2 Liver, Left Lobe 4 Gallbladder G Pancreas	Ø Open 3 Percutaneous 4 Percutaneous Endoscopic	Z No Device	Z No Qualifier
5 Hepatic Duct, Right 6 Hepatic Duct, Left 8 Cystic Duct 9 Common Bile Duct C Ampulla of Vater D Pancreatic Duct F Pancreatic Duct, Accessory	Ø Open 3 Percutaneous 4 Percutaneous Endoscopic 7 Via Natural or Artificial Opening 8 Via Natural or Artificial Opening Endoscopic	Z No Device	Z No Qualifier

New/Revised Text in Green   ~~deleted~~ Deleted   ♀ Females Only   ♂ Males Only   **Coding Clinic**
Non-covered   Limited Coverage   ⊡ Combination (See Appendix E)   DRG Non-OR   Non-OR   Hospital-Acquired Condition

SECTION: Ø MEDICAL AND SURGICAL

BODY SYSTEM: F HEPATOBILIARY SYSTEM AND PANCREAS
OPERATION: P REMOVAL: Taking out or off a device from a body part

Body Part	Approach	Device	Qualifier
Ø Liver	Ø Open 3 Percutaneous 4 Percutaneous Endoscopic X External	Ø Drainage Device 2 Monitoring Device 3 Infusion Device	Z No Qualifier
4 Gallbladder G Pancreas	Ø Open 3 Percutaneous 4 Percutaneous Endoscopic X External	Ø Drainage Device 2 Monitoring Device 3 Infusion Device D Intraluminal Device	Z No Qualifier
B Hepatobiliary Duct ⊞ D Pancreatic Duct ⊞	Ø Open 3 Percutaneous 4 Percutaneous Endoscopic 7 Via Natural or Artificial Opening 8 Via Natural or Artificial Opening Endoscopic	Ø Drainage Device 1 Radioactive Element 2 Monitoring Device 3 Infusion Device 7 Autologous Tissue Substitute C Extraluminal Device D Intraluminal Device J Synthetic Substitute K Nonautologous Tissue Substitute	Z No Qualifier
B Hepatobiliary Duct ⊞ D Pancreatic Duct ⊞	X External	Ø Drainage Device 1 Radioactive Element 2 Monitoring Device 3 Infusion Device D Intraluminal Device	Z No Qualifier

⊞ ØFPB[78]DZ
⊞ ØFPBXDZ
⊞ ØFPD[78]DZ
⊞ ØFPDXDZ
DRG Non-OR ØFP[BD]XDZ
DRG Non-OR ØFP[BD][78][Ø23D]Z

Non-OR ØFPØX[Ø23]Z
Non-OR ØFP4X[Ø23D]Z
Non-OR ØFPGX[Ø23]Z
Non-OR ØFP[BD]X[Ø123]Z

SECTION: Ø MEDICAL AND SURGICAL

BODY SYSTEM: F HEPATOBILIARY SYSTEM AND PANCREAS
OPERATION: Q REPAIR: Restoring, to the extent possible, a body part to its normal anatomic structure and function

Body Part	Approach	Device	Qualifier
Ø Liver ⊞ 1 Liver, Right Lobe 2 Liver, Left Lobe 4 Gallbladder ⊞ G Pancreas	Ø Open 3 Percutaneous 4 Percutaneous Endoscopic	Z No Device	Z No Qualifier
5 Hepatic Duct, Right 6 Hepatic Duct, Left 8 Cystic Duct 9 Common Bile Duct C Ampulla of Vater D Pancreatic Duct F Pancreatic Duct, Accessory	Ø Open 3 Percutaneous 4 Percutaneous Endoscopic 7 Via Natural or Artificial Opening 8 Via Natural or Artificial Opening Endoscopic	Z No Device	Z No Qualifier

⊞ ØFQ[Ø4][Ø34]ZZ

New/Revised Text in Green   deleted Deleted   ♀ Females Only   ♂ Males Only   **Coding Clinic**
🚫 Non-covered   🚫 Limited Coverage   ⊞ Combination (See Appendix E)   DRG Non-OR   Non-OR   🚫 Hospital-Acquired Condition

SECTION: Ø MEDICAL AND SURGICAL

BODY SYSTEM: F HEPATOBILIARY SYSTEM AND PANCREAS
OPERATION: R REPLACEMENT: Putting in or on biological or synthetic material that physically takes the place and/or function of all or a portion of a body part

Body Part	Approach	Device	Qualifier
5 Hepatic Duct, Right 6 Hepatic Duct, Left 8 Cystic Duct 9 Common Bile Duct C Ampulla of Vater D Pancreatic Duct F Pancreatic Duct, Accessory	Ø Open 4 Percutaneous Endoscopic	7 Autologous Tissue Substitute J Synthetic Substitute K Nonautologous Tissue Substitute	Z No Qualifier

SECTION: Ø MEDICAL AND SURGICAL

BODY SYSTEM: F HEPATOBILIARY SYSTEM AND PANCREAS
OPERATION: S REPOSITION: Moving to its normal location, or other suitable location, all or a portion of a body part

Body Part	Approach	Device	Qualifier
Ø Liver 4 Gallbladder 5 Hepatic Duct, Right 6 Hepatic Duct, Left 8 Cystic Duct 9 Common Bile Duct C Ampulla of Vater D Pancreatic Duct F Pancreatic Duct, Accessory G Pancreas	Ø Open 4 Percutaneous Endoscopic	Z No Device	Z No Qualifier

SECTION: Ø MEDICAL AND SURGICAL

BODY SYSTEM: F HEPATOBILIARY SYSTEM AND PANCREAS
OPERATION: T RESECTION: Cutting out or off, without replacement, all of a body part

Body Part	Approach	Device	Qualifier
Ø Liver 1 Liver, Right Lobe 2 Liver, Left Lobe 4 Gallbladder G Pancreas ⊕	Ø Open 4 Percutaneous Endoscopic	Z No Device	Z No Qualifier
5 Hepatic Duct, Right 6 Hepatic Duct, Left 8 Cystic Duct 9 Common Bile Duct C Ampulla of Vater D Pancreatic Duct F Pancreatic Duct, Accessory	Ø Open 4 Percutaneous Endoscopic 7 Via Natural or Artificial Opening 8 Via Natural or Artificial Opening Endoscopic	Z No Device	Z No Qualifier

⊕ ØFTGØZZ
Non-OR ØFT[DF][48]ZZ

Coding Clinic: 2012, Q4, P100 – ØFT00ZZ

New/Revised Text in Green   deleted Deleted   ♀ Females Only   ♂ Males Only   Coding Clinic
🔖 Non-covered   🔖 Limited Coverage   ⊕ Combination (See Appendix E)   DRG Non-OR   Non-OR   🔖 Hospital-Acquired Condition

SECTION: Ø MEDICAL AND SURGICAL
BODY SYSTEM: F HEPATOBILIARY SYSTEM AND PANCREAS
OPERATION: U SUPPLEMENT: Putting in or on biological or synthetic material that physically reinforces and/or augments the function of a portion of a body part

Body Part	Approach	Device	Qualifier
5 Hepatic Duct, Right 6 Hepatic Duct, Left 8 Cystic Duct 9 Common Bile Duct C Ampulla of Vater D Pancreatic Duct F Pancreatic Duct, Accessory	Ø Open 3 Percutaneous 4 Percutaneous Endoscopic	7 Autologous Tissue Substitute J Synthetic Substitute K Nonautologous Tissue Substitute	Z No Qualifier

SECTION: Ø MEDICAL AND SURGICAL
BODY SYSTEM: F HEPATOBILIARY SYSTEM AND PANCREAS
OPERATION: V RESTRICTION: Partially closing an orifice or the lumen of a tubular body part

Body Part	Approach	Device	Qualifier
5 Hepatic Duct, Right 6 Hepatic Duct, Left 8 Cystic Duct 9 Common Bile Duct C Ampulla of Vater D Pancreatic Duct F Pancreatic Duct, Accessory	Ø Open 3 Percutaneous 4 Percutaneous Endoscopic	C Extraluminal Device D Intraluminal Device Z No Device	Z No Qualifier
5 Hepatic Duct, Right 6 Hepatic Duct, Left 8 Cystic Duct 9 Common Bile Duct C Ampulla of Vater D Pancreatic Duct F Pancreatic Duct, Accessory	7 Via Natural or Artificial Opening 8 Via Natural or Artificial Opening Endoscopic	D Intraluminal Device Z No Device	Z No Qualifier

Non-OR ØFV[5689][34][CDZ]Z
Non-OR ØFV[5689][78][DZ]Z

SECTION: Ø MEDICAL AND SURGICAL
BODY SYSTEM: F HEPATOBILIARY SYSTEM AND PANCREAS
OPERATION: W REVISION: Correcting, to the extent possible, a portion of a malfunctioning device or the position of a displaced device

Body Part	Approach	Device	Qualifier
Ø Liver	Ø Open 3 Percutaneous 4 Percutaneous Endoscopic X External	Ø Drainage Device 2 Monitoring Device 3 Infusion Device	Z No Qualifier
4 Gallbladder G Pancreas	Ø Open 3 Percutaneous 4 Percutaneous Endoscopic X External	Ø Drainage Device 2 Monitoring Device 3 Infusion Device D Intraluminal Device	Z No Qualifier
B Hepatobiliary Duct D Pancreatic Duct	Ø Open 3 Percutaneous 4 Percutaneous Endoscopic 7 Via Natural or Artificial Opening 8 Via Natural or Artificial Opening Endoscopic X External	Ø Drainage Device 2 Monitoring Device 3 Infusion Device 7 Autologous Tissue Substitute C Extraluminal Device D Intraluminal Device J Synthetic Substitute K Nonautologous Tissue Substitute	Z No Qualifier

Non-OR   ØFWØX[Ø23]Z
Non-OR   ØFW[4G]X[Ø23D]Z
Non-OR   ØFW[BD]X[Ø237CDJK]Z

SECTION: Ø MEDICAL AND SURGICAL
BODY SYSTEM: F HEPATOBILIARY SYSTEM AND PANCREAS
OPERATION: Y TRANSPLANTATION: Putting in or on all or a portion of a living body part taken from another individual or animal to physically take the place and/or function of all or a portion of a similar body part

Body Part	Approach	Device	Qualifier
Ø Liver 🦠 G Pancreas 🦠 🦠 ⊞	Ø Open	Z No Device	Ø Allogeneic 1 Syngeneic 2 Zooplastic

🦠 ØFYGØZ2
🦠 ØFYGØZØ, ØFYGØZ1 alone [without kidney transplant codes (ØTYØØZ[Ø1], ØTY1ØZ[Ø12])], except when ØFYGØZØ or ØFYGØZ1 is combined with at least one principal or secondary diagnosis code from the following list:

E10.10	E10.321	E10.359	E10.44	E10.620	E10.649
E10.11	E10.329	E10.36	E10.49	E10.621	E10.65
E10.21	E10.331	E10.39	E10.51	E10.622	E10.69
E10.22	E10.339	E10.40	E10.52	E10.628	E10.8
E10.29	E10.341	E10.41	E10.59	E10.630	E10.9
E10.311	E10.349	E10.42	E10.610	E10.638	E89.1
E10.319	E10.351	E10.43	E10.618	E10.641	

🦠 ØFYØØZ[Ø12]
🦠 ØFYGØZ[Ø1]
⊞ ØFYGØZ[Ø12]

Coding Clinic: 2012, Q4, P100 – ØFYØØZØ

New/Revised Text in Green   ~~deleted~~ Deleted   ♀ Females Only   ♂ Males Only   **Coding Clinic**
🦠 Non-covered   🦠 Limited Coverage   ⊞ Combination (See Appendix E)   DRG Non-OR   Non-OR   🦠 Hospital-Acquired Condition

SECTION: Ø MEDICAL AND SURGICAL

BODY SYSTEM: G ENDOCRINE SYSTEM

OPERATION: 2 **CHANGE:** Taking out or off a device from a body part and putting back an identical or similar device in or on the same body part without cutting or puncturing the skin or a mucous membrane

Body Part	Approach	Device	Qualifier
Ø Pituitary Gland 1 Pineal Body 5 Adrenal Gland K Thyroid Gland R Parathyroid Gland S Endocrine Gland	X External	Ø Drainage Device Y Other Device	Z No Qualifier

Non-OR All Values

SECTION: Ø MEDICAL AND SURGICAL

BODY SYSTEM: G ENDOCRINE SYSTEM

OPERATION: 5 **DESTRUCTION:** Physical eradication of all or a portion of a body part by the direct use of energy, force, or a destructive agent

Body Part	Approach	Device	Qualifier
Ø Pituitary Gland 1 Pineal Body 2 Adrenal Gland, Left 3 Adrenal Gland, Right 4 Adrenal Glands, Bilateral 6 Carotid Body, Left 7 Carotid Body, Right 8 Carotid Bodies, Bilateral 9 Para-aortic Body B Coccygeal Glomus C Glomus Jugulare D Aortic Body F Paraganglion Extremity G Thyroid Gland Lobe, Left H Thyroid Gland Lobe, Right K Thyroid Gland L Superior Parathyroid Gland, Right M Superior Parathyroid Gland, Left N Inferior Parathyroid Gland, Right P Inferior Parathyroid Gland, Left Q Parathyroid Glands, Multiple R Parathyroid Gland	Ø Open 3 Percutaneous 4 Percutaneous Endoscopic	Z No Device	Z No Qualifier

Non-OR 0G5[6789BCDF][034]ZZ

SECTION: Ø MEDICAL AND SURGICAL

BODY SYSTEM: G ENDOCRINE SYSTEM

OPERATION: 8 **DIVISION:** Cutting into a body part, without draining fluids and/or gases from the body part, in order to separate or transect a body part

Body Part	Approach	Device	Qualifier
Ø Pituitary Gland J Thyroid Gland Isthmus	Ø Open 3 Percutaneous 4 Percutaneous Endoscopic	Z No Device	Z No Qualifier

New/Revised Text in Green   ~~deleted~~ Deleted   ♀ Females Only   ♂ Males Only   **Coding Clinic**
🚫 Non-covered   🚫 Limited Coverage   ⊡ Combination (See Appendix E)   DRG Non-OR   Non-OR   🚫 Hospital-Acquired Condition

Sidebar: 8: DIVISION   5: DESTRUCTION   2: CHANGE   G: ENDOCRINE SYSTEM   Ø: M/S

SECTION: Ø MEDICAL AND SURGICAL

BODY SYSTEM: G ENDOCRINE SYSTEM

OPERATION: 9 DRAINAGE: Taking or letting out fluids and/or gases from a body part

Body Part	Approach	Device	Qualifier
Ø Pituitary Gland 1 Pineal Body 2 Adrenal Gland, Left 3 Adrenal Gland, Right 4 Adrenal Glands, Bilateral 6 Carotid Body, Left 7 Carotid Body, Right 8 Carotid Bodies, Bilateral 9 Para-aortic Body B Coccygeal Glomus C Glomus Jugulare D Aortic Body F Paraganglion Extremity G Thyroid Gland Lobe, Left H Thyroid Gland Lobe, Right K Thyroid Gland L Superior Parathyroid Gland, Right M Superior Parathyroid Gland, Left N Inferior Parathyroid Gland, Right P Inferior Parathyroid Gland, Left Q Parathyroid Glands, Multiple R Parathyroid Gland	Ø Open 3 Percutaneous 4 Percutaneous Endoscopic	Ø Drainage Device	Z No Qualifier
Ø Pituitary Gland 1 Pineal Body 2 Adrenal Gland, Left 3 Adrenal Gland, Right 4 Adrenal Glands, Bilateral 6 Carotid Body, Left 7 Carotid Body, Right 8 Carotid Bodies, Bilateral 9 Para-aortic Body B Coccygeal Glomus C Glomus Jugulare D Aortic Body F Paraganglion Extremity G Thyroid Gland Lobe, Left H Thyroid Gland Lobe, Right K Thyroid Gland L Superior Parathyroid Gland, Right M Superior Parathyroid Gland, Left N Inferior Parathyroid Gland, Right P Inferior Parathyroid Gland, Left Q Parathyroid Glands, Multiple R Parathyroid Gland	Ø Open 3 Percutaneous 4 Percutaneous Endoscopic	Z No Device	X Diagnostic Z No Qualifier

DRG Non-OR ØG9[Ø12346789BCDF]3ØZ
DRG Non-OR ØG9[Ø12346789BCDF]3ZZ
Non-OR ØG9[6789BCDF][Ø4]ØZ
Non-OR ØG9[GHKLMNPQR][34]ØZ
Non-OR ØG9[234GHK][34]ZX
Non-OR ØG9[6789BCDF][Ø34]ZX
Non-OR ØG9[6789BCDF][Ø4]ZZ
Non-OR ØG9[GHKLMNPQR][34]ZZ

Ø: M/S

G: ENDOCRINE SYSTEM

9: DRAINAGE

B: EXCISION   C: EXTIRPATION

G: ENDOCRINE SYSTEM   0: M/S

SECTION: Ø **MEDICAL AND SURGICAL**

BODY SYSTEM: G ENDOCRINE SYSTEM

OPERATION: **B EXCISION:** Cutting out or off, without replacement, a portion of a body part

Body Part	Approach	Device	Qualifier
Ø Pituitary Gland 1 Pineal Body 2 Adrenal Gland, Left 3 Adrenal Gland, Right 4 Adrenal Glands, Bilateral 6 Carotid Body, Left 7 Carotid Body, Right 8 Carotid Bodies, Bilateral 9 Para-aortic Body B Coccygeal Glomus C Glomus Jugulare D Aortic Body F Paraganglion Extremity G Thyroid Gland Lobe, Left H Thyroid Gland Lobe, Right L Superior Parathyroid Gland, Right M Superior Parathyroid Gland, Left N Inferior Parathyroid Gland, Right P Inferior Parathyroid Gland, Left Q Parathyroid Glands, Multiple R Parathyroid Gland	Ø Open 3 Percutaneous 4 Percutaneous Endoscopic	Z No Device	X Diagnostic Z No Qualifier

Non-OR   ØGB[234GH][34]ZX
Non-OR   ØGB[6789BCDF][Ø34]Z[XZ]

SECTION: Ø **MEDICAL AND SURGICAL**

BODY SYSTEM: G ENDOCRINE SYSTEM

OPERATION: **C EXTIRPATION:** Taking or cutting out solid matter from a body part

Body Part	Approach	Device	Qualifier
Ø Pituitary Gland 1 Pineal Body 2 Adrenal Gland, Left 3 Adrenal Gland, Right 4 Adrenal Glands, Bilateral 6 Carotid Body, Left 7 Carotid Body, Right 8 Carotid Bodies, Bilateral 9 Para-aortic Body B Coccygeal Glomus C Glomus Jugulare D Aortic Body F Paraganglion Extremity G Thyroid Gland Lobe, Left H Thyroid Gland Lobe, Right K Thyroid Gland L Superior Parathyroid Gland, Right M Superior Parathyroid Gland, Left N Inferior Parathyroid Gland, Right P Inferior Parathyroid Gland, Left Q Parathyroid Glands, Multiple R Parathyroid Gland	Ø Open 3 Percutaneous 4 Percutaneous Endoscopic	Z No Device	Z No Qualifier

Non-OR   ØGC[6789BCDF][Ø34]ZZ

New/Revised Text in Green   ~~deleted~~ Deleted   ♀ Females Only   ♂ Males Only   **Coding Clinic**
🚫 Non-covered   🚫 Limited Coverage   ⊞ Combination (See Appendix E)   DRG Non-OR   Non-OR   🚫 Hospital-Acquired Condition

SECTION: Ø MEDICAL AND SURGICAL
BODY SYSTEM: G ENDOCRINE SYSTEM
OPERATION: H INSERTION: Putting in a nonbiological appliance that monitors, assists, performs, or prevents a physiological function but does not physically take the place of a body part

Body Part	Approach	Device	Qualifier
S Endocrine Gland	Ø Open 3 Percutaneous 4 Percutaneous Endoscopic	2 Monitoring Device 3 Infusion Device	Z No Qualifier

SECTION: Ø MEDICAL AND SURGICAL
BODY SYSTEM: G ENDOCRINE SYSTEM
OPERATION: J INSPECTION: Visually and/or manually exploring a body part

Body Part	Approach	Device	Qualifier
Ø Pituitary Gland 1 Pineal Body 5 Adrenal Gland K Thyroid Gland R Parathyroid Gland S Endocrine Gland	Ø Open 3 Percutaneous 4 Percutaneous Endoscopic	Z No Device	Z No Qualifier

DRG Non-OR ØGJ[Ø15KRS]3ZZ

SECTION: Ø MEDICAL AND SURGICAL
BODY SYSTEM: G ENDOCRINE SYSTEM
OPERATION: M REATTACHMENT: Putting back in or on all or a portion of a separated body part to its normal location or other suitable location

Body Part	Approach	Device	Qualifier
2 Adrenal Gland, Left 3 Adrenal Gland, Right G Thyroid Gland Lobe, Left H Thyroid Gland Lobe, Right L Superior Parathyroid Gland, Right M Superior Parathyroid Gland, Left N Inferior Parathyroid Gland, Right P Inferior Parathyroid Gland, Left Q Parathyroid Glands, Multiple R Parathyroid Gland	Ø Open 4 Percutaneous Endoscopic	Z No Device	Z No Qualifier

SECTION: Ø MEDICAL AND SURGICAL

BODY SYSTEM: G ENDOCRINE SYSTEM

OPERATION: N RELEASE: Freeing a body part from an abnormal physical constraint by cutting or by the use of force

Body Part	Approach	Device	Qualifier
Ø Pituitary Gland 1 Pineal Body 2 Adrenal Gland, Left 3 Adrenal Gland, Right 4 Adrenal Glands, Bilateral 6 Carotid Body, Left 7 Carotid Body, Right 8 Carotid Bodies, Bilateral 9 Para-aortic Body B Coccygeal Glomus C Glomus Jugulare D Aortic Body F Paraganglion Extremity G Thyroid Gland Lobe, Left H Thyroid Gland Lobe, Right K Thyroid Gland L Superior Parathyroid Gland, Right M Superior Parathyroid Gland, Left N Inferior Parathyroid Gland, Right P Inferior Parathyroid Gland, Left Q Parathyroid Glands, Multiple R Parathyroid Gland	Ø Open 3 Percutaneous 4 Percutaneous Endoscopic	Z No Device	Z No Qualifier

Non-OR ØGN[6789BCDF][Ø34]ZZ

SECTION: Ø MEDICAL AND SURGICAL

BODY SYSTEM: G ENDOCRINE SYSTEM

OPERATION: P REMOVAL: Taking out or off a device from a body part

Body Part	Approach	Device	Qualifier
Ø Pituitary Gland 1 Pineal Body 5 Adrenal Gland K Thyroid Gland R Parathyroid Gland	Ø Open 3 Percutaneous 4 Percutaneous Endoscopic X External	Ø Drainage Device	Z No Qualifier
S Endocrine Gland	Ø Open 3 Percutaneous 4 Percutaneous Endoscopic X External	Ø Drainage Device 2 Monitoring Device 3 Infusion Device	Z No Qualifier

Non-OR ØGP[Ø15KR]XØZ
Non-OR ØGPS[Ø34X][Ø23]Z

New/Revised Text in Green   ~~deleted~~ Deleted   ♀ Females Only   ♂ Males Only   **Coding Clinic**
🔖 Non-covered   🔖 Limited Coverage   ⊞ Combination (See Appendix E)   DRG Non-OR   Non-OR   🔖 Hospital-Acquired Condition

SECTION: Ø MEDICAL AND SURGICAL

BODY SYSTEM: G ENDOCRINE SYSTEM
OPERATION: Q REPAIR: Restoring, to the extent possible, a body part to its normal anatomic structure and function

Body Part	Approach	Device	Qualifier
Ø Pituitary Gland 1 Pineal Body 2 Adrenal Gland, Left 3 Adrenal Gland, Right 4 Adrenal Glands, Bilateral 6 Carotid Body, Left 7 Carotid Body, Right 8 Carotid Bodies, Bilateral 9 Para-aortic Body B Coccygeal Glomus C Glomus Jugulare D Aortic Body F Paraganglion Extremity G Thyroid Gland Lobe, Left H Thyroid Gland Lobe, Right J Thyroid Gland Isthmus K Thyroid Gland L Superior Parathyroid Gland, Right M Superior Parathyroid Gland, Left N Inferior Parathyroid Gland, Right P Inferior Parathyroid Gland, Left Q Parathyroid Glands, Multiple R Parathyroid Gland	Ø Open 3 Percutaneous 4 Percutaneous Endoscopic	Z No Device	Z No Qualifier

Non-OR   ØGQ[6789BCDF][Ø34]ZZ

SECTION: Ø MEDICAL AND SURGICAL

BODY SYSTEM: G ENDOCRINE SYSTEM
OPERATION: S REPOSITION: Moving to its normal location, or other suitable location, all or a portion of a body part

Body Part	Approach	Device	Qualifier
2 Adrenal Gland, Left 3 Adrenal Gland, Right G Thyroid Gland Lobe, Left H Thyroid Gland Lobe, Right L Superior Parathyroid Gland, Right M Superior Parathyroid Gland, Left N Inferior Parathyroid Gland, Right P Inferior Parathyroid Gland, Left Q Parathyroid Glands, Multiple R Parathyroid Gland	Ø Open 4 Percutaneous Endoscopic	Z No Device	Z No Qualifier

Ø: M/S

G: ENDOCRINE SYSTEM

Q: REPAIR   S: REPOSITION

SECTION: Ø MEDICAL AND SURGICAL

BODY SYSTEM: G ENDOCRINE SYSTEM

OPERATION: T RESECTION: Cutting out or off, without replacement, all of a body part

Body Part	Approach	Device	Qualifier
Ø Pituitary Gland 1 Pineal Body 2 Adrenal Gland, Left 3 Adrenal Gland, Right 4 Adrenal Glands, Bilateral 6 Carotid Body, Left 7 Carotid Body, Right 8 Carotid Bodies, Bilateral 9 Para-aortic Body B Coccygeal Glomus C Glomus Jugulare D Aortic Body F Paraganglion Extremity G Thyroid Gland Lobe, Left H Thyroid Gland Lobe, Right K Thyroid Gland L Superior Parathyroid Gland, Right M Superior Parathyroid Gland, Left N Inferior Parathyroid Gland, Right P Inferior Parathyroid Gland, Left Q Parathyroid Glands, Multiple R Parathyroid Gland	Ø Open 4 Percutaneous Endoscopic	Z No Device	Z No Qualifier

Non-OR ØGT[6789BCDF][04]ZZ

SECTION: Ø MEDICAL AND SURGICAL

BODY SYSTEM: G ENDOCRINE SYSTEM

OPERATION: W REVISION: Correcting, to the extent possible, a portion of a malfunctioning device or the position of a displaced device

Body Part	Approach	Device	Qualifier
Ø Pituitary Gland 1 Pineal Body 5 Adrenal Gland K Thyroid Gland R Parathyroid Gland	Ø Open 3 Percutaneous 4 Percutaneous Endoscopic X External	Ø Drainage Device	Z No Qualifier
S Endocrine Gland	Ø Open 3 Percutaneous 4 Percutaneous Endoscopic X External	Ø Drainage Device 2 Monitoring Device 3 Infusion Device	Z No Qualifier

Non-OR ØGW[Ø15KR]XØZ
Non-OR ØGWS[Ø34X][Ø23]Z

New/Revised Text in Green deleted Deleted ♀ Females Only ♂ Males Only Coding Clinic
Non-covered Limited Coverage ⊞ Combination (See Appendix E) DRG Non-OR Non-OR Hospital-Acquired Condition

Ø: ALTERATION   2: CHANGE

H: SKIN AND BREAST

Ø: M/S

SECTION: Ø MEDICAL AND SURGICAL

BODY SYSTEM: H SKIN AND BREAST

OPERATION: Ø **ALTERATION:** Modifying the anatomic structure of a body part without affecting the function of the body part

Body Part	Approach	Device	Qualifier
T Breast, Right U Breast, Left V Breast, Bilateral	Ø Open 3 Percutaneous X External	7 Autologous Tissue Substitute J Synthetic Substitute K Nonautologous Tissue Substitute Z No Device	Z No Qualifier

SECTION: Ø MEDICAL AND SURGICAL

BODY SYSTEM: H SKIN AND BREAST

OPERATION: 2 **CHANGE:** Taking out or off a device from a body part and putting back an identical or similar device in or on the same body part without cutting or puncturing the skin or a mucous membrane

Body Part	Approach	Device	Qualifier
P Skin T Breast, Right U Breast, Left	X External	Ø Drainage Device Y Other Device	Z No Qualifier

Non-OR   All Values

New/Revised Text in Green   ~~deleted~~ Deleted   ♀ Females Only   ♂ Males Only   **Coding Clinic**

🐾 Non-covered   🐾 Limited Coverage   ⊞ Combination (See Appendix E)   DRG Non-OR   Non-OR   🐾 Hospital-Acquired Condition

SECTION: Ø MEDICAL AND SURGICAL
BODY SYSTEM: H SKIN AND BREAST
OPERATION: 5 DESTRUCTION: Physical eradication of all or a portion of a body part by the direct use of energy, force, or a destructive agent

Body Part	Approach	Device	Qualifier
Ø Skin, Scalp 1 Skin, Face 2 Skin, Right Ear 3 Skin, Left Ear 4 Skin, Neck 5 Skin, Chest 6 Skin, Back 7 Skin, Abdomen 8 Skin, Buttock 9 Skin, Perineum A Skin, Genitalia B Skin, Right Upper Arm C Skin, Left Upper Arm D Skin, Right Lower Arm E Skin, Left Lower Arm F Skin, Right Hand G Skin, Left Hand H Skin, Right Upper Leg J Skin, Left Upper Leg K Skin, Right Lower Leg L Skin, Left Lower Leg M Skin, Right Foot N Skin, Left Foot	X External	Z No Device	D Multiple Z No Qualifier
Q Finger Nail R Toe Nail	X External	Z No Device	Z No Qualifier
T Breast, Right U Breast, Left V Breast, Bilateral W Nipple, Right X Nipple, Left	Ø Open 3 Percutaneous 7 Via Natural or Artificial Opening 8 Via Natural or Artificial Opening Endoscopic X External	Z No Device	Z No Qualifier

DRG Non-OR ØH5[Ø1456789ABCDEFGHJKLMN]XZ[DZ]
DRG Non-OR ØH5[QR]XZZ
Non-OR ØH5[23]XZ[DZ]

Ø: M/S

H: SKIN AND BREAST

5: DESTRUCTION

New/Revised Text in Green · deleted Deleted · ♀ Females Only · ♂ Males Only · **Coding Clinic**
🚫 Non-covered · 🚫 Limited Coverage · ⊞ Combination (See Appendix E) · DRG Non-OR · Non-OR · 🚫 Hospital-Acquired Condition

267

SECTION: Ø MEDICAL AND SURGICAL

BODY SYSTEM: H SKIN AND BREAST

OPERATION: 8 **DIVISION:** Cutting into a body part, without draining fluids and/or gases from the body part, in order to separate or transect a body part

Body Part	Approach	Device	Qualifier
Ø Skin, Scalp	X External	Z No Device	Z No Qualifier
1 Skin, Face			
2 Skin, Right Ear			
3 Skin, Left Ear			
4 Skin, Neck			
5 Skin, Chest			
6 Skin, Back			
7 Skin, Abdomen			
8 Skin, Buttock			
9 Skin, Perineum			
A Skin, Genitalia			
B Skin, Right Upper Arm			
C Skin, Left Upper Arm			
D Skin, Right Lower Arm			
E Skin, Left Lower Arm			
F Skin, Right Hand			
G Skin, Left Hand			
H Skin, Right Upper Leg			
J Skin, Left Upper Leg			
K Skin, Right Lower Leg			
L Skin, Left Lower Leg			
M Skin, Right Foot			
N Skin, Left Foot			

Non-OR ØH8[23]XZZ

8: DIVISION

H: SKIN AND BREAST

Ø: M/S

New/Revised Text in Green   ~~deleted~~ Deleted   ♀ Females Only   ♂ Males Only   **Coding Clinic**

Non-covered   Limited Coverage   ⊞ Combination (See Appendix E)   DRG Non-OR   Non-OR   Hospital-Acquired Condition

SECTION: Ø MEDICAL AND SURGICAL
BODY SYSTEM: H SKIN AND BREAST
OPERATION: 9 DRAINAGE: *(on multiple pages)*

Taking or letting out fluids and/or gases from a body part

Body Part	Approach	Device	Qualifier
Ø Skin, Scalp 1 Skin, Face 2 Skin, Right Ear 3 Skin, Left Ear 4 Skin, Neck 5 Skin, Chest 6 Skin, Back 7 Skin, Abdomen 8 Skin, Buttock 9 Skin, Perineum A Skin, Genitalia B Skin, Right Upper Arm C Skin, Left Upper Arm D Skin, Right Lower Arm E Skin, Left Lower Arm F Skin, Right Hand G Skin, Left Hand H Skin, Right Upper Leg J Skin, Left Upper Leg K Skin, Right Lower Leg L Skin, Left Lower Leg M Skin, Right Foot N Skin, Left Foot Q Finger Nail R Toe Nail	X External	Ø Drainage Device	Z No Qualifier
Ø Skin, Scalp 1 Skin, Face 2 Skin, Right Ear 3 Skin, Left Ear 4 Skin, Neck 5 Skin, Chest 6 Skin, Back 7 Skin, Abdomen 8 Skin, Buttock 9 Skin, Perineum A Skin, Genitalia B Skin, Right Upper Arm C Skin, Left Upper Arm D Skin, Right Lower Arm E Skin, Left Lower Arm F Skin, Right Hand G Skin, Left Hand H Skin, Right Upper Leg J Skin, Left Upper Leg K Skin, Right Lower Leg L Skin, Left Lower Leg M Skin, Right Foot N Skin, Left Foot Q Finger Nail R Toe Nail	X External	Z No Device	X Diagnostic Z No Qualifier

Non-OR ØH9[Ø12345678ABCDEFGHJKLMNQR]XØZ
Non-OR ØH9[Ø123456789ABCDEFGHJKLMNQR]XZX
Non-OR ØH9[Ø12345678ABCDEFGHJKLMNQR]XZZ

Ø: M/S

H: SKIN AND BREAST

9: DRAINAGE

SECTION: Ø MEDICAL AND SURGICAL

BODY SYSTEM: H SKIN AND BREAST
OPERATION: 9 DRAINAGE: *(continued)*
Taking or letting out fluids and/or gases from a body part

Body Part	Approach	Device	Qualifier
T Breast, Right U Breast, Left V Breast, Bilateral W Nipple, Right X Nipple, Left	Ø Open 3 Percutaneous 7 Via Natural or Artificial Opening 8 Via Natural or Artificial Opening Endoscopic X External	Ø Drainage Device	Z No Qualifier
T Breast, Right U Breast, Left V Breast, Bilateral W Nipple, Right X Nipple, Left	Ø Open 3 Percutaneous 7 Via Natural or Artificial Opening 8 Via Natural or Artificial Opening Endoscopic X External	Z No Device	X Diagnostic Z No Qualifier

Non-OR ØH9[TUVWX][0378X]0Z
Non-OR ØH9[TUVWX][378X]ZX
Non-OR ØH9[TUVWX][0378X]ZZ

SECTION: Ø MEDICAL AND SURGICAL

BODY SYSTEM: H SKIN AND BREAST
OPERATION: B EXCISION: *(on multiple pages)*
Cutting out or off, without replacement, a portion of a body part

Body Part	Approach	Device	Qualifier
Ø Skin, Scalp 1 Skin, Face 2 Skin, Right Ear 3 Skin, Left Ear 4 Skin, Neck 5 Skin, Chest 6 Skin, Back 7 Skin, Abdomen 8 Skin, Buttock 9 Skin, Perineum A Skin, Genitalia B Skin, Right Upper Arm C Skin, Left Upper Arm D Skin, Right Lower Arm E Skin, Left Lower Arm F Skin, Right Hand G Skin, Left Hand H Skin, Right Upper Leg J Skin, Left Upper Leg K Skin, Right Lower Leg L Skin, Left Lower Leg M Skin, Right Foot N Skin, Left Foot Q Finger Nail R Toe Nail	X External	Z No Device	X Diagnostic Z No Qualifier

DRG Non-OR ØHB9XZZ
Non-OR ØHB[Ø12456789ABCDEFGHJKLMNQR]XZX
Non-OR ØHB[23QR]XZZ

New/Revised Text in Green   ~~deleted~~ Deleted   ♀ Females Only   ♂ Males Only   **Coding Clinic**
🚫 Non-covered   🚫 Limited Coverage   ⊡ Combination (See Appendix E)   DRG Non-OR   Non-OR   🚫 Hospital-Acquired Condition

SECTION: Ø MEDICAL AND SURGICAL
BODY SYSTEM: H SKIN AND BREAST
OPERATION: B EXCISION: *(continued)*
Cutting out or off, without replacement, a portion of a body part

Body Part	Approach	Device	Qualifier
T Breast, Right U Breast, Left V Breast, Bilateral W Nipple, Right X Nipple, Left Y Supernumerary Breast	Ø Open 3 Percutaneous 7 Via Natural or Artificial Opening 8 Via Natural or Artificial Opening Endoscopic X External	Z No Device	X Diagnostic Z No Qualifier

Non-OR ØHB[TUVWXY][378X]ZX

Coding Clinic: 2015, Q3, P3 – ØHB8XZZ

SECTION: Ø MEDICAL AND SURGICAL
BODY SYSTEM: H SKIN AND BREAST
OPERATION: C EXTIRPATION: Taking or cutting out solid matter from a body part

Body Part	Approach	Device	Qualifier
Ø Skin, Scalp 1 Skin, Face 2 Skin, Right Ear 3 Skin, Left Ear 4 Skin, Neck 5 Skin, Chest 6 Skin, Back 7 Skin, Abdomen 8 Skin, Buttock 9 Skin, Perineum A Skin, Genitalia B Skin, Right Upper Arm C Skin, Left Upper Arm D Skin, Right Lower Arm E Skin, Left Lower Arm F Skin, Right Hand G Skin, Left Hand H Skin, Right Upper Leg J Skin, Left Upper Leg K Skin, Right Lower Leg L Skin, Left Lower Leg M Skin, Right Foot N Skin, Left Foot Q Finger Nail R Toe Nail	X External	Z No Device	Z No Qualifier
T Breast, Right U Breast, Left V Breast, Bilateral W Nipple, Right X Nipple, Left	Ø Open 3 Percutaneous 7 Via Natural or Artificial Opening 8 Via Natural or Artificial Opening Endoscopic X External	Z No Device	Z No Qualifier

Non-OR All Values

New/Revised Text in Green ~~deleted~~ Deleted ♀ Females Only ♂ Males Only **Coding Clinic**
🏷 Non-covered 🏷 Limited Coverage ⊞ Combination (See Appendix E) DRG Non-OR Non-OR 🏷 Hospital-Acquired Condition

SECTION: Ø MEDICAL AND SURGICAL
BODY SYSTEM: H SKIN AND BREAST

OPERATION: D EXTRACTION: Pulling or stripping out or off all or a portion of a body part by the use of force

Body Part	Approach	Device	Qualifier
Ø Skin, Scalp	X External	Z No Device	Z No Qualifier
1 Skin, Face			
2 Skin, Right Ear			
3 Skin, Left Ear			
4 Skin, Neck			
5 Skin, Chest			
6 Skin, Back			
7 Skin, Abdomen			
8 Skin, Buttock			
9 Skin, Perineum			
A Skin, Genitalia			
B Skin, Right Upper Arm			
C Skin, Left Upper Arm			
D Skin, Right Lower Arm			
E Skin, Left Lower Arm			
F Skin, Right Hand			
G Skin, Left Hand			
H Skin, Right Upper Leg			
J Skin, Left Upper Leg			
K Skin, Right Lower Leg			
L Skin, Left Lower Leg			
M Skin, Right Foot			
N Skin, Left Foot			
Q Finger Nail			
R Toe Nail			
S Hair			

Non-OR **All Values**

Coding Clinic: 2015, Q3, P5-6 – ØHD[6H]XZZ

SECTION: Ø MEDICAL AND SURGICAL
BODY SYSTEM: H SKIN AND BREAST

OPERATION: H INSERTION: Putting in a nonbiological appliance that monitors, assists, performs, or prevents a physiological function but does not physically take the place of a body part

Body Part	Approach	Device	Qualifier
T Breast, Right	Ø Open	1 Radioactive Element	Z No Qualifier
U Breast, Left	3 Percutaneous	N Tissue Expander	
V Breast, Bilateral	7 Via Natural or Artificial Opening		
W Nipple, Right	8 Via Natural or Artificial Opening Endoscopic		
X Nipple, Left			
T Breast, Right	X External	1 Radioactive Element	Z No Qualifier
U Breast, Left			
V Breast, Bilateral			
W Nipple, Right			
X Nipple, Left			

New/Revised Text in Green   ~~deleted~~ Deleted   ♀ Females Only   ♂ Males Only   **Coding Clinic**
Non-covered   Limited Coverage   ⊡ Combination (See Appendix E)   DRG Non-OR   Non-OR   Hospital-Acquired Condition

SECTION: Ø MEDICAL AND SURGICAL
BODY SYSTEM: H SKIN AND BREAST
OPERATION: J INSPECTION: Visually and/or manually exploring a body part

Body Part	Approach	Device	Qualifier
P Skin Q Finger Nail R Toe Nail	X External	Z No Device	Z No Qualifier
T Breast, Right U Breast, Left	Ø Open 3 Percutaneous 7 Via Natural or Artificial Opening 8 Via Natural or Artificial Opening Endoscopic X External	Z No Device	Z No Qualifier

Non-OR All Values

SECTION: Ø MEDICAL AND SURGICAL
BODY SYSTEM: H SKIN AND BREAST
OPERATION: M REATTACHMENT: Putting back in or on all or a portion of a separated body part to its normal location or other suitable location

Body Part	Approach	Device	Qualifier
Ø Skin, Scalp 1 Skin, Face 2 Skin, Right Ear 3 Skin, Left Ear 4 Skin, Neck 5 Skin, Chest 6 Skin, Back 7 Skin, Abdomen 8 Skin, Buttock 9 Skin, Perineum A Skin, Genitalia B Skin, Right Upper Arm C Skin, Left Upper Arm D Skin, Right Lower Arm E Skin, Left Lower Arm F Skin, Right Hand G Skin, Left Hand H Skin, Right Upper Leg J Skin, Left Upper Leg K Skin, Right Lower Leg L Skin, Left Lower Leg M Skin, Right Foot N Skin, Left Foot T Breast, Right U Breast, Left V Breast, Bilateral W Nipple, Right X Nipple, Left	X External	Z No Device	Z No Qualifier

Non-OR ØHMØXZZ

SECTION: Ø MEDICAL AND SURGICAL

BODY SYSTEM: **H SKIN AND BREAST**

OPERATION: **N RELEASE:** Freeing a body part from an abnormal physical constraint by cutting or by the use of force

Body Part	Approach	Device	Qualifier
Ø Skin, Scalp 1 Skin, Face 2 Skin, Right Ear 3 Skin, Left Ear 4 Skin, Neck 5 Skin, Chest 6 Skin, Back 7 Skin, Abdomen 8 Skin, Buttock 9 Skin, Perineum A Skin, Genitalia B Skin, Right Upper Arm C Skin, Left Upper Arm D Skin, Right Lower Arm E Skin, Left Lower Arm F Skin, Right Hand G Skin, Left Hand H Skin, Right Upper Leg J Skin, Left Upper Leg K Skin, Right Lower Leg L Skin, Left Lower Leg M Skin, Right Foot N Skin, Left Foot Q Finger Nail R Toe Nail	X External	Z No Device	Z No Qualifier

T Breast, Right
U Breast, Left
V Breast, Bilateral
W Nipple, Right
X Nipple, Left
	Ø Open
	3 Percutaneous
	7 Via Natural or Artificial
	   Opening
	8 Via Natural or Artificial
	   Opening Endoscopic
	X External
		Z No Device	Z No Qualifier

N: RELEASE

H: SKIN AND BREAST

Ø: M/S

New/Revised Text in Green   ~~deleted~~ Deleted   ♀ Females Only   ♂ Males Only   **Coding Clinic**

Non-covered   Limited Coverage   ⊞ Combination (See Appendix E)   DRG Non-OR   Non-OR   Hospital-Acquired Condition

SECTION: Ø MEDICAL AND SURGICAL

BODY SYSTEM: H SKIN AND BREAST

OPERATION: P REMOVAL: Taking out or off a device from a body part

Body Part	Approach	Device	Qualifier
P Skin Q Finger Nail R Toe Nail	X External	Ø Drainage Device 7 Autologous Tissue Substitute J Synthetic Substitute K Nonautologous Tissue Substitute	Z No Qualifier
S Hair	X External	7 Autologous Tissue Substitute J Synthetic Substitute K Nonautologous Tissue Substitute	Z No Qualifier
T Breast, Right U Breast, Left	Ø Open 3 Percutaneous 7 Via Natural or Artificial Opening 8 Via Natural or Artificial Opening Endoscopic	Ø Drainage Device 1 Radioactive Element 7 Autologous Tissue Substitute J Synthetic Substitute K Nonautologous Tissue Substitute N Tissue Expander	Z No Qualifier
T Breast, Right U Breast, Left	X External	Ø Drainage Device 1 Radioactive Element 7 Autologous Tissue Substitute J Synthetic Substitute K Nonautologous Tissue Substitute	Z No Qualifier

Non-OR   ØHP[PQR]X[Ø7JK]Z
Non-OR   ØHPSX[7JK]Z
Non-OR   ØHP[TU][Ø3][Ø17K]Z
Non-OR   ØHP[TU][78][Ø17JKN]Z
Non-OR   ØHP[TU]X[Ø17JK]Z

Coding Clinic: 2016, Q2, P27 – ØHP[TU]Ø7Z

SECTION: Ø MEDICAL AND SURGICAL
BODY SYSTEM: H SKIN AND BREAST
OPERATION: Q REPAIR: Restoring, to the extent possible, a body part to its normal anatomic structure and function

Body Part	Approach	Device	Qualifier
Ø Skin, Scalp 1 Skin, Face 2 Skin, Right Ear 3 Skin, Left Ear 4 Skin, Neck 5 Skin, Chest 6 Skin, Back 7 Skin, Abdomen 8 Skin, Buttock 9 Skin, Perineum ⊞ A Skin, Genitalia B Skin, Right Upper Arm C Skin, Left Upper Arm D Skin, Right Lower Arm E Skin, Left Lower Arm F Skin, Right Hand G Skin, Left Hand H Skin, Right Upper Leg J Skin, Left Upper Leg K Skin, Right Lower Leg L Skin, Left Lower Leg M Skin, Right Foot N Skin, Left Foot Q Finger Nail R Toe Nail	X External	Z No Device	Z No Qualifier
T Breast, Right U Breast, Left V Breast, Bilateral W Nipple, Right X Nipple, Left Y Supernumerary Breast	Ø Open 3 Percutaneous 7 Via Natural or Artificial Opening 8 Via Natural or Artificial Opening Endoscopic X External	Z No Device	Z No Qualifier

⊞ ØHQ9XZZ
`DRG Non-OR` ØHQ9XZZ
`Non-OR` ØHQ[Ø12345678ABCDEFGHJKLMN]XZZ
`Non-OR` ØHQ[TUVY]XZZ

Coding Clinic: 2016, Q1, P7 – ØHQ9XZZ

Q: REPAIR   H: SKIN AND BREAST   Ø: M/S

SECTION: Ø MEDICAL AND SURGICAL
BODY SYSTEM: H SKIN AND BREAST
OPERATION: R REPLACEMENT: *(on multiple pages)*
Putting in or on biological or synthetic material that physically takes the place and/or function of all or a portion of a body part

Body Part	Approach	Device	Qualifier
Ø Skin, Scalp 1 Skin, Face 2 Skin, Right Ear 3 Skin, Left Ear 4 Skin, Neck 5 Skin, Chest 6 Skin, Back 7 Skin, Abdomen 8 Skin, Buttock 9 Skin, Perineum A Skin, Genitalia B Skin, Right Upper Arm C Skin, Left Upper Arm D Skin, Right Lower Arm E Skin, Left Lower Arm F Skin, Right Hand G Skin, Left Hand H Skin, Right Upper Leg J Skin, Left Upper Leg K Skin, Right Lower Leg L Skin, Left Lower Leg M Skin, Right Foot N Skin, Left Foot	X External	7 Autologous Tissue Substitute K Nonautologous Tissue Substitute	3 Full Thickness 4 Partial Thickness
Ø Skin, Scalp 1 Skin, Face 2 Skin, Right Ear 3 Skin, Left Ear 4 Skin, Neck 5 Skin, Chest 6 Skin, Back 7 Skin, Abdomen 8 Skin, Buttock 9 Skin, Perineum A Skin, Genitalia B Skin, Right Upper Arm C Skin, Left Upper Arm D Skin, Right Lower Arm E Skin, Left Lower Arm F Skin, Right Hand G Skin, Left Hand H Skin, Right Upper Leg J Skin, Left Upper Leg K Skin, Right Lower Leg L Skin, Left Lower Leg M Skin, Right Foot N Skin, Left Foot	X External	J Synthetic Substitute	3 Full Thickness 4 Partial Thickness Z No Qualifier
Q Finger Nail R Toe Nail S Hair	X External	7 Autologous Tissue Substitute J Synthetic Substitute K Nonautologous Tissue Substitute	Z No Qualifier

Non-OR ØHRSX7Z

 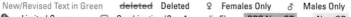

Ø: M/S

H: SKIN AND BREAST

R: REPLACEMENT

SECTION: Ø MEDICAL AND SURGICAL
BODY SYSTEM: H SKIN AND BREAST
OPERATION: R REPLACEMENT: *(continued)*
Putting in or on biological or synthetic material that physically takes the place and/or function of all or a portion of a body part

Body Part	Approach	Device	Qualifier
T Breast, Right U Breast, Left V Breast, Bilateral	Ø Open	7 Autologous Tissue Substitute	5 Latissimus Dorsi Myocutaneous Flap 6 Transverse Rectus Abdominis Myocutaneous Flap 7 Deep Inferior Epigastric Artery Perforator Flap 8 Superficial Inferior Epigastric Artery Flap 9 Gluteal Artery Perforator Flap Z No Qualifier
T Breast, Right U Breast, Left V Breast, Bilateral	Ø Open	J Synthetic Substitute K Nonautologous Tissue Substitute	Z No Qualifier
T Breast, Right ⊞ U Breast, Left ⊞ V Breast, Bilateral ⊞	3 Percutaneous X External	7 Autologous Tissue Substitute J Synthetic Substitute K Nonautologous Tissue Substitute	Z No Qualifier
W Nipple, Right X Nipple, Left	Ø Open 3 Percutaneous X External	7 Autologous Tissue Substitute J Synthetic Substitute K Nonautologous Tissue Substitute	Z No Qualifier

⊞ ØHR[TUV]37Z

SECTION: Ø MEDICAL AND SURGICAL
BODY SYSTEM: H SKIN AND BREAST
OPERATION: S REPOSITION: Moving to its normal location, or other suitable location, all or a portion of a body part

Body Part	Approach	Device	Qualifier
S Hair W Nipple, Right X Nipple, Left	X External	Z No Device	Z No Qualifier
T Breast, Right U Breast, Left V Breast, Bilateral	Ø Open	Z No Device	Z No Qualifier

Non-OR ØHSSXZZ

SECTION: Ø MEDICAL AND SURGICAL

BODY SYSTEM: H SKIN AND BREAST

OPERATION: T RESECTION: Cutting out or off, without replacement, all of a body part

Body Part	Approach	Device	Qualifier
Q Finger Nail R Toe Nail W Nipple, Right X Nipple, Left	X External	Z No Device	Z No Qualifier
T Breast, Right ⊞ U Breast, Left ⊞ V Breast, Bilateral ⊞ Y Supernumerary Breast	Ø Open	Z No Device	Z No Qualifier

⊞ ØHT[TUV]ØZZ
Non-OR ØHT[QR]XZZ

SECTION: Ø MEDICAL AND SURGICAL

BODY SYSTEM: H SKIN AND BREAST

OPERATION: U SUPPLEMENT: Putting in or on biological or synthetic material that physically reinforces and/or augments the function of a portion of a body part

Body Part	Approach	Device	Qualifier
T Breast, Right U Breast, Left V Breast, Bilateral W Nipple, Right X Nipple, Left	Ø Open 3 Percutaneous 7 Via Natural of Artificial Opening 8 Via Natural or Artificial Opening Endoscopic X External	7 Autologous Tissue Substitute J Synthetic Substitute K Nonautologous Tissue Substitute	Z No Qualifier

W: REVISION   X: TRANSFER

H: SKIN AND BREAST

Ø: M/S

SECTION: Ø MEDICAL AND SURGICAL

BODY SYSTEM: H SKIN AND BREAST

OPERATION: W REVISION: Correcting, to the extent possible, a portion of a malfunctioning device or the position of a displaced device

Body Part	Approach	Device	Qualifier
P Skin Q Finger Nail R Toe Nail	X External	Ø Drainage Device 7 Autologous Tissue Substitute J Synthetic Substitute K Nonautologous Tissue Substitute	Z No Qualifier
S Hair	X External	7 Autologous Tissue Substitute J Synthetic Substitute K Nonautologous Tissue Substitute	Z No Qualifier
T Breast, Right U Breast, Left	Ø Open 3 Percutaneous 7 Via Natural or Artificial Opening 8 Via Natural or Artificial Opening Endoscopic	Ø Drainage Device 7 Autologous Tissue Substitute J Synthetic Substitute K Nonautologous Tissue Substitute N Tissue Expander	Z No Qualifier
T Breast, Right U Breast, Left	X External	Ø Drainage Device 7 Autologous Tissue Substitute J Synthetic Substitute K Nonautologous Tissue Substitute	Z No Qualifier

Non-OR ØHW[PQR]X[Ø7JK]Z
Non-OR ØHWSX[7JK]Z
Non-OR ØHW[TU][Ø3][Ø7KN]Z

Non-OR ØHW[TU][78][Ø7JKN]Z
Non-OR ØHW[TU]X[Ø7JK]Z

SECTION: Ø MEDICAL AND SURGICAL

BODY SYSTEM: H SKIN AND BREAST

OPERATION: X TRANSFER: Moving, without taking out, all or a portion of a body part to another location to take over the function of all or a portion of a body part

Body Part	Approach	Device	Qualifier
Ø Skin, Scalp 1 Skin, Face 2 Skin, Right Ear 3 Skin, Left Ear 4 Skin, Neck 5 Skin, Chest 6 Skin, Back 7 Skin, Abdomen 8 Skin, Buttock 9 Skin, Perineum A Skin, Genitalia B Skin, Right Upper Arm C Skin, Left Upper Arm D Skin, Right Lower Arm E Skin, Left Lower Arm F Skin, Right Hand G Skin, Left Hand H Skin, Right Upper Leg J Skin, Left Upper Leg K Skin, Right Lower Leg L Skin, Left Lower Leg M Skin, Right Foot N Skin, Left Foot	X External	Z No Device	Z No Qualifier

New/Revised Text in Green   ~~deleted~~ Deleted   ♀ Females Only   ♂ Males Only   **Coding Clinic**
Non-covered   Limited Coverage   ⊞ Combination (See Appendix E)   DRG Non-OR   Non-OR   Hospital-Acquired Condition

SECTION: Ø MEDICAL AND SURGICAL
BODY SYSTEM: J SUBCUTANEOUS TISSUE AND FASCIA
OPERATION: Ø **ALTERATION:** Modifying the anatomic structure of a body part without affecting the function of the body part

Body Part	Approach	Device	Qualifier
1 Subcutaneous Tissue and Fascia, Face 4 Subcutaneous Tissue and Fascia, Anterior Neck 5 Subcutaneous Tissue and Fascia, Posterior Neck 6 Subcutaneous Tissue and Fascia, Chest 7 Subcutaneous Tissue and Fascia, Back 8 Subcutaneous Tissue and Fascia, Abdomen 9 Subcutaneous Tissue and Fascia, Buttock D Subcutaneous Tissue and Fascia, Right Upper Arm F Subcutaneous Tissue and Fascia, Left Upper Arm G Subcutaneous Tissue and Fascia, Right Lower Arm H Subcutaneous Tissue and Fascia, Left Lower Arm L Subcutaneous Tissue and Fascia, Right Upper Leg M Subcutaneous Tissue and Fascia, Left Upper Leg N Subcutaneous Tissue and Fascia, Right Lower Leg P Subcutaneous Tissue and Fascia, Left Lower Leg	Ø Open 3 Percutaneous	Z No Device	Z No Qualifier

SECTION: Ø MEDICAL AND SURGICAL
BODY SYSTEM: J SUBCUTANEOUS TISSUE AND FASCIA
OPERATION: 2 **CHANGE:** Taking out or off a device from a body part and putting back an identical or similar device in or on the same body part without cutting or puncturing the skin or a mucous membrane

Body Part	Approach	Device	Qualifier
S Subcutaneous Tissue and Fascia, Head and Neck T Subcutaneous Tissue and Fascia, Trunk V Subcutaneous Tissue and Fascia, Upper Extremity W Subcutaneous Tissue and Fascia, Lower Extremity	X External	Ø Drainage Device Y Other Device	Z No Qualifier

Non-OR All Values

New/Revised Text in Green ~~deleted~~ Deleted ♀ Females Only ♂ Males Only **Coding Clinic**
🦃 Non-covered 🦃 Limited Coverage ⊞ Combination (See Appendix E) DRG Non-OR Non-OR 🦃 Hospital-Acquired Condition

SECTION: Ø MEDICAL AND SURGICAL

BODY SYSTEM: J SUBCUTANEOUS TISSUE AND FASCIA

OPERATION: 5 DESTRUCTION: Physical eradication of all or a portion of a body part by the direct use of energy, force, or a destructive agent

Body Part	Approach	Device	Qualifier
Ø Subcutaneous Tissue and Fascia, Scalp 1 Subcutaneous Tissue and Fascia, Face 4 Subcutaneous Tissue and Fascia, Anterior Neck 5 Subcutaneous Tissue and Fascia, Posterior Neck 6 Subcutaneous Tissue and Fascia, Chest 7 Subcutaneous Tissue and Fascia, Back 8 Subcutaneous Tissue and Fascia, Abdomen 9 Subcutaneous Tissue and Fascia, Buttock B Subcutaneous Tissue and Fascia, Perineum C Subcutaneous Tissue and Fascia, Pelvic Region D Subcutaneous Tissue and Fascia, Right Upper Arm F Subcutaneous Tissue and Fascia, Left Upper Arm G Subcutaneous Tissue and Fascia, Right Lower Arm H Subcutaneous Tissue and Fascia, Left Lower Arm J Subcutaneous Tissue and Fascia, Right Hand K Subcutaneous Tissue and Fascia, Left Hand L Subcutaneous Tissue and Fascia, Right Upper Leg M Subcutaneous Tissue and Fascia, Left Upper Leg N Subcutaneous Tissue and Fascia, Right Lower Leg P Subcutaneous Tissue and Fascia, Left Lower Leg Q Subcutaneous Tissue and Fascia, Right Foot R Subcutaneous Tissue and Fascia, Left Foot	Ø Open 3 Percutaneous	Z No Device	Z No Qualifier

DRG Non-OR All Values

SECTION: Ø MEDICAL AND SURGICAL

BODY SYSTEM: J SUBCUTANEOUS TISSUE AND FASCIA

OPERATION: 8 **DIVISION:** Cutting into a body part, without draining fluids and/or gases from the body part, in order to separate or transect a body part

Body Part	Approach	Device	Qualifier
Ø Subcutaneous Tissue and Fascia, Scalp	Ø Open	Z No Device	Z No Qualifier
1 Subcutaneous Tissue and Fascia, Face	3 Percutaneous		
4 Subcutaneous Tissue and Fascia, Anterior Neck			
5 Subcutaneous Tissue and Fascia, Posterior Neck			
6 Subcutaneous Tissue and Fascia, Chest			
7 Subcutaneous Tissue and Fascia, Back			
8 Subcutaneous Tissue and Fascia, Abdomen			
9 Subcutaneous Tissue and Fascia, Buttock			
B Subcutaneous Tissue and Fascia, Perineum			
C Subcutaneous Tissue and Fascia, Pelvic Region			
D Subcutaneous Tissue and Fascia, Right Upper Arm			
F Subcutaneous Tissue and Fascia, Left Upper Arm			
G Subcutaneous Tissue and Fascia, Right Lower Arm			
H Subcutaneous Tissue and Fascia, Left Lower Arm			
J Subcutaneous Tissue and Fascia, Right Hand			
K Subcutaneous Tissue and Fascia, Left Hand			
L Subcutaneous Tissue and Fascia, Right Upper Leg			
M Subcutaneous Tissue and Fascia, Left Upper Leg			
N Subcutaneous Tissue and Fascia, Right Lower Leg			
P Subcutaneous Tissue and Fascia, Left Lower Leg			
Q Subcutaneous Tissue and Fascia, Right Foot			
R Subcutaneous Tissue and Fascia, Left Foot			
S Subcutaneous Tissue and Fascia, Head and Neck			
T Subcutaneous Tissue and Fascia, Trunk			
V Subcutaneous Tissue and Fascia, Upper Extremity			
W Subcutaneous Tissue and Fascia, Lower Extremity			

8: DIVISION

J: SUBCUTANEOUS TISSUE AND FASCIA

Ø: M/S

New/Revised Text in Green ~~deleted~~ Deleted ♀ Females Only ♂ Males Only **Coding Clinic**

🚫 Non-covered 🚫 Limited Coverage ⊡ Combination (See Appendix E) DRG Non-OR Non-OR 🚫 Hospital-Acquired Condition

SECTION: Ø MEDICAL AND SURGICAL

BODY SYSTEM: J SUBCUTANEOUS TISSUE AND FASCIA
OPERATION: 9 DRAINAGE: *(on multiple pages)*
Taking or letting out fluids and/or gases from a body part

Body Part	Approach	Device	Qualifier
Ø Subcutaneous Tissue and Fascia, Scalp	Ø Open	Ø Drainage Device	Z No Qualifier
1 Subcutaneous Tissue and Fascia, Face	3 Percutaneous		
4 Subcutaneous Tissue and Fascia, Anterior Neck			
5 Subcutaneous Tissue and Fascia, Posterior Neck			
6 Subcutaneous Tissue and Fascia, Chest			
7 Subcutaneous Tissue and Fascia, Back			
8 Subcutaneous Tissue and Fascia, Abdomen			
9 Subcutaneous Tissue and Fascia, Buttock			
B Subcutaneous Tissue and Fascia, Perineum			
C Subcutaneous Tissue and Fascia, Pelvic Region			
D Subcutaneous Tissue and Fascia, Right Upper Arm			
F Subcutaneous Tissue and Fascia, Left Upper Arm			
G Subcutaneous Tissue and Fascia, Right Lower Arm			
H Subcutaneous Tissue and Fascia, Left Lower Arm			
J Subcutaneous Tissue and Fascia, Right Hand			
K Subcutaneous Tissue and Fascia, Left Hand			
L Subcutaneous Tissue and Fascia, Right Upper Leg			
M Subcutaneous Tissue and Fascia, Left Upper Leg			
N Subcutaneous Tissue and Fascia, Right Lower Leg			
P Subcutaneous Tissue and Fascia, Left Lower Leg			
Q Subcutaneous Tissue and Fascia, Right Foot			
R Subcutaneous Tissue and Fascia, Left Foot			

DRG Non-OR ØJ9[1JK]30Z
Non-OR ØJ9[0456789BCDFGHLMNPQR][03]0Z

SECTION: Ø MEDICAL AND SURGICAL

BODY SYSTEM: J SUBCUTANEOUS TISSUE AND FASCIA
OPERATION: 9 DRAINAGE: *(continued)*

Taking or letting out fluids and/or gases from a body part

Body Part	Approach	Device	Qualifier
Ø Subcutaneous Tissue and Fascia, Scalp	Ø Open	Z No Device	X Diagnostic
1 Subcutaneous Tissue and Fascia, Face	3 Percutaneous		Z No Qualifier
4 Subcutaneous Tissue and Fascia, Anterior Neck			
5 Subcutaneous Tissue and Fascia, Posterior Neck			
6 Subcutaneous Tissue and Fascia, Chest			
7 Subcutaneous Tissue and Fascia, Back			
8 Subcutaneous Tissue and Fascia, Abdomen			
9 Subcutaneous Tissue and Fascia, Buttock			
B Subcutaneous Tissue and Fascia, Perineum			
C Subcutaneous Tissue and Fascia, Pelvic Region			
D Subcutaneous Tissue and Fascia, Right Upper Arm			
F Subcutaneous Tissue and Fascia, Left Upper Arm			
G Subcutaneous Tissue and Fascia, Right Lower Arm			
H Subcutaneous Tissue and Fascia, Left Lower Arm			
J Subcutaneous Tissue and Fascia, Right Hand			
K Subcutaneous Tissue and Fascia, Left Hand			
L Subcutaneous Tissue and Fascia, Right Upper Leg			
M Subcutaneous Tissue and Fascia, Left Upper Leg			
N Subcutaneous Tissue and Fascia, Right Lower Leg			
P Subcutaneous Tissue and Fascia, Left Lower Leg			
Q Subcutaneous Tissue and Fascia, Right Foot			
R Subcutaneous Tissue and Fascia, Left Foot			

Non-OR ØJ9[Ø1456789BCDFGHJKLMNPQR][Ø3]ZX
Non-OR ØJ9[Ø1456789BCDFGHLMNPQR]3ZZ

Coding Clinic: 2Ø15, Q3, P24 – ØJ9[6CDFLM]ØZZ

New/Revised Text in Green   ~~deleted~~ Deleted   ♀ Females Only   ♂ Males Only   **Coding Clinic**
🚫 Non-covered   🚫 Limited Coverage   ⊡ Combination (See Appendix E)   DRG Non-OR   Non-OR   🚫 Hospital-Acquired Condition

SECTION: Ø MEDICAL AND SURGICAL

BODY SYSTEM: J SUBCUTANEOUS TISSUE AND FASCIA

OPERATION: B EXCISION: Cutting out or off, without replacement, a portion of a body part

Body Part	Approach	Device	Qualifier
Ø Subcutaneous Tissue and Fascia, Scalp 1 Subcutaneous Tissue and Fascia, Face 4 Subcutaneous Tissue and Fascia, Anterior Neck 5 Subcutaneous Tissue and Fascia, Posterior Neck 6 Subcutaneous Tissue and Fascia, Chest 7 Subcutaneous Tissue and Fascia, Back 8 Subcutaneous Tissue and Fascia, Abdomen 9 Subcutaneous Tissue and Fascia, Buttock B Subcutaneous Tissue and Fascia, Perineum C Subcutaneous Tissue and Fascia, Pelvic Region D Subcutaneous Tissue and Fascia, Right Upper Arm F Subcutaneous Tissue and Fascia, Left Upper Arm G Subcutaneous Tissue and Fascia, Right Lower Arm H Subcutaneous Tissue and Fascia, Left Lower Arm J Subcutaneous Tissue and Fascia, Right Hand K Subcutaneous Tissue and Fascia, Left Hand L Subcutaneous Tissue and Fascia, Right Upper Leg ⊞ M Subcutaneous Tissue and Fascia, Left Upper Leg ⊞ N Subcutaneous Tissue and Fascia, Right Lower Leg P Subcutaneous Tissue and Fascia, Left Lower Leg Q Subcutaneous Tissue and Fascia, Right Foot R Subcutaneous Tissue and Fascia, Left Foot	Ø Open 3 Percutaneous	Z No Device	X Diagnostic Z No Qualifier

⊞ ØJB[LM]ØZZ

Non-OR ØJB[Ø1456789BCDFGHJKLMNPQR][Ø3]ZX

Non-OR ØJB[Ø456789BCDFGHLMNPQR]3ZZ

Coding Clinic: 2Ø15, Q1, P3Ø – ØJBBØZZ

Coding Clinic: 2Ø15, Q2, P13 – ØJBHØZZ

Coding Clinic: 2Ø15, Q3, P7 – ØJB9ØZZ

SECTION: Ø MEDICAL AND SURGICAL

BODY SYSTEM: J SUBCUTANEOUS TISSUE AND FASCIA

OPERATION: C EXTIRPATION: Taking or cutting out solid matter from a body part

Body Part	Approach	Device	Qualifier
Ø Subcutaneous Tissue and Fascia, Scalp	Ø Open	Z No Device	Z No Qualifier
1 Subcutaneous Tissue and Fascia, Face	3 Percutaneous		
4 Subcutaneous Tissue and Fascia, Anterior Neck			
5 Subcutaneous Tissue and Fascia, Posterior Neck			
6 Subcutaneous Tissue and Fascia, Chest			
7 Subcutaneous Tissue and Fascia, Back			
8 Subcutaneous Tissue and Fascia, Abdomen			
9 Subcutaneous Tissue and Fascia, Buttock			
B Subcutaneous Tissue and Fascia, Perineum			
C Subcutaneous Tissue and Fascia, Pelvic Region			
D Subcutaneous Tissue and Fascia, Right Upper Arm			
F Subcutaneous Tissue and Fascia, Left Upper Arm			
G Subcutaneous Tissue and Fascia, Right Lower Arm			
H Subcutaneous Tissue and Fascia, Left Lower Arm			
J Subcutaneous Tissue and Fascia, Right Hand			
K Subcutaneous Tissue and Fascia, Left Hand			
L Subcutaneous Tissue and Fascia, Right Upper Leg			
M Subcutaneous Tissue and Fascia, Left Upper Leg			
N Subcutaneous Tissue and Fascia, Right Lower Leg			
P Subcutaneous Tissue and Fascia, Left Lower Leg			
Q Subcutaneous Tissue and Fascia, Right Foot			
R Subcutaneous Tissue and Fascia, Left Foot			

Non-OR All Values

C: EXTIRPATION

J: SUBCUTANEOUS TISSUE AND FASCIA

Ø: M/S

SECTION: Ø MEDICAL AND SURGICAL
BODY SYSTEM: J SUBCUTANEOUS TISSUE AND FASCIA
OPERATION: D **EXTRACTION:** Pulling or stripping out or off all or a portion of a body part by the use of force

Body Part	Approach	Device	Qualifier
Ø Subcutaneous Tissue and Fascia, Scalp 1 Subcutaneous Tissue and Fascia, Face 4 Subcutaneous Tissue and Fascia, Anterior Neck 5 Subcutaneous Tissue and Fascia, Posterior Neck 6 Subcutaneous Tissue and Fascia, Chest ⊞ 7 Subcutaneous Tissue and Fascia, Back ⊞ 8 Subcutaneous Tissue and Fascia, Abdomen ⊞ 9 Subcutaneous Tissue and Fascia, Buttock ⊞ B Subcutaneous Tissue and Fascia, Perineum C Subcutaneous Tissue and Fascia, Pelvic Region D Subcutaneous Tissue and Fascia, Right Upper Arm F Subcutaneous Tissue and Fascia, Left Upper Arm G Subcutaneous Tissue and Fascia, Right Lower Arm H Subcutaneous Tissue and Fascia, Left Lower Arm J Subcutaneous Tissue and Fascia, Right Hand K Subcutaneous Tissue and Fascia, Left Hand L Subcutaneous Tissue and Fascia, Right Upper Leg ⊞ M Subcutaneous Tissue and Fascia, Left Upper Leg ⊞ N Subcutaneous Tissue and Fascia, Right Lower Leg P Subcutaneous Tissue and Fascia, Left Lower Leg Q Subcutaneous Tissue and Fascia, Right Foot R Subcutaneous Tissue and Fascia, Left Foot	Ø Open 3 Percutaneous	Z No Device	Z No Qualifier

⊞ ØJD[6789LM]3ZZ

Coding Clinic: 2015, Q1, P23 – ØJDCØZZ
Coding Clinic: 2016, Q1, P40 – ØJDLØZZ

H: INSERTION

J: SUBCUTANEOUS TISSUE AND FASCIA

Ø: M/S

SECTION: Ø MEDICAL AND SURGICAL

BODY SYSTEM: J SUBCUTANEOUS TISSUE AND FASCIA

OPERATION: H INSERTION: *(on multiple pages)*
Putting in a nonbiological appliance that monitors, assists, performs, or prevents a physiological function but does not physically take the place of a body part

Body Part	Approach	Device	Qualifier
Ø Subcutaneous Tissue and Fascia, Scalp 1 Subcutaneous Tissue and Fascia, Face 4 Subcutaneous Tissue and Fascia, Anterior Neck 5 Subcutaneous Tissue and Fascia, Posterior Neck 9 Subcutaneous Tissue and Fascia, Buttock B Subcutaneous Tissue and Fascia, Perineum C Subcutaneous Tissue and Fascia, Pelvic Region J Subcutaneous Tissue and Fascia, Right Hand K Subcutaneous Tissue and Fascia, Left Hand Q Subcutaneous Tissue and Fascia, Right Foot R Subcutaneous Tissue and Fascia, Left Foot	Ø Open 3 Percutaneous	N Tissue Expander	Z No Qualifer
6 Subcutaneous Tissue and Fascia, Chest ⊡ ♧ 8 Subcutaneous Tissue and Fascia, Abdomen ♧ ⊡ ♧	Ø Open 3 Percutaneous	Ø Monitoring Device, Hemodynamic 2 Monitoring Device 4 Pacemaker, Single Chamber 5 Pacemaker, Single Chamber Rate Responsive 6 Pacemaker, Dual Chamber 7 Cardiac Resynchronization Pacemaker Pulse Generator 8 Defibrillator Generator 9 Cardiac Resynchronization Defibrillator Pulse Generator A Contractility Modulation Device B Stimulator Generator, Single Array C Stimulator Generator, Single Array Rechargeable D Stimulator Generator, Multiple Array E Stimulator Generator, Multiple Array Rechargeable H Contraceptive Device M Stimulator Generator N Tissue Expander P Cardiac Rhythm Related Device V Infusion Device, Pump W Vascular Access Device, Reservoir X Vascular Access Device	Z No Qualifier

♧ ØJH8[Ø3]MZ
⊡ ØJH[68][Ø3][Ø456789ABCDEMP]Z
DRG Non-OR ØJH[68][Ø3][2456HWX]Z
♧ ØJH[68][Ø3][456789P]Z when reported with Secondary Diagnosis K68.11, T81.4XXA, T82.6XXA, or T82.7XXA, except ØJH63XZ
♧ ØJH63XZ when reported with Secondary Diagnosis J95.811

Coding Clinic: 2015, Q2, P33 – ØJH60XZ
Coding Clinic: 2015, Q4, P15 – ØJH63VZ
Coding Clinic: 2016, Q2, P16; 2015, Q4, P31-32 – ØJH63XZ

New/Revised Text in Green ~~deleted~~ Deleted ♀ Females Only ♂ Males Only **Coding Clinic**
♧ Non-covered ♧ Limited Coverage ⊡ Combination (See Appendix E) DRG Non-OR DRG Non-OR Non-OR Non-OR ♧ Hospital-Acquired Condition

SECTION: Ø MEDICAL AND SURGICAL

BODY SYSTEM: **J SUBCUTANEOUS TISSUE AND FASCIA**
OPERATION: **H INSERTION:** *(continued)*

Putting in a nonbiological appliance that monitors, assists, performs, or prevents a physiological function but does not physically take the place of a body part

Body Part	Approach	Device	Qualifier
7 Subcutaneous Tissue and Fascia, Back 🐾 ⊡	Ø Open 3 Percutaneous	B Stimulator Generator, Single Array C Stimulator Generator, Single Array Rechargeable D Stimulator Generator, Multiple Array E Stimulator Generator, Multiple Array Rechargeable M Stimulator Generator N Tissue Expander V Infusion Device, Pump	Z No Qualifier
D Subcutaneous Tissue and Fascia, Right Upper Arm F Subcutaneous Tissue and Fascia, Left Upper Arm G Subcutaneous Tissue and Fascia, Right Lower Arm H Subcutaneous Tissue and Fascia, Left Lower Arm L Subcutaneous Tissue and Fascia, Right Upper Leg M Subcutaneous Tissue and Fascia, Left Upper Leg N Subcutaneous Tissue and Fascia, Right Lower Leg P Subcutaneous Tissue and Fascia, Left Lower Leg	Ø Open 3 Percutaneous	H Contraceptive Device N Tissue Expander V Infusion Device, Pump W Vascular Access Device, Reservoir X Vascular Access Device	Z No Qualifier
S Subcutaneous Tissue and Fascia, Head and Neck V Subcutaneous Tissue and Fascia, Upper Extremity W Subcutaneous Tissue and Fascia, Lower Extremity	Ø Open 3 Percutaneous	1 Radioactive Element 3 Infusion Device	Z No Qualifier
T Subcutaneous Tissue and Fascia, Trunk	Ø Open 3 Percutaneous	1 Radioactive Element 3 Infusion Device V Infusion Device, Pump	Z No Qualifier

🐾 ØJH7[Ø3]MZ
⊡ ØJH7[Ø3][BCDEM]Z
DRG Non-OR ØJH[DFGHLM][Ø3][WX]Z
DRG Non-OR ØJHNØ[WX]Z
DRG Non-OR ØJHN3[HWX]Z
DRG Non-OR ØJHP[Ø3][HWX]Z
DRG Non-OR ØJH[SVW][Ø3]3Z
DRG Non-OR ØJHT[Ø3]3Z
Non-OR ØJH[DFGHLM][Ø3][HV]Z
Non-OR ØJHNØ[HV]Z
Non-OR ØJHN3VZ
Non-OR ØJHP[Ø3]VZ
Non-OR ØJH[SVW][Ø3]3Z
Non-OR ØJHT[Ø3]3Z

Coding Clinic: 2012, Q4, P1Ø5 – ØJH6Ø8Z & ØJH6ØPZ
Coding Clinic: 2016, Q2, P14 – ØJH8ØWZ

New/Revised Text in Green   ~~deleted~~ Deleted   ♀ Females Only   ♂ Males Only   **Coding Clinic**
🐾 Non-covered   🐾 Limited Coverage   ⊡ Combination (See Appendix E)   DRG Non-OR   Non-OR   🐾 Hospital-Acquired Condition

291

Ø: M/S

J: SUBCUTANEOUS TISSUE AND FASCIA

H: INSERTION

SECTION: Ø MEDICAL AND SURGICAL
BODY SYSTEM: J SUBCUTANEOUS TISSUE AND FASCIA
OPERATION: J INSPECTION: Visually and/or manually exploring a body part

Body Part	Approach	Device	Qualifier
S Subcutaneous Tissue and Fascia, Head and Neck T Subcutaneous Tissue and Fascia, Trunk V Subcutaneous Tissue and Fascia, Upper Extremity W Subcutaneous Tissue and Fascia, Lower Extremity	Ø Open 3 Percutaneous X External	Z No Device	Z No Qualifier

Non-OR   All Values

SECTION: Ø MEDICAL AND SURGICAL
BODY SYSTEM: J SUBCUTANEOUS TISSUE AND FASCIA
OPERATION: N RELEASE: Freeing a body part from an abnormal physical constraint by cutting or by the use of force

Body Part	Approach	Device	Qualifier
Ø Subcutaneous Tissue and Fascia, Scalp 1 Subcutaneous Tissue and Fascia, Face 4 Subcutaneous Tissue and Fascia, Anterior Neck 5 Subcutaneous Tissue and Fascia, Posterior Neck 6 Subcutaneous Tissue and Fascia, Chest 7 Subcutaneous Tissue and Fascia, Back 8 Subcutaneous Tissue and Fascia, Abdomen 9 Subcutaneous Tissue and Fascia, Buttock B Subcutaneous Tissue and Fascia, Perineum C Subcutaneous Tissue and Fascia, Pelvic Region D Subcutaneous Tissue and Fascia, Right Upper Arm F Subcutaneous Tissue and Fascia, Left Upper Arm G Subcutaneous Tissue and Fascia, Right Lower Arm H Subcutaneous Tissue and Fascia, Left Lower Arm J Subcutaneous Tissue and Fascia, Right Hand K Subcutaneous Tissue and Fascia, Left Hand L Subcutaneous Tissue and Fascia, Right Upper Leg M Subcutaneous Tissue and Fascia, Left Upper Leg N Subcutaneous Tissue and Fascia, Right Lower Leg P Subcutaneous Tissue and Fascia, Left Lower Leg Q Subcutaneous Tissue and Fascia, Right Foot R Subcutaneous Tissue and Fascia, Left Foot	Ø Open 3 Percutaneous X External	Z No Device	Z No Qualifier

Non-OR   ØJN[1456789BCDFGHJKLMNPQR]XZZ

SECTION: Ø MEDICAL AND SURGICAL
BODY SYSTEM: J SUBCUTANEOUS TISSUE AND FASCIA
OPERATION: P REMOVAL: Taking out or off a device from a body part

Body Part	Approach	Device	Qualifier
S Subcutaneous Tissue and Fascia, Head and Neck	Ø Open 3 Percutaneous	Ø Drainage Device 1 Radioactive Element 3 Infusion Device 7 Autologous Tissue Substitute J Synthetic Substitute K Nonautologous Tissue Substitute N Tissue Expander	Z No Qualifier
S Subcutaneous Tissue and Fascia, Head and Neck	X External	Ø Drainage Device 1 Radioactive Element 3 Infusion Device	Z No Qualifier
T Subcutaneous Tissue and Fascia, Trunk ⊞ ⚕	Ø Open 3 Percutaneous	Ø Drainage Device 1 Radioactive Element 2 Monitoring Device 3 Infusion Device 7 Autologous Tissue Substitute H Contraceptive Device J Synthetic Substitute K Nonautologous Tissue Substitute M Stimulator Generator N Tissue Expander P Cardiac Rhythm Related Device V Infusion Device, Pump W Vascular Access Device, Reservoir X Vascular Access Device	Z No Qualifier
T Subcutaneous Tissue and Fascia, Trunk	X External	Ø Drainage Device 1 Radioactive Element 2 Monitoring Device 3 Infusion Device H Contraceptive Device V Infusion Device, Pump X Vascular Access Device	Z No Qualifier
V Subcutaneous Tissue and Fascia, Upper Extremity W Subcutaneous Tissue and Fascia, Lower Extremity	Ø Open 3 Percutaneous	Ø Drainage Device 1 Radioactive Element 3 Infusion Device 7 Autologous Tissue Substitute H Contraceptive Device J Synthetic Substitute K Nonautologous Tissue Substitute N Tissue Expander V Infusion Device, Pump W Vascular Access Device, Reservoir X Vascular Access Device	Z No Qualifier
V Subcutaneous Tissue and Fascia, Upper Extremity W Subcutaneous Tissue and Fascia, Lower Extremity	X External	Ø Drainage Device 1 Radioactive Element 3 Infusion Device H Contraceptive Device V Infusion Pump X Vascular Access Device	Z No Qualifier

⊞ ØJPT[Ø3]PZ
Non-OR ØJPS[Ø3][Ø137JKN]Z
Non-OR ØJPSX[Ø13]Z
Non-OR ØJPT[Ø3][Ø1237HJKMNVWX]Z
Non-OR ØJPTX[Ø123HVX]Z

Non-OR ØJP[VW][Ø3][Ø137HJKNVWX]Z
Non-OR ØJP[VW]X[Ø13HVX]Z
⚕ ØJPT[Ø3]PZ when reported with Secondary Diagnosis K68.11, T81.4XXA, T82.6XXA, or T82.7XXA

Coding Clinic: 2012, Q4, P105 – ØJPTØPZ
Coding Clinic: 2016, Q2, P15; 2015, Q4, P32 – ØJPTØXZ

New/Revised Text in Green　~~deleted~~ Deleted　♀ Females Only　♂ Males Only　**Coding Clinic**
⚕ Non-covered　⚕ Limited Coverage　⊞ Combination (See Appendix E)　DRG Non-OR　Non-OR　⚕ Hospital-Acquired Condition

SECTION: Ø MEDICAL AND SURGICAL
BODY SYSTEM: J SUBCUTANEOUS TISSUE AND FASCIA
OPERATION: Q **REPAIR:** Restoring, to the extent possible, a body part to its normal anatomic structure and function

Body Part	Approach	Device	Qualifier
Ø Subcutaneous Tissue and Fascia, Scalp	Ø Open	Z No Device	Z No Qualifier
1 Subcutaneous Tissue and Fascia, Face	3 Percutaneous		
4 Subcutaneous Tissue and Fascia, Anterior Neck			
5 Subcutaneous Tissue and Fascia, Posterior Neck			
6 Subcutaneous Tissue and Fascia, Chest			
7 Subcutaneous Tissue and Fascia, Back			
8 Subcutaneous Tissue and Fascia, Abdomen			
9 Subcutaneous Tissue and Fascia, Buttock			
B Subcutaneous Tissue and Fascia, Perineum			
C Subcutaneous Tissue and Fascia, Pelvic Region			
D Subcutaneous Tissue and Fascia, Right Upper Arm			
F Subcutaneous Tissue and Fascia, Left Upper Arm			
G Subcutaneous Tissue and Fascia, Right Lower Arm			
H Subcutaneous Tissue and Fascia, Left Lower Arm			
J Subcutaneous Tissue and Fascia, Right Hand			
K Subcutaneous Tissue and Fascia, Left Hand			
L Subcutaneous Tissue and Fascia, Right Upper Leg			
M Subcutaneous Tissue and Fascia, Left Upper Leg			
N Subcutaneous Tissue and Fascia, Right Lower Leg			
P Subcutaneous Tissue and Fascia, Left Lower Leg			
Q Subcutaneous Tissue and Fascia, Right Foot			
R Subcutaneous Tissue and Fascia, Left Foot			

SECTION: Ø MEDICAL AND SURGICAL

BODY SYSTEM: J SUBCUTANEOUS TISSUE AND FASCIA

OPERATION: R REPLACEMENT: Putting in or on biological or synthetic material that physically takes the place and/or function of all or a portion of a body part

Body Part	Approach	Device	Qualifier
Ø Subcutaneous Tissue and Fascia, Scalp 1 Subcutaneous Tissue and Fascia, Face 4 Subcutaneous Tissue and Fascia, Anterior Neck 5 Subcutaneous Tissue and Fascia, Posterior Neck 6 Subcutaneous Tissue and Fascia, Chest 7 Subcutaneous Tissue and Fascia, Back 8 Subcutaneous Tissue and Fascia, Abdomen 9 Subcutaneous Tissue and Fascia, Buttock B Subcutaneous Tissue and Fascia, Perineum C Subcutaneous Tissue and Fascia, Pelvic Region D Subcutaneous Tissue and Fascia, Right Upper Arm F Subcutaneous Tissue and Fascia, Left Upper Arm G Subcutaneous Tissue and Fascia, Right Lower Arm H Subcutaneous Tissue and Fascia, Left Lower Arm J Subcutaneous Tissue and Fascia, Right Hand K Subcutaneous Tissue and Fascia, Left Hand L Subcutaneous Tissue and Fascia, Right Upper Leg M Subcutaneous Tissue and Fascia, Left Upper Leg N Subcutaneous Tissue and Fascia, Right Lower Leg P Subcutaneous Tissue and Fascia, Left Lower Leg Q Subcutaneous Tissue and Fascia, Right Foot R Subcutaneous Tissue and Fascia, Left Foot	Ø Open 3 Percutaneous	7 Autologous Tissue Substitute J Synthetic Substitute K Nonautologous Tissue Substitute	Z No Qualifier

Coding Clinic: 2Ø15, Q2, P13 – ØJR1Ø7Z

SECTION: Ø MEDICAL AND SURGICAL
BODY SYSTEM: J SUBCUTANEOUS TISSUE AND FASCIA
OPERATION: **U SUPPLEMENT:** Putting in or on biological or synthetic material that physically reinforces and/or augments the function of a portion of a body part

U: SUPPLEMENT

J: SUBCUTANEOUS TISSUE AND FASCIA

Ø: M/S

Body Part	Approach	Device	Qualifier
Ø Subcutaneous Tissue and Fascia, Scalp 1 Subcutaneous Tissue and Fascia, Face 4 Subcutaneous Tissue and Fascia, Anterior Neck 5 Subcutaneous Tissue and Fascia, Posterior Neck 6 Subcutaneous Tissue and Fascia, Chest 7 Subcutaneous Tissue and Fascia, Back 8 Subcutaneous Tissue and Fascia, Abdomen 9 Subcutaneous Tissue and Fascia, Buttock B Subcutaneous Tissue and Fascia, Perineum C Subcutaneous Tissue and Fascia, Pelvic Region D Subcutaneous Tissue and Fascia, Right Upper Arm F Subcutaneous Tissue and Fascia, Left Upper Arm G Subcutaneous Tissue and Fascia, Right Lower Arm H Subcutaneous Tissue and Fascia, Left Lower Arm J Subcutaneous Tissue and Fascia, Right Hand K Subcutaneous Tissue and Fascia, Left Hand L Subcutaneous Tissue and Fascia, Right Upper Leg M Subcutaneous Tissue and Fascia, Left Upper Leg N Subcutaneous Tissue and Fascia, Right Lower Leg P Subcutaneous Tissue and Fascia, Left Lower Leg Q Subcutaneous Tissue and Fascia, Right Foot R Subcutaneous Tissue and Fascia, Left Foot	Ø Open 3 Percutaneous	7 Autologous Tissue Substitute J Synthetic Substitute K Nonautologous Tissue Substitute	Z No Qualifier

SECTION: Ø MEDICAL AND SURGICAL

BODY SYSTEM: J SUBCUTANEOUS TISSUE AND FASCIA

OPERATION: W REVISION: Correcting, to the extent possible, a portion of a malfunctioning device or the position of a displaced device

Body Part	Approach	Device	Qualifier
S Subcutaneous Tissue and Fascia, Head and Neck	Ø Open 3 Percutaneous X External	Ø Drainage Device 3 Infusion Device 7 Autologous Tissue Substitute J Synthetic Substitute K Nonautologous Tissue Substitute N Tissue Expander	Z No Qualifier
T Subcutaneous Tissue and Fascia, Trunk 🦠	Ø Open 3 Percutaneous X External	Ø Drainage Device 2 Monitoring Device 3 Infusion Device 7 Autologous Tissue Substitute H Contraceptive Device J Synthetic Substitute K Nonautologous Tissue Substitute M Stimulator Generator N Tissue Expander P Cardiac Rhythm Related Device V Infusion Device, Pump W Vascular Access Device, Reservoir X Vascular Access Device	Z No Qualifier
V Subcutaneous Tissue and Fascia, Upper Extremity W Subcutaneous Tissue and Fascia, Lower Extremity	Ø Open 3 Percutaneous X External	Ø Drainage Device 3 Infusion Device 7 Autologous Tissue Substitute H Contraceptive Device J Synthetic Substitute K Nonautologous Tissue Substitute N Tissue Expander V Infusion Device, Pump W Vascular Access Device, Reservoir X Vascular Access Device	Z No Qualifier

DRG Non-OR ØJWS[Ø3][Ø37JKN]Z
DRG Non-OR ØJWT[Ø3][Ø237HJKNVWX]Z
DRG Non-OR ØJW[VW][Ø3][Ø37HJKNVWX]Z
Non-OR ØJWSX[Ø37JKN]Z
Non-OR ØJWTX[Ø237HJKNPVWX]Z
Non-OR ØJW[VW]X[Ø37HJKNVWX]Z
🦠 ØJWT[Ø3]PZ when reported with Secondary Diagnosis K68.11, T81.4XXA, T82.6XXA, or T82.7XXA

Coding Clinic: 2012, Q4, P106 – ØJWTØPZ
Coding Clinic: 2015, Q2, P10 – ØJWSØJZ
Coding Clinic: 2015, Q4, P33 – ØJWT33Z

SECTION: Ø MEDICAL AND SURGICAL
BODY SYSTEM: J SUBCUTANEOUS TISSUE AND FASCIA
OPERATION: X TRANSFER: Moving, without taking out, all or a portion of a body part to another location to take over the function of all or a portion of a body part

Body Part	Approach	Device	Qualifier
Ø Subcutaneous Tissue and Fascia, Scalp	Ø Open	Z No Device	B Skin and Subcutaneous Tissue
1 Subcutaneous Tissue and Fascia, Face	3 Percutaneous		C Skin, Subcutaneous Tissue and Fascia
4 Subcutaneous Tissue and Fascia, Anterior Neck			Z No Qualifier
5 Subcutaneous Tissue and Fascia, Posterior Neck			
6 Subcutaneous Tissue and Fascia, Chest			
7 Subcutaneous Tissue and Fascia, Back			
8 Subcutaneous Tissue and Fascia, Abdomen			
9 Subcutaneous Tissue and Fascia, Buttock			
B Subcutaneous Tissue and Fascia, Perineum			
C Subcutaneous Tissue and Fascia, Pelvic Region			
D Subcutaneous Tissue and Fascia, Right Upper Arm			
F Subcutaneous Tissue and Fascia, Left Upper Arm			
G Subcutaneous Tissue and Fascia, Right Lower Arm			
H Subcutaneous Tissue and Fascia, Left Lower Arm			
J Subcutaneous Tissue and Fascia, Right Hand			
K Subcutaneous Tissue and Fascia, Left Hand			
L Subcutaneous Tissue and Fascia, Right Upper Leg			
M Subcutaneous Tissue and Fascia, Left Upper Leg			
N Subcutaneous Tissue and Fascia, Right Lower Leg			
P Subcutaneous Tissue and Fascia, Left Lower Leg			
Q Subcutaneous Tissue and Fascia, Right Foot			
R Subcutaneous Tissue and Fascia, Left Foot			

New/Revised Text in Green   ~~deleted~~ Deleted   ♀ Females Only   ♂ Males Only   **Coding Clinic**
Non-covered   Limited Coverage   ⊞ Combination (See Appendix E)   DRG Non-OR   Non-OR   Hospital-Acquired Condition

SECTION: Ø MEDICAL AND SURGICAL

BODY SYSTEM: K MUSCLES

OPERATION: 2 CHANGE: Taking out or off a device from a body part and putting back an identical or similar device in or on the same body part without cutting or puncturing the skin or a mucous membrane

Body Part	Approach	Device	Qualifier
X Upper Muscle Y Lower Muscle	X External	Ø Drainage Device Y Other Device	Z No Qualifier

Non-OR   All Values

SECTION: Ø MEDICAL AND SURGICAL

BODY SYSTEM: K MUSCLES

OPERATION: 5 DESTRUCTION: Physical eradication of all or a portion of a body part by the direct use of energy, force, or a destructive agent

Body Part	Approach	Device	Qualifier
Ø Head Muscle 1 Facial Muscle 2 Neck Muscle, Right 3 Neck Muscle, Left 4 Tongue, Palate, Pharynx Muscle 5 Shoulder Muscle, Right 6 Shoulder Muscle, Left 7 Upper Arm Muscle, Right 8 Upper Arm Muscle, Left 9 Lower Arm and Wrist Muscle, Right B Lower Arm and Wrist Muscle, Left C Hand Muscle, Right D Hand Muscle, Left F Trunk Muscle, Right G Trunk Muscle, Left H Thorax Muscle, Right J Thorax Muscle, Left K Abdomen Muscle, Right L Abdomen Muscle, Left M Perineum Muscle N Hip Muscle, Right P Hip Muscle, Left Q Upper Leg Muscle, Right R Upper Leg Muscle, Left S Lower Leg Muscle, Right T Lower Leg Muscle, Left V Foot Muscle, Right W Foot Muscle, Left	Ø Open 3 Percutaneous 4 Percutaneous Endoscopic	Z No Device	Z No Qualifier

SECTION: Ø MEDICAL AND SURGICAL
BODY SYSTEM: K MUSCLES
OPERATION: 8 DIVISION: Cutting into a body part, without draining fluids and/or gases from the body part, in order to separate or transect a body part

Body Part	Approach	Device	Qualifier
Ø Head Muscle 1 Facial Muscle 2 Neck Muscle, Right 3 Neck Muscle, Left 4 Tongue, Palate, Pharynx Muscle 5 Shoulder Muscle, Right 6 Shoulder Muscle, Left 7 Upper Arm Muscle, Right 8 Upper Arm Muscle, Left 9 Lower Arm and Wrist Muscle, Right B Lower Arm and Wrist Muscle, Left C Hand Muscle, Right D Hand Muscle, Left F Trunk Muscle, Right G Trunk Muscle, Left H Thorax Muscle, Right J Thorax Muscle, Left K Abdomen Muscle, Right L Abdomen Muscle, Left M Perineum Muscle N Hip Muscle, Right P Hip Muscle, Left Q Upper Leg Muscle, Right R Upper Leg Muscle, Left S Lower Leg Muscle, Right T Lower Leg Muscle, Left V Foot Muscle, Right W Foot Muscle, Left	Ø Open 3 Percutaneous 4 Percutaneous Endoscopic	Z No Device	Z No Qualifier

SECTION: Ø MEDICAL AND SURGICAL
BODY SYSTEM: K MUSCLES
OPERATION: 9 DRAINAGE: *(on multiple pages)*
Taking or letting out fluids and/or gases from a body part

Body Part	Approach	Device	Qualifier
Ø Head Muscle	Ø Open	Ø Drainage Device	Z No Qualifier
1 Facial Muscle	3 Percutaneous		
2 Neck Muscle, Right	4 Percutaneous Endoscopic		
3 Neck Muscle, Left			
4 Tongue, Palate, Pharynx Muscle			
5 Shoulder Muscle, Right			
6 Shoulder Muscle, Left			
7 Upper Arm Muscle, Right			
8 Upper Arm Muscle, Left			
9 Lower Arm and Wrist Muscle, Right			
B Lower Arm and Wrist Muscle, Left			
C Hand Muscle, Right			
D Hand Muscle, Left			
F Trunk Muscle, Right			
G Trunk Muscle, Left			
H Thorax Muscle, Right			
J Thorax Muscle, Left			
K Abdomen Muscle, Right			
L Abdomen Muscle, Left			
M Perineum Muscle			
N Hip Muscle, Right			
P Hip Muscle, Left			
Q Upper Leg Muscle, Right			
R Upper Leg Muscle, Left			
S Lower Leg Muscle, Right			
T Lower Leg Muscle, Left			
V Foot Muscle, Right			
W Foot Muscle, Left			

DRG Non-OR   ØK9[Ø123456789BCDFGHJKLMNPQRSTVW]3ØZ

9: DRAINAGE

K: MUSCLES

Ø: M/S

New/Revised Text in Green   ~~deleted~~ Deleted   ♀ Females Only   ♂ Males Only   **Coding Clinic**
Non-covered   Limited Coverage   ⊞ Combination (See Appendix E)   DRG Non-OR   Non-OR   Hospital-Acquired Condition

SECTION: Ø MEDICAL AND SURGICAL

BODY SYSTEM: K MUSCLES

OPERATION: 9 DRAINAGE: *(continued)*
Taking or letting out fluids and/or gases from a body part

Body Part	Approach	Device	Qualifier
Ø Head Muscle	Ø Open	Z No Device	X Diagnostic
1 Facial Muscle	3 Percutaneous		Z No Qualifier
2 Neck Muscle, Right	4 Percutaneous Endoscopic		
3 Neck Muscle, Left			
4 Tongue, Palate, Pharynx Muscle			
5 Shoulder Muscle, Right			
6 Shoulder Muscle, Left			
7 Upper Arm Muscle, Right			
8 Upper Arm Muscle, Left			
9 Lower Arm and Wrist Muscle, Right			
B Lower Arm and Wrist Muscle, Left			
C Hand Muscle, Right			
D Hand Muscle, Left			
F Trunk Muscle, Right			
G Trunk Muscle, Left			
H Thorax Muscle, Right			
J Thorax Muscle, Left			
K Abdomen Muscle, Right			
L Abdomen Muscle, Left			
M Perineum Muscle			
N Hip Muscle, Right			
P Hip Muscle, Left			
Q Upper Leg Muscle, Right			
R Upper Leg Muscle, Left			
S Lower Leg Muscle, Right			
T Lower Leg Muscle, Left			
V Foot Muscle, Right			
W Foot Muscle, Left			

Non-OR ØK9[Ø123456789BFGHJKLMNPQRSTVW]3ZZ
Non-OR ØK9[CD][34]ZZ

SECTION: Ø MEDICAL AND SURGICAL

BODY SYSTEM: K MUSCLES

OPERATION: B EXCISION: Cutting out or off, without replacement, a portion of a body part

Body Part	Approach	Device	Qualifier
Ø Head Muscle	Ø Open	Z No Device	X Diagnostic
1 Facial Muscle	3 Percutaneous		Z No Qualifier
2 Neck Muscle, Right	4 Percutaneous Endoscopic		
3 Neck Muscle, Left			
4 Tongue, Palate, Pharynx Muscle			
5 Shoulder Muscle, Right			
6 Shoulder Muscle, Left			
7 Upper Arm Muscle, Right			
8 Upper Arm Muscle, Left			
9 Lower Arm and Wrist Muscle, Right			
B Lower Arm and Wrist Muscle, Left			
C Hand Muscle, Right			
D Hand Muscle, Left			
F Trunk Muscle, Right			
G Trunk Muscle, Left			
H Thorax Muscle, Right			
J Thorax Muscle, Left			
K Abdomen Muscle, Right			
L Abdomen Muscle, Left			
M Perineum Muscle			
N Hip Muscle, Right			
P Hip Muscle, Left			
Q Upper Leg Muscle, Right			
R Upper Leg Muscle, Left			
S Lower Leg Muscle, Right			
T Lower Leg Muscle, Left			
V Foot Muscle, Right			
W Foot Muscle, Left			

B: EXCISION

K: MUSCLES

Ø: M/S

New/Revised Text in Green ~~deleted~~ Deleted ♀ Females Only ♂ Males Only **Coding Clinic**

⟐ Non-covered ⟐ Limited Coverage ⊞ Combination (See Appendix E) DRG Non-OR Non-OR ⟐ Hospital-Acquired Condition

SECTION: Ø MEDICAL AND SURGICAL
BODY SYSTEM: K MUSCLES
OPERATION: C EXTIRPATION: Taking or cutting out solid matter from a body part

Body Part	Approach	Device	Qualifier
Ø Head Muscle 1 Facial Muscle 2 Neck Muscle, Right 3 Neck Muscle, Left 4 Tongue, Palate, Pharynx Muscle 5 Shoulder Muscle, Right 6 Shoulder Muscle, Left 7 Upper Arm Muscle, Right 8 Upper Arm Muscle, Left 9 Lower Arm and Wrist Muscle, Right B Lower Arm and Wrist Muscle, Left C Hand Muscle, Right D Hand Muscle, Left F Trunk Muscle, Right G Trunk Muscle, Left H Thorax Muscle, Right J Thorax Muscle, Left K Abdomen Muscle, Right L Abdomen Muscle, Left M Perineum Muscle N Hip Muscle, Right P Hip Muscle, Left Q Upper Leg Muscle, Right R Upper Leg Muscle, Left S Lower Leg Muscle, Right T Lower Leg Muscle, Left V Foot Muscle, Right W Foot Muscle, Left	Ø Open 3 Percutaneous 4 Percutaneous Endoscopic	Z No Device	Z No Qualifier

SECTION: Ø MEDICAL AND SURGICAL
BODY SYSTEM: K MUSCLES
OPERATION: H INSERTION: Putting in a nonbiological appliance that monitors, assists, performs, or prevents a physiological function but does not physically take the place of a body part

Body Part	Approach	Device	Qualifier
X Upper Muscle Y Lower Muscle	Ø Open 3 Percutaneous 4 Percutaneous Endoscopic	M Stimulator Lead	Z No Qualifier

SECTION: Ø MEDICAL AND SURGICAL

BODY SYSTEM: K MUSCLES

OPERATION: J INSPECTION: Visually and/or manually exploring a body part

Body Part	Approach	Device	Qualifier
X Upper Muscle Y Lower Muscle	Ø Open 3 Percutaneous 4 Percutaneous Endoscopic X External	Z No Device	Z No Qualifier

DRG Non-OR ØKJ[XY]3ZZ
Non-OR ØKJ[XY]XZZ

SECTION: Ø MEDICAL AND SURGICAL

BODY SYSTEM: K MUSCLES

OPERATION: M REATTACHMENT: Putting back in or on all or a portion of a separated body part to its normal location or other suitable location

Body Part	Approach	Device	Qualifier
Ø Head Muscle 1 Facial Muscle 2 Neck Muscle, Right 3 Neck Muscle, Left 4 Tongue, Palate, Pharynx Muscle 5 Shoulder Muscle, Right 6 Shoulder Muscle, Left 7 Upper Arm Muscle, Right 8 Upper Arm Muscle, Left 9 Lower Arm and Wrist Muscle, Right B Lower Arm and Wrist Muscle, Left C Hand Muscle, Right D Hand Muscle, Left F Trunk Muscle, Right G Trunk Muscle, Left H Thorax Muscle, Right J Thorax Muscle, Left K Abdomen Muscle, Right L Abdomen Muscle, Left M Perineum Muscle N Hip Muscle, Right P Hip Muscle, Left Q Upper Leg Muscle, Right R Upper Leg Muscle, Left S Lower Leg Muscle, Right T Lower Leg Muscle, Left V Foot Muscle, Right W Foot Muscle, Left	Ø Open 4 Percutaneous Endoscopic	Z No Device	Z No Qualifier

New/Revised Text in Green   ~~deleted~~ Deleted   ♀ Females Only   ♂ Males Only   **Coding Clinic**
🕭 Non-covered   🕭 Limited Coverage   ⊞ Combination (See Appendix E)   DRG Non-OR   Non-OR   🕭 Hospital-Acquired Condition

SECTION: Ø MEDICAL AND SURGICAL
BODY SYSTEM: K MUSCLES
OPERATION: N RELEASE: Freeing a body part from an abnormal physical constraint by cutting or by the use of force

Body Part	Approach	Device	Qualifier
Ø Head Muscle 1 Facial Muscle 2 Neck Muscle, Right 3 Neck Muscle, Left 4 Tongue, Palate, Pharynx Muscle 5 Shoulder Muscle, Right 6 Shoulder Muscle, Left 7 Upper Arm Muscle, Right 8 Upper Arm Muscle, Left 9 Lower Arm and Wrist Muscle, Right B Lower Arm and Wrist Muscle, Left C Hand Muscle, Right D Hand Muscle, Left F Trunk Muscle, Right G Trunk Muscle, Left H Thorax Muscle, Right J Thorax Muscle, Left K Abdomen Muscle, Right L Abdomen Muscle, Left M Perineum Muscle N Hip Muscle, Right P Hip Muscle, Left Q Upper Leg Muscle, Right R Upper Leg Muscle, Left S Lower Leg Muscle, Right T Lower Leg Muscle, Left V Foot Muscle, Right W Foot Muscle, Left	Ø Open 3 Percutaneous 4 Percutaneous Endoscopic X External	Z No Device	Z No Qualifier

Non-OR ØKN[Ø123456789BCDFGHJKLMNPQRSTVW]XZZ

Coding Clinic: 2Ø15, Q2, P22 – ØKN84ZZ

SECTION: Ø MEDICAL AND SURGICAL
BODY SYSTEM: K MUSCLES
OPERATION: P REMOVAL: Taking out or off a device from a body part

Body Part	Approach	Device	Qualifier
X Upper Muscle Y Lower Muscle	Ø Open 3 Percutaneous 4 Percutaneous Endoscopic	Ø Drainage Device 7 Autologous Tissue Substitute J Synthetic Substitute K Nonautologous Tissue Substitute M Stimulator Lead	Z No Qualifier
X Upper Muscle Y Lower Muscle	X External	Ø Drainage Device M Stimulator Lead	Z No Qualifier

Non-OR ØKP[XY]X[ØM]Z

SECTION: Ø MEDICAL AND SURGICAL
BODY SYSTEM: K MUSCLES
OPERATION: Q REPAIR: Restoring, to the extent possible, a body part to its normal anatomic structure and function

Body Part	Approach	Device	Qualifier
Ø Head Muscle	Ø Open	Z No Device	Z No Qualifier
1 Facial Muscle	3 Percutaneous		
2 Neck Muscle, Right	4 Percutaneous Endoscopic		
3 Neck Muscle, Left			
4 Tongue, Palate, Pharynx Muscle			
5 Shoulder Muscle, Right			
6 Shoulder Muscle, Left			
7 Upper Arm Muscle, Right			
8 Upper Arm Muscle, Left			
9 Lower Arm and Wrist Muscle, Right			
B Lower Arm and Wrist Muscle, Left			
C Hand Muscle, Right			
D Hand Muscle, Left			
F Trunk Muscle, Right			
G Trunk Muscle, Left			
H Thorax Muscle, Right			
J Thorax Muscle, Left			
K Abdomen Muscle, Right			
L Abdomen Muscle, Left			
M Perineum Muscle			
N Hip Muscle, Right			
P Hip Muscle, Left			
Q Upper Leg Muscle, Right			
R Upper Leg Muscle, Left			
S Lower Leg Muscle, Right			
T Lower Leg Muscle, Left			
V Foot Muscle, Right			
W Foot Muscle, Left			

Coding Clinic: 2016, Q2, P35, Q1, P7 – ØKQMØZZ

New/Revised Text in Green   ~~deleted~~ Deleted   ♀ Females Only   ♂ Males Only   **Coding Clinic**
🐾 Non-covered   🐾 Limited Coverage   ⊕ Combination (See Appendix E)   DRG Non-OR   Non-OR   🐾 Hospital-Acquired Condition

Q: REPAIR
K: MUSCLES
Ø: M/S

SECTION: Ø MEDICAL AND SURGICAL
BODY SYSTEM: K MUSCLES

OPERATION: S REPOSITION: Moving to its normal location, or other suitable location, all or a portion of a body part

Body Part	Approach	Device	Qualifier
Ø Head Muscle	Ø Open	Z No Device	Z No Qualifier
1 Facial Muscle	4 Percutaneous Endoscopic		
2 Neck Muscle, Right			
3 Neck Muscle, Left			
4 Tongue, Palate, Pharynx Muscle			
5 Shoulder Muscle, Right			
6 Shoulder Muscle, Left			
7 Upper Arm Muscle, Right			
8 Upper Arm Muscle, Left			
9 Lower Arm and Wrist Muscle, Right			
B Lower Arm and Wrist Muscle, Left			
C Hand Muscle, Right			
D Hand Muscle, Left			
F Trunk Muscle, Right			
G Trunk Muscle, Left			
H Thorax Muscle, Right			
J Thorax Muscle, Left			
K Abdomen Muscle, Right			
L Abdomen Muscle, Left			
M Perineum Muscle			
N Hip Muscle, Right			
P Hip Muscle, Left			
Q Upper Leg Muscle, Right			
R Upper Leg Muscle, Left			
S Lower Leg Muscle, Right			
T Lower Leg Muscle, Left			
V Foot Muscle, Right			
W Foot Muscle, Left			

Ø: M/S

K: MUSCLES

S: REPOSITION

SECTION: Ø MEDICAL AND SURGICAL

BODY SYSTEM: K MUSCLES

OPERATION: T RESECTION: Cutting out or off, without replacement, all of a body part

Body Part	Approach	Device	Qualifier
Ø Head Muscle 1 Facial Muscle 2 Neck Muscle, Right 3 Neck Muscle, Left 4 Tongue, Palate, Pharynx Muscle 5 Shoulder Muscle, Right 6 Shoulder Muscle, Left 7 Upper Arm Muscle, Right 8 Upper Arm Muscle, Left 9 Lower Arm and Wrist Muscle, Right B Lower Arm and Wrist Muscle, Left C Hand Muscle, Right D Hand Muscle, Left F Trunk Muscle, Right G Trunk Muscle, Left H Thorax Muscle, Right ⊞ J Thorax Muscle, Left ⊞ K Abdomen Muscle, Right L Abdomen Muscle, Left M Perineum Muscle N Hip Muscle, Right P Hip Muscle, Left Q Upper Leg Muscle, Right R Upper Leg Muscle, Left S Lower Leg Muscle, Right T Lower Leg Muscle, Left V Foot Muscle, Right W Foot Muscle, Left	Ø Open 4 Percutaneous Endoscopic	Z No Device	Z No Qualifier

⊞ ØKT[HJ]ØZZ

Coding Clinic: 2015, Q1, P38 – ØKTMØZZ
Coding Clinic: 2016, Q2, P13 – ØKT3ØZZ

New/Revised Text in Green   ~~deleted~~ Deleted   ♀ Females Only   ♂ Males Only   **Coding Clinic**
Non-covered   Limited Coverage   ⊞ Combination (See Appendix E)   DRG Non-OR   Non-OR   Hospital-Acquired Condition

SECTION: Ø MEDICAL AND SURGICAL
BODY SYSTEM: K MUSCLES
OPERATION: U SUPPLEMENT: Putting in or on biological or synthetic material that physically reinforces and/or augments the function of a portion of a body part

Body Part	Approach	Device	Qualifier
Ø Head Muscle 1 Facial Muscle 2 Neck Muscle, Right 3 Neck Muscle, Left 4 Tongue, Palate, Pharynx Muscle 5 Shoulder Muscle, Right 6 Shoulder Muscle, Left 7 Upper Arm Muscle, Right 8 Upper Arm Muscle, Left 9 Lower Arm and Wrist Muscle, Right B Lower Arm and Wrist Muscle, Left C Hand Muscle, Right D Hand Muscle, Left F Trunk Muscle, Right G Trunk Muscle, Left H Thorax Muscle, Right J Thorax Muscle, Left K Abdomen Muscle, Right L Abdomen Muscle, Left M Perineum Muscle N Hip Muscle, Right P Hip Muscle, Left Q Upper Leg Muscle, Right R Upper Leg Muscle, Left S Lower Leg Muscle, Right T Lower Leg Muscle, Left V Foot Muscle, Right W Foot Muscle, Left	Ø Open 4 Percutaneous Endoscopic	7 Autologous Tissue Substitute J Synthetic Substitute K Nonautologous Tissue Substitute	Z No Qualifier

SECTION: Ø MEDICAL AND SURGICAL
BODY SYSTEM: K MUSCLES
OPERATION: W REVISION: Correcting, to the extent possible, a portion of a malfunctioning device or the position of a displaced device

Body Part	Approach	Device	Qualifier
X Upper Muscle Y Lower Muscle	Ø Open 3 Percutaneous 4 Percutaneous Endoscopic X External	Ø Drainage Device 7 Autologous Tissue Substitute J Synthetic Substitute K Nonautologous Tissue Substitute M Stimulator Lead	Z No Qualifier

Non-OR   ØKW[XY]X[Ø7JKM]Z

SECTION: Ø MEDICAL AND SURGICAL

BODY SYSTEM: K MUSCLES

OPERATION: X TRANSFER: Moving, without taking out, all or a portion of a body part to another location to take over the function of all or a portion of a body part

Body Part	Approach	Device	Qualifier
Ø Head Muscle 1 Facial Muscle ⊞ 2 Neck Muscle, Right 3 Neck Muscle, Left 4 Tongue, Palate, Pharynx Muscle 5 Shoulder Muscle, Right 6 Shoulder Muscle, Left 7 Upper Arm Muscle, Right 8 Upper Arm Muscle, Left 9 Lower Arm and Wrist Muscle, Right B Lower Arm and Wrist Muscle, Left C Hand Muscle, Right D Hand Muscle, Left F Trunk Muscle, Right G Trunk Muscle, Left H Thorax Muscle, Right J Thorax Muscle, Left M Perineum Muscle N Hip Muscle, Right P Hip Muscle, Left Q Upper Leg Muscle, Right R Upper Leg Muscle, Left S Lower Leg Muscle, Right ⊞ T Lower Leg Muscle, Left ⊞ V Foot Muscle, Right W Foot Muscle, Left	Ø Open 4 Percutaneous Endoscopic	Z No Device	Ø Skin 1 Subcutaneous Tissue 2 Skin and Subcutaneous Tissue Z No Qualifier
K Abdomen Muscle, Right L Abdomen Muscle, Left	Ø Open 4 Percutaneous Endoscopic	Z No Device	Ø Skin 1 Subcutaneous Tissue 2 Skin and Subcutaneous Tissue 6 Transverse Rectus Abdominis Myocutaneous Flap Z No Qualifier

⊞ ØKX[1ST][Ø4]ZZ

Coding Clinic: 2Ø15, Q2, P26 – ØKX4ØZ2
Coding Clinic: 2Ø15, Q3, P33 – ØKX1ØZ2

SECTION: Ø MEDICAL AND SURGICAL

BODY SYSTEM: L TENDONS

OPERATION: 2 **CHANGE:** Taking out or off a device from a body part and putting back an identical or similar device in or on the same body part without cutting or puncturing the skin or a mucous membrane

Body Part	Approach	Device	Qualifier
X Upper Tendon Y Lower Tendon	X External	Ø Drainage Device Y Other Device	Z No Qualifier

Non-OR All Values

SECTION: Ø MEDICAL AND SURGICAL

BODY SYSTEM: L TENDONS

OPERATION: 5 **DESTRUCTION:** Physical eradication of all or a portion of a body part by the direct use of energy, force, or a destructive agent

Body Part	Approach	Device	Qualifier
Ø Head and Neck Tendon 1 Shoulder Tendon, Right 2 Shoulder Tendon, Left 3 Upper Arm Tendon, Right 4 Upper Arm Tendon, Left 5 Lower Arm and Wrist Tendon, Right 6 Lower Arm and Wrist Tendon, Left 7 Hand Tendon, Right 8 Hand Tendon, Left 9 Trunk Tendon, Right B Trunk Tendon, Left C Thorax Tendon, Right D Thorax Tendon, Left F Abdomen Tendon, Right G Abdomen Tendon, Left H Perineum Tendon J Hip Tendon, Right K Hip Tendon, Left L Upper Leg Tendon, Right M Upper Leg Tendon, Left N Lower Leg Tendon, Right P Lower Leg Tendon, Left Q Knee Tendon, Right R Knee Tendon, Left S Ankle Tendon, Right T Ankle Tendon, Left V Foot Tendon, Right W Foot Tendon, Left	Ø Open 3 Percutaneous 4 Percutaneous Endoscopic	Z No Device	Z No Qualifier

ØL2 · 2: CHANGE · 5: DESTRUCTION · L: TENDONS · Ø: M/S

SECTION: Ø MEDICAL AND SURGICAL

BODY SYSTEM: L TENDONS

OPERATION: 8 DIVISION: Cutting into a body part, without draining fluids and/or gases from the body part, in order to separate or transect a body part

Body Part	Approach	Device	Qualifier
Ø Head and Neck Tendon	Ø Open	Z No Device	Z No Qualifier
1 Shoulder Tendon, Right	3 Percutaneous		
2 Shoulder Tendon, Left	4 Percutaneous Endoscopic		
3 Upper Arm Tendon, Right			
4 Upper Arm Tendon, Left			
5 Lower Arm and Wrist Tendon, Right			
6 Lower Arm and Wrist Tendon, Left			
7 Hand Tendon, Right			
8 Hand Tendon, Left			
9 Trunk Tendon, Right			
B Trunk Tendon, Left			
C Thorax Tendon, Right			
D Thorax Tendon, Left			
F Abdomen Tendon, Right			
G Abdomen Tendon, Left			
H Perineum Tendon			
J Hip Tendon, Right			
K Hip Tendon, Left			
L Upper Leg Tendon, Right			
M Upper Leg Tendon, Left			
N Lower Leg Tendon, Right			
P Lower Leg Tendon, Left			
Q Knee Tendon, Right			
R Knee Tendon, Left			
S Ankle Tendon, Right			
T Ankle Tendon, Left			
V Foot Tendon, Right			
W Foot Tendon, Left			

SECTION: Ø MEDICAL AND SURGICAL

BODY SYSTEM: L TENDONS

OPERATION: 9 DRAINAGE: Taking or letting out fluids and/or gases from a body part

9: DRAINAGE

L: TENDONS

Ø: M/S

Body Part	Approach	Device	Qualifier
Ø Head and Neck Tendon 1 Shoulder Tendon, Right 2 Shoulder Tendon, Left 3 Upper Arm Tendon, Right 4 Upper Arm Tendon, Left 5 Lower Arm and Wrist Tendon, Right 6 Lower Arm and Wrist Tendon, Left 7 Hand Tendon, Right 8 Hand Tendon, Left 9 Trunk Tendon, Right B Trunk Tendon, Left C Thorax Tendon, Right D Thorax Tendon, Left F Abdomen Tendon, Right G Abdomen Tendon, Left H Perineum Tendon J Hip Tendon, Right K Hip Tendon, Left L Upper Leg Tendon, Right M Upper Leg Tendon, Left N Lower Leg Tendon, Right P Lower Leg Tendon, Left Q Knee Tendon, Right R Knee Tendon, Left S Ankle Tendon, Right T Ankle Tendon, Left V Foot Tendon, Right W Foot Tendon, Left	Ø Open 3 Percutaneous 4 Percutaneous Endoscopic	Ø Drainage Device	Z No Qualifier
Ø Head and Neck Tendon 1 Shoulder Tendon, Right 2 Shoulder Tendon, Left 3 Upper Arm Tendon, Right 4 Upper Arm Tendon, Left 5 Lower Arm and Wrist Tendon, Right 6 Lower Arm and Wrist Tendon, Left 7 Hand Tendon, Right 8 Hand Tendon, Left 9 Trunk Tendon, Right B Trunk Tendon, Left C Thorax Tendon, Right D Thorax Tendon, Left F Abdomen Tendon, Right G Abdomen Tendon, Left H Perineum Tendon J Hip Tendon, Right K Hip Tendon, Left L Upper Leg Tendon, Right M Upper Leg Tendon, Left N Lower Leg Tendon, Right P Lower Leg Tendon, Left Q Knee Tendon, Right R Knee Tendon, Left S Ankle Tendon, Right T Ankle Tendon, Left V Foot Tendon, Right W Foot Tendon, Left	Ø Open 3 Percutaneous 4 Percutaneous Endoscopic	Z No Device	X Diagnostic Z No Qualifier

DRG Non-OR ØL9[Ø123456789BCDFGHJKLMNPQRSTVW]3ØZ   Non-OR ØL9[78][34]ZZ
DRG Non-OR ØL9[Ø1234569BCDFGHJKLMNPQRSTVW]3ZZ

316

SECTION: Ø MEDICAL AND SURGICAL

BODY SYSTEM: L TENDONS

OPERATION: B EXCISION: Cutting out or off, without replacement, a portion of a body part

Body Part	Approach	Device	Qualifier
Ø Head and Neck Tendon	Ø Open	Z No Device	X Diagnostic
1 Shoulder Tendon, Right	3 Percutaneous		Z No Qualifier
2 Shoulder Tendon, Left	4 Percutaneous Endoscopic		
3 Upper Arm Tendon, Right			
4 Upper Arm Tendon, Left			
5 Lower Arm and Wrist Tendon, Right			
6 Lower Arm and Wrist Tendon, Left			
7 Hand Tendon, Right			
8 Hand Tendon, Left			
9 Trunk Tendon, Right			
B Trunk Tendon, Left			
C Thorax Tendon, Right			
D Thorax Tendon, Left			
F Abdomen Tendon, Right			
G Abdomen Tendon, Left			
H Perineum Tendon			
J Hip Tendon, Right			
K Hip Tendon, Left			
L Upper Leg Tendon, Right			
M Upper Leg Tendon, Left			
N Lower Leg Tendon, Right			
P Lower Leg Tendon, Left			
Q Knee Tendon, Right			
R Knee Tendon, Left			
S Ankle Tendon, Right			
T Ankle Tendon, Left			
V Foot Tendon, Right			
W Foot Tendon, Left			

Coding Clinic: 2Ø15, Q3, P27 – ØLB6ØZZ

SECTION: Ø MEDICAL AND SURGICAL

BODY SYSTEM: L TENDONS
OPERATION: C EXTIRPATION: Taking or cutting out solid matter from a body part

Body Part	Approach	Device	Qualifier
Ø Head and Neck Tendon 1 Shoulder Tendon, Right 2 Shoulder Tendon, Left 3 Upper Arm Tendon, Right 4 Upper Arm Tendon, Left 5 Lower Arm and Wrist Tendon, Right 6 Lower Arm and Wrist Tendon, Left 7 Hand Tendon, Right 8 Hand Tendon, Left 9 Trunk Tendon, Right B Trunk Tendon, Left C Thorax Tendon, Right D Thorax Tendon, Left F Abdomen Tendon, Right G Abdomen Tendon, Left H Perineum Tendon J Hip Tendon, Right K Hip Tendon, Left L Upper Leg Tendon, Right M Upper Leg Tendon, Left N Lower Leg Tendon, Right P Lower Leg Tendon, Left Q Knee Tendon, Right R Knee Tendon, Left S Ankle Tendon, Right T Ankle Tendon, Left V Foot Tendon, Right W Foot Tendon, Left	Ø Open 3 Percutaneous 4 Percutaneous Endoscopic	Z No Device	Z No Qualifier

SECTION: Ø MEDICAL AND SURGICAL

BODY SYSTEM: L TENDONS
OPERATION: J INSPECTION: Visually and/or manually exploring a body part

Body Part	Approach	Device	Qualifier
X Upper Tendon Y Lower Tendon	Ø Open 3 Percutaneous 4 Percutaneous Endoscopic X External	Z No Device	Z No Qualifier

DRG Non-OR ØLJ[XY]3ZZ
Non-OR ØLJ[XY]XZZ

SECTION: Ø MEDICAL AND SURGICAL
BODY SYSTEM: L TENDONS

OPERATION: **M REATTACHMENT:** Putting back in or on all or a portion of a separated body part to its normal location or other suitable location

Body Part	Approach	Device	Qualifier
Ø Head and Neck Tendon 1 Shoulder Tendon, Right 2 Shoulder Tendon, Left 3 Upper Arm Tendon, Right 4 Upper Arm Tendon, Left 5 Lower Arm and Wrist Tendon, Right 6 Lower Arm and Wrist Tendon, Left 7 Hand Tendon, Right 8 Hand Tendon, Left 9 Trunk Tendon, Right B Trunk Tendon, Left C Thorax Tendon, Right D Thorax Tendon, Left F Abdomen Tendon, Right G Abdomen Tendon, Left H Perineum Tendon J Hip Tendon, Right K Hip Tendon, Left L Upper Leg Tendon, Right M Upper Leg Tendon, Left N Lower Leg Tendon, Right P Lower Leg Tendon, Left Q Knee Tendon, Right R Knee Tendon, Left S Ankle Tendon, Right T Ankle Tendon, Left V Foot Tendon, Right W Foot Tendon, Left	Ø Open 4 Percutaneous Endoscopic	Z No Device	Z No Qualifier

SECTION: Ø MEDICAL AND SURGICAL

BODY SYSTEM: L TENDONS

OPERATION: N RELEASE: Freeing a body part from an abnormal physical constraint by cutting or by the use of force

Body Part	Approach	Device	Qualifier
Ø Head and Neck Tendon 1 Shoulder Tendon, Right 2 Shoulder Tendon, Left 3 Upper Arm Tendon, Right 4 Upper Arm Tendon, Left 5 Lower Arm and Wrist Tendon, Right 6 Lower Arm and Wrist Tendon, Left 7 Hand Tendon, Right 8 Hand Tendon, Left 9 Trunk Tendon, Right B Trunk Tendon, Left C Thorax Tendon, Right D Thorax Tendon, Left F Abdomen Tendon, Right G Abdomen Tendon, Left H Perineum Tendon J Hip Tendon, Right K Hip Tendon, Left L Upper Leg Tendon, Right M Upper Leg Tendon, Left N Lower Leg Tendon, Right P Lower Leg Tendon, Left Q Knee Tendon, Right R Knee Tendon, Left S Ankle Tendon, Right T Ankle Tendon, Left V Foot Tendon, Right W Foot Tendon, Left	Ø Open 3 Percutaneous 4 Percutaneous Endoscopic X External	Z No Device	Z No Qualifier

Non-OR   ØLN[Ø123456789BCDFGHJKLMNPQRSTVW]XZZ

SECTION: Ø MEDICAL AND SURGICAL

BODY SYSTEM: L TENDONS

OPERATION: P REMOVAL: Taking out or off a device from a body part

Body Part	Approach	Device	Qualifier
X Upper Tendon Y Lower Tendon	Ø Open 3 Percutaneous 4 Percutaneous Endoscopic	Ø Drainage Device 7 Autologous Tissue Substitute J Synthetic Substitute K Nonautologous Tissue Substitute	Z No Qualifier
X Upper Tendon Y Lower Tendon	X External	Ø Drainage Device	Z No Qualifier

DRG Non-OR   ØLP[XY]3ØZ

Non-OR   ØLP[XY]XØZ

SECTION: **Ø MEDICAL AND SURGICAL**
BODY SYSTEM: **L TENDONS**
OPERATION: **Q REPAIR:** Restoring, to the extent possible, a body part to its normal anatomic structure and function

Body Part	Approach	Device	Qualifier
Ø Head and Neck Tendon	Ø Open	Z No Device	Z No Qualifier
1 Shoulder Tendon, Right	3 Percutaneous		
2 Shoulder Tendon, Left	4 Percutaneous Endoscopic		
3 Upper Arm Tendon, Right			
4 Upper Arm Tendon, Left			
5 Lower Arm and Wrist Tendon, Right			
6 Lower Arm and Wrist Tendon, Left			
7 Hand Tendon, Right			
8 Hand Tendon, Left			
9 Trunk Tendon, Right			
B Trunk Tendon, Left			
C Thorax Tendon, Right			
D Thorax Tendon, Left			
F Abdomen Tendon, Right			
G Abdomen Tendon, Left			
H Perineum Tendon			
J Hip Tendon, Right			
K Hip Tendon, Left			
L Upper Leg Tendon, Right			
M Upper Leg Tendon, Left			
N Lower Leg Tendon, Right			
P Lower Leg Tendon, Left			
Q Knee Tendon, Right			
R Knee Tendon, Left			
S Ankle Tendon, Right			
T Ankle Tendon, Left			
V Foot Tendon, Right			
W Foot Tendon, Left			

Coding Clinic: 2013, Q3, P21 – ØLQ14ZZ

Ø: M/S

L: TENDONS

Q: REPAIR

SECTION: Ø MEDICAL AND SURGICAL
BODY SYSTEM: L TENDONS
OPERATION: R **REPLACEMENT:** Putting in or on biological or synthetic material that physically takes the place and/or function of all or a portion of a body part

Body Part	Approach	Device	Qualifier
Ø Head and Neck Tendon 1 Shoulder Tendon, Right 2 Shoulder Tendon, Left 3 Upper Arm Tendon, Right 4 Upper Arm Tendon, Left 5 Lower Arm and Wrist Tendon, Right 6 Lower Arm and Wrist Tendon, Left 7 Hand Tendon, Right 8 Hand Tendon, Left 9 Trunk Tendon, Right B Trunk Tendon, Left C Thorax Tendon, Right D Thorax Tendon, Left F Abdomen Tendon, Right G Abdomen Tendon, Left H Perineum Tendon J Hip Tendon, Right K Hip Tendon, Left L Upper Leg Tendon, Right M Upper Leg Tendon, Left N Lower Leg Tendon, Right P Lower Leg Tendon, Left Q Knee Tendon, Right R Knee Tendon, Left S Ankle Tendon, Right T Ankle Tendon, Left V Foot Tendon, Right W Foot Tendon, Left	Ø Open 4 Percutaneous Endoscopic	7 Autologous Tissue Substitute J Synthetic Substitute K Nonautologous Tissue Substitute	Z No Qualifier

L: TENDONS

R: REPLACEMENT

Ø: M/S

New/Revised Text in Green   ~~deleted~~ Deleted   ♀ Females Only   ♂ Males Only   **Coding Clinic**

🞍 Non-covered   🞍 Limited Coverage   ⊞ Combination (See Appendix E)   DRG Non-OR   Non-OR   🞍 Hospital-Acquired Condition

SECTION: Ø MEDICAL AND SURGICAL

BODY SYSTEM: L TENDONS

OPERATION: S REPOSITION: Moving to its normal location, or other suitable location, all or a portion of a body part

Body Part	Approach	Device	Qualifier
Ø Head and Neck Tendon	Ø Open	Z No Device	Z No Qualifier
1 Shoulder Tendon, Right	4 Percutaneous Endoscopic		
2 Shoulder Tendon, Left			
3 Upper Arm Tendon, Right			
4 Upper Arm Tendon, Left			
5 Lower Arm and Wrist Tendon, Right			
6 Lower Arm and Wrist Tendon, Left			
7 Hand Tendon, Right			
8 Hand Tendon, Left			
9 Trunk Tendon, Right			
B Trunk Tendon, Left			
C Thorax Tendon, Right			
D Thorax Tendon, Left			
F Abdomen Tendon, Right			
G Abdomen Tendon, Left			
H Perineum Tendon			
J Hip Tendon, Right			
K Hip Tendon, Left			
L Upper Leg Tendon, Right			
M Upper Leg Tendon, Left			
N Lower Leg Tendon, Right			
P Lower Leg Tendon, Left			
Q Knee Tendon, Right ⊞			
R Knee Tendon, Left ⊞			
S Ankle Tendon, Right			
T Ankle Tendon, Left			
V Foot Tendon, Right			
W Foot Tendon, Left			

⊞ ØLS[QR][Ø4]ZZ

Coding Clinic: 2Ø15, Q3, P15 – ØLS4ØZZ

SECTION: Ø MEDICAL AND SURGICAL
BODY SYSTEM: L TENDONS
OPERATION: T RESECTION: Cutting out or off, without replacement, all of a body part

Body Part	Approach	Device	Qualifier
Ø Head and Neck Tendon 1 Shoulder Tendon, Right 2 Shoulder Tendon, Left 3 Upper Arm Tendon, Right 4 Upper Arm Tendon, Left 5 Lower Arm and Wrist Tendon, Right 6 Lower Arm and Wrist Tendon, Left 7 Hand Tendon, Right 8 Hand Tendon, Left 9 Trunk Tendon, Right B Trunk Tendon, Left C Thorax Tendon, Right D Thorax Tendon, Left F Abdomen Tendon, Right G Abdomen Tendon, Left H Perineum Tendon J Hip Tendon, Right K Hip Tendon, Left L Upper Leg Tendon, Right M Upper Leg Tendon, Left N Lower Leg Tendon, Right P Lower Leg Tendon, Left Q Knee Tendon, Right R Knee Tendon, Left S Ankle Tendon, Right T Ankle Tendon, Left V Foot Tendon, Right W Foot Tendon, Left	Ø Open 4 Percutaneous Endoscopic	Z No Device	Z No Qualifier

New/Revised Text in Green ~~deleted~~ Deleted ♀ Females Only ♂ Males Only **Coding Clinic**
Non-covered Limited Coverage ⊞ Combination (See Appendix E) DRG Non-OR Non-OR Hospital-Acquired Condition

SECTION: Ø MEDICAL AND SURGICAL
BODY SYSTEM: L TENDONS
OPERATION: **U SUPPLEMENT:** Putting in or on biological or synthetic material that physically reinforces and/or augments the function of a portion of a body part

Body Part	Approach	Device	Qualifier
Ø Head and Neck Tendon 1 Shoulder Tendon, Right 2 Shoulder Tendon, Left 3 Upper Arm Tendon, Right 4 Upper Arm Tendon, Left 5 Lower Arm and Wrist Tendon, Right 6 Lower Arm and Wrist Tendon, Left 7 Hand Tendon, Right 8 Hand Tendon, Left 9 Trunk Tendon, Right B Trunk Tendon, Left C Thorax Tendon, Right D Thorax Tendon, Left F Abdomen Tendon, Right G Abdomen Tendon, Left H Perineum Tendon J Hip Tendon, Right K Hip Tendon, Left L Upper Leg Tendon, Right M Upper Leg Tendon, Left N Lower Leg Tendon, Right P Lower Leg Tendon, Left Q Knee Tendon, Right R Knee Tendon, Left S Ankle Tendon, Right T Ankle Tendon, Left V Foot Tendon, Right W Foot Tendon, Left	Ø Open 4 Percutaneous Endoscopic	7 Autologous Tissue Substitute J Synthetic Substitute K Nonautologous Tissue Substitute	Z No Qualifier

Coding Clinic: 2015, Q2, P11 – ØLU[QM]ØKZ

SECTION: Ø MEDICAL AND SURGICAL
BODY SYSTEM: L TENDONS
OPERATION: **W REVISION:** Correcting, to the extent possible, a portion of a malfunctioning device or the position of a displaced device

Body Part	Approach	Device	Qualifier
X Upper Tendon Y Lower Tendon	Ø Open 3 Percutaneous 4 Percutaneous Endoscopic X External	Ø Drainage Device 7 Autologous Tissue Substitute J Synthetic Substitute K Nonautologous Tissue Substitute	Z No Qualifier

Non-OR   ØLW[XY]X[Ø7JK]Z

SECTION: Ø MEDICAL AND SURGICAL

BODY SYSTEM: L TENDONS

OPERATION: X TRANSFER: Moving, without taking out, all or a portion of a body part to another location to take over the function of all or a portion of a body part

Body Part	Approach	Device	Qualifier
Ø Head and Neck Tendon	Ø Open	Z No Device	Z No Qualifier
1 Shoulder Tendon, Right	4 Percutaneous Endoscopic		
2 Shoulder Tendon, Left			
3 Upper Arm Tendon, Right			
4 Upper Arm Tendon, Left			
5 Lower Arm and Wrist Tendon, Right			
6 Lower Arm and Wrist Tendon, Left			
7 Hand Tendon, Right			
8 Hand Tendon, Left			
9 Trunk Tendon, Right			
B Trunk Tendon, Left			
C Thorax Tendon, Right			
D Thorax Tendon, Left			
F Abdomen Tendon, Right			
G Abdomen Tendon, Left			
H Perineum Tendon			
J Hip Tendon, Right			
K Hip Tendon, Left			
L Upper Leg Tendon, Right			
M Upper Leg Tendon, Left			
N Lower Leg Tendon, Right			
P Lower Leg Tendon, Left			
Q Knee Tendon, Right			
R Knee Tendon, Left			
S Ankle Tendon, Right			
T Ankle Tendon, Left			
V Foot Tendon, Right			
W Foot Tendon, Left			

X: TRANSFER

L: TENDONS

Ø: M/S

New/Revised Text in Green   ~~deleted~~ Deleted   ♀ Females Only   ♂ Males Only   **Coding Clinic**

Non-covered   Limited Coverage   ⊕ Combination (See Appendix E)   DRG Non-OR   Non-OR   Hospital-Acquired Condition

SECTION: Ø MEDICAL AND SURGICAL

BODY SYSTEM: M BURSAE AND LIGAMENTS

OPERATION: 2 CHANGE: Taking out or off a device from a body part and putting back an identical or similar device in or on the same body part without cutting or puncturing the skin or a mucous membrane

Body Part	Approach	Device	Qualifier
X Upper Bursa and Ligament Y Lower Bursa and Ligament	X External	Ø Drainage Device Y Other Device	Z No Qualifier

Non-OR **All Values**

SECTION: Ø MEDICAL AND SURGICAL

BODY SYSTEM: M BURSAE AND LIGAMENTS

OPERATION: 5 DESTRUCTION: Physical eradication of all or a portion of a body part by the direct use of energy, force, or a destructive agent

Body Part	Approach	Device	Qualifier
Ø Head and Neck Bursa and Ligament 1 Shoulder Bursa and Ligament, Right 2 Shoulder Bursa and Ligament, Left 3 Elbow Bursa and Ligament, Right 4 Elbow Bursa and Ligament, Left 5 Wrist Bursa and Ligament, Right 6 Wrist Bursa and Ligament, Left 7 Hand Bursa and Ligament, Right 8 Hand Bursa and Ligament, Left 9 Upper Extremity Bursa and Ligament, Right B Upper Extremity Bursa and Ligament, Left C Trunk Bursa and Ligament, Right D Trunk Bursa and Ligament, Left F Thorax Bursa and Ligament, Right G Thorax Bursa and Ligament, Left H Abdomen Bursa and Ligament, Right J Abdomen Bursa and Ligament, Left K Perineum Bursa and Ligament L Hip Bursa and Ligament, Right M Hip Bursa and Ligament, Left N Knee Bursa and Ligament, Right P Knee Bursa and Ligament, Left Q Ankle Bursa and Ligament, Right R Ankle Bursa and Ligament, Left S Foot Bursa and Ligament, Right T Foot Bursa and Ligament, Left V Lower Extremity Bursa and Ligament, Right W Lower Extremity Bursa and Ligament, Left	Ø Open 3 Percutaneous 4 Percutaneous Endoscopic	Z No Device	Z No Qualifier

Side tab: 2: CHANGE   5: DESTRUCTION   M: BURSAE AND LIGAMENTS   Ø: M/S

SECTION: Ø MEDICAL AND SURGICAL

BODY SYSTEM: M BURSAE AND LIGAMENTS

OPERATION: 8 DIVISION: Cutting into a body part, without draining fluids and/or gases from the body part, in order to separate or transect a body part

Body Part	Approach	Device	Qualifier
Ø Head and Neck Bursa and Ligament	Ø Open	Z No Device	Z No Qualifier
1 Shoulder Bursa and Ligament, Right	3 Percutaneous		
2 Shoulder Bursa and Ligament, Left	4 Percutaneous Endoscopic		
3 Elbow Bursa and Ligament, Right			
4 Elbow Bursa and Ligament, Left			
5 Wrist Bursa and Ligament, Right			
6 Wrist Bursa and Ligament, Left			
7 Hand Bursa and Ligament, Right			
8 Hand Bursa and Ligament, Left			
9 Upper Extremity Bursa and Ligament, Right			
B Upper Extremity Bursa and Ligament, Left			
C Trunk Bursa and Ligament, Right			
D Trunk Bursa and Ligament, Left			
F Thorax Bursa and Ligament, Right			
G Thorax Bursa and Ligament, Left			
H Abdomen Bursa and Ligament, Right			
J Abdomen Bursa and Ligament, Left			
K Perineum Bursa and Ligament			
L Hip Bursa and Ligament, Right			
M Hip Bursa and Ligament, Left			
N Knee Bursa and Ligament, Right			
P Knee Bursa and Ligament, Left			
Q Ankle Bursa and Ligament, Right			
R Ankle Bursa and Ligament, Left			
S Foot Bursa and Ligament, Right			
T Foot Bursa and Ligament, Left			
V Lower Extremity Bursa and Ligament, Right			
W Lower Extremity Bursa and Ligament, Left			

Non-OR ØM8[56][Ø34]ZZ

SECTION: Ø MEDICAL AND SURGICAL

BODY SYSTEM: M BURSAE AND LIGAMENTS

OPERATION: 9 DRAINAGE: Taking or letting out fluids and/or gases from a body part

Body Part	Approach	Device	Qualifier
Ø Head and Neck Bursa and Ligament 1 Shoulder Bursa and Ligament, Right 2 Shoulder Bursa and Ligament, Left 3 Elbow Bursa and Ligament, Right 4 Elbow Bursa and Ligament, Left 5 Wrist Bursa and Ligament, Right 6 Wrist Bursa and Ligament, Left 7 Hand Bursa and Ligament, Right 8 Hand Bursa and Ligament, Left 9 Upper Extremity Bursa and Ligament, Right B Upper Extremity Bursa and Ligament, Left C Trunk Bursa and Ligament, Right D Trunk Bursa and Ligament, Left F Thorax Bursa and Ligament, Right G Thorax Bursa and Ligament, Left H Abdomen Bursa and Ligament, Right J Abdomen Bursa and Ligament, Left K Perineum Bursa and Ligament L Hip Bursa and Ligament, Right M Hip Bursa and Ligament, Left N Knee Bursa and Ligament, Right P Knee Bursa and Ligament, Left Q Ankle Bursa and Ligament, Right R Ankle Bursa and Ligament, Left S Foot Bursa and Ligament, Right T Foot Bursa and Ligament, Left V Lower Extremity Bursa and Ligament, Right W Lower Extremity Bursa and Ligament, Left	Ø Open 3 Percutaneous 4 Percutaneous Endoscopic	Ø Drainage Device	Z No Qualifier
Ø Head and Neck Bursa and Ligament 1 Shoulder Bursa and Ligament, Right 2 Shoulder Bursa and Ligament, Left 3 Elbow Bursa and Ligament, Right 4 Elbow Bursa and Ligament, Left 5 Wrist Bursa and Ligament, Right 6 Wrist Bursa and Ligament, Left 7 Hand Bursa and Ligament, Right 8 Hand Bursa and Ligament, Left 9 Upper Extremity Bursa and Ligament, Right B Upper Extremity Bursa and Ligament, Left C Trunk Bursa and Ligament, Right D Trunk Bursa and Ligament, Left F Thorax Bursa and Ligament, Right G Thorax Bursa and Ligament, Left H Abdomen Bursa and Ligament, Right J Abdomen Bursa and Ligament, Left K Perineum Bursa and Ligament L Hip Bursa and Ligament, Right M Hip Bursa and Ligament, Left N Knee Bursa and Ligament, Right P Knee Bursa and Ligament, Left Q Ankle Bursa and Ligament, Right R Ankle Bursa and Ligament, Left S Foot Bursa and Ligament, Right T Foot Bursa and Ligament, Left V Lower Extremity Bursa and Ligament, Right W Lower Extremity Bursa and Ligament, Left	Ø Open 3 Percutaneous 4 Percutaneous Endoscopic	Z No Device	X Diagnostic Z No Qualifier

DRG Non-OR ØM9[056NPQRST]3ØZ

Non-OR ØM9[1234789BCDFGHJKLMVW][34]ØZ

Non-OR ØM9[Ø12345678CDFGLMNPQRST][Ø34]ZX

Non-OR ØM9[Ø56789BCDFGHJKNPQRSTVW][34]ZZ

Non-OR ØM9[1234LM]3ZZ

New/Revised Text in Green ~~deleted~~ Deleted ♀ Females Only ♂ Males Only **Coding Clinic**

⊘ Non-covered ⊘ Limited Coverage ⊞ Combination (See Appendix E) DRG Non-OR Non-OR ⊘ Hospital-Acquired Condition

SECTION: Ø MEDICAL AND SURGICAL

BODY SYSTEM: M BURSAE AND LIGAMENTS

OPERATION: B EXCISION: Cutting out or off, without replacement, a portion of a body part

Body Part	Approach	Device	Qualifier
Ø Head and Neck Bursa and Ligament	Ø Open	Z No Device	X Diagnostic
1 Shoulder Bursa and Ligament, Right	3 Percutaneous		Z No Qualifier
2 Shoulder Bursa and Ligament, Left	4 Percutaneous Endoscopic		
3 Elbow Bursa and Ligament, Right			
4 Elbow Bursa and Ligament, Left			
5 Wrist Bursa and Ligament, Right			
6 Wrist Bursa and Ligament, Left			
7 Hand Bursa and Ligament, Right			
8 Hand Bursa and Ligament, Left			
9 Upper Extremity Bursa and Ligament, Right			
B Upper Extremity Bursa and Ligament, Left			
C Trunk Bursa and Ligament, Right			
D Trunk Bursa and Ligament, Left			
F Thorax Bursa and Ligament, Right			
G Thorax Bursa and Ligament, Left			
H Abdomen Bursa and Ligament, Right			
J Abdomen Bursa and Ligament, Left			
K Perineum Bursa and Ligament			
L Hip Bursa and Ligament, Right			
M Hip Bursa and Ligament, Left			
N Knee Bursa and Ligament, Right			
P Knee Bursa and Ligament, Left			
Q Ankle Bursa and Ligament, Right			
R Ankle Bursa and Ligament, Left			
S Foot Bursa and Ligament, Right			
T Foot Bursa and Ligament, Left			
V Lower Extremity Bursa and Ligament, Right			
W Lower Extremity Bursa and Ligament, Left			

Non-OR ØMB[Ø12345678BCDFGLMNPQRST][Ø34]ZX
Non-OR ØMB94ZX

SECTION: Ø MEDICAL AND SURGICAL
BODY SYSTEM: **M BURSAE AND LIGAMENTS**
OPERATION: **C EXTIRPATION:** Taking or cutting out solid matter from a body part

Body Part	Approach	Device	Qualifier
Ø Head and Neck Bursa and Ligament 1 Shoulder Bursa and Ligament, Right 2 Shoulder Bursa and Ligament, Left 3 Elbow Bursa and Ligament, Right 4 Elbow Bursa and Ligament, Left 5 Wrist Bursa and Ligament, Right 6 Wrist Bursa and Ligament, Left 7 Hand Bursa and Ligament, Right 8 Hand Bursa and Ligament, Left 9 Upper Extremity Bursa and Ligament, Right B Upper Extremity Bursa and Ligament, Left C Trunk Bursa and Ligament, Right D Trunk Bursa and Ligament, Left F Thorax Bursa and Ligament, Right G Thorax Bursa and Ligament, Left H Abdomen Bursa and Ligament, Right J Abdomen Bursa and Ligament, Left K Perineum Bursa and Ligament L Hip Bursa and Ligament, Right M Hip Bursa and Ligament, Left N Knee Bursa and Ligament, Right P Knee Bursa and Ligament, Left Q Ankle Bursa and Ligament, Right R Ankle Bursa and Ligament, Left S Foot Bursa and Ligament, Right T Foot Bursa and Ligament, Left V Lower Extremity Bursa and Ligament, Right W Lower Extremity Bursa and Ligament, Left	Ø Open 3 Percutaneous 4 Percutaneous Endoscopic	Z No Device	Z No Qualifier

New/Revised Text in Green ~~deleted~~ Deleted ♀ Females Only ♂ Males Only **Coding Clinic**
Non-covered Limited Coverage ⊟ Combination (See Appendix E) DRG Non-OR Non-OR Hospital-Acquired Condition

SECTION: Ø MEDICAL AND SURGICAL
BODY SYSTEM: M BURSAE AND LIGAMENTS
OPERATION: D EXTRACTION: Pulling or stripping out or off all or a portion of a body part by the use of force

Body Part	Approach	Device	Qualifier
Ø Head and Neck Bursa and Ligament 1 Shoulder Bursa and Ligament, Right 2 Shoulder Bursa and Ligament, Left 3 Elbow Bursa and Ligament, Right 4 Elbow Bursa and Ligament, Left 5 Wrist Bursa and Ligament, Right 6 Wrist Bursa and Ligament, Left 7 Hand Bursa and Ligament, Right 8 Hand Bursa and Ligament, Left 9 Upper Extremity Bursa and Ligament, Right B Upper Extremity Bursa and Ligament, Left C Trunk Bursa and Ligament, Right D Trunk Bursa and Ligament, Left F Thorax Bursa and Ligament, Right G Thorax Bursa and Ligament, Left H Abdomen Bursa and Ligament, Right J Abdomen Bursa and Ligament, Left K Perineum Bursa and Ligament L Hip Bursa and Ligament, Right M Hip Bursa and Ligament, Left N Knee Bursa and Ligament, Right P Knee Bursa and Ligament, Left Q Ankle Bursa and Ligament, Right R Ankle Bursa and Ligament, Left S Foot Bursa and Ligament, Right T Foot Bursa and Ligament, Left V Lower Extremity Bursa and Ligament, Right W Lower Extremity Bursa and Ligament, Left	Ø Open 3 Percutaneous 4 Percutaneous Endoscopic	Z No Device	Z No Qualifier

SECTION: Ø MEDICAL AND SURGICAL
BODY SYSTEM: M BURSAE AND LIGAMENTS
OPERATION: J INSPECTION: Visually and/or manually exploring a body part

Body Part	Approach	Device	Qualifier
X Upper Bursa and Ligament Y Lower Bursa and Ligament	Ø Open 3 Percutaneous 4 Percutaneous Endoscopic X External	Z No Device	Z No Qualifier

DRG Non-OR ØMJ[XY]3ZZ
Non-OR ØMJ[XY]XZZ

Ø: M/S   M: BURSAE AND LIGAMENTS   D: EXTRACTION   J: INSPECTION

SECTION: Ø MEDICAL AND SURGICAL
BODY SYSTEM: M BURSAE AND LIGAMENTS
OPERATION: M REATTACHMENT: Putting back in or on all or a portion of a separated body part to its normal location or other suitable location

Body Part	Approach	Device	Qualifier
Ø Head and Neck Bursa and Ligament	Ø Open	Z No Device	Z No Qualifier
1 Shoulder Bursa and Ligament, Right	4 Percutaneous Endoscopic		
2 Shoulder Bursa and Ligament, Left			
3 Elbow Bursa and Ligament, Right			
4 Elbow Bursa and Ligament, Left			
5 Wrist Bursa and Ligament, Right			
6 Wrist Bursa and Ligament, Left			
7 Hand Bursa and Ligament, Right			
8 Hand Bursa and Ligament, Left			
9 Upper Extremity Bursa and Ligament, Right			
B Upper Extremity Bursa and Ligament, Left			
C Trunk Bursa and Ligament, Right			
D Trunk Bursa and Ligament, Left			
F Thorax Bursa and Ligament, Right			
G Thorax Bursa and Ligament, Left			
H Abdomen Bursa and Ligament, Right			
J Abdomen Bursa and Ligament, Left			
K Perineum Bursa and Ligament			
L Hip Bursa and Ligament, Right			
M Hip Bursa and Ligament, Left			
N Knee Bursa and Ligament, Right			
P Knee Bursa and Ligament, Left			
Q Ankle Bursa and Ligament, Right			
R Ankle Bursa and Ligament, Left			
S Foot Bursa and Ligament, Right			
T Foot Bursa and Ligament, Left			
V Lower Extremity Bursa and Ligament, Right			
W Lower Extremity Bursa and Ligament, Left			

Coding Clinic: 2Ø13, Q3, P22 – ØMM14ZZ

New/Revised Text in Green   deleted Deleted   ♀ Females Only   ♂ Males Only   **Coding Clinic**
🕭 Non-covered   🕭 Limited Coverage   ⊞ Combination (See Appendix E)   DRG Non-OR   Non-OR   🕭 Hospital-Acquired Condition

M: REATTACHMENT

M: BURSAE AND LIGAMENTS

Ø: M/S

SECTION: Ø MEDICAL AND SURGICAL

BODY SYSTEM: M BURSAE AND LIGAMENTS

OPERATION: N RELEASE: Freeing a body part from an abnormal physical constraint by cutting or by the use of force

Body Part	Approach	Device	Qualifier
Ø Head and Neck Bursa and Ligament 1 Shoulder Bursa and Ligament, Right 2 Shoulder Bursa and Ligament, Left 3 Elbow Bursa and Ligament, Right 4 Elbow Bursa and Ligament, Left 5 Wrist Bursa and Ligament, Right 6 Wrist Bursa and Ligament, Left 7 Hand Bursa and Ligament, Right 8 Hand Bursa and Ligament, Left 9 Upper Extremity Bursa and Ligament, Right B Upper Extremity Bursa and Ligament, Left C Trunk Bursa and Ligament, Right D Trunk Bursa and Ligament, Left F Thorax Bursa and Ligament, Right G Thorax Bursa and Ligament, Left H Abdomen Bursa and Ligament, Right J Abdomen Bursa and Ligament, Left K Perineum Bursa and Ligament L Hip Bursa and Ligament, Right M Hip Bursa and Ligament, Left N Knee Bursa and Ligament, Right P Knee Bursa and Ligament, Left Q Ankle Bursa and Ligament, Right R Ankle Bursa and Ligament, Left S Foot Bursa and Ligament, Right T Foot Bursa and Ligament, Left V Lower Extremity Bursa and Ligament, Right W Lower Extremity Bursa and Ligament, Left	Ø Open 3 Percutaneous 4 Percutaneous Endoscopic X External	Z No Device	Z No Qualifier

SECTION: Ø MEDICAL AND SURGICAL

BODY SYSTEM: M BURSAE AND LIGAMENTS

OPERATION: P REMOVAL: Taking out or off a device from a body part

Body Part	Approach	Device	Qualifier
X Upper Bursa and Ligament Y Lower Bursa and Ligament	Ø Open 3 Percutaneous 4 Percutaneous Endoscopic	Ø Drainage Device 7 Autologous Tissue Substitute J Synthetic Substitute K Nonautologous Tissue Substitute	Z No Qualifier
X Upper Bursa and Ligament Y Lower Bursa and Ligament	X External	Ø Drainage Device	Z No Qualifier

DRG Non-OR ØMP[XY]3ØZ
Non-OR ØMP[XY]XØZ

SECTION: Ø MEDICAL AND SURGICAL

BODY SYSTEM: M BURSAE AND LIGAMENTS
OPERATION: Q REPAIR: Restoring, to the extent possible, a body part to its normal anatomic structure and function

Body Part	Approach	Device	Qualifier
Ø Head and Neck Bursa and Ligament	Ø Open	Z No Device	Z No Qualifier
1 Shoulder Bursa and Ligament, Right	3 Percutaneous		
2 Shoulder Bursa and Ligament, Left	4 Percutaneous Endoscopic		
3 Elbow Bursa and Ligament, Right			
4 Elbow Bursa and Ligament, Left			
5 Wrist Bursa and Ligament, Right			
6 Wrist Bursa and Ligament, Left			
7 Hand Bursa and Ligament, Right			
8 Hand Bursa and Ligament, Left			
9 Upper Extremity Bursa and Ligament, Right			
B Upper Extremity Bursa and Ligament, Left			
C Trunk Bursa and Ligament, Right			
D Trunk Bursa and Ligament, Left			
F Thorax Bursa and Ligament, Right			
G Thorax Bursa and Ligament, Left			
H Abdomen Bursa and Ligament, Right			
J Abdomen Bursa and Ligament, Left			
K Perineum Bursa and Ligament			
L Hip Bursa and Ligament, Right			
M Hip Bursa and Ligament, Left			
N Knee Bursa and Ligament, Right ⊞			
P Knee Bursa and Ligament, Left ⊞			
Q Ankle Bursa and Ligament, Right			
R Ankle Bursa and Ligament, Left			
S Foot Bursa and Ligament, Right ⊞			
T Foot Bursa and Ligament, Left ⊞			
V Lower Extremity Bursa and Ligament, Right			
W Lower Extremity Bursa and Ligament, Left			

⊞ ØMQ[NPST][Ø34]ZZ

SECTION: Ø MEDICAL AND SURGICAL
BODY SYSTEM: M BURSAE AND LIGAMENTS
OPERATION: S REPOSITION: Moving to its normal location, or other suitable location, all or a portion of a body part

Body Part	Approach	Device	Qualifier
Ø Head and Neck Bursa and Ligament	Ø Open	Z No Device	Z No Qualifier
1 Shoulder Bursa and Ligament, Right	4 Percutaneous Endoscopic		
2 Shoulder Bursa and Ligament, Left			
3 Elbow Bursa and Ligament, Right			
4 Elbow Bursa and Ligament, Left			
5 Wrist Bursa and Ligament, Right			
6 Wrist Bursa and Ligament, Left			
7 Hand Bursa and Ligament, Right			
8 Hand Bursa and Ligament, Left			
9 Upper Extremity Bursa and Ligament, Right			
B Upper Extremity Bursa and Ligament, Left			
C Trunk Bursa and Ligament, Right			
D Trunk Bursa and Ligament, Left			
F Thorax Bursa and Ligament, Right			
G Thorax Bursa and Ligament, Left			
H Abdomen Bursa and Ligament, Right			
J Abdomen Bursa and Ligament, Left			
K Perineum Bursa and Ligament			
L Hip Bursa and Ligament, Right			
M Hip Bursa and Ligament, Left			
N Knee Bursa and Ligament, Right			
P Knee Bursa and Ligament, Left			
Q Ankle Bursa and Ligament, Right			
R Ankle Bursa and Ligament, Left			
S Foot Bursa and Ligament, Right			
T Foot Bursa and Ligament, Left			
V Lower Extremity Bursa and Ligament, Right			
W Lower Extremity Bursa and Ligament, Left			

SECTION: Ø MEDICAL AND SURGICAL
BODY SYSTEM: M BURSAE AND LIGAMENTS
OPERATION: T RESECTION: Cutting out or off, without replacement, all of a body part

Body Part	Approach	Device	Qualifier
Ø Head and Neck Bursa and Ligament	Ø Open	Z No Device	Z No Qualifier
1 Shoulder Bursa and Ligament, Right	4 Percutaneous Endoscopic		
2 Shoulder Bursa and Ligament, Left			
3 Elbow Bursa and Ligament, Right			
4 Elbow Bursa and Ligament, Left			
5 Wrist Bursa and Ligament, Right			
6 Wrist Bursa and Ligament, Left			
7 Hand Bursa and Ligament, Right			
8 Hand Bursa and Ligament, Left			
9 Upper Extremity Bursa and Ligament, Right			
B Upper Extremity Bursa and Ligament, Left			
C Trunk Bursa and Ligament, Right			
D Trunk Bursa and Ligament, Left			
F Thorax Bursa and Ligament, Right			
G Thorax Bursa and Ligament, Left			
H Abdomen Bursa and Ligament, Right			
J Abdomen Bursa and Ligament, Left			
K Perineum Bursa and Ligament			
L Hip Bursa and Ligament, Right			
M Hip Bursa and Ligament, Left			
N Knee Bursa and Ligament, Right			
P Knee Bursa and Ligament, Left			
Q Ankle Bursa and Ligament, Right			
R Ankle Bursa and Ligament, Left			
S Foot Bursa and Ligament, Right			
T Foot Bursa and Ligament, Left			
V Lower Extremity Bursa and Ligament, Right			
W Lower Extremity Bursa and Ligament, Left			

T: RESECTION

M: BURSAE AND LIGAMENTS

Ø: M/S

New/Revised Text in Green   deleted Deleted   ♀ Females Only   ♂ Males Only   **Coding Clinic**
    Non-covered   Limited Coverage   Combination (See Appendix E)   DRG Non-OR   Non-OR   Hospital-Acquired Condition

SECTION: Ø MEDICAL AND SURGICAL
BODY SYSTEM: M BURSAE AND LIGAMENTS
OPERATION: U SUPPLEMENT: Putting in or on biological or synthetic material that physically reinforces and/or augments the function of a portion of a body part

Body Part	Approach	Device	Qualifier
Ø Head and Neck Bursa and Ligament	Ø Open	7 Autologous Tissue Substitute	Z No Qualifier
1 Shoulder Bursa and Ligament, Right	4 Percutaneous Endoscopic	J Synthetic Substitute	
2 Shoulder Bursa and Ligament, Left		K Nonautologous Tissue Substitute	
3 Elbow Bursa and Ligament, Right			
4 Elbow Bursa and Ligament, Left			
5 Wrist Bursa and Ligament, Right			
6 Wrist Bursa and Ligament, Left			
7 Hand Bursa and Ligament, Right			
8 Hand Bursa and Ligament, Left			
9 Upper Extremity Bursa and Ligament, Right			
B Upper Extremity Bursa and Ligament, Left			
C Trunk Bursa and Ligament, Right			
D Trunk Bursa and Ligament, Left			
F Thorax Bursa and Ligament, Right			
G Thorax Bursa and Ligament, Left			
H Abdomen Bursa and Ligament, Right			
J Abdomen Bursa and Ligament, Left			
K Perineum Bursa and Ligament			
L Hip Bursa and Ligament, Right			
M Hip Bursa and Ligament, Left			
N Knee Bursa and Ligament, Right			
P Knee Bursa and Ligament, Left			
Q Ankle Bursa and Ligament, Right			
R Ankle Bursa and Ligament, Left			
S Foot Bursa and Ligament, Right			
T Foot Bursa and Ligament, Left			
V Lower Extremity Bursa and Ligament, Right			
W Lower Extremity Bursa and Ligament, Left			

Ø: M/S

M: BURSAE AND LIGAMENTS

U: SUPPLEMENT

SECTION: Ø MEDICAL AND SURGICAL
BODY SYSTEM: M BURSAE AND LIGAMENTS
OPERATION: W REVISION: Correcting, to the extent possible, a portion of a malfunctioning device or the position of a displaced device

Body Part	Approach	Device	Qualifier
X Upper Bursa and Ligament Y Lower Bursa and Ligament	Ø Open 3 Percutaneous 4 Percutaneous Endoscopic X External	Ø Drainage Device 7 Autologous Tissue Substitute J Synthetic Substitute K Nonautologous Tissue Substitute	Z No Qualifier

Non-OR ØMW[XY]X[Ø7JK]Z

SECTION: Ø MEDICAL AND SURGICAL
BODY SYSTEM: M BURSAE AND LIGAMENTS
OPERATION: X TRANSFER: Moving, without taking out, all or a portion of a body part to another location to take over the function of all or a portion of a body part

Body Part	Approach	Device	Qualifier
Ø Head and Neck Bursa and Ligament 1 Shoulder Bursa and Ligament, Right 2 Shoulder Bursa and Ligament, Left 3 Elbow Bursa and Ligament, Right 4 Elbow Bursa and Ligament, Left 5 Wrist Bursa and Ligament, Right 6 Wrist Bursa and Ligament, Left 7 Hand Bursa and Ligament, Right 8 Hand Bursa and Ligament, Left 9 Upper Extremity Bursa and Ligament, Right B Upper Extremity Bursa and Ligament, Left C Trunk Bursa and Ligament, Right D Trunk Bursa and Ligament, Left F Thorax Bursa and Ligament, Right G Thorax Bursa and Ligament, Left H Abdomen Bursa and Ligament, Right J Abdomen Bursa and Ligament, Left K Perineum Bursa and Ligament L Hip Bursa and Ligament, Right M Hip Bursa and Ligament, Left N Knee Bursa and Ligament, Right P Knee Bursa and Ligament, Left Q Ankle Bursa and Ligament, Right R Ankle Bursa and Ligament, Left S Foot Bursa and Ligament, Right T Foot Bursa and Ligament, Left V Lower Extremity Bursa and Ligament, Right W Lower Extremity Bursa and Ligament, Left	Ø Open 4 Percutaneous Endoscopic	Z No Device	Z No Qualifier

SECTION: Ø MEDICAL AND SURGICAL

BODY SYSTEM: N HEAD AND FACIAL BONES

OPERATION: 2 **CHANGE:** Taking out or off a device from a body part and putting back an identical or similar device in or on the same body part without cutting or puncturing the skin or a mucous membrane

Body Part	Approach	Device	Qualifier
Ø Skull B Nasal Bone W Facial Bone	X External	Ø Drainage Device Y Other Device	Z No Qualifier

Non-OR   All Values

SECTION: Ø MEDICAL AND SURGICAL

BODY SYSTEM: N HEAD AND FACIAL BONES

OPERATION: 5 **DESTRUCTION:** Physical eradication of all or a portion of a body part by the direct use of energy, force, or a destructive agent

Body Part	Approach	Device	Qualifier
Ø Skull 1 Frontal Bone, Right 2 Frontal Bone, Left 3 Parietal Bone, Right 4 Parietal Bone, Left 5 Temporal Bone, Right 6 Temporal Bone, Left 7 Occipital Bone, Right 8 Occipital Bone, Left B Nasal Bone C Sphenoid Bone, Right D Sphenoid Bone, Left F Ethmoid Bone, Right G Ethmoid Bone, Left H Lacrimal Bone, Right J Lacrimal Bone, Left K Palatine Bone, Right L Palatine Bone, Left M Zygomatic Bone, Right N Zygomatic Bone, Left P Orbit, Right Q Orbit, Left R Maxilla, Right S Maxilla, Left T Mandible, Right V Mandible, Left X Hyoid Bone	Ø Open 3 Percutaneous 4 Percutaneous Endoscopic	Z No Device	Z No Qualifier

Side tab: 2: CHANGE   5: DESTRUCTION   N: HEAD AND FACIAL BONES   Ø: M/S

SECTION: Ø MEDICAL AND SURGICAL

BODY SYSTEM: N HEAD AND FACIAL BONES

OPERATION: 8 DIVISION: Cutting into a body part, without draining fluids and/or gases from the body part, in order to separate or transect a body part

Body Part	Approach	Device	Qualifier
Ø Skull 1 Frontal Bone, Right 2 Frontal Bone, Left 3 Parietal Bone, Right 4 Parietal Bone, Left 5 Temporal Bone, Right 6 Temporal Bone, Left 7 Occipital Bone, Right 8 Occipital Bone, Left B Nasal Bone C Sphenoid Bone, Right D Sphenoid Bone, Left F Ethmoid Bone, Right G Ethmoid Bone, Left H Lacrimal Bone, Right J Lacrimal Bone, Left K Palatine Bone, Right L Palatine Bone, Left M Zygomatic Bone, Right N Zygomatic Bone, Left P Orbit, Right Q Orbit, Left R Maxilla, Right S Maxilla, Left T Mandible, Right V Mandible, Left X Hyoid Bone	Ø Open 3 Percutaneous 4 Percutaneous Endoscopic	Z No Device	Z No Qualifier

Non-OR ØN8B[Ø34]ZZ

New/Revised Text in Green   deleted Deleted   ♀ Females Only   ♂ Males Only   **Coding Clinic**
   Non-covered   Limited Coverage   ⊞ Combination (See Appendix E)   DRG Non-OR   Non-OR   Hospital-Acquired Condition

343

SECTION: Ø MEDICAL AND SURGICAL

BODY SYSTEM: N HEAD AND FACIAL BONES

OPERATION: 9 DRAINAGE: Taking or letting out fluids and/or gases from a body part

Body Part	Approach	Device	Qualifier
Ø Skull 1 Frontal Bone, Right 2 Frontal Bone, Left 3 Parietal Bone, Right 4 Parietal Bone, Left 5 Temporal Bone, Right 6 Temporal Bone, Left 7 Occipital Bone, Right 8 Occipital Bone, Left B Nasal Bone C Sphenoid Bone, Right D Sphenoid Bone, Left F Ethmoid Bone, Right G Ethmoid Bone, Left H Lacrimal Bone, Right J Lacrimal Bone, Left K Palatine Bone, Right L Palatine Bone, Left M Zygomatic Bone, Right N Zygomatic Bone, Left P Orbit, Right Q Orbit, Left R Maxilla, Right S Maxilla, Left T Mandible, Right V Mandible, Left X Hyoid Bone	Ø Open 3 Percutaneous 4 Percutaneous Endoscopic	Ø Drainage Device	Z No Qualifier
Ø Skull 1 Frontal Bone, Right 2 Frontal Bone, Left 3 Parietal Bone, Right 4 Parietal Bone, Left 5 Temporal Bone, Right 6 Temporal Bone, Left 7 Occipital Bone, Right 8 Occipital Bone, Left B Nasal Bone C Sphenoid Bone, Right D Sphenoid Bone, Left F Ethmoid Bone, Right G Ethmoid Bone, Left H Lacrimal Bone, Right J Lacrimal Bone, Left K Palatine Bone, Right L Palatine Bone, Left M Zygomatic Bone, Right N Zygomatic Bone, Left P Orbit, Right Q Orbit, Left R Maxilla, Right S Maxilla, Left T Mandible, Right V Mandible, Left X Hyoid Bone	Ø Open 3 Percutaneous 4 Percutaneous Endoscopic	Z No Device	X Diagnostic Z No Qualifier

DRG Non-OR ØN9[Ø12345678CDFGHJKLMNPQX]3ØZ
DRG Non-OR ØN9[Ø12345678CDFGHJKLMNPQX]3ZZ

Non-OR ØN9[BRSTV][Ø34]ØZ
Non-OR ØN9B[Ø34]ZX
Non-OR ØN9[BRSTV][Ø34]ZZ

9: DRAINAGE

N: HEAD AND FACIAL BONES

Ø: M/S

New/Revised Text in Green   ~~deleted~~ Deleted   ♀ Females Only   ♂ Males Only   **Coding Clinic**

🚫 Non-covered   🚫 Limited Coverage   ⊡ Combination (See Appendix E)   DRG Non-OR   Non-OR   🚫 Hospital-Acquired Condition

SECTION: Ø MEDICAL AND SURGICAL

BODY SYSTEM: N HEAD AND FACIAL BONES

OPERATION: B EXCISION: Cutting out or off, without replacement, a portion of a body part

Body Part	Approach	Device	Qualifier
Ø Skull	Ø Open	Z No Device	X Diagnostic
1 Frontal Bone, Right	3 Percutaneous		Z No Qualifier
2 Frontal Bone, Left	4 Percutaneous Endoscopic		
3 Parietal Bone, Right			
4 Parietal Bone, Left			
5 Temporal Bone, Right			
6 Temporal Bone, Left			
7 Occipital Bone, Right			
8 Occipital Bone, Left			
B Nasal Bone			
C Sphenoid Bone, Right			
D Sphenoid Bone, Left			
F Ethmoid Bone, Right			
G Ethmoid Bone, Left			
H Lacrimal Bone, Right			
J Lacrimal Bone, Left			
K Palatine Bone, Right			
L Palatine Bone, Left			
M Zygomatic Bone, Right			
N Zygomatic Bone, Left			
P Orbit, Right ⊞			
Q Orbit, Left ⊞			
R Maxilla, Right ⊞			
S Maxilla, Left ⊞			
T Mandible, Right			
V Mandible, Left			
X Hyoid Bone			

⊞ ØNB[PQ][Ø34]ZZ
⊞ ØNB[RS][Ø4]ZZ
Non-OR ØNB[BRSTV][Ø34]ZX

Coding Clinic: 2Ø15, Q2, P13 – ØNBQØZZ

SECTION: Ø MEDICAL AND SURGICAL
BODY SYSTEM: N HEAD AND FACIAL BONES
OPERATION: C EXTIRPATION: Taking or cutting out solid matter from a body part

Body Part	Approach	Device	Qualifier
1 Frontal Bone, Right 2 Frontal Bone, Left 3 Parietal Bone, Right 4 Parietal Bone, Left 5 Temporal Bone, Right 6 Temporal Bone, Left 7 Occipital Bone, Right 8 Occipital Bone, Left B Nasal Bone C Sphenoid Bone, Right D Sphenoid Bone, Left F Ethmoid Bone, Right G Ethmoid Bone, Left H Lacrimal Bone, Right J Lacrimal Bone, Left K Palatine Bone, Right L Palatine Bone, Left M Zygomatic Bone, Right N Zygomatic Bone, Left P Orbit, Right Q Orbit, Left R Maxilla, Right S Maxilla, Left T Mandible, Right V Mandible, Left X Hyoid Bone	Ø Open 3 Percutaneous 4 Percutaneous Endoscopic	Z No Device	Z No Qualifier

Non-OR ØNC[BRSTV][Ø34]ZZ

SECTION: Ø MEDICAL AND SURGICAL

BODY SYSTEM: N HEAD AND FACIAL BONES

OPERATION: H INSERTION: Putting in a nonbiological appliance that monitors, assists, performs, or prevents a physiological function but does not physically take the place of a body part

Body Part	Approach	Device	Qualifier
Ø Skull ⊞	Ø Open	4 Internal Fixation Device 5 External Fixation Device M Bone Growth Stimulator N Neurostimulator Generator	Z No Qualifier
Ø Skull	3 Percutaneous 4 Percutaneous Endoscopic	4 Internal Fixation Device 5 External Fixation Device M Bone Growth Stimulator	Z No Qualifier
1 Frontal Bone, Right 2 Frontal Bone, Left 3 Parietal Bone, Right 4 Parietal Bone, Left 7 Occipital Bone, Right 8 Occipital Bone, Left C Sphenoid Bone, Right D Sphenoid Bone, Left F Ethmoid Bone, Right G Ethmoid Bone, Left H Lacrimal Bone, Right J Lacrimal Bone, Left K Palatine Bone, Right L Palatine Bone, Left M Zygomatic Bone, Right N Zygomatic Bone, Left P Orbit, Right Q Orbit, Left X Hyoid Bone	Ø Open 3 Percutaneous 4 Percutaneous Endoscopic	4 Internal Fixation Device	Z No Qualifier
5 Temporal Bone, Right 6 Temporal Bone, Left	Ø Open 3 Percutaneous 4 Percutaneous Endoscopic	4 Internal Fixation Device S Hearing Device	Z No Qualifier
B Nasal Bone	Ø Open 3 Percutaneous 4 Percutaneous Endoscopic	4 Internal Fixation Device M Bone Growth Stimulator	Z No Qualifier
R Maxilla, Right S Maxilla, Left T Mandible, Right V Mandible, Left	Ø Open 3 Percutaneous 4 Percutaneous Endoscopic	4 Internal Fixation Device 5 External Fixation Device	Z No Qualifier
W Facial Bone	Ø Open 3 Percutaneous 4 Percutaneous Endoscopic	M Bone Growth Stimulator	Z No Qualifier

⊞ ØNHØØNZ
Non-OR ØNHØØ5Z
Non-OR ØNHØ[34]5Z
Non-OR ØNHB[Ø34][4M]Z

Coding Clinic: 2Ø15, Q3, P14 – ØNHØØ4Z

New/Revised Text in Green   ~~deleted~~ Deleted   ♀ Females Only   ♂ Males Only   **Coding Clinic**
 Non-covered   Limited Coverage   ⊞ Combination (See Appendix E)   DRG Non-OR   Non-OR   Hospital-Acquired Condition

SECTION: Ø MEDICAL AND SURGICAL

BODY SYSTEM: N HEAD AND FACIAL BONES

OPERATION: J INSPECTION: Visually and/or manually exploring a body part

Body Part	Approach	Device	Qualifier
Ø Skull B Nasal Bone W Facial Bone	Ø Open 3 Percutaneous 4 Percutaneous Endoscopic X External	Z No Device	Z No Qualifier

DRG Non-OR   ØNJ[ØBW]3ZZ
Non-OR   ØNJ[ØBW]XZZ

SECTION: Ø MEDICAL AND SURGICAL

BODY SYSTEM: N HEAD AND FACIAL BONES

OPERATION: N RELEASE: Freeing a body part from an abnormal physical constraint by cutting or by the use of force

Body Part	Approach	Device	Qualifier
1 Frontal Bone, Right 2 Frontal Bone, Left 3 Parietal Bone, Right 4 Parietal Bone, Left 5 Temporal Bone, Right 6 Temporal Bone, Left 7 Occipital Bone, Right 8 Occipital Bone, Left B Nasal Bone C Sphenoid Bone, Right D Sphenoid Bone, Left F Ethmoid Bone, Right G Ethmoid Bone, Left H Lacrimal Bone, Right J Lacrimal Bone, Left K Palatine Bone, Right L Palatine Bone, Left M Zygomatic Bone, Right N Zygomatic Bone, Left P Orbit, Right Q Orbit, Left R Maxilla, Right S Maxilla, Left T Mandible, Right V Mandible, Left X Hyoid Bone	Ø Open 3 Percutaneous 4 Percutaneous Endoscopic	Z No Device	Z No Qualifier

Non-OR   ØNNB[Ø34]ZZ

SECTION: Ø MEDICAL AND SURGICAL
BODY SYSTEM: N HEAD AND FACIAL BONES
OPERATION: P REMOVAL: Taking out or off a device from a body part

Body Part	Approach	Device	Qualifier
Ø Skull	Ø Open	Ø Drainage Device 4 Internal Fixation Device 5 External Fixation Device 7 Autologous Tissue Substitute J Synthetic Substitute K Nonautologous Tissue Substitute M Bone Growth Stimulator N Neurostimulator Generator S Hearing Device	Z No Qualifier
Ø Skull	3 Percutaneous 4 Percutaneous Endoscopic	Ø Drainage Device 4 Internal Fixation Device 5 External Fixation Device 7 Autologous Tissue Substitute J Synthetic Substitute K Nonautologous Tissue Substitute M Bone Growth Stimulator S Hearing Device	Z No Qualifier
Ø Skull	X External	Ø Drainage Device 4 Internal Fixation Device 5 External Fixation Device M Bone Growth Stimulator S Hearing Device	Z No Qualifier
B Nasal Bone W Facial Bone	Ø Open 3 Percutaneous 4 Percutaneous Endoscopic	Ø Drainage Device 4 Internal Fixation Device 7 Autologous Tissue Substitute J Synthetic Substitute K Nonautologous Tissue Substitute M Bone Growth Stimulator	Z No Qualifier
B Nasal Bone W Facial Bone	X External	Ø Drainage Device 4 Internal Fixation Device M Bone Growth Stimulator	Z No Qualifier

Non-OR ØNPØ[34]5Z
Non-OR ØNPØX[Ø5]Z
Non-OR ØNPB[Ø34][Ø47JKM]Z
Non-OR ØNPBX[Ø4M]Z
Non-OR ØNPWX[ØM]Z

Coding Clinic: 2015, Q3, P14 – ØNPØØ4Z

SECTION: Ø MEDICAL AND SURGICAL

BODY SYSTEM: N HEAD AND FACIAL BONES

OPERATION: Q **REPAIR:** Restoring, to the extent possible, a body part to its normal anatomic structure and function

Body Part	Approach	Device	Qualifier
Ø Skull	Ø Open	Z No Device	Z No Qualifier
1 Frontal Bone, Right	3 Percutaneous		
2 Frontal Bone, Left	4 Percutaneous Endoscopic		
3 Parietal Bone, Right	X External		
4 Parietal Bone, Left			
5 Temporal Bone, Right			
6 Temporal Bone, Left			
7 Occipital Bone, Right			
8 Occipital Bone, Left			
B Nasal Bone			
C Sphenoid Bone, Right			
D Sphenoid Bone, Left			
F Ethmoid Bone, Right			
G Ethmoid Bone, Left			
H Lacrimal Bone, Right			
J Lacrimal Bone, Left			
K Palatine Bone, Right			
L Palatine Bone, Left			
M Zygomatic Bone, Right			
N Zygomatic Bone, Left			
P Orbit, Right			
Q Orbit, Left			
R Maxilla, Right			
S Maxilla, Left			
T Mandible, Right			
V Mandible, Left			
X Hyoid Bone			

Q: REPAIR

N: HEAD AND FACIAL BONES

Ø: M/S

SECTION: Ø MEDICAL AND SURGICAL

BODY SYSTEM: N HEAD AND FACIAL BONES

OPERATION: R **REPLACEMENT:** Putting in or on biological or synthetic material that physically takes the place and/or function of all or a portion of a body part

Body Part	Approach	Device	Qualifier
Ø Skull	Ø Open	7 Autologous Tissue Substitute	Z No Qualifier
1 Frontal Bone, Right	3 Percutaneous	J Synthetic Substitute	
2 Frontal Bone, Left	4 Percutaneous Endoscopic	K Nonautologous Tissue	
3 Parietal Bone, Right		Substitute	
4 Parietal Bone, Left			
5 Temporal Bone, Right			
6 Temporal Bone, Left			
7 Occipital Bone, Right			
8 Occipital Bone, Left			
B Nasal Bone			
C Sphenoid Bone, Right			
D Sphenoid Bone, Left			
F Ethmoid Bone, Right			
G Ethmoid Bone, Left			
H Lacrimal Bone, Right			
J Lacrimal Bone, Left			
K Palatine Bone, Right			
L Palatine Bone, Left			
M Zygomatic Bone, Right			
N Zygomatic Bone, Left			
P Orbit, Right			
Q Orbit, Left			
R Maxilla, Right			
S Maxilla, Left			
T Mandible, Right			
V Mandible, Left			
X Hyoid Bone			

SECTION: Ø MEDICAL AND SURGICAL

BODY SYSTEM: N HEAD AND FACIAL BONES

OPERATION: S **REPOSITION:** *(on multiple pages)*
Moving to its normal location, or other suitable location, all or a portion of a body part

Body Part	Approach	Device	Qualifier
Ø Skull	Ø Open	4 Internal Fixation Device	Z No Qualifier
R Maxilla, Right	3 Percutaneous	5 External Fixation Device	
S Maxilla, Left	4 Percutaneous Endoscopic	Z No Device	
T Mandible, Right			
V Mandible, Left			
Ø Skull	X External	Z No Device	Z No Qualifier
R Maxilla, Right			
S Maxilla, Left			
T Mandible, Right			
V Mandible, Left			

Non-OR ØNS[RSTV][34][45Z]Z
Non-OR ØNS[RSTV]XZZ

Coding Clinic: 2016, Q2, P30; 2015, Q3, P18 – ØNS00ZZ

New/Revised Text in Green ~~deleted~~ Deleted ♀ Females Only ♂ Males Only **Coding Clinic**
Non-covered Limited Coverage Combination (See Appendix E) DRG Non-OR Non-OR Hospital-Acquired Condition

351

Ø: M/S

N: HEAD AND FACIAL BONES

R: REPLACEMENT S: REPOSITION

SECTION: Ø MEDICAL AND SURGICAL
BODY SYSTEM: N HEAD AND FACIAL BONES
OPERATION: S REPOSITION: *(continued)*
Moving to its normal location, or other suitable location, all or a portion of a body part

S: REPOSITION

N: HEAD AND FACIAL BONES

Ø: M/S

Body Part	Approach	Device	Qualifier
1 Frontal Bone, Right 2 Frontal Bone, Left 3 Parietal Bone, Right 4 Parietal Bone, Left 5 Temporal Bone, Right 6 Temporal Bone, Left 7 Occipital Bone, Right 8 Occipital Bone, Left B Nasal Bone C Sphenoid Bone, Right D Sphenoid Bone, Left F Ethmoid Bone, Right G Ethmoid Bone, Left H Lacrimal Bone, Right J Lacrimal Bone, Left K Palatine Bone, Right L Palatine Bone, Left M Zygomatic Bone, Right N Zygomatic Bone, Left P Orbit, Right Q Orbit, Left X Hyoid Bone	Ø Open 3 Percutaneous 4 Percutaneous Endoscopic	4 Internal Fixation Device Z No Device	Z No Qualifier
1 Frontal Bone, Right 2 Frontal Bone, Left 3 Parietal Bone, Right 4 Parietal Bone, Left 5 Temporal Bone, Right 6 Temporal Bone, Left 7 Occipital Bone, Right 8 Occipital Bone, Left B Nasal Bone C Sphenoid Bone, Right D Sphenoid Bone, Left F Ethmoid Bone, Right G Ethmoid Bone, Left H Lacrimal Bone, Right J Lacrimal Bone, Left K Palatine Bone, Right L Palatine Bone, Left M Zygomatic Bone, Right N Zygomatic Bone, Left P Orbit, Right Q Orbit, Left X Hyoid Bone	X External	Z No Device	Z No Qualifier

Non-OR ØNS[BCDFGHJKLMNPQX][34][4Z]Z
Non-OR ØNS[BCDFGHJKLMNPQX]XZZ

Coding Clinic: 2013, Q3, P25 – ØNS005Z, ØNS104Z
Coding Clinic: 2015, Q3, P28 – ØNS504Z

New/Revised Text in Green   ~~deleted~~ Deleted   ♀ Females Only   ♂ Males Only   **Coding Clinic**
🝙 Non-covered   🝙 Limited Coverage   ⊞ Combination (See Appendix E)   DRG Non-OR   Non-OR   🝙 Hospital-Acquired Condition

SECTION: Ø MEDICAL AND SURGICAL
BODY SYSTEM: N HEAD AND FACIAL BONES
OPERATION: T RESECTION: Cutting out or off, without replacement, all of a body part

Body Part	Approach	Device	Qualifier
1 Frontal Bone, Right	Ø Open	Z No Device	Z No Qualifier
2 Frontal Bone, Left			
3 Parietal Bone, Right			
4 Parietal Bone, Left			
5 Temporal Bone, Right			
6 Temporal Bone, Left			
7 Occipital Bone, Right			
8 Occipital Bone, Left			
B Nasal Bone			
C Sphenoid Bone, Right			
D Sphenoid Bone, Left			
F Ethmoid Bone, Right			
G Ethmoid Bone, Left			
H Lacrimal Bone, Right			
J Lacrimal Bone, Left			
K Palatine Bone, Right			
L Palatine Bone, Left			
M Zygomatic Bone, Right			
N Zygomatic Bone, Left			
P Orbit, Right			
Q Orbit, Left			
R Maxilla, Right			
S Maxilla, Left			
T Mandible, Right			
V Mandible, Left			
X Hyoid Bone			

Ø: M/S

N: HEAD AND FACIAL BONES

T: RESECTION

SECTION: **Ø MEDICAL AND SURGICAL**

BODY SYSTEM: N HEAD AND FACIAL BONES

OPERATION: **U SUPPLEMENT:** Putting in or on biological or synthetic material that physically reinforces and/or augments the function of a portion of a body part

Body Part	Approach	Device	Qualifier
Ø Skull 1 Frontal Bone, Right 2 Frontal Bone, Left 3 Parietal Bone, Right 4 Parietal Bone, Left 5 Temporal Bone, Right 6 Temporal Bone, Left 7 Occipital Bone, Right 8 Occipital Bone, Left B Nasal Bone C Sphenoid Bone, Right D Sphenoid Bone, Left F Ethmoid Bone, Right G Ethmoid Bone, Left H Lacrimal Bone, Right J Lacrimal Bone, Left K Palatine Bone, Right L Palatine Bone, Left M Zygomatic Bone, Right N Zygomatic Bone, Left P Orbit, Right Q Orbit, Left R Maxilla, Right S Maxilla, Left T Mandible, Right V Mandible, Left X Hyoid Bone	Ø Open 3 Percutaneous 4 Percutaneous Endoscopic	7 Autologous Tissue Substitute J Synthetic Substitute K Nonautologous Tissue Substitute	Z No Qualifier

Coding Clinic: 2013, Q3, P25 – ØNUØØJZ

U: SUPPLEMENT   N: HEAD AND FACIAL BONES   Ø: M/S

SECTION: Ø MEDICAL AND SURGICAL
BODY SYSTEM: N HEAD AND FACIAL BONES
OPERATION: W REVISION: Correcting, to the extent possible, a portion of a malfunctioning device or the position of a displaced device

Body Part	Approach	Device	Qualifier
Ø Skull	Ø Open	Ø Drainage Device 4 Internal Fixation Device 5 External Fixation Device 7 Autologous Tissue Substitute J Synthetic Substitute K Nonautologous Tissue Substitute M Bone Growth Stimulator N Neurostimulator Generator S Hearing Device	Z No Qualifier
Ø Skull	3 Percutaneous 4 Percutaneous Endoscopic X External	Ø Drainage Device 4 Internal Fixation Device 5 External Fixation Device 7 Autologous Tissue Substitute J Synthetic Substitute K Nonautologous Tissue Substitute M Bone Growth Stimulator S Hearing Device	Z No Qualifier
B Nasal Bone W Facial Bone	Ø Open 3 Percutaneous 4 Percutaneous Endoscopic X External	Ø Drainage Device 4 Internal Fixation Device 7 Autologous Tissue Substitute J Synthetic Substitute K Nonautologous Tissue Substitute M Bone Growth Stimulator	Z No Qualifier

Non-OR ØNWØX[Ø457JKMS]Z
Non-OR ØNWB[Ø34X][Ø47JKM]Z
Non-OR ØNWWX[Ø47JKM]Z

Ø: M/S

N: HEAD AND FACIAL BONES

W: REVISION

SECTION: Ø MEDICAL AND SURGICAL
BODY SYSTEM: P UPPER BONES
OPERATION: 2 CHANGE: Taking out or off a device from a body part and putting back an identical or similar device in or on the same body part without cutting or puncturing the skin or a mucous membrane

Body Part	Approach	Device	Qualifier
Y Upper Bone	X External	Ø Drainage Device Y Other Device	Z No Qualifier

Non-OR All Values

SECTION: Ø MEDICAL AND SURGICAL
BODY SYSTEM: P UPPER BONES
OPERATION: 5 DESTRUCTION: Physical eradication of all or a portion of a body part by the direct use of energy, force, or a destructive agent

Body Part	Approach	Device	Qualifier
Ø Sternum 1 Rib, Right 2 Rib, Left 3 Cervical Vertebra 4 Thoracic Vertebra 5 Scapula, Right 6 Scapula, Left 7 Glenoid Cavity, Right 8 Glenoid Cavity, Left 9 Clavicle, Right B Clavicle, Left C Humeral Head, Right D Humeral Head, Left F Humeral Shaft, Right G Humeral Shaft, Left H Radius, Right J Radius, Left K Ulna, Right L Ulna, Left M Carpal, Right N Carpal, Left P Metacarpal, Right Q Metacarpal, Left R Thumb Phalanx, Right S Thumb Phalanx, Left T Finger Phalanx, Right V Finger Phalanx, Left	Ø Open 3 Percutaneous 4 Percutaneous Endoscopic	Z No Device	Z No Qualifier

SECTION: Ø MEDICAL AND SURGICAL
BODY SYSTEM: P UPPER BONES
OPERATION: 8 DIVISION: Cutting into a body part, without draining fluids and/or gases from the body part, in order to separate or transect a body part

Body Part	Approach	Device	Qualifier
Ø Sternum	Ø Open	Z No Device	Z No Qualifier
1 Rib, Right	3 Percutaneous		
2 Rib, Left	4 Percutaneous Endoscopic		
3 Cervical Vertebra			
4 Thoracic Vertebra			
5 Scapula, Right			
6 Scapula, Left			
7 Glenoid Cavity, Right			
8 Glenoid Cavity, Left			
9 Clavicle, Right			
B Clavicle, Left			
C Humeral Head, Right			
D Humeral Head, Left			
F Humeral Shaft, Right ⊞			
G Humeral Shaft, Left ⊞			
H Radius, Right ⊞			
J Radius, Left ⊞			
K Ulna, Right ⊞			
L Ulna, Left ⊞			
M Carpal, Right ⊞			
N Carpal, Left ⊞			
P Metacarpal, Right ⊞			
Q Metacarpal, Left ⊞			
R Thumb Phalanx, Right			
S Thumb Phalanx, Left			
T Finger Phalanx, Right ⊞			
V Finger Phalanx, Left ⊞			

⊞ ØP8[FGHJKLMNPQTV][Ø34]ZZ

8: DIVISION

P: UPPER BONES

Ø: M/S

SECTION: Ø MEDICAL AND SURGICAL
BODY SYSTEM: P UPPER BONES
OPERATION: 9 DRAINAGE: Taking or letting out fluids and/or gases from a body part

Body Part	Approach	Device	Qualifier
Ø Sternum 1 Rib, Right 2 Rib, Left 3 Cervical Vertebra 4 Thoracic Vertebra 5 Scapula, Right 6 Scapula, Left 7 Glenoid Cavity, Right 8 Glenoid Cavity, Left 9 Clavicle, Right B Clavicle, Left C Humeral Head, Right D Humeral Head, Left F Humeral Shaft, Right G Humeral Shaft, Left H Radius, Right J Radius, Left K Ulna, Right L Ulna, Left M Carpal, Right N Carpal, Left P Metacarpal, Right Q Metacarpal, Left R Thumb Phalanx, Right S Thumb Phalanx, Left T Finger Phalanx, Right V Finger Phalanx, Left	Ø Open 3 Percutaneous 4 Percutaneous Endoscopic	Ø Drainage Device	Z No Qualifier
Ø Sternum 1 Rib, Right 2 Rib, Left 3 Cervical Vertebra 4 Thoracic Vertebra 5 Scapula, Right 6 Scapula, Left 7 Glenoid Cavity, Right 8 Glenoid Cavity, Left 9 Clavicle, Right B Clavicle, Left C Humeral Head, Right D Humeral Head, Left F Humeral Shaft, Right G Humeral Shaft, Left H Radius, Right J Radius, Left K Ulna, Right L Ulna, Left M Carpal, Right N Carpal, Left P Metacarpal, Right Q Metacarpal, Left R Thumb Phalanx, Right S Thumb Phalanx, Left T Finger Phalanx, Right V Finger Phalanx, Left	Ø Open 3 Percutaneous 4 Percutaneous Endoscopic	Z No Device	X Diagnostic Z No Qualifier

Ø: M/S

P: UPPER BONES

9: DRAINAGE

DRG Non-OR ØP9[Ø123456789BCDFGHJKLMNPQRSTV]3ØZ
DRG Non-OR ØP9[Ø123456789BCDFGHJKLMNPQRSTV]3ZZ

New/Revised Text in Green   deleted Deleted   ♀ Females Only   ♂ Males Only   Coding Clinic
🚫 Non-covered   🚫 Limited Coverage   ⊞ Combination (See Appendix E)   DRG Non-OR   Non-OR   🚫 Hospital-Acquired Condition

359

SECTION: Ø MEDICAL AND SURGICAL
BODY SYSTEM: P UPPER BONES
OPERATION: B EXCISION: Cutting out or off, without replacement, a portion of a body part

Body Part	Approach	Device	Qualifier
Ø Sternum	Ø Open	Z No Device	X Diagnostic
1 Rib, Right ⊞	3 Percutaneous		Z No Qualifier
2 Rib, Left ⊞	4 Percutaneous Endoscopic		
3 Cervical Vertebra			
4 Thoracic Vertebra			
5 Scapula, Right			
6 Scapula, Left			
7 Glenoid Cavity, Right			
8 Glenoid Cavity, Left			
9 Clavicle, Right			
B Clavicle, Left			
C Humeral Head, Right			
D Humeral Head, Left			
F Humeral Shaft, Right			
G Humeral Shaft, Left			
H Radius, Right			
J Radius, Left			
K Ulna, Right			
L Ulna, Left			
M Carpal, Right			
N Carpal, Left			
P Metacarpal, Right			
Q Metacarpal, Left			
R Thumb Phalanx, Right			
S Thumb Phalanx, Left			
T Finger Phalanx, Right			
V Finger Phalanx, Left			

⊞ ØPB[12]ØZZ

Coding Clinic: 2012, Q4, P101 – ØPB1ØZZ
Coding Clinic: 2013, Q3, P22 – ØPB54ZZ

B: EXCISION

P: UPPER BONES

Ø: M/S

SECTION: 0 MEDICAL AND SURGICAL
BODY SYSTEM: P UPPER BONES
OPERATION: C EXTIRPATION: Taking or cutting out solid matter from a body part

Body Part	Approach	Device	Qualifier
0 Sternum	0 Open	Z No Device	Z No Qualifier
1 Rib, Right	3 Percutaneous		
2 Rib, Left	4 Percutaneous Endoscopic		
3 Cervical Vertebra			
4 Thoracic Vertebra			
5 Scapula, Right			
6 Scapula, Left			
7 Glenoid Cavity, Right			
8 Glenoid Cavity, Left			
9 Clavicle, Right			
B Clavicle, Left			
C Humeral Head, Right			
D Humeral Head, Left			
F Humeral Shaft, Right			
G Humeral Shaft, Left			
H Radius, Right			
J Radius, Left			
K Ulna, Right			
L Ulna, Left			
M Carpal, Right			
N Carpal, Left			
P Metacarpal, Right			
Q Metacarpal, Left			
R Thumb Phalanx, Right			
S Thumb Phalanx, Left			
T Finger Phalanx, Right			
V Finger Phalanx, Left			

0: M/S

P: UPPER BONES

C: EXTIRPATION

New/Revised Text in Green   deleted Deleted   ♀ Females Only   ♂ Males Only   **Coding Clinic**
🚫 Non-covered   🚫 Limited Coverage   ⊞ Combination (See Appendix E)   DRG Non-OR   Non-OR   🚫 Hospital-Acquired Condition

361

SECTION: Ø MEDICAL AND SURGICAL
BODY SYSTEM: P UPPER BONES
OPERATION: H INSERTION: Putting in a nonbiological appliance that monitors, assists, performs, or prevents a physiological function but does not physically take the place of a body part

Body Part	Approach	Device	Qualifier
Ø Sternum	Ø Open 3 Percutaneous 4 Percutaneous Endoscopic	Ø Internal Fixation Device, Rigid Plate 4 Internal Fixation Device	Z No Qualifier
1 Rib, Right 2 Rib, Left 3 Cervical Vertebra 4 Thoracic Vertebra 5 Scapula, Right 6 Scapula, Left 7 Glenoid Cavity, Right 8 Glenoid Cavity, Left 9 Clavicle, Right B Clavicle, Left	Ø Open 3 Percutaneous 4 Percutaneous Endoscopic	4 Internal Fixation Device	Z No Qualifier
C Humeral Head, Right D Humeral Head, Left F Humeral Shaft, Right G Humeral Shaft, Left H Radius, Right J Radius, Left K Ulna, Right L Ulna, Left	Ø Open 3 Percutaneous 4 Percutaneous Endoscopic	4 Internal Fixation Device 5 External Fixation Device 6 Internal Fixation Device, Intramedullary 8 External Fixation Device, Limb Lengthening B External Fixation Device, Monoplanar C External Fixation Device, Ring D External Fixation Device, Hybrid	Z No Qualifier
M Carpal, Right N Carpal, Left P Metacarpal, Right Q Metacarpal, Left R Thumb Phalanx, Right S Thumb Phalanx, Left T Finger Phalanx, Right V Finger Phalanx, Left	Ø Open 3 Percutaneous 4 Percutaneous Endoscopic	4 Internal Fixation Device 5 External Fixation Device	Z No Qualifier
Y Upper Bone	Ø Open 3 Percutaneous 4 Percutaneous Endoscopic	M Bone Growth Stimulator	Z No Qualifier
Y Upper Bone	Ø Open 3 Percutaneous 4 Percutaneous Endoscopic X External	Z No Device	Z No Qualifier

Non-OR ØPH[CDFGHJKL][Ø34]8Z

H: INSERTION
P: UPPER BONES
Ø: M/S

New/Revised Text in Green ~~deleted~~ Deleted ♀ Females Only ♂ Males Only **Coding Clinic**
Non-covered Limited Coverage Combination (See Appendix E) DRG Non-OR Non-OR Hospital-Acquired Condition

SECTION: Ø MEDICAL AND SURGICAL
BODY SYSTEM: P UPPER BONES
OPERATION: J INSPECTION: Visually and/or manually exploring a body part

Body Part	Approach	Device	Qualifier
Y Upper Bone	Ø Open 3 Percutaneous 4 Percutaneous Endoscopic X External	Z No Device	Z No Qualifier

DRG Non-OR ØPJY3ZZ
Non-OR ØPJYXZZ

SECTION: Ø MEDICAL AND SURGICAL
BODY SYSTEM: P UPPER BONES
OPERATION: N RELEASE: Freeing a body part from an abnormal physical constraint by cutting or by the use of force

Body Part	Approach	Device	Qualifier
Ø Sternum 1 Rib, Right 2 Rib, Left 3 Cervical Vertebra 4 Thoracic Vertebra 5 Scapula, Right 6 Scapula, Left 7 Glenoid Cavity, Right 8 Glenoid Cavity, Left 9 Clavicle, Right B Clavicle, Left C Humeral Head, Right D Humeral Head, Left F Humeral Shaft, Right G Humeral Shaft, Left H Radius, Right J Radius, Left K Ulna, Right L Ulna, Left M Carpal, Right N Carpal, Left P Metacarpal, Right Q Metacarpal, Left R Thumb Phalanx, Right S Thumb Phalanx, Left T Finger Phalanx, Right V Finger Phalanx, Left	Ø Open 3 Percutaneous 4 Percutaneous Endoscopic	Z No Device	Z No Qualifier

Ø: M/S
P: UPPER BONES
J: INSPECTION   N: RELEASE

SECTION: Ø MEDICAL AND SURGICAL
BODY SYSTEM: P UPPER BONES
OPERATION: P REMOVAL: *(on multiple pages)*

Taking out or off a device from a body part

Body Part	Approach	Device	Qualifier
Ø Sternum 1 Rib, Right 2 Rib, Left 3 Cervical Vertebra 4 Thoracic Vertebra 5 Scapula, Right 6 Scapula, Left 7 Glenoid Cavity, Right 8 Glenoid Cavity, Left 9 Clavicle, Right B Clavicle, Left	Ø Open 3 Percutaneous 4 Percutaneous Endoscopic	4 Internal Fixation Device 7 Autologous Tissue Substitute J Synthetic Substitute K Nonautologous Tissue Substitute	Z No Qualifier
Ø Sternum 1 Rib, Right 2 Rib, Left 3 Cervical Vertebra 4 Thoracic Vertebra 5 Scapula, Right 6 Scapula, Left 7 Glenoid Cavity, Right 8 Glenoid Cavity, Left 9 Clavicle, Right B Clavicle, Left	X External	4 Internal Fixation Device	Z No Qualifier
C Humeral Head, Right D Humeral Head, Left F Humeral Shaft, Right G Humeral Shaft, Left H Radius, Right J Radius, Left K Ulna, Right L Ulna, Left M Carpal, Right N Carpal, Left P Metacarpal, Right Q Metacarpal, Left R Thumb Phalanx, Right S Thumb Phalanx, Left T Finger Phalanx, Right V Finger Phalanx, Left	Ø Open 3 Percutaneous 4 Percutaneous Endoscopic	4 Internal Fixation Device 5 External Fixation Device 7 Autologous Tissue Substitute J Synthetic Substitute K Nonautologous Tissue Substitute	Z No Qualifier

Non-OR ØPP[Ø123456789B]X4Z

SECTION: Ø MEDICAL AND SURGICAL
BODY SYSTEM: P UPPER BONES
OPERATION: P REMOVAL: *(continued)*
Taking out or off a device from a body part

Body Part	Approach	Device	Qualifier
C Humeral Head, Right D Humeral Head, Left F Humeral Shaft, Right G Humeral Shaft, Left H Radius, Right J Radius, Left K Ulna, Right L Ulna, Left M Carpal, Right N Carpal, Left P Metacarpal, Right Q Metacarpal, Left R Thumb Phalanx, Right S Thumb Phalanx, Left T Finger Phalanx, Right V Finger Phalanx, Left	X External	4 Internal Fixation Device 5 External Fixation Device	Z No Qualifier
Y Upper Bone	Ø Open 3 Percutaneous 4 Percutaneous Endoscopic X External	Ø Drainage Device M Bone Growth Stimulator	Z No Qualifier

DRG Non-OR ØPPY3ØZ
Non-OR ØPP[CDFGHJKLMNPQRSTV]X[45]Z
Non-OR ØPPYX[ØM]Z

SECTION: Ø MEDICAL AND SURGICAL

BODY SYSTEM: P UPPER BONES

OPERATION: Q **REPAIR:** Restoring, to the extent possible, a body part to its normal anatomic structure and function

Body Part	Approach	Device	Qualifier
Ø Sternum	Ø Open	Z No Device	Z No Qualifier
1 Rib, Right	3 Percutaneous		
2 Rib, Left	4 Percutaneous Endoscopic		
3 Cervical Vertebra	X External		
4 Thoracic Vertebra			
5 Scapula, Right			
6 Scapula, Left			
7 Glenoid Cavity, Right			
8 Glenoid Cavity, Left			
9 Clavicle, Right			
B Clavicle, Left			
C Humeral Head, Right			
D Humeral Head, Left			
F Humeral Shaft, Right			
G Humeral Shaft, Left			
H Radius, Right			
J Radius, Left			
K Ulna, Right			
L Ulna, Left			
M Carpal, Right			
N Carpal, Left			
P Metacarpal, Right			
Q Metacarpal, Left			
R Thumb Phalanx, Right			
S Thumb Phalanx, Left			
T Finger Phalanx, Right			
V Finger Phalanx, Left			

Q: REPAIR

P: UPPER BONES

Ø: M/S

New/Revised Text in Green   ~~deleted~~ Deleted   ♀ Females Only   ♂ Males Only   **Coding Clinic**

Non-covered   Limited Coverage   Combination (See Appendix E)   DRG Non-OR   Non-OR   Hospital-Acquired Condition

SECTION: Ø MEDICAL AND SURGICAL
BODY SYSTEM: P UPPER BONES
OPERATION: R **REPLACEMENT:** Putting in or on biological or synthetic material that physically takes the place and/or function of all or a portion of a body part

Body Part	Approach	Device	Qualifier
Ø Sternum 1 Rib, Right 2 Rib, Left 3 Cervical Vertebra 4 Thoracic Vertebra 5 Scapula, Right 6 Scapula, Left 7 Glenoid Cavity, Right 8 Glenoid Cavity, Left 9 Clavicle, Right B Clavicle, Left C Humeral Head, Right D Humeral Head, Left F Humeral Shaft, Right G Humeral Shaft, Left H Radius, Right J Radius, Left K Ulna, Right L Ulna, Left M Carpal, Right N Carpal, Left P Metacarpal, Right Q Metacarpal, Left R Thumb Phalanx, Right S Thumb Phalanx, Left T Finger Phalanx, Right V Finger Phalanx, Left	Ø Open 3 Percutaneous 4 Percutaneous Endoscopic	7 Autologous Tissue Substitute J Synthetic Substitute K Nonautologous Tissue Substitute	Z No Qualifier

Non-OR ØPR[CD]ØJZ

SECTION: Ø MEDICAL AND SURGICAL
BODY SYSTEM: P UPPER BONES
OPERATION: S **REPOSITION:** *(on multiple pages)*
                     Moving to its normal location, or other suitable location, all or a portion of a body part

Body Part	Approach	Device	Qualifier
Ø Sternum	Ø Open 3 Percutaneous 4 Percutaneous Endoscopic	Ø Internal Fixation Device, Rigid Plate 4 Internal Fixation Device Z No Device	Z No Qualifier
Ø Sternum	X External	Z No Device	Z No Qualifier
1 Rib, Right 2 Rib, Left 3 Cervical Vertebra ⊞ 4 Thoracic Vertebra ⊞ 5 Scapula, Right 6 Scapula, Left 7 Glenoid Cavity, Right 8 Glenoid Cavity, Left 9 Clavicle, Right B Clavicle, Left	Ø Open 3 Percutaneous 4 Percutaneous Endoscopic	4 Internal Fixation Device Z No Device	Z No Qualifier

⊞ ØPS3[34]ZZ

Non-OR ØPSØ[34]ZZ

Non-OR ØPSØXZZ

Non-OR ØPS[1256789B][34]ZZ

Coding Clinic: 2Ø15, Q4, P34 − ØPSØØZZ
Coding Clinic: 2Ø16, Q1, P21 − ØPS4XZZ

 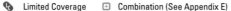
Ø: M/S
P: UPPER BONES
R: REPLACEMENT   S: REPOSITION

SECTION: Ø MEDICAL AND SURGICAL
BODY SYSTEM: P UPPER BONES
OPERATION: S REPOSITION: *(continued)*
Moving to its normal location, or other suitable location, all or a portion of a body part

Body Part	Approach	Device	Qualifier
1 Rib, Right 2 Rib, Left 3 Cervical Vertebra 4 Thoracic Vertebra 5 Scapula, Right 6 Scapula, Left 7 Glenoid Cavity, Right 8 Glenoid Cavity, Left 9 Clavicle, Right B Clavicle, Left	X External	Z No Device	Z No Qualifier
C Humeral Head, Right D Humeral Head, Left F Humeral Shaft, Right G Humeral Shaft, Left H Radius, Right J Radius, Left K Ulna, Right L Ulna, Left	Ø Open 3 Percutaneous 4 Percutaneous Endoscopic	4 Internal Fixation Device 5 External Fixation Device 6 Internal Fixation Device, Intramedullary B External Fixation Device, Monoplanar C External Fixation Device, Ring D External Fixation Device, Hybrid Z No Device	Z No Qualifier
C Humeral Head, Right D Humeral Head, Left F Humeral Shaft, Right G Humeral Shaft, Left H Radius, Right J Radius, Left K Ulna, Right L Ulna, Left	X External	Z No Device	Z No Qualifier
M Carpal, Right N Carpal, Left P Metacarpal, Right Q Metacarpal, Left R Thumb Phalanx, Right S Thumb Phalanx, Left T Finger Phalanx, Right V Finger Phalanx, Left	Ø Open 3 Percutaneous 4 Percutaneous Endoscopic	4 Internal Fixation Device 5 External Fixation Device Z No Device	Z No Qualifier
M Carpal, Right N Carpal, Left P Metacarpal, Right Q Metacarpal, Left R Thumb Phalanx, Right S Thumb Phalanx, Left T Finger Phalanx, Right V Finger Phalanx, Left	X External	Z No Device	Z No Qualifier

Non-OR ØPS[1256789B]XZZ
Non-OR ØPS[CDFGHJKL][34]ZZ
Non-OR ØPS[CDFGHJKL]XZZ
Non-OR ØPS[MNPQRSTV][34]ZZ
Non-OR ØPS[MNPQRSTV]XZZ

Coding Clinic: 2015, Q2, P35 – ØPS3XZZ

New/Revised Text in Green   ~~deleted~~ Deleted   ♀ Females Only   ♂ Males Only   **Coding Clinic**
🗞 Non-covered   🗞 Limited Coverage   ⊞ Combination (See Appendix E)   DRG Non-OR   Non-OR   🗞 Hospital-Acquired Condition

SECTION: Ø MEDICAL AND SURGICAL
BODY SYSTEM: P UPPER BONES
OPERATION: T RESECTION: Cutting out or off, without replacement, all of a body part

Body Part	Approach	Device	Qualifier
Ø Sternum	Ø Open	Z No Device	Z No Qualifier
1 Rib, Right			
2 Rib, Left			
5 Scapula, Right			
6 Scapula, Left			
7 Glenoid Cavity, Right			
8 Glenoid Cavity, Left			
9 Clavicle, Right			
B Clavicle, Left			
C Humeral Head, Right ⊞			
D Humeral Head, Left ⊞			
F Humeral Shaft, Right ⊞			
G Humeral Shaft, Left ⊞			
H Radius, Right			
J Radius, Left			
K Ulna, Right			
L Ulna, Left			
M Carpal, Right			
N Carpal, Left			
P Metacarpal, Right			
Q Metacarpal, Left			
R Thumb Phalanx, Right			
S Thumb Phalanx, Left			
T Finger Phalanx, Right			
V Finger Phalanx, Left			

⊞ ØPT[CDFG]ØZZ

Coding Clinic: 2015, Q3, P27 – ØPTNØZZ

New/Revised Text in Green   ~~deleted~~ Deleted   ♀ Females Only   ♂ Males Only   **Coding Clinic**
⊘ Non-covered   ⊘ Limited Coverage   ⊞ Combination (See Appendix E)   DRG Non-OR   Non-OR   ⊘ Hospital-Acquired Condition

369

SECTION: Ø   MEDICAL AND SURGICAL
BODY SYSTEM: P   UPPER BONES
OPERATION: U   **SUPPLEMENT:** Putting in or on biological or synthetic material that physically reinforces and/or augments the function of a portion of a body part

Body Part	Approach	Device	Qualifier
Ø Sternum	Ø Open	7 Autologous Tissue Substitute	Z No Qualifier
1 Rib, Right	3 Percutaneous	J Synthetic Substitute	
2 Rib, Left	4 Percutaneous Endoscopic	K Nonautologous Tissue	
3 Cervical Vertebra ⊞		Substitute	
4 Thoracic Vertebra ⊞			
5 Scapula, Right			
6 Scapula, Left			
7 Glenoid Cavity, Right			
8 Glenoid Cavity, Left			
9 Clavicle, Right			
B Clavicle, Left			
C Humeral Head, Right			
D Humeral Head, Left			
F Humeral Shaft, Right ⊞			
G Humeral Shaft, Left ⊞			
H Radius, Right ⊞			
J Radius, Left ⊞			
K Ulna, Right ⊞			
L Ulna, Left ⊞			
M Carpal, Right ⊞			
N Carpal, Left ⊞			
P Metacarpal, Right ⊞			
Q Metacarpal, Left ⊞			
R Thumb Phalanx, Right			
S Thumb Phalanx, Left			
T Finger Phalanx, Right ⊞			
V Finger Phalanx, Left ⊞			

⊞ ØPU[34]3JZ
⊞ ØPU[FGHJKLMNPQTV][Ø34][7K]Z

Coding Clinic: 2Ø15, Q2, P2Ø – ØPU3ØKZ

New/Revised Text in Green   ~~deleted~~ Deleted   ♀ Females Only   ♂ Males Only   **Coding Clinic**
🔖 Non-covered   🔖 Limited Coverage   ⊞ Combination (See Appendix E)   DRG Non-OR   Non-OR   🔖 Hospital-Acquired Condition

SECTION: 0 MEDICAL AND SURGICAL
BODY SYSTEM: P UPPER BONES
OPERATION: W REVISION: Correcting, to the extent possible, a portion of a malfunctioning device or the position of a displaced device

Body Part	Approach	Device	Qualifier
0 Sternum 1 Rib, Right 2 Rib, Left 3 Cervical Vertebra 4 Thoracic Vertebra 5 Scapula, Right 6 Scapula, Left 7 Glenoid Cavity, Right 8 Glenoid Cavity, Left 9 Clavicle, Right B Clavicle, Left	0 Open 3 Percutaneous 4 Percutaneous Endoscopic X External	4 Internal Fixation Device 7 Autologous Tissue Substitute J Synthetic Substitute K Nonautologous Tissue Substitute	Z No Qualifier
C Humeral Head, Right D Humeral Head, Left F Humeral Shaft, Right G Humeral Shaft, Left H Radius, Right J Radius, Left K Ulna, Right L Ulna, Left M Carpal, Right N Carpal, Left P Metacarpal, Right Q Metacarpal, Left R Thumb Phalanx, Right S Thumb Phalanx, Left T Finger Phalanx, Right V Finger Phalanx, Left	0 Open 3 Percutaneous 4 Percutaneous Endoscopic X External	4 Internal Fixation Device 5 External Fixation Device 7 Autologous Tissue Substitute J Synthetic Substitute K Nonautologous Tissue Substitute	Z No Qualifier
Y Upper Bone	0 Open 3 Percutaneous 4 Percutaneous Endoscopic X External	0 Drainage Device M Bone Growth Stimulator	Z No Qualifier

Non-OR 0PW[0123456789B]X[47JK]Z
Non-OR 0PW[CDFGHJKLMNPQRSTV]X[457JK]Z
Non-OR 0PWYX[0M]Z

New/Revised Text in Green   deleted Deleted   ♀ Females Only   ♂ Males Only   **Coding Clinic**
 Non-covered   Limited Coverage   Combination (See Appendix E)   DRG Non-OR   Non-OR   Hospital-Acquired Condition

SECTION: ❾ MEDICAL AND SURGICAL

BODY SYSTEM: Q LOWER BONES

OPERATION: 2 **CHANGE:** Taking out or off a device from a body part and putting back an identical or similar device in or on the same body part without cutting or puncturing the skin or a mucous membrane

Body Part	Approach	Device	Qualifier
Y Lower Bone	X External	❾ Drainage Device Y Other Device	Z No Qualifier

Non-OR All Values

SECTION: ❾ MEDICAL AND SURGICAL

BODY SYSTEM: Q LOWER BONES

OPERATION: 5 **DESTRUCTION:** Physical eradication of all or a portion of a body part by the direct use of energy, force, or a destructive agent

Body Part	Approach	Device	Qualifier
❾ Lumbar Vertebra 1 Sacrum 2 Pelvic Bone, Right 3 Pelvic Bone, Left 4 Acetabulum, Right 5 Acetabulum, Left 6 Upper Femur, Right 7 Upper Femur, Left 8 Femoral Shaft, Right 9 Femoral Shaft, Left B Lower Femur, Right C Lower Femur, Left D Patella, Right F Patella, Left G Tibia, Right H Tibia, Left J Fibula, Right K Fibula, Left L Tarsal, Right M Tarsal, Left N Metatarsal, Right P Metatarsal, Left Q Toe Phalanx, Right R Toe Phalanx, Left S Coccyx	❾ Open 3 Percutaneous 4 Percutaneous Endoscopic	Z No Device	Z No Qualifier

New/Revised Text in Green　　~~deleted~~ Deleted　　♀ Females Only　　♂ Males Only　　**Coding Clinic**

🐾 Non-covered　　🐾 Limited Coverage　　⊡ Combination (See Appendix E)　　DRG Non-OR　　Non-OR　　🐾 Hospital-Acquired Condition

❾: M/S

Q: LOWER BONES

2: CHANGE   5: DESTRUCTION

SECTION: Ø MEDICAL AND SURGICAL

BODY SYSTEM: Q LOWER BONES

OPERATION: 8 DIVISION: Cutting into a body part, without draining fluids and/or gases from the body part, in order to separate or transect a body part

Body Part	Approach	Device	Qualifier
Ø Lumbar Vertebra	Ø Open	Z No Device	Z No Qualifier
1 Sacrum	3 Percutaneous		
2 Pelvic Bone, Right	4 Percutaneous Endoscopic		
3 Pelvic Bone, Left			
4 Acetabulum, Right			
5 Acetabulum, Left			
6 Upper Femur, Right			
7 Upper Femur, Left			
8 Femoral Shaft, Right ⊞			
9 Femoral Shaft, Left ⊞			
B Lower Femur, Right			
C Lower Femur, Left			
D Patella, Right			
F Patella, Left			
G Tibia, Right ⊞			
H Tibia, Left ⊞			
J Fibula, Right ⊞			
K Fibula, Left ⊞			
L Tarsal, Right ⊞			
M Tarsal, Left ⊞			
N Metatarsal, Right ⊞			
P Metatarsal, Left ⊞			
Q Toe Phalanx, Right ⊞			
R Toe Phalanx, Left ⊞			
S Coccyx			

⊞ 0Q8[89GHJKLMNPQR][Ø34]ZZ

Coding Clinic: 2Ø16, Q2, P32 – ØQ83ØZZ

8: DIVISION   Q: LOWER BONES   Ø: M/S

SECTION: Ø MEDICAL AND SURGICAL

BODY SYSTEM: Q LOWER BONES

OPERATION: 9 DRAINAGE: Taking or letting out fluids and/or gases from a body part

Body Part	Approach	Device	Qualifier
Ø Lumbar Vertebra 1 Sacrum 2 Pelvic Bone, Right 3 Pelvic Bone, Left 4 Acetabulum, Right 5 Acetabulum, Left 6 Upper Femur, Right 7 Upper Femur, Left 8 Femoral Shaft, Right 9 Femoral Shaft, Left B Lower Femur, Right C Lower Femur, Left D Patella, Right F Patella, Left G Tibia, Right H Tibia, Left J Fibula, Right K Fibula, Left L Tarsal, Right M Tarsal, Left N Metatarsal, Right P Metatarsal, Left Q Toe Phalanx, Right R Toe Phalanx, Left S Coccyx	Ø Open 3 Percutaneous 4 Percutaneous Endoscopic	Ø Drainage Device	Z No Qualifier
Ø Lumbar Vertebra 1 Sacrum 2 Pelvic Bone, Right 3 Pelvic Bone, Left 4 Acetabulum, Right 5 Acetabulum, Left 6 Upper Femur, Right 7 Upper Femur, Left 8 Femoral Shaft, Right 9 Femoral Shaft, Left B Lower Femur, Right C Lower Femur, Left D Patella, Right F Patella, Left G Tibia, Right H Tibia, Left J Fibula, Right K Fibula, Left L Tarsal, Right M Tarsal, Left N Metatarsal, Right P Metatarsal, Left Q Toe Phalanx, Right R Toe Phalanx, Left S Coccyx	Ø Open 3 Percutaneous 4 Percutaneous Endoscopic	Z No Device	X Diagnostic Z No Qualifier

DRG Non-OR ØQ9[Ø123456789BCDFGHJKLMNPQRS]3ØZ
DRG Non-OR ØQ9[Ø123456789BCDFGHJKLMNPQRS]3ZZ

Ø: M/S

Q: LOWER BONES

9: DRAINAGE

SECTION: Ø MEDICAL AND SURGICAL
BODY SYSTEM: Q LOWER BONES
OPERATION: B EXCISION: Cutting out or off, without replacement, a portion of a body part

Body Part	Approach	Device	Qualifier
Ø Lumbar Vertebra 1 Sacrum 2 Pelvic Bone, Right 3 Pelvic Bone, Left 4 Acetabulum, Right 5 Acetabulum, Left 6 Upper Femur, Right 7 Upper Femur, Left 8 Femoral Shaft, Right 9 Femoral Shaft, Left B Lower Femur, Right C Lower Femur, Left D Patella, Right F Patella, Left G Tibia, Right H Tibia, Left J Fibula, Right K Fibula, Left L Tarsal, Right M Tarsal, Left N Metatarsal, Right ⊞ P Metatarsal, Left ⊞ Q Toe Phalanx, Right R Toe Phalanx, Left S Coccyx	Ø Open 3 Percutaneous 4 Percutaneous Endoscopic	Z No Device	X Diagnostic Z No Qualifier

⊞ ØQB[NP][Ø34]ZZ

Coding Clinic: 2Ø13, Q2, P4Ø – ØQBKØZZ
Coding Clinic: 2Ø15, Q3, P4 – ØQBSØZZ

SECTION: Ø MEDICAL AND SURGICAL

BODY SYSTEM: Q LOWER BONES

OPERATION: C EXTIRPATION: Taking or cutting out solid matter from a body part

Body Part	Approach	Device	Qualifier
Ø Lumbar Vertebra	Ø Open	Z No Device	Z No Qualifier
1 Sacrum	3 Percutaneous		
2 Pelvic Bone, Right	4 Percutaneous Endoscopic		
3 Pelvic Bone, Left			
4 Acetabulum, Right			
5 Acetabulum, Left			
6 Upper Femur, Right			
7 Upper Femur, Left			
8 Femoral Shaft, Right			
9 Femoral Shaft, Left			
B Lower Femur, Right			
C Lower Femur, Left			
D Patella, Right			
F Patella, Left			
G Tibia, Right			
H Tibia, Left			
J Fibula, Right			
K Fibula, Left			
L Tarsal, Right			
M Tarsal, Left			
N Metatarsal, Right			
P Metatarsal, Left			
Q Toe Phalanx, Right			
R Toe Phalanx, Left			
S Coccyx			

Ø: M/S

Q: LOWER BONES

C: EXTIRPATION

SECTION: Ø MEDICAL AND SURGICAL

BODY SYSTEM: Q LOWER BONES

OPERATION: H **INSERTION:** Putting in a nonbiological appliance that monitors, assists, performs, or prevents a physiological function but does not physically take the place of a body part

Body Part	Approach	Device	Qualifier
Ø Lumbar Vertebra 1 Sacrum 2 Pelvic Bone, Right 3 Pelvic Bone, Left 4 Acetabulum, Right 5 Acetabulum, Left D Patella, Right F Patella, Left L Tarsal, Right M Tarsal, Left N Metatarsal, Right P Metatarsal, Left Q Toe Phalanx, Right R Toe Phalanx, Left S Coccyx	Ø Open 3 Percutaneous 4 Percutaneous Endoscopic	4 Internal Fixation Device 5 External Fixation Device	Z No Qualifier
6 Upper Femur, Right 7 Upper Femur, Left 8 Femoral Shaft, Right 9 Femoral Shaft, Left B Lower Femur, Right C Lower Femur, Left G Tibia, Right H Tibia, Left J Fibula, Right K Fibula, Left	Ø Open 3 Percutaneous 4 Percutaneous Endoscopic	4 Internal Fixation Device 5 External Fixation Device 6 Internal Fixation Device, Intramedullary 8 External Fixation Device, Limb Lengthening B External Fixation Device, Monoplanar C External Fixation Device, Ring D External Fixation Device, Hybrid	Z No Qualifier
Y Lower Bone	Ø Open 3 Percutaneous 4 Percutaneous Endoscopic	M Bone Growth Stimulator	Z No Qualifier

Non-OR ØQH[6789BCGHJK][Ø34]8Z

New/Revised Text in Green ~~deleted~~ Deleted ♀ Females Only ♂ Males Only **Coding Clinic**

⊘ Non-covered ⊗ Limited Coverage ⊞ Combination (See Appendix E) DRG Non-OR Non-OR ⊘ Hospital-Acquired Condition

SECTION: 0 MEDICAL AND SURGICAL
BODY SYSTEM: Q LOWER BONES
OPERATION: **J INSPECTION:** Visually and/or manually exploring a body part

Body Part	Approach	Device	Qualifier
Y Lower Bone	0 Open 3 Percutaneous 4 Percutaneous Endoscopic X External	Z No Device	Z No Qualifier

DRG Non-OR 0QJY3ZZ
Non-OR 0QJYXZZ

SECTION: 0 MEDICAL AND SURGICAL
BODY SYSTEM: Q LOWER BONES
OPERATION: **N RELEASE:** Freeing a body part from an abnormal physical constraint by cutting or by the use of force

Body Part	Approach	Device	Qualifier
0 Lumbar Vertebra 1 Sacrum 2 Pelvic Bone, Right 3 Pelvic Bone, Left 4 Acetabulum, Right 5 Acetabulum, Left 6 Upper Femur, Right 7 Upper Femur, Left 8 Femoral Shaft, Right 9 Femoral Shaft, Left B Lower Femur, Right C Lower Femur, Left D Patella, Right F Patella, Left G Tibia, Right H Tibia, Left J Fibula, Right K Fibula, Left L Tarsal, Right M Tarsal, Left N Metatarsal, Right P Metatarsal, Left Q Toe Phalanx, Right R Toe Phalanx, Left S Coccyx	0 Open 3 Percutaneous 4 Percutaneous Endoscopic	Z No Device	Z No Qualifier

0: M/S

Q: LOWER BONES

J: INSPECTION N: RELEASE

SECTION: 0 MEDICAL AND SURGICAL

BODY SYSTEM: Q LOWER BONES
OPERATION: P REMOVAL: *(on multiple pages)*
Taking out or off a device from a body part

P: REMOVAL

Q: LOWER BONES

0: M/S

Body Part	Approach	Device	Qualifier
0 Lumbar Vertebra 1 Sacrum 4 Acetabulum, Right 5 Acetabulum, Left S Coccyx	0 Open 3 Percutaneous 4 Percutaneous Endoscopic	4 Internal Fixation Device 7 Autologous Tissue Substitute J Synthetic Substitute K Nonautologous Tissue Substitute	Z No Qualifier
0 Lumbar Vertebra 1 Sacrum 4 Acetabulum, Right 5 Acetabulum, Left S Coccyx	X External	4 Internal Fixation Device	Z No Qualifier
2 Pelvic Bone, Right 3 Pelvic Bone, Left 6 Upper Femur, Right 7 Upper Femur, Left 8 Femoral Shaft, Right 9 Femoral Shaft, Left B Lower Femur, Right C Lower Femur, Left D Patella, Right ⊞ F Patella, Left ⊞ G Tibia, Right H Tibia, Left J Fibula, Right K Fibula, Left L Tarsal, Right M Tarsal, Left N Metatarsal, Right P Metatarsal, Left Q Toe Phalanx, Right R Toe Phalanx, Left	0 Open 3 Percutaneous 4 Percutaneous Endoscopic	4 Internal Fixation Device 5 External Fixation Device 7 Autologous Tissue Substitute J Synthetic Substitute K Nonautologous Tissue Substitute	Z No Qualifier
2 Pelvic Bone, Right 3 Pelvic Bone, Left 6 Upper Femur, Right 7 Upper Femur, Left 8 Femoral Shaft, Right 9 Femoral Shaft, Left B Lower Femur, Right C Lower Femur, Left D Patella, Right F Patella, Left G Tibia, Right H Tibia, Left J Fibula, Right K Fibula, Left L Tarsal, Right M Tarsal, Left N Metatarsal, Right P Metatarsal, Left Q Toe Phalanx, Right R Toe Phalanx, Left	X External	4 Internal Fixation Device 5 External Fixation Device	Z No Qualifier

⊞ 0QP[DF][034]JZ
Non-OR 0QP[0145S]X4Z

Non-OR 0QP[236789BCDFGHJKLMNPQR]X[45]Z

Coding Clinic: 2015, Q2, P6 – 0QPG04Z

New/Revised Text in Green   ~~deleted~~ Deleted   ♀ Females Only   ♂ Males Only   **Coding Clinic**
🚫 Non-covered   🚫 Limited Coverage   ⊞ Combination (See Appendix E)   DRG Non-OR   Non-OR   🚫 Hospital-Acquired Condition

SECTION: Ø MEDICAL AND SURGICAL

BODY SYSTEM: Q LOWER BONES

OPERATION: P REMOVAL: *(continued)*
Taking out or off a device from a body part

Body Part	Approach	Device	Qualifier
Y Lower Bone	Ø Open 3 Percutaneous 4 Percutaneous Endoscopic X External	Ø Drainage Device M Bone Growth Stimulator	Z No Qualifier

DRG Non-OR ØQPY3ØZ
Non-OR ØQPYX[ØM]Z

SECTION: Ø MEDICAL AND SURGICAL

BODY SYSTEM: Q LOWER BONES

OPERATION: Q REPAIR: Restoring, to the extent possible, a body part to its normal anatomic structure and function

Body Part	Approach	Device	Qualifier
Ø Lumbar Vertebra 1 Sacrum 2 Pelvic Bone, Right 3 Pelvic Bone, Left 4 Acetabulum, Right 5 Acetabulum, Left 6 Upper Femur, Right 7 Upper Femur, Left 8 Femoral Shaft, Right 9 Femoral Shaft, Left B Lower Femur, Right C Lower Femur, Left D Patella, Right F Patella, Left G Tibia, Right H Tibia, Left J Fibula, Right K Fibula, Left L Tarsal, Right M Tarsal, Left N Metatarsal, Right P Metatarsal, Left Q Toe Phalanx, Right R Toe Phalanx, Left S Coccyx	Ø Open 3 Percutaneous 4 Percutaneous Endoscopic X External	Z No Device	Z No Qualifier

New/Revised Text in Green ~~deleted~~ Deleted ♀ Females Only ♂ Males Only **Coding Clinic**
⬮ Non-covered ⬮ Limited Coverage ⊕ Combination (See Appendix E) DRG Non-OR Non-OR ⬮ Hospital-Acquired Condition

381

SECTION: Ø MEDICAL AND SURGICAL

BODY SYSTEM: Q LOWER BONES

OPERATION: R REPLACEMENT: Putting in or on biological or synthetic material that physically takes the place and/or function of all or a portion of a body part

Body Part	Approach	Device	Qualifier
Ø Lumbar Vertebra	Ø Open	7 Autologous Tissue Substitute	Z No Qualifier
1 Sacrum	3 Percutaneous	J Synthetic Substitute	
2 Pelvic Bone, Right	4 Percutaneous Endoscopic	K Nonautologous Tissue	
3 Pelvic Bone, Left		Substitute	
4 Acetabulum, Right			
5 Acetabulum, Left			
6 Upper Femur, Right			
7 Upper Femur, Left			
8 Femoral Shaft, Right ⊞			
9 Femoral Shaft, Left ⊞			
B Lower Femur, Right			
C Lower Femur, Left			
D Patella, Right ⊞			
F Patella, Left ⊞			
G Tibia, Right ⊞			
H Tibia, Left ⊞			
J Fibula, Right ⊞			
K Fibula, Left ⊞			
L Tarsal, Right ⊞			
M Tarsal, Left ⊞			
N Metatarsal, Right ⊞			
P Metatarsal, Left ⊞			
Q Toe Phalanx, Right ⊞			
R Toe Phalanx, Left ⊞			
S Coccyx			

⊞ ØQR[89GHJKLMNPQR][Ø34][7K]Z
⊞ ØQR[DF][Ø34]JZ

SECTION: Ø MEDICAL AND SURGICAL
BODY SYSTEM: Q LOWER BONES
OPERATION: S REPOSITION: *(on multiple pages)*
Moving to its normal location, or other suitable location, all or a portion of a body part

Body Part	Approach	Device	Qualifier
Ø Lumbar Vertebra ⊞ 1 Sacrum ⊞ 4 Acetabulum, Right 5 Acetabulum, Left S Coccyx ⊞	Ø Open 3 Percutaneous 4 Percutaneous Endoscopic	4 Internal Fixation Device Z No Device	Z No Qualifier
Ø Lumbar Vertebra 1 Sacrum 4 Acetabulum, Right 5 Acetabulum, Left S Coccyx	X External	Z No Device	Z No Qualifier
2 Pelvic Bone, Right 3 Pelvic Bone, Left D Patella, Right F Patella, Left L Tarsal, Right M Tarsal, Left N Metatarsal, Right P Metatarsal, Left Q Toe Phalanx, Right R Toe Phalanx, Left	Ø Open 3 Percutaneous 4 Percutaneous Endoscopic	4 Internal Fixation Device 5 External Fixation Device Z No Device	Z No Qualifier
2 Pelvic Bone, Right 3 Pelvic Bone, Left D Patella, Right F Patella, Left L Tarsal, Right M Tarsal, Left N Metatarsal, Right P Metatarsal, Left Q Toe Phalanx, Right R Toe Phalanx, Left	X External	Z No Device	Z No Qualifier
6 Upper Femur, Right 7 Upper Femur, Left 8 Femoral Shaft, Right 9 Femoral Shaft, Left B Lower Femur, Right C Lower Femur, Left G Tibia, Right H Tibia, Left J Fibula, Right K Fibula, Left	Ø Open 3 Percutaneous 4 Percutaneous Endoscopic	4 Internal Fixation Device 5 External Fixation Device 6 Internal Fixation Device, Intramedullary B External Fixation Device, Monoplanar C External Fixation Device, Ring D External Fixation Device, Hybrid Z No Device	Z No Qualifier

⊞ ØQS[Ø1S]3ZZ
Non-OR ØQS[45][34]ZZ
Non-OR ØQS[45]XZZ
Non-OR ØQS[23DFLMNPQR][34]ZZ
Non-OR ØQS[23DFLMNPQR]XZZ
Non-OR ØQS[6789BCGHJK][34]ZZ

SECTION: **Ø MEDICAL AND SURGICAL**

BODY SYSTEM: Q LOWER BONES

OPERATION: **S REPOSITION:** *(continued)*

Moving to its normal location, or other suitable location, all or a portion of a body part

Body Part	Approach	Device	Qualifier
6 Upper Femur, Right 7 Upper Femur, Left 8 Femoral Shaft, Right 9 Femoral Shaft, Left B Lower Femur, Right C Lower Femur, Left G Tibia, Right H Tibia, Left J Fibula, Right K Fibula, Left	X External	Z No Device	Z No Qualifier

Non-OR   ØQS[6789BCGHJK]XZZ

SECTION: **Ø MEDICAL AND SURGICAL**

BODY SYSTEM: Q LOWER BONES

OPERATION: **T RESECTION:** Cutting out or off, without replacement, all of a body part

Body Part	Approach	Device	Qualifier
2 Pelvic Bone, Right 3 Pelvic Bone, Left 4 Acetabulum, Right 5 Acetabulum, Left 6 Upper Femur, Right ⊞ 7 Upper Femur, Left ⊞ 8 Femoral Shaft, Right ⊞ 9 Femoral Shaft, Left ⊞ B Lower Femur, Right ⊞ C Lower Femur, Left ⊞ D Patella, Right F Patella, Left G Tibia, Right H Tibia, Left J Fibula, Right K Fibula, Left L Tarsal, Right M Tarsal, Left N Metatarsal, Right P Metatarsal, Left Q Toe Phalanx, Right R Toe Phalanx, Left S Coccyx	Ø Open	Z No Device	Z No Qualifier

⊞ ØQT[6789BC]ØZZ

Coding Clinic: 2Ø15, Q3, P26 – ØQT7ØZZ

New/Revised Text in Green   ~~deleted~~ Deleted   ♀ Females Only   ♂ Males Only   **Coding Clinic**

🚫 Non-covered   🚫 Limited Coverage   ⊞ Combination (See Appendix E)   DRG Non-OR   Non-OR   🚫 Hospital-Acquired Condition

SECTION: 0 MEDICAL AND SURGICAL

BODY SYSTEM: Q LOWER BONES

OPERATION: U SUPPLEMENT: Putting in or on biological or synthetic material that physically reinforces and/or augments the function of a portion of a body part

Body Part	Approach	Device	Qualifier
0 Lumbar Vertebra ⊞	0 Open	7 Autologous Tissue Substitute	Z No Qualifier
1 Sacrum ⊞	3 Percutaneous	J Synthetic Substitute	
2 Pelvic Bone, Right	4 Percutaneous Endoscopic	K Nonautologous Tissue	
3 Pelvic Bone, Left		Substitute	
4 Acetabulum, Right			
5 Acetabulum, Left			
6 Upper Femur, Right			
7 Upper Femur, Left			
8 Femoral Shaft, Right ⊞			
9 Femoral Shaft, Left ⊞			
B Lower Femur, Right			
C Lower Femur, Left			
D Patella, Right ⊞			
F Patella, Left ⊞			
G Tibia, Right ⊞			
H Tibia, Left ⊞			
J Fibula, Right ⊞			
K Fibula, Left ⊞			
L Tarsal, Right ⊞			
M Tarsal, Left ⊞			
N Metatarsal, Right ⊞			
P Metatarsal, Left ⊞			
Q Toe Phalanx, Right ⊞			
R Toe Phalanx, Left ⊞			
S Coccyx ⊞			

⊞ 0QU[01S]3JZ
⊞ 0QU[89GHJKLMNPQR][034][7K]Z
⊞ 0QU[DF][034]JZ

Coding Clinic: 2013, Q2, P36 – 0QU20JZ
Coding Clinic: 2015, Q3, P19 – 0QU50JZ

New/Revised Text in Green   deleted Deleted   ♀ Females Only   ♂ Males Only   Coding Clinic
🚫 Non-covered   🚫 Limited Coverage   ⊞ Combination (See Appendix E)   DRG Non-OR   Non-OR   🚫 Hospital-Acquired Condition

385

SECTION: Ø MEDICAL AND SURGICAL

BODY SYSTEM: Q LOWER BONES

OPERATION: W **REVISION:** Correcting, to the extent possible, a portion of a malfunctioning device or the position of a displaced device

Body Part	Approach	Device	Qualifier
Ø Lumbar Vertebra 1 Sacrum 4 Acetabulum, Right 5 Acetabulum, Left S Coccyx	Ø Open 3 Percutaneous 4 Percutaneous Endoscopic X External	4 Internal Fixation Device 7 Autologous Tissue Substitute J Synthetic Substitute K Nonautologous Tissue Substitute	Z No Qualifier
2 Pelvic Bone, Right 3 Pelvic Bone, Left 6 Upper Femur, Right 7 Upper Femur, Left 8 Femoral Shaft, Right 9 Femoral Shaft, Left B Lower Femur, Right C Lower Femur, Left D Patella, Right F Patella, Left G Tibia, Right H Tibia, Left J Fibula, Right K Fibula, Left L Tarsal, Right M Tarsal, Left N Metatarsal, Right P Metatarsal, Left Q Toe Phalanx, Right R Toe Phalanx, Left	Ø Open 3 Percutaneous 4 Percutaneous Endoscopic X External	4 Internal Fixation Device 5 External Fixation Device 7 Autologous Tissue Substitute J Synthetic Substitute K Nonautologous Tissue Substitute	Z No Qualifier
Y Lower Bone	Ø Open 3 Percutaneous 4 Percutaneous Endoscopic X External	Ø Drainage Device M Bone Growth Stimulator	Z No Qualifier

Non-OR ØQW[Ø145S]X[47JK]Z
Non-OR ØQW[236789BCDFGHJKLMNPQR]X[457JK]Z
Non-OR ØQWYX[ØM]Z

W: REVISION

Q: LOWER BONES

Ø: M/S

New/Revised Text in Green ~~deleted~~ Deleted ♀ Females Only ♂ Males Only **Coding Clinic**
🔗 Non-covered 🔗 Limited Coverage ⊞ Combination (See Appendix E) DRG Non-OR Non-OR 🔗 Hospital-Acquired Condition

SECTION: Ø MEDICAL AND SURGICAL

BODY SYSTEM: R UPPER JOINTS

OPERATION: 2 **CHANGE:** Taking out or off a device from a body part and putting back an identical or similar device in or on the same body part without cutting or puncturing the skin or a mucous membrane

Body Part	Approach	Device	Qualifier
Y Upper Joint	X External	Ø Drainage Device Y Other Device	Z No Qualifier

Non-OR All Values

SECTION: Ø MEDICAL AND SURGICAL

BODY SYSTEM: R UPPER JOINTS

OPERATION: 5 **DESTRUCTION:** Physical eradication of all or a portion of a body part by the direct use of energy, force, or destructive agent

Body Part	Approach	Device	Qualifier
Ø Occipital-cervical Joint 1 Cervical Vertebral Joint 3 Cervical Vertebral Disc 4 Cervicothoracic Vertebral Joint 5 Cervicothoracic Vertebral Disc 6 Thoracic Vertebral Joint 9 Thoracic Vertebral Disc A Thoracolumbar Vertebral Joint B Thoracolumbar Vertebral Disc C Temporomandibular Joint, Right D Temporomandibular Joint, Left E Sternoclavicular Joint, Right F Sternoclavicular Joint, Left G Acromioclavicular Joint, Right H Acromioclavicular Joint, Left J Shoulder Joint, Right K Shoulder Joint, Left L Elbow Joint, Right M Elbow Joint, Left N Wrist Joint, Right P Wrist Joint, Left Q Carpal Joint, Right R Carpal Joint, Left S Metacarpocarpal Joint, Right T Metacarpocarpal Joint, Left U Metacarpophalangeal Joint, Right V Metacarpophalangeal Joint, Left W Finger Phalangeal Joint, Right X Finger Phalangeal Joint, Left	Ø Open 3 Percutaneous 4 Percutaneous Endoscopic	Z No Device	Z No Qualifier

Non-OR ØR5[359B][34]ZZ

SECTION: Ø MEDICAL AND SURGICAL
BODY SYSTEM: R UPPER JOINTS
OPERATION: 9 DRAINAGE: *(on multiple pages)*
Taking or letting out fluids and/or gases from a body part

Body Part	Approach	Device	Qualifier
Ø Occipital-cervical Joint	Ø Open	Ø Drainage Device	Z No Qualifier
1 Cervical Vertebral Joint	3 Percutaneous		
3 Cervical Vertebral Disc	4 Percutaneous Endoscopic		
4 Cervicothoracic Vertebral Joint			
5 Cervicothoracic Vertebral Disc			
6 Thoracic Vertebral Joint			
9 Thoracic Vertebral Disc			
A Thoracolumbar Vertebral Joint			
B Thoracolumbar Vertebral Disc			
C Temporomandibular Joint, Right			
D Temporomandibular Joint, Left			
E Sternoclavicular Joint, Right			
F Sternoclavicular Joint, Left			
G Acromioclavicular Joint, Right			
H Acromioclavicular Joint, Left			
J Shoulder Joint, Right			
K Shoulder Joint, Left			
L Elbow Joint, Right			
M Elbow Joint, Left			
N Wrist Joint, Right			
P Wrist Joint, Left			
Q Carpal Joint, Right			
R Carpal Joint, Left			
S Metacarpocarpal Joint, Right			
T Metacarpocarpal Joint, Left			
U Metacarpophalangeal Joint, Right			
V Metacarpophalangeal Joint, Left			
W Finger Phalangeal Joint, Right			
X Finger Phalangeal Joint, Left			

DRG Non-OR ØR9[CD]3ØZ
Non-OR ØR9[Ø134569ABEFGHJKLMNPQRSTUVWX][34]ØZ

Ø: M/S

R: UPPER JOINTS

9: DRAINAGE

SECTION: Ø MEDICAL AND SURGICAL

BODY SYSTEM: R UPPER JOINTS

OPERATION: 9 DRAINAGE: *(continued)*
Taking or letting out fluids and/or gases from a body part

Body Part	Approach	Device	Qualifier
Ø Occipital-cervical Joint	Ø Open	Z No Device	X Diagnostic
1 Cervical Vertebral Joint	3 Percutaneous		Z No Qualifier
3 Cervical Vertebral Disc	4 Percutaneous Endoscopic		
4 Cervicothoracic Vertebral Joint			
5 Cervicothoracic Vertebral Disc			
6 Thoracic Vertebral Joint			
9 Thoracic Vertebral Disc			
A Thoracolumbar Vertebral Joint			
B Thoracolumbar Vertebral Disc			
C Temporomandibular Joint, Right			
D Temporomandibular Joint, Left			
E Sternoclavicular Joint, Right			
F Sternoclavicular Joint, Left			
G Acromioclavicular Joint, Right			
H Acromioclavicular Joint, Left			
J Shoulder Joint, Right			
K Shoulder Joint, Left			
L Elbow Joint, Right			
M Elbow Joint, Left			
N Wrist Joint, Right			
P Wrist Joint, Left			
Q Carpal Joint, Right			
R Carpal Joint, Left			
S Metacarpocarpal Joint, Right			
T Metacarpocarpal Joint, Left			
U Metacarpophalangeal Joint, Right			
V Metacarpophalangeal Joint, Left			
W Finger Phalangeal Joint, Right			
X Finger Phalangeal Joint, Left			

DRG Non-OR ØR9[CD]3ZZ
Non-OR ØR9[Ø134569ABEFGHJKLMNPQRSTUVWX][Ø34]ZX
Non-OR ØR9[Ø134569ABEFGHJKLMNPQRSTUVWX][34]ZZ

New/Revised Text in Green   ~~deleted~~ Deleted   ♀ Females Only   ♂ Males Only   **Coding Clinic**
Non-covered   Limited Coverage   Combination (See Appendix E)   DRG Non-OR   Non-OR   Hospital-Acquired Condition

SECTION: Ø MEDICAL AND SURGICAL

BODY SYSTEM: R UPPER JOINTS

OPERATION: B EXCISION: Cutting out or off, without replacement, a portion of a body part

Body Part	Approach	Device	Qualifier
Ø Occipital-cervical Joint 1 Cervical Vertebral Joint 3 Cervical Vertebral Disc 4 Cervicothoracic Vertebral Joint 5 Cervicothoracic Vertebral Disc 6 Thoracic Vertebral Joint 9 Thoracic Vertebral Disc A Thoracolumbar Vertebral Joint B Thoracolumbar Vertebral Disc C Temporomandibular Joint, Right D Temporomandibular Joint, Left E Sternoclavicular Joint, Right F Sternoclavicular Joint, Left G Acromioclavicular Joint, Right H Acromioclavicular Joint, Left J Shoulder Joint, Right K Shoulder Joint, Left L Elbow Joint, Right M Elbow Joint, Left N Wrist Joint, Right P Wrist Joint, Left Q Carpal Joint, Right R Carpal Joint, Left S Metacarpocarpal Joint, Right T Metacarpocarpal Joint, Left U Metacarpophalangeal Joint, Right V Metacarpophalangeal Joint, Left W Finger Phalangeal Joint, Right X Finger Phalangeal Joint, Left	Ø Open 3 Percutaneous 4 Percutaneous Endoscopic	Z No Device	X Diagnostic Z No Qualifier

Non-OR ØRB[Ø134569ABEFGHJKLMNPQRSTUVWX][Ø34]ZX

Ø: M/S

R: UPPER JOINTS

B: EXCISION

SECTION: Ø MEDICAL AND SURGICAL
BODY SYSTEM: R UPPER JOINTS
OPERATION: C EXTIRPATION: Taking or cutting out solid matter from a body part

Body Part	Approach	Device	Qualifier
Ø Occipital-cervical Joint	Ø Open	Z No Device	Z No Qualifier
1 Cervical Vertebral Joint	3 Percutaneous		
3 Cervical Vertebral Disc	4 Percutaneous Endoscopic		
4 Cervicothoracic Vertebral Joint			
5 Cervicothoracic Vertebral Disc			
6 Thoracic Vertebral Joint			
9 Thoracic Vertebral Disc			
A Thoracolumbar Vertebral Joint			
B Thoracolumbar Vertebral Disc			
C Temporomandibular Joint, Right			
D Temporomandibular Joint, Left			
E Sternoclavicular Joint, Right			
F Sternoclavicular Joint, Left			
G Acromioclavicular Joint, Right			
H Acromioclavicular Joint, Left			
J Shoulder Joint, Right			
K Shoulder Joint, Left			
L Elbow Joint, Right			
M Elbow Joint, Left			
N Wrist Joint, Right			
P Wrist Joint, Left			
Q Carpal Joint, Right			
R Carpal Joint, Left			
S Metacarpocarpal Joint, Right			
T Metacarpocarpal Joint, Left			
U Metacarpophalangeal Joint, Right			
V Metacarpophalangeal Joint, Left			
W Finger Phalangeal Joint, Right			
X Finger Phalangeal Joint, Left			

C: EXTIRPATION

R: UPPER JOINTS

Ø: M/S

New/Revised Text in Green ~~deleted~~ Deleted ♀ Females Only ♂ Males Only **Coding Clinic**

🔖 Non-covered 🔖 Limited Coverage ⊞ Combination (See Appendix E) DRG Non-OR Non-OR 🔖 Hospital-Acquired Condition

SECTION: Ø MEDICAL AND SURGICAL
BODY SYSTEM: R UPPER JOINTS
OPERATION: G FUSION: Joining together portions of an articular body part, rendering the articular body part immobile

Body Part	Approach	Device	Qualifier
Ø Occipital-cervical Joint 🔖 1 Cervical Vertebral Joint 🔖 2 Cervical Vertebral Joints, 2 or more 🔖 4 Cervicothoracic Vertebral Joint 🔖 6 Thoracic Vertebral Joint 🔖 7 Thoracic Vertebral Joint, 2 to 7 ⊞ 🔖 8 Thoracic Vertebral Joint, 8 or more 🔖 A Thoracolumbar Vertebral Joint 🔖	Ø Open 3 Percutaneous 4 Percutaneous Endoscopic	7 Autologous Tissue Substitute A Interbody Fusion Device J Synthetic Substitute K Nonautologous Tissue Substitute Z No Device	Ø Anterior Approach, Anterior Column 1 Posterior Approach, Posterior Column J Posterior Approach, Anterior Column
C Temporomandibular Joint, Right D Temporomandibular Joint, Left E Sternoclavicular Joint, Right 🔖 F Sternoclavicular Joint, Left 🔖 G Acromioclavicular Joint, Right 🔖 H Acromioclavicular Joint, Left 🔖 J Shoulder Joint, Right 🔖 K Shoulder Joint, Left 🔖	Ø Open 3 Percutaneous 4 Percutaneous Endoscopic	4 Internal Fixation Device 7 Autologous Tissue Substitute J Synthetic Substitute K Nonautologous Tissue Substitute Z No Device	Z No Qualifier
L Elbow Joint, Right 🔖 M Elbow Joint, Left 🔖 N Wrist Joint, Right P Wrist Joint, Left Q Carpal Joint, Right R Carpal Joint, Left S Metacarpocarpal Joint, Right T Metacarpocarpal Joint, Left U Metacarpophalangeal Joint, Right V Metacarpophalangeal Joint, Left W Finger Phalangeal Joint, Right X Finger Phalangeal Joint, Left	Ø Open 3 Percutaneous 4 Percutaneous Endoscopic	4 Internal Fixation Device 5 External Fixation Device 7 Autologous Tissue Substitute J Synthetic Substitute K Nonautologous Tissue Substitute Z No Device	Z No Qualifier

⊞ ØRG7[Ø34][7AJKZ][Ø1J]
🔖 ØRG[Ø124678A][Ø34][7AJKZ][Ø1J] when reported with Secondary Diagnosis K68.11, T81.4XXA, or T84.6ØXA-T84.7XXA
🔖 ØRG[EFGHJK][Ø34][47JKZ]Z when reported with Secondary Diagnosis K68.11, T81.4XXA, or T84.6ØXA-T84.7XXA
🔖 ØRG[LM][Ø34][457JKZ]Z when reported with Secondary Diagnosis K68.11, T81.4XXA, or T84.6ØXA-T84.7XXA

Coding Clinic: 2013, Q1, P29 – ØRG4ØAØ
Coding Clinic: 2013, Q1, P22 – ØRG7Ø71, ØRGAØ71

SECTION: Ø MEDICAL AND SURGICAL
BODY SYSTEM: R UPPER JOINTS
OPERATION: H INSERTION: Putting in a nonbiological appliance that monitors, assists, performs, or prevents a physiological function but does not physically take the place of a body part

Body Part	Approach	Device	Qualifier
Ø Occipital-cervical Joint 1 Cervical Vertebral Joint 4 Cervicothoracic Vertebral Joint 6 Thoracic Vertebral Joint A Thoracolumbar Vertebral Joint	Ø Open 3 Percutaneous 4 Percutaneous Endoscopic	3 Infusion Device 4 Internal Fixation Device 8 Spacer B Spinal Stabilization Device, Interspinous Process C Spinal Stabilization Device, Pedicle-Based D Spinal Stabilization Device, Facet Replacement	Z No Qualifier
3 Cervical Vertebral Disc 5 Cervicothoracic Vertebral Disc 9 Thoracic Vertebral Disc B Thoracolumbar Vertebral Disc	Ø Open 3 Percutaneous 4 Percutaneous Endoscopic	3 Infusion Device	Z No Qualifier
C Temporomandibular Joint, Right D Temporomandibular Joint, Left E Sternoclavicular Joint, Right F Sternoclavicular Joint, Left G Acromioclavicular Joint, Right H Acromioclavicular Joint, Left J Shoulder Joint, Right K Shoulder Joint, Left	Ø Open 3 Percutaneous 4 Percutaneous Endoscopic	3 Infusion Device 4 Internal Fixation Device 8 Spacer	Z No Qualifier
L Elbow Joint, Right M Elbow Joint, Left N Wrist Joint, Right P Wrist Joint, Left Q Carpal Joint, Right R Carpal Joint, Left S Metacarpocarpal Joint, Right T Metacarpocarpal Joint, Left U Metacarpophalangeal Joint, Right V Metacarpophalangeal Joint, Left W Finger Phalangeal Joint, Right X Finger Phalangeal Joint, Left	Ø Open 3 Percutaneous 4 Percutaneous Endoscopic	3 Infusion Device 4 Internal Fixation Device 5 External Fixation Device 8 Spacer	Z No Qualifier

DRG Non-OR ØRH[0146A][34]3Z
DRG Non-OR ØRH[359B][34]3Z
DRG Non-OR ØRH[CD]33Z
DRG Non-OR ØRH[EFGHJK][34]3Z
DRG Non-OR ØRH[LMNPQRSTUVWX][34]3Z

Non-OR ØRH[0146A][034][38]Z
Non-OR ØRH[359B][034]3Z
Non-OR ØRH[CD][034]8Z
Non-OR ØRH[EFGHJK][034][38]Z
Non-OR ØRH[LMNPQRSTUVWX][034][38]Z

New/Revised Text in Green ~~deleted~~ Deleted ♀ Females Only ♂ Males Only **Coding Clinic**
Non-covered Limited Coverage ⊞ Combination (See Appendix E) DRG Non-OR Non-OR Hospital-Acquired Condition

H: INSERTION
R: UPPER JOINTS
Ø: M/S

SECTION: Ø MEDICAL AND SURGICAL
BODY SYSTEM: R UPPER JOINTS
OPERATION: J INSPECTION: Visually and/or manually exploring a body part

Body Part	Approach	Device	Qualifier
Ø Occipital-cervical Joint 1 Cervical Vertebral Joint 3 Cervical Vertebral Disc 4 Cervicothoracic Vertebral Joint 5 Cervicothoracic Vertebral Disc 6 Thoracic Vertebral Joint 9 Thoracic Vertebral Disc A Thoracolumbar Vertebral Joint B Thoracolumbar Vertebral Disc C Temporomandibular Joint, Right D Temporomandibular Joint, Left E Sternoclavicular Joint, Right F Sternoclavicular Joint, Left G Acromioclavicular Joint, Right H Acromioclavicular Joint, Left J Shoulder Joint, Right K Shoulder Joint, Left L Elbow Joint, Right M Elbow Joint, Left N Wrist Joint, Right P Wrist Joint, Left Q Carpal Joint, Right R Carpal Joint, Left S Metacarpocarpal Joint, Right T Metacarpocarpal Joint, Left U Metacarpophalangeal Joint, Right V Metacarpophalangeal Joint, Left W Finger Phalangeal Joint, Right X Finger Phalangeal Joint, Left	Ø Open 3 Percutaneous 4 Percutaneous Endoscopic X External	Z No Device	Z No Qualifier

DRG Non-OR ØRJ[Ø134569ABCDEFGHJKLMNPQRSTUVWX]3ZZ
Non-OR ØRJ[Ø134569ABCDEFGHJKLMNPQRSTUVWX]XZZ

New/Revised Text in Green deleted Deleted ♀ Females Only ♂ Males Only Coding Clinic
Non-covered Limited Coverage Combination (See Appendix E) DRG Non-OR Non-OR Hospital-Acquired Condition

395

Ø: M/S R: UPPER JOINTS J: INSPECTION

SECTION: Ø MEDICAL AND SURGICAL

BODY SYSTEM: R UPPER JOINTS

OPERATION: N RELEASE: Freeing a body part from an abnormal physical constraint by cutting or by the use of force

Body Part	Approach	Device	Qualifier
Ø Occipital-cervical Joint	Ø Open	Z No Device	Z No Qualifier
1 Cervical Vertebral Joint	3 Percutaneous		
3 Cervical Vertebral Disc	4 Percutaneous Endoscopic		
4 Cervicothoracic Vertebral Joint	X External		
5 Cervicothoracic Vertebral Disc			
6 Thoracic Vertebral Joint			
9 Thoracic Vertebral Disc			
A Thoracolumbar Vertebral Joint			
B Thoracolumbar Vertebral Disc			
C Temporomandibular Joint, Right			
D Temporomandibular Joint, Left			
E Sternoclavicular Joint, Right			
F Sternoclavicular Joint, Left			
G Acromioclavicular Joint, Right			
H Acromioclavicular Joint, Left			
J Shoulder Joint, Right			
K Shoulder Joint, Left			
L Elbow Joint, Right			
M Elbow Joint, Left			
N Wrist Joint, Right			
P Wrist Joint, Left			
Q Carpal Joint, Right			
R Carpal Joint, Left			
S Metacarpocarpal Joint, Right			
T Metacarpocarpal Joint, Left			
U Metacarpophalangeal Joint, Right			
V Metacarpophalangeal Joint, Left			
W Finger Phalangeal Joint, Right			
X Finger Phalangeal Joint, Left			

Non-OR ØRN[Ø134569ABCDEFGHJKLMNPQRSTUVWX]XZZ

Coding Clinic: 2015, Q2, P23 – ØRNK4ZZ

SECTION: Ø MEDICAL AND SURGICAL

BODY SYSTEM: R UPPER JOINTS

OPERATION: P REMOVAL: *(on multiple pages)*
Taking out or off a device from a body part

Body Part	Approach	Device	Qualifier
Ø Occipital-cervical Joint	Ø Open	Ø Drainage Device	Z No Qualifier
1 Cervical Vertebral Joint	3 Percutaneous	3 Infusion Device	
4 Cervicothoracic Vertebral Joint	4 Percutaneous Endoscopic	4 Internal Fixation Device	
6 Thoracic Vertebral Joint		7 Autologous Tissue Substitute	
A Thoracolumbar Vertebral Joint		8 Spacer	
		A Interbody Fusion Device	
		J Synthetic Substitute	
		K Nonautologous Tissue Substitute	

DRG Non-OR ØRP[Ø146A]3[Ø3]Z
Non-OR ØRP[Ø146A][Ø34]8Z

New/Revised Text in Green ~~deleted~~ Deleted ♀ Females Only ♂ Males Only **Coding Clinic**
🐾 Non-covered 🐾 Limited Coverage ⊞ Combination (See Appendix E) DRG Non-OR Non-OR 🐾 Hospital-Acquired Condition

SECTION: Ø MEDICAL AND SURGICAL
BODY SYSTEM: R UPPER JOINTS
OPERATION: P REMOVAL: *(continued)*
Taking out or off a device from a body part

Body Part	Approach	Device	Qualifier
Ø Occipital-cervical Joint 1 Cervical Vertebral Joint 4 Cervicothoracic Vertebral Joint 6 Thoracic Vertebral Joint A Thoracolumbar Vertebral Joint	X External	Ø Drainage Device 3 Infusion Device 4 Internal Fixation Device	Z No Qualifier
3 Cervical Vertebral Disc 5 Cervicothoracic Vertebral Disc 9 Thoracic Vertebral Disc B Thoracolumbar Vertebral Disc	Ø Open 3 Percutaneous 4 Percutaneous Endoscopic	Ø Drainage Device 3 Infusion Device 7 Autologous Tissue Substitute J Synthetic Substitute K Nonautologous Tissue Substitute	Z No Qualifier
3 Cervical Vertebral Disc 5 Cervicothoracic Vertebral Disc 9 Thoracic Vertebral Disc B Thoracolumbar Vertebral Disc	X External	Ø Drainage Device 3 Infusion Device	Z No Qualifier
C Temporomandibular Joint, Right D Temporomandibular Joint, Left E Sternoclavicular Joint, Right F Sternoclavicular Joint, Left G Acromioclavicular Joint, Right H Acromioclavicular Joint, Left J Shoulder Joint, Right K Shoulder Joint, Left	Ø Open 3 Percutaneous 4 Percutaneous Endoscopic	Ø Drainage Device 3 Infusion Device 4 Internal Fixation Device 7 Autologous Tissue Substitute 8 Spacer J Synthetic Substitute K Nonautologous Tissue Substitute	Z No Qualifier
C Temporomandibular Joint, Right D Temporomandibular Joint, Left E Sternoclavicular Joint, Right F Sternoclavicular Joint, Left G Acromioclavicular Joint, Right H Acromioclavicular Joint, Left J Shoulder Joint, Right K Shoulder Joint, Left	X External	Ø Drainage Device 3 Infusion Device 4 Internal Fixation Device	Z No Qualifier
L Elbow Joint, Right M Elbow Joint, Left N Wrist Joint, Right P Wrist Joint, Left Q Carpal Joint, Right R Carpal Joint, Left S Metacarpocarpal Joint, Right T Metacarpocarpal Joint, Left U Metacarpophalangeal Joint, Right V Metacarpophalangeal Joint, Left W Finger Phalangeal Joint, Right X Finger Phalangeal Joint, Left	Ø Open 3 Percutaneous 4 Percutaneous Endoscopic	Ø Drainage Device 3 Infusion Device 4 Internal Fixation Device 5 External Fixation Device 7 Autologous Tissue Substitute 8 Spacer J Synthetic Substitute K Nonautologous Tissue Substitute	Z No Qualifier

DRG Non-OR   ØRP[359B]3[Ø3]Z
DRG Non-OR   ØRP[CDEFGHJK]3[Ø3]Z
DRG Non-OR   ØRP[LMNPQRSTUVWX]3[Ø3]Z
Non-OR   ØRP[Ø146A]X[Ø34]Z
Non-OR   ØRP[359B]X[Ø3]Z
Non-OR   ØRP[CDEFGHJK][Ø34]8Z
Non-OR   ØRP[CD]X[Ø3]Z
Non-OR   ØRP[EFGHJK]X[Ø34]Z
Non-OR   ØRP[LMNPQRSTUVWX][Ø34]8Z

Ø: M/S   R: UPPER JOINTS   P: REMOVAL

New/Revised Text in Green   ~~deleted~~ Deleted   ♀ Females Only   ♂ Males Only   **Coding Clinic**
🐾 Non-covered   🐾 Limited Coverage   ⊞ Combination (See Appendix E)   DRG Non-OR   Non-OR   🐾 Hospital-Acquired Condition

SECTION: Ø MEDICAL AND SURGICAL

BODY SYSTEM: R UPPER JOINTS

OPERATION: P REMOVAL: *(continued)*
Taking out or off a device from a body part

Body Part	Approach	Device	Qualifier
L Elbow Joint, Right M Elbow Joint, Left N Wrist Joint, Right P Wrist Joint, Left Q Carpal Joint, Right R Carpal Joint, Left S Metacarpocarpal Joint, Right T Metacarpocarpal Joint, Left U Metacarpophalangeal Joint, Right V Metacarpophalangeal Joint, Left W Finger Phalangeal Joint, Right X Finger Phalangeal Joint, Left	X External	Ø Drainage Device 3 Infusion Device 4 Internal Fixation Device 5 External Fixation Device	Z No Qualifier

Non-OR ØRP[LMNPQRSTUVWX]X[Ø345]Z

SECTION: Ø MEDICAL AND SURGICAL

BODY SYSTEM: R UPPER JOINTS

OPERATION: Q REPAIR: Restoring, to the extent possible, a body part to its normal anatomic structure and function

Body Part	Approach	Device	Qualifier
Ø Occipital-cervical Joint 1 Cervical Vertebral Joint 3 Cervical Vertebral Disc 4 Cervicothoracic Vertebral Joint 5 Cervicothoracic Vertebral Disc 6 Thoracic Vertebral Joint 9 Thoracic Vertebral Disc A Thoracolumbar Vertebral Joint B Thoracolumbar Vertebral Disc C Temporomandibular Joint, Right D Temporomandibular Joint, Left E Sternoclavicular Joint, Right ⚕ F Sternoclavicular Joint, Left ⚕ G Acromioclavicular Joint, Right ⚕ H Acromioclavicular Joint, Left ⚕ J Shoulder Joint, Right ⚕ K Shoulder Joint, Left ⚕ L Elbow Joint, Right ⚕ M Elbow Joint, Left ⚕ N Wrist Joint, Right P Wrist Joint, Left Q Carpal Joint, Right R Carpal Joint, Left S Metacarpocarpal Joint, Right T Metacarpocarpal Joint, Left U Metacarpophalangeal Joint, Right V Metacarpophalangeal Joint, Left W Finger Phalangeal Joint, Right X Finger Phalangeal Joint, Left	Ø Open 3 Percutaneous 4 Percutaneous Endoscopic X External	Z No Device	Z No Qualifier

Non-OR ØRQ[CD]XZZ

⚕ ØRQ[EFGHJKLM][Ø34X]ZZ when reported with Secondary Diagnosis K68.11, T81.4XXA, or T84.60XA-T84.7XXA

Coding Clinic: 2Ø16, Q1, P3Ø – ØRQJ4ZZ

New/Revised Text in Green   deleted Deleted   ♀ Females Only   ♂ Males Only   Coding Clinic

⚕ Non-covered   ⚕ Limited Coverage   ⊞ Combination (See Appendix E)   DRG Non-OR   Non-OR   ⚕ Hospital-Acquired Condition

SECTION: Ø MEDICAL AND SURGICAL

BODY SYSTEM: R UPPER JOINTS

OPERATION: R REPLACEMENT: Putting in or on biological or synthetic material that physically takes the place and/or function of all or a portion of a body part

Body Part	Approach	Device	Qualifier
Ø Occipital-cervical Joint 1 Cervical Vertebral Joint 3 Cervical Vertebral Disc 4 Cervicothoracic Vertebral Joint 5 Cervicothoracic Vertebral Disc 6 Thoracic Vertebral Joint 9 Thoracic Vertebral Disc A Thoracolumbar Vertebral Joint B Thoracolumbar Vertebral Disc C Temporomandibular Joint, Right D Temporomandibular Joint, Left E Sternoclavicular Joint, Right F Sternoclavicular Joint, Left G Acromioclavicular Joint, Right H Acromioclavicular Joint, Left L Elbow Joint, Right M Elbow Joint, Left N Wrist Joint, Right P Wrist Joint, Left Q Carpal Joint, Right R Carpal Joint, Left S Metacarpocarpal Joint, Right T Metacarpocarpal Joint, Left U Metacarpophalangeal Joint, Right V Metacarpophalangeal Joint, Left W Finger Phalangeal Joint, Right X Finger Phalangeal Joint, Left	Ø Open	7 Autologous Tissue Substitute J Synthetic Substitute K Nonautologous Tissue Substitute	Z No Qualifier
J Shoulder Joint, Right K Shoulder Joint, Left	Ø Open	Ø Synthetic Substitute, Reverse Ball and Socket 7 Autologous Tissue Substitute K Nonautologous Tissue Substitute	Z No Qualifier
J Shoulder Joint, Right K Shoulder Joint, Left	Ø Open	J Synthetic Substitute	6 Humeral Surface 7 Glenoid Surface Z No Qualifier

Coding Clinic: 2015, Q1, P27 – ØRRJ00Z
Coding Clinic: 2015, Q3, P15 – ØRRKØJ6

SECTION: Ø MEDICAL AND SURGICAL

BODY SYSTEM: R UPPER JOINTS

OPERATION: S REPOSITION: Moving to its normal location, or other suitable location, all or a portion of a body part

Body Part	Approach	Device	Qualifier
Ø Occipital-cervical Joint 1 Cervical Vertebral Joint 4 Cervicothoracic Vertebral Joint 6 Thoracic Vertebral Joint A Thoracolumbar Vertebral Joint C Temporomandibular Joint, Right D Temporomandibular Joint, Left E Sternoclavicular Joint, Right F Sternoclavicular Joint, Left G Acromioclavicular Joint, Right H Acromioclavicular Joint, Left J Shoulder Joint, Right K Shoulder Joint, Left	Ø Open 3 Percutaneous 4 Percutaneous Endoscopic X External	4 Internal Fixation Device Z No Device	Z No Qualifier
L Elbow Joint, Right M Elbow Joint, Left N Wrist Joint, Right P Wrist Joint, Left Q Carpal Joint, Right R Carpal Joint, Left S Metacarpocarpal Joint, Right T Metacarpocarpal Joint, Left U Metacarpophalangeal Joint, Right V Metacarpophalangeal Joint, Left W Finger Phalangeal Joint, Right X Finger Phalangeal Joint, Left	Ø Open 3 Percutaneous 4 Percutaneous Endoscopic X External	4 Internal Fixation Device 5 External Fixation Device Z No Device	Z No Qualifier

Non-OR ØRS[Ø146ACDEFGHJK][34X][4Z]Z
Non-OR ØRS[LMNPQRSTUVWX][34X][45Z]Z

Coding Clinic: 2015, Q2, P35; 2013, Q2, P39 – ØRS1XZZ

New/Revised Text in Green ~~deleted~~ Deleted ♀ Females Only ♂ Males Only **Coding Clinic**

🔖 Non-covered 🔖 Limited Coverage ⊞ Combination (See Appendix E) DRG Non-OR Non-OR 🔖 Hospital-Acquired Condition

S: REPOSITION

R: UPPER JOINTS

Ø: M/S

SECTION: Ø MEDICAL AND SURGICAL

BODY SYSTEM: R UPPER JOINTS

OPERATION: T RESECTION: Cutting out or off, without replacement, all of a body part

Body Part	Approach	Device	Qualifier
3 Cervical Vertebral Disc	Ø Open	Z No Device	Z No Qualifier
4 Cervicothoracic Vertebral Joint			
5 Cervicothoracic Vertebral Disc			
9 Thoracic Vertebral Disc			
B Thoracolumbar Vertebral Disc			
C Temporomandibular Joint, Right			
D Temporomandibular Joint, Left			
E Sternoclavicular Joint, Right			
F Sternoclavicular Joint, Left			
G Acromioclavicular Joint, Right			
H Acromioclavicular Joint, Left			
J Shoulder Joint, Right			
K Shoulder Joint, Left			
L Elbow Joint, Right			
M Elbow Joint, Left			
N Wrist Joint, Right			
P Wrist Joint, Left			
Q Carpal Joint, Right			
R Carpal Joint, Left			
S Metacarpocarpal Joint, Right			
T Metacarpocarpal Joint, Left			
U Metacarpophalangeal Joint, Right			
V Metacarpophalangeal Joint, Left			
W Finger Phalangeal Joint, Right			
X Finger Phalangeal Joint, Left			

Ø: M/S

R: UPPER JOINTS

T: RESECTION

SECTION: Ø MEDICAL AND SURGICAL
BODY SYSTEM: R UPPER JOINTS
OPERATION: U SUPPLEMENT: Putting in or on biological or synthetic material that physically reinforces and/or augments the function of a portion of a body part

Body Part	Approach	Device	Qualifier
Ø Occipital-cervical Joint	Ø Open	7 Autologous Tissue Substitute	Z No Qualifier
1 Cervical Vertebral Joint	3 Percutaneous	J Synthetic Substitute	
3 Cervical Vertebral Disc	4 Percutaneous Endoscopic	K Nonautologous Tissue	
4 Cervicothoracic Vertebral Joint		Substitute	
5 Cervicothoracic Vertebral Disc			
6 Thoracic Vertebral Joint			
9 Thoracic Vertebral Disc			
A Thoracolumbar Vertebral Joint			
B Thoracolumbar Vertebral Disc			
C Temporomandibular Joint, Right			
D Temporomandibular Joint, Left			
E Sternoclavicular Joint, Right ◔			
F Sternoclavicular Joint, Left ◔			
G Acromioclavicular Joint, Right ◔			
H Acromioclavicular Joint, Left ◔			
J Shoulder Joint, Right ◔			
K Shoulder Joint, Left ◔			
L Elbow Joint, Right ◔			
M Elbow Joint, Left ◔			
N Wrist Joint, Right			
P Wrist Joint, Left			
Q Carpal Joint, Right			
R Carpal Joint, Left			
S Metacarpocarpal Joint, Right			
T Metacarpocarpal Joint, Left			
U Metacarpophalangeal Joint, Right			
V Metacarpophalangeal Joint, Left			
W Finger Phalangeal Joint, Right			
X Finger Phalangeal Joint, Left			

◔ ØRU[EFGHJKLM][Ø34][7JK]Z when reported with Secondary Diagnosis K68.11, T81.4XXA, or T84.6ØXA-T84.7XXA

Coding Clinic: 2Ø15, Q3, P27 – ØRUTØ7Z

SECTION: Ø MEDICAL AND SURGICAL

BODY SYSTEM: R UPPER JOINTS

OPERATION: W REVISION: Correcting, to the extent possible, a portion of a malfunctioning device or the position of a displaced device

Body Part	Approach	Device	Qualifier
Ø Occipital-cervical Joint 1 Cervical Vertebral Joint 4 Cervicothoracic Vertebral Joint 6 Thoracic Vertebral Joint A Thoracolumbar Vertebral Joint	Ø Open 3 Percutaneous 4 Percutaneous Endoscopic X External	Ø Drainage Device 3 Infusion Device 4 Internal Fixation Device 7 Autologous Tissue Substitute 8 Spacer A Interbody Fusion Device J Synthetic Substitute K Nonautologous Tissue Substitute	Z No Qualifier
3 Cervical Vertebral Disc 5 Cervicothoracic Vertebral Disc 9 Thoracic Vertebral Disc B Thoracolumbar Vertebral Disc	Ø Open 3 Percutaneous 4 Percutaneous Endoscopic X External	Ø Drainage Device 3 Infusion Device 7 Autologous Tissue Substitute J Synthetic Substitute K Nonautologous Tissue Substitute	Z No Qualifier
C Temporomandibular Joint, Right D Temporomandibular Joint, Left E Sternoclavicular Joint, Right F Sternoclavicular Joint, Left G Acromioclavicular Joint, Right H Acromioclavicular Joint, Left J Shoulder Joint, Right K Shoulder Joint, Left	Ø Open 3 Percutaneous 4 Percutaneous Endoscopic X External	Ø Drainage Device 3 Infusion Device 4 Internal Fixation Device 7 Autologous Tissue Substitute 8 Spacer J Synthetic Substitute K Nonautologous Tissue Substitute	Z No Qualifier
L Elbow Joint, Right M Elbow Joint, Left N Wrist Joint, Right P Wrist Joint, Left Q Carpal Joint, Right R Carpal Joint, Left S Metacarpocarpal Joint, Right T Metacarpocarpal Joint, Left U Metacarpophalangeal Joint, Right V Metacarpophalangeal Joint, Left W Finger Phalangeal Joint, Right X Finger Phalangeal Joint, Left	Ø Open 3 Percutaneous 4 Percutaneous Endoscopic X External	Ø Drainage Device 3 Infusion Device 4 Internal Fixation Device 5 External Fixation Device 7 Autologous Tissue Substitute 8 Spacer J Synthetic Substitute K Nonautologous Tissue Substitute	Z No Qualifier

Non-OR ØRW[Ø146A]X[Ø3478AJK]Z
Non-OR ØRW[359B]X[Ø37JK]Z
Non-OR ØRW[CDEFGHJK]X[Ø3478JK]Z
Non-OR ØRW[LMNPQRSTUVWX]X[Ø34578JK]Z

New/Revised Text in Green ~~deleted~~ Deleted ♀ Females Only ♂ Males Only **Coding Clinic**
🐾 Non-covered 🐾 Limited Coverage ⊡ Combination (See Appendix E) DRG Non-OR Non-OR 🐾 Hospital-Acquired Condition

SECTION:　0　MEDICAL AND SURGICAL

BODY SYSTEM: S LOWER JOINTS

OPERATION:　2　CHANGE: Taking out or off a device from a body part and putting back an identical or similar device in or on the same body part without cutting or puncturing the skin or a mucous membrane

Body Part	Approach	Device	Qualifier
Y Lower Joint	X External	Ø Drainage Device Y Other Device	Z No Qualifier

Non-OR　All Values

SECTION:　0　MEDICAL AND SURGICAL

BODY SYSTEM: S LOWER JOINTS

OPERATION:　5　DESTRUCTION: Physical eradication of all or a portion of a body part by the direct use of energy, force, or destructive agent

Body Part	Approach	Device	Qualifier
Ø Lumbar Vertebral Joint 2 Lumbar Vertebral Disc 3 Lumbosacral Joint 4 Lumbosacral Disc 5 Sacrococcygeal Joint 6 Coccygeal Joint 7 Sacroiliac Joint, Right 8 Sacroiliac Joint, Left 9 Hip Joint, Right B Hip Joint, Left C Knee Joint, Right D Knee Joint, Left F Ankle Joint, Right G Ankle Joint, Left H Tarsal Joint, Right J Tarsal Joint, Left K Metatarsal-Tarsal Joint, Right L Metatarsal-Tarsal Joint, Left M Metatarsal-Phalangeal Joint, Right N Metatarsal-Phalangeal Joint, Left P Toe Phalangeal Joint, Right Q Toe Phalangeal Joint, Left	Ø Open 3 Percutaneous 4 Percutaneous Endoscopic	Z No Device	Z No Qualifier

SECTION: Ø MEDICAL AND SURGICAL

BODY SYSTEM: S LOWER JOINTS

OPERATION: 9 DRAINAGE: Taking or letting out fluids and/or gases from a body part

Body Part	Approach	Device	Qualifier
Ø Lumbar Vertebral Joint 2 Lumbar Vertebral Disc 3 Lumbosacral Joint 4 Lumbosacral Disc 5 Sacrococcygeal Joint 6 Coccygeal Joint 7 Sacroiliac Joint, Right 8 Sacroiliac Joint, Left 9 Hip Joint, Right B Hip Joint, Left C Knee Joint, Right D Knee Joint, Left F Ankle Joint, Right G Ankle Joint, Left H Tarsal Joint, Right J Tarsal Joint, Left K Metatarsal-Tarsal Joint, Right L Metatarsal-Tarsal Joint, Left M Metatarsal-Phalangeal Joint, Right N Metatarsal-Phalangeal Joint, Left P Toe Phalangeal Joint, Right Q Toe Phalangeal Joint, Left	Ø Open 3 Percutaneous 4 Percutaneous Endoscopic	Ø Drainage Device	Z No Qualifier
Ø Lumbar Vertebral Joint 2 Lumbar Vertebral Disc 3 Lumbosacral Joint 4 Lumbosacral Disc 5 Sacrococcygeal Joint 6 Coccygeal Joint 7 Sacroiliac Joint, Right 8 Sacroiliac Joint, Left 9 Hip Joint, Right B Hip Joint, Left C Knee Joint, Right D Knee Joint, Left F Ankle Joint, Right G Ankle Joint, Left H Tarsal Joint, Right J Tarsal Joint, Left K Metatarsal-Tarsal Joint, Right L Metatarsal-Tarsal Joint, Left M Metatarsal-Phalangeal Joint, Right N Metatarsal-Phalangeal Joint, Left P Toe Phalangeal Joint, Right Q Toe Phalangeal Joint, Left	Ø Open 3 Percutaneous 4 Percutaneous Endoscopic	Z No Device	X Diagnostic Z No Qualifier

Non-OR ØS9[Ø23456789BCDFGHJKLMNPQ][34]ØZ
Non-OR ØS9[Ø23456789BCDFGHJKLMNPQ][Ø34]ZX
Non-OR ØS9[Ø23456789BCDFGHJKLMNPQ][34]ZZ

9: DRAINAGE

S: LOWER JOINTS

Ø: M/S

New/Revised Text in Green ~~deleted~~ Deleted ♀ Females Only ♂ Males Only **Coding Clinic**
🚫 Non-covered 🚫 Limited Coverage ⊞ Combination (See Appendix E) DRG Non-OR Non-OR 🚫 Hospital-Acquired Condition

SECTION: Ø MEDICAL AND SURGICAL

BODY SYSTEM: S LOWER JOINTS

OPERATION: B EXCISION: Cutting out or off, without replacement, a portion of a body part

Body Part	Approach	Device	Qualifier
Ø Lumbar Vertebral Joint 2 Lumbar Vertebral Disc 3 Lumbosacral Joint 4 Lumbosacral Disc 5 Sacrococcygeal Joint 6 Coccygeal Joint 7 Sacroiliac Joint, Right 8 Sacroiliac Joint, Left 9 Hip Joint, Right B Hip Joint, Left C Knee Joint, Right ⊞ D Knee Joint, Left ⊞ F Ankle Joint, Right G Ankle Joint, Left H Tarsal Joint, Right J Tarsal Joint, Left K Metatarsal-Tarsal Joint, Right L Metatarsal-Tarsal Joint, Left M Metatarsal-Phalangeal Joint, Right N Metatarsal-Phalangeal Joint, Left P Toe Phalangeal Joint, Right Q Toe Phalangeal Joint, Left	Ø Open 3 Percutaneous 4 Percutaneous Endoscopic	Z No Device	X Diagnostic Z No Qualifier

⊞ ØSB[CD][Ø34]ZZ
Non-OR ØSB[Ø23456789BCDFGHJKLMNPQ][Ø34]ZX

Coding Clinic: 2015, Q1, P34 – ØSBD4ZZ
Coding Clinic: 2016, Q2, P16 – ØSB2ØZZ

SECTION: Ø MEDICAL AND SURGICAL

BODY SYSTEM: S LOWER JOINTS

OPERATION: C EXTIRPATION: Taking or cutting out solid matter from a body part

Body Part	Approach	Device	Qualifier
Ø Lumbar Vertebral Joint 2 Lumbar Vertebral Disc 3 Lumbosacral Joint 4 Lumbosacral Disc 5 Sacrococcygeal Joint 6 Coccygeal Joint 7 Sacroiliac Joint, Right 8 Sacroiliac Joint, Left 9 Hip Joint, Right B Hip Joint, Left C Knee Joint, Right D Knee Joint, Left F Ankle Joint, Right G Ankle Joint, Left H Tarsal Joint, Right J Tarsal Joint, Left K Metatarsal-Tarsal Joint, Right L Metatarsal-Tarsal Joint, Left M Metatarsal-Phalangeal Joint, Right N Metatarsal-Phalangeal Joint, Left P Toe Phalangeal Joint, Right Q Toe Phalangeal Joint, Left	Ø Open 3 Percutaneous 4 Percutaneous Endoscopic	Z No Device	Z No Qualifier

New/Revised Text in Green   ~~deleted~~ Deleted   ♀ Females Only   ♂ Males Only   **Coding Clinic**
🔖 Non-covered   🔖 Limited Coverage   ⊞ Combination (See Appendix E)   DRG Non-OR   Non-OR   🔖 Hospital-Acquired Condition

SECTION: Ø MEDICAL AND SURGICAL

BODY SYSTEM: S LOWER JOINTS

OPERATION: G FUSION: Joining together portions of an articular body part, rendering the articular body part immobile

Body Part	Approach	Device	Qualifier
Ø Lumbar Vertebral Joint 🦰 1 Lumbar Vertebral Joints, 2 or more ⊞ 🦰 3 Lumbosacral Joint 🦰	Ø Open 3 Percutaneous 4 Percutaneous Endoscopic	7 Autologous Tissue Substitute A Interbody Fusion Device J Synthetic Substitute K Nonautologous Tissue Substitute Z No Device	Ø Anterior Approach, Anterior Column 1 Posterior Approach, Posterior Column J Posterior Approach, Anterior Column
5 Sacrococcygeal Joint 6 Coccygeal Joint 7 Sacroiliac Joint, Right 🦰 8 Sacroiliac Joint, Left 🦰	Ø Open 3 Percutaneous 4 Percutaneous Endoscopic	4 Internal Fixation Device 7 Autologous Tissue Substitute J Synthetic Substitute K Nonautologous Tissue Substitute Z No Device	Z No Qualifier
9 Hip Joint, Right B Hip Joint, Left C Knee Joint, Right D Knee Joint, Left F Ankle Joint, Right G Ankle Joint, Left H Tarsal Joint, Right J Tarsal Joint, Left K Metatarsal-Tarsal Joint, Right L Metatarsal-Tarsal Joint, Left M Metatarsal-Phalangeal Joint, Right ⊞ N Metatarsal-Phalangeal Joint, Left ⊞ P Toe Phalangeal Joint, Right Q Toe Phalangeal Joint, Left	Ø Open 3 Percutaneous 4 Percutaneous Endoscopic	4 Internal Fixation Device 5 External Fixation Device 7 Autologous Tissue Substitute J Synthetic Substitute K Nonautologous Tissue Substitute Z No Device	Z No Qualifier

⊞ ØSG1[Ø34][7AJKZ][Ø1J]

⊞ ØSG[MN][Ø34]ZZ

🦰 ØSG[Ø13][Ø34][7AJKZ][Ø1J] when reported with Secondary Diagnosis K68.11, T81.4XXA, or T84.6ØXA-T84.7XXA

🦰 ØSG[78][Ø34][47JKZ]Z when reported with Secondary Diagnosis K68.11, T81.4XXA, or T84.6ØXA-T84.7XXA

Coding Clinic: 2013, Q3, P26, Q1, P23 – ØSGØØ71

Coding Clinic: 2013, Q3, P26 – ØSGØØAJ

Coding Clinic: 2013, Q2, P4Ø – ØSGGØ4Z, ØSGGØ7Z

New/Revised Text in Green   ~~deleted~~ Deleted   ♀ Females Only   ♂ Males Only   **Coding Clinic**

🦰 Non-covered   🦰 Limited Coverage   ⊞ Combination (See Appendix E)   DRG Non-OR   Non-OR   🦰 Hospital-Acquired Condition

G: FUSION

S: LOWER JOINTS

Ø: M/S

SECTION: Ø MEDICAL AND SURGICAL

BODY SYSTEM: S LOWER JOINTS

OPERATION: H INSERTION: Putting in a nonbiological appliance that monitors, assists, performs, or prevents a physiological function but does not physically take the place of a body part

Body Part	Approach	Device	Qualifier
Ø Lumbar Vertebral Joint 3 Lumbosacral Joint	Ø Open 3 Percutaneous 4 Percutaneous Endoscopic	3 Infusion Device 4 Internal Fixation Device 8 Spacer B Spinal Stabilization Device, Interspinous Process C Spinal Stabilization Device, Pedicle-Based D Spinal Stabilization Device, Facet Replacement	Z No Qualifier
2 Lumbar Vertebral Disc 4 Lumbosacral Disc	Ø Open 3 Percutaneous 4 Percutaneous Endoscopic	3 Infusion Device 8 Spacer	Z No Qualifier
5 Sacrococcygeal Joint 6 Coccygeal Joint 7 Sacroiliac Joint, Right 8 Sacroiliac Joint, Left	Ø Open 3 Percutaneous 4 Percutaneous Endoscopic	3 Infusion Device 4 Internal Fixation Device 8 Spacer	Z No Qualifier
9 Hip Joint, Right B Hip Joint, Left C Knee Joint, Right D Knee Joint, Left F Ankle Joint, Right G Ankle Joint, Left H Tarsal Joint, Right J Tarsal Joint, Left K Metatarsal-Tarsal Joint, Right L Metatarsal-Tarsal Joint, Left M Metatarsal-Phalangeal Joint, Right N Metatarsal-Phalangeal Joint, Left P Toe Phalangeal Joint, Right Q Toe Phalangeal Joint, Left	Ø Open 3 Percutaneous 4 Percutaneous Endoscopic	3 Infusion Device 4 Internal Fixation Device 5 External Fixation Device 8 Spacer	Z No Qualifier

DRG Non-OR   ØSH[Ø3][34]3Z
DRG Non-OR   ØSH[24][34]3Z
DRG Non-OR   ØSH[5678][34]3Z
DRG Non-OR   ØSH[9BCDFGHJKLMNPQ][34]3Z
Non-OR   ØSH[Ø3]Ø3Z
Non-OR   ØSH[Ø3][Ø34]8Z
Non-OR   ØSH[24]Ø3Z
Non-OR   ØSH[24][Ø34]8Z
Non-OR   ØSH[5678]Ø3Z
Non-OR   ØSH[5678][Ø34]8Z
Non-OR   ØSH[9BCDFGHJKLMNPQ]Ø3Z
Non-OR   ØSH[9BCDFGHJKLMNPQ][Ø34]8Z

Ø: M/S

S: LOWER JOINTS

H: INSERTION

SECTION: Ø MEDICAL AND SURGICAL

BODY SYSTEM: S LOWER JOINTS
OPERATION: J INSPECTION: Visually and/or manually exploring a body part

Body Part	Approach	Device	Qualifier
Ø Lumbar Vertebral Joint 2 Lumbar Vertebral Disc 3 Lumbosacral Joint 4 Lumbosacral Disc 5 Sacrococcygeal Joint 6 Coccygeal Joint 7 Sacroiliac Joint, Right 8 Sacroiliac Joint, Left 9 Hip Joint, Right B Hip Joint, Left C Knee Joint, Right D Knee Joint, Left F Ankle Joint, Right G Ankle Joint, Left H Tarsal Joint, Right J Tarsal Joint, Left K Metatarsal-Tarsal Joint, Right L Metatarsal-Tarsal Joint, Left M Metatarsal-Phalangeal Joint, Right N Metatarsal-Phalangeal Joint, Left P Toe Phalangeal Joint, Right Q Toe Phalangeal Joint, Left	Ø Open 3 Percutaneous 4 Percutaneous Endoscopic X External	Z No Device	Z No Qualifier

DRG Non-OR ØSJ[Ø23456789BCDFGHJKLMNPQ]3ZZ
Non-OR ØSJ[Ø23456789BCDFGHJKLMNPQ]XZZ

SECTION: Ø MEDICAL AND SURGICAL

BODY SYSTEM: S LOWER JOINTS
OPERATION: N RELEASE: Freeing a body part from an abnormal physical constraint by cutting or by the use of force

Body Part	Approach	Device	Qualifier
Ø Lumbar Vertebral Joint 2 Lumbar Vertebral Disc 3 Lumbosacral Joint 4 Lumbosacral Disc 5 Sacrococcygeal Joint 6 Coccygeal Joint 7 Sacroiliac Joint, Right 8 Sacroiliac Joint, Left 9 Hip Joint, Right B Hip Joint, Left C Knee Joint, Right D Knee Joint, Left F Ankle Joint, Right G Ankle Joint, Left H Tarsal Joint, Right J Tarsal Joint, Left K Metatarsal-Tarsal Joint, Right L Metatarsal-Tarsal Joint, Left M Metatarsal-Phalangeal Joint, Right N Metatarsal-Phalangeal Joint, Left P Toe Phalangeal Joint, Right Q Toe Phalangeal Joint, Left	Ø Open 3 Percutaneous 4 Percutaneous Endoscopic X External	Z No Device	Z No Qualifier

Non-OR ØSN[Ø23456789BCDFGHJKLMNPQ]XZZ

J: INSPECTION N: RELEASE
S: LOWER JOINTS
Ø: M/S

SECTION: Ø MEDICAL AND SURGICAL
BODY SYSTEM: S LOWER JOINTS
OPERATION: P REMOVAL: *(on multiple pages)*
Taking out or off a device from a body part

Body Part	Approach	Device	Qualifier
Ø Lumbar Vertebral Joint 3 Lumbosacral Joint	Ø Open 3 Percutaneous 4 Percutaneous Endoscopic	Ø Drainage Device 3 Infusion Device 4 Internal Fixation Device 7 Autologous Tissue Substitute 8 Spacer A Interbody Fusion Device J Synthetic Substitute K Nonautologous Tissue Substitute	Z No Qualifier
Ø Lumbar Vertebral Joint 3 Lumbosacral Joint	X External	Ø Drainage Device 3 Infusion Device 4 Internal Fixation Device	Z No Qualifier
2 Lumbar Vertebral Disc 4 Lumbosacral Disc	Ø Open 3 Percutaneous 4 Percutaneous Endoscopic	Ø Drainage Device 3 Infusion Device 7 Autologous Tissue Substitute J Synthetic Substitute K Nonautologous Tissue Substitute	Z No Qualifier
2 Lumbar Vertebral Disc 4 Lumbosacral Disc	X External	Ø Drainage Device 3 Infusion Device	Z No Qualifier
5 Sacrococcygeal Joint 6 Coccygeal Joint 7 Sacroiliac Joint, Right 8 Sacroiliac Joint, Left	Ø Open 3 Percutaneous 4 Percutaneous Endoscopic	Ø Drainage Device 3 Infusion Device 4 Internal Fixation Device 7 Autologous Tissue Substitute 8 Spacer J Synthetic Substitute K Nonautologous Tissue Substitute	Z No Qualifier
5 Sacrococcygeal Joint 6 Coccygeal Joint 7 Sacroiliac Joint, Right 8 Sacroiliac Joint, Left	X External	Ø Drainage Device 3 Infusion Device 4 Internal Fixation Device	Z No Qualifier
9 Hip Joint, Right ⊞ B Hip Joint, Left ⊞	Ø Open	Ø Drainage Device 3 Infusion Device 4 Internal Fixation Device 5 External Fixation Device 7 Autologous Tissue Substitute 8 Spacer 9 Liner B Resurfacing Device J Synthetic Substitute K Nonautologous Tissue Substitute	Z No Qualifier
9 Hip Joint, Right ⊞ B Hip Joint, Left ⊞	3 Percutaneous 4 Percutaneous Endoscopic	Ø Drainage Device 3 Infusion Device 4 Internal Fixation Device 5 External Fixation Device 7 Autologous Tissue Substitute 8 Spacer J Synthetic Substitute K Nonautologous Tissue Substitute	Z No Qualifier

⊞ ØSP[9B]Ø[89BJ]Z
⊞ ØSP[9B]4[8J]Z
DRG Non-OR ØSP[Ø3]3[Ø3]Z
DRG Non-OR ØSP[24]3[Ø3]Z
DRG Non-OR ØSP[5678]3[Ø3]Z

DRG Non-OR ØSP[9B]Ø8Z
DRG Non-OR ØSP[9B]3[Ø3]Z
DRG Non-OR ØSP[9B]48Z
Non-OR ØSP[Ø3][Ø34]8Z
Non-OR ØSP[Ø3]X[Ø34]Z

Non-OR ØSP[24]X[Ø3]Z
Non-OR ØSP[5678][Ø34]8Z
Non-OR ØSP[5678]X[Ø34]Z
Non-OR ØSP[9B]38Z

Coding Clinic: 2Ø15, Q2, P2Ø – ØSP9Ø9Z

SECTION: Ø MEDICAL AND SURGICAL
BODY SYSTEM: S LOWER JOINTS
OPERATION: P REMOVAL: *(continued)*
Taking out or off a device from a body part

Body Part	Approach	Device	Qualifier
9 Hip Joint, Right B Hip Joint, Left	X External	Ø Drainage Device 3 Infusion Device 4 Internal Fixation Device 5 External Fixation Device	Z No Qualifier
A Hip Joint, Acetabular Surface, Right E Hip Joint, Acetabular Surface, Left R Hip Joint, Femoral Surface, Right S Hip Joint, Femoral Surface, Left T Knee Joint, Femoral Surface, Right U Knee Joint, Femoral Surface, Left V Knee Joint, Tibial Surface, Right W Knee Joint, Tibial Surface, Left	Ø Open 3 Percutaneous 4 Percutaneous Endoscopic	J Synthetic Substitute	Z No Qualifier
C Knee Joint, Right ⊕ D Knee Joint, Left ⊕	Ø Open	Ø Drainage Device 3 Infusion Device 4 Internal Fixation Device 5 External Fixation Device 7 Autologous Tissue Substitute 8 Spacer 9 Liner J Synthetic Substitute K Nonautologous Tissue Substitute	Z No Qualifier
C Knee Joint, Right D Knee Joint, Left	Ø Open	J Synthetic Substitute	C Patellar Surface Z No Qualifier
C Knee Joint, Right ⊕ D Knee Joint, Left ⊕	3 Percutaneous 4 Percutaneous Endoscopic	Ø Drainage Device 3 Infusion Device 4 Internal Fixation Device 5 External Fixation Device 7 Autologous Tissue Substitute 8 Spacer J Synthetic Substitute K Nonautologous Tissue Substitute	Z No Qualifier
C Knee Joint, Right D Knee Joint, Left	3 Percutaneous 4 Percutaneous Endoscopic	J Synthetic Substitute	C Patellar Surface Z No Qualifier
C Knee Joint, Right D Knee Joint, Left	X External	Ø Drainage Device 3 Infusion Device 4 Internal Fixation Device 5 External Fixation Device	Z No Qualifier

⊕ ØSP[CD]Ø[9J]Z
⊕ ØSP[CD]4JZ
DRG Non-OR ØSP[CD]3[Ø3]Z

Non-OR ØSP[9B]X[Ø345]Z
Non-OR ØSP[CD]Ø8Z
Non-OR ØSP[CD][34]8Z
Non-OR ØSP[CD]X[Ø345]Z

Coding Clinic: 2Ø15, Q2, P18 – ØSPCØJZ
Coding Clinic: 2Ø15, Q2, P2Ø – ØSP9ØJZ

New/Revised Text in Green   ~~deleted~~ Deleted   ♀ Females Only   ♂ Males Only   **Coding Clinic**
🚫 Non-covered   🚫 Limited Coverage   ⊕ Combination (See Appendix E)   DRG Non-OR   Non-OR   🚫 Hospital-Acquired Condition

SECTION: Ø MEDICAL AND SURGICAL
BODY SYSTEM: S LOWER JOINTS
OPERATION: P REMOVAL: *(continued)*
Taking out or off a device from a body part

Body Part	Approach	Device	Qualifier
F Ankle Joint, Right G Ankle Joint, Left H Tarsal Joint, Right J Tarsal Joint, Left K Metatarsal-Tarsal Joint, Right L Metatarsal-Tarsal Joint, Left M Metatarsal-Phalangeal Joint, Right N Metatarsal-Phalangeal Joint, Left P Toe Phalangeal Joint, Right Q Toe Phalangeal Joint, Left	Ø Open 3 Percutaneous 4 Percutaneous Endoscopic	Ø Drainage Device 3 Infusion Device 4 Internal Fixation Device 5 External Fixation Device 7 Autologous Tissue Substitute 8 Spacer J Synthetic Substitute K Nonautologous Tissue Substitute	Z No Qualifier
F Ankle Joint, Right G Ankle Joint, Left H Tarsal Joint, Right J Tarsal Joint, Left K Metatarsal-Tarsal Joint, Right L Metatarsal-Tarsal Joint, Left M Metatarsal-Phalangeal Joint, Right N Metatarsal-Phalangeal Joint, Left P Toe Phalangeal Joint, Right Q Toe Phalangeal Joint, Left	X External	Ø Drainage Device 3 Infusion Device 4 Internal Fixation Device 5 External Fixation Device	Z No Qualifier

DRG Non-OR   ØSP[FGHJKLMNPQ]3[Ø3]Z
Non-OR   ØSP[FGHJKLMNPQ][Ø34]8Z
Non-OR   ØSP[FGHJKLMNPQ]X[Ø345]Z

Coding Clinic: 2Ø13, Q2, P4Ø – ØSPGØ4Z

New/Revised Text in Green   ~~deleted~~ Deleted   ♀ Females Only   ♂ Males Only   **Coding Clinic**
Non-covered   Limited Coverage   Combination (See Appendix E)   DRG Non-OR   Non-OR   Hospital-Acquired Condition

Ø: M/S   S: LOWER JOINTS   P: REMOVAL

413

SECTION: Ø MEDICAL AND SURGICAL

BODY SYSTEM: S LOWER JOINTS

OPERATION: Q **REPAIR:** Restoring, to the extent possible, a body part to its normal anatomic structure and function

Body Part	Approach	Device	Qualifier
Ø Lumbar Vertebral Joint 2 Lumbar Vertebral Disc 3 Lumbosacral Joint 4 Lumbosacral Disc 5 Sacrococcygeal Joint 6 Coccygeal Joint 7 Sacroiliac Joint, Right 8 Sacroiliac Joint, Left 9 Hip Joint, Right B Hip Joint, Left C Knee Joint, Right D Knee Joint, Left F Ankle Joint, Right G Ankle Joint, Left H Tarsal Joint, Right J Tarsal Joint, Left K Metatarsal-Tarsal Joint, Right L Metatarsal-Tarsal Joint, Left M Metatarsal-Phalangeal Joint, Right N Metatarsal-Phalangeal Joint, Left P Toe Phalangeal Joint, Right Q Toe Phalangeal Joint, Left	Ø Open 3 Percutaneous 4 Percutaneous Endoscopic X External	Z No Device	Z No Qualifier

SECTION: Ø MEDICAL AND SURGICAL
BODY SYSTEM: S LOWER JOINTS
OPERATION: R REPLACEMENT: *(on multiple pages)*
Putting in or on biological or synthetic material that physically takes the place and/or function of all or a portion of a body part

Body Part	Approach	Device	Qualifier
Ø Lumbar Vertebral Joint 2 Lumbar Vertebral Disc 🜲 3 Lumbosacral Joint 4 Lumbosacral Disc 🜲 5 Sacrococcygeal Joint 6 Coccygeal Joint 7 Sacroiliac Joint, Right 8 Sacroiliac Joint, Left H Tarsal Joint, Right J Tarsal Joint, Left K Metatarsal-Tarsal Joint, Right L Metatarsal-Tarsal Joint, Left M Metatarsal-Phalangeal Joint, Right N Metatarsal-Phalangeal Joint, Left P Toe Phalangeal Joint, Right Q Toe Phalangeal Joint, Left	Ø Open	7 Autologous Tissue Substitute J Synthetic Substitute K Nonautologous Tissue Substitute	Z No Qualifier
9 Hip Joint, Right ⊞ 🜲 B Hip Joint, Left ⊞ 🜲	Ø Open	1 Synthetic Substitute, Metal 2 Synthetic Substitute, Metal on Polyethylene 3 Synthetic Substitute, Ceramic 4 Synthetic Substitute, Ceramic on Polyethylene J Synthetic Substitute	9 Cemented A Uncemented Z No Qualifier
9 Hip Joint, Right 🜲 B Hip Joint, Left 🜲	Ø Open	7 Autologous Tissue Substitute K Nonautologous Tissue Substitute	Z No Qualifier
A Hip Joint, Acetabular Surface, Right ⊞ 🜲 E Hip Joint, Acetabular Surface, Left ⊞ 🜲	Ø Open	Ø Synthetic Substitute, Polyethylene 1 Synthetic Substitute, Metal 3 Synthetic Substitute, Ceramic J Synthetic Substitute	9 Cemented A Uncemented Z No Qualifier
A Hip Joint, Acetabular Surface, Right 🜲 E Hip Joint, Acetabular Surface, Left 🜲	Ø Open	7 Autologous Tissue Substitute K Nonautologous Tissue Substitute	Z No Qualifier

🜲 ØSR[24]Ø[7JK]Z when the beneficiary is over age 6Ø
🜲 ØSR[24]ØJZ when beneficiary is over age 6Ø
⊞ ØSR[9B]Ø[1234J][9AZ]
⊞ ØSR[AE]Ø[Ø13J][9AZ]
🜲 ØSR[9B]Ø[1234J][9AZ] when reported with Secondary Diagnosis from I26.Ø2-I26.Ø9, I26.92-I26.99, or I82.4Ø1-I82.4Z9

🜲 ØSR[9B]Ø[7K]Z when reported with Secondary Diagnosis from I26.Ø2-I26.Ø9, I26.92-I26.99, or I82.4Ø1-I82.4Z9
🜲 ØSR[AE]Ø[Ø13J][9AZ] when reported with Secondary Diagnosis from I26.Ø2-I26.Ø9, I26.92-I26.99, or I82.4Ø1-I82.4Z9
🜲 ØSR[AE]Ø[7K]Z when reported with Secondary Diagnosis from I26.Ø2-I26.Ø9, I26.92-I26.99, or I82.4Ø1-I82.4Z9

SECTION: Ø MEDICAL AND SURGICAL

BODY SYSTEM: S LOWER JOINTS

OPERATION: R REPLACEMENT: *(continued)*
Putting in or on biological or synthetic material that physically takes the place and/or function of all or a portion of a body part

Body Part	Approach	Device	Qualifier
C Knee Joint, Right 🐾 D Knee Joint, Left 🐾	Ø Open	7 Autologous Tissue Substitute K Nonautologous Tissue Substitute	Z No Qualifier
C Knee Joint, Right ⊞ 🐾 D Knee Joint, Left ⊞ 🐾	Ø Open	J Synthetic Substitute L Synthetic Substitute, Unicondylar	9 Cemented A Uncemented Z No Qualifier
F Ankle Joint, Right G Ankle Joint, Left T Knee Joint, Femoral Surface, Right 🐾 U Knee Joint, Femoral Surface, Left 🐾 V Knee Joint, Tibial Surface, Right 🐾 W Knee Joint, Tibial Surface, Left 🐾	Ø Open	7 Autologous Tissue Substitute K Nonautologous Tissue Substitute	Z No Qualifier
F Ankle Joint, Right G Ankle Joint, Left T Knee Joint, Femoral Surface, Right ⊞ 🐾 U Knee Joint, Femoral Surface, Left ⊞ 🐾 V Knee Joint, Tibial Surface, Right ⊞ 🐾 W Knee Joint, Tibial Surface, Left ⊞ 🐾	Ø Open	J Synthetic Substitute	9 Cemented A Uncemented Z No Qualifier
R Hip Joint, Femoral Surface, Right ⊞ 🐾 S Hip Joint, Femoral Surface, Left ⊞ 🐾	Ø Open	1 Synthetic Substitute, Metal 3 Synthetic Substitute, Ceramic J Synthetic Substitute	9 Cemented A Uncemented Z No Qualifier
R Hip Joint, Femoral Surface, Right 🐾 S Hip Joint, Femoral Surface, Left 🐾	Ø Open	7 Autologous Tissue Substitute K Nonautologous Tissue Substitute	Z No Qualifier

⊞ ØSR[CDTUVW]ØJ[9AZ]

⊞ ØSR[RS]Ø[13J][9AZ]

🐾 ØSR[CD]Ø[7K]Z when reported with Secondary Diagnosis from I26.Ø2-I26.Ø9, I26.92-I26.99, or I82.4Ø1-I82.4Z9

🐾 ØSR[TUVW]Ø[7K]Z when reported with Secondary Diagnosis from I26.Ø2-I26.Ø9, I26.92-I26.99, or I82.4Ø1-I82.4Z9

🐾 ØSR[CD]ØJ[9AZ] when reported with Secondary Diagnosis from I26.Ø2-I26.Ø9, I26.92-I26.99, or I82.4Ø1-I82.4Z9

🐾 ØSR[TUVW]ØJ[9AZ] when reported with Secondary Diagnosis from I26.Ø2-I26.Ø9, I26.92-I26.99, or I82.4Ø1-I82.4Z9

🐾 ØSR[RS]Ø[13J][9AZ] when reported with Secondary Diagnosis from I26.Ø2-I26.Ø9, I26.92-I26.99, or I82.4Ø1-I82.4Z9

🐾 ØSR[RS]Ø[7K]Z when reported with Secondary Diagnosis from I26.Ø2-I26.Ø9, I26.92-I26.99, or I82.4Ø1-I82.4Z9

Coding Clinic: 2015, Q2, P18 – ØSRCØJ9

Coding Clinic: 2015, Q2, P2Ø – ØSRRØ3A

Coding Clinic: 2015, Q3, P19 – ØSRBØJ9

New/Revised Text in Green   ~~deleted~~ Deleted   ♀ Females Only   ♂ Males Only   **Coding Clinic**

🐾 Non-covered   🐾 Limited Coverage   ⊞ Combination (See Appendix E)   DRG Non-OR   Non-OR   🐾 Hospital-Acquired Condition

R: REPLACEMENT

S: LOWER JOINTS

Ø: M/S

SECTION: Ø   MEDICAL AND SURGICAL

BODY SYSTEM: S   LOWER JOINTS

OPERATION: **S   REPOSITION:** Moving to its normal location, or other suitable location, all or a portion of a body part

Body Part	Approach	Device	Qualifier
Ø Lumbar Vertebral Joint 3 Lumbosacral Joint 5 Sacrococcygeal Joint 6 Coccygeal Joint 7 Sacroiliac Joint, Right 8 Sacroiliac Joint, Left	Ø Open 3 Percutaneous 4 Percutaneous Endoscopic X External	4 Internal Fixation Device Z No Device	Z No Qualifier
9 Hip Joint, Right B Hip Joint, Left C Knee Joint, Right D Knee Joint, Left F Ankle Joint, Right G Ankle Joint, Left H Tarsal Joint, Right J Tarsal Joint, Left K Metatarsal-Tarsal Joint, Right L Metatarsal-Tarsal Joint, Left M Metatarsal-Phalangeal Joint, Right N Metatarsal-Phalangeal Joint, Left P Toe Phalangeal Joint, Right Q Toe Phalangeal Joint, Left	Ø Open 3 Percutaneous 4 Percutaneous Endoscopic X External	4 Internal Fixation Device 5 External Fixation Device Z No Device	Z No Qualifier

Non-OR   ØSS[Ø35678][34X][4Z]Z
Non-OR   ØSS[9BCDFGHJKLMNPQ][34X][45Z]Z

Coding Clinic: 2Ø16, Q2, P32 – ØSSBØ4Z

SECTION: Ø   MEDICAL AND SURGICAL

BODY SYSTEM: S   LOWER JOINTS

OPERATION: **T   RESECTION:** Cutting out or off, without replacement, all of a body part

Body Part	Approach	Device	Qualifier
2 Lumbar Vertebral Disc 4 Lumbosacral Disc 5 Sacrococcygeal Joint 6 Coccygeal Joint 7 Sacroiliac Joint, Right 8 Sacroiliac Joint, Left 9 Hip Joint, Right B Hip Joint, Left C Knee Joint, Right D Knee Joint, Left F Ankle Joint, Right G Ankle Joint, Left H Tarsal Joint, Right J Tarsal Joint, Left K Metatarsal-Tarsal Joint, Right L Metatarsal-Tarsal Joint, Left M Metatarsal-Phalangeal Joint, Right N Metatarsal-Phalangeal Joint, Left P Toe Phalangeal Joint, Right Q Toe Phalangeal Joint, Left	Ø Open	Z No Device	Z No Qualifier

Coding Clinic: 2Ø16, Q1, P2Ø – ØSTMØZZ

Ø: M/S   S: LOWER JOINTS   S: REPOSITION   T: RESECTION

SECTION: Ø MEDICAL AND SURGICAL

BODY SYSTEM: S LOWER JOINTS

OPERATION: U SUPPLEMENT: Putting in or on biological or synthetic material that physically reinforces and/or augments the function of a portion of a body part

Body Part	Approach	Device	Qualifier
2 Lumbar Vertebral Joint 4 Lumbosacral Disc 5 Sacrococcygeal Joint 6 Coccygeal Joint 7 Sacroiliac Joint, Right 8 Sacroiliac Joint, Left F Ankle Joint, Right G Ankle Joint, Left H Tarsal Joint, Right J Tarsal Joint, Left K Metatarsal-Tarsal Joint, Right L Metatarsal-Tarsal Joint, Left M Metatarsal-Phalangeal Joint, Right N Metatarsal-Phalangeal Joint, Left P Toe Phalangeal Joint, Right Q Toe Phalangeal Joint, Left	Ø Open 3 Percutaneous 4 Percutaneous Endoscopic	7 Autologous Tissue Substitute J Synthetic Substitute K Nonautologous Tissue Substitute	Z No Qualifier
9 Hip Joint, Right ⊞ ◔ B Hip Joint, Left ⊞ ◔	Ø Open	7 Autologous Tissue Substitute 9 Liner B Resurfacing Device J Synthetic Substitute K Nonautologous Tissue Substitute	Z No Qualifier
9 Hip Joint, Right B Hip Joint, Left	3 Percutaneous 4 Percutaneous Endoscopic	7 Autologous Tissue Substitute J Synthetic Substitute K Nonautologous Tissue Substitute	Z No Qualifier
A Hip Joint, Acetabular Surface, Right ⊞ ◔ E Hip Joint, Acetabular Surface, Left ⊞ ◔ R Hip Joint, Femoral Surface, Right ⊞ ◔ S Hip Joint, Femoral Surface, Left ⊞ ◔	Ø Open	9 Liner B Resurfacing Device	Z No Qualifier
C Knee Joint, Right ⊞ D Knee Joint, Left ⊞	Ø Open	7 Autologous Tissue Substitute J Synthetic Substitute K Nonautologous Tissue Substitute	Z No Qualifier
C Knee Joint, Right ⊞ D Knee Joint, Left ⊞	Ø Open	9 Liner	C Patellar Surface Z No Qualifier
C Knee Joint, Right ⊞ D Knee Joint, Left ⊞	3 Percutaneous 4 Percutaneous Endoscopic	7 Autologous Tissue Substitute J Synthetic Substitute K Nonautologous Tissue Substitute	Z No Qualifier
T Knee Joint, Femoral Surface, Right ⊞ U Knee Joint, Femoral Surface, Left ⊞ V Knee Joint, Tibial Surface, Right ⊞ W Knee Joint, Tibial Surface, Left ⊞	Ø Open	9 Liner	Z No Qualifier

⊞ ØSU[9B]Ø9Z

⊞ ØSU[AERS]Ø9Z

⊞ ØSU[CD]ØJZ

⊞ ØSUCØ9Z

⊞ ØSUDØ9C

⊞ ØSU[CD]4JZ

⊞ ØSU[TUVW]Ø9Z

◔ ØSU[9B]ØBZ when reported with Secondary Diagnosis from I26.Ø2-I26.Ø9, I26.92-I26.99, or I82.4Ø1-I82.4Z9

◔ ØSU[AERS]ØBZ when reported with Secondary Diagnosis from I26.Ø2-I26.Ø9, I26.92-I26.99, or I82.4Ø1-I82.4Z9

Coding Clinic: 2Ø15, Q2, P2Ø – ØSUAØ9Z

SECTION: Ø MEDICAL AND SURGICAL
BODY SYSTEM: S LOWER JOINTS
OPERATION: W REVISION: *(on multiple pages)*
Correcting, to the extent possible, a portion of a malfunctioning device or the position of a displaced device

Body Part	Approach	Device	Qualifier
Ø Lumbar Vertebral Joint 3 Lumbosacral Joint	Ø Open 3 Percutaneous 4 Percutaneous Endoscopic X External	Ø Drainage Device 3 Infusion Device 4 Internal Fixation Device 7 Autologous Tissue Substitute 8 Spacer A Interbody Fusion Device J Synthetic Substitute K Nonautologous Tissue Substitute	Z No Qualifier
2 Lumbar Vertebral Disc 4 Lumbosacral Disc	Ø Open 3 Percutaneous 4 Percutaneous Endoscopic X External	Ø Drainage Device 3 Infusion Device 7 Autologous Tissue Substitute J Synthetic Substitute K Nonautologous Tissue Substitute	Z No Qualifier
5 Sacrococcygeal Joint 6 Coccygeal Joint 7 Sacroiliac Joint, Right 8 Sacroiliac Joint, Left	Ø Open 3 Percutaneous 4 Percutaneous Endoscopic X External	Ø Drainage Device 3 Infusion Device 4 Internal Fixation Device 7 Autologous Tissue Substitute 8 Spacer J Synthetic Substitute K Nonautologous Tissue Substitute	Z No Qualifier
9 Hip Joint, Right B Hip Joint, Left	Ø Open	Ø Drainage Device 3 Infusion Device 4 Internal Fixation Device 5 External Fixation Device 7 Autologous Tissue Substitute 8 Spacer 9 Liner B Resurfacing Device J Synthetic Substitute K Nonautologous Tissue Substitute	Z No Qualifier
9 Hip Joint, Right B Hip Joint, Left	3 Percutaneous 4 Percutaneous Endoscopic X External	Ø Drainage Device 3 Infusion Device 4 Internal Fixation Device 5 External Fixation Device 7 Autologous Tissue Substitute 8 Spacer J Synthetic Substitute K Nonautologous Tissue Substitute	Z No Qualifier

Non-OR ØSW[Ø3]X[Ø3478AJK]Z
Non-OR ØSW[24]X[Ø37JK]Z
Non-OR ØSW[5678]X[Ø3478JK]Z
Non-OR ØSW[9B]X[Ø34578JK]Z

Ø: M/S

S: LOWER JOINTS

W: REVISION

New/Revised Text in Green   ~~deleted~~ Deleted   ♀ Females Only   ♂ Males Only   **Coding Clinic**
Non-covered   Limited Coverage   ⊞ Combination (See Appendix E)   DRG Non-OR   Non-OR   Hospital-Acquired Condition

SECTION: Ø MEDICAL AND SURGICAL
BODY SYSTEM: S LOWER JOINTS
OPERATION: W REVISION: *(continued)*
Correcting, to the extent possible, a portion of a malfunctioning device or the position of a displaced device

Body Part	Approach	Device	Qualifier
A Hip Joint, Acetabular Surface, Right E Hip Joint, Acetabular Surface, Left R Hip Joint, Femoral Surface, Right S Hip Joint, Femoral Surface, Left T Knee Joint, Femoral Surface, Right U Knee Joint, Femoral Surface, Left V Knee Joint, Tibial Surface, Right W Knee Joint, Tibial Surface, Left	Ø Open 3 Percutaneous 4 Percutaneous Endoscopic X External	J Synthetic Substitute	Z No Qualifier
C Knee Joint, Right D Knee Joint, Left	Ø Open	Ø Drainage Device 3 Infusion Device 4 Internal Fixation Device 5 External Fixation Device 7 Autologous Tissue Substitute 8 Spacer 9 Liner J Synthetic Substitute K Nonautologous Tissue Substitute	Z No Qualifier
C Knee Joint, Right D Knee Joint, Left	Ø Open	J Synthetic Substitute	C Patellar Surface Z No Qualifier
C Knee Joint, Right D Knee Joint, Left	3 Percutaneous 4 Percutaneous Endoscopic X External	Ø Drainage Device 3 Infusion Device 4 Internal Fixation Device 5 External Fixation Device 7 Autologous Tissue Substitute 8 Spacer J Synthetic Substitute K Nonautologous Tissue Substitute	Z No Qualifier
C Knee Joint, Right D Knee Joint, Left	3 Percutaneous 4 Percutaneous Endoscopic X External	J Synthetic Substitute	C Patellar Surface Z No Qualifier
F Ankle Joint, Right G Ankle Joint, Left H Tarsal Joint, Right J Tarsal Joint, Left K Metatarsal-Tarsal Joint, Right L Metatarsal-Tarsal Joint, Left M Metatarsal-Phalangeal Joint, Right N Metatarsal-Phalangeal Joint, Left P Toe Phalangeal Joint, Right Q Toe Phalangeal Joint, Left	Ø Open 3 Percutaneous 4 Percutaneous Endoscopic X External	Ø Drainage Device 3 Infusion Device 4 Internal Fixation Device 5 External Fixation Device 7 Autologous Tissue Substitute 8 Spacer J Synthetic Substitute K Nonautologous Tissue Substitute	Z No Qualifier

Non-OR ØSW[CD]X[Ø34578K]Z
Non-OR ØSW[CD]XJZ
Non-OR ØSW[FGHJKLMNPQ]X[Ø34578JK]Z

New/Revised Text in Green   ~~deleted~~ Deleted   ♀ Females Only   ♂ Males Only   **Coding Clinic**
🔹 Non-covered   🔹 Limited Coverage   ⊞ Combination (See Appendix E)   DRG Non-OR   Non-OR   🔹 Hospital-Acquired Condition

SECTION: Ø MEDICAL AND SURGICAL
BODY SYSTEM: T URINARY SYSTEM
OPERATION: 1 **BYPASS:** Altering the route of passage of the contents of a tubular body part

Body Part	Approach	Device	Qualifier
3 Kidney Pelvis, Right 4 Kidney Pelvis, Left	Ø Open 4 Percutaneous Endoscopic	7 Autologous Tissue Substitute J Synthetic Substitute K Nonautologous Tissue Substitute Z No Device	3 Kidney Pelvis, Right 4 Kidney Pelvis, Left 6 Ureter, Right 7 Ureter, Left 8 Colon 9 Colocutaneous A Ileum B Bladder C Ileocutaneous D Cutaneous
3 Kidney Pelvis, Right 4 Kidney Pelvis, Left	3 Percutaneous	J Synthetic Substitute	D Cutaneous
6 Ureter, Right 7 Ureter, Left 8 Ureters, Bilateral	Ø Open 4 Percutaneous Endoscopic	7 Autologous Tissue Substitute J Synthetic Substitute K Nonautologous Tissue Substitute Z No Device	6 Ureter, Right 7 Ureter, Left 8 Colon 9 Colocutaneous A Ileum B Bladder C Ileocutaneous D Cutaneous
6 Ureter, Right 7 Ureter, Left 8 Ureters, Bilateral	3 Percutaneous	J Synthetic Substitute	D Cutaneous
B Bladder	Ø Open 4 Percutaneous Endoscopic	7 Autologous Tissue Substitute J Synthetic Substitute K Nonautologous Tissue Substitute Z No Device	9 Colocutaneous C Ileocutaneous D Cutaneous
B Bladder	3 Percutaneous	J Synthetic Substitute	D Cutaneous

Coding Clinic: 2Ø15, Q3, P35 – ØT17ØZB

SECTION: Ø MEDICAL AND SURGICAL
BODY SYSTEM: T URINARY SYSTEM
OPERATION: 2 **CHANGE:** Taking out or off a device from a body part and putting back an identical or similar device in or on the same body part without cutting or puncturing the skin or a mucous membrane

Body Part	Approach	Device	Qualifier
5 Kidney 9 Ureter B Bladder D Urethra	X External	Ø Drainage Device Y Other Device	Z No Qualifier

Non-OR   All Values

SECTION: Ø MEDICAL AND SURGICAL

BODY SYSTEM: T URINARY SYSTEM

OPERATION: 5 DESTRUCTION: Physical eradication of all or a portion of a body part by the direct use of energy, force, or a destructive agent

Body Part	Approach	Device	Qualifier
Ø Kidney, Right 1 Kidney, Left 3 Kidney Pelvis, Right 4 Kidney Pelvis, Left 6 Ureter, Right 7 Ureter, Left B Bladder C Bladder Neck	Ø Open 3 Percutaneous 4 Percutaneous Endoscopic 7 Via Natural or Artificial Opening 8 Via Natural or Artificial Opening Endoscopic	Z No Device	Z No Qualifier
D Urethra	Ø Open 3 Percutaneous 4 Percutaneous Endoscopic 7 Via Natural or Artificial Opening 8 Via Natural or Artificial Opening Endoscopic X External	Z No Device	Z No Qualifier

Non-OR ØT5D[Ø3478X]ZZ

SECTION: Ø MEDICAL AND SURGICAL

BODY SYSTEM: T URINARY SYSTEM

OPERATION: 7 DILATION: Expanding an orifice or the lumen of a tubular body part

Body Part	Approach	Device	Qualifier
3 Kidney Pelvis, Right 4 Kidney Pelvis, Left 6 Ureter, Right 7 Ureter, Left 8 Ureters, Bilateral B Bladder C Bladder Neck D Urethra	Ø Open 3 Percutaneous 4 Percutaneous Endoscopic 7 Via Natural or Artificial Opening 8 Via Natural or Artificial Opening Endoscopic	D Intraluminal Device Z No Device	Z No Qualifier

Non-OR ØT7[67][Ø3478]DZ
Non-OR ØT7[8D][Ø34]DZ
Non-OR ØT7[8D][78][DZ]Z
Non-OR ØT7C[Ø3478][DZ]Z

Coding Clinic: 2016, Q2, P28 – ØT767DZ

SECTION: Ø MEDICAL AND SURGICAL

BODY SYSTEM: T URINARY SYSTEM

OPERATION: 8 DIVISION: Cutting into a body part, without draining fluids and/or gases from the body part, in order to separate or transect a body part

Body Part	Approach	Device	Qualifier
2 Kidneys, Bilateral C Bladder Neck	Ø Open 3 Percutaneous 4 Percutaneous Endoscopic	Z No Device	Z No Qualifier

Ø: M/S

T: URINARY SYSTEM

5: DESTRUCTION 7: DILATION 8: DIVISION

New/Revised Text in Green   ~~deleted~~ Deleted   ♀ Females Only   ♂ Males Only   **Coding Clinic**

🚫 Non-covered   🚫 Limited Coverage   ⊞ Combination (See Appendix E)   DRG Non-OR   Non-OR   🚫 Hospital-Acquired Condition

SECTION: Ø MEDICAL AND SURGICAL

BODY SYSTEM: T URINARY SYSTEM

OPERATION: 9 DRAINAGE: Taking or letting out fluids and/or gases from a body part

Body Part	Approach	Device	Qualifier
Ø Kidney, Right 1 Kidney, Left 3 Kidney Pelvis, Right 4 Kidney Pelvis, Left 6 Ureter, Right 7 Ureter, Left 8 Ureters, Bilateral B Bladder C Bladder Neck	Ø Open 3 Percutaneous 4 Percutaneous Endoscopic 7 Via Natural or Artificial Opening 8 Via Natural or Artificial Opening Endoscopic	Ø Drainage Device	Z No Qualifier
Ø Kidney, Right 1 Kidney, Left 3 Kidney Pelvis, Right 4 Kidney Pelvis, Left 6 Ureter, Right 7 Ureter, Left 8 Ureters, Bilateral B Bladder C Bladder Neck	Ø Open 3 Percutaneous 4 Percutaneous Endoscopic 7 Via Natural or Artificial Opening 8 Via Natural or Artificial Opening Endoscopic	Z No Device	X Diagnostic Z No Qualifier
D Urethra	Ø Open 3 Percutaneous 4 Percutaneous Endoscopic 7 Via Natural or Artificial Opening 8 Via Natural or Artificial Opening Endoscopic X External	Ø Drainage Device	Z No Qualifier
D Urethra	Ø Open 3 Percutaneous 4 Percutaneous Endoscopic 7 Via Natural or Artificial Opening 8 Via Natural or Artificial Opening Endoscopic X External	Z No Device	X Diagnostic Z No Qualifier

DRG Non-OR ØT9[0134]30Z
DRG Non-OR ØT9[678]3ZZ
DRG Non-OR ØT9D30Z
DRG Non-OR ØT9D3ZZ

Non-OR ØT9[678][03478]0Z
Non-OR ØT9[BC][3478]0Z
Non-OR ØT9[0134678][3478]ZX

Non-OR ØT9[0134][34]ZZ
Non-OR ØT9[BC][3478]ZZ
Non-OR ØT9D[03478X]ZX

9: DRAINAGE

T: URINARY SYSTEM

Ø: M/S

New/Revised Text in Green   deleted Deleted   ♀ Females Only   ♂ Males Only   **Coding Clinic**

🔖 Non-covered   🔖 Limited Coverage   ⊡ Combination (See Appendix E)   DRG Non-OR   Non-OR   🔖 Hospital-Acquired Condition

SECTION: Ø MEDICAL AND SURGICAL

BODY SYSTEM: T URINARY SYSTEM

OPERATION: B EXCISION: Cutting out or off, without replacement, a portion of a body part

Body Part	Approach	Device	Qualifier
Ø Kidney, Right 1 Kidney, Left 3 Kidney Pelvis, Right 4 Kidney Pelvis, Left 6 Ureter, Right 7 Ureter, Left B Bladder C Bladder Neck	Ø Open 3 Percutaneous 4 Percutaneous Endoscopic 7 Via Natural or Artificial Opening 8 Via Natural or Artificial Opening Endoscopic	Z No Device	X Diagnostic Z No Qualifier
D Urethra	Ø Open 3 Percutaneous 4 Percutaneous Endoscopic 7 Via Natural or Artificial Opening 8 Via Natural or Artificial Opening Endoscopic X External	Z No Device	X Diagnostic Z No Qualifier

Non-OR ØTB[013467][3478]ZX
Non-OR ØTBD[03478X]ZX

Coding Clinic: 2015, Q3, P34 – ØTBD8ZZ
Coding Clinic: 2016, Q1, P19 – ØTBB8ZX

SECTION: Ø MEDICAL AND SURGICAL

BODY SYSTEM: T URINARY SYSTEM

OPERATION: C EXTIRPATION: Taking or cutting out solid matter from a body part

Body Part	Approach	Device	Qualifier
Ø Kidney, Right 1 Kidney, Left 3 Kidney Pelvis, Right 4 Kidney Pelvis, Left 6 Ureter, Right 7 Ureter, Left B Bladder C Bladder Neck	Ø Open 3 Percutaneous 4 Percutaneous Endoscopic 7 Via Natural or Artificial Opening 8 Via Natural or Artificial Opening Endoscopic	Z No Device	Z No Qualifier
D Urethra	Ø Open 3 Percutaneous 4 Percutaneous Endoscopic 7 Via Natural or Artificial Opening 8 Via Natural or Artificial Opening Endoscopic X External	Z No Device	Z No Qualifier

Non-OR ØTC[BC][78]ZZ
Non-OR ØTCD[78X]ZZ

Coding Clinic: 2015, Q2, P8 – ØTC48ZZ
Coding Clinic: 2015, Q2, P9 – ØTC18ZZ, ØTC78ZZ, ØTCB8ZZ, ØTC78DZ

SECTION: Ø MEDICAL AND SURGICAL

BODY SYSTEM: T URINARY SYSTEM

OPERATION: D EXTRACTION: Pulling or stripping out or off all or a portion of a body part by the use of force

Body Part	Approach	Device	Qualifier
Ø Kidney, Right 1 Kidney, Left	Ø Open 3 Percutaneous 4 Percutaneous Endoscopic	Z No Device	Z No Qualifier

Ø: M/S
T: URINARY SYSTEM
B: EXCISION   C: EXTIRPATION   D: EXTRACTION

SECTION: Ø MEDICAL AND SURGICAL

BODY SYSTEM: T URINARY SYSTEM

OPERATION: F FRAGMENTATION: Breaking solid matter in a body part into pieces

Body Part	Approach	Device	Qualifier
3 Kidney Pelvis, Right 4 Kidney Pelvis, Left 6 Ureter, Right 7 Ureter, Left B Bladder C Bladder Neck D Urethra 🔾	Ø Open 3 Percutaneous 4 Percutaneous Endoscopic 7 Via Natural or Artificial Opening 8 Via Natural or Artificial Opening Endoscopic X External	Z No Device	Z No Qualifier

🔾 ØTFDXZZ

DRG Non-OR ØTF[3467BC]XZZ

Non-OR ØTF[34][Ø78]ZZ

Non-OR ØTF[67BC][Ø3478]ZZ

Non-OR ØTFD[Ø3478X]ZZ

SECTION: Ø MEDICAL AND SURGICAL

BODY SYSTEM: T URINARY SYSTEM

OPERATION: H INSERTION: Putting in a nonbiological appliance that monitors, assists, performs, or prevents a physiological function but does not physically take the place of a body part

Body Part	Approach	Device	Qualifier
5 Kidney	Ø Open 3 Percutaneous 4 Percutaneous Endoscopic 7 Via Natural or Artificial Opening 8 Via Natural or Artificial Opening Endoscopic	2 Monitoring Device 3 Infusion Device	Z No Qualifier
9 Ureter ⊞	Ø Open 3 Percutaneous 4 Percutaneous Endoscopic 7 Via Natural or Artificial Opening 8 Via Natural or Artificial Opening Endoscopic	2 Monitoring Device 3 Infusion Device M Stimulator Lead	Z No Qualifier
B Bladder 🔾 ⊞	Ø Open 3 Percutaneous 4 Percutaneous Endoscopic 7 Via Natural or Artificial Opening 8 Via Natural or Artificial Opening Endoscopic	2 Monitoring Device 3 Infusion Device L Artificial Sphincter M Stimulator Lead	Z No Qualifier
C Bladder Neck	Ø Open 3 Percutaneous 4 Percutaneous Endoscopic 7 Via Natural or Artificial Opening 8 Via Natural or Artificial Opening Endoscopic	L Artificial Sphincter	Z No Qualifier
D Urethra	Ø Open 3 Percutaneous 4 Percutaneous Endoscopic 7 Via Natural or Artificial Opening 8 Via Natural or Artificial Opening Endoscopic X External	2 Monitoring Device 3 Infusion Device L Artificial Sphincter	Z No Qualifier

🔾 ØTHB[Ø3478]MZ

⊞ ØTH9[Ø3478]MZ

⊞ ØTHB[Ø3478]MZ

DRG Non-OR ØTH5[Ø3478]3Z

DRG Non-OR ØTH5[78]2Z

DRG Non-OR ØTH9[Ø3478]3Z

DRG Non-OR ØTH9[78]2Z

DRG Non-OR ØTHB[Ø3478]3Z

DRG Non-OR ØTHB[78]2Z

DRG Non-OR ØTHD[Ø3478X]3Z

DRG Non-OR ØTHD[78]2Z

New/Revised Text in Green ~~deleted~~ Deleted ♀ Females Only ♂ Males Only **Coding Clinic**

🔾 Non-covered 🔾 Limited Coverage ⊞ Combination (See Appendix E) DRG Non-OR Non-OR 🔾 Hospital-Acquired Condition

(left margin) F: FRAGMENTATION H: INSERTION T: URINARY SYSTEM Ø: M/S

SECTION: Ø MEDICAL AND SURGICAL
BODY SYSTEM: T URINARY SYSTEM
OPERATION: J INSPECTION: Visually and/or manually exploring a body part

Body Part	Approach	Device	Qualifier
5 Kidney 9 Ureter B Bladder D Urethra	Ø Open 3 Percutaneous 4 Percutaneous Endoscopic 7 Via Natural or Artificial Opening 8 Via Natural or Artificial Opening Endoscopic X External	Z No Device	Z No Qualifier

DRG Non-OR ØTJ[59B][37]ZZ
Non-OR ØTJ[59][48X]ZZ
Non-OR ØTJB[8X]ZZ
Non-OR ØTJD[3478X]ZZ

SECTION: Ø MEDICAL AND SURGICAL
BODY SYSTEM: T URINARY SYSTEM
OPERATION: L OCCLUSION: Completely closing an orifice or the lumen of a tubular body part

Body Part	Approach	Device	Qualifier
3 Kidney Pelvis, Right 4 Kidney Pelvis, Left 6 Ureter, Right 7 Ureter, Left B Bladder C Bladder Neck	Ø Open 3 Percutaneous 4 Percutaneous Endoscopic	C Extraluminal Device D Intraluminal Device Z No Device	Z No Qualifier
3 Kidney Pelvis, Right 4 Kidney Pelvis, Left 6 Ureter, Right 7 Ureter, Left B Bladder C Bladder Neck	7 Via Natural or Artificial Opening 8 Via Natural or Artificial Opening Endoscopic	D Intraluminal Device Z No Device	Z No Qualifier
D Urethra	Ø Open 3 Percutaneous 4 Percutaneous Endoscopic X External	C Extraluminal Device D Intraluminal Device Z No Device	Z No Qualifier
D Urethra	7 Via Natural or Artificial Opening 8 Via Natural or Artificial Opening Endoscopic	D Intraluminal Device Z No Device	Z No Qualifier

SECTION: Ø MEDICAL AND SURGICAL
BODY SYSTEM: T URINARY SYSTEM
OPERATION: M REATTACHMENT: Putting back in or on all or a portion of a separated body part to its normal location or other suitable location

Body Part	Approach	Device	Qualifier
Ø Kidney, Right 1 Kidney, Left 2 Kidneys, Bilateral 3 Kidney Pelvis, Right 4 Kidney Pelvis, Left 6 Ureter, Right 7 Ureter, Left 8 Ureters, Bilateral B Bladder C Bladder Neck D Urethra	Ø Open 4 Percutaneous Endoscopic	Z No Device	Z No Qualifier

SECTION: Ø MEDICAL AND SURGICAL
BODY SYSTEM: T URINARY SYSTEM
OPERATION: N RELEASE: Freeing a body part from an abnormal physical constraint by cutting or by the use of force

Body Part	Approach	Device	Qualifier
Ø Kidney, Right 1 Kidney, Left 3 Kidney Pelvis, Right 4 Kidney Pelvis, Left 6 Ureter, Right 7 Ureter, Left B Bladder C Bladder Neck	Ø Open 3 Percutaneous 4 Percutaneous Endoscopic 7 Via Natural or Artificial Opening 8 Via Natural or Artificial Opening Endoscopic	Z No Device	Z No Qualifier
D Urethra	Ø Open 3 Percutaneous 4 Percutaneous Endoscopic 7 Via Natural or Artificial Opening 8 Via Natural or Artificial Opening Endoscopic X External	Z No Device	Z No Qualifier

New/Revised Text in Green   ~~deleted~~ Deleted   ♀ Females Only   ♂ Males Only   **Coding Clinic**
 Non-covered   Limited Coverage   ⊕ Combination (See Appendix E)   DRG Non-OR   Non-OR   Hospital-Acquired Condition

SECTION: Ø MEDICAL AND SURGICAL

BODY SYSTEM: T URINARY SYSTEM

OPERATION: P REMOVAL: *(on multiple pages)*

Taking out or off a device from a body part

Body Part	Approach	Device	Qualifier
5 Kidney	Ø Open 3 Percutaneous 4 Percutaneous Endoscopic 7 Via Natural or Artificial Opening 8 Via Natural or Artificial Opening Endoscopic	Ø Drainage Device 2 Monitoring Device 3 Infusion Device 7 Autologous Tissue Substitute C Extraluminal Device D Intraluminal Device J Synthetic Substitute K Nonautologous Tissue Substitute	Z No Qualifier
5 Kidney	X External	Ø Drainage Device 2 Monitoring Device 3 Infusion Device D Intraluminal Device	Z No Qualifier
9 Ureter ⊞	Ø Open 3 Percutaneous 4 Percutaneous Endoscopic 7 Via Natural or Artificial Opening 8 Via Natural or Artificial Opening Endoscopic	Ø Drainage Device 2 Monitoring Device 3 Infusion Device 7 Autologous Tissue Substitute C Extraluminal Device D Intraluminal Device J Synthetic Substitute K Nonautologous Tissue Substitute M Stimulator Lead	Z No Qualifier
9 Ureter	X External	Ø Drainage Device 2 Monitoring Device 3 Infusion Device D Intraluminal Device M Stimulator Lead	Z No Qualifier
B Bladder ⌖ ⊞	Ø Open 3 Percutaneous 4 Percutaneous Endoscopic 7 Via Natural or Artificial Opening 8 Via Natural or Artificial Opening Endoscopic	Ø Drainage Device 2 Monitoring Device 3 Infusion Device 7 Autologous Tissue Substitute C Extraluminal Device D Intraluminal Device J Synthetic Substitute K Nonautologous Tissue Substitute L Artificial Sphincter M Stimulator Lead	Z No Qualifier
B Bladder	X External	Ø Drainage Device 2 Monitoring Device 3 Infusion Device D Intraluminal Device L Artificial Sphincter M Stimulator Lead	Z No Qualifier

⌖ ØTPB[Ø3478]MZ
⊞ ØTP9[Ø3478]MZ
⊞ ØTPB[Ø3478]MZ
DRG Non-OR ØTP5[78][Ø23D]Z
DRG Non-OR ØTP9[78][Ø23D]Z
DRG Non-OR ØTPB[78][Ø23D]Z

Non-OR ØTP5X[Ø23D]Z
Non-OR ØTP9X[Ø23D]Z
Non-OR ØTPBX[Ø23DL]Z

Coding Clinic: 2016, Q2, P28 – Ø2P98DZ

Ø: M/S

T: URINARY SYSTEM

P: REMOVAL

SECTION: Ø MEDICAL AND SURGICAL
BODY SYSTEM: T URINARY SYSTEM
OPERATION: P REMOVAL: *(continued)*
Taking out or off a device from a body part

Body Part	Approach	Device	Qualifier
D Urethra	Ø Open 3 Percutaneous 4 Percutaneous Endoscopic 7 Via Natural or Artificial Opening 8 Via Natural or Artificial Opening Endoscopic	Ø Drainage Device 2 Monitoring Device 3 Infusion Device 7 Autologous Tissue Substitute C Extraluminal Device D Intraluminal Device J Synthetic Substitute K Nonautologous Tissue Substitute L Artificial Sphincter	Z No Qualifier
D Urethra	X External	Ø Drainage Device 2 Monitoring Device 3 Infusion Device D Intraluminal Device L Artificial Sphincter	Z No Qualifier

DRG Non-OR ØTPD[78][Ø23D]Z
Non-OR ØTPDX[Ø23D]Z

SECTION: Ø MEDICAL AND SURGICAL
BODY SYSTEM: T URINARY SYSTEM
OPERATION: Q REPAIR: Restoring, to the extent possible, a body part to its normal anatomic structure and function

Body Part	Approach	Device	Qualifier
Ø Kidney, Right ⊞ 1 Kidney, Left ⊞ 3 Kidney Pelvis, Right ⊞ 4 Kidney Pelvis, Left ⊞ 6 Ureter, Right ⊞ 7 Ureter, Left ⊞ B Bladder ⊞ C Bladder Neck	Ø Open 3 Percutaneous 4 Percutaneous Endoscopic 7 Via Natural or Artificial Opening 8 Via Natural or Artificial Opening Endoscopic	Z No Device	Z No Qualifier
D Urethra ⊞	Ø Open 3 Percutaneous 4 Percutaneous Endoscopic 7 Via Natural or Artificial Opening 8 Via Natural or Artificial Opening Endoscopic X External	Z No Device	Z No Qualifier

⊞ ØTQ[Ø13467B][Ø34]ZZ
⊞ ØTQD[Ø34]ZZ
Non-OR ØTQC[Ø3478]ZZ

P: REMOVAL   Q: REPAIR
T: URINARY SYSTEM
Ø: M/S

SECTION: 0 MEDICAL AND SURGICAL
BODY SYSTEM: T URINARY SYSTEM
OPERATION: R REPLACEMENT: Putting in or on biological or synthetic material that physically takes the place and/or function of all or a portion of a body part

Body Part	Approach	Device	Qualifier
3 Kidney Pelvis, Right 4 Kidney Pelvis, Left 6 Ureter, Right 7 Ureter, Left B Bladder ⊞ C Bladder Neck	0 Open 4 Percutaneous Endoscopic 7 Via Natural or Artificial Opening 8 Via Natural or Artificial Opening Endoscopic	7 Autologous Tissue Substitute J Synthetic Substitute K Nonautologous Tissue Substitute	Z No Qualifier
D Urethra	0 Open 4 Percutaneous Endoscopic 7 Via Natural or Artificial Opening 8 Via Natural or Artificial Opening Endoscopic X External	7 Autologous Tissue Substitute J Synthetic Substitute K Nonautologous Tissue Substitute	Z No Qualifier

⊞ 0TRB07Z

SECTION: 0 MEDICAL AND SURGICAL
BODY SYSTEM: T URINARY SYSTEM
OPERATION: S REPOSITION: Moving to its normal location, or other suitable location, all or a portion of a body part

Body Part	Approach	Device	Qualifier
0 Kidney, Right 1 Kidney, Left 2 Kidneys, Bilateral 3 Kidney Pelvis, Right 4 Kidney Pelvis, Left 6 Ureter, Right 7 Ureter, Left 8 Ureters, Bilateral B Bladder C Bladder Neck D Urethra	0 Open 4 Percutaneous Endoscopic	Z No Device	Z No Qualifier

Coding Clinic: 2016, Q1, P15 – 0TSD0ZZ

New/Revised Text in Green ~~deleted~~ Deleted ♀ Females Only ♂ Males Only **Coding Clinic**
☜ Non-covered ☜ Limited Coverage ⊞ Combination (See Appendix E) DRG Non-OR Non-OR ☜ Hospital-Acquired Condition

431

0: M/S

T: URINARY SYSTEM

R: REPLACEMENT S: REPOSITION

SECTION: Ø MEDICAL AND SURGICAL

BODY SYSTEM: T URINARY SYSTEM

OPERATION: T RESECTION: Cutting out or off, without replacement, all of a body part

Body Part	Approach	Device	Qualifier
Ø Kidney, Right 1 Kidney, Left 2 Kidneys, Bilateral	Ø Open 4 Percutaneous Endoscopic	Z No Device	Z No Qualifier
3 Kidney Pelvis, Right 4 Kidney Pelvis, Left 6 Ureter, Right 7 Ureter, Left B Bladder ⊞ C Bladder Neck D Urethra ⊞	Ø Open 4 Percutaneous Endoscopic 7 Via Natural or Artificial Opening 8 Via Natural or Artificial Opening Endoscopic	Z No Device	Z No Qualifier

⊞ ØTTB[Ø478]ZZ
⊞ ØTTDØZZ
`DRG Non-OR` ØTTDØZZ
`Non-OR` ØTTD[478]ZZ

SECTION: Ø MEDICAL AND SURGICAL

BODY SYSTEM: T URINARY SYSTEM

OPERATION: U SUPPLEMENT: Putting in or on biological or synthetic material that physically reinforces and/or augments the function of a portion of a body part

Body Part	Approach	Device	Qualifier
3 Kidney Pelvis, Right 4 Kidney Pelvis, Left 6 Ureter, Right 7 Ureter, Left B Bladder C Bladder Neck	Ø Open 4 Percutaneous Endoscopic 7 Via Natural or Artificial Opening 8 Via Natural or Artificial Opening Endoscopic	7 Autologous Tissue Substitute J Synthetic Substitute K Nonautologous Tissue Substitute	Z No Qualifier
D Urethra	Ø Open 4 Percutaneous Endoscopic 7 Via Natural or Artificial Opening 8 Via Natural or Artificial Opening Endoscopic X External	7 Autologous Tissue Substitute J Synthetic Substitute K Nonautologous Tissue Substitute	Z No Qualifier

SECTION: Ø MEDICAL AND SURGICAL

BODY SYSTEM: T URINARY SYSTEM

OPERATION: V RESTRICTION: Partially closing an orifice or the lumen of a tubular body part

Body Part	Approach	Device	Qualifier
3 Kidney Pelvis, Right 4 Kidney Pelvis, Left 6 Ureter, Right 7 Ureter, Left B Bladder C Bladder Neck	Ø Open 3 Percutaneous 4 Percutaneous Endoscopic	C Extraluminal Device D Intraluminal Device Z No Device	Z No Qualifier
3 Kidney Pelvis, Right 4 Kidney Pelvis, Left 6 Ureter, Right 7 Ureter, Left B Bladder C Bladder Neck	7 Via Natural or Artificial Opening 8 Via Natural or Artificial Opening Endoscopic	D Intraluminal Device Z No Device	Z No Qualifier
D Urethra	Ø Open 3 Percutaneous 4 Percutaneous Endoscopic	C Extraluminal Device D Intraluminal Device Z No Device	Z No Qualifier
D Urethra	7 Via Natural or Artificial Opening 8 Via Natural or Artificial Opening Endoscopic	D Intraluminal Device Z No Device	Z No Qualifier
D Urethra	X External	Z No Device	Z No Qualifier

Coding Clinic: 2015, Q2, P12 – ØTV[67]8ZZ

SECTION: Ø MEDICAL AND SURGICAL

BODY SYSTEM: T URINARY SYSTEM

OPERATION: W REVISION: (on multiple pages)

Correcting, to the extent possible, a portion of a malfunctioning device or the position of a displaced device

Body Part	Approach	Device	Qualifier
5 Kidney	Ø Open 3 Percutaneous 4 Percutaneous Endoscopic 7 Via Natural or Artificial Opening 8 Via Natural or Artificial Opening Endoscopic X External	Ø Drainage Device 2 Monitoring Device 3 Infusion Device 7 Autologous Tissue Substitute C Extraluminal Device D Intraluminal Device J Synthetic Substitute K Nonautologous Tissue Substitute	Z No Qualifier

Non-OR ØTW5X[0237CDJK]Z

SECTION: Ø MEDICAL AND SURGICAL

BODY SYSTEM: T URINARY SYSTEM
OPERATION: W REVISION: *(continued)*
Correcting, to the extent possible, a portion of a malfunctioning device or the position of a displaced device

Body Part	Approach	Device	Qualifier
9 Ureter	0 Open 3 Percutaneous 4 Percutaneous Endoscopic 7 Via Natural or Artificial Opening 8 Via Natural or Artificial Opening Endoscopic X External	0 Drainage Device 2 Monitoring Device 3 Infusion Device 7 Autologous Tissue Substitute C Extraluminal Device D Intraluminal Device J Synthetic Substitute K Nonautologous Tissue Substitute M Stimulator Lead	Z No Qualifier
B Bladder	0 Open 3 Percutaneous 4 Percutaneous Endoscopic 7 Via Natural or Artificial Opening 8 Via Natural or Artificial Opening Endoscopic X External	0 Drainage Device 2 Monitoring Device 3 Infusion Device 7 Autologous Tissue Substitute C Extraluminal Device D Intraluminal Device J Synthetic Substitute K Nonautologous Tissue Substitute L Artificial Sphincter M Stimulator Lead	Z No Qualifier
D Urethra	0 Open 3 Percutaneous 4 Percutaneous Endoscopic 7 Via Natural or Artificial Opening 8 Via Natural or Artificial Opening Endoscopic X External	0 Drainage Device 2 Monitoring Device 3 Infusion Device 7 Autologous Tissue Substitute C Extraluminal Device D Intraluminal Device J Synthetic Substitute K Nonautologous Tissue Substitute L Artificial Sphincter	Z No Qualifier

Non-OR ØTW9X[0237CDJKM]Z
Non-OR ØTWBX[0237CDJKLM]Z
Non-OR ØTWDX[0237CDJKL]Z

SECTION: Ø MEDICAL AND SURGICAL

BODY SYSTEM: T URINARY SYSTEM
OPERATION: Y TRANSPLANTATION: Putting in or on all or a portion of a living body part taken from another individual or animal to physically take the place and/or function of all or a portion of a similar body part

Body Part	Approach	Device	Qualifier
0 Kidney, Right 🐾 ⊞ 1 Kidney, Left 🐾 ⊞	0 Open	Z No Device	0 Allogeneic 1 Syngeneic 2 Zooplastic

🐾 ØTY[01]0Z[012]
⊞ ØTY[01]0Z[012]

1: BYPASS   2: CHANGE

U: FEMALE REPRODUCTIVE SYSTEM

0: M/S

SECTION: 0 MEDICAL AND SURGICAL
BODY SYSTEM: U FEMALE REPRODUCTIVE SYSTEM
OPERATION: 1 BYPASS: Altering the route of passage of the contents of a tubular body part

Body Part	Approach	Device	Qualifier
5 Fallopian Tube, Right ♀ 6 Fallopian Tube, Left ♀	0 Open 4 Percutaneous Endoscopic	7 Autologous Tissue Substitute J Synthetic Substitute K Nonautologous Tissue Substitute Z No Device	5 Fallopian Tube, Right 6 Fallopian Tube, Left 9 Uterus

SECTION: 0 MEDICAL AND SURGICAL
BODY SYSTEM: U FEMALE REPRODUCTIVE SYSTEM
OPERATION: 2 CHANGE: Taking out or off a device from a body part and putting back an identical or similar device in or on the same body part without cutting or puncturing the skin or a mucous membrane

Body Part	Approach	Device	Qualifier
3 Ovary ♀ 8 Fallopian Tube ♀ M Vulva ♀	X External	0 Drainage Device Y Other Device	Z No Qualifier
D Uterus and Cervix ♀	X External	0 Drainage Device H Contraceptive Device Y Other Device	Z No Qualifier
H Vagina and Cul-de-sac ♀	X External	0 Drainage Device G Intraluminal Device, Pessary Y Other Device	Z No Qualifier

Non-OR   All Values

New/Revised Text in Green   deleted Deleted   ♀ Females Only   ♂ Males Only   **Coding Clinic**
Non-covered   Limited Coverage   Combination (See Appendix E)   DRG Non-OR   Non-OR   Hospital-Acquired Condition

SECTION: 0 MEDICAL AND SURGICAL

BODY SYSTEM: U FEMALE REPRODUCTIVE SYSTEM

OPERATION: 5 **DESTRUCTION:** Physical eradication of all or a portion of a body part by the direct use of energy, force, or a destructive agent

Body Part	Approach	Device	Qualifier
0 Ovary, Right ♀ 1 Ovary, Left ♀ 2 Ovaries, Bilateral ♀ 4 Uterine Supporting Structure ♀	0 Open 3 Percutaneous 4 Percutaneous Endoscopic	Z No Device	Z No Qualifier
5 Fallopian Tube, Right ♀ 6 Fallopian Tube, Left ♀ 7 Fallopian Tubes, Bilateral ♀ ⓠ 9 Uterus ♀ B Endometrium ♀ C Cervix ♀ F Cul-de-sac ♀	0 Open 3 Percutaneous 4 Percutaneous Endoscopic 7 Via Natural or Artificial Opening 8 Via Natural or Artificial Opening Endoscopic	Z No Device	Z No Qualifier
G Vagina ♀ K Hymen ♀	0 Open 3 Percutaneous 4 Percutaneous Endoscopic 7 Via Natural or Artificial Opening 8 Via Natural or Artificial Opening Endoscopic X External	Z No Device	Z No Qualifier
J Clitoris ♀ L Vestibular Gland ♀ M Vulva ♀	0 Open X External	Z No Device	Z No Qualifier

ⓠ 0U57[03478]ZZ when Z30.2 is listed as the principal diagnosis

0: M/S

U: FEMALE REPRODUCTIVE SYSTEM

5: DESTRUCTION

SECTION: Ø MEDICAL AND SURGICAL

BODY SYSTEM: U FEMALE REPRODUCTIVE SYSTEM
OPERATION: 7 DILATION: Expanding an orifice or the lumen of a tubular body part

Body Part	Approach	Device	Qualifier
5 Fallopian Tube, Right ♀ 6 Fallopian Tube, Left ♀ 7 Fallopian Tubes, Bilateral ♀ 9 Uterus ♀ C Cervix ♀ G Vagina ♀	Ø Open 3 Percutaneous 4 Percutaneous Endoscopic 7 Via Natural or Artificial Opening 8 Via Natural or Artificial Opening Endoscopic	D Intraluminal Device Z No Device	Z No Qualifier
K Hymen ♀	Ø Open 3 Percutaneous 4 Percutaneous Endoscopic 7 Via Natural or Artificial Opening 8 Via Natural or Artificial Opening Endoscopic X External	D Intraluminal Device Z No Device	Z No Qualifier

Non-OR ØU7C[Ø3478][DZ]Z
Non-OR ØU7G[78][DZ]Z

SECTION: Ø MEDICAL AND SURGICAL

BODY SYSTEM: U FEMALE REPRODUCTIVE SYSTEM
OPERATION: 8 DIVISION: Cutting into a body part, without draining fluids and/or gases from the body part, in order to separate or transect a body part

Body Part	Approach	Device	Qualifier
Ø Ovary, Right ♀ 1 Ovary, Left ♀ 2 Ovaries, Bilateral ♀ 4 Uterine Supporting Structure ♀	Ø Open 3 Percutaneous 4 Percutaneous Endoscopic	Z No Device	Z No Qualifier
K Hymen ♀	7 Via Natural or Artificial Opening 8 Via Natural or Artificial Opening Endoscopic X External	Z No Device	Z No Qualifier

Non-OR ØU8K[78X]ZZ

New/Revised Text in Green ~~deleted~~ Deleted ♀ Females Only ♂ Males Only **Coding Clinic**
Non-covered Limited Coverage Combination (See Appendix E) DRG Non-OR Non-OR Hospital-Acquired Condition

SECTION: Ø MEDICAL AND SURGICAL

BODY SYSTEM: U FEMALE REPRODUCTIVE SYSTEM

OPERATION: 9 DRAINAGE: *(on multiple pages)*
Taking or letting out fluids and/or gases from a body part

Body Part	Approach	Device	Qualifier
Ø Ovary, Right ♀ 1 Ovary, Left ♀ 2 Ovaries, Bilateral ♀	Ø Open 3 Percutaneous 4 Percutaneous Endoscopic	Ø Drainage Device	Z No Qualifier
Ø Ovary, Right ♀ 1 Ovary, Left ♀ 2 Ovaries, Bilateral ♀	Ø Open 3 Percutaneous 4 Percutaneous Endoscopic	Z No Device	X Diagnostic Z No Qualifier
Ø Ovary, Right ♀ 1 Ovary, Left ♀ 2 Ovaries, Bilateral ♀	X External	Z No Device	Z No Qualifier
4 Uterine Supporting Structure ♀	Ø Open 3 Percutaneous 4 Percutaneous Endoscopic	Ø Drainage Device	Z No Qualifier
4 Uterine Supporting Structure ♀	Ø Open 3 Percutaneous 4 Percutaneous Endoscopic	Z No Device	X Diagnostic Z No Qualifier
5 Fallopian Tube, Right ♀ 6 Fallopian Tube, Left ♀ 7 Fallopian Tubes, Bilateral ♀ 9 Uterus ♀ C Cervix ♀ F Cul-de-sac ♀	Ø Open 3 Percutaneous 4 Percutaneous Endoscopic 7 Via Natural or Artificial Opening 8 Via Natural or Artificial Opening Endoscopic	Ø Drainage Device	Z No Qualifier
5 Fallopian Tube, Right ♀ 6 Fallopian Tube, Left ♀ 7 Fallopian Tubes, Bilateral ♀ 9 Uterus ♀ C Cervix ♀ F Cul-de-sac ♀	Ø Open 3 Percutaneous 4 Percutaneous Endoscopic 7 Via Natural or Artificial Opening 8 Via Natural or Artificial Opening Endoscopic	Z No Device	X Diagnostic Z No Qualifier
G Vagina ♀ K Hymen ♀	Ø Open 3 Percutaneous 4 Percutaneous Endoscopic 7 Via Natural or Artificial Opening 8 Via Natural or Artificial Opening Endoscopic X External	Ø Drainage Device	Z No Qualifier
G Vagina ♀ K Hymen ♀	Ø Open 3 Percutaneous 4 Percutaneous Endoscopic 7 Via Natural or Artificial Opening 8 Via Natural or Artificial Opening Endoscopic X External	Z No Device	X Diagnostic Z No Qualifier

DRG Non-OR ØU9[012]3ØZ
DRG Non-OR ØU9[012]3ZZ
DRG Non-OR ØU943ØZ
DRG Non-OR ØU943ZZ

DRG Non-OR ØU9[5679C]3ØZ
DRG Non-OR ØU9[9C]3ZZ
DRG Non-OR ØU9G3ØZ
DRG Non-OR ØU9G3ZZ

Non-OR ØU9F[34]ØZ
Non-OR ØU9[567][3478]ZZ
Non-OR ØU9F[34]ZZ
Non-OR ØU9K[Ø3478X]ØZ
Non-OR ØU9K[Ø3478X]ZZ

New/Revised Text in Green   ~~deleted~~ Deleted   ♀ Females Only   ♂ Males Only   **Coding Clinic**
Non-covered   Limited Coverage   Combination (See Appendix E)   DRG Non-OR   Non-OR   Hospital-Acquired Condition

Ø: M/S

U: FEMALE REPRODUCTIVE SYSTEM

9: DRAINAGE

9: DRAINAGE　　B: EXCISION

U: FEMALE REPRODUCTIVE SYSTEM

0: M/S

SECTION: 0 MEDICAL AND SURGICAL

BODY SYSTEM: U FEMALE REPRODUCTIVE SYSTEM

OPERATION: 9 DRAINAGE: *(continued)*
Taking or letting out fluids and/or gases from a body part

Body Part	Approach	Device	Qualifier
J Clitoris ♀ L Vestibular Gland ♀ M Vulva ♀	0 Open X External	0 Drainage Device	Z No Qualifier
J Clitoris ♀ L Vestibular Gland ♀ M Vulva ♀	0 Open X External	Z No Device	X Diagnostic Z No Qualifier

Non-OR　0U9L[0X]0Z
Non-OR　0U9L[0X]ZZ

SECTION: 0 MEDICAL AND SURGICAL

BODY SYSTEM: U FEMALE REPRODUCTIVE SYSTEM

OPERATION: B EXCISION: Cutting out or off, without replacement, a portion of a body part

Body Part	Approach	Device	Qualifier
0 Ovary, Right ♀ 1 Ovary, Left ♀ 2 Ovaries, Bilateral ♀ 4 Uterine Supporting Structure ♀ 5 Fallopian Tube, Right ♀ 6 Fallopian Tube, Left ♀ 7 Fallopian Tubes, Bilateral ♀ 9 Uterus ♀ C Cervix ♀ F Cul-de-sac ♀	0 Open 3 Percutaneous 4 Percutaneous Endoscopic 7 Via Natural or Artificial Opening 8 Via Natural or Artificial Opening Endoscopic	Z No Device	X Diagnostic Z No Qualifier
G Vagina ♀ K Hymen ♀	0 Open 3 Percutaneous 4 Percutaneous Endoscopic 7 Via Natural or Artificial Opening 8 Via Natural or Artificial Opening Endoscopic X External	Z No Device	X Diagnostic Z No Qualifier
J Clitoris ♀ L Vestibular Gland ♀ M Vulva ♀	0 Open X External	Z No Device	X Diagnostic Z No Qualifier

Coding Clinic: 2015, Q3, P31 – 0UB70ZZ
Coding Clinic: 2015, Q3, P32 – 0UB64ZZ

New/Revised Text in Green　　~~deleted~~ Deleted　　♀ Females Only　　♂ Males Only　　**Coding Clinic**
　Non-covered　　　Limited Coverage　　⊡ Combination (See Appendix E)　　DRG Non-OR　　Non-OR　　　Hospital-Acquired Condition

SECTION: Ø MEDICAL AND SURGICAL
BODY SYSTEM: U FEMALE REPRODUCTIVE SYSTEM
OPERATION: C EXTIRPATION: Taking or cutting out solid matter from a body part

Body Part	Approach	Device	Qualifier
Ø Ovary, Right ♀ 1 Ovary, Left ♀ 2 Ovaries, Bilateral ♀ 4 Uterine Supporting Structure ♀	Ø Open 3 Percutaneous 4 Percutaneous Endoscopic	Z No Device	Z No Qualifier
5 Fallopian Tube, Right ♀ 6 Fallopian Tube, Left ♀ 7 Fallopian Tubes, Bilateral ♀ 9 Uterus ♀ B Endometrium ♀ C Cervix ♀ F Cul-de-sac ♀	Ø Open 3 Percutaneous 4 Percutaneous Endoscopic 7 Via Natural or Artificial Opening 8 Via Natural or Artificial Opening Endoscopic	Z No Device	Z No Qualifier
G Vagina ♀ K Hymen ♀	Ø Open 3 Percutaneous 4 Percutaneous Endoscopic 7 Via Natural or Artificial Opening 8 Via Natural or Artificial Opening Endoscopic X External	Z No Device	Z No Qualifier
J Clitoris ♀ L Vestibular Gland ♀ M Vulva ♀	Ø Open X External	Z No Device	Z No Qualifier

Non-OR ØUC9[78]ZZ
Non-OR ØUCG[78X]ZZ
Non-OR ØUCK[Ø3478X]ZZ
Non-OR ØUCMXZZ

Coding Clinic: 2013, Q2, P38 – ØUC97ZZ
Coding Clinic: 2015, Q3, P3Ø-31 – ØUCC[78]ZZ

SECTION: Ø MEDICAL AND SURGICAL

BODY SYSTEM: U FEMALE REPRODUCTIVE SYSTEM

OPERATION: D **EXTRACTION:** Pulling or stripping out or off all or a portion of a body part by the use of force

Body Part	Approach	Device	Qualifier
B Endometrium ♀	7 Via Natural or Artificial Opening 8 Via Natural or Artificial Opening Endoscopic	Z No Device	X Diagnostic Z No Qualifier
N Ova ♀	Ø Open 3 Percutaneous 4 Percutaneous Endoscopic	Z No Device	Z No Qualifier

SECTION: Ø MEDICAL AND SURGICAL

BODY SYSTEM: U FEMALE REPRODUCTIVE SYSTEM

OPERATION: F **FRAGMENTATION:** Breaking solid matter in a body part into pieces

Body Part	Approach	Device	Qualifier
5 Fallopian Tube, Right ♀ 🦠 6 Fallopian Tube, Left ♀ 🦠 7 Fallopian Tubes, Bilateral ♀ 🦠 9 Uterus ♀ 🦠	Ø Open 3 Percutaneous 4 Percutaneous Endoscopic 7 Via Natural or Artificial Opening 8 Via Natural or Artificial Opening Endoscopic X External	Z No Device	Z No Qualifier

🦠 ØUF[5679]XZZ

Non-OR ØUF[5679]XZZ

SECTION: Ø MEDICAL AND SURGICAL

BODY SYSTEM: U FEMALE REPRODUCTIVE SYSTEM

OPERATION: H INSERTION: Putting in a nonbiological appliance that monitors, assists, performs, or prevents a physiological function but does not physically take the place of a body part

Body Part	Approach	Device	Qualifier
3 Ovary ♀	Ø Open 3 Percutaneous 4 Percutaneous Endoscopic	3 Infusion Device	Z No Qualifier
8 Fallopian Tube ♀ D Uterus and Cervix ♀ H Vagina and Cul-de-sac ♀	Ø Open 3 Percutaneous 4 Percutaneous Endoscopic 7 Via Natural or Artificial Opening 8 Via Natural or Artificial Opening Endoscopic	3 Infusion Device	Z No Qualifier
9 Uterus ♀	7 Via Natural or Artificial Opening 8 Via Natural or Artificial Opening Endoscopic	H Contraceptive Device	Z No Qualifier
C Cervix ♀	Ø Open 3 Percutaneous 4 Percutaneous Endoscopic	1 Radioactive Element	Z No Qualifier
C Cervix ♀	7 Via Natural or Artificial Opening 8 Via Natural or Artificial Opening Endoscopic	1 Radioactive Element H Contraceptive Device	Z No Qualifier
F Cul-de-sac ♀	7 Via Natural or Artificial Opening 8 Via Natural or Artificial Opening Endoscopic	G Intraluminal Device, Pessary	Z No Qualifier
G Vagina ♀	Ø Open 3 Percutaneous 4 Percutaneous Endoscopic X External	1 Radioactive Element	Z No Qualifier
G Vagina ♀	7 Via Natural or Artificial Opening 8 Via Natural or Artificial Opening Endoscopic	1 Radioactive Element G Intraluminal Device, Pessary	Z No Qualifier

DRG Non-OR   ØUH3[Ø34]3Z
DRG Non-OR   ØUH8[Ø3478]3Z
DRG Non-OR   ØUHH[78]3Z
Non-OR   ØUH3[Ø34]3Z
Non-OR   ØUHD[Ø3478]3Z
Non-OR   ØUH9[78]HZ
Non-OR   ØUHC[78]HZ
Non-OR   ØUHF[78]GZ
Non-OR   ØUHG[78]GZ

Coding Clinic: 2013, Q2, P34 – ØUH97HZ

SECTION: Ø MEDICAL AND SURGICAL

BODY SYSTEM: U FEMALE REPRODUCTIVE SYSTEM
OPERATION: J INSPECTION: Visually and/or manually exploring a body part

Body Part	Approach	Device	Qualifier
3 Ovary ♀	Ø Open 3 Percutaneous 4 Percutaneous Endoscopic X External	Z No Device	Z No Qualifier
8 Fallopian Tube ♀ D Uterus and Cervix ♀ H Vagina and Cul-de-sac ♀	Ø Open 3 Percutaneous 4 Percutaneous Endoscopic 7 Via Natural or Artificial Opening 8 Via Natural or Artificial Opening Endoscopic X External	Z No Device	Z No Qualifier
M Vulva ♀	Ø Open X External	Z No Device	Z No Qualifier

DRG Non-OR ØUJ33ZZ
DRG Non-OR ØUJ8[378]ZZ
DRG Non-OR ØUJD3ZZ
DRG Non-OR ØUJH[37]ZZ
Non-OR ØUJ3XZZ
Non-OR ØUJ8XZZ
Non-OR ØUJD[78X]ZZ
Non-OR ØUJH[8X]ZZ
Non-OR ØUJMXZZ

Coding Clinic: 2Ø15, Q1, P34 – ØUJD4ZZ

SECTION: Ø MEDICAL AND SURGICAL

BODY SYSTEM: U FEMALE REPRODUCTIVE SYSTEM
OPERATION: L OCCLUSION: Completely closing an orifice or the lumen of a tubular body part

Body Part	Approach	Device	Qualifier
5 Fallopian Tube, Right ♀ 6 Fallopian Tube, Left ♀ 7 Fallopian Tubes, Bilateral ♀	Ø Open 3 Percutaneous 4 Percutaneous Endoscopic	C Extraluminal Device D Intraluminal Device Z No Device	Z No Qualifier
5 Fallopian Tube, Right ♀ 6 Fallopian Tube, Left ♀ 7 Fallopian Tubes, Bilateral ♀	7 Via Natural or Artificial Opening 8 Via Natural or Artificial Opening Endoscopic	D Intraluminal Device Z No Device	Z No Qualifier
F Cul-de-sac ♀ G Vagina ♀	7 Via Natural or Artificial Opening 8 Via Natural or Artificial Opening Endoscopic	D Intraluminal Device Z No Device	Z No Qualifier

ØUL7[Ø34][CDZ]Z when Z3Ø.2 is listed as the principal diagnosis
ØUL7[78][DZ]Z when Z3Ø.2 is listed as the principal diagnosis

J: INSPECTION   L: OCCLUSION
U: FEMALE REPRODUCTIVE SYSTEM   Ø: M/S

SECTION: Ø MEDICAL AND SURGICAL

BODY SYSTEM: U FEMALE REPRODUCTIVE SYSTEM

OPERATION: M REATTACHMENT: Putting back in or on all or a portion of a separated body part to its normal location or other suitable location

Body Part	Approach	Device	Qualifier
Ø Ovary, Right ♀ 1 Ovary, Left ♀ 2 Ovaries, Bilateral ♀ 4 Uterine Supporting Structure ♀ 5 Fallopian Tube, Right ♀ 6 Fallopian Tube, Left ♀ 7 Fallopian Tubes, Bilateral ♀ 9 Uterus ♀ C Cervix ♀ F Cul-de-sac ♀ G Vagina ♀	Ø Open 4 Percutaneous Endoscopic	Z No Device	Z No Qualifier
J Clitoris ♀ M Vulva ♀	X External	Z No Device	Z No Qualifier
K Hymen ♀	Ø Open 4 Percutaneous Endoscopic X External	Z No Device	Z No Qualifier

SECTION: Ø MEDICAL AND SURGICAL

BODY SYSTEM: U FEMALE REPRODUCTIVE SYSTEM

OPERATION: N RELEASE: Freeing a body part from an abnormal physical constraint by cutting or by the use of force

Body Part	Approach	Device	Qualifier
Ø Ovary, Right ♀ 1 Ovary, Left ♀ 2 Ovaries, Bilateral ♀ 4 Uterine Supporting Structure ♀	Ø Open 3 Percutaneous 4 Percutaneous Endoscopic	Z No Device	Z No Qualifier
5 Fallopian Tube, Right ♀ 6 Fallopian Tube, Left ♀ 7 Fallopian Tubes, Bilateral ♀ 9 Uterus ♀ C Cervix ♀ F Cul-de-sac ♀	Ø Open 3 Percutaneous 4 Percutaneous Endoscopic 7 Via Natural or Artificial Opening 8 Via Natural or Artificial Opening Endoscopic	Z No Device	Z No Qualifier
G Vagina ♀ K Hymen ♀	Ø Open 3 Percutaneous 4 Percutaneous Endoscopic 7 Via Natural or Artificial Opening 8 Via Natural or Artificial Opening Endoscopic X External	Z No Device	Z No Qualifier
J Clitoris ♀ L Vestibular Gland ♀ M Vulva ♀	Ø Open X External	Z No Device	Z No Qualifier

Ø: M/S   U: FEMALE REPRODUCTIVE SYSTEM   M: REATTACHMENT   N: RELEASE

New/Revised Text in Green ~~deleted~~ Deleted ♀ Females Only ♂ Males Only **Coding Clinic**
Non-covered · Limited Coverage · Combination (See Appendix E) · DRG Non-OR · Non-OR · Hospital-Acquired Condition

445

SECTION: Ø MEDICAL AND SURGICAL
BODY SYSTEM: U FEMALE REPRODUCTIVE SYSTEM
OPERATION: P REMOVAL: Taking out or off a device from a body part

Body Part	Approach	Device	Qualifier
3 Ovary ♀	Ø Open 3 Percutaneous 4 Percutaneous Endoscopic X External	Ø Drainage Device 3 Infusion Device	Z No Qualifier
8 Fallopian Tube ♀	Ø Open 3 Percutaneous 4 Percutaneous Endoscopic 7 Via Natural or Artificial Opening 8 Via Natural or Artificial Opening Endoscopic	Ø Drainage Device 3 Infusion Device 7 Autologous Tissue Substitute C Extraluminal Device D Intraluminal Device J Synthetic Substitute K Nonautologous Tissue Substitute	Z No Qualifier
8 Fallopian Tube ♀	X External	Ø Drainage Device 3 Infusion Device D Intraluminal Device	Z No Qualifier
D Uterus and Cervix ♀	Ø Open 3 Percutaneous 4 Percutaneous Endoscopic 7 Via Natural or Artificial Opening 8 Via Natural or Artificial Opening Endoscopic	Ø Drainage Device 1 Radioactive Element 3 Infusion Device 7 Autologous Tissue Substitute C Extraluminal Device D Intraluminal Device H Contraceptive Device J Synthetic Substitute K Nonautologous Tissue Substitute	Z No Qualifier
D Uterus and Cervix ♀	X External	Ø Drainage Device 3 Infusion Device D Intraluminal Device H Contraceptive Device	Z No Qualifier
H Vagina and Cul-de-sac ♀	Ø Open 3 Percutaneous 4 Percutaneous Endoscopic 7 Via Natural or Artificial Opening 8 Via Natural or Artificial Opening Endoscopic	Ø Drainage Device 1 Radioactive Element 3 Infusion Device 7 Autologous Tissue Substitute D Intraluminal Device J Synthetic Substitute K Nonautologous Tissue Substitute	Z No Qualifier
H Vagina and Cul-de-sac ♀	X External	Ø Drainage Device 1 Radioactive Element 3 Infusion Device D Intraluminal Device	Z No Qualifier
M Vulva ♀	Ø Open	Ø Drainage Device 7 Autologous Tissue Substitute J Synthetic Substitute K Nonautologous Tissue Substitute	Z No Qualifier
M Vulva ♀	X External	Ø Drainage Device	Z No Qualifier

DRG Non-OR ØUP8[78][Ø3D]Z
DRG Non-OR ØUPD[78][Ø3D]Z
DRG Non-OR ØUPH[78][Ø3D]Z

Non-OR ØUP3X[Ø3]Z
Non-OR ØUP8X[Ø3D]Z
Non-OR ØUPD[34]CZ
Non-OR ØUPD[78][CH]Z

Non-OR ØUPDX[Ø3DH]Z
Non-OR ØUPHX[Ø13D]Z
Non-OR ØUPMXØZ

New/Revised Text in Green   deleted Deleted   ♀ Females Only   ♂ Males Only   **Coding Clinic**
Non-covered   Limited Coverage   ⊞ Combination (See Appendix E)   DRG Non-OR   Non-OR   Hospital-Acquired Condition

SECTION: Ø MEDICAL AND SURGICAL

BODY SYSTEM: U FEMALE REPRODUCTIVE SYSTEM
OPERATION: Q REPAIR: Restoring, to the extent possible, a body part to its normal anatomic structure and function

Body Part	Approach	Device	Qualifier
Ø Ovary, Right ♀ ⊞ 1 Ovary, Left ♀ ⊞ 2 Ovaries, Bilateral ♀ ⊞ 4 Uterine Supporting Structure ♀	Ø Open 3 Percutaneous 4 Percutaneous Endoscopic	Z No Device	Z No Qualifier
5 Fallopian Tube, Right ♀ ⊞ 6 Fallopian Tube, Left ♀ ⊞ 7 Fallopian Tubes, Bilateral ♀ ⊞ 9 Uterus ♀ C Cervix ♀ F Cul-de-sac ♀	Ø Open 3 Percutaneous 4 Percutaneous Endoscopic 7 Via Natural or Artificial Opening 8 Via Natural or Artificial Opening Endoscopic	Z No Device	Z No Qualifier
G Vagina ♀ K Hymen ♀	Ø Open 3 Percutaneous 4 Percutaneous Endoscopic 7 Via Natural or Artificial Opening 8 Via Natural or Artificial Opening Endoscopic X External	Z No Device	Z No Qualifier
J Clitoris ♀ L Vestibular Gland ♀ M Vulva ♀ ⊞	Ø Open X External	Z No Device	Z No Qualifier

⊞ ØUQ[Ø12][Ø34]ZZ
⊞ ØUQ[567][Ø34]ZZ
⊞ ØUQM[ØX]ZZ

SECTION: Ø MEDICAL AND SURGICAL

BODY SYSTEM: U FEMALE REPRODUCTIVE SYSTEM
OPERATION: S REPOSITION: Moving to its normal location, or other suitable location, all or a portion of a body part

Body Part	Approach	Device	Qualifier
Ø Ovary, Right ♀ 1 Ovary, Left ♀ 2 Ovaries, Bilateral ♀ 4 Uterine Supporting Structure ♀ 5 Fallopian Tube, Right ♀ 6 Fallopian Tube, Left ♀ 7 Fallopian Tubes, Bilateral ♀ C Cervix ♀ F Cul-de-sac ♀	Ø Open 4 Percutaneous Endoscopic	Z No Device	Z No Qualifier
9 Uterus ♀ G Vagina ♀	Ø Open 4 Percutaneous Endoscopic X External	Z No Device	Z No Qualifier

Non-OR ØUS9XZZ

Coding Clinic: 2Ø16, Q1, P9 – ØUS9XZZ

SECTION: Ø MEDICAL AND SURGICAL

BODY SYSTEM: U FEMALE REPRODUCTIVE SYSTEM

OPERATION: T RESECTION: Cutting out or off, without replacement, all of a body part

Body Part	Approach	Device	Qualifier
Ø Ovary, Right ♀ ⊞ 1 Ovary, Left ♀ ⊞ 2 Ovaries, Bilateral ♀ ⊞ 5 Fallopian Tube, Right ♀ ⊞ 6 Fallopian Tube, Left ♀ ⊞ 7 Fallopian Tubes, Bilateral ♀ ⊞ 9 Uterus ♀ ⊞	Ø Open 4 Percutaneous Endoscopic 7 Via Natural or Artificial Opening 8 Via Natural or Artificial Opening Endoscopic F Via Natural or Artificial Opening With Percutaneous Endoscopic Assistance	Z No Device	Z No Qualifier
4 Uterine Supporting Structure ♀ ⊞ C Cervix ♀ ⊞ F Cul-de-sac ♀ G Vagina ♀ ⊞	Ø Open 4 Percutaneous Endoscopic 7 Via Natural or Artificial Opening 8 Via Natural or Artificial Opening Endoscopic	Z No Device	Z No Qualifier
J Clitoris ♀ L Vestibular Gland ♀ M Vulva ♀ ⊞	Ø Open X External	Z No Device	Z No Qualifier
K Hymen ♀	Ø Open 4 Percutaneous Endoscopic 7 Via Natural or Artificial Opening 8 Via Natural or Artificial Opening Endoscopic X External	Z No Device	Z No Qualifier

⊞ ØUT[012567][04]ZZ
⊞ ØUT9[0478F]ZZ
⊞ ØUT[4C][0478]ZZ
⊞ ØUTGØZZ
⊞ ØUTM[ØX]ZZ

Coding Clinic: 2013, Q1, P24 – ØUTØØZZ
Coding Clinic: 2015, Q1, P33-34; 2013, Q3, P28 – ØUT9ØZZ, ØUTCØZZ
Coding Clinic: 2015, Q1, P34 – ØUT2ØZZ, ØUT7ØZZ

SECTION: Ø MEDICAL AND SURGICAL

BODY SYSTEM: U FEMALE REPRODUCTIVE SYSTEM

OPERATION: U SUPPLEMENT: Putting in or on biological or synthetic material that physically reinforces and/or augments the function of a portion of a body part

Body Part	Approach	Device	Qualifier
4 Uterine Supporting Structure ♀	Ø Open 4 Percutaneous Endoscopic	7 Autologous Tissue Substitute J Synthetic Substitute K Nonautologous Tissue Substitute	Z No Qualifier
5 Fallopian Tube Right ♀ 6 Fallopian Tube, Left ♀ 7 Fallopian Tubes, Bilateral ♀ F Cul-de-sac ♀	Ø Open 4 Percutaneous Endoscopic 7 Via Natural or Artificial Opening 8 Via Natural or Artificial Opening Endoscopic	7 Autologous Tissue Substitute J Synthetic Substitute K Nonautologous Tissue Substitute	Z No Qualifier
G Vagina ♀ K Hymen ♀	Ø Open 4 Percutaneous Endoscopic 7 Via Natural or Artificial Opening 8 Via Natural or Artificial Opening Endoscopic X External	7 Autologous Tissue Substitute J Synthetic Substitute K Nonautologous Tissue Substitute	Z No Qualifier
J Clitoris ♀ M Vulva ♀	Ø Open X External	7 Autologous Tissue Substitute J Synthetic Substitute K Nonautologous Tissue Substitute	Z No Qualifier

New/Revised Text in Green   deleted Deleted   ♀ Females Only   ♂ Males Only   **Coding Clinic**
⚬ Non-covered   ⚬ Limited Coverage   ⊞ Combination (See Appendix E)   DRG Non-OR   Non-OR   ⚬ Hospital-Acquired Condition

Vertical side text: T: RESECTION   U: SUPPLEMENT   U: FEMALE REPRODUCTIVE SYSTEM   Ø: M/S

SECTION: Ø MEDICAL AND SURGICAL

BODY SYSTEM: U FEMALE REPRODUCTIVE SYSTEM

OPERATION: V RESTRICTION: Partially closing an orifice or the lumen of a tubular body part

Body Part	Approach	Device	Qualifier
C Cervix ♀	Ø Open 3 Percutaneous 4 Percutaneous Endoscopic	C Extraluminal Device D Intraluminal Device Z No Device	Z No Qualifier
C Cervix ♀	7 Via Natural or Artificial Opening 8 Via Natural or Artificial Opening Endoscopic	D Intraluminal Device Z No Device	Z No Qualifier

Coding Clinic: 2015, Q3, P30 – ØUVC7ZZ

SECTION: Ø MEDICAL AND SURGICAL

BODY SYSTEM: U FEMALE REPRODUCTIVE SYSTEM

OPERATION: W REVISION: *(on multiple pages)*
Correcting, to the extent possible, a portion of a malfunctioning device or the position of a displaced device

Body Part	Approach	Device	Qualifier
3 Ovary ♀	Ø Open 3 Percutaneous 4 Percutaneous Endoscopic X External	Ø Drainage Device 3 Infusion Device	Z No Qualifier
8 Fallopian Tube ♀	Ø Open 3 Percutaneous 4 Percutaneous Endoscopic 7 Via Natural or Artificial Opening 8 Via Natural or Artificial Opening Endoscopic X External	Ø Drainage Device 3 Infusion Device 7 Autologous Tissue Substitute C Extraluminal Device D Intraluminal Device J Synthetic Substitute K Nonautologous Tissue Substitute	Z No Qualifier
D Uterus and Cervix ♀	Ø Open 3 Percutaneous 4 Percutaneous Endoscopic 7 Via Natural or Artificial Opening 8 Via Natural or Artificial Opening Endoscopic	Ø Drainage Device 1 Radioactive Element 3 Infusion Device 7 Autologous Tissue Substitute C Extraluminal Device D Intraluminal Device H Contraceptive Device J Synthetic Substitute K Nonautologous Tissue Substitute	Z No Qualifier
D Uterus and Cervix ♀	X External	Ø Drainage Device 3 Infusion Device 7 Autologous Tissue Substitute C Extraluminal Device D Intraluminal Device H Contraceptive Device J Synthetic Substitute K Nonautologous Tissue Substitute	Z No Qualifier

Non-OR ØUW3X[Ø3]Z
Non-OR ØUW8X[Ø37CDJK]Z
Non-OR ØUWDX[Ø37CDHJK]Z

SECTION: Ø MEDICAL AND SURGICAL
BODY SYSTEM: U FEMALE REPRODUCTIVE SYSTEM
OPERATION: W REVISION: *(continued)*
Correcting, to the extent possible, a portion of a malfunctioning device or the position of a displaced device

Body Part	Approach	Device	Qualifier
H Vagina and Cul-de-sac ♀	Ø Open 3 Percutaneous 4 Percutaneous Endoscopic 7 Via Natural or Artificial Opening 8 Via Natural or Artificial Opening Endoscopic	Ø Drainage Device 1 Radioactive Element 3 Infusion Device 7 Autologous Tissue Substitute D Intraluminal Device J Synthetic Substitute K Nonautologous Tissue Substitute	Z No Qualifier
H Vagina and Cul-de-sac ♀	X External	Ø Drainage Device 3 Infusion Device 7 Autologous Tissue Substitute D Intraluminal Device J Synthetic Substitute K Nonautologous Tissue Substitute	Z No Qualifier
M Vulva ♀	Ø Open X External	Ø Drainage Device 7 Autologous Tissue Substitute J Synthetic Substitute K Nonautologous Tissue Substitute	Z No Qualifier

Non-OR ØUWHX[Ø37DJK]Z
Non-OR ØUWMX[Ø7JK]Z

SECTION: Ø MEDICAL AND SURGICAL
BODY SYSTEM: U FEMALE REPRODUCTIVE SYSTEM
OPERATION: Y TRANSPLANTATION: Putting in or on all or a portion of a living body part taken from another individual or animal to physically take the place and/or function of all or a portion of a similar body part

Body Part	Approach	Device	Qualifier
Ø Ovary, Right ♀ 1 Ovary, Left ♀	Ø Open	Z No Device	Ø Allogeneic 1 Syngeneic 2 Zooplastic

1: BYPASS   2: CHANGE

V: MALE REPRODUCTIVE SYSTEM

Ø: M/S

SECTION: Ø MEDICAL AND SURGICAL
BODY SYSTEM: V MALE REPRODUCTIVE SYSTEM
OPERATION: 1 **BYPASS:** Altering the route of passage of the contents of a tubular body part

Body Part	Approach	Device	Qualifier
N Vas Deferens, Right ♂ P Vas Deferens, Left ♂ Q Vas Deferens, Bilateral ♂	Ø Open 4 Percutaneous Endoscopic	7 Autologous Tissue Substitute J Synthetic Substitute K Nonautologous Tissue Substitute Z No Device	J Epididymis, Right K Epididymis, Left N Vas Deferens, Right P Vas Deferens, Left

SECTION: Ø MEDICAL AND SURGICAL
BODY SYSTEM: V MALE REPRODUCTIVE SYSTEM
OPERATION: 2 **CHANGE:** Taking out or off a device from a body part and putting back an identical or similar device in or on the same body part without cutting or puncturing the skin or a mucous membrane

Body Part	Approach	Device	Qualifier
4 Prostate and Seminal Vesicles ♂ 8 Scrotum and Tunica Vaginalis ♂ D Testis ♂ M Epididymis and Spermatic Cord ♂ R Vas Deferens ♂ S Penis ♂	X External	Ø Drainage Device Y Other Device	Z No Qualifier

Non-OR   All Values

SECTION: Ø MEDICAL AND SURGICAL
BODY SYSTEM: V MALE REPRODUCTIVE SYSTEM
OPERATION: 5 DESTRUCTION: Physical eradication of all or a portion of a body part by the direct use of energy, force, or a destructive agent

Body Part	Approach	Device	Qualifier
Ø Prostate ♂	Ø Open 3 Percutaneous 4 Percutaneous Endoscopic 7 Via Natural or Artificial Opening 8 Via Natural or Artificial Opening Endoscopic	Z No Device	Z No Qualifier
1 Seminal Vesicle, Right ♂ 2 Seminal Vesicle, Left ♂ 3 Seminal Vesicles, Bilateral ♂ 6 Tunica Vaginalis, Right ♂ 7 Tunica Vaginalis, Left ♂ 9 Testis, Right ♂ B Testis, Left ♂ C Testes, Bilateral ♂ F Spermatic Cord, Right ♂ G Spermatic Cord, Left ♂ H Spermatic Cords, Bilateral ♂ J Epididymis, Right ♂ K Epididymis, Left ♂ L Epididymis, Bilateral ♂ N Vas Deferens, Right ♂ 🚱 P Vas Deferens, Left ♂ 🚱 Q Vas Deferens, Bilateral ♂ 🚱	Ø Open 3 Percutaneous 4 Percutaneous Endoscopic	Z No Device	Z No Qualifier
5 Scrotum ♂ S Penis ♂ T Prepuce ♂	Ø Open 3 Percutaneous 4 Percutaneous Endoscopic X External	Z No Device	Z No Qualifier

🚱 ØV5[NPQ][Ø34]ZZ when Z3Ø.2 is listed as the principal diagnosis
Non-OR ØV5[NPQ][Ø34]ZZ
Non-OR ØV55[Ø34X]ZZ

SECTION: Ø MEDICAL AND SURGICAL
BODY SYSTEM: V MALE REPRODUCTIVE SYSTEM
OPERATION: 7 DILATION: Expanding an orifice or the lumen of a tubular body part

Body Part	Approach	Device	Qualifier
N Vas Deferens, Right ♂ P Vas Deferens, Left ♂ Q Vas Deferens, Bilateral ♂	Ø Open 3 Percutaneous 4 Percutaneous Endoscopic	D Intraluminal Device Z No Device	Z No Qualifier

New/Revised Text in Green   ~~deleted~~ Deleted   ♀ Females Only   ♂ Males Only   **Coding Clinic**
🚱 Non-covered   🚱 Limited Coverage   ⊞ Combination (See Appendix E)   DRG Non-OR   Non-OR   🚱 Hospital-Acquired Condition

453

SECTION: Ø MEDICAL AND SURGICAL
BODY SYSTEM: V MALE REPRODUCTIVE SYSTEM
OPERATION: 9 DRAINAGE: *(on multiple pages)*
Taking or letting out fluids and/or gases from a body part

9: DRAINAGE

V: MALE REPRODUCTIVE SYSTEM

Ø: M/S

Body Part	Approach	Device	Qualifier
Ø Prostate ♂	Ø Open 3 Percutaneous 4 Percutaneous Endoscopic 7 Via Natural or Artificial Opening 8 Via Natural or Artificial Opening Endoscopic	Ø Drainage Device	Z No Qualifier
Ø Prostate ♂	Ø Open 3 Percutaneous 4 Percutaneous Endoscopic 7 Via Natural or Artificial Opening 8 Via Natural or Artificial Opening Endoscopic	Z No Device	X Diagnostic Z No Qualifier
1 Seminal Vesicle, Right ♂ 2 Seminal Vesicle, Left ♂ 3 Seminal Vesicles, Bilateral ♂ 6 Tunica Vaginalis, Right ♂ 7 Tunica Vaginalis, Left ♂ 9 Testis, Right ♂ B Testis, Left ♂ C Testes, Bilateral ♂ F Spermatic Cord, Right ♂ G Spermatic Cord, Left ♂ H Spermatic Cords, Bilateral ♂ J Epididymis, Right ♂ K Epididymis, Left ♂ L Epididymis, Bilateral ♂ N Vas Deferens, Right ♂ P Vas Deferens, Left ♂ Q Vas Deferens, Bilateral ♂	Ø Open 3 Percutaneous 4 Percutaneous Endoscopic	Ø Drainage Device	Z No Qualifier
1 Seminal Vesicle, Right ♂ 2 Seminal Vesicle, Left ♂ 3 Seminal Vesicles, Bilateral ♂ 6 Tunica Vaginalis, Right ♂ 7 Tunica Vaginalis, Left ♂ 9 Testis, Right ♂ B Testis, Left ♂ C Testes, Bilateral ♂ F Spermatic Cord, Right ♂ G Spermatic Cord, Left ♂ H Spermatic Cords, Bilateral ♂ J Epididymis, Right ♂ K Epididymis, Left ♂ L Epididymis, Bilateral ♂ N Vas Deferens, Right ♂ P Vas Deferens, Left ♂ Q Vas Deferens, Bilateral ♂	Ø Open 3 Percutaneous 4 Percutaneous Endoscopic	Z No Device	X Diagnostic Z No Qualifier

DRG Non-OR ØV9[JKL]3ØZ
DRG Non-OR ØV9[JKL]3ZZ
Non-OR ØV9Ø[34]ØZ
Non-OR ØV9Ø[34]ZZ
Non-OR ØV9Ø[3478]ZX

Non-OR ØV9[1239BC][34]ØZ
Non-OR ØV9[67FGHNPQ][Ø34]ØZ
Non-OR ØV9[1239BC][34]Z[XZ]
Non-OR ØV9[67FGHJKLNPQ][Ø34]ZX
Non-OR ØV9[67FGHNPQ][Ø34]ZZ

New/Revised Text in Green   ~~deleted~~ Deleted   ♀ Females Only   ♂ Males Only   **Coding Clinic**
🖉 Non-covered   🖉 Limited Coverage   ⊞ Combination (See Appendix E)   DRG Non-OR   Non-OR   🖉 Hospital-Acquired Condition

SECTION: Ø MEDICAL AND SURGICAL
BODY SYSTEM: V MALE REPRODUCTIVE SYSTEM
OPERATION: 9 DRAINAGE: *(continued)*
Taking or letting out fluids and/or gases from a body part

Body Part	Approach	Device	Qualifier
5 Scrotum ♂ S Penis ♂ T Prepuce ♂	Ø Open 3 Percutaneous 4 Percutaneous Endoscopic X External	Ø Drainage Device	Z No Qualifier
5 Scrotum ♂ S Penis ♂ T Prepuce ♂	Ø Open 3 Percutaneous 4 Percutaneous Endoscopic X External	Z No Device	X Diagnostic Z No Qualifier

DRG Non-OR ØV9[ST]3ØZ
DRG Non-OR ØV9[ST]3ZZ

Non-OR ØV9[ST]3ØZ
Non-OR ØV95[Ø34X]Z[XZ]

SECTION: Ø MEDICAL AND SURGICAL
BODY SYSTEM: V MALE REPRODUCTIVE SYSTEM
OPERATION: B EXCISION: Cutting out or off, without replacement, a portion of a body part

Body Part	Approach	Device	Qualifier
Ø Prostate ♂	Ø Open 3 Percutaneous 4 Percutaneous Endoscopic 7 Via Natural or Artificial Opening 8 Via Natural or Artificial Opening Endoscopic	Z No Device	X Diagnostic Z No Qualifier
1 Seminal Vesicle, Right ♂ 2 Seminal Vesicle, Left ♂ 3 Seminal Vesicles, Bilateral ♂ 6 Tunica Vaginalis, Right ♂ 7 Tunica Vaginalis, Left ♂ 9 Testis, Right ♂ B Testis, Left ♂ C Testes, Bilateral ♂ F Spermatic Cord, Right ♂ G Spermatic Cord, Left ♂ H Spermatic Cords, Bilateral ♂ J Epididymis, Right ♂ K Epididymis, Left ♂ L Epididymis, Bilateral ♂ N Vas Deferens, Right ♂ 🐾 P Vas Deferens, Left ♂ 🐾 Q Vas Deferens, Bilateral ♂ 🐾	Ø Open 3 Percutaneous 4 Percutaneous Endoscopic	Z No Device	X Diagnostic Z No Qualifier
5 Scrotum ♂ S Penis ♂ T Prepuce ♂	Ø Open 3 Percutaneous 4 Percutaneous Endoscopic X External	Z No Device	X Diagnostic Z No Qualifier

🐾 ØVB[NPQ][Ø34]ZZ when Z3Ø.2 is listed as the principal diagnosis
Non-OR ØVBØ[3478]ZX
Non-OR ØVB[1239BC][34]ZX
Non-OR ØVB[67FGHJKL][Ø34]ZX
Non-OR ØVB[NPQ][Ø34]Z[XZ]
Non-OR ØVB5[Ø34X]Z[XZ]

Coding Clinic: 2Ø16, Q1, P23 – ØVBQ4ZZ

New/Revised Text in Green   ~~deleted~~ Deleted   ♀ Females Only   ♂ Males Only   **Coding Clinic**
🐾 Non-covered   🐾 Limited Coverage   ⊞ Combination (See Appendix E)   DRG Non-OR   Non-OR   🐾 Hospital-Acquired Condition

SECTION: Ø MEDICAL AND SURGICAL
BODY SYSTEM: V MALE REPRODUCTIVE SYSTEM
OPERATION: C EXTIRPATION: Taking or cutting out solid matter from a body part

Body Part	Approach	Device	Qualifier
Ø Prostate ♂	Ø Open 3 Percutaneous 4 Percutaneous Endoscopic 7 Via Natural or Artificial Opening 8 Via Natural or Artificial Opening Endoscopic	Z No Device	Z No Qualifier
1 Seminal Vesicle, Right ♂ 2 Seminal Vesicle, Left ♂ 3 Seminal Vesicles, Bilateral ♂ 6 Tunica Vaginalis, Right ♂ 7 Tunica Vaginalis, Left ♂ 9 Testis, Right ♂ B Testis, Left ♂ C Testes, Bilateral ♂ F Spermatic Cord, Right ♂ G Spermatic Cord, Left ♂ H Spermatic Cords, Bilateral ♂ J Epididymis, Right ♂ K Epididymis, Left ♂ L Epididymis, Bilateral ♂ N Vas Deferens, Right ♂ P Vas Deferens, Left ♂ Q Vas Deferens, Bilateral ♂	Ø Open 3 Percutaneous 4 Percutaneous Endoscopic	Z No Device	Z No Qualifier
5 Scrotum ♂ S Penis ♂ T Prepuce ♂	Ø Open 3 Percutaneous 4 Percutaneous Endoscopic X External	Z No Device	Z No Qualifier

Non-OR ØVC[67NPQ][Ø34]ZZ
Non-OR ØVC5[Ø34X]ZZ
Non-OR ØVCSXZZ

C: EXTIRPATION

V: MALE REPRODUCTIVE SYSTEM

Ø: M/S

New/Revised Text in Green   ~~deleted~~ Deleted   ♀ Females Only   ♂ Males Only   **Coding Clinic**

Non-covered   Limited Coverage   ⊕ Combination (See Appendix E)   DRG Non-OR   Non-OR   Hospital-Acquired Condition

SECTION: Ø MEDICAL AND SURGICAL

BODY SYSTEM: V MALE REPRODUCTIVE SYSTEM

OPERATION: H INSERTION: Putting in a nonbiological appliance that monitors, assists, performs, or prevents a physiological function but does not physically take the place of a body part

Body Part	Approach	Device	Qualifier
Ø Prostate ♂	Ø Open 3 Percutaneous 4 Percutaneous Endoscopic 7 Via Natural or Artificial Opening 8 Via Natural or Artificial Opening Endoscopic	1 Radioactive Element	Z No Qualifier
4 Prostate and Seminal Vesicles ♂ 8 Scrotum and Tunica Vaginalis ♂ D Testis ♂ M Epididymis and Spermatic Cord ♂ R Vas Deferens ♂	Ø Open 3 Percutaneous 4 Percutaneous Endoscopic 7 Via Natural or Artificial Opening 8 Via Natural or Artificial Opening Endoscopic	3 Infusion Device	Z No Qualifier
S Penis ♂	Ø Open 3 Percutaneous 4 Percutaneous Endoscopic X External	3 Infusion Device	Z No Qualifier

DRG Non-OR ØVH[48DMR][Ø3478]3Z
DRG Non-OR ØVHS[Ø34X]3Z

SECTION: Ø MEDICAL AND SURGICAL

BODY SYSTEM: V MALE REPRODUCTIVE SYSTEM

OPERATION: J INSPECTION: Visually and/or manually exploring a body part

Body Part	Approach	Device	Qualifier
4 Prostate and Seminal Vesicles ♂ 8 Scrotum and Tunica Vaginalis ♂ D Testis ♂ M Epididymis and Spermatic Cord ♂ R Vas Deferens ♂ S Penis ♂	Ø Open 3 Percutaneous 4 Percutaneous Endoscopic X External	Z No Device	Z No Qualifier

DRG Non-OR ØVJ[4DMR]3ZZ
Non-OR ØVJ[4DMR]XZZ
Non-OR ØVJ[8S][Ø34X]ZZ

SECTION: Ø MEDICAL AND SURGICAL
BODY SYSTEM: V MALE REPRODUCTIVE SYSTEM
OPERATION: L **OCCLUSION:** Completely closing an orifice or the lumen of a tubular body part

Body Part	Approach	Device	Qualifier
F Spermatic Cord, Right ♂ ⊘ G Spermatic Cord, Left ♂ ⊘ H Spermatic Cords, Bilateral ♂ ⊘ N Vas Deferens, Right ♂ ⊘ P Vas Deferens, Left ♂ ⊘ Q Vas Deferens, Bilateral ♂ ⊘	Ø Open 3 Percutaneous 4 Percutaneous Endoscopic	C Extraluminal Device D Intraluminal Device Z No Device	Z No Qualifier

⊘ ØVL[FGH][Ø34][CDZ]Z when Z3Ø.2 is listed as the principal diagnosis
⊘ ØVL[NPQ][Ø34][CZ]Z when Z3Ø.2 is listed as the principal diagnosis
Non-OR ØVL[FGH][Ø34][CDZ]Z
Non-OR ØVL[NPQ][Ø34][CZ]Z

SECTION: Ø MEDICAL AND SURGICAL
BODY SYSTEM: V MALE REPRODUCTIVE SYSTEM
OPERATION: M **REATTACHMENT:** Putting back in or on all or a portion of a separated body part to its normal location or other suitable location

Body Part	Approach	Device	Qualifier
5 Scrotum ♂ S Penis ♂	X External	Z No Device	Z No Qualifier
6 Tunica Vaginalis, Right ♂ 7 Tunica Vaginalis, Left ♂ 9 Testis, Right ♂ B Testis, Left ♂ C Testes, Bilateral ♂ F Spermatic Cord, Right ♂ G Spermatic Cord, Left ♂ H Spermatic Cords, Bilateral ♂	Ø Open 4 Percutaneous Endoscopic	Z No Device	Z No Qualifier

SECTION: Ø MEDICAL AND SURGICAL
BODY SYSTEM: V MALE REPRODUCTIVE SYSTEM
OPERATION: N RELEASE: Freeing a body part from an abnormal physical restraint by cutting or by the use of force

Body Part	Approach	Device	Qualifier
Ø Prostate ♂	Ø Open 3 Percutaneous 4 Percutaneous Endoscopic 7 Via Natural or Artificial Opening 8 Via Natural or Artificial Opening Endoscopic	Z No Device	Z No Qualifier
1 Seminal Vesicle, Right ♂ 2 Seminal Vesicle, Left ♂ 3 Seminal Vesicles, Bilateral ♂ 6 Tunica Vaginalis, Right ♂ 7 Tunica Vaginalis, Left ♂ 9 Testis, Right ♂ B Testis, Left ♂ C Testes, Bilateral ♂ F Spermatic Cord, Right ♂ G Spermatic Cord, Left ♂ H Spermatic Cords, Bilateral ♂ J Epididymis, Right ♂ K Epididymis, Left ♂ L Epididymis, Bilateral ♂ N Vas Deferens, Right ♂ P Vas Deferens, Left ♂ Q Vas Deferens, Bilateral ♂	Ø Open 3 Percutaneous 4 Percutaneous Endoscopic	Z No Device	Z No Qualifier
5 Scrotum ♂ S Penis ♂ T Prepuce ♂	Ø Open 3 Percutaneous 4 Percutaneous Endoscopic X External	Z No Device	Z No Qualifier

Non-OR ØVN[9BC][Ø34]ZZ
Non-OR ØVNT[Ø34X]ZZ

SECTION: Ø MEDICAL AND SURGICAL

BODY SYSTEM: V MALE REPRODUCTIVE SYSTEM
OPERATION: P REMOVAL: Taking out or off a device from a body part

Body Part	Approach	Device	Qualifier
4 Prostate and Seminal Vesicles ♂	Ø Open 3 Percutaneous 4 Percutaneous Endoscopic 7 Via Natural or Artificial Opening 8 Via Natural or Artificial Opening Endoscopic	Ø Drainage Device 1 Radioactive Element 3 Infusion Device 7 Autologous Tissue Substitute J Synthetic Substitute K Nonautologous Tissue Substitute	Z No Qualifier
4 Prostate and Seminal Vesicles ♂	X External	Ø Drainage Device 1 Radioactive Element 3 Infusion Device	Z No Qualifier
8 Scrotum and Tunica Vaginalis ♂ D Testis ♂ S Penis ♂	Ø Open 3 Percutaneous 4 Percutaneous Endoscopic 7 Via Natural or Artificial Opening 8 Via Natural or Artificial Opening Endoscopic	Ø Drainage Device 3 Infusion Device 7 Autologous Tissue Substitute J Synthetic Substitute K Nonautologous Tissue Substitute	Z No Qualifier
8 Scrotum and Tunica Vaginalis ♂ D Testis ♂ S Penis ♂	X External	Ø Drainage Device 3 Infusion Device	Z No Qualifier
M Epididymis and Spermatic Cord ♂	Ø Open 3 Percutaneous 4 Percutaneous Endoscopic 7 Via Natural or Artificial Opening 8 Via Natural or Artificial Opening Endoscopic	Ø Drainage Device 3 Infusion Device 7 Autologous Tissue Substitute C Extraluminal Device J Synthetic Substitute K Nonautologous Tissue Substitute	Z No Qualifier
M Epididymis and Spermatic Cord ♂	X External	Ø Drainage Device 3 Infusion Device	Z No Qualifier
R Vas Deferens ♂	Ø Open 3 Percutaneous 4 Percutaneous Endoscopic 7 Via Natural or Artificial Opening 8 Via Natural or Artificial Opening Endoscopic	Ø Drainage Device 3 Infusion Device 7 Autologous Tissue Substitute C Extraluminal Device D Intraluminal Device J Synthetic Substitute K Nonautologous Tissue Substitute	Z No Qualifier
R Vas Deferens ♂	X External	Ø Drainage Device 3 Infusion Device D Intraluminal Device	Z No Qualifier

DRG Non-OR ØVP4[78][Ø3]Z
DRG Non-OR ØVPD[78][Ø3]Z
DRG Non-OR ØVPS[78][Ø3]Z
DRG Non-OR ØVPM[78][Ø3]Z
DRG Non-OR ØVPR[78]DZ
Non-OR ØVP4X[Ø13]Z
Non-OR ØVP8[Ø3478][Ø37JK]Z
Non-OR ØVP[8DS]X[Ø3]Z
Non-OR ØVPMX[Ø3]Z
Non-OR ØVPR[Ø3478][Ø37CDJK]Z
Non-OR ØVPRX[Ø3D]Z

Coding Clinic: 2Ø16, Q2, P28 – ØVPSØJZ

SECTION: Ø MEDICAL AND SURGICAL
BODY SYSTEM: V MALE REPRODUCTIVE SYSTEM
OPERATION: Q REPAIR: Restoring, to the extent possible, a body part to its normal anatomic structure and function

Body Part	Approach	Device	Qualifier
Ø Prostate ♂	Ø Open 3 Percutaneous 4 Percutaneous Endoscopic 7 Via Natural or Artificial Opening 8 Via Natural or Artificial Opening Endoscopic	Z No Device	Z No Qualifier
1 Seminal Vesicle, Right ♂ 2 Seminal Vesicle, Left ♂ 3 Seminal Vesicles, Bilateral ♂ 6 Tunica Vaginalis, Right ♂ 7 Tunica Vaginalis, Left ♂ 9 Testis, Right ♂ B Testis, Left ♂ C Testes, Bilateral ♂ F Spermatic Cord, Right ♂ G Spermatic Cord, Left ♂ H Spermatic Cords, Bilateral ♂ J Epididymis, Right ♂ K Epididymis, Left ♂ L Epididymis, Bilateral ♂ N Vas Deferens, Right ♂ P Vas Deferens, Left ♂ Q Vas Deferens, Bilateral ♂	Ø Open 3 Percutaneous 4 Percutaneous Endoscopic	Z No Device	Z No Qualifier
5 Scrotum ♂ S Penis ♂ T Prepuce ♂	Ø Open 3 Percutaneous 4 Percutaneous Endoscopic X External	Z No Device	Z No Qualifier

Non-OR ØVQ[67][Ø34]ZZ
Non-OR ØVQ5[Ø34X]ZZ

SECTION: Ø MEDICAL AND SURGICAL
BODY SYSTEM: V MALE REPRODUCTIVE SYSTEM
OPERATION: R REPLACEMENT: Putting in or on biological or synthetic material that physically takes the place and/or function of all or a portion of a body part

Body Part	Approach	Device	Qualifier
9 Testis, Right ♂ B Testis, Left ♂ C Testis, Bilateral ♂	Ø Open	J Synthetic Substitute	Z No Qualifier

New/Revised Text in Green deleted Deleted ♀ Females Only ♂ Males Only Coding Clinic
Non-covered Limited Coverage Combination (See Appendix E) DRG Non-OR Non-OR Hospital-Acquired Condition

461

SECTION: Ø MEDICAL AND SURGICAL

BODY SYSTEM: V MALE REPRODUCTIVE SYSTEM

OPERATION: S REPOSITION: Moving to its normal location or other suitable location all or a portion of a body part

Body Part	Approach	Device	Qualifier
9 Testis, Right ♂ B Testis, Left ♂ C Testes, Bilateral ♂ F Spermatic Cord, Right ♂ G Spermatic Cord, Left ♂ H Spermatic Cords, Bilateral ♂	Ø Open 3 Percutaneous 4 Percutaneous Endoscopic	Z No Device	Z No Qualifier

SECTION: Ø MEDICAL AND SURGICAL

BODY SYSTEM: V MALE REPRODUCTIVE SYSTEM

OPERATION: T RESECTION: Cutting out or off, without replacement, all of a body part

Body Part	Approach	Device	Qualifier
Ø Prostate ♂ ⊞	Ø Open 4 Percutaneous Endoscopic 7 Via Natural or Artificial Opening 8 Via Natural or Artificial Opening Endoscopic	Z No Device	Z No Qualifier
1 Seminal Vesicle, Right ♂ 2 Seminal Vesicle, Left ♂ 3 Seminal Vesicles, Bilateral ♂ ⊞ 6 Tunica Vaginalis, Right ♂ 7 Tunica Vaginalis, Left ♂ 9 Testis, Right ♂ B Testis, Left ♂ C Testes, Bilateral ♂ F Spermatic Cord, Right ♂ G Spermatic Cord, Left ♂ H Spermatic Cords, Bilateral ♂ J Epididymis, Right ♂ K Epididymis, Left ♂ L Epididymis, Bilateral ♂ N Vas Deferens, Right ♂ ⚕ P Vas Deferens, Left ♂ ⚕ Q Vas Deferens, Bilateral ♂ ⚕	Ø Open 4 Percutaneous Endoscopic	Z No Device	Z No Qualifier
5 Scrotum ♂ S Penis ♂ T Prepuce ♂	Ø Open 4 Percutaneous Endoscopic X External	Z No Device	Z No Qualifier

⚕ ØVT[NPQ][Ø4]ZZ when Z30.2 is listed as the principal diagnosis
⊞ ØVTØ[Ø478]ZZ
⊞ ØVT3[Ø4]ZZ
Non-OR ØVT[NPQ][Ø4]ZZ
Non-OR ØVT[5T][Ø4X]ZZ

SECTION: Ø MEDICAL AND SURGICAL
BODY SYSTEM: V MALE REPRODUCTIVE SYSTEM
OPERATION: U SUPPLEMENT: Putting in or on biological or synthetic material that physically reinforces and/or augments the function of a portion of a body part

Body Part	Approach	Device	Qualifier
1 Seminal Vesicle, Right ♂ 2 Seminal Vesicle, Left ♂ 3 Seminal Vesicles, Bilateral ♂ 6 Tunica Vaginalis, Right ♂ 7 Tunica Vaginalis, Left ♂ F Spermatic Cord, Right ♂ G Spermatic Cord, Left ♂ H Spermatic Cords, Bilateral ♂ J Epididymis, Right ♂ K Epididymis, Left ♂ L Epididymis, Bilateral ♂ N Vas Deferens, Right ♂ P Vas Deferens, Left ♂ Q Vas Deferens, Bilateral ♂	Ø Open 4 Percutaneous Endoscopic	7 Autologous Tissue Substitute J Synthetic Substitute K Nonautologous Tissue Substitute	Z No Qualifier
5 Scrotum ♂ S Penis ♂ T Prepuce ♂	Ø Open 4 Percutaneous Endoscopic X External	7 Autologous Tissue Substitute J Synthetic Substitute K Nonautologous Tissue Substitute	Z No Qualifier
9 Testis, Right ♂ B Testis, Left ♂ C Testis, Bilateral ♂	Ø Open	7 Autologous Tissue Substitute J Synthetic Substitute K Nonautologous Tissue Substitute	Z No Qualifier

Non-OR ØVUSX[7JK]Z

Coding Clinic: 2016, Q2, P29; 2015, Q3, P25 – ØVUSØJZ

SECTION: Ø MEDICAL AND SURGICAL
BODY SYSTEM: V MALE REPRODUCTIVE SYSTEM
OPERATION: W REVISION: Correcting, to the extent possible, a portion of a malfunctioning device or the position of a displaced device

Body Part	Approach	Device	Qualifier
4 Prostate and Seminal Vesicles ♂ 8 Scrotum and Tunica Vaginalis ♂ D Testis ♂ S Penis ♂	Ø Open 3 Percutaneous 4 Percutaneous Endoscopic 7 Via Natural or Artificial Opening 8 Via Natural or Artificial Opening Endoscopic X External	Ø Drainage Device 3 Infusion Device 7 Autologous Tissue Substitute J Synthetic Substitute K Nonautologous Tissue Substitute	Z No Qualifier
M Epididymis and Spermatic Cord ♂	Ø Open 3 Percutaneous 4 Percutaneous Endoscopic 7 Via Natural or Artificial Opening 8 Via Natural or Artificial Opening Endoscopic X External	Ø Drainage Device 3 Infusion Device 7 Autologous Tissue Substitute C Extraluminal Device J Synthetic Substitute K Nonautologous Tissue Substitute	Z No Qualifier
R Vas Deferens ♂	Ø Open 3 Percutaneous 4 Percutaneous Endoscopic 7 Via Natural or Artificial Opening 8 Via Natural or Artificial Opening Endoscopic X External	Ø Drainage Device 3 Infusion Device 7 Autologous Tissue Substitute C Extraluminal Device D Intraluminal Device J Synthetic Substitute K Nonautologous Tissue Substitute	Z No Qualifier

Non-OR ØVW[4DS]X[Ø37JK]Z
Non-OR ØVW8[Ø3478X][Ø37JK]Z
Non-OR ØVWMX[Ø37CJK]Z
Non-OR ØVWR[Ø3478X][Ø37CDJK]Z

W: REVISION

V: MALE REPRODUCTIVE SYSTEM

Ø: M/S

New/Revised Text in Green   ~~deleted~~ Deleted   ♀ Females Only   ♂ Males Only   **Coding Clinic**
🔾 Non-covered   🔾 Limited Coverage   ⊞ Combination (See Appendix E)   DRG Non-OR   Non-OR   🔾 Hospital-Acquired Condition

SECTION: Ø MEDICAL AND SURGICAL

BODY SYSTEM: W ANATOMICAL REGIONS, GENERAL

OPERATION: Ø ALTERATION: Modifying the anatomic structure of a body part without affecting the function of the body part

Body Part	Approach	Device	Qualifier
Ø Head 2 Face 4 Upper Jaw 5 Lower Jaw 6 Neck 8 Chest Wall F Abdominal Wall K Upper Back L Lower Back M Perineum, Male ♂ N Perineum, Female ♀	Ø Open 3 Percutaneous 4 Percutaneous Endoscopic	7 Autologous Tissue Substitute J Synthetic Substitute K Nonautologous Tissue Substitute Z No Device	Z No Qualifier

Coding Clinic: 2Ø15, Q1, P31 – ØWØ2ØZZ

SECTION: Ø MEDICAL AND SURGICAL

BODY SYSTEM: W ANATOMICAL REGIONS, GENERAL

OPERATION: 1 BYPASS: Altering the route of passage of the contents of a tubular body part

Body Part	Approach	Device	Qualifier
1 Cranial Cavity	Ø Open	J Synthetic Substitute	9 Pleural Cavity, Right B Pleural Cavity, Left G Peritoneal Cavity J Pelvic Cavity
9 Pleural Cavity, Right B Pleural Cavity, Left G Peritoneal Cavity J Pelvic Cavity	Ø Open 4 Percutaneous Endoscopic	J Synthetic Substitute	4 Cutaneous 9 Pleural Cavity, Right B Pleural Cavity, Left G Peritoneal Cavity J Pelvic Cavity Y Lower Vein
9 Pleural Cavity, Right B Pleural Cavity, Left G Peritoneal Cavity J Pelvic Cavity	3 Percutaneous	J Synthetic Substitute	4 Cutaneous

Non-OR ØW1[9B][Ø4]J[4GY]
Non-OR ØW1G[Ø4]J[9BGJ]
Non-OR ØW1J[Ø4]J[4Y]
Non-OR ØW1[9BJ]3J4

New/Revised Text in Green   ~~deleted~~ Deleted   ♀ Females Only   ♂ Males Only   **Coding Clinic**

Non-covered   Limited Coverage   Combination (See Appendix E)   DRG Non-OR   Non-OR   Hospital-Acquired Condition

Ø: ALTERATION   1: BYPASS

W: ANATOMICAL REGIONS, GENERAL

Ø: M/S

SECTION: Ø MEDICAL AND SURGICAL

BODY SYSTEM: W ANATOMICAL REGIONS, GENERAL

OPERATION: 2 CHANGE: Taking out or off a device from a body part and putting back an identical or similar device in or on the same body part without cutting or puncturing the skin or a mucous membrane

Body Part	Approach	Device	Qualifier
Ø Head	X External	Ø Drainage Device	Z No Qualifier
1 Cranial Cavity		Y Other Device	
2 Face			
4 Upper Jaw			
5 Lower Jaw			
6 Neck			
8 Chest Wall			
9 Pleural Cavity, Right			
B Pleural Cavity, Left			
C Mediastinum			
D Pericardial Cavity			
F Abdominal Wall			
G Peritoneal Cavity			
H Retroperitoneum			
J Pelvic Cavity			
K Upper Back			
L Lower Back			
M Perineum, Male ♂			
N Perineum, Female ♀			

Non-OR All Values

SECTION: Ø MEDICAL AND SURGICAL

BODY SYSTEM: W ANATOMICAL REGIONS, GENERAL

OPERATION: 3 CONTROL: *(on multiple pages)*
Stopping, or attempting to stop, postprocedure or other acute bleeding

Body Part	Approach	Device	Qualifier
Ø Head	Ø Open	Z No Device	Z No Qualifier
1 Cranial Cavity	3 Percutaneous		
2 Face	4 Percutaneous Endoscopic		
3 Oral Cavity and Throat			
4 Upper Jaw			
5 Lower Jaw			
6 Neck			
8 Chest Wall			
9 Pleural Cavity, Right			
B Pleural Cavity, Left			
C Mediastinum			
D Pericardial Cavity			
F Abdominal Wall			
G Peritoneal Cavity			
H Retroperitoneum			
J Pelvic Cavity			
K Upper Back			
L Lower Back			
M Perineum, Male ♂			
N Perineum, Female ♀			

Non-OR ØW3GØZZ

Ø: M/S

W: ANATOMICAL REGIONS, GENERAL

2: CHANGE   3: CONTROL

SECTION: Ø MEDICAL AND SURGICAL

BODY SYSTEM: W ANATOMICAL REGIONS, GENERAL

OPERATION: 3 CONTROL: *(continued)*
Stopping, or attempting to stop, postprocedure or other acute bleeding

Body Part	Approach	Device	Qualifier
3 Oral Cavity and Throat	Ø Open 3 Percutaneous 4 Percutaneous Endoscopic 7 Via Natural or Artificial Opening 8 Via Natural or Artificial Opening Endoscopic X External	Z No Device	Z No Qualifier
P Gastrointestinal Tract Q Respiratory Tract R Genitourinary Tract	Ø Open 3 Percutaneous 4 Percutaneous Endoscopic 7 Via Natural or Artificial Opening 8 Via Natural or Artificial Opening Endoscopic	Z No Device	Z No Qualifier

Non-OR ØW3P8ZZ

SECTION: Ø MEDICAL AND SURGICAL

BODY SYSTEM: W ANATOMICAL REGIONS, GENERAL

OPERATION: 4 CREATION: Putting in or on biological or synthetic material to form a new body part that to the extent possible replicates the anatomic structure or function of an absent body part

Body Part	Approach	Device	Qualifier
M Perineum, Male ♂ 🗞	Ø Open	7 Autologous Tissue Substitute J Synthetic Substitute K Nonautologous Tissue Substitute Z No Device	Ø Vagina
N Perineum, Female ♀ 🗞	Ø Open	7 Autologous Tissue Substitute J Synthetic Substitute K Nonautologous Tissue Substitute Z No Device	1 Penis

🗞 ØW4MØ[7JKZ]Ø
🗞 ØW4NØ[7JKZ]1

SECTION: Ø MEDICAL AND SURGICAL

BODY SYSTEM: W ANATOMICAL REGIONS, GENERAL

OPERATION: 8 DIVISION: Cutting into a body part, without draining fluids and/or gases from the body part, in order to separate or transect a body part

Body Part	Approach	Device	Qualifier
N Perineum, Female ♀	X External	Z No Device	Z No Qualifier

Non-OR ØW8NXZZ

New/Revised Text in Green   ~~deleted~~ Deleted   ♀ Females Only   ♂ Males Only   **Coding Clinic**
🗞 Non-covered   🗞 Limited Coverage   ⊞ Combination (See Appendix E)   DRG Non-OR   Non-OR   🗞 Hospital-Acquired Condition

SECTION: Ø MEDICAL AND SURGICAL

BODY SYSTEM: W ANATOMICAL REGIONS, GENERAL

OPERATION: 9 DRAINAGE: Taking or letting out fluids and/or gases from a body part

Body Part	Approach	Device	Qualifier
Ø Head 1 Cranial Cavity 2 Face 3 Oral Cavity and Throat 4 Upper Jaw 5 Lower Jaw 6 Neck 8 Chest Wall 9 Pleural Cavity, Right B Pleural Cavity, Left C Mediastinum D Pericardial Cavity F Abdominal Wall G Peritoneal Cavity H Retroperitoneum J Pelvic Cavity K Upper Back L Lower Back M Perineum, Male ♂ N Perineum, Female ♀	Ø Open 3 Percutaneous 4 Percutaneous Endoscopic	Ø Drainage Device	Z No Qualifier
Ø Head 1 Cranial Cavity 2 Face 3 Oral Cavity and Throat 4 Upper Jaw 5 Lower Jaw 6 Neck 8 Chest Wall 9 Pleural Cavity, Right B Pleural Cavity, Left C Mediastinum D Pericardial Cavity F Abdominal Wall G Peritoneal Cavity H Retroperitoneum J Pelvic Cavity K Upper Back L Lower Back M Perineum, Male ♂ N Perineum, Female ♀	Ø Open 3 Percutaneous 4 Percutaneous Endoscopic	Z No Device	X Diagnostic Z No Qualifier

DRG Non-OR ØW9[23456CHN]3ØZ
DRG Non-OR ØW9[23456CHN]3ZZ
Non-OR ØW9[Ø8KLM][Ø34]ØZ
Non-OR ØW9[9B][Ø3]ØZ
Non-OR ØW9[1DFG][34]ØZ
Non-OR ØW9J3ØZ
Non-OR ØW9[Ø234568KLMN][Ø34]ZX
Non-OR ØW9[9B][Ø3]ZZ
Non-OR ØW9[Ø89BKLM][Ø34]ZZ
Non-OR ØW9[1CD][34]ZX
Non-OR ØW9[1DFG][34]ZZ
Non-OR ØW9J3ZZ

SECTION: Ø MEDICAL AND SURGICAL
BODY SYSTEM: W ANATOMICAL REGIONS, GENERAL
OPERATION: B EXCISION: Cutting out or off, without replacement, a portion of a body part

Body Part	Approach	Device	Qualifier
Ø Head 2 Face 4 Upper Jaw 5 Lower Jaw 8 Chest Wall K Upper Back L Lower Back M Perineum, Male ♂ N Perineum, Female ♀	Ø Open 3 Percutaneous 4 Percutaneous Endoscopic X External	Z No Device	X Diagnostic Z No Qualifier
6 Neck F Abdominal Wall	Ø Open 3 Percutaneous 4 Percutaneous Endoscopic	Z No Device	X Diagnostic Z No Qualifier
6 Neck F Abdominal Wall	X External	Z No Device	2 Stoma X Diagnostic Z No Qualifier
C Mediastinum H Retroperitoneum	Ø Open 3 Percutaneous 4 Percutaneous Endoscopic	Z No Device	X Diagnostic Z No Qualifier

Non-OR ØWB[Ø2458KLM][Ø34X]ZX
Non-OR ØWB6[Ø34]ZX
Non-OR ØWB6XZX
Non-OR ØWB[CH][34]ZX

Coding Clinic: 2Ø16, Q1, P22 – ØWBF4ZZ

SECTION: Ø MEDICAL AND SURGICAL
BODY SYSTEM: W ANATOMICAL REGIONS, GENERAL
OPERATION: C EXTIRPATION: Taking or cutting out solid matter from a body part

Body Part	Approach	Device	Qualifier
1 Cranial Cavity 3 Oral Cavity and Throat 9 Pleural Cavity, Right B Pleural Cavity, Left C Mediastinum D Pericardial Cavity G Peritoneal Cavity J Pelvic Cavity	Ø Open 3 Percutaneous 4 Percutaneous Endoscopic X External	Z No Device	Z No Qualifier
P Gastrointestinal Tract Q Respiratory Tract R Genitourinary Tract	Ø Open 3 Percutaneous 4 Percutaneous Endoscopic 7 Via Natural or Artificial Opening 8 Via Natural or Artificial Opening Endoscopic X External	Z No Device	Z No Qualifier

Non-OR ØWC[13]XZZ
Non-OR ØWC[9B][Ø34X]ZZ
Non-OR ØWC[CDGJ]XZZ
Non-OR ØWCP[78X]ZZ
Non-OR ØWCQ[Ø34X]ZZ
Non-OR ØWCR[78X]ZZ

New/Revised Text in Green   ~~deleted~~ Deleted   ♀ Females Only   ♂ Males Only   **Coding Clinic**
🚫 Non-covered   🚫 Limited Coverage   ⊞ Combination (See Appendix E)   DRG Non-OR   Non-OR   🚫 Hospital-Acquired Condition

SECTION: Ø MEDICAL AND SURGICAL

BODY SYSTEM: W ANATOMICAL REGIONS, GENERAL

OPERATION: F FRAGMENTATION: Breaking solid matter in a body part into pieces

Body Part	Approach	Device	Qualifier
1 Cranial Cavity 🔖 3 Oral Cavity and Throat 🔖 9 Pleural Cavity, Right 🔖 B Pleural Cavity, Left 🔖 C Mediastinum 🔖 D Pericardial Cavity G Peritoneal Cavity 🔖 J Pelvic Cavity 🔖	Ø Open 3 Percutaneous 4 Percutaneous Endoscopic X External	Z No Device	Z No Qualifier

P Gastrointestinal Tract 🔖
Q Respiratory Tract 🔖
R Genitourinary Tract
	Ø Open
	3 Percutaneous
	4 Percutaneous Endoscopic
	7 Via Natural or Artificial
	  Opening
	8 Via Natural or Artificial
	  Opening Endoscopic
	X External
		Z No Device	Z No Qualifier

🔖 ØWF[139BCGJ]XZZ
🔖 ØWF[PQ]XZZ
DRG Non-OR ØWFRXZZ
Non-OR ØWF[139BCG]XZZ
Non-OR ØWFJ[Ø34X]ZZ
Non-OR ØWFP[Ø3478X]ZZ
Non-OR ØWFQXZZ
Non-OR ØWFR[Ø3478]ZZ

SECTION: Ø MEDICAL AND SURGICAL
BODY SYSTEM: W ANATOMICAL REGIONS, GENERAL
OPERATION: H INSERTION: Putting in a nonbiological appliance that monitors, assists, performs, or prevents a physiological function but does not physically take the place of a body part

Body Part	Approach	Device	Qualifier
Ø Head 1 Cranial Cavity 2 Face 3 Oral Cavity and Throat 4 Upper Jaw 5 Lower Jaw 6 Neck 8 Chest Wall 9 Pleural Cavity, Right B Pleural Cavity, Left C Mediastinum D Pericardial Cavity F Abdominal Wall G Peritoneal Cavity H Retroperitoneum J Pelvic Cavity K Upper Back L Lower Back M Perineum, Male ♂ N Perineum, Female ♀	Ø Open 3 Percutaneous 4 Percutaneous Endoscopic	1 Radioactive Element 3 Infusion Device Y Other Device	Z No Qualifier
P Gastrointestinal Tract Q Respiratory Tract R Genitourinary Tract	Ø Open 3 Percutaneous 4 Percutaneous Endoscopic 7 Via Natural or Artificial Opening 8 Via Natural or Artificial Opening Endoscopic	1 Radioactive Element 3 Infusion Device Y Other Device	Z No Qualifier

DRG Non-OR   ØWH[02456KLM][034][3Y]Z
Non-OR   ØWH1[034]3Z
Non-OR   ØWH[89B][034][3Y]Z
Non-OR   ØWHPØYZ
Non-OR   ØWHP[3478][3Y]Z
Non-OR   ØWHQ[078][3Y]Z
Non-OR   ØWHR[03478][3Y]Z

Coding Clinic: 2Ø16, Q2, P14 – ØWHG33Z

New/Revised Text in Green   ~~deleted~~ Deleted   ♀ Females Only   ♂ Males Only   Coding Clinic
Non-covered   Limited Coverage   ⊡ Combination (See Appendix E)   DRG Non-OR   Non-OR   Hospital-Acquired Condition

SECTION: Ø MEDICAL AND SURGICAL
BODY SYSTEM: W ANATOMICAL REGIONS, GENERAL
OPERATION: J INSPECTION: Visually and/or manually exploring a body part

Body Part	Approach	Device	Qualifier
Ø Head 2 Face 3 Oral Cavity and Throat 4 Upper Jaw 5 Lower Jaw 6 Neck 8 Chest Wall F Abdominal Wall K Upper Back L Lower Back M Perineum, Male ♂ N Perineum, Female ♀	Ø Open 3 Percutaneous 4 Percutaneous Endoscopic X External	Z No Device	Z No Qualifier
1 Cranial Cavity 9 Pleural Cavity, Right B Pleural Cavity, Left C Mediastinum D Pericardial Cavity G Peritoneal Cavity H Retroperitoneum J Pelvic Cavity	Ø Open 3 Percutaneous 4 Percutaneous Endoscopic	Z No Device	Z No Qualifier
P Gastrointestinal Tract Q Respiratory Tract R Genitourinary Tract	Ø Open 3 Percutaneous 4 Percutaneous Endoscopic 7 Via Natural or Artificial Opening 8 Via Natural or Artificial Opening Endoscopic	Z No Device	Z No Qualifier

DRG Non-OR ØWJ[Ø245KL]ØZZ
DRG Non-OR ØWJ[68FN]3ZZ
DRG Non-OR ØWJM[Ø4]ZZ
DRG Non-OR ØWJ[19BCGHJ]3ZZ
DRG Non-OR ØWJ[PQR][378]ZZ

Non-OR ØWJ[Ø245KL][34X]ZZ
Non-OR ØWJ3[Ø34X]ZZ
Non-OR ØWJ[68FN]XZZ

Non-OR OWJM[3X]ZZ
Non-OR ØWJD[Ø3]ZZ

Coding Clinic: 2013, Q2, P37 – ØWJG4ZZ

SECTION: Ø MEDICAL AND SURGICAL
BODY SYSTEM: W ANATOMICAL REGIONS, GENERAL
OPERATION: M REATTACHMENT: Putting back in or on all or a portion of a separated body part to its normal location or other suitable location

Body Part	Approach	Device	Qualifier
2 Face 4 Upper Jaw 5 Lower Jaw 6 Neck 8 Chest Wall F Abdominal Wall K Upper Back L Lower Back M Perineum, Male ♂ N Perineum, Female ♀	Ø Open	Z No Device	Z No Qualifier

SECTION: Ø MEDICAL AND SURGICAL

BODY SYSTEM: W ANATOMICAL REGIONS, GENERAL

OPERATION: P REMOVAL: Taking out or off a device from a body part

Body Part	Approach	Device	Qualifier
Ø Head 2 Face 4 Upper Jaw 5 Lower Jaw 6 Neck 8 Chest Wall C Mediastinum F Abdominal Wall K Upper Back L Lower Back M Perineum, Male ♂ N Perineum, Female ♀	Ø Open 3 Percutaneous 4 Percutaneous Endoscopic X External	Ø Drainage Device 1 Radioactive Element 3 Infusion Device 7 Autologous Tissue Substitute J Synthetic Substitute K Nonautologous Tissue Substitute Y Other Device	Z No Qualifier
1 Cranial Cavity 9 Pleural Cavity, Right B Pleural Cavity, Left G Peritoneal Cavity J Pelvic Cavity	Ø Open 3 Percutaneous 4 Percutaneous Endoscopic	Ø Drainage Device 1 Radioactive Element 3 Infusion Device J Synthetic Substitute Y Other Device	Z No Qualifier
1 Cranial Cavity 9 Pleural Cavity, Right B Pleural Cavity, Left G Peritoneal Cavity J Pelvic Cavity	X External	Ø Drainage Device 1 Radioactive Element 3 Infusion Device	Z No Qualifier
D Pericardial Cavity H Retroperitoneum	Ø Open 3 Percutaneous 4 Percutaneous Endoscopic	Ø Drainage Device 1 Radioactive Element 3 Infusion Device Y Other Device	Z No Qualifier
D Pericardial Cavity H Retroperitoneum	X External	Ø Drainage Device 1 Radioactive Element 3 Infusion Device	Z No Qualifier
P Gastrointestinal Tract Q Respiratory Tract R Genitourinary Tract	Ø Open 3 Percutaneous 4 Percutaneous Endoscopic 7 Via Natural or Artificial Opening 8 Via Natural or Artificial Opening Endoscopic X External	1 Radioactive Element 3 Infusion Device Y Other Device	Z No Qualifier

DRG Non-OR ØWPQ73Z
Non-OR OWP[Ø24568KL][Ø34X][Ø137JKY]Z
Non-OR OWPM[Ø34][Ø13JY]Z
Non-OR OWPMX[Ø13Y]Z
Non-OR OWP[CFN]X[Ø137JKY]Z
Non-OR OWP1[Ø34]3Z
Non-OR OWP[9BJ][Ø34][Ø13JY]Z
Non-OR OWP[19BGJ]X[Ø13]Z
Non-OR OWP[DH]X[Ø13]Z
Non-OR OWPP[3478X][13Y]Z
Non-OR OWPQ8[3Y]Z
Non-OR OWPQ[ØX][13Y]Z
Non-OR OWPR[Ø3478X][13Y]Z

New/Revised Text in Green deleted Deleted ♀ Females Only ♂ Males Only Coding Clinic
Non-covered Limited Coverage Combination (See Appendix E) DRG Non-OR Non-OR Hospital-Acquired Condition

SECTION: Ø MEDICAL AND SURGICAL

BODY SYSTEM: W ANATOMICAL REGIONS, GENERAL

OPERATION: Q REPAIR: Restoring, to the extent possible, a body part to its normal anatomic structure and function

Body Part	Approach	Device	Qualifier
Ø Head 2 Face 4 Upper Jaw 5 Lower Jaw 8 Chest Wall ⊞ K Upper Back L Lower Back M Perineum, Male ♂ N Perineum, Female ♀ ⊞	Ø Open 3 Percutaneous 4 Percutaneous Endoscopic X External	Z No Device	Z No Qualifier
6 Neck F Abdominal Wall	Ø Open 3 Percutaneous 4 Percutaneous Endoscopic	Z No Device	Z No Qualifier
6 Neck F Abdominal Wall ⊞	X External	Z No Device	2 Stoma Z No Qualifier
C Mediastinum ⊞	Ø Open 3 Percutaneous 4 Percutaneous Endoscopic	Z No Device	Z No Qualifier

⊞ ØWQ[8N][Ø34]ZZ
⊞ ØWQFXZ[2Z]
⊞ ØWQC[Ø34]ZZ
Non-OR ØWQNXZZ

SECTION: Ø MEDICAL AND SURGICAL

BODY SYSTEM: W ANATOMICAL REGIONS, GENERAL

OPERATION: U SUPPLEMENT: Putting in or on biological or synthetic material that physically reinforces and/or augments the function of a portion of a body part

Body Part	Approach	Device	Qualifier
Ø Head 2 Face 4 Upper Jaw 5 Lower Jaw 6 Neck 8 Chest Wall C Mediastinum F Abdominal Wall K Upper Back L Lower Back M Perineum, Male ♂ N Perineum, Female ♀	Ø Open 4 Percutaneous Endoscopic	7 Autologous Tissue Substitute J Synthetic Substitute K Nonautologous Tissue Substitute	Z No Qualifier

Coding Clinic: 2012, Q4, P101 – ØWU80JZ

SECTION: Ø MEDICAL AND SURGICAL

BODY SYSTEM: W ANATOMICAL REGIONS, GENERAL

OPERATION: W **REVISION:** Correcting, to the extent possible, a portion of a malfunctioning device or the position of a displaced device

Body Part	Approach	Device	Qualifier
Ø Head 2 Face 4 Upper Jaw 5 Lower Jaw 6 Neck 8 Chest Wall C Mediastinum F Abdominal Wall K Upper Back L Lower Back M Perineum, Male ♂ N Perineum, Female ♀	Ø Open 3 Percutaneous 4 Percutaneous Endoscopic X External	Ø Drainage Device 1 Radioactive Element 3 Infusion Device 7 Autologous Tissue Substitute J Synthetic Substitute K Nonautologous Tissue Substitute Y Other Device	Z No Qualifier
1 Cranial Cavity 9 Pleural Cavity, Right B Pleural Cavity, Left G Peritoneal Cavity J Pelvic Cavity	Ø Open 3 Percutaneous 4 Percutaneous Endoscopic X External	Ø Drainage Device 1 Radioactive Element 3 Infusion Device J Synthetic Substitute Y Other Device	Z No Qualifier
D Pericardial Cavity H Retroperitoneum	Ø Open 3 Percutaneous 4 Percutaneous Endoscopic X External	Ø Drainage Device 1 Radioactive Element 3 Infusion Device Y Other Device	Z No Qualifier
P Gastrointestinal Tract Q Respiratory Tract R Genitourinary Tract	Ø Open 3 Percutaneous 4 Percutaneous Endoscopic 7 Via Natural or Artificial Opening 8 Via Natural or Artificial Opening Endoscopic X External	1 Radioactive Element 3 Infusion Device Y Other Device	Z No Qualifier

DRG Non-OR ØWW[02456KL][034][0137JKY]Z
DRG Non-OR ØWWM[034][013JY]Z
Non-OR OWW[02456CFKLMN]X[0137JKY]Z
Non-OR OWW8[034X][0137JKY]Z
Non-OR OWW[1GJ]X[013JY]Z
Non-OR OWW[9B][034X][013JY]Z

Non-OR OWW[DH]X[013Y]Z
Non-OR OWWP[3478X][13Y]Z
Non-OR OWWQ[ØX][13Y]Z
Non-OR OWWR[03478X][13Y]Z

Coding Clinic: 2Ø15, Q2, P1Ø – ØWWG4JZ

SECTION: Ø MEDICAL AND SURGICAL

BODY SYSTEM: W ANATOMICAL REGIONS, GENERAL

OPERATION: Y **TRANSPLANTATION:** Putting in or on all or a portion of a living body part taken from another individual or animal to physically take the place and/or function of all or a portion of a similar body part

Body Part	Approach	Device	Qualifier
2 Face	Ø Open	Z No Device	Ø Allogeneic 1 Syngeneic

New/Revised Text in Green   ~~deleted~~ Deleted   ♀ Females Only   ♂ Males Only   **Coding Clinic**

🏷 Non-covered   🏷 Limited Coverage   ⊞ Combination (See Appendix E)   DRG Non-OR   Non-OR   🏷 Hospital-Acquired Condition

SECTION: Ø MEDICAL AND SURGICAL
BODY SYSTEM: X ANATOMICAL REGIONS, UPPER EXTREMITIES
OPERATION: Ø ALTERATION: Modifying the anatomic structure of a body part without affecting the function of the body part

Body Part	Approach	Device	Qualifier
2 Shoulder Region, Right 3 Shoulder Region, Left 4 Axilla, Right 5 Axilla, Left 6 Upper Extremity, Right 7 Upper Extremity, Left 8 Upper Arm, Right 9 Upper Arm, Left B Elbow Region, Right C Elbow Region, Left D Lower Arm, Right F Lower Arm, Left G Wrist Region, Right H Wrist Region, Left	Ø Open 3 Percutaneous 4 Percutaneous Endoscopic	7 Autologous Tissue Substitute J Synthetic Substitute K Nonautologous Tissue Substitute Z No Device	Z No Qualifier

SECTION: Ø MEDICAL AND SURGICAL
BODY SYSTEM: X ANATOMICAL REGIONS, UPPER EXTREMITIES
OPERATION: 2 CHANGE: Taking out or off a device from a body part and putting back an identical or similar device in or on the same body part without cutting or puncturing the skin or a mucous membrane

Body Part	Approach	Device	Qualifier
6 Upper Extremity, Right 7 Upper Extremity, Left	X External	Ø Drainage Device Y Other Device	Z No Qualifier

Non-OR   All Values

SECTION: Ø MEDICAL AND SURGICAL
BODY SYSTEM: X ANATOMICAL REGIONS, UPPER EXTREMITIES
OPERATION: 3 CONTROL: Stopping, or attempting to stop, postprocedure or other acute bleeding

Body Part	Approach	Device	Qualifier
2 Shoulder Region, Right 3 Shoulder Region, Left 4 Axilla, Right 5 Axilla, Left 6 Upper Extremity, Right 7 Upper Extremity, Left 8 Upper Arm, Right 9 Upper Arm, Left B Elbow Region, Right C Elbow Region, Left D Lower Arm, Right F Lower Arm, Left G Wrist Region, Right H Wrist Region, Left J Hand, Right K Hand, Left	Ø Open 3 Percutaneous 4 Percutaneous Endoscopic	Z No Device	Z No Qualifier

Coding Clinic: 2015, Q1, P35 – ØX37ØZZ

New/Revised Text in Green   ~~deleted~~ Deleted   ♀ Females Only   ♂ Males Only   **Coding Clinic**
🔲 Non-covered   🔲 Limited Coverage   ⊡ Combination (See Appendix E)   DRG Non-OR   Non-OR   🔲 Hospital-Acquired Condition

SECTION: Ø MEDICAL AND SURGICAL

BODY SYSTEM: X ANATOMICAL REGIONS, UPPER EXTREMITIES

OPERATION: 6 **DETACHMENT:** Cutting off all or a portion of the upper or lower extremities

Body Part	Approach	Device	Qualifier
Ø Forequarter, Right 1 Forequarter, Left 2 Shoulder Region, Right 3 Shoulder Region, Left B Elbow Region, Right C Elbow Region, Left	Ø Open	Z No Device	Z No Qualifier
8 Upper Arm, Right 9 Upper Arm, Left D Lower Arm, Right F Lower Arm, Left	Ø Open	Z No Device	1 High 2 Mid 3 Low
J Hand, Right K Hand, Left	Ø Open	Z No Device	Ø Complete 4 Complete 1st Ray 5 Complete 2nd Ray 6 Complete 3rd Ray 7 Complete 4th Ray 8 Complete 5th Ray 9 Partial 1st Ray B Partial 2nd Ray C Partial 3rd Ray D Partial 4th Ray F Partial 5th Ray
L Thumb, Right M Thumb, Left N Index Finger, Right P Index Finger, Left Q Middle Finger, Right R Middle Finger, Left S Ring Finger, Right T Ring Finger, Left V Little Finger, Right W Little Finger, Left	Ø Open	Z No Device	Ø Complete 1 High 2 Mid 3 Low

New/Revised Text in Green   ~~deleted~~ Deleted   ♀ Females Only   ♂ Males Only   **Coding Clinic**

🚫 Non-covered   🚫 Limited Coverage   ⊞ Combination (See Appendix E)   DRG Non-OR   Non-OR   🚫 Hospital-Acquired Condition

SECTION: Ø MEDICAL AND SURGICAL

BODY SYSTEM: X ANATOMICAL REGIONS, UPPER EXTREMITIES
OPERATION: 9 DRAINAGE: Taking or letting out fluids and/or gases from a body part

Body Part	Approach	Device	Qualifier
2 Shoulder Region, Right 3 Shoulder Region, Left 4 Axilla, Right 5 Axilla, Left 6 Upper Extremity, Right 7 Upper Extremity, Left 8 Upper Arm, Right 9 Upper Arm, Left B Elbow Region, Right C Elbow Region, Left D Lower Arm, Right F Lower Arm, Left G Wrist Region, Right H Wrist Region, Left J Hand, Right K Hand, Left	Ø Open 3 Percutaneous 4 Percutaneous Endoscopic	Ø Drainage Device	Z No Qualifier
2 Shoulder Region, Right 3 Shoulder Region, Left 4 Axilla, Right 5 Axilla, Left 6 Upper Extremity, Right 7 Upper Extremity, Left 8 Upper Arm, Right 9 Upper Arm, Left B Elbow Region, Right C Elbow Region, Left D Lower Arm, Right F Lower Arm, Left G Wrist Region, Right H Wrist Region, Left J Hand, Right K Hand, Left	Ø Open 3 Percutaneous 4 Percutaneous Endoscopic	Z No Device	X Diagnostic Z No Qualifier

Non-OR All Values

SECTION: Ø MEDICAL AND SURGICAL

BODY SYSTEM: X ANATOMICAL REGIONS, UPPER EXTREMITIES

OPERATION: B EXCISION: Cutting out or off, without replacement, a portion of a body part

Body Part	Approach	Device	Qualifier
2 Shoulder Region, Right 3 Shoulder Region, Left 4 Axilla, Right 5 Axilla, Left 6 Upper Extremity, Right 7 Upper Extremity, Left 8 Upper Arm, Right 9 Upper Arm, Left B Elbow Region, Right C Elbow Region, Left D Lower Arm, Right F Lower Arm, Left G Wrist Region, Right H Wrist Region, Left J Hand, Right K Hand, Left	Ø Open 3 Percutaneous 4 Percutaneous Endoscopic	Z No Device	X Diagnostic Z No Qualifier

Non-OR ØXB[23456789BCDFGHJK][Ø34]ZX

SECTION: Ø MEDICAL AND SURGICAL

BODY SYSTEM: X ANATOMICAL REGIONS, UPPER EXTREMITIES

OPERATION: H INSERTION: Putting in a nonbiological appliance that monitors, assists, performs, or prevents a physiological function but does not physically take the place of a body part

Body Part	Approach	Device	Qualifier
2 Shoulder Region, Right 3 Shoulder Region, Left 4 Axilla, Right 5 Axilla, Left 6 Upper Extremity, Right 7 Upper Extremity, Left 8 Upper Arm, Right 9 Upper Arm, Left B Elbow Region, Right C Elbow Region, Left D Lower Arm, Right F Lower Arm, Left G Wrist Region, Right H Wrist Region, Left J Hand, Right K Hand, Left	Ø Open 3 Percutaneous 4 Percutaneous Endoscopic	1 Radioactive Element 3 Infusion Device Y Other Device	Z No Qualifier

DRG Non-OR ØXH[23456789BCDFGHJK][Ø34][3Y]Z

New/Revised Text in Green ~~deleted~~ Deleted ♀ Females Only ♂ Males Only **Coding Clinic**

Non-covered Limited Coverage ⊕ Combination (See Appendix E) DRG Non-OR Non-OR Hospital-Acquired Condition

SECTION: Ø MEDICAL AND SURGICAL

BODY SYSTEM: X ANATOMICAL REGIONS, UPPER EXTREMITIES

OPERATION: J INSPECTION: Visually and/or manually exploring a body part

Body Part	Approach	Device	Qualifier
2 Shoulder Region, Right	Ø Open	Z No Device	Z No Qualifier
3 Shoulder Region, Left	3 Percutaneous		
4 Axilla, Right	4 Percutaneous Endoscopic		
5 Axilla, Left	X External		
6 Upper Extremity, Right			
7 Upper Extremity, Left			
8 Upper Arm, Right			
9 Upper Arm, Left			
B Elbow Region, Right			
C Elbow Region, Left			
D Lower Arm, Right			
F Lower Arm, Left			
G Wrist Region, Right			
H Wrist Region, Left			
J Hand, Right			
K Hand, Left			

DRG Non-OR ØXJ[23456789BCDFGHJK]ØZZ   Non-OR ØXJ[23456789BCDFGH][34X]ZZ   Non-OR ØXJ[JK]XZZ

DRG Non-OR ØXJ[JK]3ZZ

SECTION: Ø MEDICAL AND SURGICAL

BODY SYSTEM: X ANATOMICAL REGIONS, UPPER EXTREMITIES

OPERATION: M REATTACHMENT: Putting back in or on all or a portion of a separated body part to its normal location or other suitable location

Body Part	Approach	Device	Qualifier
Ø Forequarter, Right	Ø Open	Z No Device	Z No Qualifier
1 Forequarter, Left			
2 Shoulder Region, Right			
3 Shoulder Region, Left			
4 Axilla, Right			
5 Axilla, Left			
6 Upper Extremity, Right			
7 Upper Extremity, Left			
8 Upper Arm, Right			
9 Upper Arm, Left			
B Elbow Region, Right			
C Elbow Region, Left			
D Lower Arm, Right			
F Lower Arm, Left			
G Wrist Region, Right			
H Wrist Region, Left			
J Hand, Right			
K Hand, Left			
L Thumb, Right			
M Thumb, Left			
N Index Finger, Right			
P Index Finger, Left			
Q Middle Finger, Right			
R Middle Finger, Left			
S Ring Finger, Right			
T Ring Finger, Left			
V Little Finger, Right			
W Little Finger, Left			

New/Revised Text in Green   deleted Deleted   ♀ Females Only   ♂ Males Only   **Coding Clinic**

Non-covered   Limited Coverage   ⊞ Combination (See Appendix E)   DRG Non-OR   Non-OR   Hospital-Acquired Condition

SECTION: Ø MEDICAL AND SURGICAL

BODY SYSTEM: X ANATOMICAL REGIONS, UPPER EXTREMITIES

OPERATION: P **REMOVAL:** Taking out or off a device from a body part

Body Part	Approach	Device	Qualifier
6 Upper Extremity, Right 7 Upper Extremity, Left	Ø Open 3 Percutaneous 4 Percutaneous Endoscopic X External	Ø Drainage Device 1 Radioactive Element 3 Infusion Device 7 Autologous Tissue Substitute J Synthetic Substitute K Nonautologous Tissue Substitute Y Other Device	Z No Qualifier

Non-OR   All Values

SECTION: Ø MEDICAL AND SURGICAL

BODY SYSTEM: X ANATOMICAL REGIONS, UPPER EXTREMITIES

OPERATION: Q **REPAIR:** Restoring, to the extent possible, a body part to its normal anatomic structure and function

Body Part	Approach	Device	Qualifier
2 Shoulder Region, Right 3 Shoulder Region, Left 4 Axilla, Right 5 Axilla, Left 6 Upper Extremity, Right 7 Upper Extremity, Left 8 Upper Arm, Right 9 Upper Arm, Left B Elbow Region, Right C Elbow Region, Left D Lower Arm, Right F Lower Arm, Left G Wrist Region, Right H Wrist Region, Left J Hand, Right K Hand, Left L Thumb, Right M Thumb, Left N Index Finger, Right P Index Finger, Left Q Middle Finger, Right R Middle Finger, Left S Ring Finger, Right T Ring Finger, Left V Little Finger, Right W Little Finger, Left	Ø Open 3 Percutaneous 4 Percutaneous Endoscopic X External	Z No Device	Z No Qualifier

SECTION: Ø MEDICAL AND SURGICAL

BODY SYSTEM: X ANATOMICAL REGIONS, UPPER EXTREMITIES

OPERATION: R REPLACEMENT: Putting in or on biological or synthetic material that physically takes the place and/or function of all or a portion of a body part

Body Part	Approach	Device	Qualifier
L Thumb, Right M Thumb, Left	Ø Open 4 Percutaneous Endoscopic	7 Autologous Tissue Substitute	N Toe, Right P Toe, Left

SECTION: Ø MEDICAL AND SURGICAL

BODY SYSTEM: X ANATOMICAL REGIONS, UPPER EXTREMITIES

OPERATION: U SUPPLEMENT: Putting in or on biological or synthetic material that physically reinforces and/or augments the function of a portion of a body part

Body Part	Approach	Device	Qualifier
2 Shoulder Region, Right 3 Shoulder Region, Left 4 Axilla, Right 5 Axilla, Left 6 Upper Extremity, Right 7 Upper Extremity, Left 8 Upper Arm, Right 9 Upper Arm, Left B Elbow Region, Right C Elbow Region, Left D Lower Arm, Right F Lower Arm, Left G Wrist Region, Right H Wrist Region, Left J Hand, Right K Hand, Left L Thumb, Right M Thumb, Left N Index Finger, Right P Index Finger, Left Q Middle Finger, Right R Middle Finger, Left S Ring Finger, Right T Ring Finger, Left V Little Finger, Right W Little Finger, Left	Ø Open 4 Percutaneous Endoscopic	7 Autologous Tissue Substitute J Synthetic Substitute K Nonautologous Tissue Substitute	Z No Qualifier

Side tab: U: SUPPLEMENT   R: REPLACEMENT   X: ANATOMICAL REGIONS, UPPER EXTREMITIES   Ø: M/S

SECTION: Ø MEDICAL AND SURGICAL

BODY SYSTEM: X ANATOMICAL REGIONS, UPPER EXTREMITIES

OPERATION: W REVISION: Correcting, to the extent possible, a portion of a malfunctioning device or the position of displaced device

Body Part	Approach	Device	Qualifier
6 Upper Extremity, Right 7 Upper Extremity, Left	Ø Open 3 Percutaneous 4 Percutaneous Endoscopic X External	Ø Drainage Device 3 Infusion Device 7 Autologous Tissue Substitute J Synthetic Substitute K Nonautologous Tissue Substitute Y Other Device	Z No Qualifier

DRG Non-OR ØXW[67][Ø34][Ø37JKY]Z
Non-OR ØXW[67]X[Ø37JKY]Z

SECTION: Ø MEDICAL AND SURGICAL

BODY SYSTEM: X ANATOMICAL REGIONS, UPPER EXTREMITIES

OPERATION: X TRANSFER: Moving, without taking out, all or a portion of a body part to another location to take over the function of all or a portion of a body part

Body Part	Approach	Device	Qualifier
N Index Finger, Right	Ø Open	Z No Device	L Thumb, Right
P Index Finger, Left	Ø Open	Z No Device	M Thumb, Left

SECTION: Ø MEDICAL AND SURGICAL

BODY SYSTEM: X ANATOMICAL REGIONS, UPPER EXTREMITIES

OPERATION: Y TRANSPLANTATION: Putting in or on all or a portion of a living body part taken from another individual or animal to physically take the place and/or function of all or a portion of a similar body part

Body Part	Approach	Device	Qualifier
J Hand, Right K Hand, Left	Ø Open	Z No Device	Ø Allogeneic 1 Syngeneic

SECTION: Ø MEDICAL AND SURGICAL

BODY SYSTEM: Y ANATOMICAL REGIONS, LOWER EXTREMITIES

OPERATION: Ø ALTERATION: Modifying the anatomic structure of a body part without affecting the function of the body part

Body Part	Approach	Device	Qualifier
Ø Buttock, Right 1 Buttock, Left 9 Lower Extremity, Right B Lower Extremity, Left C Upper Leg, Right D Upper Leg, Left F Knee Region, Right G Knee Region, Left H Lower Leg, Right J Lower Leg, Left K Ankle Region, Right L Ankle Region, Left	Ø Open 3 Percutaneous 4 Percutaneous Endoscopic	7 Autologous Tissue Substitute J Synthetic Substitute K Nonautologous Tissue Substitute Z No Device	Z No Qualifier

SECTION: Ø MEDICAL AND SURGICAL

BODY SYSTEM: Y ANATOMICAL REGIONS, LOWER EXTREMITIES

OPERATION: 2 CHANGE: Taking out or off a device from a body part and putting back an identical or similar device in or on the same body part without cutting or puncturing the skin or a mucous membrane

Body Part	Approach	Device	Qualifier
9 Lower Extremity, Right B Lower Extremity, Left	X External	Ø Drainage Device Y Other Device	Z No Qualifier

Non-OR All Values

SECTION: Ø MEDICAL AND SURGICAL

BODY SYSTEM: Y ANATOMICAL REGIONS, LOWER EXTREMITIES

OPERATION: 3 CONTROL: Stopping, or attempting to stop, postprocedure or other acute bleeding

Body Part	Approach	Device	Qualifier
Ø Buttock, Right 1 Buttock, Left 5 Inguinal Region, Right 6 Inguinal Region, Left 7 Femoral Region, Right 8 Femoral Region, Left 9 Lower Extremity, Right B Lower Extremity, Left C Upper Leg, Right D Upper Leg, Left F Knee Region, Right G Knee Region, Left H Lower Leg, Right J Lower Leg, Left K Ankle Region, Right L Ankle Region, Left M Foot, Right N Foot, Left	Ø Open 3 Percutaneous 4 Percutaneous Endoscopic	Z No Device	Z No Qualifier

SECTION: Ø MEDICAL AND SURGICAL

BODY SYSTEM: Y ANATOMICAL REGIONS, LOWER EXTREMITIES

OPERATION: 6 DETACHMENT: Cutting off all or a portion of the upper or lower extremities

Body Part	Approach	Device	Qualifier
2 Hindquarter, Right 3 Hindquarter, Left 4 Hindquarter, Bilateral 7 Femoral Region, Right 8 Femoral Region, Left F Knee Region, Right G Knee Region, Left	Ø Open	Z No Device	Z No Qualifier
C Upper Leg, Right D Upper Leg, Left H Lower Leg, Right J Lower Leg, Left	Ø Open	Z No Device	1 High 2 Mid 3 Low
M Foot, Right N Foot, Left	Ø Open	Z No Device	Ø Complete 4 Complete 1st Ray 5 Complete 2nd Ray 6 Complete 3rd Ray 7 Complete 4th Ray 8 Complete 5th Ray 9 Partial 1st Ray B Partial 2nd Ray C Partial 3rd Ray D Partial 4th Ray F Partial 5th Ray
P 1st Toe, Right Q 1st Toe, Left R 2nd Toe, Right S 2nd Toe, Left T 3rd Toe, Right U 3rd Toe, Left V 4th Toe, Right W 4th Toe, Left X 5th Toe, Right Y 5th Toe, Left	Ø Open	Z No Device	Ø Complete 1 High 2 Mid 3 Low

Coding Clinic: 2Ø15, Q1, P28 – ØY6NØZØ
Coding Clinic: 2Ø15, Q2, P29 – ØY6[PQ]ØZ3

New/Revised Text in Green ~~deleted~~ Deleted ♀ Females Only ♂ Males Only **Coding Clinic**
Non-covered Limited Coverage ⊞ Combination (See Appendix E) DRG Non-OR Non-OR Hospital-Acquired Condition

SECTION: Ø MEDICAL AND SURGICAL

BODY SYSTEM: Y ANATOMICAL REGIONS, LOWER EXTREMITIES

OPERATION: 9 DRAINAGE: Taking or letting out fluids and/or gases from a body part

Body Part	Approach	Device	Qualifier
Ø Buttock, Right 1 Buttock, Left 5 Inguinal Region, Right 6 Inguinal Region, Left 7 Femoral Region, Right 8 Femoral Region, Left 9 Lower Extremity, Right B Lower Extremity, Left C Upper Leg, Right D Upper Leg, Left F Knee Region, Right G Knee Region, Left H Lower Leg, Right J Lower Leg, Left K Ankle Region, Right L Ankle Region, Left M Foot, Right N Foot, Left	Ø Open 3 Percutaneous 4 Percutaneous Endoscopic	Ø Drainage Device	Z No Qualifier
Ø Buttock, Right 1 Buttock, Left 5 Inguinal Region, Right 6 Inguinal Region, Left 7 Femoral Region, Right 8 Femoral Region, Left 9 Lower Extremity, Right B Lower Extremity, Left C Upper Leg, Right D Upper Leg, Left F Knee Region, Right G Knee Region, Left H Lower Leg, Right J Lower Leg, Left K Ankle Region, Right L Ankle Region, Left M Foot, Right N Foot, Left	Ø Open 3 Percutaneous 4 Percutaneous Endoscopic	Z No Device	X Diagnostic Z No Qualifier

DRG Non-OR ØY9[56]3ØZ
DRG Non-OR ØY9[56]3ZZ
Non-OR ØY9[Ø1789BCDFGHJKLMN][Ø34]ØZ
Non-OR ØY9[Ø1789BCDFGHJKLMN][Ø34]Z[XZ]

Coding Clinic: 2Ø15, Q1, P22-23 – ØY98ØZZ

SECTION: Ø MEDICAL AND SURGICAL

BODY SYSTEM: Y ANATOMICAL REGIONS, LOWER EXTREMITIES

OPERATION: B EXCISION: Cutting out or off, without replacement, a portion of a body part

Body Part	Approach	Device	Qualifier
Ø Buttock, Right 1 Buttock, Left 5 Inguinal Region, Right 6 Inguinal Region, Left 7 Femoral Region, Right 8 Femoral Region, Left 9 Lower Extremity, Right B Lower Extremity, Left C Upper Leg, Right D Upper Leg, Left F Knee Region, Right G Knee Region, Left H Lower Leg, Right J Lower Leg, Left K Ankle Region, Right L Ankle Region, Left M Foot, Right N Foot, Left	Ø Open 3 Percutaneous 4 Percutaneous Endoscopic	Z No Device	X Diagnostic Z No Qualifier

Non-OR ØYB[Ø19BCDFGHJKLMN][Ø34]ZX

SECTION: Ø MEDICAL AND SURGICAL

BODY SYSTEM: Y ANATOMICAL REGIONS, LOWER EXTREMITIES

OPERATION: H INSERTION: Putting in a nonbiological appliance that monitors, assists, performs, or prevents a physiological function but does not physically take the place of a body part

Body Part	Approach	Device	Qualifier
Ø Buttock, Right 1 Buttock, Left 5 Inguinal Region, Right 6 Inguinal Region, Left 7 Femoral Region, Right 8 Femoral Region, Left 9 Lower Extremity, Right B Lower Extremity, Left C Upper Leg, Right D Upper Leg, Left F Knee Region, Right G Knee Region, Left H Lower Leg, Right J Lower Leg, Left K Ankle Region, Right L Ankle Region, Left M Foot, Right N Foot, Left	Ø Open 3 Percutaneous 4 Percutaneous Endoscopic	1 Radioactive Element 3 Infusion Device Y Other Device	Z No Qualifier

DRG Non-OR ØYH[Ø156789BCDFGHJKLMN][Ø34][3Y]Z

New/Revised Text in Green   deleted Deleted   ♀ Females Only   ♂ Males Only   **Coding Clinic**

Non-covered   Limited Coverage   ⊞ Combination (See Appendix E)   DRG Non-OR   Non-OR   Hospital-Acquired Condition

B: EXCISION   H: INSERTION

Y: ANATOMICAL REGIONS, LOWER EXTREMITIES

Ø: M/S

SECTION: Ø MEDICAL AND SURGICAL

BODY SYSTEM: Y ANATOMICAL REGIONS, LOWER EXTREMITIES
OPERATION: J INSPECTION: Visually and/or manually exploring a body part

Body Part	Approach	Device	Qualifier
Ø Buttock, Right 1 Buttock, Left 5 Inguinal Region, Right 6 Inguinal Region, Left 7 Femoral Region, Right 8 Femoral Region, Left 9 Lower Extremity, Right A Inguinal Region, Bilateral B Lower Extremity, Left C Upper Leg, Right D Upper Leg, Left E Femoral Region, Bilateral F Knee Region, Right G Knee Region, Left H Lower Leg, Right J Lower Leg, Left K Ankle Region, Right L Ankle Region, Left M Foot, Right N Foot, Left	Ø Open 3 Percutaneous 4 Percutaneous Endoscopic X External	Z No Device	Z No Qualifier

DRG Non-OR ØYJ[Ø19BCDFGHJKLMN]ØZZ
DRG Non-OR ØYJ[567A]3ZZ
DRG Non-OR ØYJ[8E][Ø3]ZZ
Non-OR ØYJ[Ø19BCDFGHJKLMN][34X]ZZ
Non-OR ØYJ[5678AE]XZZ

SECTION: Ø MEDICAL AND SURGICAL

BODY SYSTEM: Y ANATOMICAL REGIONS, LOWER EXTREMITIES

OPERATION: M REATTACHMENT: Putting back in or on all or a portion of a separated body part to its normal location or other suitable location

Body Part	Approach	Device	Qualifier
Ø Buttock, Right	Ø Open	Z No Device	Z No Qualifier
1 Buttock, Left			
2 Hindquarter, Right			
3 Hindquarter, Left			
4 Hindquarter, Bilateral			
5 Inguinal Region, Right			
6 Inguinal Region, Left			
7 Femoral Region, Right			
8 Femoral Region, Left			
9 Lower Extremity, Right			
B Lower Extremity, Left			
C Upper Leg, Right			
D Upper Leg, Left			
F Knee Region, Right			
G Knee Region, Left			
H Lower Leg, Right			
J Lower Leg, Left			
K Ankle Region, Right			
L Ankle Region, Left			
M Foot, Right			
N Foot, Left			
P 1st Toe, Right			
Q 1st Toe, Left			
R 2nd Toe, Right			
S 2nd Toe, Left			
T 3rd Toe, Right			
U 3rd Toe, Left			
V 4th Toe, Right			
W 4th Toe, Left			
X 5th Toe, Right			
Y 5th Toe, Left			

SECTION: Ø MEDICAL AND SURGICAL

BODY SYSTEM: Y ANATOMICAL REGIONS, LOWER EXTREMITIES

OPERATION: P REMOVAL: Taking out or off a device from a body part

Body Part	Approach	Device	Qualifier
9 Lower Extremity, Right	Ø Open	Ø Drainage Device	Z No Qualifier
B Lower Extremity, Left	3 Percutaneous	1 Radioactive Element	
	4 Percutaneous Endoscopic	3 Infusion Device	
	X External	7 Autologous Tissue Substitute	
		J Synthetic Substitute	
		K Nonautologous Tissue Substitute	
		Y Other Device	

Non-OR All Values

SECTION: Ø MEDICAL AND SURGICAL

BODY SYSTEM: Y ANATOMICAL REGIONS, LOWER EXTREMITIES

OPERATION: Q REPAIR: Restoring, to the extent possible, a body part to its normal anatomic structure and function

Body Part	Approach	Device	Qualifier
Ø Buttock, Right	Ø Open	Z No Device	Z No Qualifier
1 Buttock, Left	3 Percutaneous		
5 Inguinal Region, Right	4 Percutaneous Endoscopic		
6 Inguinal Region, Left	X External		
7 Femoral Region, Right			
8 Femoral Region, Left			
9 Lower Extremity, Right			
A Inguinal Region, Bilateral			
B Lower Extremity, Left			
C Upper Leg, Right			
D Upper Leg, Left			
E Femoral Region, Bilateral			
F Knee Region, Right			
G Knee Region, Left			
H Lower Leg, Right			
J Lower Leg, Left			
K Ankle Region, Right			
L Ankle Region, Left			
M Foot, Right			
N Foot, Left			
P 1st Toe, Right			
Q 1st Toe, Left			
R 2nd Toe, Right			
S 2nd Toe, Left			
T 3rd Toe, Right			
U 3rd Toe, Left			
V 4th Toe, Right			
W 4th Toe, Left			
X 5th Toe, Right			
Y 5th Toe, Left			

Non-OR ØYQ[5678AE]XZZ

Ø: M/S

Y: ANATOMICAL REGIONS, LOWER EXTREMITIES

Q: REPAIR

U: SUPPLEMENT W: REVISION

Y: ANATOMICAL REGIONS, LOWER EXTREMITIES

Ø: M/S

SECTION: Ø MEDICAL AND SURGICAL
BODY SYSTEM: Y ANATOMICAL REGIONS, LOWER EXTREMITIES
OPERATION: U SUPPLEMENT: Putting in or on biological or synthetic material that physically reinforces and/or augments the function of a portion of a body part

Body Part	Approach	Device	Qualifier
Ø Buttock, Right 1 Buttock, Left 5 Inguinal Region, Right 6 Inguinal Region, Left 7 Femoral Region, Right 8 Femoral Region, Left 9 Lower Extremity, Right A Inguinal Region, Bilateral B Lower Extremity, Left C Upper Leg, Right D Upper Leg, Left E Femoral Region, Bilateral F Knee Region, Right G Knee Region, Left H Lower Leg, Right J Lower Leg, Left K Ankle Region, Right L Ankle Region, Left M Foot, Right N Foot, Left P 1st Toe, Right Q 1st Toe, Left R 2nd Toe, Right S 2nd Toe, Left T 3rd Toe, Right U 3rd Toe, Left V 4th Toe, Right W 4th Toe, Left X 5th Toe, Right Y 5th Toe, Left	Ø Open 4 Percutaneous Endoscopic	7 Autologous Tissue Substitute J Synthetic Substitute K Nonautologous Tissue Substitute	Z No Qualifier

SECTION: Ø MEDICAL AND SURGICAL
BODY SYSTEM: Y ANATOMICAL REGIONS, LOWER EXTREMITIES
OPERATION: W REVISION: Correcting, to the extent possible, a portion of a malfunctioning device or the position of a displaced device

Body Part	Approach	Device	Qualifier
9 Lower Extremity, Right B Lower Extremity, Left	Ø Open 3 Percutaneous 4 Percutaneous Endoscopic X External	Ø Drainage Device 3 Infusion Device 7 Autologous Tissue Substitute J Synthetic Substitute K Nonautologous Tissue Substitute Y Other Device	Z No Qualifier

DRG Non-OR ØYW[9B][Ø34][Ø37JKY]Z
Non-OR ØYW[9B]X[Ø37JKY]Z

ICD-10-PCS Coding Guidelines

Obstetric Section Guidelines (section 1)

C. Obstetrics Section

Products of conception

C1

Procedures performed on the products of conception are coded to the Obstetrics section. Procedures performed on the pregnant female other than the products of conception are coded to the appropriate root operation in the Medical and Surgical section.

Example: Amniocentesis is coded to the products of conception body part in the Obstetrics section. Repair of obstetric urethral laceration is coded to the urethra body part in the Medical and Surgical section.

Procedures following delivery or abortion

C2

Procedures performed following a delivery or abortion for curettage of the endometrium or evacuation of retained products of conception are all coded in the Obstetrics section, to the root operation Extraction and the body part Products of Conception, Retained. Diagnostic or therapeutic dilation and curettage performed during times other than the postpartum or post-abortion period are all coded in the Medical and Surgical section, to the root operation Extraction and the body part Endometrium.

SECTION: 1 OBSTETRICS
BODY SYSTEM: Ø PREGNANCY
OPERATION: 2 CHANGE: Taking out or off a device from a body part and putting back an identical or similar device in or on the same body part without cutting or puncturing the skin or a mucous membrane

Body Part	Approach	Device	Qualifier
Ø Products of Conception ♀	7 Via Natural or Artificial Opening	3 Monitoring Electrode Y Other Device	Z No Qualifier

Non-OR   All Values

SECTION: 1 OBSTETRICS
BODY SYSTEM: Ø PREGNANCY
OPERATION: 9 DRAINAGE: Taking or letting out fluids and/or gases from a body part

Body Part	Approach	Device	Qualifier
Ø Products of Conception ♀	Ø Open 3 Percutaneous 4 Percutaneous Endoscopic 7 Via Natural or Artificial Opening 8 Via Natural or Artificial Opening Endoscopic	Z No Device	9 Fetal Blood A Fetal Cerebrospinal Fluid B Fetal Fluid, Other C Amniotic Fluid, Therapeutic D Fluid, Other U Amniotic Fluid, Diagnostic

Non-OR   All Values

SECTION: 1 OBSTETRICS
BODY SYSTEM: Ø PREGNANCY
OPERATION: A ABORTION: Artificially terminating a pregnancy

Body Part	Approach	Device	Qualifier
Ø Products of Conception ♀	Ø Open 3 Percutaneous 4 Percutaneous Endoscopic 8 Via Natural or Artificial Opening Endoscopic	Z No Device	Z No Qualifier
Ø Products of Conception ♀	7 Via Natural or Artificial Opening	Z No Device	6 Vacuum W Laminaria X Abortifacient Z No Qualifier

DRG Non-OR   10AØ7Z6
Non-OR   10AØ7Z[WX]

Sidebar: 0: PREGNANCY   2: CHANGE   9: DRAINAGE   A: ABORTION   1: OBSTETRICS

SECTION: 1 OBSTETRICS

BODY SYSTEM: Ø PREGNANCY

OPERATION: D EXTRACTION: Pulling or stripping out or off all or a portion of a body part by the use of force

Body Part	Approach	Device	Qualifier
Ø Products of Conception ♀	Ø Open	Z No Device	Ø Classical 1 Low Cervical 2 Extraperitoneal
Ø Products of Conception ♀ ⊞	7 Via Natural or Artificial Opening	Z No Device	3 Low Forceps 4 Mid Forceps 5 High Forceps 6 Vacuum 7 Internal Version 8 Other
1 Products of Conception, Retained ♀ 2 Products of Conception, Ectopic ♀	7 Via Natural or Artificial Opening 8 Via Natural or Artificial Opening Endoscopic	Z No Device	Z No Qualifier

⊞ 10D07Z[3456]
DRG Non-OR 10D07Z[345678]

Coding Clinic: 2016, Q1, P10 – 10D07Z3

SECTION: 1 OBSTETRICS

BODY SYSTEM: Ø PREGNANCY

OPERATION: E DELIVERY: Assisting the passage of the products of conception from the genital canal

Body Part	Approach	Device	Qualifier
Ø Products of Conception ♀ ⊞	X External	Z No Device	Z No Qualifier

⊞ 10E0XZZ
DRG Non-OR 10E0XZZ

Coding Clinic: 2016, Q2, P34-35 – 10E0XZZ

SECTION: 1 OBSTETRICS

BODY SYSTEM: Ø PREGNANCY

OPERATION: H INSERTION: Putting in a nonbiological appliance that monitors, assists, performs, or prevents a physiological function but does not physically take the place of a body part

Body Part	Approach	Device	Qualifier
Ø Products of Conception ♀	Ø Open 7 Via Natural or Artificial Opening	3 Monitoring Electrode Y Other Device	Z No Qualifier

Non-OR 10H07[3Y]Z

Coding Clinic: 2013, Q2, P36 – 10H07YZ

New/Revised Text in Green — deleted Deleted — ♀ Females Only — ♂ Males Only — **Coding Clinic**
🚫 Non-covered — 🚫 Limited Coverage — ⊞ Combination (See Appendix E) — DRG Non-OR — Non-OR — 🚫 Hospital-Acquired Condition

SECTION: 1 OBSTETRICS

BODY SYSTEM: Ø PREGNANCY

OPERATION: J INSPECTION: Visually and/or manually exploring a body part

Body Part	Approach	Device	Qualifier
Ø Products of Conception ♀ 1 Products of Conception, Retained ♀ 2 Products of Conception, Ectopic ♀	Ø Open 3 Percutaneous 4 Percutaneous Endoscopic 7 Via Natural or Artificial Opening 8 Via Natural or Artificial Opening Endoscopic X External	Z No Device	Z No Qualifier

Non-OR   All Values

SECTION: 1 OBSTETRICS

BODY SYSTEM: Ø PREGNANCY

OPERATION: P REMOVAL: Taking out or off a device from a body part, region or orifice

Body Part	Approach	Device	Qualifier
Ø Products of Conception ♀	Ø Open 7 Via Natural or Artificial Opening	3 Monitoring Electrode Y Other Device	Z No Qualifier

SECTION: 1 OBSTETRICS

BODY SYSTEM: Ø PREGNANCY

OPERATION: Q REPAIR: Restoring, to the extent possible, a body part to its normal anatomic structure and function

Body Part	Approach	Device	Qualifier
Ø Products of Conception ♀	Ø Open 3 Percutaneous 4 Percutaneous Endoscopic 7 Via Natural or Artificial Opening 8 Via Natural or Artificial Opening Endoscopic	Y Other Device Z No Device	E Nervous System F Cardiovascular System G Lymphatics and Hemic H Eye J Ear, Nose, and Sinus K Respiratory System L Mouth and Throat M Gastrointestinal System N Hepatobiliary and Pancreas P Endocrine System Q Skin R Musculoskeletal System S Urinary System T Female Reproductive System V Male Reproductive System Y Other Body System

Non-OR   All Values

SECTION: 1 OBSTETRICS

BODY SYSTEM: Ø PREGNANCY

OPERATION: S REPOSITION: Moving to its normal location or other suitable location all or a portion of a body part

Body Part	Approach	Device	Qualifier
Ø Products of Conception ♀	7 Via Natural or Artificial Opening X External	Z No Device	Z No Qualifier
2 Products of Conception, Ectopic ♀	Ø Open 3 Percutaneous 4 Percutaneous Endoscopic 7 Via Natural or Artificial Opening 8 Via Natural or Artificial Opening Endoscopic	Z No Device	Z No Qualifier

DRG Non-OR 10S07ZZ
Non-OR 10S0XZZ

SECTION: 1 OBSTETRICS

BODY SYSTEM: Ø PREGNANCY

OPERATION: T RESECTION: Cutting out or off, without replacement, all of a body part

Body Part	Approach	Device	Qualifier
2 Products of Conception, Ectopic ♀	Ø Open 3 Percutaneous 4 Percutaneous Endoscopic 7 Via Natural or Artificial Opening 8 Via Natural or Artificial Opening Endoscopic	Z No Device	Z No Qualifier

Coding Clinic: 2015, Q3, P32 – 10T24ZZ

SECTION: 1 OBSTETRICS

BODY SYSTEM: Ø PREGNANCY

OPERATION: Y TRANSPLANTATION: Putting in or on all or a portion of a living body part taken from another individual or animal to physically take the place and/or function of all or a portion of a similar body part

Body Part	Approach	Device	Qualifier
Ø Products of Conception ♀	3 Percutaneous 4 Percutaneous Endoscopic 7 Via Natural or Artificial Opening	Z No Device	E Nervous System F Cardiovascular System G Lymphatics and Hemic H Eye J Ear, Nose, and Sinus K Respiratory System L Mouth and Throat M Gastrointestinal System N Hepatobiliary and Pancreas P Endocrine System Q Skin R Musculoskeletal System S Urinary System T Female Reproductive System V Male Reproductive System Y Other Body System

Non-OR All Values

New/Revised Text in Green ~~deleted~~ Deleted ♀ Females Only ♂ Males Only **Coding Clinic**

  Non-covered   Limited Coverage   Combination (See Appendix E)   DRG Non-OR   Non-OR   Hospital-Acquired Condition

SECTION: 2 PLACEMENT
BODY SYSTEM: W ANATOMICAL REGIONS
OPERATION: Ø CHANGE: Taking out or off a device from a body part and putting back an identical or similar device in or on the same body part without cutting or puncturing the skin or a mucous membrane

Body Region	Approach	Device	Qualifier
Ø Head 2 Neck 3 Abdominal Wall 4 Chest Wall 5 Back 6 Inguinal Region, Right 7 Inguinal Region, Left 8 Upper Extremity, Right 9 Upper Extremity, Left A Upper Arm, Right B Upper Arm, Left C Lower Arm, Right D Lower Arm, Left E Hand, Right F Hand, Left G Thumb, Right H Thumb, Left J Finger, Right K Finger, Left L Lower Extremity, Right M Lower Extremity, Left N Upper Leg, Right P Upper Leg, Left Q Lower Leg, Right R Lower Leg, Left S Foot, Right T Foot, Left U Toe, Right V Toe, Left	X External	Ø Traction Apparatus 1 Splint 2 Cast 3 Brace 4 Bandage 5 Packing Material 6 Pressure Dressing 7 Intermittent Pressure Device Y Other Device	Z No Qualifier
1 Face	X External	Ø Traction Apparatus 1 Splint 2 Cast 3 Brace 4 Bandage 5 Packing Material 6 Pressure Dressing 7 Intermittent Pressure Device 9 Wire Y Other Device	Z No Qualifier

2: PLACEMENT

W: ANATOMICAL REGIONS

Ø: CHANGE

SECTION: 2 PLACEMENT

BODY SYSTEM: W ANATOMICAL REGIONS

OPERATION: 1 **COMPRESSION:** Putting pressure on a body region

Body Region	Approach	Device	Qualifier
Ø Head 1 Face 2 Neck 3 Abdominal Wall 4 Chest Wall 5 Back 6 Inguinal Region, Right 7 Inguinal Region, Left 8 Upper Extremity, Right 9 Upper Extremity, Left A Upper Arm, Right B Upper Arm, Left C Lower Arm, Right D Lower Arm, Left E Hand, Right F Hand, Left G Thumb, Right H Thumb, Left J Finger, Right K Finger, Left L Lower Extremity, Right M Lower Extremity, Left N Upper Leg, Right P Upper Leg, Left Q Lower Leg, Right R Lower Leg, Left S Foot, Right T Foot, Left U Toe, Right V Toe, Left	X External	6 Pressure Dressing 7 Intermittent Pressure Device	Z No Qualifier

1: COMPRESSION

W: ANATOMICAL REGIONS

2: PLACEMENT

New/Revised Text in Green   ~~deleted~~ Deleted   ♀ Females Only   ♂ Males Only   **Coding Clinic**

Non-covered   Limited Coverage   ⊟ Combination (See Appendix E)   DRG Non-OR   Non-OR   Hospital-Acquired Condition

SECTION: 2 PLACEMENT

BODY SYSTEM: W ANATOMICAL REGIONS

OPERATION: 2 DRESSING: Putting material on a body region for protection

Body Region	Approach	Device	Qualifier
Ø Head	X External	4 Bandage	Z No Qualifier
1 Face			
2 Neck			
3 Abdominal Wall			
4 Chest Wall			
5 Back			
6 Inguinal Region, Right			
7 Inguinal Region, Left			
8 Upper Extremity, Right			
9 Upper Extremity, Left			
A Upper Arm, Right			
B Upper Arm, Left			
C Lower Arm, Right			
D Lower Arm, Left			
E Hand, Right			
F Hand, Left			
G Thumb, Right			
H Thumb, Left			
J Finger, Right			
K Finger, Left			
L Lower Extremity, Right			
M Lower Extremity, Left			
N Upper Leg, Right			
P Upper Leg, Left			
Q Lower Leg, Right			
R Lower Leg, Left			
S Foot, Right			
T Foot, Left			
U Toe, Right			
V Toe, Left			

2: PLACEMENT

W: ANATOMICAL REGIONS

2: DRESSING

SECTION: 2 PLACEMENT
BODY SYSTEM: W ANATOMICAL REGIONS
OPERATION: 3 **IMMOBILIZATION:** Limiting or preventing motion of a body region

Body Region	Approach	Device	Qualifier
Ø Head 2 Neck 3 Abdominal Wall 4 Chest Wall 5 Back 6 Inguinal Region, Right 7 Inguinal Region, Left 8 Upper Extremity, Right 9 Upper Extremity, Left A Upper Arm, Right B Upper Arm, Left C Lower Arm, Right D Lower Arm, Left E Hand, Right F Hand, Left G Thumb, Right H Thumb, Left J Finger, Right K Finger, Left L Lower Extremity, Right M Lower Extremity, Left N Upper Leg, Right P Upper Leg, Left Q Lower Leg, Right R Lower Leg, Left S Foot, Right T Foot, Left U Toe, Right V Toe, Left	X External	1 Splint 2 Cast 3 Brace Y Other Device	Z No Qualifier
1 Face	X External	1 Splint 2 Cast 3 Brace 9 Wire Y Other Device	Z No Qualifier

3: IMMOBILIZATION
W: ANATOMICAL REGIONS
2: PLACEMENT

SECTION: 2 PLACEMENT

BODY SYSTEM: W ANATOMICAL REGIONS

OPERATION: 4 PACKING: Putting material in a body region or orifice

Body Region	Approach	Device	Qualifier
Ø Head	X External	5 Packing Material	Z No Qualifier
1 Face			
2 Neck			
3 Abdominal Wall			
4 Chest Wall			
5 Back			
6 Inguinal Region, Right			
7 Inguinal Region, Left			
8 Upper Extremity, Right			
9 Upper Extremity, Left			
A Upper Arm, Right			
B Upper Arm, Left			
C Lower Arm, Right			
D Lower Arm, Left			
E Hand, Right			
F Hand, Left			
G Thumb, Right			
H Thumb, Left			
J Finger, Right			
K Finger, Left			
L Lower Extremity, Right			
M Lower Extremity, Left			
N Upper Leg, Right			
P Upper Leg, Left			
Q Lower Leg, Right			
R Lower Leg, Left			
S Foot, Right			
T Foot, Left			
U Toe, Right			
V Toe, Left			

SECTION: 2 PLACEMENT

BODY SYSTEM: W ANATOMICAL REGIONS

OPERATION: 5 REMOVAL: Taking out or off a device from a body part

Body Region	Approach	Device	Qualifier
Ø Head 2 Neck 3 Abdominal Wall 4 Chest Wall 5 Back 6 Inguinal Region, Right 7 Inguinal Region, Left 8 Upper Extremity, Right 9 Upper Extremity, Left A Upper Arm, Right B Upper Arm, Left C Lower Arm, Right D Lower Arm, Left E Hand, Right F Hand, Left G Thumb, Right H Thumb, Left J Finger, Right K Finger, Left L Lower Extremity, Right M Lower Extremity, Left N Upper Leg, Right P Upper Leg, Left Q Lower Leg, Right R Lower Leg, Left S Foot, Right T Foot, Left U Toe, Right V Toe, Left	X External	Ø Traction Apparatus 1 Splint 2 Cast 3 Brace 4 Bandage 5 Packing Material 6 Pressure Dressing 7 Intermittent Pressure Device Y Other Device	Z No Qualifier
1 Face	X External	Ø Traction Apparatus 1 Splint 2 Cast 3 Brace 4 Bandage 5 Packing Material 6 Pressure Dressing 7 Intermittent Pressure Device 9 Wire Y Other Device	Z No Qualifier

SECTION: 2 PLACEMENT
BODY SYSTEM: W ANATOMICAL REGIONS
OPERATION: 6 **TRACTION:** Exerting a pulling force on a body region in a distal direction

Body Region	Approach	Device	Qualifier
0 Head	X External	0 Traction Apparatus	Z No Qualifier
1 Face		Z No Device	
2 Neck			
3 Abdominal Wall			
4 Chest Wall			
5 Back			
6 Inguinal Region, Right			
7 Inguinal Region, Left			
8 Upper Extremity, Right			
9 Upper Extremity, Left			
A Upper Arm, Right			
B Upper Arm, Left			
C Lower Arm, Right			
D Lower Arm, Left			
E Hand, Right			
F Hand, Left			
G Thumb, Right			
H Thumb, Left			
J Finger, Right			
K Finger, Left			
L Lower Extremity, Right			
M Lower Extremity, Left			
N Upper Leg, Right			
P Upper Leg, Left			
Q Lower Leg, Right			
R Lower Leg, Left			
S Foot, Right			
T Foot, Left			
U Toe, Right			
V Toe, Left			

Coding Clinic: 2015, Q2, P35; 2013, Q2, P39 – 2W60X0Z
Coding Clinic: 2015, Q2, P35 – 2W62X0Z

New/Revised Text in Green   ~~deleted~~ Deleted   ♀ Females Only   ♂ Males Only   **Coding Clinic**
Non-covered   Limited Coverage   ⊞ Combination (See Appendix E)   DRG Non-OR   Non-OR   Hospital-Acquired Condition

SECTION: 2 PLACEMENT

BODY SYSTEM: Y ANATOMICAL ORIFICES

OPERATION: Ø CHANGE: Taking out or off a device from a body part and putting back an identical or similar device in or on the same body part without cutting or puncturing the skin or a mucous membrane

Body Region	Approach	Device	Qualifier
Ø Mouth and Pharynx 1 Nasal 2 Ear 3 Anorectal 4 Female Genital Tract ♀ 5 Urethra	X External	5 Packing Material	Z No Qualifier

SECTION: 2 PLACEMENT

BODY SYSTEM: Y ANATOMICAL ORIFICES

OPERATION: 4 PACKING: Putting material in a body region or orifice

Body Region	Approach	Device	Qualifier
Ø Mouth and Pharynx 1 Nasal 2 Ear 3 Anorectal 4 Female Genital Tract ♀ 5 Urethra	X External	5 Packing Material	Z No Qualifier

SECTION: 2 PLACEMENT

BODY SYSTEM: Y ANATOMICAL ORIFICES

OPERATION: 5 REMOVAL: Taking out or off a device from a body part

Body Region	Approach	Device	Qualifier
Ø Mouth and Pharynx 1 Nasal 2 Ear 3 Anorectal 4 Female Genital Tract ♀ 5 Urethra	X External	5 Packing Material	Z No Qualifier

Side tab: 2: PLACEMENT   Y: ANATOMICAL ORIFICES   Ø: CHANGE   4: PACKING   5: REMOVAL

SECTION: 3 ADMINISTRATION
BODY SYSTEM: Ø **CIRCULATORY**
OPERATION: 2 **TRANSFUSION:** *(on multiple pages)*
Putting in blood or blood products

Body System / Region	Approach	Substance	Qualifier
3 Peripheral Vein 🐾 4 Central Vein 🐾	Ø Open 3 Percutaneous	A Stem Cells, Embryonic	Z No Qualifier
3 Peripheral Vein 4 Central Vein	Ø Open 3 Percutaneous	G Bone Marrow X Stem Cells, Cord Blood Y Stem Cells, Hematopoietic	Ø Autologous 2 Allogeneic, Related 3 Allogeneic, Unrelated 4 Allogeneic, Unspecified
3 Peripheral Vein 🐾 4 Central Vein 🐾	Ø Open 3 Percutaneous	G~~ Bone Marrow~~ H Whole Blood J Serum Albumin K Frozen Plasma L Fresh Plasma M Plasma Cryoprecipitate N Red Blood Cells P Frozen Red Cells Q White Cells R Platelets S Globulin T Fibrinogen V Antihemophilic Factors W Factor IX X ~~Stem Cells, Cord Blood~~ Y ~~Stem Cells, Hematopoietic~~	Ø Autologous 1 Nonautologous
5 Peripheral Artery 🐾 6 Central Artery 🐾	Ø Open 3 Percutaneous	G Bone Marrow H Whole Blood J Serum Albumin K Frozen Plasma L Fresh Plasma M Plasma Cryoprecipitate N Red Blood Cells P Frozen Red Cells Q White Cells R Platelets S Globulin T Fibrinogen V Antihemophilic Factors W Factor IX X Stem Cells, Cord Blood Y Stem Cells, Hematopoietic	Ø Autologous 1 Nonautologous

🐾 3Ø2[34][Ø3]AZ, 3Ø2[34][Ø3][GY]Ø, and 3Ø2[56][Ø3][GY]Ø are identified as non-covered when a code from the diagnosis list below is present as a principal or secondary diagnosis

C91ØØ	C924Ø	C93ØØ
C92ØØ	C925Ø	C94ØØ
C921Ø	C926Ø	C95ØØ
C9211	C92AØ	

🐾 3Ø2[56][Ø3][GY]1 is identified as non-covered when C90.00 or C90.01 are present as a principal or secondary diagnosis

New/Revised Text in Green ~~deleted~~ Deleted ♀ Females Only ♂ Males Only **Coding Clinic**
🐾 Non-covered 🐾 Limited Coverage ⊞ Combination (See Appendix E) DRG Non-OR Non-OR 🐾 Hospital-Acquired Condition

SECTION: 3 ADMINISTRATION
BODY SYSTEM: Ø CIRCULATORY
OPERATION: 2 TRANSFUSION: *(continued)*
Putting in blood or blood products

Body System / Region	Approach	Substance	Qualifier
7 Products of Conception, Circulatory ♀	3 Percutaneous 7 Via Natural or Artificial Opening	H Whole Blood J Serum Albumin K Frozen Plasma L Fresh Plasma M Plasma Cryoprecipitate N Red Blood Cells P Frozen Red Cells Q White Cells R Platelets S Globulin T Fibrinogen V Antihemophilic Factors W Factor IX	1 Nonautologous
8 Vein	Ø Open 3 Percutaneous	B 4-Factor Prothrombin Complex Concentrate	1 Nonautologous

SECTION: 3 ADMINISTRATION
BODY SYSTEM: C INDWELLING DEVICE
OPERATION: 1 IRRIGATION: Putting in or on a cleansing substance

Body System / Region	Approach	Substance	Qualifier
Z None	X External	8 Irrigating Substance	Z No Qualifier

SECTION: 3 ADMINISTRATION
BODY SYSTEM: E PHYSIOLOGICAL SYSTEMS AND ANATOMICAL REGIONS
OPERATION: Ø INTRODUCTION: *(on multiple pages)*
Putting in or on a therapeutic, diagnostic, nutritional, physiological, or prophylactic substance except blood or blood products

Body System / Region	Approach	Substance	Qualifier
Ø Skin and Mucous Membranes	X External	Ø Antineoplastic	5 Other Antineoplastic M Monoclonal Antibody
Ø Skin and Mucous Membranes	X External	2 Anti-infective	8 Oxazolidinones 9 Other Anti-infective
Ø Skin and Mucous Membranes	X External	3 Anti-inflammatory 4 Serum, Toxoid and Vaccine B Local Anesthetic K Other Diagnostic Substance M Pigment N Analgesics, Hypnotics, Sedatives T Destructive Agent	Z No Qualifier
Ø Skin and Mucous Membranes	X External	G Other Therapeutic Substance	C Other Substance
1 Subcutaneous Tissue	Ø Open	2 Anti-infective	A Anti-Infective Envelope
1 Subcutaneous Tissue	3 Percutaneous	Ø Antineoplastic	5 Other Antineoplastic M Monoclonal Antibody
1 Subcutaneous Tissue	3 Percutaneous	2 Anti-infective	8 Oxazolidinones 9 Other Anti-infective A Anti-Infective Envelope
1 Subcutaneous Tissue	3 Percutaneous	3 Anti-inflammatory 4 Serum, Toxoid, and Vaccine 6 Nutritional Substance 7 Electrolytic and Water Balance Substance B Local Anesthetic H Radioactive Substance K Other Diagnostic Substance N Analgesics, Hypnotics, Sedatives T Destructive Agent	Z No Qualifier
1 Subcutaneous Tissue	3 Percutaneous	G Other Therapeutic Substance	C Other Substance
1 Subcutaneous Tissue	3 Percutaneous	V Hormone	G Insulin J Other Hormone
2 Muscle	3 Percutaneous	Ø Antineoplastic	5 Other Antineoplastic M Monoclonal Antibody

New/Revised Text in Green ~~deleted~~ Deleted ♀ Females Only ♂ Males Only **Coding Clinic**
Non-covered   Limited Coverage   Combination (See Appendix E)   DRG Non-OR   Non-OR   Hospital-Acquired Condition

SECTION: 3 ADMINISTRATION
BODY SYSTEM: E PHYSIOLOGICAL SYSTEMS AND ANATOMICAL REGIONS
OPERATION: 0 INTRODUCTION: *(continued)*

Putting in or on a therapeutic, diagnostic, nutritional, physiological, or prophylactic substance except blood or blood products

Body System / Region	Approach	Substance	Qualifier
2 Muscle	3 Percutaneous	2 Anti-infective	8 Oxazolidinones 9 Other Anti-infective
2 Muscle	3 Percutaneous	3 Anti-inflammatory 4 Serum, Toxoid and Vaccine 6 Nutritional Substance 7 Electrolytic and Water Balance Substance B Local Anesthetic H Radioactive Substance K Other Diagnostic Substance N Analgesics, Hypnotics, Sedatives T Destructive Agent	Z No Qualifier
2 Muscle	3 Percutaneous	G Other Therapeutic Substance	C Other Substance
3 Peripheral Vein	0 Open	0 Antineoplastic	2 High-dose Interleukin-2 3 Low-dose Interleukin-2 5 Other Antineoplastic M Monoclonal Antibody P Clofarabine
3 Peripheral Vein	0 Open	1 Thrombolytic	6 Recombinant Human-activated Protein C 7 Other Thrombolytic
3 Peripheral Vein	0 Open	2 Anti-infective	8 Oxazolidinones 9 Other Anti-infective
3 Peripheral Vein	0 Open	3 Anti-inflammatory 4 Serum, Toxoid and Vaccine 6 Nutritional Substance 7 Electrolytic and Water Balance Substance F Intracirculatory Anesthetic H Radioactive Substance K Other Diagnostic Substance N Analgesics, Hypnotics, Sedatives P Platelet Inhibitor R Antiarrhythmic T Destructive Agent X Vasopressor	Z No Qualifier
3 Peripheral Vein	0 Open	G Other Therapeutic Substance	C Other Substance N Blood Brain Barrier Disruption
3 Peripheral Vein	0 Open	U Pancreatic Islet Cells	0 Autologous 1 Nonautologous
3 Peripheral Vein	0 Open	V Hormone	G Insulin H Human B-type Natriuretic Peptide J Other Hormone
3 Peripheral Vein	0 Open	W Immunotherapeutic	K Immunostimulator L Immunosuppressive

DRG Non-OR 3E03002
DRG Non-OR 3E03017
DRG Non-OR 3E030U[01]

3: ADMINISTRATION   E: PHYSIOLOGICAL SYSTEMS AND ANATOMICAL REGIONS   0: INTRODUCTION

SECTION: 3 ADMINISTRATION

BODY SYSTEM: E PHYSIOLOGICAL SYSTEMS AND ANATOMICAL REGIONS
OPERATION: Ø INTRODUCTION: *(continued)*

Putting in or on a therapeutic, diagnostic, nutritional, physiological, or prophylactic substance except blood or blood products

Body System / Region	Approach	Substance	Qualifier
3 Peripheral Vein	3 Percutaneous	Ø Antineoplastic	2 High-dose Interleukin-2 3 Low-dose Interleukin-2 5 Other Antineoplastic M Monoclonal Antibody P Clofarabine
3 Peripheral Vein	3 Percutaneous	1 Thrombolytic	6 Recombinant Human-activated Protein C 7 Other Thrombolytic
3 Peripheral Vein	3 Percutaneous	2 Anti-infective	8 Oxazolidinones 9 Other Anti-infective
3 Peripheral Vein	3 Percutaneous	3 Anti-inflammatory 4 Serum, Toxoid and Vaccine 6 Nutritional Substance 7 Electrolytic and Water Balance Substance F Intracirculatory Anesthetic H Radioactive Substance K Other Diagnostic Substance N Analgesics, Hypnotics, Sedatives P Platelet Inhibitor R Antiarrhythmic T Destructive Agent X Vasopressor	Z No Qualifier
3 Peripheral Vein	3 Percutaneous	G Other Therapeutic Substance	C Other Substance N Blood Brain Barrier Disruption Q Glucarpidase
3 Peripheral Vein	3 Percutaneous	U Pancreatic Islet Cells	Ø Autologous 1 Nonautologous
3 Peripheral Vein	3 Percutaneous	V Hormone	G Insulin H Human B-type Natriuretic Peptide J Other Hormone
3 Peripheral Vein	3 Percutaneous	W Immunotherapeutic	K Immunostimulator L Immunosuppressive
4 Central Vein	Ø Open	Ø Antineoplastic	2 High-dose Interleukin-2 3 Low-dose Interleukin-2 5 Other Antineoplastic M Monoclonal Antibody P Clofarabine
4 Central Vein	Ø Open	1 Thrombolytic	6 Recombinant Human-activated Protein C 7 Other Thrombolytic
4 Central Vein	Ø Open	2 Anti-infective	8 Oxazolidinones 9 Other Anti-infective

DRG Non-OR 3EØ33Ø2
DRG Non-OR 3EØ3317
DRG Non-OR 3EØ33U[Ø1]
DRG Non-OR 3EØ4ØØ2
DRG Non-OR 3EØ417

New/Revised Text in Green   ~~deleted~~ Deleted   ♀ Females Only   ♂ Males Only   **Coding Clinic**
⬡ Non-covered   ⬡ Limited Coverage   ⊞ Combination (See Appendix E)   DRG Non-OR   Non-OR   ⬡ Hospital-Acquired Condition

0: INTRODUCTION

E: PHYSIOLOGICAL SYSTEMS AND ANATOMICAL REGIONS

3: ADMINISTRATION

SECTION: 3 ADMINISTRATION
BODY SYSTEM: E PHYSIOLOGICAL SYSTEMS AND ANATOMICAL REGIONS
OPERATION: 0 INTRODUCTION: *(continued)*
Putting in or on a therapeutic, diagnostic, nutritional, physiological, or prophylactic substance except blood or blood products

Body System / Region	Approach	Substance	Qualifier
4 Central Vein	0 Open	3 Anti-inflammatory 4 Serum, Toxoid and Vaccine 6 Nutritional Substance 7 Electrolytic and Water Balance Substance F Intracirculatory Anesthetic H Radioactive Substance K Other Diagnostic Substance N Analgesics, Hypnotics, Sedatives P Platelet Inhibitor R Antiarrhythmic T Destructive Agent X Vasopressor	Z No Qualifier
4 Central Vein	0 Open	G Other Therapeutic Substance	C Other Substance N Blood Brain Barrier Disruption
4 Central Vein	0 Open	V Hormone	G Insulin H Human B-type Natriuretic Peptide J Other Hormone
4 Central Vein	0 Open	W Immunotherapeutic	K Immunostimulator L Immunosuppressive
4 Central Vein	3 Percutaneous	0 Antineoplastic	2 High-dose Interleukin-2 3 Low-dose Interleukin-2 5 Other Antineoplastic M Monoclonal Antibody P Clofarabine
4 Central Vein	3 Percutaneous	1 Thrombolytic	6 Recombinant Human-activated Protein C 7 Other Thrombolytic
4 Central Vein	3 Percutaneous	2 Anti-infective	8 Oxazolidinones 9 Other Anti-infective
4 Central Vein	3 Percutaneous	3 Anti-inflammatory 4 Serum, Toxoid and Vaccine 6 Nutritional Substance 7 Electrolytic and Water Balance Substance F Intracirculatory Anesthetic H Radioactive Substance K Other Diagnostic Substance N Analgesics, Hypnotics, Sedatives P Platelet Inhibitor R Antiarrhythmic T Destructive Agent X Vasopressor	Z No Qualifier
4 Central Vein	3 Percutaneous	G Other Therapeutic Substance	C Other Substance N Blood Brain Barrier Disruption Q Glucarpidase
4 Central Vein	3 Percutaneous	V Hormone	G Insulin H Human B-type Natriuretic Peptide J Other Hormone

DRG Non-OR 3E04302
DRG Non-OR 3E04317

New/Revised Text in Green ~~deleted~~ Deleted ♀ Females Only ♂ Males Only **Coding Clinic**
Non-covered Limited Coverage ⊞ Combination (See Appendix E) DRG Non-OR Non-OR Hospital-Acquired Condition

515

SECTION: 3 ADMINISTRATION
BODY SYSTEM: E PHYSIOLOGICAL SYSTEMS AND ANATOMICAL REGIONS
OPERATION: Ø INTRODUCTION: *(continued)*
Putting in or on a therapeutic, diagnostic, nutritional, physiological, or prophylactic substance except blood or blood products

Body System / Region	Approach	Substance	Qualifier
4 Central Vein	3 Percutaneous	W Immunotherapeutic	K Immunostimulator L Immunosuppressive
5 Peripheral Artery 6 Central Artery	Ø Open 3 Percutaneous	Ø Antineoplastic	2 High-dose Interleukin-2 3 Low-dose Interleukin-2 5 Other Antineoplastic M Monoclonal Antibody P Clofarabine
5 Peripheral Artery 6 Central Artery	Ø Open 3 Percutaneous	1 Thrombolytic	6 Recombinant Human-activated Protein C 7 Other Thrombolytic
5 Peripheral Artery 6 Central Artery	Ø Open 3 Percutaneous	2 Anti-infective	8 Oxazolidinones 9 Other Anti-infective
5 Peripheral Artery 6 Central Artery	Ø Open 3 Percutaneous	3 Anti-inflammatory 4 Serum, Toxoid and Vaccine 6 Nutritional Substance 7 Electrolytic and Water Balance Substance F Intracirculatory Anesthetic H Radioactive Substance K Other Diagnostic Substance N Analgesics, Hypnotics, Sedatives P Platelet Inhibitor R Antiarrhythmic T Destructive Agent X Vasopressor	Z No Qualifier
5 Peripheral Artery 6 Central Artery	Ø Open 3 Percutaneous	G Other Therapeutic Substance	C Other Substance N Blood Brain Barrier Disruption
5 Peripheral Artery 6 Central Artery	Ø Open 3 Percutaneous	V Hormone	G Insulin H Human B-type Natriuretic Peptide J Other Hormone
5 Peripheral Artery 6 Central Artery	Ø Open 3 Percutaneous	W Immunotherapeutic	K Immunostimulator L Immunosuppressive
7 Coronary Artery 8 Heart	Ø Open 3 Percutaneous	1 Thrombolytic	6 Recombinant Human-activated Protein C 7 Other Thrombolytic
7 Coronary Artery 8 Heart	Ø Open 3 Percutaneous	G Other Therapeutic Substance	C Other Substance
7 Coronary Artery 8 Heart	Ø Open 3 Percutaneous	K Other Diagnostic Substance P Platelet Inhibitor	Z No Qualifier
9 Nose	3 Percutaneous 7 Via Natural or Artificial Opening X External	Ø Antineoplastic	5 Other Antineoplastic M Monoclonal Antibody
9 Nose	3 Percutaneous 7 Via Natural or Artificial Opening X External	2 Anti-infective	8 Oxazolidinones 9 Other Anti-infective

DRG Non-OR 3EØ[56][Ø3]Ø2
DRG Non-OR 3EØ[56][Ø3]17
DRG Non-OR 3EØ8[Ø3]17

New/Revised Text in Green ~~deleted~~ Deleted ♀ Females Only ♂ Males Only **Coding Clinic**
🚫 Non-covered 🚫 Limited Coverage ⊡ Combination (See Appendix E) DRG Non-OR Non-OR 🚫 Hospital-Acquired Condition

SECTION: 3 ADMINISTRATION

BODY SYSTEM: E PHYSIOLOGICAL SYSTEMS AND ANATOMICAL REGIONS
OPERATION: Ø INTRODUCTION: *(continued)*
Putting in or on a therapeutic, diagnostic, nutritional, physiological, or prophylactic substance except blood or blood products

Body System / Region	Approach	Substance	Qualifier
9 Nose	3 Percutaneous 7 Via Natural or Artificial Opening X External	3 Anti-inflammatory 4 Serum, Toxoid and Vaccine B Local Anesthetic H Radioactive Substance K Other Diagnostic Substance N Analgesics, Hypnotics, Sedatives T Destructive Agent	Z No Qualifier
9 Nose	3 Percutaneous 7 Via Natural or Artificial Opening X External	G Other Therapeutic Substance	C Other Substance
A Bone Marrow	3 Percutaneous	Ø Antineoplastic	5 Other Antineoplastic M Monoclonal Antibody
A Bone Marrow	3 Percutaneous	G Other Therapeutic Substance	C Other Substance
B Ear	3 Percutaneous 7 Via Natural or Artificial Opening X External	Ø Antineoplastic	4 Liquid Brachytherapy Radioisotope 5 Other Antineoplastic M Monoclonal Antibody
B Ear	3 Percutaneous 7 Via Natural or Artificial Opening X External	2 Anti-infective	8 Oxazolidinones 9 Other Anti-infective
B Ear	3 Percutaneous 7 Via Natural or Artificial Opening X External	3 Anti-inflammatory B Local Anesthetic H Radioactive Substance K Other Diagnostic Substance N Analgesics, Hypnotics, Sedatives T Destructive Agent	Z No Qualifier
B Ear	3 Percutaneous 7 Via Natural or Artificial Opening X External	G Other Therapeutic Substance	C Other Substance
C Eye	3 Percutaneous 7 Via Natural or Artificial Opening X External	Ø Antineoplastic	4 Liquid Brachytherapy Radioisotope 5 Other Antineoplastic M Monoclonal Antibody
C Eye	3 Percutaneous 7 Via Natural or Artificial Opening X External	2 Anti-infective	8 Oxazolidinones 9 Other Anti-infective
C Eye	3 Percutaneous 7 Via Natural or Artificial Opening X External	3 Anti-inflammatory B Local Anesthetic H Radioactive Substance K Other Diagnostic Substance M Pigment N Analgesics, Hypnotics, Sedatives T Destructive Agent	Z No Qualifier
C Eye	3 Percutaneous 7 Via Natural or Artificial Opening X External	G Other Therapeutic Substance	C Other Substance
C Eye	3 Percutaneous 7 Via Natural or Artificial Opening X External	S Gas	F Other Gas

0: INTRODUCTION

E: PHYSIOLOGICAL SYSTEMS AND ANATOMICAL REGIONS

3: ADMINISTRATION

SECTION: 3 ADMINISTRATION
BODY SYSTEM: E PHYSIOLOGICAL SYSTEMS AND ANATOMICAL REGIONS
OPERATION: 0 INTRODUCTION: *(continued)*
Putting in or on a therapeutic, diagnostic, nutritional, physiological, or prophylactic substance except blood or blood products

Body System / Region	Approach	Substance	Qualifier
D Mouth and Pharynx	3 Percutaneous 7 Via Natural or Artificial Opening X External	0 Antineoplastic	4 Liquid Brachytherapy Radioisotope 5 Other Antineoplastic M Monoclonal Antibody
D Mouth and Pharynx	3 Percutaneous 7 Via Natural or Artificial Opening X External	2 Anti-infective	8 Oxazolidinones 9 Other Anti-infective
D Mouth and Pharynx	3 Percutaneous 7 Via Natural or Artificial Opening X External	3 Anti-inflammatory 4 Serum, Toxoid and Vaccine 6 Nutritional Substance 7 Electrolytic and Water Balance Substance B Local Anesthetic H Radioactive Substance K Other Diagnostic Substance N Analgesics, Hypnotics, Sedatives R Antiarrhythmic T Destructive Agent	Z No Qualifier
D Mouth and Pharynx	3 Percutaneous 7 Via Natural or Artificial Opening X External	G Other Therapeutic Substance	C Other Substance
E Products of Conception ♀ G Upper GI H Lower GI K Genitourinary Tract N Male Reproductive ♂	3 Percutaneous 7 Via Natural or Artificial Opening 8 Via Natural or Artificial Opening Endoscopic	0 Antineoplastic	4 Liquid Brachytherapy Radioisotope 5 Other Antineoplastic M Monoclonal Antibody
E Products of Conception ♀ G Upper GI H Lower GI K Genitourinary Tract N Male Reproductive ♂	3 Percutaneous 7 Via Natural or Artificial Opening 8 Via Natural or Artificial Opening Endoscopic	2 Anti-infective	8 Oxazolidinones 9 Other Anti-infective
E Products of Conception ♀ G Upper GI H Lower GI K Genitourinary Tract N Male Reproductive ♂	3 Percutaneous 7 Via Natural or Artificial Opening 8 Via Natural or Artificial Opening Endoscopic	3 Anti-inflammatory 6 Nutritional Substance 7 Electrolytic and Water Balance Substance B Local Anesthetic H Radioactive Substance K Other Diagnostic Substance N Analgesics, Hypnotics, Sedatives T Destructive Agent	Z No Qualifier
E Products of Conception ♀ G Upper GI H Lower GI K Genitourinary Tract N Male Reproductive ♂	3 Percutaneous 7 Via Natural or Artificial Opening 8 Via Natural or Artificial Opening Endoscopic	G Other Therapeutic Substance	C Other Substance
E Products of Conception ♀ G Upper GI H Lower GI K Genitourinary Tract N Male Reproductive ♂	3 Percutaneous 7 Via Natural or Artificial Opening 8 Via Natural or Artificial Opening Endoscopic	S Gas	F Other Gas

Coding Clinic: 2015, Q2, P29 – 3E0G76Z
Coding Clinic: 2015, Q3, P25 – 3E0G8GC

New/Revised Text in Green   ~~deleted~~ Deleted   ♀ Females Only   ♂ Males Only   **Coding Clinic**
Non-covered   Limited Coverage   ⊞ Combination (See Appendix E)   DRG Non-OR   Non-OR   Hospital-Acquired Condition

SECTION: 3 ADMINISTRATION
BODY SYSTEM: E PHYSIOLOGICAL SYSTEMS AND ANATOMICAL REGIONS
OPERATION: Ø INTRODUCTION: *(continued)*

Putting in or on a therapeutic, diagnostic, nutritional, physiological, or prophylactic substance except blood or blood products

Body System / Region	Approach	Substance	Qualifier
F Respiratory Tract	3 Percutaneous	Ø Antineoplastic	4 Liquid Brachytherapy Radioisotope 5 Other Antineoplastic M Monoclonal Antibody
F Respiratory Tract	3 Percutaneous	2 Anti-infective	8 Oxazolidinones 9 Other Anti-infective
F Respiratory Tract	3 Percutaneous	3 Anti-inflammatory 6 Nutritional Substance 7 Electrolytic and Water Balance Substance B Local Anesthetic H Radioactive Substance K Other Diagnostic Substance N Analgesics, Hypnotics, Sedatives T Destructive Agent	Z No Qualifier
F Respiratory Tract	3 Percutaneous	G Other Therapeutic Substance	C Other Substance
F Respiratory Tract	3 Percutaneous	S Gas	D Nitric Oxide F Other Gas
F Respiratory Tract	7 Via Natural or Artificial Opening 8 Via Natural or Artificial Opening Endoscopic	Ø Antineoplastic	4 Liquid Brachytherapy Radioisotope 5 Other Antineoplastic M Monoclonal Antibody
F Respiratory Tract	7 Via Natural or Artificial Opening 8 Via Natural or Artificial Opening Endoscopic	2 Anti-infective	8 Oxazolidinones 9 Other Anti-infective
F Respiratory Tract	7 Via Natural or Artificial Opening 8 Via Natural or Artificial Opening Endoscopic	3 Anti-inflammatory 6 Nutritional Substance 7 Electrolytic and Water Balance Substance B Local Anesthetic D Inhalation Anesthetic H Radioactive Substance K Other Diagnostic Substance N Analgesics, Hypnotics, Sedatives T Destructive Agent	Z No Qualifier
F Respiratory Tract	7 Via Natural or Artificial Opening 8 Via Natural or Artificial Opening Endoscopic	G Other Therapeutic Substance	C Other Substance
F Respiratory Tract	7 Via Natural or Artificial Opening 8 Via Natural or Artificial Opening Endoscopic	S Gas	D Nitric Oxide F Other Gas
J Biliary and Pancreatic Tract	3 Percutaneous 7 Via Natural or Artificial Opening 8 Via Natural or Artificial Opening Endoscopic	Ø Antineoplastic	4 Liquid Brachytherapy Radioisotope 5 Other Antineoplastic M Monoclonal Antibody
J Biliary and Pancreatic Tract	3 Percutaneous 7 Via Natural or Artificial Opening 8 Via Natural or Artificial Opening Endoscopic	2 Anti-infective	8 Oxazolidinones 9 Other Anti-infective

SECTION: 3 ADMINISTRATION
BODY SYSTEM: E PHYSIOLOGICAL SYSTEMS AND ANATOMICAL REGIONS
OPERATION: 0 INTRODUCTION: *(continued)*
Putting in or on a therapeutic, diagnostic, nutritional, physiological, or prophylactic substance except blood or blood products

Body System / Region	Approach	Substance	Qualifier
J Biliary and Pancreatic Tract	3 Percutaneous 7 Via Natural or Artificial Opening 8 Via Natural or Artificial Opening Endoscopic	3 Anti-inflammatory 6 Nutritional Substance 7 Electrolytic and Water Balance Substance B Local Anesthetic H Radioactive Substance K Other Diagnostic Substance N Analgesics, Hypnotics, Sedatives T Destructive Agent	Z No Qualifier
J Biliary and Pancreatic Tract	3 Percutaneous 7 Via Natural or Artificial Opening 8 Via Natural or Artificial Opening Endoscopic	G Other Therapeutic Substance	C Other Substance
J Biliary and Pancreatic Tract	3 Percutaneous 7 Via Natural or Artificial Opening 8 Via Natural or Artificial Opening Endoscopic	S Gas	F Other Gas
J Biliary and Pancreatic Tract	3 Percutaneous 7 Via Natural or Artificial Opening 8 Via Natural or Artificial Opening Endoscopic	U Pancreatic Islet Cells	0 Autologous 1 Nonautologous
L Pleural Cavity M Peritoneal Cavity	0 Open	5 Adhesion Barrier	Z No Qualifier
L Pleural Cavity M Peritoneal Cavity	3 Percutaneous	0 Antineoplastic	4 Liquid Brachytherapy Radioisotope 5 Other Antineoplastic M Monoclonal Antibody
L Pleural Cavity M Peritoneal Cavity	3 Percutaneous	2 Anti-infective	8 Oxazolidinones 9 Other Anti-infective
L Pleural Cavity M Peritoneal Cavity	3 Percutaneous	3 Anti-inflammatory 6 Nutritional Substance 7 Electrolytic and Water Balance Substance B Local Anesthetic H Radioactive Substance K Other Diagnostic Substance N Analgesics, Hypnotics, Sedatives T Destructive Agent	Z No Qualifier
L Pleural Cavity M Peritoneal Cavity	3 Percutaneous	G Other Therapeutic Substance	C Other Substance
L Pleural Cavity M Peritoneal Cavity	3 Percutaneous	S Gas	F Other Gas
L Pleural Cavity M Peritoneal Cavity	7 Via Natural or Artificial Opening	0 Antineoplastic	4 Liquid Brachytherapy Radioisotope 5 Other Antineoplastic M Monoclonal Antibody
L Pleural Cavity M Peritoneal Cavity	7 Via Natural or Artificial Opening	S Gas	F Other Gas
P Female Reproductive ♀	0 Open	5 Adhesion Barrier	Z No Qualifier

DRG Non-OR   3E0J[378]U[01]

Coding Clinic: 2015, Q2, P31 – 3E0L3GC

New/Revised Text in Green   ~~deleted~~ Deleted   ♀ Females Only   ♂ Males Only   **Coding Clinic**
🚫 Non-covered   🚫 Limited Coverage   ⊞ Combination (See Appendix E)   DRG Non-OR   Non-OR   🚫 Hospital-Acquired Condition

SECTION: 3 ADMINISTRATION
BODY SYSTEM: E PHYSIOLOGICAL SYSTEMS AND ANATOMICAL REGIONS
OPERATION: Ø INTRODUCTION: *(continued)*

Putting in or on a therapeutic, diagnostic, nutritional, physiological, or prophylactic substance except blood or blood products

Body System / Region	Approach	Substance	Qualifier
P Female Reproductive ♀	3 Percutaneous 7 Via Natural or Artificial Opening	Ø Antineoplastic	4 Liquid Brachytherapy Radioisotope 5 Other Antineoplastic M Monoclonal Antibody
P Female Reproductive ♀	3 Percutaneous 7 Via Natural or Artificial Opening	2 Anti-infective	8 Oxazolidinones 9 Other Anti-infective
P Female Reproductive ♀	3 Percutaneous 7 Via Natural or Artificial Opening	3 Anti-inflammatory 6 Nutritional Substance 7 Electrolytic and Water Balance Substance B Local Anesthetic H Radioactive Substance K Other Diagnostic Substance L Sperm N Analgesics, Hypnotics, Sedatives T Destructive Agent	Z No Qualifier
P Female Reproductive ♀	3 Percutaneous 7 Via Natural or Artificial Opening	G Other Therapeutic Substance	C Other Substance
P Female Reproductive ♀	3 Percutaneous 7 Via Natural or Artificial Opening	Q Fertilized Ovum	Ø Autologous 1 Nonautologous
P Female Reproductive ♀	3 Percutaneous 7 Via Natural or Artificial Opening	S Gas	F Other Gas
P Female Reproductive ♀	8 Via Natural or Artificial Opening Endoscopic	Ø Antineoplastic	4 Liquid Brachytherapy Radioisotope 5 Other Antineoplastic M Monoclonal Antibody
P Female Reproductive ♀	8 Via Natural or Artificial Opening Endoscopic	2 Anti-infective	8 Oxazolidinones 9 Other Anti-infective
P Female Reproductive ♀	8 Via Natural or Artificial Opening Endoscopic	3 Anti-inflammatory 6 Nutritional Substance 7 Electrolytic and Water Balance Substance B Local Anesthetic H Radioactive Substance K Other Diagnostic Substance N Analgesics, Hypnotics, Sedatives T Destructive Agent	Z No Qualifier
P Female Reproductive ♀	8 Via Natural or Artificial Opening Endoscopic	G Other Therapeutic Substance	C Other Substance
P Female Reproductive ♀	8 Via Natural or Artificial Opening Endoscopic	S Gas	F Other Gas
~~Q Cranial Cavity and Brain~~	~~Ø Open~~	~~A Stem Cells, Embryonic~~	~~Z No Qualifier~~
~~Q Cranial Cavity and Brain~~	~~Ø Open~~	~~E Stem Cells, Somatic~~	~~Ø Autologous~~ ~~1 Nonautologous~~
Q Cranial Cavity and Brain	Ø Open 3 Percutaneous	Ø Antineoplastic	4 Liquid Brachytherapy Radioisotope 5 Other Antineoplastic M Monoclonal Antibody
Q Cranial Cavity and Brain	Ø Open 3 Percutaneous	2 Anti-infective	8 Oxazolidinones 9 Other Anti-infective

New/Revised Text in Green   ~~deleted~~ Deleted   ♀ Females Only   ♂ Males Only   **Coding Clinic**
Non-covered   Limited Coverage   ⊞ Combination (See Appendix E)   DRG Non-OR   Non-OR   Hospital-Acquired Condition

SECTION: 3 ADMINISTRATION
BODY SYSTEM: E **PHYSIOLOGICAL SYSTEMS AND ANATOMICAL REGIONS**
OPERATION: Ø **INTRODUCTION:** *(continued)*
Putting in or on a therapeutic, diagnostic, nutritional, physiological, or prophylactic substance except blood or blood products

Body System / Region	Approach	Substance	Qualifier
Q Cranial Cavity and Brain	Ø Open 3 Percutaneous	3 Anti-inflammatory 6 Nutritional Substance 7 Electrolytic and Water Balance Substance A Stem Cells, Embryonic B Local Anesthetic H Radioactive Substance K Other Diagnostic Substance N Analgesics, Hypnotics, Sedatives T Destructive Agent	Z No Qualifier
Q Cranial Cavity and Brain	Ø Open 3 Percutaneous	E Stem Cells, Somatic	Ø Autologous 1 Nonautologous
Q Cranial Cavity and Brain	Ø Open 3 Percutaneous	G Other Therapeutic Substance	C Other Substance
Q Cranial Cavity and Brain	Ø Open 3 Percutaneous	S Gas	F Other Gas
Q Cranial Cavity and Brain	7 Via Natural or Artificial Opening	Ø Antineoplastic	4 Liquid Brachytherapy Radioisotope 5 Other Antineoplastic M Monoclonal Antibody
Q Cranial Cavity and Brain	7 Via Natural or Artificial Opening	S Gas	F Other Gas
R Spinal Canal	Ø Open	A Stem Cells, Embryonic	Z No Qualifier
R Spinal Canal	Ø Open	A Stem Cells, Somatic	Ø Autologous 1 Nonautologous
R Spinal Canal	3 Percutaneous	Ø Antineoplastic	2 High-dose Interleukin-2 3 Low-dose Interleukin-2 4 Liquid Brachytherapy Radioisotope 5 Other Antineoplastic M Monoclonal Antibody
R Spinal Canal	3 Percutaneous	2 Anti-infective	8 Oxazolidinones 9 Other Anti-infective
R Spinal Canal	3 Percutaneous	3 Anti-inflammatory 6 Nutritional Substance 7 Electrolytic and Water Balance Substance A Stem Cells, Embryonic B Local Anesthetic C Regional Anesthetic H Radioactive Substance K Other Diagnostic Substance N Analgesics, Hypnotics, Sedatives T Destructive Agent	Z No Qualifier
R Spinal Canal	3 Percutaneous	E Stem Cells, Somatic	Ø Autologous 1 Nonautologous
R Spinal Canal	3 Percutaneous	G Other Therapeutic Substance	C Other Substance
R Spinal Canal	3 Percutaneous	S Gas	F Other Gas
R Spinal Canal	7 Via Natural or Artificial Opening	S Gas	F Other Gas

DRG Non-OR 3EØQ7Ø5
DRG Non-OR 3EØR3Ø2

New/Revised Text in Green   ~~deleted~~ Deleted   ♀ Females Only   ♂ Males Only   **Coding Clinic**
Non-covered   Limited Coverage   ⊞ Combination (See Appendix E)   DRG Non-OR   Non-OR   Hospital-Acquired Condition

SECTION: 3 ADMINISTRATION
BODY SYSTEM: E PHYSIOLOGICAL SYSTEMS AND ANATOMICAL REGIONS
OPERATION: Ø INTRODUCTION: *(continued)*
Putting in or on a therapeutic, diagnostic, nutritional, physiological, or prophylactic substance except blood or blood products

Body System / Region	Approach	Substance	Qualifier
S Epidural Space	3 Percutaneous	Ø Antineoplastic	2 High-dose Interleukin-2 3 Low-dose Interleukin-2 4 Liquid Brachytherapy Radioisotope 5 Other Antineoplastic M Monoclonal Antibody
S Epidural Space	3 Percutaneous	2 Anti-infective	8 Oxazolidinones 9 Other Anti-infective
S Epidural Space	3 Percutaneous	3 Anti-inflammatory 6 Nutritional Substance 7 Electrolytic and Water Balance Substance B Local Anesthetic C Regional Anesthetic H Radioactive Substance K Other Diagnostic Substance N Analgesics, Hypnotics, Sedatives T Destructive Agent	Z No Qualifier
S Epidural Space	3 Percutaneous	G Other Therapeutic Substance	C Other Substance
S Epidural Space	3 Percutaneous	S Gas	F Other Gas
S Epidural Space	7 Via Natural or Artificial Opening	S Gas	F Other Gas
T Peripheral Nerves and Plexi X Cranial Nerves	3 Percutaneous	3 Anti-inflammatory B Local Anesthetic C Regional Anesthetic T Destructive Agent	Z No Qualifier
T Peripheral Nerves and Plexi X Cranial Nerves	3 Percutaneous	G Other Therapeutic Substance	C Other Substance
U Joints	Ø Open	2 Anti-infective	8 Oxazolidinones 9 Other Anti-infective
U Joints	Ø Open	G Other Therapeutic Substance	B Recombinant Bone Morphogenetic Protein
U Joints	3 Percutaneous	Ø Antineoplastic	4 Liquid Brachytherapy Radioisotope 5 Other Antineoplastic M Monoclonal Antibody
U Joints	3 Percutaneous	2 Anti-infective	8 Oxazolidinones 9 Other Anti-infective
U Joints	3 Percutaneous	3 Anti-inflammatory 6 Nutritional Substance 7 Electrolytic and Water Balance Substance B Local Anesthetic H Radioactive Substance K Other Diagnostic Substance N Analgesics, Hypnotics, Sedatives T Destructive Agent	Z No Qualifier
U Joints	3 Percutaneous	G Other Therapeutic Substance	B Recombinant Bone Morphogenetic Protein C Other Substance

DRG Non-OR 3EØS3Ø2

SECTION: 3 ADMINISTRATION
BODY SYSTEM: E PHYSIOLOGICAL SYSTEMS AND ANATOMICAL REGIONS
OPERATION: Ø INTRODUCTION: *(continued)*
Putting in or on a therapeutic, diagnostic, nutritional, physiological, or prophylactic substance except blood or blood products

Body System / Region	Approach	Substance	Qualifier
U Joints	3 Percutaneous	S Gas	F Other Gas
V Bones	Ø Open	G Other Therapeutic Substance	B Recombinant Bone Morphogenetic Protein
V Bones	3 Percutaneous	Ø Antineoplastic	5 Other Antineoplastic M Monoclonal Antibody
V Bones	3 Percutaneous	2 Anti-infective	8 Oxazolidinones 9 Other Anti-infective
V Bones	3 Percutaneous	3 Anti-inflammatory 6 Nutritional Substance 7 Electrolytic and Water Balance Substance B Local Anesthetic H Radioactive Substance K Other Diagnostic Substance N Analgesics, Hypnotics, Sedatives T Destructive Agent	Z No Qualifier
V Bones	3 Percutaneous	G Other Therapeutic Substance	B Recombinant Bone Morphogenetic Protein C Other Substance
W Lymphatics	3 Percutaneous	Ø Antineoplastic	5 Other Antineoplastic M Monoclonal Antibody
W Lymphatics	3 Percutaneous	2 Anti-infective	8 Oxazolidinones 9 Other Anti-infective
W Lymphatics	3 Percutaneous	3 Anti-inflammatory 6 Nutritional Substance 7 Electrolytic and Water Balance Substance B Local Anesthetic H Radioactive Substance K Other Diagnostic Substance N Analgesics, Hypnotics, Sedatives T Destructive Agent	Z No Qualifier

New/Revised Text in Green   ~~deleted~~ Deleted   ♀ Females Only   ♂ Males Only   **Coding Clinic**
🚫 Non-covered   🚫 Limited Coverage   ⊞ Combination (See Appendix E)   DRG Non-OR   Non-OR   🚫 Hospital-Acquired Condition

SECTION: 3 ADMINISTRATION

BODY SYSTEM: E **PHYSIOLOGICAL SYSTEMS AND ANATOMICAL REGIONS**
OPERATION: 0 **INTRODUCTION:** *(continued)*
Putting in or on a therapeutic, diagnostic, nutritional, physiological, or prophylactic substance except blood or blood products

Body System / Region	Approach	Substance	Qualifier
W Lymphatics	3 Percutaneous	G Other Therapeutic Substance	C Other Substance
Y Pericardial Cavity	3 Percutaneous	0 Antineoplastic	4 Liquid Brachytherapy Radioisotope 5 Other Antineoplastic M Monoclonal Antibody
Y Pericardial Cavity	3 Percutaneous	2 Anti-infective	8 Oxazolidinones 9 Other Anti-infective
Y Pericardial Cavity	3 Percutaneous	3 Anti-inflammatory 6 Nutritional Substance 7 Electrolytic and Water Balance Substance B Local Anesthetic H Radioactive Substance K Other Diagnostic Substance N Analgesics, Hypnotics, Sedatives T Destructive Agent	Z No Qualifier
Y Pericardial Cavity	3 Percutaneous	G Other Therapeutic Substance	C Other Substance
Y Pericardial Cavity	3 Percutaneous	S Gas	F Other Gas
Y Pericardial Cavity	7 Via Natural or Artificial Opening	0 Antineoplastic	4 Liquid Brachytherapy Radioisotope 5 Other Antineoplastic M Monoclonal Antibody
Y Pericardial Cavity	7 Via Natural or Artificial Opening	S Gas	F Other Gas

Coding Clinic: 2013, Q1, P27 – 3E0G8TZ

Coding Clinic: 2015, Q1, P31 – 3E0R305

Coding Clinic: 2015, Q1, P38 – 3E05305

SECTION: 3 ADMINISTRATION

BODY SYSTEM: E PHYSIOLOGICAL SYSTEMS AND ANATOMICAL REGIONS

OPERATION: 1 IRRIGATION: Putting in or on a cleansing substance

Body System / Region	Approach	Substance	Qualifier
Ø Skin and Mucous Membranes C Eye	3 Percutaneous X External	8 Irrigating Substance	X Diagnostic Z No Qualifier
9 Nose B Ear F Respiratory Tract G Upper GI H Lower GI J Biliary and Pancreatic Tract K Genitourinary Tract N Male Reproductive ♂ P Female Reproductive ♀	3 Percutaneous 7 Via Natural or Artificial Opening 8 Via Natural or Artificial Opening Endoscopic	8 Irrigating Substance	X Diagnostic Z No Qualifier
L Pleural Cavity Q Cranial Cavity and Brain R Spinal Canal S Epidural Space U Joints Y Pericardial Cavity	3 Percutaneous	8 Irrigating Substance	X Diagnostic Z No Qualifier
M Peritoneal Cavity	3 Percutaneous	8 Irrigating Substance	X Diagnostic Z No Qualifier
M Peritoneal Cavity	3 Percutaneous	9 Dialysate	Z No Qualifier

New/Revised Text in Green   deleted Deleted   ♀ Females Only   ♂ Males Only   **Coding Clinic**

🜂 Non-covered   🜂 Limited Coverage   ⊞ Combination (See Appendix E)   DRG Non-OR   Non-OR   🜂 Hospital-Acquired Condition

SECTION: 4 MEASUREMENT AND MONITORING
BODY SYSTEM: A PHYSIOLOGICAL SYSTEMS
OPERATION: 0 **MEASUREMENT:** *(on multiple pages)*
Determining the level of a physiological or physical function
at a point in time

Body System	Approach	Function / Device	Qualifier
0 Central Nervous	0 Open	2 Conductivity 4 Electrical Activity B Pressure	Z No Qualifier
0 Central Nervous	3 Percutaneous	4 Electrical Activity	Z No Qualifier
0 Central Nervous	3 Percutaneous	B Pressure K Temperature R Saturation	D Intracranial
0 Central Nervous	7 Via Natural or Artificial Opening	B Pressure K Temperature R Saturation	D Intracranial
0 Central Nervous	X External	2 Conductivity 4 Electrical Activity	Z No Qualifier
1 Peripheral Nervous	0 Open 3 Percutaneous X External	2 Conductivity	9 Sensory B Motor
1 Peripheral Nervous	0 Open 3 Percutaneous X External	4 Electrical Activity	Z No Qualifier
2 Cardiac	0 Open 3 Percutaneous	4 Electrical Activity 9 Output C Rate F Rhythm H Sound P Action Currents	Z No Qualifier
2 Cardiac	0 Open 3 Percutaneous	N Sampling and Pressure	6 Right Heart 7 Left Heart 8 Bilateral
2 Cardiac ⊞	X External	4 Electrical Activity	A Guidance Z No Qualifier
2 Cardiac	X External	9 Output C Rate F Rhythm H Sound P Action Currents	Z No Qualifier
2 Cardiac	X External	M Total Activity	4 Stress
3 Arterial	0 Open 3 Percutaneous	5 Flow J Pulse	1 Peripheral 3 Pulmonary C Coronary
3 Arterial	0 Open 3 Percutaneous	B Pressure	1 Peripheral 3 Pulmonary C Coronary F Other Thoracic
3 Arterial	0 Open 3 Percutaneous	H Sound R Saturation	1 Peripheral

⊞ 4A02X4A

DRG Non-OR 4A023FZ

DRG Non-OR 4A02[03]N[678]

DRG Non-OR 4A02X4A

Coding Clinic: 2015, Q3, P29 – 4A02X4Z

New/Revised Text in Green   ~~deleted~~ Deleted   ♀ Females Only   ♂ Males Only   **Coding Clinic**
Non-covered   Limited Coverage   ⊞ Combination (See Appendix E)   DRG Non-OR   Non-OR   Hospital-Acquired Condition

SECTION: 4 MEASUREMENT AND MONITORING
BODY SYSTEM: A PHYSIOLOGICAL SYSTEMS
OPERATION: Ø MEASUREMENT: *(continued)*
Determining the level of a physiological or physical function
at a point in time

Body System	Approach	Function / Device	Qualifier
3 Arterial	X External	5 Flow B Pressure H Sound J Pulse R Saturation	1 Peripheral
4 Venous	Ø Open 3 Percutaneous	5 Flow B Pressure J Pulse	Ø Central 1 Peripheral 2 Portal 3 Pulmonary
4 Venous	Ø Open 3 Percutaneous	R Saturation	1 Peripheral
4 Venous	X External	5 Flow B Pressure J Pulse R Saturation	1 Peripheral
5 Circulatory	X External	L Volume	Z No Qualifier
6 Lymphatic	Ø Open 3 Percutaneous	5 Flow B Pressure	Z No Qualifier
7 Visual	X External	Ø Acuity 7 Mobility B Pressure	Z No Qualifier
8 Olfactory	X External	Ø Acuity	Z No Qualifier
9 Respiratory	7 Via Natural or Artificial Opening 8 Via Natural or Artificial Opening Endoscopic X External	1 Capacity 5 Flow C Rate D Resistance L Volume M Total Activity	Z No Qualifier
B Gastrointestinal	7 Via Natural or Artificial Opening 8 Via Natural or Artificial Opening Endoscopic	8 Motility B Pressure G Secretion	Z No Qualifier
C Biliary	3 Percutaneous 4 Percutaneous Endoscopic 7 Via Natural or Artificial Opening 8 Via Natural or Artificial Opening Endoscopic	5 Flow B Pressure	Z No Qualifier
D Urinary	7 Via Natural or Artificial Opening	3 Contractility 5 Flow B Pressure D Resistance L Volume	Z No Qualifier
F Musculoskeletal	3 Percutaneous X External	3 Contractility	Z No Qualifier
H Products of Conception, Cardiac ♀	7 Via Natural or Artificial Opening 8 Via Natural or Artificial Opening Endoscopic X External	4 Electrical Activity C Rate F Rhythm H Sound	Z No Qualifier

SECTION: 4 MEASUREMENT AND MONITORING

BODY SYSTEM: **A PHYSIOLOGICAL SYSTEMS**
OPERATION: **Ø MEASUREMENT:** *(continued)*
Determining the level of a physiological or physical function
at a point in time

Body System	Approach	Function / Device	Qualifier
J Products of Conception, Nervous ♀	7 Via Natural or Artificial Opening 8 Via Natural or Artificial Opening Endoscopic X External	2 Conductivity 4 Electrical Activity B Pressure	Z No Qualifier
Z None	7 Via Natural or Artificial Opening	6 Metabolism K Temperature	Z No Qualifier
Z None	X External	6 Metabolism K Temperature Q Sleep	Z No Qualifier

SECTION: 4 MEASUREMENT AND MONITORING

BODY SYSTEM: **A PHYSIOLOGICAL SYSTEMS**
OPERATION: **1 MONITORING:** *(on multiple pages)*
Determining the level of a physiological or physical function repetitively
over a period of time

Body System	Approach	Function / Device	Qualifier
Ø Central Nervous	Ø Open	2 Conductivity B Pressure	Z No Qualifier
Ø Central Nervous	Ø Open	4 Electrical Activity	G Intraoperative Z No Qualifier
Ø Central Nervous	3 Percutaneous	4 Electrical Activity	G Intraoperative Z No Qualifier
Ø Central Nervous	3 Percutaneous	B Pressure K Temperature R Saturation	D Intracranial
Ø Central Nervous	7 Via Natural or Artificial Opening	B Pressure K Temperature R Saturation	D Intracranial
Ø Central Nervous	X External	2 Conductivity	Z No Qualifier
Ø Central Nervous	X External	4 Electrical Activity	G Intraoperative Z No Qualifier
1 Peripheral Nervous	Ø Open 3 Percutaneous X External	2 Conductivity	9 Sensory B Motor
1 Peripheral Nervous	Ø Open 3 Percutaneous X External	4 Electrical Activity	G Intraoperative Z No Qualifier

Coding Clinic: 2015, Q2, P14 – 4A11X4G
Coding Clinic: 2016, Q2, P29 – 4A103BD

New/Revised Text in Green   ~~deleted~~ Deleted   ♀ Females Only   ♂ Males Only   **Coding Clinic**
🔖 Non-covered   🔖 Limited Coverage   ⊞ Combination (See Appendix E)   DRG Non-OR   Non-OR   🔖 Hospital-Acquired Condition

SECTION: 4 MEASUREMENT AND MONITORING
BODY SYSTEM: A PHYSIOLOGICAL SYSTEMS
OPERATION: 1 MONITORING: *(continued)*
Determining the level of a physiological or physical function repetitively over a period of time

Body System	Approach	Function / Device	Qualifier
2 Cardiac	Ø Open 3 Percutaneous	4 Electrical Activity 9 Output C Rate F Rhythm H Sound	Z No Qualifier
2 Cardiac	X External	4 Electrical Activity	5 Ambulatory Z No Qualifier
2 Cardiac	X External	9 Output C Rate F Rhythm H Sound	Z No Qualifier
2 Cardiac	X External	M Total Activity	4 Stress
2 Cardiac	X External	S Vascular Perfusion	H Indocyanine Green Dye
3 Arterial	Ø Open 3 Percutaneous	5 Flow B Pressure J Pulse	1 Peripheral 3 Pulmonary C Coronary
3 Arterial	Ø Open 3 Percutaneous	H Sound R Saturation	1 Peripheral
3 Arterial	X External	5 Flow B Pressure H Sound J Pulse R Saturation	1 Peripheral
4 Venous	Ø Open 3 Percutaneous	5 Flow B Pressure J Pulse	Ø Central 1 Peripheral 2 Portal 3 Pulmonary
4 Venous	Ø Open 3 Percutaneous	R Saturation	Ø Central 2 Portal 3 Pulmonary
4 Venous	X External	5 Flow B Pressure J Pulse	1 Peripheral
6 Lymphatic	Ø Open 3 Percutaneous	5 Flow B Pressure	Z No Qualifier
9 Respiratory	7 Via Natural or Artificial Opening X External	1 Capacity 5 Flow C Rate D Resistance L Volume	Z No Qualifier
B Gastrointestinal	7 Via Natural or Artificial Opening 8 Via Natural or Artificial Opening Endoscopic	8 Motility B Pressure G Secretion	Z No Qualifier
B Gastrointestinal	X External	S Vascular Perfusion	H Indocyanine Green Dye

Coding Clinic: 2015, Q3, P35 – 4A1239Z, 4A133B3
Coding Clinic: 2016, Q2, P33 – 4A133[BJ]1

New/Revised Text in Green ~~deleted~~ Deleted ♀ Females Only ♂ Males Only **Coding Clinic**

⬡ Non-covered ⬡ Limited Coverage ⊡ Combination (See Appendix E) DRG Non-OR Non-OR ⬡ Hospital-Acquired Condition

SECTION: 4 MEASUREMENT AND MONITORING

BODY SYSTEM: A PHYSIOLOGICAL SYSTEMS

OPERATION: 1 MONITORING: *(continued)*
Determining the level of a physiological or physical function repetitively over a period of time

Body System	Approach	Function / Device	Qualifier
D Urinary	7 Via Natural or Artificial Opening	3 Contractility 5 Flow B Pressure D Resistance L Volume	Z No Qualifier
G Skin and Breast	X External	S Vascular Perfusion	H Indocyanine Green Dye
H Products of Conception, Cardiac ♀	7 Via Natural or Artificial Opening 8 Via Natural or Artificial Opening Endoscopic X External	4 Electrical Activity C Rate F Rhythm H Sound	Z No Qualifier
J Products of Conception, Nervous ♀	7 Via Natural or Artificial Opening 8 Via Natural or Artificial Opening Endoscopic X External	2 Conductivity 4 Electrical Activity B Pressure	Z No Qualifier
Z None	7 Via Natural or Artificial Opening	K Temperature	Z No Qualifier
Z None	X External	K Temperature Q Sleep	Z No Qualifier

Coding Clinic: 2015, Q1, P26 – 4A11X4G

SECTION: 4 MEASUREMENT AND MONITORING

BODY SYSTEM: B PHYSIOLOGICAL DEVICES

OPERATION: 0 MEASUREMENT: Determining the level of a physiological or physical function at a point in time

Body System	Approach	Function / Device	Qualifier
0 Central Nervous 1 Peripheral Nervous F Musculoskeletal	X External	V Stimulator	Z No Qualifier
2 Cardiac	X External	S Pacemaker T Defibrillator	Z No Qualifier
9 Respiratory	X External	S Pacemaker	Z No Qualifier

New/Revised Text in Green   ~~deleted~~ Deleted   ♀ Females Only   ♂ Males Only   **Coding Clinic**
🔖 Non-covered   🔖 Limited Coverage   ⊕ Combination (See Appendix E)   DRG Non-OR   Non-OR   🔖 Hospital-Acquired Condition

Side tab text: 4: MEASUREMENT AND MONITORING   A: PHYSIOLOGICAL SYSTEMS   B: PHYSIOLOGICAL DEVICES   1; 0

SECTION: 5 EXTRACORPOREAL ASSISTANCE AND PERFORMANCE

BODY SYSTEM: A PHYSIOLOGICAL SYSTEMS
OPERATION: Ø **ASSISTANCE:** Taking over a portion of a physiological function by extracorporeal means

Body System	Duration	Function	Qualifier
2 Cardiac	1 Intermittent 2 Continuous	1 Output	Ø Balloon Pump 5 Pulsatile Compression 6 Pump D Impeller Pump
5 Circulatory	1 Intermittent 2 Continuous	2 Oxygenation	1 Hyperbaric C Supersaturated
9 Respiratory	3 Less than 24 Consecutive Hours 4 24-96 Consecutive Hours 5 Greater than 96 Consecutive Hours	5 Ventilation	7 Continuous Positive Airway Pressure 8 Intermittent Positive Airway Pressure 9 Continuous Negative Airway Pressure B Intermittent Negative Airway Pressure Z No Qualifier

Coding Clinic: 2Ø13, Q3, P19 – 5AØ221Ø

SECTION: 5 EXTRACORPOREAL ASSISTANCE AND PERFORMANCE

BODY SYSTEM: A PHYSIOLOGICAL SYSTEMS

OPERATION: 1 PERFORMANCE: Completely taking over a physiological function by extracorporeal means

Body System	Duration	Function	Qualifier
2 Cardiac	Ø Single	1 Output	2 Manual
2 Cardiac	1 Intermittent	3 Pacing	Z No Qualifier
2 Cardiac	2 Continuous	1 Output 3 Pacing	Z No Qualifier
5 Circulatory	2 Continuous	2 Oxygenation	3 Membrane
9 Respiratory	Ø Single	5 Ventilation	4 Nonmechanical
9 Respiratory	3 Less than 24 Consecutive Hours 4 24-96 Consecutive Hours 5 Greater than 96 Consecutive Hours	5 Ventilation	Z No Qualifier
C Biliary D Urinary	Ø Single 6 Multiple	Ø Filtration	Z No Qualifier

DRG Non-OR 5A19[345]5Z

NOTE: **5A1955Z** should only be coded on claims when the respiratory ventilation is provided for greater than four consecutive days during the length of stay.

Coding Clinic: 2013, Q3, P19 – 5A1223Z
Coding Clinic: 2015, Q4, P23-25; 2013, Q3, P19 – 5A1221Z
Coding Clinic: 2016, Q1, P28 – 5A1221Z
Coding Clinic: 2016, Q1, P29 – 5A1C00Z, 5A1D60Z

SECTION: 5 EXTRACORPOREAL ASSISTANCE AND PERFORMANCE

BODY SYSTEM: A PHYSIOLOGICAL SYSTEMS

OPERATION: 2 RESTORATION: Returning, or attempting to return, a physiological function to its original state by extracorporeal means

Body System	Duration	Function	Qualifier
2 Cardiac	Ø Single	4 Rhythm	Z No Qualifier

SECTION: 6 EXTRACORPOREAL THERAPIES
BODY SYSTEM: A PHYSIOLOGICAL SYSTEMS
OPERATION: Ø **ATMOSPHERIC CONTROL:** Extracorporeal control of atmospheric pressure and composition

Body System	Duration	Qualifier	Qualifier
Z None	Ø Single 1 Multiple	Z No Qualifier	Z No Qualifier

SECTION: 6 EXTRACORPOREAL THERAPIES
BODY SYSTEM: A PHYSIOLOGICAL SYSTEMS
OPERATION: 1 **DECOMPRESSION:** Extracorporeal elimination of undissolved gas from body fluids

Body System	Duration	Qualifier	Qualifier
5 Circulatory	Ø Single 1 Multiple	Z No Qualifier	Z No Qualifier

SECTION: 6 EXTRACORPOREAL THERAPIES
BODY SYSTEM: A PHYSIOLOGICAL SYSTEMS
OPERATION: 2 **ELECTROMAGNETIC THERAPY:** Extracorporeal treatment by electromagnetic rays

Body System	Duration	Qualifier	Qualifier
1 Urinary 2 Central Nervous	Ø Single 1 Multiple	Z No Qualifier	Z No Qualifier

SECTION: 6 EXTRACORPOREAL THERAPIES
BODY SYSTEM: A PHYSIOLOGICAL SYSTEMS
OPERATION: 3 **HYPERTHERMIA:** Extracorporeal raising of body temperature

Body System	Duration	Qualifier	Qualifier
Z None	Ø Single 1 Multiple	Z No Qualifier	Z No Qualifier

SECTION: 6 EXTRACORPOREAL THERAPIES
BODY SYSTEM: A PHYSIOLOGICAL SYSTEMS
OPERATION: 4 **HYPOTHERMIA:** Extracorporeal lowering of body temperature

Body System	Duration	Qualifier	Qualifier
Z None	Ø Single 1 Multiple	Z No Qualifier	Z No Qualifier

SECTION: 6 EXTRACORPOREAL THERAPIES
BODY SYSTEM: A PHYSIOLOGICAL SYSTEMS
OPERATION: 5 **PHERESIS:** Extracorporeal separation of blood products

Body System	Duration	Qualifier	Qualifier
5 Circulatory	Ø Single 1 Multiple	Z No Qualifier	Ø Erythrocytes 1 Leukocytes 2 Platelets 3 Plasma T Stem Cells, Cord Blood V Stem Cells, Hematopoietic

SECTION: 6 EXTRACORPOREAL THERAPIES
BODY SYSTEM: A PHYSIOLOGICAL SYSTEMS
OPERATION: 6 **PHOTOTHERAPY:** Extracorporeal treatment by light rays

Body System	Duration	Qualifier	Qualifier
Ø Skin 5 Circulatory	Ø Single 1 Multiple	Z No Qualifier	Z No Qualifier

SECTION: 6 EXTRACORPOREAL THERAPIES
BODY SYSTEM: A PHYSIOLOGICAL SYSTEMS
OPERATION: 7 **ULTRASOUND THERAPY:** Extracorporeal treatment by ultrasound

Body System	Duration	Qualifier	Qualifier
5 Circulatory	Ø Single 1 Multiple	Z No Qualifier	4 Head and Neck Vessels 5 Heart 6 Peripheral Vessels 7 Other Vessels Z No Qualifier

SECTION: 6 EXTRACORPOREAL THERAPIES
BODY SYSTEM: A PHYSIOLOGICAL SYSTEMS
OPERATION: 8 **ULTRAVIOLET LIGHT THERAPY:** Extracorporeal treatment by ultraviolet light

Body System	Duration	Qualifier	Qualifier
Ø Skin	Ø Single 1 Multiple	Z No Qualifier	Z No Qualifier

New/Revised Text in Green   ~~deleted~~ Deleted   ♀ Females Only   ♂ Males Only   **Coding Clinic**
🚫 Non-covered   🚫 Limited Coverage   ⊞ Combination (See Appendix E)   DRG Non-OR   Non-OR   🚫 Hospital-Acquired Condition

SECTION: 6 EXTRACORPOREAL THERAPIES
BODY SYSTEM: A PHYSIOLOGICAL SYSTEMS
OPERATION: 9 SHOCK WAVE THERAPY: Extracorporeal treatment by shock waves

Body System	Duration	Qualifier	Qualifier
3 Musculoskeletal	Ø Single 1 Multiple	Z No Qualifier	Z No Qualifier

SECTION: 6 EXTRACORPOREAL THERAPIES
BODY SYSTEM: A PHYSIOLOGICAL SYSTEMS
OPERATION: B PERFUSION: Extracorporeal treatment by diffusion of therapeutic fluid

Body System	Duration	Qualifier	Qualifier
5 Circulatory B Respiratory System F Hepatobiliary System and Pancreas T Urinary System	Ø Single	B Donor Organ	Z No Qualifier

6:EXTRACORPOREALTHERAPIES   A:PHYSIOLOGICALSYSTEMS   9:SHOCKWAVETHERAPY   B:SHOCKWAVETHERAPY

SECTION: 7 OSTEOPATHIC
BODY SYSTEM: W ANATOMICAL REGIONS
OPERATION: Ø **TREATMENT:** Manual treatment to eliminate or alleviate somatic dysfunction and related disorders

Body Region	Approach	Method	Qualifier
Ø Head	X External	Ø Articulatory-Raising	Z None
1 Cervical		1 Fascial Release	
2 Thoracic		2 General Mobilization	
3 Lumbar		3 High Velocity-Low Amplitude	
4 Sacrum		4 Indirect	
5 Pelvis		5 Low Velocity-High Amplitude	
6 Lower Extremities		6 Lymphatic Pump	
7 Upper Extremities		7 Muscle Energy-Isometric	
8 Rib Cage		8 Muscle Energy-Isotonic	
9 Abdomen		9 Other Method	

7: OSTEOPATHIC

W: ANATOMICAL REGIONS

Ø: TREATMENT

New/Revised Text in Green ~~deleted~~ Deleted ♀ Females Only ♂ Males Only **Coding Clinic**
⬡ Non-covered ⬡ Limited Coverage ⊞ Combination (See Appendix E) DRG Non-OR Non-OR ⬡ Hospital-Acquired Condition

SECTION: 8 OTHER PROCEDURES
BODY SYSTEM: C INDWELLING DEVICE
OPERATION: Ø OTHER PROCEDURES: Methodologies which attempt to remediate or cure a disorder or disease

Body Region	Approach	Method	Qualifier
1 Nervous System	X External	6 Collection	J Cerebrospinal Fluid L Other Fluid
2 Circulatory System	X External	6 Collection	K Blood L Other Fluid

SECTION: 8 OTHER PROCEDURES
BODY SYSTEM: E PHYSIOLOGICAL SYSTEMS AND ANATOMICAL REGIONS
OPERATION: 0 OTHER PROCEDURES: Methodologies which attempt to remediate or cure a disorder or disease

Body Region	Approach	Method	Qualifier
1 Nervous System U Female Reproductive System ♀	X External	Y Other Method	7 Examination
2 Circulatory System	3 Percutaneous	D Near Infrared Spectroscopy	Z No Qualifier
9 Head and Neck Region W Trunk Region	0 Open 3 Percutaneous 4 Percutaneous Endoscopic 7 Via Natural or Artificial Opening 8 Via Natural or Artificial Opening Endoscopic	C Robotic Assisted Procedure	Z No Qualifier
9 Head and Neck Region W Trunk Region	X External	B Computer Assisted Procedure	F With Fluoroscopy G With Computerized Tomography H With Magnetic Resonance Imaging Z No Qualifier
9 Head and Neck Region W Trunk Region	X External	C Robotic Assisted Procedure	Z No Qualifier
9 Head and Neck Region W Trunk Region	X External	Y Other Method	8 Suture Removal
H Integumentary System and Breast	3 Percutaneous	0 Acupuncture	0 Anesthesia Z No Qualifier
H Integumentary System and Breast	X External	6 Collection	2 Breast Milk ♀
H Integumentary System and Breast	X External	Y Other Method	9 Piercing
K Musculoskeletal System	X External	1 Therapeutic Massage	Z No Qualifier
K Musculoskeletal System	X External	Y Other Method	7 Examination
V Male Reproductive System ♂	X External	1 Therapeutic Massage	C Prostate D Rectum
V Male Reproductive System ♂	X External	6 Collection	3 Sperm
X Upper Extremity Y Lower Extremity	0 Open 3 Percutaneous 4 Percutaneous Endoscopic	C Robotic Assisted Procedure	Z No Qualifier
X Upper Extremity Y Lower Extremity	X External	B Computer Assisted Procedure	F With Fluoroscopy G With Computerized Tomography H With Magnetic Resonance Imaging Z No Qualifier
X Upper Extremity Y Lower Extremity	X External	C Robotic Assisted Procedure	Z No Qualifier
X Upper Extremity Y Lower Extremity	X External	Y Other Method	8 Suture Removal
Z None	X External	Y Other Method	1 In Vitro Fertilization 4 Yoga Therapy 5 Meditation 6 Isolation

Coding Clinic: 2015, Q1, P34 – 8E0W4CZ

SECTION: 9 CHIROPRACTIC
BODY SYSTEM: W ANATOMICAL REGIONS
OPERATION: B MANIPULATION: Manual procedure that involves a directed thrust to move a joint past the physiological range of motion, without exceeding the anatomical limit

Body Region	Approach	Method	Qualifier
Ø Head	X External	B Non-Manual	Z None
1 Cervical		C Indirect Visceral	
2 Thoracic		D Extra-Articular	
3 Lumbar		F Direct Visceral	
4 Sacrum		G Long Lever Specific Contact	
5 Pelvis		H Short Lever Specific Contact	
6 Lower Extremities		J Long and Short Lever Specific Contact	
7 Upper Extremities		K Mechanically Assisted	
8 Rib Cage		L Other Method	
9 Abdomen			

B: MANIPULATION

W: ANATOMICAL REGIONS

9: CHIROPRACTIC

New/Revised Text in Green   ~~deleted~~ Deleted   ♀ Females Only   ♂ Males Only   **Coding Clinic**

🚫 Non-covered   🚫 Limited Coverage   ⊞ Combination (See Appendix E)   DRG Non-OR   Non-OR   🚫 Hospital-Acquired Condition

SECTION: B IMAGING
BODY SYSTEM: Ø CENTRAL NERVOUS SYSTEM
TYPE: Ø **PLAIN RADIOGRAPHY:** Planar display of an image developed from the capture of external ionizing radiation on photographic or photoconductive plate

Body Part	Contrast	Qualifier	Qualifier
B Spinal Cord	Ø High Osmolar 1 Low Osmolar Y Other Contrast Z None	Z None	Z None

SECTION: B IMAGING
BODY SYSTEM: Ø CENTRAL NERVOUS SYSTEM
TYPE: 1 **FLUOROSCOPY:** Single plane or bi-plane real time display of an image developed from the capture of external ionizing radiation on a fluorescent screen. The image may also be stored by either digital or analog means

Body Part	Contrast	Qualifier	Qualifier
B Spinal Cord	Ø High Osmolar 1 Low Osmolar Y Other Contrast Z None	Z None	Z None

SECTION: B IMAGING
BODY SYSTEM: Ø CENTRAL NERVOUS SYSTEM
TYPE: 2 **COMPUTERIZED TOMOGRAPHY (CT SCAN):** Computer reformatted digital display of multiplanar images developed from the capture of multiple exposures of external ionizing radiation

Body Part	Contrast	Qualifier	Qualifier
Ø Brain 7 Cisterna 8 Cerebral Ventricle(s) 9 Sella Turcica/Pituitary Gland B Spinal Cord	Ø High Osmolar 1 Low Osmolar Y Other Contrast	Ø Unenhanced and Enhanced Z None	Z None
Ø Brain 7 Cisterna 8 Cerebral Ventricle(s) 9 Sella Turcica/Pituitary Gland B Spinal Cord	Z None	Z None	Z None

SECTION: B IMAGING
BODY SYSTEM: Ø CENTRAL NERVOUS SYSTEM
TYPE: 3 **MAGNETIC RESONANCE IMAGING (MRI):** Computer reformatted digital display of multiplanar images developed from the capture of radiofrequency signals emitted by nuclei in a body site excited within a magnetic field

Body Part	Contrast	Qualifier	Qualifier
Ø Brain 9 Sella Turcica/Pituitary Gland B Spinal Cord C Acoustic Nerves	Y Other Contrast	Ø Unenhanced and Enhanced Z None	Z None
Ø Brain 9 Sella Turcica/Pituitary Gland B Spinal Cord C Acoustic Nerves	Z None	Z None	Z None

SECTION: B IMAGING
BODY SYSTEM: Ø CENTRAL NERVOUS SYSTEM
TYPE: 4 **ULTRASONOGRAPHY:** Real time display of images of anatomy or flow information developed from the capture of reflected and attenuated high frequency sound waves

Body Part	Contrast	Qualifier	Qualifier
Ø Brain B Spinal Cord	Z None	Z None	Z None

3; 4

Ø: CENTRAL NERVOUS SYSTEM

B: IMAGING

SECTION: B IMAGING

BODY SYSTEM: 2 HEART

TYPE: Ø **PLAIN RADIOGRAPHY:** Planar display of an image developed from the capture of external ionizing radiation on photographic or photoconductive plate

Body Part	Contrast	Qualifier	Qualifier
Ø Coronary Artery, Single 1 Coronary Arteries, Multiple 2 Coronary Artery Bypass Graft, Single 3 Coronary Artery Bypass Grafts, Multiple 4 Heart, Right 5 Heart, Left 6 Heart, Right and Left 7 Internal Mammary Bypass Graft, Right 8 Internal Mammary Bypass Graft, Left F Bypass Graft, Other	Ø High Osmolar 1 Low Osmolar Y Other Contrast	Z None	Z None

DRG Non-OR   All Values

SECTION: B IMAGING

BODY SYSTEM: 2 HEART

TYPE: 1 **FLUOROSCOPY:** Single plane or bi-plane real time display of an image developed from the capture of external ionizing radiation on a fluorescent screen. The image may also be stored by either digital or analog means

Body Part	Contrast	Qualifier	Qualifier
Ø Coronary Artery, Single 1 Coronary Arteries, Multiple 2 Coronary Artery Bypass Graft, Single 3 Coronary Artery Bypass Grafts, Multiple	Ø High Osmolar 1 Low Osmolar Y Other Contrast	1 Laser	Ø Intraoperative
Ø Coronary Artery, Single 1 Coronary Arteries, Multiple 2 Coronary Artery Bypass Graft, Single 3 Coronary Artery Bypass Grafts, Multiple	Ø High Osmolar 1 Low Osmolar Y Other Contrast	Z None	Z None
4 Heart, Right 5 Heart, Left 6 Heart, Right and Left 7 Internal Mammary Bypass Graft, Right 8 Internal Mammary Bypass Graft, Left F Bypass Graft, Other	Ø High Osmolar 1 Low Osmolar Y Other Contrast	Z None	Z None

DRG Non-OR   B21[Ø123][Ø1Y]ZZ
DRG Non-OR   B21[45678F][Ø1Y]ZZ

B: IMAGING   2: HEART   Ø: PLAIN RADIOGRAPHY   1: FLUOROSCOPY

SECTION: B IMAGING

BODY SYSTEM: 2 HEART

TYPE: 2 COMPUTERIZED TOMOGRAPHY (CT SCAN): Computer reformatted digital display of multiplanar images developed from the capture of multiple exposures of external ionizing radiation

Body Part	Contrast	Qualifier	Qualifier
1 Coronary Arteries, Multiple 3 Coronary Artery Bypass Grafts, Multiple 6 Heart, Right and Left	Ø High Osmolar 1 Low Osmolar Y Other Contrast	Ø Unenhanced and Enhanced Z None	Z None
1 Coronary Arteries, Multiple 3 Coronary Artery Bypass Grafts, Multiple 6 Heart, Right and Left	Z None	2 Intravascular Optical Coherence Z None	Z None

SECTION: B IMAGING

BODY SYSTEM: 2 HEART

TYPE: 3 MAGNETIC RESONANCE IMAGING (MRI): Computer reformatted digital display of multiplanar images developed from the capture of radiofrequency signals emitted by nuclei in a body site excited within a magnetic field

Body Part	Contrast	Qualifier	Qualifier
1 Coronary Arteries, Multiple 3 Coronary Artery Bypass Grafts, Multiple 6 Heart, Right and Left	Y Other Contrast	Ø Unenhanced and Enhanced Z None	Z None
1 Coronary Arteries, Multiple 3 Coronary Artery Bypass Grafts, Multiple 6 Heart, Right and Left	Z None	Z None	Z None

SECTION: B IMAGING

BODY SYSTEM: 2 HEART

TYPE: **4 ULTRASONOGRAPHY:** Real time display of images of anatomy or flow information developed from the capture of reflected and attenuated high frequency sound waves

Body Part	Contrast	Qualifier	Qualifier
Ø Coronary Artery, Single 1 Coronary Arteries, Multiple 4 Heart, Right 5 Heart, Left 6 Heart, Right and Left B Heart with Aorta C Pericardium D Pediatric Heart	Y Other Contrast	Z None	Z None
Ø Coronary Artery, Single 1 Coronary Arteries, Multiple 4 Heart, Right 5 Heart, Left 6 Heart, Right and Left B Heart with Aorta C Pericardium D Pediatric Heart	Z None	Z None	3 Intravascular 4 Transesophageal Z None

SECTION: B IMAGING

BODY SYSTEM: 3 UPPER ARTERIES

TYPE: Ø **PLAIN RADIOGRAPHY:** Planar display of an image developed from the capture of external ionizing radiation on photographic or photoconductive plate

Body Part	Contrast	Qualifier	Qualifier
Ø Thoracic Aorta	Ø High Osmolar	Z None	Z None
1 Brachiocephalic-Subclavian Artery, Right	1 Low Osmolar		
2 Subclavian Artery, Left	Y Other Contrast		
3 Common Carotid Artery, Right	Z None		
4 Common Carotid Artery, Left			
5 Common Carotid Arteries, Bilateral			
6 Internal Carotid Artery, Right			
7 Internal Carotid Artery, Left			
8 Internal Carotid Arteries, Bilateral			
9 External Carotid Artery, Right			
B External Carotid Artery, Left			
C External Carotid Arteries, Bilateral			
D Vertebral Artery, Right			
F Vertebral Artery, Left			
G Vertebral Arteries, Bilateral			
H Upper Extremity Arteries, Right			
J Upper Extremity Arteries, Left			
K Upper Extremity Arteries, Bilateral			
L Intercostal and Bronchial Arteries			
M Spinal Arteries			
N Upper Arteries, Other			
P Thoraco-Abdominal Aorta			
Q Cervico-Cerebral Arch			
R Intracranial Arteries			
S Pulmonary Artery, Right			
T Pulmonary Artery, Left			

Ø: PLAIN RADIOGRAPHY

3: UPPER ARTERIES

B: IMAGING

New/Revised Text in Green   deleted Deleted   ♀ Females Only   ♂ Males Only   **Coding Clinic**

Non-covered   Limited Coverage   ⊞ Combination (See Appendix E)   DRG Non-OR   Non-OR   Hospital-Acquired Condition

SECTION: **B IMAGING**

BODY SYSTEM: 3 **UPPER ARTERIES**

TYPE: 1 **FLUOROSCOPY:** *(on multiple pages)*

Single plane or bi-plane real time display of an image developed from the capture of external ionizing radiation on a fluorescent screen. The image may also be stored by either digital or analog means

Body Part	Contrast	Qualifier	Qualifier
Ø Thoracic Aorta	Ø High Osmolar	1 Laser	Ø Intraoperative
1 Brachiocephalic-Subclavian Artery, Right	1 Low Osmolar		
2 Subclavian Artery, Left	Y Other Contrast		
3 Common Carotid Artery, Right			
4 Common Carotid Artery, Left			
5 Common Carotid Arteries, Bilateral			
6 Internal Carotid Artery, Right			
7 Internal Carotid Artery, Left			
8 Internal Carotid Arteries, Bilateral			
9 External Carotid Artery, Right			
B External Carotid Artery, Left			
C External Carotid Arteries, Bilateral			
D Vertebral Artery, Right			
F Vertebral Artery, Left			
G Vertebral Arteries, Bilateral			
H Upper Extremity Arteries, Right			
J Upper Extremity Arteries, Left			
K Upper Extremity Arteries, Bilateral			
L Intercostal and Bronchial Arteries			
M Spinal Arteries			
N Upper Arteries, Other			
P Thoraco-Abdominal Aorta			
Q Cervico-Cerebral Arch			
R Intracranial Arteries			
S Pulmonary Artery, Right			
T Pulmonary Artery, Left			

B: IMAGING

3: UPPER ARTERIES

1: FLUOROSCOPY

SECTION: B IMAGING

BODY SYSTEM: 3 UPPER ARTERIES

TYPE: 1 FLUOROSCOPY: *(continued)*

Single plane or bi-plane real time display of an image developed from the capture of external ionizing radiation on a fluorescent screen. The image may also be stored by either digital or analog means

Body Part	Contrast	Qualifier	Qualifier
Ø Thoracic Aorta	Ø High Osmolar	Z None	Z None
1 Brachiocephalic-Subclavian Artery, Right	1 Low Osmolar		
2 Subclavian Artery, Left	Y Other Contrast		
3 Common Carotid Artery, Right			
4 Common Carotid Artery, Left			
5 Common Carotid Arteries, Bilateral			
6 Internal Carotid Artery, Right			
7 Internal Carotid Artery, Left			
8 Internal Carotid Arteries, Bilateral			
9 External Carotid Artery, Right			
B External Carotid Artery, Left			
C External Carotid Arteries, Bilateral			
D Vertebral Artery, Right			
F Vertebral Artery, Left			
G Vertebral Arteries, Bilateral			
H Upper Extremity Arteries, Right			
J Upper Extremity Arteries, Left			
K Upper Extremity Arteries, Bilateral			
L Intercostal and Bronchial Arteries			
M Spinal Arteries			
N Upper Arteries, Other			
P Thoraco-Abdominal Aorta			
Q Cervico-Cerebral Arch			
R Intracranial Arteries			
S Pulmonary Artery, Right			
T Pulmonary Artery, Left			

1: FLUOROSCOPY

3: UPPER ARTERIES

B: IMAGING

SECTION: B IMAGING
BODY SYSTEM: 3 UPPER ARTERIES
TYPE: 1 FLUOROSCOPY: *(continued)*
Single plane or bi-plane real time display of an image developed from the capture of external ionizing radiation on a fluorescent screen. The image may also be stored by either digital or analog means

Body Part	Contrast	Qualifier	Qualifier
Ø Thoracic Aorta 1 Brachiocephalic-Subclavian Artery, Right 2 Subclavian Artery, Left 3 Common Carotid Artery, Right 4 Common Carotid Artery, Left 5 Common Carotid Arteries, Bilateral 6 Internal Carotid Artery, Right 7 Internal Carotid Artery, Left 8 Internal Carotid Arteries, Bilateral 9 External Carotid Artery, Right B External Carotid Artery, Left C External Carotid Arteries, Bilateral D Vertebral Artery, Right F Vertebral Artery, Left G Vertebral Arteries, Bilateral H Upper Extremity Arteries, Right J Upper Extremity Arteries, Left K Upper Extremity Arteries, Bilateral L Intercostal and Bronchial Arteries M Spinal Arteries N Upper Arteries, Other P Thoraco-Abdominal Aorta Q Cervico-Cerebral Arch R Intracranial Arteries S Pulmonary Artery, Right T Pulmonary Artery, Left	Z None	Z None	Z None

SECTION: B IMAGING
BODY SYSTEM: 3 UPPER ARTERIES
TYPE: 2 COMPUTERIZED TOMOGRAPHY (CT SCAN): Computer reformatted digital display of multiplanar images developed from the capture of multiple exposures of external ionizing radiation

Body Part	Contrast	Qualifier	Qualifier
Ø Thoracic Aorta 5 Common Carotid Arteries, Bilateral 8 Internal Carotid Arteries, Bilateral G Vertebral Arteries, Bilateral R Intracranial Arteries S Pulmonary Artery, Right T Pulmonary Artery, Left	Ø High Osmolar 1 Low Osmolar Y Other Contrast	Z None	Z None
Ø Thoracic Aorta 5 Common Carotid Arteries, Bilateral 8 Internal Carotid Arteries, Bilateral G Vertebral Arteries, Bilateral R Intracranial Arteries S Pulmonary Artery, Right T Pulmonary Artery, Left	Z None	2 Intravascular Optical Coherence Z None	Z None

SECTION: B IMAGING

BODY SYSTEM: 3 UPPER ARTERIES

TYPE: 3 **MAGNETIC RESONANCE IMAGING (MRI):** Computer reformatted digital display of multiplanar images developed from the capture of radiofrequency signals emitted by nuclei in a body site excited within a magnetic field

Body Part	Contrast	Qualifier	Qualifier
Ø Thoracic Aorta 5 Common Carotid Arteries, Bilateral 8 Internal Carotid Arteries, Bilateral G Vertebral Arteries, Bilateral H Upper Extremity Arteries, Right J Upper Extremity Arteries, Left K Upper Extremity Arteries, Bilateral M Spinal Arteries Q Cervico-Cerebral Arch R Intracranial Arteries	Y Other Contrast	Ø Unenhanced and Enhanced Z None	Z None
Ø Thoracic Aorta 5 Common Carotid Arteries, Bilateral 8 Internal Carotid Arteries, Bilateral G Vertebral Arteries, Bilateral H Upper Extremity Arteries, Right J Upper Extremity Arteries, Left K Upper Extremity Arteries, Bilateral M Spinal Arteries Q Cervico-Cerebral Arch R Intracranial Arteries	Z None	Z None	Z None

SECTION: B IMAGING

BODY SYSTEM: 3 UPPER ARTERIES

TYPE: 4 **ULTRASONOGRAPHY:** Real time display of images of anatomy or flow information developed from the capture of reflected and attenuated high frequency sound waves

Body Part	Contrast	Qualifier	Qualifier
Ø Thoracic Aorta 1 Brachiocephalic-Subclavian Artery, Right 2 Subclavian Artery, Left 3 Common Carotid Artery, Right 4 Common Carotid Artery, Left 5 Common Carotid Arteries, Bilateral 6 Internal Carotid Artery, Right 7 Internal Carotid Artery, Left 8 Internal Carotid Arteries, Bilateral H Upper Extremity Arteries, Right J Upper Extremity Arteries, Left K Upper Extremity Arteries, Bilateral R Intracranial Arteries S Pulmonary Artery, Right T Pulmonary Artery, Left V Ophthalmic Arteries	Z None	Z None	3 Intravascular Z None

SECTION: B IMAGING

BODY SYSTEM: 4 LOWER ARTERIES

TYPE: Ø **PLAIN RADIOGRAPHY:** Planar display of an image developed from the capture of external ionizing radiation on photographic or photoconductive plate

Body Part	Contrast	Qualifier	Qualifier
Ø Abdominal Aorta	Ø High Osmolar	Z None	Z None
2 Hepatic Artery	1 Low Osmolar		
3 Splenic Arteries	Y Other Contrast		
4 Superior Mesenteric Artery			
5 Inferior Mesenteric Artery			
6 Renal Artery, Right			
7 Renal Artery, Left			
8 Renal Arteries, Bilateral			
9 Lumbar Arteries			
B Intra-Abdominal Arteries, Other			
C Pelvic Arteries			
D Aorta and Bilateral Lower Extremity Arteries			
F Lower Extremity Arteries, Right			
G Lower Extremity Arteries, Left			
J Lower Arteries, Other			
M Renal Artery Transplant			

SECTION: B IMAGING
BODY SYSTEM: 4 LOWER ARTERIES
TYPE: 1 FLUOROSCOPY: Single plane or bi-plane real time display of an image developed from the capture of external ionizing radiation on a fluorescent screen. The image may also be stored by either digital or analog means

1: FLUOROSCOPY

4: LOWER ARTERIES

B: IMAGING

Body Part	Contrast	Qualifier	Qualifier
0 Abdominal Aorta 2 Hepatic Artery 3 Splenic Arteries 4 Superior Mesenteric Artery 5 Inferior Mesenteric Artery 6 Renal Artery, Right 7 Renal Artery, Left 8 Renal Arteries, Bilateral 9 Lumbar Arteries B Intra-Abdominal Arteries, Other C Pelvic Arteries D Aorta and Bilateral Lower Extremity Arteries F Lower Extremity Arteries, Right G Lower Extremity Arteries, Left J Lower Arteries, Other	0 High Osmolar 1 Low Osmolar Y Other Contrast	1 Laser	0 Intraoperative
0 Abdominal Aorta 2 Hepatic Artery 3 Splenic Arteries 4 Superior Mesenteric Artery 5 Inferior Mesenteric Artery 6 Renal Artery, Right 7 Renal Artery, Left 8 Renal Arteries, Bilateral 9 Lumbar Arteries B Intra-Abdominal Arteries, Other C Pelvic Arteries D Aorta and Bilateral Lower Extremity Arteries F Lower Extremity Arteries, Right G Lower Extremity Arteries, Left J Lower Arteries, Other	0 High Osmolar 1 Low Osmolar Y Other Contrast	Z None	Z None
0 Abdominal Aorta 2 Hepatic Artery 3 Splenic Arteries 4 Superior Mesenteric Artery 5 Inferior Mesenteric Artery 6 Renal Artery, Right 7 Renal Artery, Left 8 Renal Arteries, Bilateral 9 Lumbar Arteries B Intra-Abdominal Arteries, Other C Pelvic Arteries D Aorta and Bilateral Lower Extremity Arteries F Lower Extremity Arteries, Right G Lower Extremity Arteries, Left J Lower Arteries, Other	Z None	Z None	Z None

New/Revised Text in Green   ~~deleted~~ Deleted   ♀ Females Only   ♂ Males Only   **Coding Clinic**

🚫 Non-covered   🚫 Limited Coverage   ⊕ Combination (See Appendix E)   DRG Non-OR   Non-OR   🚫 Hospital-Acquired Condition

SECTION: B IMAGING

BODY SYSTEM: 4 LOWER ARTERIES

TYPE: 2 COMPUTERIZED TOMOGRAPHY (CT SCAN): Computer reformatted digital display of multiplanar images developed from the capture of multiple exposures of external ionizing radiation

Body Part	Contrast	Qualifier	Qualifier
Ø Abdominal Aorta 1 Celiac Artery 4 Superior Mesenteric Artery 8 Renal Arteries, Bilateral C Pelvic Arteries F Lower Extremity Arteries, Right G Lower Extremity Arteries, Left H Lower Extremity Arteries, Bilateral M Renal Artery Transplant	Ø High Osmolar 1 Low Osmolar Y Other Contrast	Z None	Z None
Ø Abdominal Aorta 1 Celiac Artery 4 Superior Mesenteric Artery 8 Renal Arteries, Bilateral C Pelvic Arteries F Lower Extremity Arteries, Right G Lower Extremity Arteries, Left H Lower Extremity Arteries, Bilateral M Renal Artery Transplant	Z None	2 Intravascular Optical Coherence Z None	Z None

SECTION: B IMAGING

BODY SYSTEM: 4 LOWER ARTERIES

TYPE: 3 MAGNETIC RESONANCE IMAGING (MRI): Computer reformatted digital display of multiplanar images developed from the capture of radiofrequency signals emitted by nuclei in a body site excited within a magnetic field

Body Part	Contrast	Qualifier	Qualifier
Ø Abdominal Aorta 1 Celiac Artery 4 Superior Mesenteric Artery 8 Renal Arteries, Bilateral C Pelvic Arteries F Lower Extremity Arteries, Right G Lower Extremity Arteries, Left H Lower Extremity Arteries, Bilateral	Y Other Contrast	Ø Unenhanced and Enhanced Z None	Z None
Ø Abdominal Aorta 1 Celiac Artery 4 Superior Mesenteric Artery 8 Renal Arteries, Bilateral C Pelvic Arteries F Lower Extremity Arteries, Right G Lower Extremity Arteries, Left H Lower Extremity Arteries, Bilateral	Z None	Z None	Z None

B: IMAGING

4: LOWER ARTERIES

2: COMPUTERIZED TOMOGRAPHY

3: MAGNETIC RESONANCE IMAGING

SECTION: B IMAGING

BODY SYSTEM: 4 LOWER ARTERIES

TYPE: 4 **ULTRASONOGRAPHY:** Real time display of images of anatomy or flow information developed from the capture of reflected and attenuated high frequency sound waves

Body Part	Contrast	Qualifier	Qualifier
Ø Abdominal Aorta	Z None	Z None	3 Intravascular
4 Superior Mesenteric Artery			Z None
5 Inferior Mesenteric Artery			
6 Renal Artery, Right			
7 Renal Artery, Left			
8 Renal Arteries, Bilateral			
B Intra-Abdominal Arteries, Other			
F Lower Extremity Arteries, Right			
G Lower Extremity Arteries, Left			
H Lower Extremity Arteries, Bilateral			
K Celiac and Mesenteric Arteries			
L Femoral Artery			
N Penile Arteries			

4: ULTRASONOGRAPHY

4: LOWER ARTERIES

B: IMAGING

SECTION: B IMAGING
BODY SYSTEM: 5 VEINS
TYPE: Ø **PLAIN RADIOGRAPHY:** Planar display of an image developed from the capture of external ionizing radiation on photographic or photoconductive plate

Body Part	Contrast	Qualifier	Qualifier
Ø Epidural Veins	Ø High Osmolar	Z None	Z None
1 Cerebral and Cerebellar Veins	1 Low Osmolar		
2 Intracranial Sinuses	Y Other Contrast		
3 Jugular Veins, Right			
4 Jugular Veins, Left			
5 Jugular Veins, Bilateral			
6 Subclavian Vein, Right			
7 Subclavian Vein, Left			
8 Superior Vena Cava			
9 Inferior Vena Cava			
B Lower Extremity Veins, Right			
C Lower Extremity Veins, Left			
D Lower Extremity Veins, Bilateral			
F Pelvic (Iliac) Veins, Right			
G Pelvic (Iliac) Veins, Left			
H Pelvic (Iliac) Veins, Bilateral			
J Renal Vein, Right			
K Renal Vein, Left			
L Renal Veins, Bilateral			
M Upper Extremity Veins, Right			
N Upper Extremity Veins, Left			
P Upper Extremity Veins, Bilateral			
Q Pulmonary Vein, Right			
R Pulmonary Vein, Left			
S Pulmonary Veins, Bilateral			
T Portal and Splanchnic Veins			
V Veins, Other			
W Dialysis Shunt/Fistula			

B: IMAGING

5: VEINS

Ø: PLAIN RADIOGRAPHY

SECTION: B IMAGING

BODY SYSTEM: 5 VEINS

TYPE: 1 **FLUOROSCOPY:** Single plane or bi-plane real time display of an image developed from the capture of external ionizing radiation on a fluorescent screen. The image may also be stored by either digital or analog means

Body Part	Contrast	Qualifier	Qualifier
Ø Epidural Veins	Ø High Osmolar	Z None	A Guidance
1 Cerebral and Cerebellar Veins	1 Low Osmolar		Z None
2 Intracranial Sinuses	Y Other Contrast		
3 Jugular Veins, Right ⊞	Z None		
4 Jugular Veins, Left ⊞			
5 Jugular Veins, Bilateral ⊞			
6 Subclavian Vein, Right ⊞			
7 Subclavian Vein, Left ⊞			
8 Superior Vena Cava			
9 Inferior Vena Cava			
B Lower Extremity Veins, Right ⊞			
C Lower Extremity Veins, Left ⊞			
D Lower Extremity Veins, Bilateral ⊞			
F Pelvic (Iliac) Veins, Right			
G Pelvic (Iliac) Veins, Left			
H Pelvic (Iliac) Veins, Bilateral			
J Renal Vein, Right			
K Renal Vein, Left			
L Renal Veins, Bilateral			
M Upper Extremity Veins, Right			
N Upper Extremity Veins, Left			
P Upper Extremity Veins, Bilateral			
Q Pulmonary Vein, Right			
R Pulmonary Vein, Left			
S Pulmonary Veins, Bilateral			
T Portal and Splanchnic Veins			
V Veins, Other			
W Dialysis Shunt/Fistula			

⊞ B51[34567BCD][Ø1YZ]ZA

DRG Non-OR B51[34567BCD][Ø1YZ]ZA

Coding Clinic: 2Ø15, Q4, P3Ø – B518ZZA

New/Revised Text in Green   ~~deleted~~ Deleted   ♀ Females Only   ♂ Males Only   **Coding Clinic**

🐾 Non-covered   🐾 Limited Coverage   ⊞ Combination (See Appendix E)   DRG Non-OR   Non-OR   🐾 Hospital-Acquired Condition

SECTION: B IMAGING
BODY SYSTEM: 5 VEINS
TYPE: 2 **COMPUTERIZED TOMOGRAPHY (CT SCAN):** Computer reformatted digital display of multiplanar images developed from the capture of multiple exposures of external ionizing radiation

Body Part	Contrast	Qualifier	Qualifier
2 Intracranial Sinuses 8 Superior Vena Cava 9 Inferior Vena Cava F Pelvic (Iliac) Veins, Right G Pelvic (Iliac) Veins, Left H Pelvic (Iliac) Veins, Bilateral J Renal Vein, Right K Renal Vein, Left L Renal Veins, Bilateral Q Pulmonary Vein, Right R Pulmonary Vein, Left S Pulmonary Veins, Bilateral T Portal and Splanchnic Veins	Ø High Osmolar 1 Low Osmolar Y Other Contrast	Ø Unenhanced and Enhanced Z None	Z None
2 Intracranial Sinuses 8 Superior Vena Cava 9 Inferior Vena Cava F Pelvic (Iliac) Veins, Right G Pelvic (Iliac) Veins, Left H Pelvic (Iliac) Veins, Bilateral J Renal Vein, Right K Renal Vein, Left L Renal Veins, Bilateral Q Pulmonary Vein, Right R Pulmonary Vein, Left S Pulmonary Veins, Bilateral T Portal and Splanchnic Veins	Z None	2 Intravascular Optical Coherence Z None	Z None

SECTION: B IMAGING
BODY SYSTEM: 5 VEINS
TYPE: **3 MAGNETIC RESONANCE IMAGING (MRI):** Computer reformatted digital display of multiplanar images developed from the capture of radiofrequency signals emitted by nuclei in a body site excited within a magnetic field

Body Part	Contrast	Qualifier	Qualifier
1 Cerebral and Cerebellar Veins 2 Intracranial Sinuses 5 Jugular Veins, Bilateral 8 Superior Vena Cava 9 Inferior Vena Cava B Lower Extremity Veins, Right C Lower Extremity Veins, Left D Lower Extremity Veins, Bilateral H Pelvic (Iliac) Veins, Bilateral L Renal Veins, Bilateral M Upper Extremity Veins, Right N Upper Extremity Veins, Left P Upper Extremity Veins, Bilateral S Pulmonary Veins, Bilateral T Portal and Splanchnic Veins V Veins, Other	Y Other Contrast	Ø Unenhanced and Enhanced Z None	Z None
1 Cerebral and Cerebellar Veins 2 Intracranial Sinuses 5 Jugular Veins, Bilateral 8 Superior Vena Cava 9 Inferior Vena Cava B Lower Extremity Veins, Right C Lower Extremity Veins, Left D Lower Extremity Veins, Bilateral H Pelvic (Iliac) Veins, Bilateral L Renal Veins, Bilateral M Upper Extremity Veins, Right N Upper Extremity Veins, Left P Upper Extremity Veins, Bilateral S Pulmonary Veins, Bilateral T Portal and Splanchnic Veins V Veins, Other	Z None	Z None	Z None

3: MAGNETIC RESONANCE IMAGING (MRI)

5: VEINS

B: IMAGING

New/Revised Text in Green   ~~deleted~~ Deleted   ♀ Females Only   ♂ Males Only   **Coding Clinic**
🦚 Non-covered   🦚 Limited Coverage   ⊟ Combination (See Appendix E)   DRG Non-OR   Non-OR   🦚 Hospital-Acquired Condition

SECTION: B IMAGING

BODY SYSTEM: 5 VEINS

TYPE: 4 **ULTRASONOGRAPHY:** Real time display of images of anatomy or flow information developed from the capture of reflected and attenuated high frequency sound waves

Body Part	Contrast	Qualifier	Qualifier
3 Jugular Veins, Right ⊞ 4 Jugular Veins, Left ⊞ 6 Subclavian Vein, Right ⊞ 7 Subclavian Vein, Left ⊞ 9 Inferior Vena Cava B Lower Extremity Veins, Right ⊞ C Lower Extremity Veins, Left ⊞ D Lower Extremity Veins, Bilateral ⊞ J Renal Vein, Right K Renal Vein, Left L Renal Veins, Bilateral M Upper Extremity Veins, Right N Upper Extremity Veins, Left P Upper Extremity Veins, Bilateral T Portal and Splanchnic Veins	Z None	Z None	3 Intravascular A Guidance Z None

⊞ B54[3467BCD]ZZA

DRG Non-OR B54[3467BCD]ZZA

B: IMAGING

5: VEINS

4: ULTRASONOGRAPHY

SECTION: B IMAGING

BODY SYSTEM: 7 LYMPHATIC SYSTEM

TYPE: Ø **PLAIN RADIOGRAPHY:** Planar display of an image developed from the capture of external ionizing radiation on photographic or photoconductive plate

Body Part	Contrast	Qualifier	Qualifier
Ø Abdominal/Retroperitoneal Lymphatics, Unilateral	Ø High Osmolar	Z None	Z None
1 Abdominal/Retroperitoneal Lymphatics, Bilateral	1 Low Osmolar		
4 Lymphatics, Head and Neck	Y Other Contrast		
5 Upper Extremity Lymphatics, Right			
6 Upper Extremity Lymphatics, Left			
7 Upper Extremity Lymphatics, Bilateral			
8 Lower Extremity Lymphatics, Right			
9 Lower Extremity Lymphatics, Left			
B Lower Extremity Lymphatics, Bilateral			
C Lymphatics, Pelvic			

Ø: PLAIN RADIOGRAPHY

7: LYMPHATIC SYSTEM

B: IMAGING

New/Revised Text in Green   ~~deleted~~ Deleted   ♀ Females Only   ♂ Males Only   **Coding Clinic**

Non-covered   Limited Coverage   ⊞ Combination (See Appendix E)   DRG Non-OR   Non-OR   Hospital-Acquired Condition

SECTION: B IMAGING

BODY SYSTEM: 8 EYE

TYPE: Ø **PLAIN RADIOGRAPHY:** Planar display of an image developed from the capture of external ionizing radiation on photographic or photoconductive plate

Body Part	Contrast	Qualifier	Qualifier
Ø Lacrimal Duct, Right 1 Lacrimal Duct, Left 2 Lacrimal Ducts, Bilateral	Ø High Osmolar 1 Low Osmolar Y Other Contrast	Z None	Z None
3 Optic Foramina, Right 4 Optic Foramina, Left 5 Eye, Right 6 Eye, Left 7 Eyes, Bilateral	Z None	Z None	Z None

SECTION: B IMAGING

BODY SYSTEM: 8 EYE

TYPE: 2 **COMPUTERIZED TOMOGRAPHY (CT SCAN):** Computer reformatted digital display of multiplanar images developed from the capture of multiple exposures of external ionizing radiation

Body Part	Contrast	Qualifier	Qualifier
5 Eye, Right 6 Eye, Left 7 Eyes, Bilateral	Ø High Osmolar 1 Low Osmolar Y Other Contrast	Ø Unenhanced and Enhanced Z None	Z None
5 Eye, Right 6 Eye, Left 7 Eyes, Bilateral	Z None	Z None	Z None

B: IMAGING 8: EYE Ø: PLAIN RADIOGRAPHY 2: COMPUTERIZED TOMOGRAPHY (CT SCAN)

SECTION: B IMAGING

BODY SYSTEM: 8 EYE

TYPE: 3 **MAGNETIC RESONANCE IMAGING (MRI):** Computer reformatted digital display of multiplanar images developed from the capture of radiofrequency signals emitted by nuclei in a body site excited within a magnetic field

Body Part	Contrast	Qualifier	Qualifier
5 Eye, Right 6 Eye, Left 7 Eyes, Bilateral	Y Other Contrast	Ø Unenhanced and Enhanced Z None	Z None
5 Eye, Right 6 Eye, Left 7 Eyes, Bilateral	Z None	Z None	Z None

SECTION: B IMAGING

BODY SYSTEM: 8 EYE

TYPE: 4 **ULTRASONOGRAPHY:** Real time display of images of anatomy or flow information developed from the capture of reflected and attenuated high frequency sound waves

Body Part	Contrast	Qualifier	Qualifier
5 Eye, Right 6 Eye, Left 7 Eyes, Bilateral	Z None	Z None	Z None

New/Revised Text in Green ~~deleted~~ Deleted ♀ Females Only ♂ Males Only **Coding Clinic**

Non-covered Limited Coverage Combination (See Appendix E) DRG Non-OR Non-OR Hospital-Acquired Condition

SECTION: B IMAGING

BODY SYSTEM: 9 EAR, NOSE, MOUTH, AND THROAT

TYPE: Ø PLAIN RADIOGRAPHY: Planar display of an image developed from the capture of external ionizing radiation on photographic or photoconductive plate

Body Part	Contrast	Qualifier	Qualifier
2 Paranasal Sinuses F Nasopharynx/Oropharynx H Mastoids	Z None	Z None	Z None
4 Parotid Gland, Right 5 Parotid Gland, Left 6 Parotid Glands, Bilateral 7 Submandibular Gland, Right 8 Submandibular Gland, Left 9 Submandibular Glands, Bilateral B Salivary Gland, Right C Salivary Gland, Left D Salivary Glands, Bilateral	Ø High Osmolar 1 Low Osmolar Y Other Contrast	Z None	Z None

SECTION: B IMAGING

BODY SYSTEM: 9 EAR, NOSE, MOUTH, AND THROAT

TYPE: 1 FLUOROSCOPY: Single plane or bi-plane real time display of an image developed from the capture of external ionizing radiation on a fluorescent screen. The image may also be stored by either digital or analog means

Body Part	Contrast	Qualifier	Qualifier
G Pharynx and Epiglottis J Larynx	Y Other Contrast Z None	Z None	Z None

New/Revised Text in Green   ~~deleted~~ Deleted   ♀ Females Only   ♂ Males Only   **Coding Clinic**

🚫 Non-covered   🚫 Limited Coverage   ⊞ Combination (See Appendix E)   DRG Non-OR   Non-OR   🚫 Hospital-Acquired Condition

SECTION: B IMAGING

BODY SYSTEM: 9 EAR, NOSE, MOUTH, AND THROAT

TYPE: 2 COMPUTERIZED TOMOGRAPHY (CT SCAN): Computer reformatted digital display of multiplanar images developed from the capture of multiple exposures of external ionizing radiation

Body Part	Contrast	Qualifier	Qualifier
Ø Ear 2 Paranasal Sinuses 6 Parotid Glands, Bilateral 9 Submandibular Glands, Bilateral D Salivary Glands, Bilateral F Nasopharynx/Oropharynx J Larynx	Ø High Osmolar 1 Low Osmolar Y Other Contrast	Ø Unenhanced and Enhanced Z None	Z None
Ø Ear 2 Paranasal Sinuses 6 Parotid Glands, Bilateral 9 Submandibular Glands, Bilateral D Salivary Glands, Bilateral F Nasopharynx/Oropharynx J Larynx	Z None	Z None	Z None

SECTION: B IMAGING

BODY SYSTEM: 9 EAR, NOSE, MOUTH, AND THROAT

TYPE: 3 MAGNETIC RESONANCE IMAGING (MRI): Computer reformatted digital display of multiplanar images developed from the capture of radiofrequency signals emitted by nuclei in a body site excited within a magnetic field

Body Part	Contrast	Qualifier	Qualifier
Ø Ear 2 Paranasal Sinuses 6 Parotid Glands, Bilateral 9 Submandibular Glands, Bilateral D Salivary Glands, Bilateral F Nasopharynx/Oropharynx J Larynx	Y Other Contrast	Ø Unenhanced and Enhanced Z None	Z None
Ø Ear 2 Paranasal Sinuses 6 Parotid Glands, Bilateral 9 Submandibular Glands, Bilateral D Salivary Glands, Bilateral F Nasopharynx/Oropharynx J Larynx	Z None	Z None	Z None

2: CT SCAN 3: MRI

9: EAR, NOSE, MOUTH, AND THROAT

B: IMAGING

New/Revised Text in Green   ~~deleted~~ Deleted   ♀ Females Only   ♂ Males Only   **Coding Clinic**

Non-covered   Limited Coverage   ⊕ Combination (See Appendix E)   DRG Non-OR   Non-OR   Hospital-Acquired Condition

SECTION: B IMAGING

BODY SYSTEM: B RESPIRATORY SYSTEM

TYPE: Ø **PLAIN RADIOGRAPHY:** Planar display of an image developed from the capture of external ionizing radiation on photographic or photoconductive plate

Body Part	Contrast	Qualifier	Qualifier
7 Tracheobronchial Tree, Right 8 Tracheobronchial Tree, Left 9 Tracheobronchial Trees, Bilateral	Y Other Contrast	Z None	Z None
D Upper Airways	Z None	Z None	Z None

SECTION: B IMAGING

BODY SYSTEM: B RESPIRATORY SYSTEM

TYPE: 1 **FLUOROSCOPY:** Single plane or bi-plane real time display of an image developed from the capture of external ionizing radiation on a fluorescent screen. The image may also be stored by either digital or analog means

Body Part	Contrast	Qualifier	Qualifier
2 Lung, Right 3 Lung, Left 4 Lungs, Bilateral 6 Diaphragm C Mediastinum D Upper Airways	Z None	Z None	Z None
7 Tracheobronchial Tree, Right 8 Tracheobronchial Tree, Left 9 Tracheobronchial Trees, Bilateral	Y Other Contrast	Z None	Z None

SECTION: B IMAGING

BODY SYSTEM: B RESPIRATORY SYSTEM

TYPE: 2 **COMPUTERIZED TOMOGRAPHY (CT SCAN):** Computer reformatted digital display of multiplanar images developed from the capture of multiple exposures of external ionizing radiation

Body Part	Contrast	Qualifier	Qualifier
4 Lungs, Bilateral 7 Tracheobronchial Tree, Right 8 Tracheobronchial Tree, Left 9 Tracheobronchial Trees, Bilateral F Trachea/Airways	Ø High Osmolar 1 Low Osmolar Y Other Contrast	Ø Unenhanced and Enhanced Z None	Z None
4 Lungs, Bilateral 7 Tracheobronchial Tree, Right 8 Tracheobronchial Tree, Left 9 Tracheobronchial Trees, Bilateral F Trachea/Airways	Z None	Z None	Z None

B: IMAGING

B: RESPIRATORY SYSTEM

Ø: PLAIN RADIOGRAPHY   1: FLUOROSCOPY   2: CT SCAN

SECTION: B IMAGING

BODY SYSTEM: B RESPIRATORY SYSTEM

TYPE: **3 MAGNETIC RESONANCE IMAGING (MRI):** Computer reformatted digital display of multiplanar images developed from the capture of radiofrequency signals emitted by nuclei in a body site excited within a magnetic field

Body Part	Contrast	Qualifier	Qualifier
G Lung Apices	Y Other Contrast	Ø Unenhanced and Enhanced Z None	Z None
G Lung Apices	Z None	Z None	Z None

SECTION: B IMAGING

BODY SYSTEM: B RESPIRATORY SYSTEM

TYPE: **4 ULTRASONOGRAPHY:** Real time display of images of anatomy or flow information developed from the capture of reflected and attenuated high frequency sound waves

Body Part	Contrast	Qualifier	Qualifier
B Pleura C Mediastinum	Z None	Z None	Z None

Side tabs: 4: ULTRASONOGRAPHY   3: MRI   B: RESPIRATORY SYSTEM   B: IMAGING

SECTION: **B IMAGING**
BODY SYSTEM: D GASTROINTESTINAL SYSTEM
TYPE: **1 FLUOROSCOPY:** Single plane or bi-plane real time display of an image developed from the capture of external ionizing radiation on a fluorescent screen. The image may also be stored by either digital or analog means

Body Part	Contrast	Qualifier	Qualifier
1 Esophagus 2 Stomach 3 Small Bowel 4 Colon 5 Upper GI 6 Upper GI and Small Bowel 9 Duodenum B Mouth/Oropharynx	Y Other Contrast Z None	Z None	Z None

SECTION: **B IMAGING**
BODY SYSTEM: D GASTROINTESTINAL SYSTEM
TYPE: **2 COMPUTERIZED TOMOGRAPHY (CT SCAN):** Computer reformatted digital display of multiplanar images developed from the capture of multiple exposures of external ionizing radiation

Body Part	Contrast	Qualifier	Qualifier
4 Colon	Ø High Osmolar 1 Low Osmolar Y Other Contrast	Ø Unenhanced and Enhanced Z None	Z None
4 Colon	Z None	Z None	Z None

SECTION: **B IMAGING**
BODY SYSTEM: D GASTROINTESTINAL SYSTEM
TYPE: **4 ULTRASONOGRAPHY:** Real time display of images of anatomy or flow information developed from the capture of reflected and attenuated high frequency sound waves

Body Part	Contrast	Qualifier	Qualifier
1 Esophagus 2 Stomach 7 Gastrointestinal Tract 8 Appendix 9 Duodenum C Rectum	Z None	Z None	Z None

1: FLUOROSCOPY

0: PLAIN RADIOGRAPHY

F: HEPATOBILIARY SYSTEM AND PANCREAS

B: IMAGING

SECTION: B IMAGING
BODY SYSTEM: F **HEPATOBILIARY SYSTEM AND PANCREAS**
TYPE: 0 **PLAIN RADIOGRAPHY:** Planar display of an image developed from the capture of external ionizing radiation on photographic or photoconductive plate

Body Part	Contrast	Qualifier	Qualifier
0 Bile Ducts	0 High Osmolar	Z None	Z None
3 Gallbladder and Bile Ducts	1 Low Osmolar		
C Hepatobiliary System, All	Y Other Contrast		

SECTION: B IMAGING
BODY SYSTEM: F **HEPATOBILIARY SYSTEM AND PANCREAS**
TYPE: 1 **FLUOROSCOPY:** Single plane or bi-plane real time display of an image developed from the capture of external ionizing radiation on a fluorescent screen. The image may also be stored by either digital or analog means

Body Part	Contrast	Qualifier	Qualifier
0 Bile Ducts	0 High Osmolar	Z None	Z None
1 Biliary and Pancreatic Ducts	1 Low Osmolar		
2 Gallbladder	Y Other Contrast		
3 Gallbladder and Bile Ducts			
4 Gallbladder, Bile Ducts, and Pancreatic Ducts			
8 Pancreatic Ducts			

SECTION: B IMAGING
BODY SYSTEM: F HEPATOBILIARY SYSTEM AND PANCREAS
TYPE: 2 **COMPUTERIZED TOMOGRAPHY (CT SCAN):** Computer reformatted digital display of multiplanar images developed from the capture of multiple exposures of external ionizing radiation

Body Part	Contrast	Qualifier	Qualifier
5 Liver 6 Liver and Spleen 7 Pancreas C Hepatobiliary System, All	Ø High Osmolar 1 Low Osmolar Y Other Contrast	Ø Unenhanced and Enhanced Z None	Z None
5 Liver 6 Liver and Spleen 7 Pancreas C Hepatobiliary System, All	Z None	Z None	Z None

SECTION: B IMAGING
BODY SYSTEM: F HEPATOBILIARY SYSTEM AND PANCREAS
TYPE: 3 **MAGNETIC RESONANCE IMAGING (MRI):** Computer reformatted digital display of multiplanar images developed from the capture of radiofrequency signals emitted by nuclei in a body site excited within a magnetic field

Body Part	Contrast	Qualifier	Qualifier
5 Liver 6 Liver and Spleen 7 Pancreas	Y Other Contrast	Ø Unenhanced and Enhanced Z None	Z None
5 Liver 6 Liver and Spleen 7 Pancreas	Z None	Z None	Z None

SECTION: B IMAGING
BODY SYSTEM: F HEPATOBILIARY SYSTEM AND PANCREAS
TYPE: 4 **ULTRASONOGRAPHY:** Real time display of images of anatomy or flow information developed from the capture of reflected and attenuated high frequency sound waves

Body Part	Contrast	Qualifier	Qualifier
Ø Bile Ducts 2 Gallbladder 3 Gallbladder and Bile Ducts 5 Liver 6 Liver and Spleen 7 Pancreas C Hepatobiliary System, All	Z None	Z None	Z None

SECTION: B IMAGING
BODY SYSTEM: G ENDOCRINE SYSTEM
TYPE: 2 **COMPUTERIZED TOMOGRAPHY (CT SCAN):** Computer reformatted digital display of multiplanar images developed from the capture of multiple exposures of external ionizing radiation

Body Part	Contrast	Qualifier	Qualifier
2 Adrenal Glands, Bilateral 3 Parathyroid Glands 4 Thyroid Gland	Ø High Osmolar 1 Low Osmolar Y Other Contrast	Ø Unenhanced and Enhanced Z None	Z None
2 Adrenal Glands, Bilateral 3 Parathyroid Glands 4 Thyroid Gland	Z None	Z None	Z None

SECTION: B IMAGING
BODY SYSTEM: G ENDOCRINE SYSTEM
TYPE: 3 **MAGNETIC RESONANCE IMAGING (MRI):** Computer reformatted digital display of multiplanar images developed from the capture of radiofrequency signals emitted by nuclei in a body site excited within a magnetic field

Body Part	Contrast	Qualifier	Qualifier
2 Adrenal Glands, Bilateral 3 Parathyroid Glands 4 Thyroid Gland	Y Other Contrast	Ø Unenhanced and Enhanced Z None	Z None
2 Adrenal Glands, Bilateral 3 Parathyroid Glands 4 Thyroid Gland	Z None	Z None	Z None

SECTION: B IMAGING
BODY SYSTEM: G ENDOCRINE SYSTEM
TYPE: 4 **ULTRASONOGRAPHY:** Real time display of images of anatomy or flow information developed from the capture of reflected and attenuated high frequency sound waves

Body Part	Contrast	Qualifier	Qualifier
Ø Adrenal Gland, Right 1 Adrenal Gland, Left 2 Adrenal Glands, Bilateral 3 Parathyroid Glands 4 Thyroid Gland	Z None	Z None	Z None

New/Revised Text in Green ~~deleted~~ Deleted ♀ Females Only ♂ Males Only **Coding Clinic**
Non-covered Limited Coverage ⊡ Combination (See Appendix E) DRG Non-OR Non-OR Hospital-Acquired Condition

SECTION: B IMAGING

BODY SYSTEM: H SKIN, SUBCUTANEOUS TISSUE AND BREAST

TYPE: Ø **PLAIN RADIOGRAPHY:** Planar display of an image developed from the capture of external ionizing radiation on photographic or photoconductive plate

Body Part	Contrast	Qualifier	Qualifier
Ø Breast, Right 1 Breast, Left 2 Breasts, Bilateral	Z None	Z None	Z None
3 Single Mammary Duct, Right 4 Single Mammary Duct, Left 5 Multiple Mammary Ducts, Right 6 Multiple Mammary Ducts, Left	Ø High Osmolar 1 Low Osmolar Y Other Contrast Z None	Z None	Z None

SECTION: B IMAGING

BODY SYSTEM: H SKIN, SUBCUTANEOUS TISSUE AND BREAST

TYPE: 3 **MAGNETIC RESONANCE IMAGING (MRI):** Computer reformatted digital display of multiplanar images developed from the capture of radiofrequency signals emitted by nuclei in a body site excited within a magnetic field

Body Part	Contrast	Qualifier	Qualifier
Ø Breast, Right 1 Breast, Left 2 Breasts, Bilateral D Subcutaneous Tissue, Head/Neck F Subcutaneous Tissue, Upper Extremity G Subcutaneous Tissue, Thorax H Subcutaneous Tissue, Abdomen and Pelvis J Subcutaneous Tissue, Lower Extremity	Y Other Contrast	Ø Unenhanced and Enhanced Z None	Z None
Ø Breast, Right 1 Breast, Left 2 Breasts, Bilateral D Subcutaneous Tissue, Head/Neck F Subcutaneous Tissue, Upper Extremity G Subcutaneous Tissue, Thorax H Subcutaneous Tissue, Abdomen and Pelvis J Subcutaneous Tissue, Lower Extremity	Z None	Z None	Z None

SECTION: B IMAGING

BODY SYSTEM: H SKIN, SUBCUTANEOUS TISSUE AND BREAST

TYPE: 4 **ULTRASONOGRAPHY:** Real time display of images of anatomy or flow information developed from the capture of reflected and attenuated high frequency sound waves

Body Part	Contrast	Qualifier	Qualifier
Ø Breast, Right 1 Breast, Left 2 Breasts, Bilateral 7 Extremity, Upper 8 Extremity, Lower 9 Abdominal Wall B Chest Wall C Head and Neck	Z None	Z None	Z None

4: ULTRASONOGRAPHY

H: SKIN, SUBCUTANEOUS TISSUE AND BREAST

B: IMAGING

SECTION: B IMAGING
BODY SYSTEM: L CONNECTIVE TISSUE
TYPE: 3 **MAGNETIC RESONANCE IMAGING (MRI):** Computer reformatted digital display of multiplanar images developed from the capture of radiofrequency signals emitted by nuclei in a body site excited within a magnetic field

Body Part	Contrast	Qualifier	Qualifier
Ø Connective Tissue, Upper Extremity 1 Connective Tissue, Lower Extremity 2 Tendons, Upper Extremity 3 Tendons, Lower Extremity	Y Other Contrast	Ø Unenhanced and Enhanced Z None	Z None
Ø Connective Tissue, Upper Extremity 1 Connective Tissue, Lower Extremity 2 Tendons, Upper Extremity 3 Tendons, Lower Extremity	Z None	Z None	Z None

SECTION: B IMAGING
BODY SYSTEM: L CONNECTIVE TISSUE
TYPE: 4 **ULTRASONOGRAPHY:** Real time display of images of anatomy or flow information developed from the capture of reflected and attenuated high frequency sound waves

Body Part	Contrast	Qualifier	Qualifier
Ø Connective Tissue, Upper Extremity 1 Connective Tissue, Lower Extremity 2 Tendons, Upper Extremity 3 Tendons, Lower Extremity	Z None	Z None	Z None

SECTION: B IMAGING

BODY SYSTEM: N SKULL AND FACIAL BONES

TYPE: Ø **PLAIN RADIOGRAPHY:** Planar display of an image developed from the capture of external ionizing radiation on photographic or photoconductive plate

Body Part	Contrast	Qualifier	Qualifier
Ø Skull 1 Orbit, Right 2 Orbit, Left 3 Orbits, Bilateral 4 Nasal Bones 5 Facial Bones 6 Mandible B Zygomatic Arch, Right C Zygomatic Arch, Left D Zygomatic Arches, Bilateral G Tooth, Single H Teeth, Multiple J Teeth, All	Z None	Z None	Z None
7 Temporomandibular Joint, Right 8 Temporomandibular Joint, Left 9 Temporomandibular Joints, Bilateral	Ø High Osmolar 1 Low Osmolar Y Other Contrast Z None	Z None	Z None

SECTION: B IMAGING

BODY SYSTEM: N SKULL AND FACIAL BONES

TYPE: 1 **FLUOROSCOPY:** Single plane or bi-plane real time display of an image developed from the capture of external ionizing radiation on a fluorescent screen. The image may also be stored by either digital or analog means

Body Part	Contrast	Qualifier	Qualifier
7 Temporomandibular Joint, Right 8 Temporomandibular Joint, Left 9 Temporomandibular Joints, Bilateral	Ø High Osmolar 1 Low Osmolar Y Other Contrast Z None	Z None	Z None

Ø: PLAIN RADIOGRAPHY   1: FLUOROSCOPY

N: SKULL AND FACIAL BONES

B: IMAGING

New/Revised Text in Green   deleted Deleted   ♀ Females Only   ♂ Males Only   **Coding Clinic**

Non-covered   Limited Coverage   ⊕ Combination (See Appendix E)   DRG Non-OR   Non-OR   Hospital-Acquired Condition

SECTION: B IMAGING

BODY SYSTEM: N SKULL AND FACIAL BONES

TYPE: 2 **COMPUTERIZED TOMOGRAPHY (CT SCAN):** Computer reformatted digital display of multiplanar images developed from the capture of multiple exposures of external ionizing radiation

Body Part	Contrast	Qualifier	Qualifier
Ø Skull 3 Orbits, Bilateral 5 Facial Bones 6 Mandible 9 Temporomandibular Joints, Bilateral F Temporal Bones	Ø High Osmolar 1 Low Osmolar Y Other Contrast Z None	Z None	Z None

SECTION: B IMAGING

BODY SYSTEM: N SKULL AND FACIAL BONES

TYPE: 3 **MAGNETIC RESONANCE IMAGING (MRI):** Computer reformatted digital display of multiplanar images developed from the capture of radiofrequency signals emitted by nuclei in a body site excited within a magnetic field

Body Part	Contrast	Qualifier	Qualifier
9 Temporomandibular Joints, Bilateral	Y Other Contrast Z None	Z None	Z None

B: IMAGING

N: SKULL AND FACIAL BONES

2: CT SCAN   3: MRI

SECTION: B IMAGING
BODY SYSTEM: P NON-AXIAL UPPER BONES
TYPE: Ø **PLAIN RADIOGRAPHY:** Planar display of an image developed from the capture of external ionizing radiation on photographic or photoconductive plate

Body Part	Contrast	Qualifier	Qualifier
Ø Sternoclavicular Joint, Right 1 Sternoclavicular Joint, Left 2 Sternoclavicular Joints, Bilateral 3 Acromioclavicular Joints, Bilateral 4 Clavicle, Right 5 Clavicle, Left 6 Scapula, Right 7 Scapula, Left A Humerus, Right B Humerus, Left E Upper Arm, Right F Upper Arm, Left J Forearm, Right K Forearm, Left N Hand, Right P Hand, Left R Finger(s), Right S Finger(s), Left X Ribs, Right Y Ribs, Left	Z None	Z None	Z None
8 Shoulder, Right 9 Shoulder, Left C Hand/Finger Joint, Right D Hand/Finger Joint, Left G Elbow, Right H Elbow, Left L Wrist, Right M Wrist, Left	Ø High Osmolar 1 Low Osmolar Y Other Contrast Z None	Z None	Z None

Ø: PLAIN RADIOGRAPHY

P: NON-AXIAL UPPER BONES

B: IMAGING

SECTION: B IMAGING
BODY SYSTEM: P NON-AXIAL UPPER BONES
TYPE: 1 **FLUOROSCOPY:** Single plane or bi-plane real time display of an image developed from the capture of external ionizing radiation on a fluorescent screen. The image may also be stored by either digital or analog means

Body Part	Contrast	Qualifier	Qualifier
Ø Sternoclavicular Joint, Right 1 Sternoclavicular Joint, Left 2 Sternoclavicular Joints, Bilateral 3 Acromioclavicular Joints, Bilateral 4 Clavicle, Right 5 Clavicle, Left 6 Scapula, Right 7 Scapula, Left A Humerus, Right B Humerus, Left E Upper Arm, Right F Upper Arm, Left J Forearm, Right K Forearm, Left N Hand, Right P Hand, Left R Finger(s), Right S Finger(s), Left X Ribs, Right Y Ribs, Left	Z None	Z None	Z None
8 Shoulder, Right 9 Shoulder, Left L Wrist, Right M Wrist, Left	Ø High Osmolar 1 Low Osmolar Y Other Contrast Z None	Z None	Z None
C Hand/Finger Joint, Right D Hand/Finger Joint, Left G Elbow, Right H Elbow, Left	Ø High Osmolar 1 Low Osmolar Y Other Contrast	Z None	Z None

SECTION: B IMAGING
BODY SYSTEM: P NON-AXIAL UPPER BONES
TYPE: 2 COMPUTERIZED TOMOGRAPHY (CT SCAN): Computer reformatted digital display of multiplanar images developed from the capture of multiple exposures of external ionizing radiation

2: COMPUTERIZED TOMOGRAPHY (CT SCAN)

P: NON-AXIAL UPPER BONES

B: IMAGING

Body Part	Contrast	Qualifier	Qualifier
Ø Sternoclavicular Joint, Right 1 Sternoclavicular Joint, Left W Thorax	Ø High Osmolar 1 Low Osmolar Y Other Contrast	Z None	Z None
2 Sternoclavicular Joints, Bilateral 3 Acromioclavicular Joints, Bilateral 4 Clavicle, Right 5 Clavicle, Left 6 Scapula, Right 7 Scapula, Left 8 Shoulder, Right 9 Shoulder, Left A Humerus, Right B Humerus, Left E Upper Arm, Right F Upper Arm, Left G Elbow, Right H Elbow, Left J Forearm, Right K Forearm, Left L Wrist, Right M Wrist, Left N Hand, Right P Hand, Left Q Hands and Wrists, Bilateral R Finger(s), Right S Finger(s), Left T Upper Extremity, Right U Upper Extremity, Left V Upper Extremities, Bilateral X Ribs, Right Y Ribs, Left	Ø High Osmolar 1 Low Osmolar Y Other Contrast Z None	Z None	Z None
C Hand/Finger Joint, Right D Hand/Finger Joint, Left	Z None	Z None	Z None

New/Revised Text in Green   ~~deleted~~ Deleted   ♀ Females Only   ♂ Males Only   **Coding Clinic**
Non-covered   Limited Coverage   ⊞ Combination (See Appendix E)   DRG Non-OR   Non-OR   Hospital-Acquired Condition

SECTION: B IMAGING

BODY SYSTEM: P NON-AXIAL UPPER BONES

TYPE: 3 MAGNETIC RESONANCE IMAGING (MRI): Computer reformatted digital display of multiplanar images developed from the capture of radiofrequency signals emitted by nuclei in a body site excited within a magnetic field

Body Part	Contrast	Qualifier	Qualifier
8 Shoulder, Right 9 Shoulder, Left C Hand/Finger Joint, Right D Hand/Finger Joint, Left E Upper Arm, Right F Upper Arm, Left G Elbow, Right H Elbow, Left J Forearm, Right K Forearm, Left L Wrist, Right M Wrist, Left	Y Other Contrast	Ø Unenhanced and Enhanced Z None	Z None
8 Shoulder, Right 9 Shoulder, Left C Hand/Finger Joint, Right D Hand/Finger Joint, Left E Upper Arm, Right F Upper Arm, Left G Elbow, Right H Elbow, Left J Forearm, Right K Forearm, Left L Wrist, Right M Wrist, Left	Z None	Z None	Z None

SECTION: B IMAGING

BODY SYSTEM: P NON-AXIAL UPPER BONES

TYPE: 4 ULTRASONOGRAPHY: Real time display of images of anatomy or flow information developed from the capture of reflected and attenuated high frequency sound waves

Body Part	Contrast	Qualifier	Qualifier
8 Shoulder, Right 9 Shoulder, Left G Elbow, Right H Elbow, Left L Wrist, Right M Wrist, Left N Hand, Right P Hand, Left	Z None	Z None	1 Densitometry Z None

SECTION: B IMAGING

BODY SYSTEM: Q NON-AXIAL LOWER BONES

TYPE: 0 **PLAIN RADIOGRAPHY:** Planar display of an image developed from the capture of external ionizing radiation on photographic or photoconductive plate

Body Part	Contrast	Qualifier	Qualifier
0 Hip, Right 1 Hip, Left	0 High Osmolar 1 Low Osmolar Y Other Contrast	Z None	Z None
0 Hip, Right 1 Hip, Left	Z None	Z None	1 Densitometry Z None
3 Femur, Right 4 Femur, Left	Z None	Z None	1 Densitometry Z None
7 Knee, Right 8 Knee, Left G Ankle, Right H Ankle, Left	0 High Osmolar 1 Low Osmolar Y Other Contrast Z None	Z None	Z None
D Lower Leg, Right F Lower Leg, Left J Calcaneus, Right K Calcaneus, Left L Foot, Right M Foot, Left P Toe(s), Right Q Toe(s), Left V Patella, Right W Patella, Left	Z None	Z None	Z None
X Foot/Toe Joint, Right Y Foot/Toe Joint, Left	0 High Osmolar 1 Low Osmolar Y Other Contrast	Z None	Z None

0: PLAIN RADIOGRAPHY

Q: NON-AXIAL LOWER BONES

B: IMAGING

New/Revised Text in Green   deleted Deleted   ♀ Females Only   ♂ Males Only   **Coding Clinic**

Non-covered   Limited Coverage   ⊞ Combination (See Appendix E)   DRG Non-OR   Non-OR   Hospital-Acquired Condition

SECTION: B IMAGING
BODY SYSTEM: Q NON-AXIAL LOWER BONES
TYPE: 1 **FLUOROSCOPY:** Single plane or bi-plane real time display of an image developed from the capture of external ionizing radiation on a fluorescent screen. The image may also be stored by either digital or analog means

Body Part	Contrast	Qualifier	Qualifier
Ø Hip, Right 1 Hip, Left 7 Knee, Right 8 Knee, Left G Ankle, Right H Ankle, Left X Foot/Toe Joint, Right Y Foot/Toe Joint, Left	Ø High Osmolar 1 Low Osmolar Y Other Contrast Z None	Z None	Z None
3 Femur, Right 4 Femur, Left D Lower Leg, Right F Lower Leg, Left J Calcaneus, Right K Calcaneus, Left L Foot, Right M Foot, Left P Toe(s), Right Q Toe(s), Left V Patella, Right W Patella, Left	Z None	Z None	Z None

SECTION: B IMAGING

BODY SYSTEM: Q NON-AXIAL LOWER BONES

TYPE: 2 **COMPUTERIZED TOMOGRAPHY (CT SCAN):** Computer reformatted digital display of multiplanar images developed from the capture of multiple exposures of external ionizing radiation

Body Part	Contrast	Qualifier	Qualifier
Ø Hip, Right 1 Hip, Left 3 Femur, Right 4 Femur, Left 7 Knee, Right 8 Knee, Left D Lower Leg, Right F Lower Leg, Left G Ankle, Right H Ankle, Left J Calcaneus, Right K Calcaneus, Left L Foot, Right M Foot, Left P Toe(s), Right Q Toe(s), Left R Lower Extremity, Right S Lower Extremity, Left V Patella, Right W Patella, Left X Foot/Toe Joint, Right Y Foot/Toe Joint, Left	Ø High Osmolar 1 Low Osmolar Y Other Contrast Z None	Z None	Z None
B Tibia/Fibula, Right C Tibia/Fibula, Left	Ø High Osmolar 1 Low Osmolar Y Other Contrast	Z None	Z None

Left margin: 2: COMPUTERIZED TOMOGRAPHY (CT SCAN)   Q: NON-AXIAL LOWER BONES   B: IMAGING

SECTION: B IMAGING

BODY SYSTEM: Q NON-AXIAL LOWER BONES

TYPE: 3 **MAGNETIC RESONANCE IMAGING (MRI):** Computer reformatted digital display of multiplanar images developed from the capture of radiofrequency signals emitted by nuclei in a body site excited within a magnetic field

Body Part	Contrast	Qualifier	Qualifier
Ø Hip, Right 1 Hip, Left 3 Femur, Right 4 Femur, Left 7 Knee, Right 8 Knee, Left D Lower Leg, Right F Lower Leg, Left G Ankle, Right H Ankle, Left J Calcaneus, Right K Calcaneus, Left L Foot, Right M Foot, Left P Toe(s), Right Q Toe(s), Left V Patella, Right W Patella, Left	Y Other Contrast	Ø Unenhanced and Enhanced Z None	Z None
Ø Hip, Right 1 Hip, Left 3 Femur, Right 4 Femur, Left 7 Knee, Right 8 Knee, Left D Lower Leg, Right F Lower Leg, Left G Ankle, Right H Ankle, Left J Calcaneus, Right K Calcaneus, Left L Foot, Right M Foot, Left P Toe(s), Right Q Toe(s), Left V Patella, Right W Patella, Left	Z None	Z None	Z None

SECTION: B IMAGING
BODY SYSTEM: Q NON-AXIAL LOWER BONES
TYPE: 4 **ULTRASONOGRAPHY:** Real time display of images of anatomy or flow information developed from the capture of reflected and attenuated high frequency sound waves

Body Part	Contrast	Qualifier	Qualifier
Ø Hip, Right 1 Hip, Left 2 Hips, Bilateral 7 Knee, Right 8 Knee, Left 9 Knees, Bilateral	Z None	Z None	Z None

SECTION: B IMAGING

BODY SYSTEM: R AXIAL SKELETON, EXCEPT SKULL AND FACIAL BONES
TYPE: Ø **PLAIN RADIOGRAPHY:** Planar display of an image developed from the capture of external ionizing radiation on photographic or photoconductive plate

Body Part	Contrast	Qualifier	Qualifier
Ø Cervical Spine 7 Thoracic Spine 9 Lumbar Spine G Whole Spine	Z None	Z None	1 Densitometry Z None
1 Cervical Disc(s) 2 Thoracic Disc(s) 3 Lumbar Disc(s) 4 Cervical Facet Joint(s) 5 Thoracic Facet Joint(s) 6 Lumbar Facet Joint(s) D Sacroiliac Joints	Ø High Osmolar 1 Low Osmolar Y Other Contrast Z None	Z None	Z None
8 Thoracolumbar Joint B Lumbosacral Joint C Pelvis F Sacrum and Coccyx H Sternum	Z None	Z None	Z None

SECTION: B IMAGING

BODY SYSTEM: R AXIAL SKELETON, EXCEPT SKULL AND FACIAL BONES
TYPE: 1 **FLUOROSCOPY:** Single plane or bi-plane real time display of an image developed from the capture of external ionizing radiation on a fluorescent screen. The image may also be stored by either digital or analog means

Body Part	Contrast	Qualifier	Qualifier
Ø Cervical Spine 1 Cervical Disc(s) 2 Thoracic Disc(s) 3 Lumbar Disc(s) 4 Cervical Facet Joint(s) 5 Thoracic Facet Joint(s) 6 Lumbar Facet Joint(s) 7 Thoracic Spine 8 Thoracolumbar Joint 9 Lumbar Spine B Lumbosacral Joint C Pelvis D Sacroiliac Joints F Sacrum and Coccyx G Whole Spine H Sternum	Ø High Osmolar 1 Low Osmolar Y Other Contrast Z None	Z None	Z None

SECTION: B IMAGING
BODY SYSTEM: R AXIAL SKELETON, EXCEPT SKULL AND FACIAL BONES
TYPE: 2 **COMPUTERIZED TOMOGRAPHY (CT SCAN):** Computer reformatted digital display of multiplanar images developed from the capture of multiple exposures of external ionizing radiation

Body Part	Contrast	Qualifier	Qualifier
Ø Cervical Spine 7 Thoracic Spine 9 Lumbar Spine C Pelvis D Sacroiliac Joints F Sacrum and Coccyx	Ø High Osmolar 1 Low Osmolar Y Other Contrast Z None	Z None	Z None

SECTION: B IMAGING
BODY SYSTEM: R AXIAL SKELETON, EXCEPT SKULL AND FACIAL BONES
TYPE: 3 **MAGNETIC RESONANCE IMAGING (MRI):** Computer reformatted digital display of multiplanar images developed from the capture of radiofrequency signals emitted by nuclei in a body site excited within a magnetic field

Body Part	Contrast	Qualifier	Qualifier
Ø Cervical Spine 1 Cervical Disc(s) 2 Thoracic Disc(s) 3 Lumbar Disc(s) 7 Thoracic Spine 9 Lumbar Spine C Pelvis F Sacrum and Coccyx	Y Other Contrast	Ø Unenhanced and Enhanced Z None	Z None
Ø Cervical Spine 1 Cervical Disc(s) 2 Thoracic Disc(s) 3 Lumbar Disc(s) 7 Thoracic Spine 9 Lumbar Spine C Pelvis F Sacrum and Coccyx	Z None	Z None	Z None

SECTION: B IMAGING
BODY SYSTEM: R AXIAL SKELETON, EXCEPT SKULL AND FACIAL BONES
TYPE: 4 **ULTRASONOGRAPHY:** Real time display of images of anatomy or flow information developed from the capture of reflected and attenuated high frequency sound waves

Body Part	Contrast	Qualifier	Qualifier
Ø Cervical Spine 7 Thoracic Spine 9 Lumbar Spine F Sacrum and Coccyx	Z None	Z None	Z None

New/Revised Text in Green ~~deleted~~ Deleted ♀ Females Only ♂ Males Only **Coding Clinic**
🔖 Non-covered 🔖 Limited Coverage ⊡ Combination (See Appendix E) DRG Non-OR Non-OR 🔖 Hospital-Acquired Condition

SECTION: B IMAGING

BODY SYSTEM: T URINARY SYSTEM

TYPE: Ø **PLAIN RADIOGRAPHY:** Planar display of an image developed from the capture of external ionizing radiation on photographic or photoconductive plate

Body Part	Contrast	Qualifier	Qualifier
Ø Bladder	Ø High Osmolar	Z None	Z None
1 Kidney, Right	1 Low Osmolar		
2 Kidney, Left	Y Other Contrast		
3 Kidneys, Bilateral	Z None		
4 Kidneys, Ureters, and Bladder			
5 Urethra			
6 Ureter, Right			
7 Ureter, Left			
8 Ureters, Bilateral			
B Bladder and Urethra			
C Ileal Diversion Loop			

SECTION: B IMAGING

BODY SYSTEM: T URINARY SYSTEM

TYPE: 1 **FLUOROSCOPY:** Single plane or bi-plane real time display of an image developed from the capture of external ionizing radiation on a fluorescent screen. The image may also be stored by either digital or analog means

Body Part	Contrast	Qualifier	Qualifier
Ø Bladder	Ø High Osmolar	Z None	Z None
1 Kidney, Right	1 Low Osmolar		
2 Kidney, Left	Y Other Contrast		
3 Kidneys, Bilateral	Z None		
4 Kidneys, Ureters, and Bladder			
5 Urethra			
6 Ureter, Right			
7 Ureter, Left			
B Bladder and Urethra			
C Ileal Diversion Loop			
D Kidney, Ureter, and Bladder, Right			
F Kidney, Ureter, and Bladder, Left			
G Ileal Loop, Ureters, and Kidneys			

SECTION: B IMAGING

BODY SYSTEM: T URINARY SYSTEM

TYPE: 2 **COMPUTERIZED TOMOGRAPHY (CT SCAN):** Computer reformatted digital display of multiplanar images developed from the capture of multiple exposures of external ionizing radiation

Body Part	Contrast	Qualifier	Qualifier
Ø Bladder 1 Kidney, Right 2 Kidney, Left 3 Kidneys, Bilateral 9 Kidney Transplant	Ø High Osmolar 1 Low Osmolar Y Other Contrast	Ø Unenhanced and Enhanced Z None	Z None
Ø Bladder 1 Kidney, Right 2 Kidney, Left 3 Kidneys, Bilateral 9 Kidney Transplant	Z None	Z None	Z None

SECTION: B IMAGING

BODY SYSTEM: T URINARY SYSTEM

TYPE: 3 **MAGNETIC RESONANCE IMAGING (MRI):** Computer reformatted digital display of multiplanar images developed from the capture of radiofrequency signals emitted by nuclei in a body site excited within a magnetic field

Body Part	Contrast	Qualifier	Qualifier
Ø Bladder 1 Kidney, Right 2 Kidney, Left 3 Kidneys, Bilateral 9 Kidney Transplant	Y Other Contrast	Ø Unenhanced and Enhanced Z None	Z None
Ø Bladder 1 Kidney, Right 2 Kidney, Left 3 Kidneys, Bilateral 9 Kidney Transplant	Z None	Z None	Z None

New/Revised Text in Green   deleted Deleted   ♀ Females Only   ♂ Males Only   **Coding Clinic**

Non-covered   Limited Coverage   ⊕ Combination (See Appendix E)   DRG Non-OR   Non-OR   Hospital-Acquired Condition

2: CT SCAN   3: MRI

T: URINARY SYSTEM

B: IMAGING

SECTION: B IMAGING
BODY SYSTEM: T URINARY SYSTEM
TYPE: 4 **ULTRASONOGRAPHY:** Real time display of images of anatomy or flow information developed from the capture of reflected and attenuated high frequency sound waves

Body Part	Contrast	Qualifier	Qualifier
Ø Bladder	Z None	Z None	Z None
1 Kidney, Right			
2 Kidney, Left			
3 Kidneys, Bilateral			
5 Urethra			
6 Ureter, Right			
7 Ureter, Left			
8 Ureters, Bilateral			
9 Kidney Transplant			
J Kidneys and Bladder			

New/Revised Text in Green   ~~deleted~~ Deleted   ♀ Females Only   ♂ Males Only   **Coding Clinic**
🚫 Non-covered   🚫 Limited Coverage   ⊡ Combination (See Appendix E)   DRG Non-OR   Non-OR   🚫 Hospital-Acquired Condition

597

SECTION: B IMAGING

BODY SYSTEM: U FEMALE REPRODUCTIVE SYSTEM

TYPE: Ø **PLAIN RADIOGRAPHY:** Planar display of an image developed from the capture of external ionizing radiation on photographic or photoconductive plate

Body Part	Contrast	Qualifier	Qualifier
Ø Fallopian Tube, Right ♀ 1 Fallopian Tube, Left ♀ 2 Fallopian Tubes, Bilateral ♀ 6 Uterus ♀ 8 Uterus and Fallopian Tubes ♀ 9 Vagina ♀	Ø High Osmolar 1 Low Osmolar Y Other Contrast	Z None	Z None

SECTION: B IMAGING

BODY SYSTEM: U FEMALE REPRODUCTIVE SYSTEM

TYPE: 1 **FLUOROSCOPY:** Single plane or bi-plane real time display of an image developed from the capture of external ionizing radiation on a fluorescent screen. The image may also be stored by either digital or analog means

Body Part	Contrast	Qualifier	Qualifier
Ø Fallopian Tube, Right ♀ 1 Fallopian Tube, Left ♀ 2 Fallopian Tubes, Bilateral ♀ 6 Uterus ♀ 8 Uterus and Fallopian Tubes ♀ 9 Vagina ♀	Ø High Osmolar 1 Low Osmolar Y Other Contrast Z None	Z None	Z None

SECTION: B IMAGING

BODY SYSTEM: U FEMALE REPRODUCTIVE SYSTEM

TYPE: 3 MAGNETIC RESONANCE IMAGING (MRI): Computer reformatted digital display of multiplanar images developed from the capture of radiofrequency signals emitted by nuclei in a body site excited within a magnetic field

Body Part	Contrast	Qualifier	Qualifier
3 Ovary, Right ♀ 4 Ovary, Left ♀ 5 Ovaries, Bilateral ♀ 6 Uterus ♀ 9 Vagina ♀ B Pregnant Uterus ♀ C Uterus and Ovaries ♀	Y Other Contrast	Ø Unenhanced and Enhanced Z None	Z None
3 Ovary, Right ♀ 4 Ovary, Left ♀ 5 Ovaries, Bilateral ♀ 6 Uterus ♀ 9 Vagina ♀ B Pregnant Uterus ♀ C Uterus and Ovaries ♀	Z None	Z None	Z None

SECTION: B IMAGING

BODY SYSTEM: U FEMALE REPRODUCTIVE SYSTEM

TYPE: 4 ULTRASONOGRAPHY: Real time display of images of anatomy or flow information developed from the capture of reflected and attenuated high frequency sound waves

Body Part	Contrast	Qualifier	Qualifier
Ø Fallopian Tube, Right ♀ 1 Fallopian Tube, Left ♀ 2 Fallopian Tubes, Bilateral ♀ 3 Ovary, Right ♀ 4 Ovary, Left ♀ 5 Ovaries, Bilateral ♀ 6 Uterus ♀ C Uterus and Ovaries ♀	Y Other Contrast Z None	Z None	Z None

New/Revised Text in Green   deleted Deleted   ♀ Females Only   ♂ Males Only   **Coding Clinic**
🚫 Non-covered   🚫 Limited Coverage   ⊡ Combination (See Appendix E)   DRG Non-OR   Non-OR   🚫 Hospital-Acquired Condition

SECTION: B IMAGING

BODY SYSTEM: V MALE REPRODUCTIVE SYSTEM

TYPE: Ø **PLAIN RADIOGRAPHY:** Planar display of an image developed from the capture of external ionizing radiation on photographic or photoconductive plate

Body Part	Contrast	Qualifier	Qualifier
Ø Corpora Cavernosa ♂ 1 Epididymis, Right ♂ 2 Epididymis, Left ♂ 3 Prostate ♂ 5 Testicle, Right ♂ 6 Testicle, Left ♂ 8 Vasa Vasorum ♂	Ø High Osmolar 1 Low Osmolar Y Other Contrast	Z None	Z None

SECTION: B IMAGING

BODY SYSTEM: V MALE REPRODUCTIVE SYSTEM

TYPE: 1 **FLUOROSCOPY:** Single plane or bi-plane real time display of an image developed from the capture of external ionizing radiation on a fluorescent screen. The image may also be stored by either digital or analog means

Body Part	Contrast	Qualifier	Qualifier
Ø Corpora Cavernosa ♂ 8 Vasa Vasorum ♂	Ø High Osmolar 1 Low Osmolar Y Other Contrast Z None	Z None	Z None

SECTION: B IMAGING

BODY SYSTEM: V MALE REPRODUCTIVE SYSTEM

TYPE: **2 COMPUTERIZED TOMOGRAPHY (CT SCAN):** Computer reformatted digital display of multiplanar images developed from the capture of multiple exposures of external ionizing radiation

Body Part	Contrast	Qualifier	Qualifier
3 Prostate ♂	Ø High Osmolar 1 Low Osmolar Y Other Contrast	Ø Unenhanced and Enhanced Z None	Z None
3 Prostate ♂	Z None	Z None	Z None

SECTION: B IMAGING

BODY SYSTEM: V MALE REPRODUCTIVE SYSTEM

TYPE: **3 MAGNETIC RESONANCE IMAGING (MRI):** Computer reformatted digital display of multiplanar images developed from the capture of radiofrequency signals emitted by nuclei in a body site excited within a magnetic field

Body Part	Contrast	Qualifier	Qualifier
Ø Corpora Cavernosa ♂ 3 Prostate ♂ 4 Scrotum ♂ 5 Testicle, Right ♂ 6 Testicle, Left ♂ 7 Testicles, Bilateral ♂	Y Other Contrast	Ø Unenhanced and Enhanced Z None	Z None
Ø Corpora Cavernosa ♂ 3 Prostate ♂ 4 Scrotum ♂ 5 Testicle, Right ♂ 6 Testicle, Left ♂ 7 Testicles, Bilateral ♂	Z None	Z None	Z None

SECTION: B IMAGING

BODY SYSTEM: V MALE REPRODUCTIVE SYSTEM

TYPE: **4 ULTRASONOGRAPHY:** Real time display of images of anatomy or flow information developed from the capture of reflected and attenuated high frequency sound waves

Body Part	Contrast	Qualifier	Qualifier
4 Scrotum ♂ 9 Prostate and Seminal Vesicles ♂ B Penis ♂	Z None	Z None	Z None

0: PLAIN RADIOGRAPHY 1: FLUOROSCOPY 2: CT SCAN

W: ANATOMICAL REGIONS

B: IMAGING

SECTION: B IMAGING
BODY SYSTEM: W ANATOMICAL REGIONS
TYPE: Ø **PLAIN RADIOGRAPHY:** Planar display of an image developed from the capture of external ionizing radiation on photographic or photoconductive plate

Body Part	Contrast	Qualifier	Qualifier
Ø Abdomen 1 Abdomen and Pelvis 3 Chest B Long Bones, All C Lower Extremity J Upper Extremity K Whole Body L Whole Skeleton M Whole Body, Infant	Z None	Z None	Z None

SECTION: B IMAGING
BODY SYSTEM: W ANATOMICAL REGIONS
TYPE: 1 **FLUOROSCOPY:** Single plane or bi-plane real time display of an image developed from the capture of external ionizing radiation on a fluorescent screen. The image may also be stored by either digital or analog means

Body Part	Contrast	Qualifier	Qualifier
1 Abdomen and Pelvis 9 Head and Neck C Lower Extremity J Upper Extremity	Ø High Osmolar 1 Low Osmolar Y Other Contrast Z None	Z None	Z None

SECTION: B IMAGING
BODY SYSTEM: W ANATOMICAL REGIONS
TYPE: 2 **COMPUTERIZED TOMOGRAPHY (CT SCAN):** Computer reformatted digital display of multiplanar images developed from the capture of multiple exposures of external ionizing radiation

Body Part	Contrast	Qualifier	Qualifier
Ø Abdomen 1 Abdomen and Pelvis 4 Chest and Abdomen 5 Chest, Abdomen, and Pelvis 8 Head 9 Head and Neck F Neck G Pelvic Region	Ø High Osmolar 1 Low Osmolar Y Other Contrast	Ø Unenhanced and Enhanced Z None	Z None
Ø Abdomen 1 Abdomen and Pelvis 4 Chest and Abdomen 5 Chest, Abdomen, and Pelvis 8 Head 9 Head and Neck F Neck G Pelvic Region	Z None	Z None	Z None

New/Revised Text in Green ~~deleted~~ Deleted ♀ Females Only ♂ Males Only **Coding Clinic** Non-covered Limited Coverage ⊞ Combination (See Appendix E) DRG Non-OR Non-OR Hospital-Acquired Condition

SECTION: B IMAGING

BODY SYSTEM: W ANATOMICAL REGIONS

TYPE: 3 **MAGNETIC RESONANCE IMAGING (MRI):** Computer reformatted digital display of multiplanar images developed from the capture of radiofrequency signals emitted by nuclei in a body site excited within a magnetic field

Body Part	Contrast	Qualifier	Qualifier
Ø Abdomen 8 Head F Neck G Pelvic Region H Retroperitoneum P Brachial Plexus	Y Other Contrast	Ø Unenhanced and Enhanced Z None	Z None
Ø Abdomen 8 Head F Neck G Pelvic Region H Retroperitoneum P Brachial Plexus	Z None	Z None	Z None
3 Chest	Y Other Contrast	Ø Unenhanced and Enhanced Z None	Z None

SECTION: B IMAGING

BODY SYSTEM: W ANATOMICAL REGIONS

TYPE: 4 **ULTRASONOGRAPHY:** Real time display of images of anatomy or flow information developed from the capture of reflected and attenuated high frequency sound waves

Body Part	Contrast	Qualifier	Qualifier
Ø Abdomen 1 Abdomen and Pelvis F Neck G Pelvic Region	Z None	Z None	Z None

SECTION: B IMAGING

BODY SYSTEM: Y FETUS AND OBSTETRICAL
TYPE: **3 MAGNETIC RESONANCE IMAGING (MRI):** Computer reformatted digital display of multiplanar images developed from the capture of radiofrequency signals emitted by nuclei in a body site excited within a magnetic field

Body Part	Contrast	Qualifier	Qualifier
0 Fetal Head ♀ 1 Fetal Heart ♀ 2 Fetal Thorax ♀ 3 Fetal Abdomen ♀ 4 Fetal Spine ♀ 5 Fetal Extremities ♀ 6 Whole Fetus ♀	Y Other Contrast	0 Unenhanced and Enhanced Z None	Z None
0 Fetal Head ♀ 1 Fetal Heart ♀ 2 Fetal Thorax ♀ 3 Fetal Abdomen ♀ 4 Fetal Spine ♀ 5 Fetal Extremities ♀ 6 Whole Fetus ♀	Z None	Z None	Z None

SECTION: B IMAGING

BODY SYSTEM: Y FETUS AND OBSTETRICAL
TYPE: **4 ULTRASONOGRAPHY:** Real time display of images of anatomy or flow information developed from the capture of reflected and attenuated high frequency sound waves

Body Part	Contrast	Qualifier	Qualifier
7 Fetal Umbilical Cord ♀ 8 Placenta ♀ 9 First Trimester, Single Fetus ♀ B First Trimester, Multiple Gestation ♀ C Second Trimester, Single Fetus ♀ D Second Trimester, Multiple Gestation ♀ F Third Trimester, Single Fetus ♀ G Third Trimester, Multiple Gestation ♀	Z None	Z None	Z None

SECTION: **C NUCLEAR MEDICINE**
BODY SYSTEM: Ø **CENTRAL NERVOUS SYSTEM**
TYPE: 1 **PLANAR NUCLEAR MEDICINE IMAGING:** Introduction of radioactive materials into the body for single plane display of images developed from the capture of radioactive emissions

Body Part	Radionuclide	Qualifier	Qualifier
Ø Brain	1 Technetium 99m (Tc-99m) Y Other Radionuclide	Z None	Z None
5 Cerebrospinal Fluid	D Indium 111 (In-111) Y Other Radionuclide	Z None	Z None
Y Central Nervous System	Y Other Radionuclide	Z None	Z None

SECTION: **C NUCLEAR MEDICINE**
BODY SYSTEM: Ø **CENTRAL NERVOUS SYSTEM**
TYPE: 2 **TOMOGRAPHIC (TOMO) NUCLEAR MEDICINE IMAGING:** Introduction of radioactive materials into the body for three dimensional display of images developed from the capture of radioactive emissions

Body Part	Radionuclide	Qualifier	Qualifier
Ø Brain	1 Technetium 99m (Tc-99m) F Iodine 123 (I-123) S Thallium 2Ø1 (Tl-2Ø1) Y Other Radionuclide	Z None	Z None
5 Cerebrospinal Fluid	D Indium 111 (In-111) Y Other Radionuclide	Z None	Z None
Y Central Nervous System	Y Other Radionuclide	Z None	Z None

1; 2

Ø: CENTRAL NERVOUS SYSTEM

C: NUCLEAR MEDICINE

SECTION: C NUCLEAR MEDICINE
BODY SYSTEM: Ø CENTRAL NERVOUS SYSTEM
TYPE: 3 **POSITRON EMISSION TOMOGRAPHIC (PET) IMAGING:** Introduction of radioactive materials into the body for three dimensional display of images developed from the simultaneous capture, 18Ø degrees apart, of radioactive emissions

Body Part	Radionuclide	Qualifier	Qualifier
Ø Brain	B Carbon 11 (C-11) K Fluorine 18 (F-18) M Oxygen 15 (O-15) Y Other Radionuclide	Z None	Z None
Y Central Nervous System	Y Other Radionuclide	Z None	Z None

SECTION: C NUCLEAR MEDICINE
BODY SYSTEM: Ø CENTRAL NERVOUS SYSTEM
TYPE: 5 **NONIMAGING NUCLEAR MEDICINE PROBE:** Introduction of radioactive materials into the body for the study of distribution and fate of certain substances by the detection of radioactive emissions; or, alternatively, measurement of absorption of radioactive emissions from an external source

Body Part	Radionuclide	Qualifier	Qualifier
Ø Brain	V Xenon 133 (Xe-133) Y Other Radionuclide	Z None	Z None
Y Central Nervous System	Y Other Radionuclide	Z None	Z None

New/Revised Text in Green   deleted Deleted   ♀ Females Only   ♂ Males Only   **Coding Clinic**
🚫 Non-covered   🚫 Limited Coverage   ⊟ Combination (See Appendix E)   DRG Non-OR   Non-OR   🚫 Hospital-Acquired Condition

6Ø7

SECTION: C NUCLEAR MEDICINE

BODY SYSTEM: 2 HEART

TYPE: 1 **PLANAR NUCLEAR MEDICINE IMAGING:** Introduction of radioactive materials into the body for single plane display of images developed from the capture of radioactive emissions

Body Part	Radionuclide	Qualifier	Qualifier
6 Heart, Right and Left	1 Technetium 99m (Tc-99m) Y Other Radionuclide	Z None	Z None
G Myocardium	1 Technetium 99m (Tc-99m) D Indium 111 (In-111) S Thallium 201 (Tl-201) Y Other Radionuclide Z None	Z None	Z None
Y Heart	Y Other Radionuclide	Z None	Z None

SECTION: C NUCLEAR MEDICINE

BODY SYSTEM: 2 HEART

TYPE: 2 **TOMOGRAPHIC (TOMO) NUCLEAR MEDICINE IMAGING:** Introduction of radioactive materials into the body for three dimensional display of images developed from the capture of radioactive emissions

Body Part	Radionuclide	Qualifier	Qualifier
6 Heart, Right and Left	1 Technetium 99m (Tc-99m) Y Other Radionuclide	Z None	Z None
G Myocardium	1 Technetium 99m (Tc-99m) D Indium 111 (In-111) K Fluorine 18 (F-18) S Thallium 201 (Tl-201) Y Other Radionuclide Z None	Z None	Z None
Y Heart	Y Other Radionuclide	Z None	Z None

SECTION: C NUCLEAR MEDICINE
BODY SYSTEM: 2 HEART
TYPE: 3 **POSITRON EMISSION TOMOGRAPHIC (PET) IMAGING:** Introduction of radioactive materials into the body for three dimensional display of images developed from the simultaneous capture, 18Ø degrees apart, of radioactive emissions

Body Part	Radionuclide	Qualifier	Qualifier
G Myocardium	K Fluorine 18 (F-18) M Oxygen 15 (O-15) Q Rubidium 82 (Rb-82) R Nitrogen 13 (N-13) Y Other Radionuclide	Z None	Z None
Y Heart	Y Other Radionuclide	Z None	Z None

SECTION: C NUCLEAR MEDICINE
BODY SYSTEM: 2 HEART
TYPE: 5 **NONIMAGING NUCLEAR MEDICINE PROBE:** Introduction of radioactive materials into the body for the study of distribution and fate of certain substances by the detection of radioactive emissions; or, alternatively, measurement of absorption of radioactive emissions from an external source

Body Part	Radionuclide	Qualifier	Qualifier
6 Heart, Right and Left	1 Technetium 99m (Tc-99m) Y Other Radionuclide	Z None	Z None
Y Heart	Y Other Radionuclide	Z None	Z None

SECTION: C NUCLEAR MEDICINE

BODY SYSTEM: 5 VEINS

TYPE: 1 PLANAR NUCLEAR MEDICINE IMAGING: Introduction of radioactive materials into the body for single plane display of images developed from the capture of radioactive emissions

Body Part	Radionuclide	Qualifier	Qualifier
B Lower Extremity Veins, Right C Lower Extremity Veins, Left D Lower Extremity Veins, Bilateral N Upper Extremity Veins, Right P Upper Extremity Veins, Left Q Upper Extremity Veins, Bilateral R Central Veins	1 Technetium 99m (Tc-99m) Y Other Radionuclide	Z None	Z None
Y Veins	Y Other Radionuclide	Z None	Z None

SECTION: C NUCLEAR MEDICINE

BODY SYSTEM: 7 LYMPHATIC AND HEMATOLOGIC SYSTEM

TYPE: 1 **PLANAR NUCLEAR MEDICINE IMAGING:** Introduction of radioactive materials into the body for single plane display of images developed from the capture of radioactive emissions

Body Part	Radionuclide	Qualifier	Qualifier
Ø Bone Marrow	1 Technetium 99m (Tc-99m) D Indium 111 (In-111) Y Other Radionuclide	Z None	Z None
2 Spleen 5 Lymphatics, Head and Neck D Lymphatics, Pelvic J Lymphatics, Head K Lymphatics, Neck L Lymphatics, Upper Chest M Lymphatics, Trunk N Lymphatics, Upper Extremity P Lymphatics, Lower Extremity	1 Technetium 99m (Tc-99m) Y Other Radionuclide	Z None	Z None
3 Blood	D Indium 111 (In-111) Y Other Radionuclide	Z None	Z None
Y Lymphatic and Hematologic System	Y Other Radionuclide	Z None	Z None

SECTION: C NUCLEAR MEDICINE

BODY SYSTEM: 7 LYMPHATIC AND HEMATOLOGIC SYSTEM

TYPE: 2 **TOMOGRAPHIC (TOMO) NUCLEAR MEDICINE IMAGING:** Introduction of radioactive materials into the body for three dimensional display of images developed from the capture of radioactive emissions

Body Part	Radionuclide	Qualifier	Qualifier
2 Spleen	1 Technetium 99m (Tc-99m) Y Other Radionuclide	Z None	Z None
Y Lymphatic and Hematologic System	Y Other Radionuclide	Z None	Z None

C: NUCLEAR MEDICINE

7: LYMPHATIC AND HEMATOLOGIC SYSTEM

1; 2

SECTION: C NUCLEAR MEDICINE
BODY SYSTEM: 7 LYMPHATIC AND HEMATOLOGIC SYSTEM
TYPE: 5 NONIMAGING NUCLEAR MEDICINE PROBE: Introduction of radioactive materials into the body for the study of distribution and fate of certain substances by the detection of radioactive emissions; or, alternatively, measurement of absorption of radioactive emissions from an external source

Body Part	Radionuclide	Qualifier	Qualifier
5 Lymphatics, Head and Neck D Lymphatics, Pelvic J Lymphatics, Head K Lymphatics, Neck L Lymphatics, Upper Chest M Lymphatics, Trunk N Lymphatics, Upper Extremity P Lymphatics, Lower Extremity	1 Technetium 99m (Tc-99m) Y Other Radionuclide	Z None	Z None
Y Lymphatic and Hematologic System	Y Other Radionuclide	Z None	Z None

SECTION: C NUCLEAR MEDICINE
BODY SYSTEM: 7 LYMPHATIC AND HEMATOLOGIC SYSTEM
TYPE: 6 NONIMAGING NUCLEAR MEDICINE ASSAY: Introduction of radioactive materials into the body for the study of body fluids and blood elements, by the detection of radioactive emissions

Body Part	Radionuclide	Qualifier	Qualifier
3 Blood	1 Technetium 99m (Tc-99m) 7 Cobalt 58 (Co-58) C Cobalt 57 (Co-57) D Indium 111 (In-111) H Iodine 125 (I-125) W Chromium (Cr-51) Y Other Radionuclide	Z None	Z None
Y Lymphatic and Hematologic System	Y Other Radionuclide	Z None	Z None

SECTION: C NUCLEAR MEDICINE
BODY SYSTEM: 8   EYE
TYPE: **1   PLANAR NUCLEAR MEDICINE IMAGING:** Introduction of radioactive materials into the body for single plane display of images developed from the capture of radioactive emissions

Body Part	Radionuclide	Qualifier	Qualifier
9 Lacrimal Ducts, Bilateral	1 Technetium 99m (Tc-99m) Y Other Radionuclide	Z None	Z None
Y Eye	Y Other Radionuclide	Z None	Z None

SECTION: C NUCLEAR MEDICINE
BODY SYSTEM: 9 EAR, NOSE, MOUTH, AND THROAT
TYPE: **1 PLANAR NUCLEAR MEDICINE IMAGING:** Introduction of radioactive materials into the body for single plane display of images developed from the capture of radioactive emissions

Body Part	Radionuclide	Qualifier	Qualifier
B Salivary Glands, Bilateral	1 Technetium 99m (Tc-99m) Y Other Radionuclide	Z None	Z None
Y Ear, Nose, Mouth and Throat	Y Other Radionuclide	Z None	Z None

SECTION: C NUCLEAR MEDICINE
BODY SYSTEM: B RESPIRATORY SYSTEM
TYPE: 1 **PLANAR NUCLEAR MEDICINE IMAGING:** Introduction of radioactive materials into the body for single plane display of images developed from the capture of radioactive emissions

Body Part	Radionuclide	Qualifier	Qualifier
2 Lungs and Bronchi	1 Technetium 99m (Tc-99m) 9 Krypton (Kr-81m) T Xenon 127 (Xe-127) V Xenon 133 (Xe-133) Y Other Radionuclide	Z None	Z None
Y Respiratory System	Y Other Radionuclide	Z None	Z None

SECTION: C NUCLEAR MEDICINE
BODY SYSTEM: B RESPIRATORY SYSTEM
TYPE: 2 **TOMOGRAPHIC (TOMO) NUCLEAR MEDICINE IMAGING:** Introduction of radioactive materials into the body for three dimensional display of images developed from the capture of radioactive emissions

Body Part	Radionuclide	Qualifier	Qualifier
2 Lungs and Bronchi	1 Technetium 99m (Tc-99m) 9 Krypton (Kr-81m) Y Other Radionuclide	Z None	Z None
Y Respiratory System	Y Other Radionuclide	Z None	Z None

SECTION: C NUCLEAR MEDICINE
BODY SYSTEM: B RESPIRATORY SYSTEM
TYPE: 3 **POSITRON EMISSION TOMOGRAPHIC (PET) IMAGING:** Introduction of radioactive materials into the body for three dimensional display of images developed from the simultaneous capture, 18Ø degrees apart, of radioactive emissions

Body Part	Radionuclide	Qualifier	Qualifier
2 Lungs and Bronchi	K Fluorine 18 (F-18) Y Other Radionuclide	Z None	Z None
Y Respiratory System	Y Other Radionuclide	Z None	Z None

SECTION: C NUCLEAR MEDICINE
BODY SYSTEM: D GASTROINTESTINAL SYSTEM
TYPE: 1 **PLANAR NUCLEAR MEDICINE IMAGING:** Introduction of radioactive materials into the body for single plane display of images developed from the capture of radioactive emissions

Body Part	Radionuclide	Qualifier	Qualifier
5 Upper Gastrointestinal Tract 7 Gastrointestinal Tract	1 Technetium 99m (Tc-99m) D Indium 111 (In-111) Y Other Radionuclide	Z None	Z None
Y Digestive System	Y Other Radionuclide	Z None	Z None

SECTION: C NUCLEAR MEDICINE
BODY SYSTEM: D GASTROINTESTINAL SYSTEM
TYPE: 2 **TOMOGRAPHIC (TOMO) NUCLEAR MEDICINE IMAGING:** Introduction of radioactive materials into the body for three dimensional display of images developed from the capture of radioactive emissions

Body Part	Radionuclide	Qualifier	Qualifier
7 Gastrointestinal Tract	1 Technetium 99m (Tc-99m) D Indium 111 (In-111) Y Other Radionuclide	Z None	Z None
Y Digestive System	Y Other Radionuclide	Z None	Z None

D: GASTROINTESTINAL SYSTEM

C: NUCLEAR MEDICINE

1; 2

New/Revised Text in Green ~~deleted~~ Deleted ♀ Females Only ♂ Males Only **Coding Clinic**
Non-covered Limited Coverage ⊟ Combination (See Appendix E) DRG Non-OR Non-OR Hospital-Acquired Condition

SECTION: C NUCLEAR MEDICINE

BODY SYSTEM: F HEPATOBILIARY SYSTEM AND PANCREAS

TYPE: 1 PLANAR NUCLEAR MEDICINE IMAGING: Introduction of radioactive materials into the body for single plane display of images developed from the capture of radioactive emissions

Body Part	Radionuclide	Qualifier	Qualifier
4 Gallbladder 5 Liver 6 Liver and Spleen C Hepatobiliary System, All	1 Technetium 99m (Tc-99m) Y Other Radionuclide	Z None	Z None
Y Hepatobiliary System and Pancreas	Y Other Radionuclide	Z None	Z None

SECTION: C NUCLEAR MEDICINE

BODY SYSTEM: F HEPATOBILIARY SYSTEM AND PANCREAS

TYPE: 2 TOMOGRAPHIC (TOMO) NUCLEAR MEDICINE IMAGING: Introduction of radioactive materials into the body for three dimensional display of images developed from the capture of radioactive emissions

Body Part	Radionuclide	Qualifier	Qualifier
4 Gallbladder 5 Liver 6 Liver and Spleen	1 Technetium 99m (Tc-99m) Y Other Radionuclide	Z None	Z None
Y Hepatobiliary System and Pancreas	Y Other Radionuclide	Z None	Z None

SECTION: C NUCLEAR MEDICINE
BODY SYSTEM: G ENDOCRINE SYSTEM
TYPE: **1 PLANAR NUCLEAR MEDICINE IMAGING:** Introduction of radioactive materials into the body for single plane display of images developed from the capture of radioactive emissions

Body Part	Radionuclide	Qualifier	Qualifier
1 Parathyroid Glands	1 Technetium 99m (Tc-99m) S Thallium 201 (Tl-201) Y Other Radionuclide	Z None	Z None
2 Thyroid Gland	1 Technetium 99m (Tc-99m) F Iodine 123 (I-123) G Iodine 131 (I-131) Y Other Radionuclide	Z None	Z None
4 Adrenal Glands, Bilateral	G Iodine 131 (I-131) Y Other Radionuclide	Z None	Z None
Y Endocrine System	Y Other Radionuclide	Z None	Z None

SECTION: C NUCLEAR MEDICINE
BODY SYSTEM: G ENDOCRINE SYSTEM
TYPE: **2 TOMOGRAPHIC (TOMO) NUCLEAR MEDICINE IMAGING:** Introduction of radioactive materials into the body for three dimensional display of images developed from the capture of radioactive emissions

Body Part	Radionuclide	Qualifier	Qualifier
1 Parathyroid Glands	1 Technetium 99m (Tc-99m) S Thallium 201 (Tl-201) Y Other Radionuclide	Z None	Z None
Y Endocrine System	Y Other Radionuclide	Z None	Z None

SECTION: C NUCLEAR MEDICINE
BODY SYSTEM: G ENDOCRINE SYSTEM
TYPE: **4 NONIMAGING NUCLEAR MEDICINE UPTAKE:** Introduction of radioactive materials into the body for measurements of organ function, from the detection of radioactive emissions

Body Part	Radionuclide	Qualifier	Qualifier
2 Thyroid Gland	1 Technetium 99m (Tc-99m) F Iodine 123 (I-123) G Iodine 131 (I-131) Y Other Radionuclide	Z None	Z None
Y Endocrine System	Y Other Radionuclide	Z None	Z None

New/Revised Text in Green　~~deleted~~ Deleted　♀ Females Only　♂ Males Only　**Coding Clinic**
🦘 Non-covered　🦘 Limited Coverage　⊡ Combination (See Appendix E)　DRG Non-OR　Non-OR　🦘 Hospital-Acquired Condition

C: NUCLEAR MEDICINE　G: ENDOCRINE SYSTEM　1; 2; 4

SECTION: C NUCLEAR MEDICINE

BODY SYSTEM: H SKIN, SUBCUTANEOUS TISSUE AND BREAST

TYPE: 1 **PLANAR NUCLEAR MEDICINE IMAGING:** Introduction of radioactive materials into the body for single plane display of images developed from the capture of radioactive emissions

Body Part	Radionuclide	Qualifier	Qualifier
Ø Breast, Right 1 Breast, Left 2 Breasts, Bilateral	1 Technetium 99m (Tc-99m) S Thallium 201 (Tl-201) Y Other Radionuclide	Z None	Z None
Y Skin, Subcutaneous Tissue, and Breast	Y Other Radionuclide	Z None	Z None

SECTION: C NUCLEAR MEDICINE

BODY SYSTEM: H SKIN, SUBCUTANEOUS TISSUE AND BREAST

TYPE: 2 **TOMOGRAPHIC (TOMO) NUCLEAR MEDICINE IMAGING:** Introduction of radioactive materials into the body for three dimensional display of images developed from the capture of radioactive emissions

Body Part	Radionuclide	Qualifier	Qualifier
Ø Breast, Right 1 Breast, Left 2 Breasts, Bilateral	1 Technetium 99m (Tc-99m) S Thallium 201 (Tl-201) Y Other Radionuclide	Z None	Z None
Y Skin, Subcutaneous Tissue, and Breast	Y Other Radionuclide	Z None	Z None

C: NUCLEAR MEDICINE

H: SKIN, SUBCUTANEOUS TISSUE AND BREAST

1; 2

SECTION: **C NUCLEAR MEDICINE**
BODY SYSTEM: P MUSCULOSKELETAL SYSTEM
TYPE: **1 PLANAR NUCLEAR MEDICINE IMAGING:** Introduction of radioactive materials into the body for single plane display of images developed from the capture of radioactive emissions

Body Part	Radionuclide	Qualifier	Qualifier
1 Skull 4 Thorax 5 Spine 6 Pelvis 7 Spine and Pelvis 8 Upper Extremity, Right 9 Upper Extremity, Left B Upper Extremities, Bilateral C Lower Extremity, Right D Lower Extremity, Left F Lower Extremities, Bilateral Z Musculoskeletal System, All	1 Technetium 99m (Tc-99m) Y Other Radionuclide	Z None	Z None
Y Musculoskeletal System, Other	Y Other Radionuclide	Z None	Z None

SECTION: **C NUCLEAR MEDICINE**
BODY SYSTEM: P MUSCULOSKELETAL SYSTEM
TYPE: **2 TOMOGRAPHIC (TOMO) NUCLEAR MEDICINE IMAGING:** Introduction of radioactive materials into the body for three dimensional display of images developed from the capture of radioactive emissions

Body Part	Radionuclide	Qualifier	Qualifier
1 Skull 2 Cervical Spine 3 Skull and Cervical Spine 4 Thorax 6 Pelvis 7 Spine and Pelvis 8 Upper Extremity, Right 9 Upper Extremity, Left B Upper Extremities, Bilateral C Lower Extremity, Right D Lower Extremity, Left F Lower Extremities, Bilateral G Thoracic Spine H Lumbar Spine J Thoracolumbar Spine	1 Technetium 99m (Tc-99m) Y Other Radionuclide	Z None	Z None
Y Musculoskeletal System, Other	Y Other Radionuclide	Z None	Z None

SECTION: C NUCLEAR MEDICINE
BODY SYSTEM: P MUSCULOSKELETAL SYSTEM
TYPE: 5 NONIMAGING NUCLEAR MEDICINE PROBE: Introduction of radioactive materials into the body for the study of distribution and fate of certain substances by the detection of radioactive emissions; or, alternatively, measurement of absorption of radioactive emissions from an external source

Body Part	Radionuclide	Qualifier	Qualifier
5 Spine N Upper Extremities P Lower Extremities	Z None	Z None	Z None
Y Musculoskeletal System, Other	Y Other Radionuclide	Z None	Z None

SECTION: C NUCLEAR MEDICINE
BODY SYSTEM: T URINARY SYSTEM
TYPE: 1 **PLANAR NUCLEAR MEDICINE IMAGING:** Introduction of radioactive materials into the body for single plane display of images developed from the capture of radioactive emissions

Body Part	Radionuclide	Qualifier	Qualifier
3 Kidneys, Ureters, and Bladder	1 Technetium 99m (Tc-99m) F Iodine 123 (I-123) G Iodine 131 (I-131) Y Other Radionuclide	Z None	Z None
H Bladder and Ureters	1 Technetium 99m (Tc-99m) Y Other Radionuclide	Z None	Z None
Y Urinary System	Y Other Radionuclide	Z None	Z None

SECTION: C NUCLEAR MEDICINE
BODY SYSTEM: T URINARY SYSTEM
TYPE: 2 **TOMOGRAPHIC (TOMO) NUCLEAR MEDICINE IMAGING:** Introduction of radioactive materials into the body for three dimensional display of images developed from the capture of radioactive emissions

Body Part	Radionuclide	Qualifier	Qualifier
3 Kidneys, Ureters, and Bladder	1 Technetium 99m (Tc-99m) Y Other Radionuclide	Z None	Z None
Y Urinary System	Y Other Radionuclide	Z None	Z None

SECTION: C NUCLEAR MEDICINE
BODY SYSTEM: T URINARY SYSTEM
TYPE: 6 **NONIMAGING NUCLEAR MEDICINE ASSAY:** Introduction of radioactive materials into the body for the study of body fluids and blood elements, by the detection of radioactive emissions

Body Part	Radionuclide	Qualifier	Qualifier
3 Kidneys, Ureters, and Bladder	1 Technetium 99m (Tc-99m) F Iodine 123 (I-123) G Iodine 131 (I-131) H Iodine 125 (I-125) Y Other Radionuclide	Z None	Z None
Y Urinary System	Y Other Radionuclide	Z None	Z None

SECTION: C NUCLEAR MEDICINE
BODY SYSTEM: V MALE REPRODUCTIVE SYSTEM
TYPE: 1 **PLANAR NUCLEAR MEDICINE IMAGING:** Introduction of radioactive materials into the body for single plane display of images developed from the capture of radioactive emissions

Body Part	Radionuclide	Qualifier	Qualifier
9 Testicles, Bilateral ♂	1 Technetium 99m (Tc-99m) Y Other Radionuclide	Z None	Z None
Y Male Reproductive System ♂	Y Other Radionuclide	Z None	Z None

SECTION: **C NUCLEAR MEDICINE**

BODY SYSTEM: **W ANATOMICAL REGIONS**

TYPE: **1 PLANAR NUCLEAR MEDICINE IMAGING:** Introduction of radioactive materials into the body for single plane display of images developed from the capture of radioactive emissions

Body Part	Radionuclide	Qualifier	Qualifier
Ø Abdomen 1 Abdomen and Pelvis 4 Chest and Abdomen 6 Chest and Neck B Head and Neck D Lower Extremity J Pelvic Region M Upper Extremity N Whole Body	1 Technetium 99m (Tc-99m) D Indium 111 (In-111) F Iodine 123 (I-123) G Iodine 131 (I-131) L Gallium 67 (Ga-67) S Thallium 201 (Tl-201) Y Other Radionuclide	Z None	Z None
3 Chest	1 Technetium 99m (Tc-99m) D Indium 111 (In-111) F Iodine 123 (I-123) G Iodine 131 (I-131) K Fluorine 18 (F-18) L Gallium 67 (Ga-67) S Thallium 201 (Tl-201) Y Other Radionuclide	Z None	Z None
Y Anatomical Regions, Multiple	Y Other Radionuclide	Z None	Z None
Z Anatomical Region, Other	Z None	Z None	Z None

SECTION: **C NUCLEAR MEDICINE**

BODY SYSTEM: **W ANATOMICAL REGIONS**

TYPE: **2 TOMOGRAPHIC (TOMO) NUCLEAR MEDICINE IMAGING:** Introduction of radioactive materials into the body for three dimensional display of images developed from the capture of radioactive emissions

Body Part	Radionuclide	Qualifier	Qualifier
Ø Abdomen 1 Abdomen and Pelvis 3 Chest 4 Chest and Abdomen 6 Chest and Neck B Head and Neck D Lower Extremity J Pelvic Region M Upper Extremity	1 Technetium 99m (Tc-99m) D Indium 111 (In-111) F Iodine 123 (I-123) G Iodine 131 (I-131) K Fluorine 18 (F-18) L Gallium 67 (Ga-67) S Thallium 201 (Tl-201) Y Other Radionuclide	Z None	Z None
Y Anatomical Regions, Multiple	Y Other Radionuclide	Z None	Z None

New/Revised Text in Green   ~~deleted~~ Deleted   ♀ Females Only   ♂ Males Only   **Coding Clinic**

⬥ Non-covered   ⬥ Limited Coverage   ⊞ Combination (See Appendix E)   DRG Non-OR   Non-OR   ⬥ Hospital-Acquired Condition

SECTION: C NUCLEAR MEDICINE

BODY SYSTEM: W ANATOMICAL REGIONS
TYPE: 3 **POSITRON EMISSION TOMOGRAPHIC (PET) IMAGING:** Introduction of radioactive materials into the body for three dimensional display of images developed from the simultaneous capture, 18Ø degrees apart, of radioactive emissions

Body Part	Radionuclide	Qualifier	Qualifier
N Whole Body	Y Other Radionuclide	Z None	Z None

SECTION: C NUCLEAR MEDICINE

BODY SYSTEM: W ANATOMICAL REGIONS
TYPE: 5 **NONIMAGING NUCLEAR MEDICINE PROBE:** Introduction of radioactive materials into the body for the study of distribution and fate of certain substances by the detection of radioactive emissions; or, alternatively, measurement of absorption of radioactive emissions from an external source

Body Part	Radionuclide	Qualifier	Qualifier
Ø Abdomen 1 Abdomen and Pelvis 3 Chest 4 Chest and Abdomen 6 Chest and Neck B Head and Neck D Lower Extremity J Pelvic Region M Upper Extremity	1 Technetium 99m (Tc-99m) D Indium 111 (In-111) Y Other Radionuclide	Z None	Z None

SECTION: C NUCLEAR MEDICINE

BODY SYSTEM: W ANATOMICAL REGIONS
TYPE: 7 **SYSTEMIC NUCLEAR MEDICINE THERAPY:** Introduction of unsealed radioactive materials into the body for treatment

Body Part	Radionuclide	Qualifier	Qualifier
Ø Abdomen 3 Chest	N Phosphorus 32 (P-32) Y Other Radionuclide	Z None	Z None
G Thyroid	G Iodine 131 (I-131) Y Other Radionuclide	Z None	Z None
N Whole Body	8 Samarium 153 (Sm-153) G Iodine 131 (I-131) N Phosphorus 32 (P-32) P Strontium 89 (Sr-89) Y Other Radionuclide	Z None	Z None
Y Anatomical Regions, Multiple	Y Other Radionuclide	Z None	Z None

New/Revised Text in Green ~~deleted~~ Deleted ♀ Females Only ♂ Males Only **Coding Clinic**

🔖 Non-covered 🔖 Limited Coverage ⊡ Combination (See Appendix E) DRG Non-OR Non-OR 🔖 Hospital-Acquired Condition

SECTION: D RADIATION THERAPY

BODY SYSTEM: 0 CENTRAL AND PERIPHERAL NERVOUS SYSTEM
MODALITY: 0 BEAM RADIATION

Treatment Site	Modality Qualifier	Isotope	Qualifier
0 Brain 1 Brain Stem 6 Spinal Cord 7 Peripheral Nerve	0 Photons <1 MeV 1 Photons 1 - 10 MeV 2 Photons >10 MeV 4 Heavy Particles (Protons, Ions) 5 Neutrons 6 Neutron Capture	Z None	Z None
0 Brain 1 Brain Stem 6 Spinal Cord 7 Peripheral Nerve	3 Electrons	Z None	0 Intraoperative Z None

SECTION: D RADIATION THERAPY

BODY SYSTEM: 0 CENTRAL AND PERIPHERAL NERVOUS SYSTEM
MODALITY: 1 BRACHYTHERAPY

Treatment Site	Modality Qualifier	Isotope	Qualifier
0 Brain 1 Brain Stem 6 Spinal Cord 7 Peripheral Nerve	9 High Dose Rate (HDR) B Low Dose Rate (LDR)	7 Cesium 137 (Cs-137) 8 Iridium 192 (Ir-192) 9 Iodine 125 (I-125) B Palladium 103 (Pd-103) C Californium 252 (Cf-252) Y Other Isotope	Z None

SECTION: D RADIATION THERAPY

BODY SYSTEM: 0 CENTRAL AND PERIPHERAL NERVOUS SYSTEM
MODALITY: 2 STEREOTACTIC RADIOSURGERY

Treatment Site	Modality Qualifier	Isotope	Qualifier
0 Brain 1 Brain Stem 6 Spinal Cord 7 Peripheral Nerve	D Stereotactic Other Photon Radiosurgery H Stereotactic Particulate Radiosurgery J Stereotactic Gamma Beam Radiosurgery	Z None	Z None

DRG Non-OR All Values

SECTION: D RADIATION THERAPY

BODY SYSTEM: 0 CENTRAL AND PERIPHERAL NERVOUS SYSTEM
MODALITY: Y OTHER RADIATION

Treatment Site	Modality Qualifier	Isotope	Qualifier
0 Brain 1 Brain Stem 6 Spinal Cord 7 Peripheral Nerve	7 Contact Radiation 8 Hyperthermia F Plaque Radiation K Laser Interstitial Thermal Therapy	Z None	Z None

New/Revised Text in Green ~~deleted~~ Deleted ♀ Females Only ♂ Males Only **Coding Clinic**
🔖 Non-covered 🔖 Limited Coverage ⊡ Combination (See Appendix E) DRG Non-OR Non-OR 🔖 Hospital-Acquired Condition

SECTION: D RADIATION THERAPY

BODY SYSTEM: 7 LYMPHATIC AND HEMATOLOGIC SYSTEM
MODALITY: Ø BEAM RADIATION

Treatment Site	Modality Qualifier	Isotope	Qualifier
Ø Bone Marrow 1 Thymus 2 Spleen 3 Lymphatics, Neck 4 Lymphatics, Axillary 5 Lymphatics, Thorax 6 Lymphatics, Abdomen 7 Lymphatics, Pelvis 8 Lymphatics, Inguinal	Ø Photons <1 MeV 1 Photons 1 - 10 MeV 2 Photons >10 MeV 4 Heavy Particles (Protons, Ions) 5 Neutrons 6 Neutron Capture	Z None	Z None
Ø Bone Marrow 1 Thymus 2 Spleen 3 Lymphatics, Neck 4 Lymphatics, Axillary 5 Lymphatics, Thorax 6 Lymphatics, Abdomen 7 Lymphatics, Pelvis 8 Lymphatics, Inguinal	3 Electrons	Z None	Ø Intraoperative Z None

SECTION: D RADIATION THERAPY

BODY SYSTEM: 7 LYMPHATIC AND HEMATOLOGIC SYSTEM
MODALITY: 1 BRACHYTHERAPY

Treatment Site	Modality Qualifier	Isotope	Qualifier
Ø Bone Marrow 1 Thymus 2 Spleen 3 Lymphatics, Neck 4 Lymphatics, Axillary 5 Lymphatics, Thorax 6 Lymphatics, Abdomen 7 Lymphatics, Pelvis 8 Lymphatics, Inguinal	9 High Dose Rate (HDR) B Low Dose Rate (LDR)	7 Cesium 137 (Cs-137) 8 Iridium 192 (Ir-192) 9 Iodine 125 (I-125) B Palladium 103 (Pd-103) C Californium 252 (Cf-252) Y Other Isotope	Z None

SECTION: D RADIATION THERAPY
BODY SYSTEM: 7 LYMPHATIC AND HEMATOLOGIC SYSTEM
MODALITY: 2 STEREOTACTIC RADIOSURGERY

Treatment Site	Modality Qualifier	Isotope	Qualifier

Ø Bone Marrow
1 Thymus
2 Spleen
3 Lymphatics, Neck
4 Lymphatics, Axillary
5 Lymphatics, Thorax
6 Lymphatics, Abdomen
7 Lymphatics, Pelvis
8 Lymphatics, Inguinal
	D Stereotactic Other Photon
	  Radiosurgery
	H Stereotactic Particulate
	  Radiosurgery
	J Stereotactic Gamma Beam
	  Radiosurgery
		Z None	Z None

`DRG Non-OR` All Values

SECTION: D RADIATION THERAPY
BODY SYSTEM: 7 LYMPHATIC AND HEMATOLOGIC SYSTEM
MODALITY: Y OTHER RADIATION

Treatment Site	Modality Qualifier	Isotope	Qualifier
Ø Bone Marrow 1 Thymus 2 Spleen 3 Lymphatics, Neck 4 Lymphatics, Axillary 5 Lymphatics, Thorax 6 Lymphatics, Abdomen 7 Lymphatics, Pelvis 8 Lymphatics, Inguinal	8 Hyperthermia F Plaque Radiation	Z None	Z None

SECTION: D RADIATION THERAPY
BODY SYSTEM: 8 EYE
MODALITY: Ø BEAM RADIATION

Treatment Site	Modality Qualifier	Isotope	Qualifier
Ø Eye	Ø Photons <1 MeV 1 Photons 1 - 1Ø MeV 2 Photons >1Ø MeV 4 Heavy Particles (Protons, Ions) 5 Neutrons 6 Neutron Capture	Z None	Z None
Ø Eye	3 Electrons	Z None	Ø Intraoperative Z None

SECTION: D RADIATION THERAPY
BODY SYSTEM: 8 EYE
MODALITY: 1 BRACHYTHERAPY

Treatment Site	Modality Qualifier	Isotope	Qualifier
Ø Eye	9 High Dose Rate (HDR) B Low Dose Rate (LDR)	7 Cesium 137 (Cs-137) 8 Iridium 192 (Ir-192) 9 Iodine 125 (I-125) B Palladium 1Ø3 (Pd-1Ø3) C Californium 252 (Cf-252) Y Other Isotope	Z None

SECTION: D RADIATION THERAPY
BODY SYSTEM: 8 EYE
MODALITY: 2 STEREOTACTIC RADIOSURGERY

Treatment Site	Modality Qualifier	Isotope	Qualifier
Ø Eye	D Stereotactic Other Photon Radiosurgery H Stereotactic Particulate Radiosurgery J Stereotactic Gamma Beam Radiosurgery	Z None	Z None

`DRG Non-OR` All Values

SECTION: D RADIATION THERAPY
BODY SYSTEM: 8 EYE
MODALITY: Y OTHER RADIATION

Treatment Site	Modality Qualifier	Isotope	Qualifier
Ø Eye	7 Contact Radiation 8 Hyperthermia F Plaque Radiation	Z None	Z None

New/Revised Text in Green ~~deleted~~ Deleted ♀ Females Only ♂ Males Only **Coding Clinic**
🚫 Non-covered 🚫 Limited Coverage ⊡ Combination (See Appendix E) `DRG Non-OR` Non-OR 🚫 Hospital-Acquired Condition

SECTION: D RADIATION THERAPY

BODY SYSTEM: 9 EAR, NOSE, MOUTH, AND THROAT
MODALITY: Ø BEAM RADIATION

Treatment Site	Modality Qualifier	Isotope	Qualifier
Ø Ear 1 Nose 3 Hypopharynx 4 Mouth 5 Tongue 6 Salivary Glands 7 Sinuses 8 Hard Palate 9 Soft Palate B Larynx D Nasopharynx F Oropharynx	Ø Photons <1 MeV 1 Photons 1 - 1Ø MeV 2 Photons >1Ø MeV 4 Heavy Particles (Protons, Ions) 5 Neutrons 6 Neutron Capture	Z None	Z None
Ø Ear 1 Nose 3 Hypopharynx 4 Mouth 5 Tongue 6 Salivary Glands 7 Sinuses 8 Hard Palate 9 Soft Palate B Larynx D Nasopharynx F Oropharynx	3 Electrons	Z None	Ø Intraoperative Z None

SECTION: D RADIATION THERAPY

BODY SYSTEM: 9 EAR, NOSE, MOUTH, AND THROAT
MODALITY: 1 BRACHYTHERAPY

Treatment Site	Modality Qualifier	Isotope	Qualifier
Ø Ear 1 Nose 3 Hypopharynx 4 Mouth 5 Tongue 6 Salivary Glands 7 Sinuses 8 Hard Palate 9 Soft Palate B Larynx D Nasopharynx F Oropharynx	9 High Dose Rate (HDR) B Low Dose Rate (LDR)	7 Cesium 137 (Cs-137) 8 Iridium 192 (Ir-192) 9 Iodine 125 (I-125) B Palladium 1Ø3 (Pd-1Ø3) C Californium 252 (Cf-252) Y Other Isotope	Z None

New/Revised Text in Green   ~~deleted~~ Deleted   ♀ Females Only   ♂ Males Only   **Coding Clinic**
Non-covered   Limited Coverage   ⊞ Combination (See Appendix E)   DRG Non-OR   Non-OR   Hospital-Acquired Condition

SECTION: D RADIATION THERAPY
BODY SYSTEM: 9 EAR, NOSE, MOUTH, AND THROAT
MODALITY: 2 STEREOTACTIC RADIOSURGERY

Treatment Site	Modality Qualifier	Isotope	Qualifier

Ø Ear
1 Nose
4 Mouth
5 Tongue
6 Salivary Glands
7 Sinuses
8 Hard Palate
9 Soft Palate
B Larynx
C Pharynx
D Nasopharynx
	D Stereotactic Other Photon
	  Radiosurgery
	H Stereotactic Particulate
	  Radiosurgery
	J Stereotactic Gamma Beam
	  Radiosurgery
		Z None	Z None

DRG Non-OR All Values

SECTION: D RADIATION THERAPY
BODY SYSTEM: 9 EAR, NOSE, MOUTH, AND THROAT
MODALITY: Y OTHER RADIATION

Treatment Site	Modality Qualifier	Isotope	Qualifier
Ø Ear 1 Nose 5 Tongue 6 Salivary Glands 7 Sinuses 8 Hard Palate 9 Soft Palate	7 Contact Radiation 8 Hyperthermia F Plaque Radiation	Z None	Z None
3 Hypopharynx F Oropharynx	7 Contact Radiation 8 Hyperthermia	Z None	Z None
4 Mouth B Larynx D Nasopharynx	7 Contact Radiation 8 Hyperthermia C Intraoperative Radiation Therapy (IORT) F Plaque Radiation	Z None	Z None
C Pharynx	C Intraoperative Radiation Therapy (IORT) F Plaque Radiation	Z None	Z None

New/Revised Text in Green   deleted Deleted   ♀ Females Only   ♂ Males Only   Coding Clinic
🚫 Non-covered   🚫 Limited Coverage   ⊕ Combination (See Appendix E)   DRG Non-OR   Non-OR   🚫 Hospital-Acquired Condition

633

SECTION: D RADIATION THERAPY

BODY SYSTEM: B RESPIRATORY SYSTEM
MODALITY: Ø BEAM RADIATION

Treatment Site	Modality Qualifier	Isotope	Qualifier
Ø Trachea 1 Bronchus 2 Lung 5 Pleura 6 Mediastinum 7 Chest Wall 8 Diaphragm	Ø Photons <1 MeV 1 Photons 1 - 1Ø MeV 2 Photons >1Ø MeV 4 Heavy Particles (Protons, Ions) 5 Neutrons 6 Neutron Capture	Z None	Z None
Ø Trachea 1 Bronchus 2 Lung 5 Pleura 6 Mediastinum 7 Chest Wall 8 Diaphragm	3 Electrons	Z None	Ø Intraoperative Z None

SECTION: D RADIATION THERAPY

BODY SYSTEM: B RESPIRATORY SYSTEM
MODALITY: 1 BRACHYTHERAPY

Treatment Site	Modality Qualifier	Isotope	Qualifier
Ø Trachea 1 Bronchus 2 Lung 5 Pleura 6 Mediastinum 7 Chest Wall 8 Diaphragm	9 High Dose Rate (HDR) B Low Dose Rate (LDR)	7 Cesium 137 (Cs-137) 8 Iridium 192 (Ir-192) 9 Iodine 125 (I-125) B Palladium 1Ø3 (Pd-1Ø3) C Californium 252 (Cf-252) Y Other Isotope	Z None

B: RESPIRATORY SYSTEM

Ø; 1

D: RADIATION THERAPY

SECTION: D RADIATION THERAPY
BODY SYSTEM: B RESPIRATORY SYSTEM
MODALITY: 2 STEREOTACTIC RADIOSURGERY

Treatment Site	Modality Qualifier	Isotope	Qualifier

Ø Trachea
1 Bronchus
2 Lung
5 Pleura
6 Mediastinum
7 Chest Wall
8 Diaphragm
	D Stereotactic Other Photon
	  Radiosurgery
	H Stereotactic Particulate
	  Radiosurgery
	J Stereotactic Gamma Beam
	  Radiosurgery
		Z None	Z None

`DRG Non-OR` All Values

SECTION: D RADIATION THERAPY
BODY SYSTEM: B RESPIRATORY SYSTEM
MODALITY: Y OTHER RADIATION

Treatment Site	Modality Qualifier	Isotope	Qualifier
Ø Trachea 1 Bronchus 2 Lung 5 Pleura 6 Mediastinum 7 Chest Wall 8 Diaphragm	7 Contact Radiation 8 Hyperthermia F Plaque Radiation K Laser Interstitial Thermal Therapy	Z None	Z None

D: RADIATION THERAPY

B: RESPIRATORY SYSTEM

2; Y

SECTION: D RADIATION THERAPY
BODY SYSTEM: D GASTROINTESTINAL SYSTEM
MODALITY: Ø BEAM RADIATION

Treatment Site	Modality Qualifier	Isotope	Qualifier
Ø Esophagus 1 Stomach 2 Duodenum 3 Jejunum 4 Ileum 5 Colon 7 Rectum	Ø Photons <1 MeV 1 Photons 1 - 1Ø MeV 2 Photons >1Ø MeV 4 Heavy Particles (Protons, Ions) 5 Neutrons 6 Neutron Capture	Z None	Z None
Ø Esophagus 1 Stomach 2 Duodenum 3 Jejunum 4 Ileum 5 Colon 7 Rectum	3 Electrons	Z None	Ø Intraoperative Z None

SECTION: D RADIATION THERAPY
BODY SYSTEM: D GASTROINTESTINAL SYSTEM
MODALITY: 1 BRACHYTHERAPY

Treatment Site	Modality Qualifier	Isotope	Qualifier
Ø Esophagus 1 Stomach 2 Duodenum 3 Jejunum 4 Ileum 5 Colon 7 Rectum	9 High Dose Rate (HDR) B Low Dose Rate (LDR)	7 Cesium 137 (Cs-137) 8 Iridium 192 (Ir-192) 9 Iodine 125 (I-125) B Palladium 1Ø3 (Pd-1Ø3) C Californium 252 (Cf-252) Y Other Isotope	Z None

New/Revised Text in Green ~~deleted~~ Deleted ♀ Females Only ♂ Males Only **Coding Clinic**
Non-covered Limited Coverage ⊞ Combination (See Appendix E) DRG Non-OR Non-OR Hospital-Acquired Condition

D: GASTROINTESTINAL SYSTEM
D: RADIATION THERAPY
Ø; 1

SECTION: D RADIATION THERAPY
BODY SYSTEM: D GASTROINTESTINAL SYSTEM
MODALITY: 2 STEREOTACTIC RADIOSURGERY

Treatment Site	Modality Qualifier	Isotope	Qualifier

Ø Esophagus
1 Stomach
2 Duodenum
3 Jejunum
4 Ileum
5 Colon
7 Rectum
	D Stereotactic Other Photon
	  Radiosurgery
	H Stereotactic Particulate
	  Radiosurgery
	J Stereotactic Gamma Beam
	  Radiosurgery
		Z None	Z None

DRG Non-OR All Values

SECTION: D RADIATION THERAPY
BODY SYSTEM: D GASTROINTESTINAL SYSTEM
MODALITY: Y OTHER RADIATION

Treatment Site	Modality Qualifier	Isotope	Qualifier
Ø Esophagus	7 Contact Radiation 8 Hyperthermia F Plaque Radiation K Laser Interstitial Thermal Therapy	Z None	Z None

1 Stomach
2 Duodenum
3 Jejunum
4 Ileum
5 Colon
7 Rectum
	7 Contact Radiation
	8 Hyperthermia
	C Intraoperative Radiation
	  Therapy (IORT)
	F Plaque Radiation
	K Laser Interstitial Thermal
	  Therapy
		Z None	Z None

8 Anus	C Intraoperative Radiation
	  Therapy (IORT)
	F Plaque Radiation
	K Laser Interstitial Thermal
	  Therapy
		Z None	Z None

SECTION: D RADIATION THERAPY
BODY SYSTEM: F HEPATOBILIARY SYSTEM AND PANCREAS
MODALITY: Ø BEAM RADIATION

Treatment Site	Modality Qualifier	Isotope	Qualifier
Ø Liver 1 Gallbladder 2 Bile Ducts 3 Pancreas	Ø Photons <1 MeV 1 Photons 1 - 1Ø MeV 2 Photons >1Ø MeV 4 Heavy Particles (Protons, Ions) 5 Neutrons 6 Neutron Capture	Z None	Z None
Ø Liver 1 Gallbladder 2 Bile Ducts 3 Pancreas	3 Electrons	Z None	Ø Intraoperative Z None

SECTION: D RADIATION THERAPY
BODY SYSTEM: F HEPATOBILIARY SYSTEM AND PANCREAS
MODALITY: 1 BRACHYTHERAPY

Treatment Site	Modality Qualifier	Isotope	Qualifier
Ø Liver 1 Gallbladder 2 Bile Ducts 3 Pancreas	9 High Dose Rate (HDR) B Low Dose Rate (LDR)	7 Cesium 137 (Cs-137) 8 Iridium 192 (Ir-192) 9 Iodine 125 (I-125) B Palladium 1Ø3 (Pd-1Ø3) C Californium 252 (Cf-252) Y Other Isotope	Z None

SECTION: D RADIATION THERAPY
BODY SYSTEM: F HEPATOBILIARY SYSTEM AND PANCREAS
MODALITY: 2 STEREOTACTIC RADIOSURGERY

Treatment Site	Modality Qualifier	Isotope	Qualifier
Ø Liver 1 Gallbladder 2 Bile Ducts 3 Pancreas	D Stereotactic Other Photon Radiosurgery H Stereotactic Particulate Radiosurgery J Stereotactic Gamma Beam Radiosurgery	Z None	Z None

DRG Non-OR   All Values

SECTION: D RADIATION THERAPY
BODY SYSTEM: F HEPATOBILIARY SYSTEM AND PANCREAS
MODALITY: Y OTHER RADIATION

Treatment Site	Modality Qualifier	Isotope	Qualifier
Ø Liver 1 Gallbladder 2 Bile Ducts 3 Pancreas	7 Contact Radiation 8 Hyperthermia C Intraoperative Radiation Therapy (IORT) F Plaque Radiation K Laser Interstitial Thermal Therapy	Z None	Z None

SECTION: D RADIATION THERAPY
BODY SYSTEM: G ENDOCRINE SYSTEM
MODALITY: Ø BEAM RADIATION

Treatment Site	Modality Qualifier	Isotope	Qualifier
Ø Pituitary Gland 1 Pineal Body 2 Adrenal Glands 4 Parathyroid Glands 5 Thyroid	Ø Photons <1 MeV 1 Photons 1 - 1Ø MeV 2 Photons >1Ø MeV 5 Neutrons 6 Neutron Capture	Z None	Z None
Ø Pituitary Gland 1 Pineal Body 2 Adrenal Glands 4 Parathyroid Glands 5 Thyroid	3 Electrons	Z None	Ø Intraoperative Z None

SECTION: D RADIATION THERAPY
BODY SYSTEM: G ENDOCRINE SYSTEM
MODALITY: 1 BRACHYTHERAPY

Treatment Site	Modality Qualifier	Isotope	Qualifier
Ø Pituitary Gland 1 Pineal Body 2 Adrenal Glands 4 Parathyroid Glands 5 Thyroid	9 High Dose Rate (HDR) B Low Dose Rate (LDR)	7 Cesium 137 (Cs-137) 8 Iridium 192 (Ir-192) 9 Iodine 125 (I-125) B Palladium 1Ø3 (Pd-1Ø3) C Californium 252 (Cf-252) Y Other Isotope	Z None

SECTION: D RADIATION THERAPY
BODY SYSTEM: G ENDOCRINE SYSTEM
MODALITY: 2 STEREOTACTIC RADIOSURGERY

Treatment Site	Modality Qualifier	Isotope	Qualifier
Ø Pituitary Gland 1 Pineal Body 2 Adrenal Glands 4 Parathyroid Glands 5 Thyroid	D Stereotactic Other Photon Radiosurgery H Stereotactic Particulate Radiosurgery J Stereotactic Gamma Beam Radiosurgery	Z None	Z None

DRG Non-OR   All Values

SECTION: D RADIATION THERAPY
BODY SYSTEM: G ENDOCRINE SYSTEM
MODALITY: Y OTHER RADIATION

Treatment Site	Modality Qualifier	Isotope	Qualifier
Ø Pituitary Gland 1 Pineal Body 2 Adrenal Glands 4 Parathyroid Glands 5 Thyroid	7 Contact Radiation 8 Hyperthermia F Plaque Radiation K Laser Interstitial Thermal Therapy	Z None	Z None

SECTION: D RADIATION THERAPY
BODY SYSTEM: H SKIN
MODALITY: Ø BEAM RADIATION

Treatment Site	Modality Qualifier	Isotope	Qualifier
2 Skin, Face 3 Skin, Neck 4 Skin, Arm 6 Skin, Chest 7 Skin, Back 8 Skin, Abdomen 9 Skin, Buttock B Skin, Leg	Ø Photons <1 MeV 1 Photons 1 - 1Ø MeV 2 Photons >1Ø MeV 4 Heavy Particles (Protons, Ions) 5 Neutrons 6 Neutron Capture	Z None	Z None
2 Skin, Face 3 Skin, Neck 4 Skin, Arm 6 Skin, Chest 7 Skin, Back 8 Skin, Abdomen 9 Skin, Buttock B Skin, Leg	3 Electrons	Z None	Ø Intraoperative Z None

SECTION: D RADIATION THERAPY
BODY SYSTEM: H SKIN
MODALITY: Y OTHER RADIATION

Treatment Site	Modality Qualifier	Isotope	Qualifier
2 Skin, Face 3 Skin, Neck 4 Skin, Arm 6 Skin, Chest 7 Skin, Back 8 Skin, Abdomen 9 Skin, Buttock B Skin, Leg	7 Contact Radiation 8 Hyperthermia F Plaque Radiation	Z None	Z None
5 Skin, Hand C Skin, Foot	F Plaque Radiation	Z None	Z None

SECTION: D RADIATION THERAPY
BODY SYSTEM: M BREAST
MODALITY: Ø BEAM RADIATION

Treatment Site	Modality Qualifier	Isotope	Qualifier
Ø Breast, Left 1 Breast, Right	Ø Photons <1 MeV 1 Photons 1 - 1Ø MeV 2 Photons >1Ø MeV 4 Heavy Particles (Protons, Ions) 5 Neutrons 6 Neutron Capture	Z None	Z None
Ø Breast, Left 1 Breast, Right	3 Electrons	Z None	Ø Intraoperative Z None

SECTION: D RADIATION THERAPY
BODY SYSTEM: M BREAST
MODALITY: 1 BRACHYTHERAPY

Treatment Site	Modality Qualifier	Isotope	Qualifier
Ø Breast, Left 1 Breast, Right	9 High Dose Rate (HDR) B Low Dose Rate (LDR)	7 Cesium 137 (Cs-137) 8 Iridium 192 (Ir-192) 9 Iodine 125 (I-125) B Palladium 1Ø3 (Pd-1Ø3) C Californium 252 (Cf-252) Y Other Isotope	Z None

SECTION: D RADIATION THERAPY
BODY SYSTEM: M BREAST
MODALITY: 2 STEREOTACTIC RADIOSURGERY

Treatment Site	Modality Qualifier	Isotope	Qualifier
Ø Breast, Left 1 Breast, Right	D Stereotactic Other Photon Radiosurgery H Stereotactic Particulate Radiosurgery J Stereotactic Gamma Beam Radiosurgery	Z None	Z None

DRG Non-OR All Values

SECTION: D RADIATION THERAPY
BODY SYSTEM: M BREAST
MODALITY: Y OTHER RADIATION

Treatment Site	Modality Qualifier	Isotope	Qualifier
Ø Breast, Left 1 Breast, Right	7 Contact Radiation 8 Hyperthermia F Plaque Radiation K Laser Interstitial Thermal Therapy	Z None	Z None

D: RADIATION THERAPY

M: BREAST

Ø; 1; 2; Y

SECTION: D RADIATION THERAPY
BODY SYSTEM: P MUSCULOSKELETAL SYSTEM
MODALITY: Ø BEAM RADIATION

Treatment Site	Modality Qualifier	Isotope	Qualifier
Ø Skull 2 Maxilla 3 Mandible 4 Sternum 5 Rib(s) 6 Humerus 7 Radius/Ulna 8 Pelvic Bones 9 Femur B Tibia/Fibula C Other Bone	Ø Photons <1 MeV 1 Photons 1 - 1Ø MeV 2 Photons >1Ø MeV 4 Heavy Particles (Protons, Ions) 5 Neutrons 6 Neutron Capture	Z None	Z None
Ø Skull 2 Maxilla 3 Mandible 4 Sternum 5 Rib(s) 6 Humerus 7 Radius/Ulna 8 Pelvic Bones 9 Femur B Tibia/Fibula C Other Bone	3 Electrons	Z None	Ø Intraoperative Z None

SECTION: D RADIATION THERAPY
BODY SYSTEM: P MUSCULOSKELETAL SYSTEM
MODALITY: Y OTHER RADIATION

Treatment Site	Modality Qualifier	Isotope	Qualifier
Ø Skull 2 Maxilla 3 Mandible 4 Sternum 5 Rib(s) 6 Humerus 7 Radius/Ulna 8 Pelvic Bones 9 Femur B Tibia/Fibula C Other Bone	7 Contact Radiation 8 Hyperthermia F Plaque Radiation	Z None	Z None

SECTION: **D RADIATION THERAPY**
BODY SYSTEM: T URINARY SYSTEM
MODALITY: Ø BEAM RADIATION

Treatment Site	Modality Qualifier	Isotope	Qualifier
Ø Kidney 1 Ureter 2 Bladder 3 Urethra	Ø Photons <1 MeV 1 Photons 1 - 1Ø MeV 2 Photons >1Ø MeV 4 Heavy Particles (Protons, Ions) 5 Neutrons 6 Neutron Capture	Z None	Z None
Ø Kidney 1 Ureter 2 Bladder 3 Urethra	3 Electrons	Z None	Ø Intraoperative Z None

SECTION: **D RADIATION THERAPY**
BODY SYSTEM: T URINARY SYSTEM
MODALITY: 1 BRACHYTHERAPY

Treatment Site	Modality Qualifier	Isotope	Qualifier
Ø Kidney 1 Ureter 2 Bladder 3 Urethra	9 High Dose Rate (HDR) B Low Dose Rate (LDR)	7 Cesium 137 (Cs-137) 8 Iridium 192 (Ir-192) 9 Iodine 125 (I-125) B Palladium 1Ø3 (Pd-1Ø3) C Californium 252 (Cf-252) Y Other Isotope	Z None

SECTION: **D RADIATION THERAPY**
BODY SYSTEM: T URINARY SYSTEM
MODALITY: 2 STEREOTACTIC RADIOSURGERY

Treatment Site	Modality Qualifier	Isotope	Qualifier
Ø Kidney 1 Ureter 2 Bladder 3 Urethra	D Stereotactic Other Photon Radiosurgery H Stereotactic Particulate Radiosurgery J Stereotactic Gamma Beam Radiosurgery	Z None	Z None

DRG Non-OR All Values

SECTION: **D RADIATION THERAPY**
BODY SYSTEM: T URINARY SYSTEM
MODALITY: Y OTHER RADIATION

Treatment Site	Modality Qualifier	Isotope	Qualifier
Ø Kidney 1 Ureter 2 Bladder 3 Urethra	7 Contact Radiation 8 Hyperthermia C Intraoperative Radiation Therapy (IORT) F Plaque Radiation	Z None	Z None

SECTION: D RADIATION THERAPY
BODY SYSTEM: U FEMALE REPRODUCTIVE SYSTEM
MODALITY: Ø BEAM RADIATION

Treatment Site	Modality Qualifier	Isotope	Qualifier
Ø Ovary ♀ 1 Cervix ♀ 2 Uterus ♀	Ø Photons <1 MeV 1 Photons 1 - 1Ø MeV 2 Photons >1Ø MeV 4 Heavy Particles (Protons, Ions) 5 Neutrons 6 Neutron Capture	Z None	Z None
Ø Ovary ♀ 1 Cervix ♀ 2 Uterus ♀	3 Electrons	Z None	Ø Intraoperative Z None

SECTION: D RADIATION THERAPY
BODY SYSTEM: U FEMALE REPRODUCTIVE SYSTEM
MODALITY: 1 BRACHYTHERAPY

Treatment Site	Modality Qualifier	Isotope	Qualifier
Ø Ovary ♀ 1 Cervix ♀ 2 Uterus ♀	9 High Dose Rate (HDR) B Low Dose Rate (LDR)	7 Cesium 137 (Cs-137) 8 Iridium 192 (Ir-192) 9 Iodine 125 (I-125) B Palladium 1Ø3 (Pd-1Ø3) C Californium 252 (Cf-252) Y Other Isotope	Z None

New/Revised Text in Green ~~deleted~~ Deleted ♀ Females Only ♂ Males Only **Coding Clinic**
🚫 Non-covered 🚫 Limited Coverage ⊞ Combination (See Appendix E) DRG Non-OR Non-OR 🚫 Hospital-Acquired Condition

Ø: 1

U: FEMALE REPRODUCTIVE SYSTEM

D: RADIATION THERAPY

SECTION: D RADIATION THERAPY
BODY SYSTEM: U FEMALE REPRODUCTIVE SYSTEM
MODALITY: 2 STEREOTACTIC RADIOSURGERY

Treatment Site	Modality Qualifier	Isotope	Qualifier
Ø Ovary ♀ 1 Cervix ♀ 2 Uterus ♀	D Stereotactic Other Photon Radiosurgery H Stereotactic Particulate Radiosurgery J Stereotactic Gamma Beam Radiosurgery	Z None	Z None

DRG Non-OR   All Values

SECTION: D RADIATION THERAPY
BODY SYSTEM: U FEMALE REPRODUCTIVE SYSTEM
MODALITY: Y OTHER RADIATION

Treatment Site	Modality Qualifier	Isotope	Qualifier
Ø Ovary ♀ 1 Cervix ♀ 2 Uterus ♀	7 Contact Radiation 8 Hyperthermia C Intraoperative Radiation Therapy (IORT) F Plaque Radiation	Z None	Z None

D: RADIATION THERAPY

U: FEMALE REPRODUCTIVE SYSTEM

2; Y

SECTION: D RADIATION THERAPY
BODY SYSTEM: V MALE REPRODUCTIVE SYSTEM
MODALITY: Ø BEAM RADIATION

Treatment Site	Modality Qualifier	Isotope	Qualifier
Ø Prostate ♂ 1 Testis ♂	Ø Photons <1 MeV 1 Photons 1 - 1Ø MeV 2 Photons >1Ø MeV 4 Heavy Particles (Protons, Ions) 5 Neutrons 6 Neutron Capture	Z None	Z None
Ø Prostate ♂ 1 Testis ♂	3 Electrons	Z None	Ø Intraoperative Z None

SECTION: D RADIATION THERAPY
BODY SYSTEM: V MALE REPRODUCTIVE SYSTEM
MODALITY: 1 BRACHYTHERAPY

Treatment Site	Modality Qualifier	Isotope	Qualifier
Ø Prostate ♂ 1 Testis ♂	9 High Dose Rate (HDR) B Low Dose Rate (LDR)	7 Cesium 137 (Cs-137) 8 Iridium 192 (Ir-192) 9 Iodine 125 (I-125) B Palladium 1Ø3 (Pd-1Ø3) C Californium 252 (Cf-252) Y Other Isotope	Z None

Ø; 1

V: MALE REPRODUCTIVE SYSTEM

D: RADIATION THERAPY

New/Revised Text in Green deleted Deleted ♀ Females Only ♂ Males Only **Coding Clinic**
Non-covered Limited Coverage Combination (See Appendix E) DRG Non-OR Non-OR Hospital-Acquired Condition

SECTION: **D RADIATION THERAPY**
BODY SYSTEM: V MALE REPRODUCTIVE SYSTEM
MODALITY: 2 STEREOTACTIC RADIOSURGERY

Treatment Site	Modality Qualifier	Isotope	Qualifier
Ø Prostate ♂ 1 Testis ♂	D Stereotactic Other Photon Radiosurgery H Stereotactic Particulate Radiosurgery J Stereotactic Gamma Beam Radiosurgery	Z None	Z None

DRG Non-OR   All Values

SECTION: **D RADIATION THERAPY**
BODY SYSTEM: V MALE REPRODUCTIVE SYSTEM
MODALITY: Y OTHER RADIATION

Treatment Site	Modality Qualifier	Isotope	Qualifier
Ø Prostate ♂	7 Contact Radiation 8 Hyperthermia C Intraoperative Radiation Therapy (IORT) F Plaque Radiation K Laser Interstitial Thermal Therapy	Z None	Z None
1 Testis ♂	7 Contact Radiation 8 Hyperthermia F Plaque Radiation	Z None	Z None

SECTION: D RADIATION THERAPY
BODY SYSTEM: W ANATOMICAL REGIONS
MODALITY: Ø BEAM RADIATION

Treatment Site	Modality Qualifier	Isotope	Qualifier
1 Head and Neck 2 Chest 3 Abdomen 4 Hemibody 5 Whole Body 6 Pelvic Region	Ø Photons <1 MeV 1 Photons 1 - 1Ø MeV 2 Photons >1Ø MeV 4 Heavy Particles (Protons, Ions) 5 Neutrons 6 Neutron Capture	Z None	Z None
1 Head and Neck 2 Chest 3 Abdomen 4 Hemibody 5 Whole Body 6 Pelvic Region	3 Electrons	Z None	Ø Intraoperative Z None

SECTION: D RADIATION THERAPY
BODY SYSTEM: W ANATOMICAL REGIONS
MODALITY: 1 BRACHYTHERAPY

Treatment Site	Modality Qualifier	Isotope	Qualifier
1 Head and Neck 2 Chest 3 Abdomen 6 Pelvic Region	9 High Dose Rate (HDR) B Low Dose Rate (LDR)	7 Cesium 137 (Cs-137) 8 Iridium 192 (Ir-192) 9 Iodine 125 (I-125) B Palladium 1Ø3 (Pd-1Ø3) C Californium 252 (Cf-252) Y Other Isotope	Z None

W: ANATOMICAL REGIONS

Ø; 1

D: RADIATION THERAPY

New/Revised Text in Green ~~deleted~~ Deleted ♀ Females Only ♂ Males Only **Coding Clinic**
Non-covered Limited Coverage ⊞ Combination (See Appendix E) DRG Non-OR Non-OR Hospital-Acquired Condition

SECTION: D RADIATION THERAPY
BODY SYSTEM: W ANATOMICAL REGIONS
MODALITY: 2 STEREOTACTIC RADIOSURGERY

Treatment Site	Modality Qualifier	Isotope	Qualifier
1 Head and Neck 2 Chest 3 Abdomen 6 Pelvic Region	D Stereotactic Other Photon Radiosurgery H Stereotactic Particulate Radiosurgery J Stereotactic Gamma Beam Radiosurgery	Z None	Z None

DRG Non-OR All Values

SECTION: D RADIATION THERAPY
BODY SYSTEM: W ANATOMICAL REGIONS
MODALITY: Y OTHER RADIATION

Treatment Site	Modality Qualifier	Isotope	Qualifier
1 Head and Neck 2 Chest 3 Abdomen 4 Hemibody 6 Pelvic Region	7 Contact Radiation 8 Hyperthermia F Plaque Radiation	Z None	Z None
5 Whole Body	7 Contact Radiation 8 Hyperthermia F Plaque Radiation	Z None	Z None
5 Whole Body	G Isotope Administration	D Iodine 131 (I-131) F Phosphorus 32 (P-32) G Strontium 89 (Sr-89) H Strontium 90 (Sr-90) Y Other Isotope	Z None

New/Revised Text in Green   ~~deleted~~ Deleted   ♀ Females Only   ♂ Males Only   **Coding Clinic**

  Non-covered   Limited Coverage   Combination (See Appendix E)   DRG Non-OR   Non-OR   Hospital-Acquired Condition

SECTION: F PHYSICAL REHABILITATION AND DIAGNOSTIC AUDIOLOGY

SECTION QUALIFIER: Ø REHABILITATION

TYPE: Ø SPEECH ASSESSMENT: *(on multiple pages)*

Measurement of speech and related functions

Body System – Body Region	Type Qualifier	Equipment	Qualifier
3 Neurological System - Whole Body	G Communicative/Cognitive Integration Skills	K Audiovisual M Augmentative/Alternative Communication P Computer Y Other Equipment Z None	Z None
Z None	Ø Filtered Speech 3 Staggered Spondaic Word Q Performance Intensity Phonetically Balanced Speech Discrimination R Brief Tone Stimuli S Distorted Speech T Dichotic Stimuli V Temporal Ordering of Stimuli W Masking Patterns	1 Audiometer 2 Sound Field/Booth K Audiovisual Z None	Z None
Z None	1 Speech Threshold 2 Speech/Word Recognition	1 Audiometer 2 Sound Field/Booth 9 Cochlear Implant K Audiovisual Z None	Z None
Z None	4 Sensorineural Acuity Level	1 Audiometer 2 Sound Field/Booth Z None	Z None
Z None	5 Synthetic Sentence Identification	1 Audiometer 2 Sound Field/Booth 9 Cochlear Implant K Audiovisual	Z None
Z None	6 Speech and/or Language Screening 7 Nonspoken Language 8 Receptive/Expressive Language C Aphasia G Communicative/Cognitive Integration Skills L Augmentative/Alternative Communication System	K Audiovisual M Augmentative/Alternative Communication P Computer Y Other Equipment Z None	Z None
Z None	9 Articulation/Phonology	K Audiovisual P Computer Q Speech Analysis Y Other Equipment Z None	Z None
Z None	B Motor Speech	K Audiovisual N Biosensory Feedback P Computer Q Speech Analysis T Aerodynamic Function Y Other Equipment Z None	Z None

DRG Non-OR **All Values**

Ø: SPEECH ASSESSMENT

Ø: REHABILITATION

F: PHYSICAL REHABILITATION AND DIAGNOSTIC AUDIOLOGY

SECTION: F PHYSICAL REHABILITATION AND DIAGNOSTIC AUDIOLOGY

SECTION QUALIFIER: Ø REHABILITATION
TYPE: Ø SPEECH ASSESSMENT: *(continued)*
Measurement of speech and related functions

Body System – Body Region	Type Qualifier	Equipment	Qualifier
Z None	D Fluency	K Audiovisual N Biosensory Feedback P Computer Q Speech Analysis S Voice Analysis T Aerodynamic Function Y Other Equipment Z None	Z None
Z None	F Voice	K Audiovisual N Biosensory Feedback P Computer S Voice Analysis T Aerodynamic Function Y Other Equipment Z None	Z None
Z None	H Bedside Swallowing and Oral Function P Oral Peripheral Mechanism	Y Other Equipment Z None	Z None
Z None	J Instrumental Swallowing and Oral Function	T Aerodynamic Function W Swallowing Y Other Equipment	Z None
Z None	K Orofacial Myofunctional	K Audiovisual P Computer Y Other Equipment Z None	Z None
Z None	M Voice Prosthetic	K Audiovisual P Computer S Voice Analysis V Speech Prosthesis Y Other Equipment Z None	Z None
Z None	N Non-invasive Instrumental Status	N Biosensory Feedback P Computer Q Speech Analysis S Voice Analysis T Aerodynamic Function Y Other Equipment	Z None
Z None	X Other Specified Central Auditory Processing	Z None	Z None

DRG Non-OR All Values

New/Revised Text in Green   ~~deleted~~ Deleted   ♀ Females Only   ♂ Males Only   **Coding Clinic**

Non-covered   Limited Coverage   Combination (See Appendix E)   DRG Non-OR   Non-OR   Hospital-Acquired Condition

SECTION: F PHYSICAL REHABILITATION AND DIAGNOSTIC AUDIOLOGY

SECTION QUALIFIER: 0 REHABILITATION
TYPE: 1 MOTOR AND/OR NERVE FUNCTION
ASSESSMENT: *(on multiple pages)*
Measurement of motor, nerve, and related functions

Body System – Body Region	Type Qualifier	Equipment	Qualifier
0 Neurological System - Head and Neck 1 Neurological System - Upper Back/Upper Extremity 2 Neurological System - Lower Back/Lower Extremity 3 Neurological System - Whole Body	0 Muscle Performance	E Orthosis F Assistive, Adaptive, Supportive or Protective U Prosthesis Y Other Equipment Z None	Z None
0 Neurological System - Head and Neck 1 Neurological System - Upper Back/Upper Extremity 2 Neurological System - Lower Back/Lower Extremity 3 Neurological System - Whole Body	1 Integumentary Integrity 3 Coordination/Dexterity 4 Motor Function G Reflex Integrity	Z None	Z None
0 Neurological System - Head and Neck 1 Neurological System - Upper Back/Upper Extremity 2 Neurological System - Lower Back/Lower Extremity 3 Neurological System - Whole Body	5 Range of Motion and Joint Integrity 6 Sensory Awareness/Processing/Integrity	Y Other Equipment Z None	Z None
D Integumentary System - Head and Neck F Integumentary System - Upper Back/Upper Extremity G Integumentary System - Lower Back/Lower Extremity H Integumentary System - Whole Body J Musculoskeletal System - Head and Neck K Musculoskeletal System - Upper Back/Upper Extremity L Musculoskeletal System - Lower Back/Lower Extremity M Musculoskeletal System - Whole Body	0 Muscle Performance	E Orthosis F Assistive, Adaptive, Supportive or Protective U Prosthesis Y Other Equipment Z None	Z None
D Integumentary System - Head and Neck F Integumentary System - Upper Back/Upper Extremity G Integumentary System - Lower Back/Lower Extremity H Integumentary System - Whole Body J Musculoskeletal System - Head and Neck K Musculoskeletal System - Upper Back/Upper Extremity L Musculoskeletal System - Lower Back/Lower Extremity M Musculoskeletal System - Whole Body	1 Integumentary Integrity	Z None	Z None
D Integumentary System - Head and Neck F Integumentary System - Upper Back/Upper Extremity G Integumentary System - Lower Back/Lower Extremity H Integumentary System - Whole Body J Musculoskeletal System - Head and Neck K Musculoskeletal System - Upper Back/Upper Extremity L Musculoskeletal System - Lower Back/Lower Extremity M Musculoskeletal System - Whole Body	5 Range of Motion and Joint Integrity 6 Sensory Awareness/Processing/Integrity	Y Other Equipment Z None	Z None

DRG Non-OR All Values

SECTION: F PHYSICAL REHABILITATION AND DIAGNOSTIC AUDIOLOGY

SECTION QUALIFIER: Ø REHABILITATION
TYPE: 1 MOTOR AND/OR NERVE FUNCTION ASSESSMENT: *(continued)*

Measurement of motor, nerve, and related functions

Body System – Body Region	Type Qualifier	Equipment	Qualifier
N Genitourinary System	Ø Muscle Performance	E Orthosis F Assistive, Adaptive, Supportive or Protective U Prosthesis Y Other Equipment Z None	Z None
Z None	2 Visual Motor Integration	K Audiovisual M Augmentative/Alternative Communication N Biosensory Feedback P Computer Q Speech Analysis S Voice Analysis Y Other Equipment Z None	Z None
Z None	7 Facial Nerve Function	7 Electrophysiologic	Z None
Z None	9 Somatosensory Evoked Potentials	J Somatosensory	Z None
Z None	B Bed Mobility C Transfer F Wheelchair Mobility	E Orthosis F Assistive, Adaptive, Supportive or Protective U Prosthesis Z None	Z None
Z None	D Gait and/or Balance	E Orthosis F Assistive, Adaptive, Supportive or Protective U Prosthesis Y Other Equipment Z None	Z None

DRG Non-OR All Values

SECTION: F PHYSICAL REHABILITATION AND DIAGNOSTIC AUDIOLOGY

SECTION QUALIFIER: Ø REHABILITATION

TYPE: 2 ACTIVITIES OF DAILY LIVING ASSESSMENT: *(on multiple pages)*
Measurement of functional level for activities of daily living

Body System – Body Region	Type Qualifier	Equipment	Qualifier
Ø Neurological System - Head and Neck	9 Cranial Nerve Integrity D Neuromotor Development	Y Other Equipment Z None	Z None
1 Neurological System - Upper Back/Upper Extremity 2 Neurological System - Lower Back/Lower Extremity 3 Neurological System - Whole Body	D Neuromotor Development	Y Other Equipment Z None	Z None
4 Circulatory System - Head and Neck 5 Circulatory System - Upper Back/Upper Extremity 6 Circulatory System - Lower Back/Lower Extremity 8 Respiratory System - Head and Neck 9 Respiratory System - Upper Back/Upper Extremity B Respiratory System - Lower Back/Lower Extremity	G Ventilation, Respiration and Circulation	C Mechanical G Aerobic Endurance and Conditioning Y Other Equipment Z None	Z None
7 Circulatory System - Whole Body C Respiratory System - Whole Body	7 Aerobic Capacity and Endurance	E Orthosis G Aerobic Endurance and Conditioning U Prosthesis Y Other Equipment Z None	Z None
7 Circulatory System - Whole Body C Respiratory System - Whole Body	G Ventilation, Respiration and Circulation	C Mechanical G Aerobic Endurance and Conditioning Y Other Equipment Z None	Z None

DRG Non-OR All Values

New/Revised Text in Green   ~~deleted~~ Deleted   ♀ Females Only   ♂ Males Only   **Coding Clinic**

Non-covered   Limited Coverage   Combination (See Appendix E)   DRG Non-OR   Non-OR   Hospital-Acquired Condition

SECTION: **F PHYSICAL REHABILITATION AND DIAGNOSTIC AUDIOLOGY**

SECTION QUALIFIER: Ø   **REHABILITATION**

TYPE: **2 ACTIVITIES OF DAILY LIVING ASSESSMENT:** *(continued)*

Measurement of functional level for activities of daily living

Body System – Body Region	Type Qualifier	Equipment	Qualifier
Z None	Ø Bathing/Showering 1 Dressing 3 Grooming/Personal Hygiene 4 Home Management	E Orthosis F Assistive, Adaptive, Supportive or Protective U Prosthesis Z None	Z None
Z None	2 Feeding/Eating 8 Anthropometric Characteristics F Pain	Y Other Equipment Z None	Z None
Z None	5 Perceptual Processing	K Audiovisual M Augmentative/Alternative Communication N Biosensory Feedback P Computer Q Speech Analysis S Voice Analysis Y Other Equipment Z None	Z None
Z None	6 Psychosocial Skills	Z None	Z None
Z None	B Environmental, Home and Work Barriers C Ergonomics and Body Mechanics	E Orthosis F Assistive, Adaptive, Supportive or Protective U Prosthesis Y Other Equipment Z None	Z None
Z None	H Vocational Activities and Functional Community or Work Reintegration Skills	E Orthosis F Assistive, Adaptive, Supportive or Protective G Aerobic Endurance and Conditioning U Prosthesis Y Other Equipment Z None	Z None

DRG Non-OR   All Values

New/Revised Text in Green   ~~deleted~~ Deleted   ♀ Females Only   ♂ Males Only   **Coding Clinic**

⊘ Non-covered   ⊘ Limited Coverage   ⊞ Combination (See Appendix E)   DRG Non-OR   Non-OR   ⊘ Hospital-Acquired Condition

SECTION: F PHYSICAL REHABILITATION AND DIAGNOSTIC AUDIOLOGY

SECTION QUALIFIER: Ø REHABILITATION
TYPE: 6 SPEECH TREATMENT: *(on multiple pages)*
Application of techniques to improve, augment, or compensate for speech and related functional impairment

Body System – Body Region	Type Qualifier	Equipment	Qualifier
3 Neurological System - Whole Body	6 Communicative/Cognitive Integration Skills	K Audiovisual M Augmentative/Alternative Communication P Computer Y Other Equipment Z None	Z None
Z None	Ø Nonspoken Language 3 Aphasia 6 Communicative/Cognitive Integration Skills	K Audiovisual M Augmentative/Alternative Communication P Computer Y Other Equipment Z None	Z None
Z None	1 Speech-Language Pathology and Related Disorders Counseling 2 Speech-Language Pathology and Related Disorders Prevention	K Audiovisual Z None	Z None
Z None	4 Articulation/Phonology	K Audiovisual P Computer Q Speech Analysis T Aerodynamic Function Y Other Equipment Z None	Z None
Z None	5 Aural Rehabilitation	K Audiovisual L Assistive Listening M Augmentative/Alternative Communication N Biosensory Feedback P Computer Q Speech Analysis S Voice Analysis Y Other Equipment Z None	Z None
Z None	7 Fluency	4 Electroacoustic Immitance/ Acoustic Reflex K Audiovisual N Biosensory Feedback Q Speech Analysis S Voice Analysis T Aerodynamic Function Y Other Equipment Z None	Z None

DRG Non-OR   All Values

New/Revised Text in Green   ~~deleted~~ Deleted   ♀ Females Only   ♂ Males Only   **Coding Clinic**
🚫 Non-covered   🚫 Limited Coverage   ⊡ Combination (See Appendix E)   DRG Non-OR   Non-OR   🚫 Hospital-Acquired Condition

SECTION: F PHYSICAL REHABILITATION AND DIAGNOSTIC AUDIOLOGY

SECTION QUALIFIER: 0 REHABILITATION
TYPE: 6 SPEECH TREATMENT: *(continued)*

Application of techniques to improve, augment, or compensate for speech and related functional impairment

Body System – Body Region	Type Qualifier	Equipment	Qualifier
Z None	8 Motor Speech	K Audiovisual N Biosensory Feedback P Computer Q Speech Analysis S Voice Analysis T Aerodynamic Function Y Other Equipment Z None	Z None
Z None	9 Orofacial Myofunctional	K Audiovisual P Computer Y Other Equipment Z None	Z None
Z None	B Receptive/Expressive Language	K Audiovisual L Assistive Listening M Augmentative/Alternative Communication P Computer Y Other Equipment Z None	Z None
Z None	C Voice	K Audiovisual N Biosensory Feedback P Computer S Voice Analysis T Aerodynamic Function V Speech Prosthesis Y Other Equipment Z None	Z None
Z None	D Swallowing Dysfunction	M Augmentative/Alternative Communication T Aerodynamic Function V Speech Prosthesis Y Other Equipment Z None	Z None

DRG Non-OR   All Values

SECTION: F PHYSICAL REHABILITATION AND DIAGNOSTIC AUDIOLOGY

SECTION QUALIFIER: Ø REHABILITATION

TYPE: 7 MOTOR TREATMENT: *(on multiple pages)*

Exercise or activities to increase or facilitate motor function

Body System – Body Region	Type Qualifier	Equipment	Qualifier
Ø Neurological System - Head and Neck 1 Neurological System - Upper Back/Upper Extremity 2 Neurological System - Lower Back/Lower Extremity 3 Neurological System - Whole Body D Integumentary System - Head and Neck F Integumentary System - Upper Back/Upper Extremity G Integumentary System - Lower Back/Lower Extremity H Integumentary System - Whole Body J Musculoskeletal System - Head and Neck K Musculoskeletal System - Upper Back/Upper Extremity L Musculoskeletal System - Lower Back/Lower Extremity M Musculoskeletal System - Whole Body	Ø Range of Motion and Joint Mobility 1 Muscle Performance 2 Coordination/Dexterity 3 Motor Function	E Orthosis F Assistive, Adaptive, Supportive or Protective U Prosthesis Y Other Equipment Z None	Z None
Ø Neurological System - Head and Neck 1 Neurological System - Upper Back/Upper Extremity 2 Neurological System - Lower Back/Lower Extremity 3 Neurological System - Whole Body D Integumentary System - Head and Neck F Integumentary System - Upper Back/Upper Extremity G Integumentary System - Lower Back/Lower Extremity H Integumentary System - Whole Body J Musculoskeletal System - Head and Neck K Musculoskeletal System - Upper Back/Upper Extremity L Musculoskeletal System - Lower Back/Lower Extremity M Musculoskeletal System - Whole Body	6 Therapeutic Exercise	B Physical Agents C Mechanical D Electrotherapeutic E Orthosis F Assistive, Adaptive, Supportive or Protective G Aerobic Endurance and Conditioning H Mechanical or Electromechanical U Prosthesis Y Other Equipment Z None	Z None
Ø Neurological System - Head and Neck 1 Neurological System - Upper Back/Upper Extremity 2 Neurological System - Lower Back/Lower Extremity 3 Neurological System - Whole Body D Integumentary System - Head and Neck F Integumentary System - Upper Back/Upper Extremity G Integumentary System - Lower Back/Lower Extremity H Integumentary System - Whole Body J Musculoskeletal System - Head and Neck K Musculoskeletal System - Upper Back/Upper Extremity L Musculoskeletal System - Lower Back/Lower Extremity M Musculoskeletal System - Whole Body	7 Manual Therapy Techniques	Z None	Z None

DRG Non-OR All Values

SECTION: F PHYSICAL REHABILITATION AND DIAGNOSTIC AUDIOLOGY

SECTION QUALIFIER: Ø REHABILITATION

TYPE: 7 MOTOR TREATMENT: *(continued)*

Exercise or activities to increase or facilitate motor function

Body System – Body Region	Type Qualifier	Equipment	Qualifier
4 Circulatory System - Head and Neck 5 Circulatory System - Upper Back/Upper Extremity 6 Circulatory System - Lower Back/Lower Extremity 7 Circulatory System - Whole Body 8 Respiratory System - Head and Neck 9 Respiratory System - Upper Back/Upper Extremity B Respiratory System - Lower Back/Lower Extremity C Respiratory System - Whole Body	6 Therapeutic Exercise	B Physical Agents C Mechanical D Electrotherapeutic E Orthosis F Assistive, Adaptive, Supportive or Protective G Aerobic Endurance and Conditioning H Mechanical or Electromechanical U Prosthesis Y Other Equipment Z None	Z None
N Genitourinary System	1 Muscle Performance	E Orthosis F Assistive, Adaptive, Supportive or Protective U Prosthesis Y Other Equipment Z None	Z None
N Genitourinary System	6 Therapeutic Exercise	B Physical Agents C Mechanical D Electrotherapeutic E Orthosis F Assistive, Adaptive, Supportive or Protective G Aerobic Endurance and Conditioning H Mechanical or Electromechanical U Prosthesis Y Other Equipment Z None	Z None
Z None	4 Wheelchair Mobility	D Electrotherapeutic E Orthosis F Assistive, Adaptive, Supportive or Protective U Prosthesis Y Other Equipment Z None	Z None
Z None	5 Bed Mobility	C Mechanical E Orthosis F Assistive, Adaptive, Supportive or Protective U Prosthesis Y Other Equipment Z None	Z None
Z None	8 Transfer Training	C Mechanical D Electrotherapeutic E Orthosis F Assistive, Adaptive, Supportive or Protective U Prosthesis Y Other Equipment Z None	Z None
Z None	9 Gait Training/Functional Ambulation	C Mechanical D Electrotherapeutic E Orthosis F Assistive, Adaptive, Supportive or Protective G Aerobic Endurance and Conditioning U Prosthesis Y Other Equipment Z None	Z None

7: MOTOR TREATMENT

Ø: REHABILITATION

F: PHYSICAL REHABILITATION AND DIAGNOSTIC AUDIOLOGY

DRG Non-OR   All Values

New/Revised Text in Green   ~~deleted~~ Deleted   ♀ Females Only   ♂ Males Only   **Coding Clinic**

Non-covered   Limited Coverage   Combination (See Appendix E)   DRG Non-OR   Non-OR   Hospital-Acquired Condition

SECTION: F PHYSICAL REHABILITATION AND DIAGNOSTIC AUDIOLOGY

SECTION QUALIFIER: Ø REHABILITATION

TYPE: 8 ACTIVITIES OF DAILY LIVING TREATMENT: Exercise or activities to facilitate functional competence for activities of daily living

Body System – Body Region	Type Qualifier	Equipment	Qualifier
D Integumentary System - Head and Neck F Integumentary System - Upper Back/Upper Extremity G Integumentary System - Lower Back/Lower Extremity H Integumentary System - Whole Body J Musculoskeletal System - Head and Neck K Musculoskeletal System - Upper Back/Upper Extremity L Musculoskeletal System - Lower Back/Lower Extremity M Musculoskeletal System - Whole Body	5 Wound Management	B Physical Agents C Mechanical D Electrotherapeutic E Orthosis F Assistive, Adaptive, Supportive or Protective U Prosthesis Y Other Equipment Z None	Z None
Z None	Ø Bathing/Showering Techniques 1 Dressing Techniques 2 Grooming/Personal Hygiene	E Orthosis F Assistive, Adaptive, Supportive or Protective U Prosthesis Y Other Equipment Z None	Z None
Z None	3 Feeding/Eating	C Mechanical D Electrotherapeutic E Orthosis F Assistive, Adaptive, Supportive or Protective U Prosthesis Y Other Equipment Z None	Z None
Z None	4 Home Management	D Electrotherapeutic E Orthosis F Assistive, Adaptive, Supportive or Protective U Prosthesis Y Other Equipment Z None	Z None
Z None	6 Psychosocial Skills	Z None	Z None
Z None	7 Vocational Activities and Functional Community or Work Reintegration Skills	B Physical Agents C Mechanical D Electrotherapeutic E Orthosis F Assistive, Adaptive, Supportive or Protective G Aerobic Endurance and Conditioning U Prosthesis Y Other Equipment Z None	Z None

DRG Non-OR   All Values

SECTION: F PHYSICAL REHABILITATION AND DIAGNOSTIC AUDIOLOGY

SECTION QUALIFIER: Ø REHABILITATION

TYPE: 9 **HEARING TREATMENT:** Application of techniques to improve, augment, or compensate for hearing and related functional impairment

Body System – Body Region	Type Qualifier	Equipment	Qualifier
Z None	Ø Hearing and Related Disorders Counseling 1 Hearing and Related Disorders Prevention	K Audiovisual Z None	Z None
Z None	2 Auditory Processing	K Audiovisual L Assistive Listening P Computer Y Other Equipment Z None	Z None
Z None	3 Cerumen Management	X Cerumen Management Z None	Z None

DRG Non-OR All Values

SECTION: F PHYSICAL REHABILITATION AND DIAGNOSTIC AUDIOLOGY

SECTION QUALIFIER: Ø REHABILITATION

TYPE: B **COCHLEAR IMPLANT TREATMENT:** Application of techniques to improve the communication abilities of individuals with cochlear implant

Body System – Body Region	Type Qualifier	Equipment	Qualifier
Z None	Ø Cochlear Implant Rehabilitation	1 Audiometer 2 Sound Field/Booth 9 Cochlear Implant K Audiovisual P Computer Y Other Equipment	Z None

DRG Non-OR All Values

New/Revised Text in Green ~~deleted~~ Deleted ♀ Females Only ♂ Males Only **Coding Clinic**
🚫 Non-covered 🚫 Limited Coverage ⊕ Combination (See Appendix E) DRG Non-OR Non-OR 🚫 Hospital-Acquired Condition

SECTION:

F PHYSICAL REHABILITATION AND DIAGNOSTIC AUDIOLOGY

SECTION QUALIFIER: Ø REHABILITATION

TYPE: **C VESTIBULAR TREATMENT:** Application of techniques to improve, augment, or compensate for vestibular and related functional impairment

Body System – Body Region	Type Qualifier	Equipment	Qualifier
3 Neurological System - Whole Body H Integumentary System - Whole Body M Musculoskeletal System - Whole Body	3 Postural Control	E Orthosis F Assistive, Adaptive, Supportive or Protective U Prosthesis Y Other Equipment Z None	Z None
Z None	Ø Vestibular	8 Vestibular/Balance Z None	Z None
Z None	1 Perceptual Processing 2 Visual Motor Integration	K Audiovisual L Assistive Listening N Biosensory Feedback P Computer Q Speech Analysis S Voice Analysis T Aerodynamic Function Y Other Equipment Z None	Z None

DRG Non-OR All Values

SECTION:

F PHYSICAL REHABILITATION AND DIAGNOSTIC AUDIOLOGY

SECTION QUALIFIER: Ø REHABILITATION

TYPE: **D DEVICE FITTING:** Fitting of a device designed to facilitate or support achievement of a higher level of function

Body System – Body Region	Type Qualifier	Equipment	Qualifier
Z None	Ø Tinnitus Masker	5 Hearing Aid Selection/Fitting/Test Z None	Z None
Z None	1 Monaural Hearing Aid 2 Binaural Hearing Aid 5 Assistive Listening Device	1 Audiometer 2 Sound Field/Booth 5 Hearing Aid Selection/Fitting/Test K Audiovisual L Assistive Listening Z None	Z None
Z None	3 Augmentative/Alternative Communication System	M Augmentative/Alternative Communication	Z None
Z None	4 Voice Prosthetic	S Voice Analysis V Speech Prosthesis	Z None
Z None	6 Dynamic Orthosis 7 Static Orthosis 8 Prosthesis 9 Assistive, Adaptive, Supportive or Protective Devices	E Orthosis F Assistive, Adaptive, Supportive or Protective U Prosthesis Z None	Z None

DRG Non-OR FØDZØ[5Z]Z
DRG Non-OR FØDZ[125][125KLZ]Z
DRG Non-OR FØDZ3MZ

DRG Non-OR FØDZ4[SV]Z
DRG Non-OR FØDZ[67][EFUZ]Z
DRG Non-OR FØDZ8[EFU]Z

New/Revised Text in Green   deleted Deleted   ♀ Females Only   ♂ Males Only   **Coding Clinic**
🚫 Non-covered   🚫 Limited Coverage   ⊕ Combination (See Appendix E)   DRG Non-OR   Non-OR   🚫 Hospital-Acquired Condition

663

SECTION: F PHYSICAL REHABILITATION AND DIAGNOSTIC AUDIOLOGY

SECTION QUALIFIER: Ø **REHABILITATION**

TYPE: F **CAREGIVER TRAINING:** Training in activities to support patient's optimal level of function

Body System – Body Region	Type Qualifier	Equipment	Qualifier
Z None	Ø Bathing/Showering Technique 1 Dressing 2 Feeding and Eating 3 Grooming/Personal Hygiene 4 Bed Mobility 5 Transfer 6 Wheelchair Mobility 7 Therapeutic Exercise 8 Airway Clearance Techniques 9 Wound Management B Vocational Activities and Functional Community or Work Reintegration Skills C Gait Training/Functional Ambulation D Application, Proper Use and Care Devices F Application, Proper Use and Care of Orthoses G Application, Proper Use and Care of Prosthesis H Home Management	E Orthosis F Assistive, Adaptive, Supportive or Protective U Prosthesis Z None	Z None
Z None	J Communication Skills	K Audiovisual L Assistive Listening M Augmentative/Alternative Communication P Computer Z None	Z None

DRG Non-OR   All Values

SECTION: F PHYSICAL REHABILITATION AND DIAGNOSTIC AUDIOLOGY

SECTION QUALIFIER: 1 DIAGNOSTIC AUDIOLOGY
TYPE: 3 HEARING ASSESSMENT: Measurement of hearing and related functions

Body System – Body Region	Type Qualifier	Equipment	Qualifier
Z None	Ø Hearing Screening	Ø Occupational Hearing 1 Audiometer 2 Sound Field/Booth 3 Tympanometer 8 Vestibular/Balance 9 Cochlear Implant Z None	Z None
Z None	1 Pure Tone Audiometry, Air 2 Pure Tone Audiometry, Air and Bone	Ø Occupational Hearing 1 Audiometer 2 Sound Field/Booth Z None	Z None
Z None	3 Bekesy Audiometry 6 Visual Reinforcement Audiometry 9 Short Increment Sensitivity Index B Stenger C Pure Tone Stenger	1 Audiometer 2 Sound Field/Booth Z None	Z None
Z None	4 Conditioned Play Audiometry 5 Select Picture Audiometry	1 Audiometer 2 Sound Field/Booth K Audiovisual Z None	Z None
Z None	7 Alternate Binaural or Monaural Loudness Balance	1 Audiometer K Audiovisual Z None	Z None
Z None	8 Tone Decay D Tympanometry F Eustachian Tube Function G Acoustic Reflex Patterns H Acoustic Reflex Threshold J Acoustic Reflex Decay	3 Tympanometer 4 Electroacoustic Immitance/ Acoustic Reflex Z None	Z None
Z None	K Electrocochleography L Auditory Evoked Potentials	7 Electrophysiologic Z None	Z None
Z None	M Evoked Otoacoustic Emissions, Screening N Evoked Otoacoustic Emissions, Diagnostic	6 Otoacoustic Emission (OAE) Z None	Z None
Z None	P Aural Rehabilitation Status	1 Audiometer 2 Sound Field/Booth 4 Electroacoustic Immitance/ Acoustic Reflex 9 Cochlear Implant K Audiovisual L Assistive Listening P Computer Z None	Z None
Z None	Q Auditory Processing	K Audiovisual P Computer Y Other Equipment Z None	Z None

New/Revised Text in Green   deleted Deleted   ♀ Females Only   ♂ Males Only   **Coding Clinic**
Non-covered   Limited Coverage   Combination (See Appendix E)   DRG Non-OR   Non-OR   Hospital-Acquired Condition

SECTION: F PHYSICAL REHABILITATION AND DIAGNOSTIC AUDIOLOGY

SECTION QUALIFIER: 1 DIAGNOSTIC AUDIOLOGY

TYPE: 4 **HEARING AID ASSESSMENT:** Measurement of the appropriateness and/or effectiveness of a hearing device

Body System – Body Region	Type Qualifier	Equipment	Qualifier

Z None	Ø Cochlear Implant	1 Audiometer
		2 Sound Field/Booth
		3 Tympanometer
		4 Electroacoustic Immitance/
		  Acoustic Reflex
		5 Hearing Aid Selection/
		  Fitting/Test
		7 Electrophysiologic
		9 Cochlear Implant
		K Audiovisual
		L Assistive Listening
		P Computer
		Y Other Equipment
		Z None
			Z None

Z None	1 Ear Canal Probe Microphone
	6 Binaural Electroacoustic
	  Hearing Aid Check
	8 Monaural Electroacoustic
	  Hearing Aid Check
		5 Hearing Aid Selection/
		  Fitting/Test
		Z None
			Z None

Z None	2 Monaural Hearing Aid
	3 Binaural Hearing Aid
		1 Audiometer
		2 Sound Field/Booth
		3 Tympanometer
		4 Electroacoustic Immitance/
		  Acoustic Reflex
		5 Hearing Aid Selection/
		  Fitting/Test
		K Audiovisual
		L Assistive Listening
		P Computer
		Z None
			Z None

Z None	4 Assistive Listening System/
	  Device Selection
		1 Audiometer
		2 Sound Field/Booth
		3 Tympanometer
		4 Electroacoustic Immitance/
		  Acoustic Reflex
		K Audiovisual
		L Assistive Listening
		Z None
			Z None

Z None	5 Sensory Aids	1 Audiometer
		2 Sound Field/Booth
		3 Tympanometer
		4 Electroacoustic Immitance/
		  Acoustic Reflex
		5 Hearing Aid Selection/
		  Fitting/Test
		K Audiovisual
		L Assistive Listening
		Z None
			Z None

Z None	7 Ear Protector Attentuation	Ø Occupational Hearing Z None	Z None

SECTION: F PHYSICAL REHABILITATION AND DIAGNOSTIC AUDIOLOGY

SECTION QUALIFIER: 1 DIAGNOSTIC AUDIOLOGY

TYPE: 5 **VESTIBULAR ASSESSMENT:** Measurement of the vestibular system and related functions

Body System – Body Region	Type Qualifier	Equipment	Qualifier
Z None	Ø Bithermal, Binaural Caloric Irrigation 1 Bithermal, Monaural Caloric Irrigation 2 Unithermal Binaural Screen 3 Oscillating Tracking 4 Sinusoidal Vertical Axis Rotational 5 Dix-Hallpike Dynamic 6 Computerized Dynamic Posturography	8 Vestibular/Balance Z None	Z None
Z None	7 Tinnitus Masker	5 Hearing Aid Selection/ Fitting/Test Z None	Z None

SECTION: **G MENTAL HEALTH**

SECTION QUALIFIER: Z　NONE

TYPE: 1　**PSYCHOLOGICAL TESTS:** The administration and interpretation of standardized psychological tests and measurement instruments for the assessment of psychological function

Qualifier	Qualifier	Qualifier	Qualifier
Ø Developmental 1 Personality and Behavioral 2 Intellectual and Psychoeducational 3 Neuropsychological 4 Neurobehavioral and Cognitive Status	Z None	Z None	Z None

SECTION: **G MENTAL HEALTH**

SECTION QUALIFIER: Z　NONE

TYPE: 2　**CRISIS INTERVENTION:** Treatment of a traumatized, acutely disturbed or distressed individual for the purpose of short-term stabilization

Qualifier	Qualifier	Qualifier	Qualifier
Z None	Z None	Z None	Z None

SECTION: **G MENTAL HEALTH**

SECTION QUALIFIER: Z　NONE

TYPE: 3　**MEDICATION MANAGEMENT:** Monitoring and adjusting the use of medications for the treatment of a mental health disorder

Qualifier	Qualifier	Qualifier	Qualifier
Z None	Z None	Z None	Z None

SECTION: **G MENTAL HEALTH**

SECTION QUALIFIER: Z　NONE

TYPE: 5　**INDIVIDUAL PSYCHOTHERAPY:** Treatment of an individual with a mental health disorder by behavioral, cognitive, psychoanalytic, psychodynamic or psychophysiological means to improve functioning or well-being

Qualifier	Qualifier	Qualifier	Qualifier
Ø Interactive 1 Behavioral 2 Cognitive 3 Interpersonal 4 Psychoanalysis 5 Psychodynamic 6 Supportive 8 Cognitive-Behavioral 9 Psychophysiological	Z None	Z None	Z None

SECTION: G MENTAL HEALTH

SECTION QUALIFIER: Z NONE

TYPE: 6 **COUNSELING:** The application of psychological methods to treat an individual with normal developmental issues and psychological problems in order to increase function, improve well-being, alleviate distress, maladjustment or resolve crises

Qualifier	Qualifier	Qualifier	Qualifier
Ø Educational 1 Vocational 3 Other Counseling	Z None	Z None	Z None

SECTION: G MENTAL HEALTH

SECTION QUALIFIER: Z NONE

TYPE: 7 **FAMILY PSYCHOTHERAPY:** Treatment that includes one or more family members of an individual with a mental health disorder by behavioral, cognitive, psychoanalytic, psychodynamic or psychophysiological means to improve functioning or well-being

Qualifier	Qualifier	Qualifier	Qualifier
2 Other Family Psychotherapy	Z None	Z None	Z None

SECTION: G MENTAL HEALTH

SECTION QUALIFIER: Z NONE

TYPE: B **ELECTROCONVULSIVE THERAPY:** The application of controlled electrical voltages to treat a mental health disorder

Qualifier	Qualifier	Qualifier	Qualifier
Ø Unilateral-Single Seizure 1 Unilateral-Multiple Seizure 2 Bilateral-Single Seizure 3 Bilateral-Multiple Seizure 4 Other Electroconvulsive Therapy	Z None	Z None	Z None

SECTION: G MENTAL HEALTH

SECTION QUALIFIER: Z NONE

TYPE: C **BIOFEEDBACK:** Provision of information from the monitoring and regulating of physiological processes in conjunction with cognitive-behavioral techniques to improve patient functioning or well-being

Qualifier	Qualifier	Qualifier	Qualifier
9 Other Biofeedback	Z None	Z None	Z None

C; B; 7; 6;   Z: NONE   G: MENTAL HEALTH

SECTION: **G MENTAL HEALTH**

SECTION QUALIFIER: Z   NONE

TYPE: **F HYPNOSIS:** Induction of a state of heightened suggestibility by auditory, visual, and tactile techniques to elicit an emotional or behavioral response

Qualifier	Qualifier	Qualifier	Qualifier
Z None	Z None	Z None	Z None

SECTION: **G MENTAL HEALTH**

SECTION QUALIFIER: Z   NONE

TYPE: **G NARCOSYNTHESIS:** Administration of intravenous barbiturates in order to release suppressed or repressed thoughts

Qualifier	Qualifier	Qualifier	Qualifier
Z None	Z None	Z None	Z None

SECTION: **G MENTAL HEALTH**

SECTION QUALIFIER: Z   NONE

TYPE: **H GROUP PSYCHOTHERAPY:** Treatment of two or more individuals with a mental health disorder by behavioral, cognitive, psychoanalytic, psychodynamic, or psychophysiological means to improve functioning or well-being

Qualifier	Qualifier	Qualifier	Qualifier
Z None	Z None	Z None	Z None

SECTION: **G MENTAL HEALTH**

SECTION QUALIFIER: Z   NONE

TYPE: **J LIGHT THERAPY:** Application of specialized light treatments to improve functioning or well-being

Qualifier	Qualifier	Qualifier	Qualifier
Z None	Z None	Z None	Z None

SECTION: H SUBSTANCE ABUSE TREATMENT
SECTION QUALIFIER: Z NONE
TYPE: 2 **DETOXIFICATION SERVICES:** Detoxification from alcohol and/or drugs

Qualifier	Qualifier	Qualifier	Qualifier
Z None	Z None	Z None	Z None

SECTION: H SUBSTANCE ABUSE TREATMENT
SECTION QUALIFIER: Z NONE
TYPE: 3 **INDIVIDUAL COUNSELING:** The application of psychological methods to treat an individual with addictive behavior

Qualifier	Qualifier	Qualifier	Qualifier
Ø Cognitive 1 Behavioral 2 Cognitive-Behavioral 3 12-Step 4 Interpersonal 5 Vocational 6 Psychoeducation 7 Motivational Enhancement 8 Confrontational 9 Continuing Care B Spiritual C Pre/Post-Test Infectious Disease	Z None	Z None	Z None

DRG Non-OR HZ3[Ø123456789B]ZZZ

SECTION: H SUBSTANCE ABUSE TREATMENT
SECTION QUALIFIER: Z NONE
TYPE: 4 **GROUP COUNSELING:** The application of psychological methods to treat two or more individuals with addictive behavior

Qualifier	Qualifier	Qualifier	Qualifier
Ø Cognitive 1 Behavioral 2 Cognitive-Behavioral 3 12-Step 4 Interpersonal 5 Vocational 6 Psychoeducation 7 Motivational Enhancement 8 Confrontational 9 Continuing Care B Spiritual C Pre/Post-Test Infectious Disease	Z None	Z None	Z None

DRG Non-OR HZ4[Ø123456789B]ZZZ

SECTION: H SUBSTANCE ABUSE TREATMENT
SECTION QUALIFIER: Z NONE
TYPE: 5 INDIVIDUAL PSYCHOTHERAPY: Treatment of an individual with addictive behavior by behavioral, cognitive, psychoanalytic, psychodynamic, or psychophysiological means

Qualifier	Qualifier	Qualifier	Qualifier
Ø Cognitive 1 Behavioral 2 Cognitive-Behavioral 3 12-Step 4 Interpersonal 5 Interactive 6 Psychoeducation 7 Motivational Enhancement 8 Confrontational 9 Supportive B Psychoanalysis C Psychodynamic D Psychophysiological	Z None	Z None	Z None

DRG Non-OR All Values

SECTION: H SUBSTANCE ABUSE TREATMENT
SECTION QUALIFIER: Z NONE
TYPE: 6 FAMILY COUNSELING: The application of psychological methods that includes one or more family members to treat an individual with addictive behavior

Qualifier	Qualifier	Qualifier	Qualifier
3 Other Family Counseling	Z None	Z None	Z None

SECTION: H SUBSTANCE ABUSE TREATMENT
SECTION QUALIFIER: Z NONE
TYPE: 8 MEDICATION MANAGEMENT: Monitoring and adjusting the use of replacement medications for the treatment of addiction

Qualifier	Qualifier	Qualifier	Qualifier
Ø Nicotine Replacement 1 Methadone Maintenance 2 Levo-alpha-acetyl-methadol (LAAM) 3 Antabuse 4 Naltrexone 5 Naloxone 6 Clonidine 7 Bupropion 8 Psychiatric Medication 9 Other Replacement Medication	Z None	Z None	Z None

H: SUBSTANCE ABUSE TREATMENT   Z: NONE   5; 6; 8

New/Revised Text in Green   ~~deleted~~ Deleted   ♀ Females Only   ♂ Males Only   Coding Clinic
🔖 Non-covered   🔖 Limited Coverage   ⊞ Combination (See Appendix E)   DRG Non-OR   Non-OR   🔖 Hospital-Acquired Condition

SECTION: H SUBSTANCE ABUSE TREATMENT

SECTION QUALIFIER: Z NONE

TYPE: 9 **PHARMACOTHERAPY:** The use of replacement medications for the treatment of addiction

Qualifier	Qualifier	Qualifier	Qualifier
Ø Nicotine Replacement	Z None	Z None	Z None
1 Methadone Maintenance			
2 Levo-alpha-acetyl-methadol (LAAM)			
3 Antabuse			
4 Naltrexone			
5 Naloxone			
6 Clonidine			
7 Bupropion			
8 Psychiatric Medication			
9 Other Replacement Medication			

ICD-10-PCS Coding Guidelines

New Technology Section Guidelines (section X)

D. New Technology Section

General guidelines

D1

Section X codes are standalone codes. They are not supplemental codes. Section X codes fully represent the specific procedure described in the code title, and do not require any additional codes from other sections of ICD-10-PCS. When section X contains a code title which describes a specific new technology procedure, only that X code is reported for the procedure. There is no need to report a broader, non-specific code in another section of ICD-10-PCS.

Example: XWØ4321 Introduction of Ceftazidime-Avibactam Anti-infective into Central Vein, Percutaneous Approach, New Technology Group 1, can be coded to indicate that Ceftazidime-Avibactam Anti-infective was administered via a central vein. A separate code from table 3EØ in the Administration section of ICD-10-PCS is not coded in addition to this code.

Selection of Principal Procedure

The following instructions should be applied in the selection of principal procedure and clarification on the importance of the relation to the principal diagnosis when more than one procedure is performed:

1. Procedure performed for definitive treatment of both principal diagnosis and secondary diagnosis

   a. Sequence procedure performed for definitive treatment most related to principal diagnosis as principal procedure.

2. Procedure performed for definitive treatment and diagnostic procedures performed for both principal diagnosis and secondary diagnosis

   a. Sequence procedure performed for definitive treatment most related to principal diagnosis as principal procedure

3. A diagnostic procedure was performed for the principal diagnosis and a procedure is performed for definitive treatment of a secondary diagnosis.

   a. Sequence diagnostic procedure as principal procedure, since the procedure most related to the principal diagnosis takes precedence.

4. No procedures performed that are related to principal diagnosis; procedures performed for definitive treatment and diagnostic procedures were performed for secondary diagnosis

   a. Sequence procedure performed for definitive treatment of secondary diagnosis as principal procedure, since there are no procedures (definitive or nondefinitive treatment) related to principal diagnosis.

New/Revised Text in Green   ~~deleted~~ Deleted   ♀ Females Only   ♂ Males Only   **Coding Clinic**

  Non-covered   Limited Coverage   ⊕ Combination (See Appendix E)   DRG Non-OR   Non-OR   Hospital-Acquired Condition

SECTION: X NEW TECHNOLOGY
BODY SYSTEM: 2 CARDIOVASCULAR SYSTEM
OPERATION: A ASSISTANCE: Taking over a portion of a physiological function by extracorporeal means

Body Part	Approach	Device / Substance / Technology	Qualifier
5 Innominate Artery and Left Common Carotid Artery	3 Percutaneous	1 Cerebral Embolic Filtration, Dual Filter	2 New Technology Group 2

SECTION: X NEW TECHNOLOGY
BODY SYSTEM: 2 CARDIOVASCULAR SYSTEM
OPERATION: C EXTIRPATION: Taking or cutting out solid matter from a body part

Body Part	Approach	Device / Substance / Technology	Qualifier
Ø Coronary Artery, One Artery 1 Coronary Artery, Two Arteries 2 Coronary Artery, Three Arteries 3 Coronary Artery, Four or More Arteries	3 Percutaneous	6 Orbital Atherectomy Technology	1 New Technology Group 1

Coding Clinic: 2015, Q4, P14 – X2C0361

SECTION: X NEW TECHNOLOGY
BODY SYSTEM: 2 CARDIOVASCULAR SYSTEM
OPERATION: R REPLACEMENT: Putting in or on biological or synthetic material that physically takes the place and/or function of all or a portion of a body part

Body Part	Approach	Device / Substance / Technology	Qualifier
F Aortic Valve	Ø Open 3 Percutaneous 4 Percutaneous Endoscopic	3 Zooplastic Tissue, Rapid Deployment Technique	2 New Technology Group 2

SECTION: **X NEW TECHNOLOGY**
BODY SYSTEM: **H SKIN, SUBCUTANEOUS TISSUE, FASCIA AND BREAST**
OPERATION: **R REPLACEMENT:** Putting in or on biological or synthetic material that physically takes the place and/or function of all or a portion of a body part

Body Part	Approach	Device / Substance / Technology	Qualifier
P Skin	X External	L Skin Substitute, Porcine Liver Derived	2 New Technology Group 2

SECTION: **X NEW TECHNOLOGY**
BODY SYSTEM: **N BONES**
OPERATION: **S REPOSITION:** Moving to its normal location, or other suitable location, all or a portion of a body part

Body Part	Approach	Device / Substance / Technology	Qualifier
Ø Lumbar Vertebra 3 Cervical Vertebra 4 Thoracic Vertebra	Ø Open 4 Percutaneous Endoscopic	3 Magnetically Controlled Growth Rod(s)	2 New Technology Group 2

SECTION: X NEW TECHNOLOGY
BODY SYSTEM: R JOINTS
OPERATION: 2 MONITORING: Determining the level of a physiological or physical function repetitively over a period of time

Body Part	Approach	Device / Substance / Technology	Qualifier
G Knee Joint, Right H Knee Joint, Left	Ø Open	2 Intraoperative Knee Replacement Sensor	1 New Technology Group 1

SECTION: X NEW TECHNOLOGY
BODY SYSTEM: R JOINTS
OPERATION: G FUSION: Joining together portions of an articular body part rendering the articular body part immobile

Body Part	Approach	Device / Substance / Technology	Qualifier
Ø Occipital-cervical Joint 1 Cervical Vertebral Joint 2 Cervical Vertebral Joints, 2 or more 4 Cervicothoracic Vertebral Joint 6 Thoracic Vertebral Joint 7 Thoracic Vertebral Joints, 2 to 7 8 Thoracic Vertebral Joints, 8 or more A Thoracolumbar Vertebral Joint B Lumbar Vertebral Joint C Lumbar Vertebral Joints, 2 or more D Lumbosacral Joint	Ø Open	9 Interbody Fusion Device, Nanotextured Surface	2 New Technology Group 2

New/Revised Text in Green   deleted Deleted   ♀ Females Only   ♂ Males Only   **Coding Clinic**

⦿ Non-covered   ⦿ Limited Coverage   ⊡ Combination (See Appendix E)   DRG Non-OR   Non-OR   ⦿ Hospital-Acquired Condition

SECTION: X NEW TECHNOLOGY
BODY SYSTEM: W ANATOMICAL REGIONS
OPERATION: Ø INTRODUCTION: Putting in or on a therapeutic, diagnostic, nutritional, physiological, or prophylactic substance except blood or blood products

Body Part	Approach	Device / Substance / Technology	Qualifier
3 Peripheral Vein ~~4 Central Vein~~	3 Percutaneous	2 Ceftazidime-Avibactam Anti-infective 3 Idarucizumab, Dabigatran Reversal Agent 4 Isavuconazole Anti-infective 5 Blinatumomab Antineoplastic Immunotherapy	1 New Technology Group 1
3 Peripheral Vein	3 Percutaneous	7 Andexanet Alfa, Factor Xa Inhibitor Reversal Agent 9 Defibrotide Sodium Anticoagulant	2 New Technology Group 2
4 Central Vein	3 Percutaneous	2 Ceftazidime-Avibactam Anti-infective 3 Idarucizumab, Dabigatran Reversal Agent 4 Isavuconazole Antiinfective 5 Blinatumomab Antineoplastic Immunotherapy	1 New Technology Group 1
4 Central Vein	3 Percutaneous	7 Andexanet Alfa, Factor Xa Inhibitor Reversal Agent 9 Defibrotide Sodium Anticoagulant	2 New Technology Group 2
D Mouth and Pharynx	X External	8 Uridine Triacetate	2 New Technology Group 2

Coding Clinic: 2Ø15, Q4, P13, P15 – XWØ4331, XWØ4351

New/Revised Text in Green ~~deleted~~ Deleted ♀ Females Only ♂ Males Only **Coding Clinic**
🚫 Non-covered 🚫 Limited Coverage ⊞ Combination (See Appendix E) DRG Non-OR Non-OR 🚫 Hospital-Acquired Condition

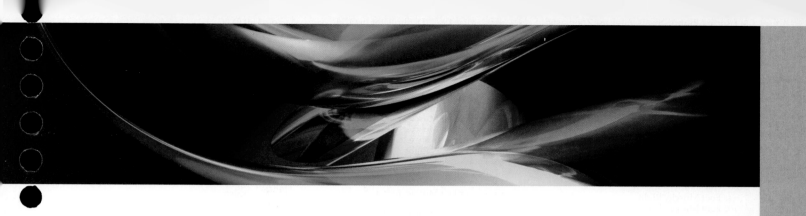

◄ New   ◄⁞⁞ Revised   ~~deleted~~ Deleted

Alveolotomy
  see Division, Head and Facial Bones ØN8
  see Drainage, Head and Facial Bones ØN9
Ambulatory cardiac monitoring 4A12X45
Amniocentesis see Drainage, Products of
  Conception 1Ø9Ø
Amnioinfusion see Introduction of substance in
  or on, Products of Conception 3EØE
Amnioscopy 1ØJØ8ZZ
Amniotomy see Drainage, Products of
  Conception 1Ø9Ø
AMPLATZER® Muscular VSD Occluder use
  Synthetic Substitute
Amputation see Detachment
AMS 800® Urinary Control System use
  Artificial Sphincter in Urinary System
Anal orifice use Anus
Analog radiography see Plain Radiography
Analog radiology see Plain Radiography
Anastomosis see Bypass
Anatomical snuffbox
  use Lower Arm and Wrist Muscle, Right
  use Lower Arm and Wrist Muscle, Left
Andexanet Alfa, Factor Xa Inhibitor Reversal
  Agent XWØ ◄
AneuRx® AAA Advantage® use Intraluminal
  Device
Angiectomy
  see Excision, Heart and Great Vessels 02B
  see Excision, Upper Arteries 03B
  see Excision, Lower Arteries 04B
  see Excision, Upper Veins 05B
  see Excision, Lower Veins 06B
Angiocardiography
  Combined right and left heart see
    Fluoroscopy, Heart, Right and Left B216
  Left Heart see Fluoroscopy, Heart, Left B215
  Right Heart see Fluoroscopy, Heart, Right B214
  SPY system intravascular fluorescence
    see Monitoring, Physiological Systems
    4A1 ◄〰
Angiography
  see Plain Radiography, Heart B20
  see Fluoroscopy, Heart B21
Angioplasty
  see Dilation, Heart and Great Vessels 027
  see Repair, Heart and Great Vessels 02Q
  see Replacement, Heart and Great Vessels 02R
  see Supplement, Heart and Great Vessels 02U
  see Dilation, Upper Arteries 037
  see Repair, Upper Arteries 03Q
  see Replacement, Upper Arteries 03R
  see Supplement, Upper Arteries 03U
  see Dilation, Lower Arteries 047
  see Repair, Lower Arteries 04Q
  see Replacement, Lower Arteries 04R
  see Supplement, Lower Arteries 04U
Angiorrhaphy
  see Repair, Heart and Great Vessels 02Q
  see Repair, Upper Arteries 03Q
  see Repair, Lower Arteries 04Q
Angioscopy
  02JY4ZZ
  03JY4ZZ
  04JY4ZZ
Angiotripsy
  see Occlusion, Upper Arteries 03L
  see Occlusion, Lower Arteries 04L
Angular artery use Face Artery
Angular vein
  use Face Vein, Right
  use Face Vein, Left
Annular ligament
  use Elbow Bursa and Ligament, Right
  use Elbow Bursa and Ligament, Left
Annuloplasty
  see Repair, Heart and Great Vessels 02Q
  see Supplement, Heart and Great Vessels 02U
Annuloplasty ring use Synthetic Substitute
Anoplasty
  see Repair, Anus ØDQQ
  see Supplement, Anus ØDUQ

Anorectal junction use Rectum
Anoscopy ØDJD8ZZ
Ansa cervicalis use Cervical Plexus
Antabuse therapy HZ93ZZZ
Antebrachial fascia
  use Subcutaneous Tissue and Fascia, Right
    Lower Arm
  use Subcutaneous Tissue and Fascia, Left
    Lower Arm
Anterior (pectoral) lymph node
  use Lymphatic, Right Axillary
  use Lymphatic, Left Axillary
Anterior cerebral artery use Intracranial
  Artery
Anterior cerebral vein use Intracranial Vein
Anterior choroidal artery use Intracranial
  Artery
Anterior circumflex humeral artery
  use Axillary Artery, Right
  use Axillary Artery, Left
Anterior communicating artery use Intracranial
  Artery
Anterior cruciate ligament (ACL)
  use Knee Bursa and Ligament, Right
  use Knee Bursa and Ligament, Left
Anterior crural nerve use Femoral Nerve
Anterior facial vein
  use Face Vein, Right
  use Face Vein, Left
Anterior intercostal artery
  use Internal Mammary Artery, Right
  use Internal Mammary Artery, Left
Anterior interosseous nerve use Median
  Nerve
Anterior lateral malleolar artery
  use Anterior Tibial Artery, Right
  use Anterior Tibial Artery, Left
Anterior lingual gland use Minor Salivary
  Gland
Anterior medial malleolar artery
  use Anterior Tibial Artery, Right
  use Anterior Tibial Artery, Left
Anterior spinal artery
  use Vertebral Artery, Right
  use Vertebral Artery, Left
Anterior tibial recurrent artery
  use Anterior Tibial Artery, Right
  use Anterior Tibial Artery, Left
Anterior ulnar recurrent artery
  use Ulnar Artery, Right
  use Ulnar Artery, Left
Anterior vagal trunk use Vagus Nerve
Anterior vertebral muscle
  use Neck Muscle, Right
  use Neck Muscle, Left
Antihelix
  use External Ear, Right
  use External Ear, Left
  use External Ear, Bilateral
Antimicrobial envelope use Anti-Infective
  Envelope
Antitragus
  use External Ear, Right
  use External Ear, Left
  use External Ear, Bilateral
Antrostomy see Drainage, Ear, Nose, Sinus
  Ø99
Antrotomy see Drainage, Ear, Nose, Sinus
  Ø99
Antrum of Highmore
  use Maxillary Sinus, Right
  use Maxillary Sinus, Left
Aortic annulus use Aortic Valve
Aortic arch use Thoracic Aorta, Ascending/
  Arch ◄〰
Aortic intercostal artery use Upper Artery ◄〰
Aortography
  see Plain Radiography, Upper Arteries B30
  see Fluoroscopy, Upper Arteries B31
  see Plain Radiography, Lower Arteries B40
  see Fluoroscopy, Lower Arteries B41

Aortoplasty
  ~~see Repair, Aorta, Thoracic 02QW~~
  ~~see Replacement, Aorta, Thoracic 02RW~~
  ~~see Supplement, Aorta, Thoracic 02UW~~
  see Repair, Aorta, Thoracic, Descending
    02QW ◄
  see Repair, Aorta, Thoracic, Ascending/Arch
    02QX ◄
  see Replacement, Aorta, Thoracic, Descending
    02RW ◄
  see Replacement, Aorta, Thoracic, Ascending/
    Arch 02RX ◄
  see Supplement, Aorta, Thoracic, Descending
    02UW ◄
  see Supplement, Aorta, Thoracic, Ascending/
    Arch 02UX ◄
  see Repair, Aorta, Abdominal 04Q0
  see Replacement, Aorta, Abdominal 04R0
  see Supplement, Aorta, Abdominal 04U0
Apical (subclavicular) lymph node
  use Lymphatic, Axillary, Right
  use Lymphatic, Axillary, Left
Apneustic center use Pons
Appendectomy
  see Excision, Appendix ØDBJ
  see Resection, Appendix ØDTJ
Appendicolysis see Release, Appendix ØDNJ
Appendicotomy see Drainage, Appendix ØD9J
Application see Introduction of substance in
  or on
Aquapheresis 6A550Z3
Aqueduct of Sylvius use Cerebral Ventricle
Aqueous humour
  use Anterior Chamber, Right
  use Anterior Chamber, Left
Arachnoid mater, intracranial use Cerebral
  Meninges
Arachnoid mater, spinal use Spinal Meninges
Arcuate artery
  use Foot Artery, Right
  use Foot Artery, Left
Areola
  use Nipple, Right
  use Nipple, Left
AROM (artificial rupture of membranes)
  10907ZC
Arterial canal (duct) use Pulmonary Artery, Left
Arterial pulse tracing see Measurement,
  Arterial 4A03
Arteriectomy
  see Excision, Heart and Great Vessels 02B
  see Excision, Upper Arteries 03B
  see Excision, Lower Arteries 04B
Arteriography
  see Plain Radiography, Heart B20
  see Fluoroscopy, Heart B21
  see Plain Radiography, Upper Arteries B30
  see Fluoroscopy, Upper Arteries B31
  see Plain Radiography, Lower Arteries B40
  see Fluoroscopy, Lower Arteries B41
Arterioplasty
  see Repair, Heart and Great Vessels 02Q
  see Replacement, Heart and Great Vessels 02R
  see Supplement, Heart and Great Vessels 02U
  see Repair, Upper Arteries 03Q
  see Replacement, Upper Arteries 03R
  see Supplement, Upper Arteries 03U
  see Repair, Lower Arteries 04Q
  see Replacement, Lower Arteries 04R
  see Supplement, Lower Arteries 04U
Arteriorrhaphy
  see Repair, Heart and Great Vessels 02Q
  see Repair, Upper Arteries 03Q
  see Repair, Lower Arteries 04Q
Arterioscopy
  ~~02JY4ZZ~~
  ~~03JY4ZZ~~
  ~~04JY4ZZ~~
  see Inspection, Great Vessel 02JY ◄
  see Inspection, Artery, Upper 03JY ◄
  see Inspection, Artery, Lower 04JY ◄

Arthrectomy
see Excision, Upper Joints ØRB
see Resection, Upper Joints ØRT
see Excision, Lower Joints ØSB
see Resection, Lower Joints ØST
Arthrocentesis
see Drainage, Upper Joints ØR9
see Drainage, Lower Joints ØS9
Arthrodesis
see Fusion, Upper Joints ØRG
see Fusion, Lower Joints ØSG
Arthrography
see Plain Radiography, Skull and Facial Bones BNØ
see Plain Radiography, Non-Axial Upper Bones BPØ
see Plain Radiography, Non-Axial Lower Bones BQØ
Arthrolysis
see Release, Upper Joints ØRN
see Release, Lower Joints ØSN
Arthropexy
see Repair, Upper Joints ØRQ
see Reposition, Upper Joints ØRS
see Repair, Lower Joints ØSQ
see Reposition, Lower Joints ØSS
Arthroplasty
see Repair, Upper Joints ØRQ
see Replacement, Upper Joints ØRR
see Supplement, Upper Joints ØRU
see Repair, Lower Joints ØSQ
see Replacement, Lower Joints ØSR
see Supplement, Lower Joints ØSU
Arthroscopy
see Inspection, Upper Joints ØRJ
see Inspection, Lower Joints ØSJ
Arthrotomy
see Drainage, Upper Joints ØR9
see Drainage, Lower Joints ØS9
Artificial anal sphincter (AAS) use Artificial Sphincter in Gastrointestinal System
Artificial bowel sphincter (neosphincter) use Artificial Sphincter in Gastrointestinal System
Artificial Sphincter
Insertion of device in
Anus ØDHQ
Bladder ØTHB
Bladder Neck ØTHC
Urethra ØTHD
Removal of device from
Anus ØDPQ
Bladder ØTPB
Urethra ØTPD
Revision of device in
Anus ØDWQ
Bladder ØTWB
Urethra ØTWD
Artificial urinary sphincter (AUS) use Artificial Sphincter in Urinary System
Aryepiglottic fold use Larynx
Arytenoid cartilage use Larynx
Arytenoid muscle
use Neck Muscle, Right
use Neck Muscle, Left
Arytenoidectomy see Excision, Larynx ØCBS
Arytenoidopexy see Repair, Larynx ØCQS
Ascenda Intrathecal Catheter use Infusion Device
Ascending aorta use Thoracic Aorta, Ascending/Arch ◄▥
Ascending palatine artery use Face Artery
Ascending pharyngeal artery
use External Carotid Artery, Right
use External Carotid Artery, Left
Aspiration, fine needle
fluid or gas see Drainage
tissue see Excision

Assessment
Activities of daily living see Activities of Daily Living Assessment, Rehabilitation F02
Hearing see Hearing Assessment, Diagnostic Audiology F13
Hearing aid see Hearing Aid Assessment, Diagnostic Audiology F14
Intravascular perfusion, using indocyanine green (ICG) dye see Monitoring, Physiological Systems 4A1 ◄
Motor function see Motor Function Assessment, Rehabilitation F01
Nerve function see Motor Function Assessment, Rehabilitation F01
Speech see Speech Assessment, Rehabilitation F00
Vestibular see Vestibular Assessment, Diagnostic Audiology F15
Vocational see Activities of Daily Living Treatment, Rehabilitation F08
Assistance
Cardiac
Continuous
Balloon Pump 5A02210
Impeller Pump 5A0221D
Other Pump 5A02216
Pulsatile Compression 5A02215
Intermittent
Balloon Pump 5A02110
Impeller Pump 5A0211D
Other Pump 5A02116
Pulsatile Compression 5A02115
Circulatory
Continuous
Hyperbaric 5A05221
Supersaturated 5A0522C
Intermittent
Hyperbaric 5A05121
Supersaturated 5A0512C
Respiratory
24-96 Consecutive Hours
Continuous Negative Airway Pressure 5A09459
Continuous Positive Airway Pressure 5A09457
Intermittent Negative Airway Pressure 5A0945B
Intermittent Positive Airway Pressure 5A09458
No Qualifier 5A0945Z
Greater than 96 Consecutive Hours
Continuous Negative Airway Pressure 5A09559
Continuous Positive Airway Pressure 5A09557
Intermittent Negative Airway Pressure 5A0955B
Intermittent Positive Airway Pressure 5A09558
No Qualifier 5A0955Z
Less than 24 Consecutive Hours
Continuous Negative Airway Pressure 5A09359
Continuous Positive Airway Pressure 5A09357
Intermittent Negative Airway Pressure 5A0935B
Intermittent Positive Airway Pressure 5A09358
No Qualifier 5A0935Z
Assurant (Cobalt) stent use Intraluminal Device
Atherectomy
see Extirpation, Heart and Great Vessels 02C
see Extirpation, Upper Arteries 03C
see Extirpation, Lower Arteries 04C
Atlantoaxial joint use Cervical Vertebral Joint
Atmospheric Control 6A0Z

Atrioseptoplasty
see Repair, Heart and Great Vessels 02Q
see Replacement, Heart and Great Vessels 02R
see Supplement, Heart and Great Vessels 02U
Atrioventricular node use Conduction Mechanism
Atrium dextrum cordis use Atrium, Right
Atrium pulmonale use Atrium, Left
Attain Ability® lead
use Cardiac Lead, Pacemaker in 02H
use Cardiac Lead, Defibrillator in 02H
Attain StarFix® (OTW) lead
use Cardiac Lead, Pacemaker in 02H
use Cardiac Lead, Defibrillator in O2H
Audiology, diagnostic
see Hearing Assessment, Diagnostic Audiology F13
see Hearing Aid Assessment, Diagnostic Audiology F14
see Vestibular Assessment, Diagnostic Audiology F15
Audiometry see Hearing Assessment, Diagnostic Audiology F13
Auditory tube
use Eustachian Tube, Right
use Eustachian Tube, Left
Auerbach's (myenteric) plexus use Nerve, Abdominal Sympathetic
Auricle
use External Ear, Right
use External Ear, Left
use External Ear, Bilateral
Auricularis muscle use Head Muscle
Autograft use Autologous Tissue Substitute
Autologous artery graft
use Autologous Arterial Tissue in Heart and Great Vessels
use Autologous Arterial Tissue in Upper Arteries
use Autologous Arterial Tissue in Lower Arteries
use Autologous Arterial Tissue in Upper Veins
use Autologous Arterial Tissue in Lower Veins
Autologous vein graft
use Autologous Venous Tissue in Heart and Great Vessels
use Autologous Venous Tissue in Upper Arteries
use Autologous Venous Tissue in Lower Arteries
use Autologous Venous Tissue in Upper Veins
use Autologous Venous Tissue in Lower Veins
Autotransfusion see Transfusion
Autotransplant
Adrenal tissue see Reposition, Endocrine System ØGS
Kidney
see Reposition, Urinary System ØTS
Pancreatic tissue see Reposition, Pancreas ØFSG
Parathyroid tissue see Reposition, Endocrine System ØGS
Thyroid tissue see Reposition, Endocrine System ØGS
Tooth see Reattachment, Mouth and Throat ØCM
Avulsion see Extraction
Axial Lumbar Interbody Fusion System use Interbody Fusion Device in Lower Joints
AxiaLIF® System use Interbody Fusion Device in Lower Joints
Axillary fascia
use Subcutaneous Tissue and Fascia, Right Upper Arm
use Subcutaneous Tissue and Fascia, Left Upper Arm
Axillary nerve use Brachial Plexus

INDEX TO PROCEDURES / Biceps femoris muscle

B

BAK/C® Interbody Cervical Fusion System *use*
 Interbody Fusion Device in Upper Joints
BAL (bronchial alveolar lavage), diagnostic *see*
 Drainage, Respiratory System ØB9
Balanoplasty
 see Repair, Penis ØVQS
 see Supplement, Penis ØVUS
Balloon Pump
 Continuous, Output 5AØ2210
 Intermittent, Output 5AØ2110
Bandage, Elastic *see* Compression
Banding
 see Occlusion
 see Restriction
Bard® Composix® (E/X) (LP) mesh *use* Synthetic
 Substitute
Bard® Composix® Kugel® patch *use* Synthetic
 Substitute
Bard® Dulex™ mesh *use* Synthetic Substitute
Bard® Ventralex™ hernia patch *use* Synthetic
 Substitute
Barium swallow *see* Fluoroscopy,
 Gastrointestinal System BD1
Baroreflex Activation Therapy® (BAT®)
 use Stimulator Generator in Subcutaneous
 Tissue and Fascia
 use Stimulator Lead in Upper Arteries
Bartholin's (greater vestibular) gland *use*
 Vestibular Gland
Basal (internal) cerebral vein *use* Intracranial
 Vein
Basal metabolic rate (BMR) *see*
 Measurement, Physiological
 Systems 4AØZ
Basal nuclei *use* Basal Ganglia
Base of Tongue *use* Pharynx ◀
Basilar artery *use* Intracranial Artery
Basis pontis *use* Pons
Beam Radiation
 Abdomen DWØ3
 Intraoperative DWØ33ZØ
 Adrenal Gland DGØ2
 Intraoperative DGØ23ZØ
 Bile Ducts DFØ2
 Intraoperative DFØ23ZØ
 Bladder DTØ2
 Intraoperative DTØ23ZØ
 Bone
 Other DPØC
 Intraoperative DPØC3ZØ
 Bone Marrow D7ØØ
 Intraoperative D7ØØ3ZØ
 Brain DØØØ
 Intraoperative DØØØ3ZØ
 Brain Stem DØØ1
 Intraoperative DØØ13ZØ
 Breast
 Left DMØØ
 Intraoperative DMØØ3ZØ
 Right DMØ1
 Intraoperative DMØ13ZØ
 Bronchus DBØ1
 Intraoperative DBØ13ZØ
 Cervix DUØ1
 Intraoperative DUØ13ZØ
 Chest DWØ2
 Intraoperative DWØ23ZØ
 Chest Wall DBØ7
 Intraoperative DBØ73ZØ
 Colon DDØ5
 Intraoperative DDØ53ZØ
 Diaphragm DBØ8
 Intraoperative DBØ83ZØ
 Duodenum DDØ2
 Intraoperative DDØ23ZØ
 Ear D9ØØ
 Intraoperative D9ØØ3ZØ
 Esophagus DDØØ
 Intraoperative DDØØ3ZØ

Beam Radiation *(Continued)*
 Eye D8ØØ
 Intraoperative D8ØØ3ZØ
 Femur DPØ9
 Intraoperative DPØ93ZØ
 Fibula DPØB
 Intraoperative DPØB3ZØ
 Gallbladder DFØ1
 Intraoperative DFØ13ZØ
 Gland
 Adrenal DGØ2
 Intraoperative DGØ23ZØ
 Parathyroid DGØ4
 Intraoperative DGØ43ZØ
 Pituitary DGØØ
 Intraoperative DGØØ3ZØ
 Thyroid DGØ5
 Intraoperative DGØ53ZØ
 Glands
 Salivary D9Ø6
 Intraoperative D9Ø63ZØ
 Head and Neck DWØ1
 Intraoperative DWØ13ZØ
 Hemibody DWØ4
 Intraoperative DWØ43ZØ
 Humerus DPØ6
 Intraoperative DPØ63ZØ
 Hypopharynx D9Ø3
 Intraoperative D9Ø33ZØ
 Ileum DDØ4
 Intraoperative DDØ43ZØ
 Jejunum DDØ3
 Intraoperative DDØ33ZØ
 Kidney DTØØ
 Intraoperative DTØØ3ZØ
 Larynx D9ØB
 Intraoperative D9ØB3ZØ
 Liver DFØØ
 Intraoperative DFØØ3ZØ
 Lung DBØ2
 Intraoperative DBØ23ZØ
 Lymphatics
 Abdomen D7Ø6
 Intraoperative D7Ø63ZØ
 Axillary D7Ø4
 Intraoperative D7Ø43ZØ
 Inguinal D7Ø8
 Intraoperative D7Ø83ZØ
 Neck D7Ø3
 Intraoperative D7Ø33ZØ
 Pelvis D7Ø7
 Intraoperative D7Ø73ZØ
 Thorax D7Ø5
 Intraoperative D7Ø53ZØ
 Mandible DPØ3
 Intraoperative DPØ33ZØ
 Maxilla DPØ2
 Intraoperative DPØ23ZØ
 Mediastinum DBØ6
 Intraoperative DBØ63ZØ
 Mouth D9Ø4
 Intraoperative D9Ø43ZØ
 Nasopharynx D9ØD
 Intraoperative D9ØD3ZØ
 Neck and Head DWØ1
 Intraoperative DWØ13ZØ
 Nerve
 Peripheral DØØ7
 Intraoperative DØØ73ZØ
 Nose D9Ø1
 Intraoperative D9Ø13ZØ
 Oropharynx D9ØF
 Intraoperative D9ØF3ZØ
 Ovary DUØØ
 Intraoperative DUØØ3ZØ
 Palate
 Hard D9Ø8
 Intraoperative D9Ø83ZØ
 Soft D9Ø9
 Intraoperative D9Ø93ZØ
 Pancreas DFØ3
 Intraoperative DFØ33ZØ

Beam Radiation *(Continued)*
 Parathyroid Gland DGØ4
 Intraoperative DGØ43ZØ
 Pelvic Bones DPØ8
 Intraoperative DPØ83ZØ
 Pelvic Region DWØ6
 Intraoperative DWØ63ZØ
 Pineal Body DGØ1
 Intraoperative DGØ13ZØ
 Pituitary Gland DGØØ
 Intraoperative DGØØ3ZØ
 Pleura DBØ5
 Intraoperative DBØ53ZØ
 Prostate DVØØ
 Intraoperative DVØØ3ZØ
 Radius DPØ7
 Intraoperative DPØ73ZØ
 Rectum DDØ7
 Intraoperative DDØ73ZØ
 Rib DPØ5
 Intraoperative DPØ53ZØ
 Sinuses D9Ø7
 Intraoperative D9Ø73ZØ
 Skin
 Abdomen DHØ8
 Intraoperative DHØ83ZØ
 Arm DHØ4
 Intraoperative DHØ43ZØ
 Back DHØ7
 Intraoperative DHØ73ZØ
 Buttock DHØ9
 Intraoperative DHØ93ZØ
 Chest DHØ6
 Intraoperative DHØ63ZØ
 Face DHØ2
 Intraoperative DHØ23ZØ
 Leg DHØB
 Intraoperative DHØB3ZØ
 Neck DHØ3
 Intraoperative DHØ33ZØ
 Skull DPØØ
 Intraoperative DPØØ3ZØ
 Spinal Cord DØØ6
 Intraoperative DØØ63ZØ
 Spleen D7Ø2
 Intraoperative D7Ø23ZØ
 Sternum DPØ4
 Intraoperative DPØ43ZØ
 Stomach DDØ1
 Intraoperative DDØ13ZØ
 Testis DVØ1
 Intraoperative DVØ13ZØ
 Thymus D7Ø1
 Intraoperative D7Ø13ZØ
 Thyroid Gland DGØ5
 Intraoperative DGØ53ZØ
 Tibia DPØB
 Intraoperative DPØB3ZØ
 Tongue D9Ø5
 Intraoperative D9Ø53ZØ
 Trachea DBØØ
 Intraoperative DBØØ3ZØ
 Ulna DPØ7
 Intraoperative DPØ73ZØ
 Ureter DTØ1
 Intraoperative DTØ13ZØ
 Urethra DTØ3
 Intraoperative DTØ33ZØ
 Uterus DUØ2
 Intraoperative DUØ23ZØ
 Whole Body DWØ5
 Intraoperative DWØ53ZØ
Bedside swallow FØØZJWZ
Berlin Heart Ventricular Assist Device *use*
 Implantable Heart Assist System in Heart
 and Great Vessels
Biceps brachii muscle
 use Upper Arm Muscle, Right
 use Upper Arm Muscle, Left
Biceps femoris muscle
 use Upper Leg Muscle, Right
 use Upper Leg Muscle, Left

◀ New   ◀◀◀ Revised   ~~deleted~~ Deleted   685

◀ New　◀▥ Revised　~~deleted~~ Deleted

Bypass *(Continued)*
  Artery
    Axillary
      Left 0316Ø
      Right 0315Ø
    Brachial
      Left 0318Ø
      Right 0317Ø
    Common Carotid
      Left 031JØ
      Right 031HØ
    Common Iliac
      Left 041D
      Right 041C
    Coronary
      ~~Four or More Sites 0213~~
      ~~One Site 0210~~
      ~~Three Sites 0212~~
      ~~Two Sites 0211~~
      Four or More Arteries 0213 ◄
      One Artery 0210 ◄
      Three Arteries 0212 ◄
      Two Arteries 0211 ◄
    External Carotid
      Left 031NØ
      Right 031MØ
    External Iliac
      Left 041J
      Right 041H
    Femoral
      Left 041L
      Right 041K
    Innominate 0312Ø
    Internal Carotid
      Left 031LØ
      Right 031KØ
    Internal Iliac
      Left 041F
      Right 041E
    Intracranial 031GØ
    Popliteal
      Left 041N
      Right 041M
    Pulmonary ◄
      Left 021R ◄
      Right 021Q ◄
    Pulmonary Trunk 021P ◄
    Radial
      Left 031CØ
      Right 031BØ
    Splenic 0414
    Subclavian
      Left 0314Ø
      Right 0313Ø
    Temporal
      Left 031TØ
      Right 031SØ
    Ulnar
      Left 031AØ
      Right 0319Ø
  Atrium
    Left 0217
    Right 0216
  Bladder 0T1B
  Cavity, Cranial 0W110J
  Cecum ØD1H
  Cerebral Ventricle 0016

Bypass *(Continued)*
  Colon
    Ascending ØD1K
    Descending ØD1M
    Sigmoid ØD1N
    Transverse ØD1L
  Duct
    Common Bile ØF19
    Cystic ØF18
    Hepatic
      Left ØF16
      Right ØF15
    Lacrimal
      Left 081Y
      Right 081X
    Pancreatic ØF1D
      Accessory ØF1F
  Duodenum ØD19
  Ear
    Left 091EØ
    Right 091DØ
  Esophagus ØD15
    Lower ØD13
    Middle ØD12
    Upper ØD11
  Fallopian Tube
    Left ØU16
    Right ØU15
  Gallbladder ØF14
  Ileum ØD1B
  Jejunum ØD1A
  Kidney Pelvis
    Left ØT14
    Right ØT13
  Pancreas ØF1G
  Pelvic Cavity ØW1J
  Peritoneal Cavity ØW1G
  Pleural Cavity
    Left ØW1B
    Right ØW19
  Spinal Canal 001U
  Stomach ØD16
  Trachea 0B11
  Ureter
    Left ØT17
    Right ØT16
  Ureters, Bilateral ØT18
  Vas Deferens
    Bilateral ØV1Q
    Left ØV1P
    Right ØV1N
  Vein
    Axillary
      Left 0518
      Right 0517
    Azygos 0510
    Basilic
      Left 051C
      Right 051B
    Brachial
      Left 051A
      Right 0519
    Cephalic
      Left 051F
      Right 051D

Bypass *(Continued)*
  Vein *(Continued)*
    Colic 0617
    Common Iliac
      Left 061D
      Right 061C
    Esophageal 0613
    External Iliac
      Left 061G
      Right 061F
    External Jugular
      Left 051Q
      Right 051P
    Face
      Left 051V
      Right 051T
    Femoral
      Left 061N
      Right 061M
    Foot
      Left 061V
      Right 061T
    Gastric 0612
    Greater Saphenous
      Left 061Q
      Right 061P
    Hand
      Left 051H
      Right 051G
    Hemiazygos 0511
    Hepatic 0614
    Hypogastric
      Left 061J
      Right 061H
    Inferior Mesenteric 0616
    Innominate
      Left 0514
      Right 0513
    Internal Jugular
      Left 051N
      Right 051M
    Intracranial 051L
    Lesser Saphenous
      Left 061S
      Right 061R
    Portal 0618
    Renal
      Left 061B
      Right 0619
    Splenic 0611
    Subclavian
      Left 0516
      Right 0515
    Superior Mesenteric 0615
    Vertebral
      Left 051S
      Right 051R
  Vena Cava
    Inferior 0610
    Superior 021V
  Ventricle
    Left 021L
    Right 021K
Bypass, cardiopulmonary 5A1221Z

C

Caesarean section *see* Extraction, Products of Conception 10D0
Calcaneocuboid joint
 use Tarsal Joint, Right
 use Tarsal Joint, Left
Calcaneocuboid ligament
 use Foot Bursa and Ligament, Right
 use Foot Bursa and Ligament, Left
Calcaneofibular ligament
 use Ankle Bursa and Ligament, Right
 use Ankle Bursa and Ligament, Left
Calcaneus
 use Tarsal, Right
 use Tarsal, Left
Cannulation
 see Bypass
 see Dilation
 see Drainage
 see Irrigation
Canthorrhaphy *see* Repair, Eye 08Q
Canthotomy *see* Release, Eye 08N
Capitate bone
 use Carpal, Right
 use Carpal, Left
Capsulectomy, lens *see* Excision, Eye 08B
Capsulorrhaphy, joint
 see Repair, Upper Joints 0RQ
 see Repair, Lower Joints 0SQ
Cardia *use* Esophagogastric Junction
Cardiac contractility modulation lead *use* Cardiac Lead in Heart and Great Vessels
Cardiac event recorder *use* Monitoring Device
Cardiac Lead
 Defibrillator
  Atrium
   Left 02H7
   Right 02H6
  Pericardium 02HN
  Vein, Coronary 02H4
  Ventricle
   Left 02HL
   Right 02HK
 Insertion of device in
  Atrium
   Left 02H7
   Right 02H6
  Pericardium 02HN
  Vein, Coronary 02H4
  Ventricle
   Left 02HL
   Right 02HK
 Pacemaker
  Atrium
   Left 02H7
   Right 02H6
  Pericardium 02HN
  Vein, Coronary 02H4
  Ventricle
   Left 02HL
   Right 02HK
 Removal of device from, Heart 02PA
 Revision of device in, Heart 02WA
Cardiac plexus *use* Nerve, Thoracic Sympathetic
Cardiac Resynchronization Defibrillator Pulse Generator
 Abdomen 0JH8
 Chest 0JH6
Cardiac Resynchronization Pacemaker Pulse Generator
 Abdomen 0JH8
 Chest 0JH6
Cardiac resynchronization therapy (CRT) lead
 use Cardiac Lead, Pacemaker in 02H
 use Cardiac Lead, Defibrillator in 02H
Cardiac Rhythm Related Device
 Insertion of device in
  Abdomen 0JH8
  Chest 0JH6

Cardiac Rhythm Related Device *(Continued)*
 Removal of device from, Subcutaneous Tissue and Fascia, Trunk 0JPT
 Revision of device in, Subcutaneous Tissue and Fascia, Trunk 0JWT
Cardiocentesis *see* Drainage, Pericardial Cavity 0W9D
Cardioesophageal junction *use* Esophagogastric Junction
Cardiolysis *see* Release, Heart and Great Vessels 02N
CardioMEMS® pressure sensor *use* Monitoring Device, Pressure Sensor in 02H
Cardiomyotomy *see* Division, Esophagogastric Junction 0D84
Cardioplegia *see* Introduction of substance in or on, Heart 3E08
Cardiorrhaphy *see* Repair, Heart and Great Vessels 02Q
Cardioversion 5A2204Z
Caregiver Training F0FZ
Caroticotympanic artery
 use Internal Carotid Artery, Right
 use Internal Carotid Artery, Left
Carotid (artery) sinus (baroreceptor) lead *use* Stimulator Lead in Upper Arteries
Carotid glomus
 use Carotid Body, Left
 use Carotid Body, Right
 use Carotid Bodies, Bilateral
Carotid sinus
 use Internal Carotid Artery, Right
 use Internal Carotid Artery, Left
Carotid sinus nerve *use* Glossopharyngeal Nerve
Carotid WALLSTENT® Monorail® Endoprosthesis *use* Intraluminal Device
Carpectomy
 see Excision, Upper Bones 0PB
 see Resection, Upper Bones 0PT
Carpometacarpal (CMC) joint
 use Metacarpocarpal Joint, Right
 use Metacarpocarpal Joint, Left
Carpometacarpal ligament
 use Hand Bursa and Ligament, Right
 use Hand Bursa and Ligament, Left
Casting *see* Immobilization
CAT scan *see* Computerized Tomography (CT Scan)
Catheterization
 see Dilation
 see Drainage
 see Insertion of device in
 see Irrigation
 Heart *see* Measurement, Cardiac 4A02
 Umbilical vein, for infusion 06H033T
Cauda equina *use* Lumbar Spinal Cord
Cauterization
 see Destruction
 see Repair
Cavernous plexus *use* Head and Neck Sympathetic Nerve
Cecectomy
 see Excision, Cecum 0DBH
 see Resection, Cecum 0DTH
Cecocolostomy
 see Bypass, Gastrointestinal System 0D1
 see Drainage, Gastrointestinal System 0D9
Cecopexy
 see Repair, Cecum 0DQH
 see Reposition, Cecum 0DSH
Cecoplication *see* Restriction, Cecum 0DVH
Cecorrhaphy *see* Repair, Cecum 0DQH
Cecostomy
 see Bypass, Cecum 0D1H
 see Drainage, Cecum 0D9H
Cecotomy *see* Drainage, Cecum 0D9H
Ceftazidime-Avibactam Anti-infective XW0
Celiac (solar) plexus *use* Abdominal Sympathetic Nerve

Celiac ganglion *use* Abdominal Sympathetic Nerve
Celiac lymph node *use* Lymphatic, Aortic
Celiac trunk *use* Celiac Artery
Central axillary lymph node
 use Lymphatic, Right Axillary
 use Lymphatic, Left Axillary
Central venous pressure *see* Measurement, Venous 4A04
Centrimag® Blood Pump *use* External Heart Assist System in Heart and Great Vessels
Cephalogram BN00ZZZ
Ceramic on ceramic bearing surface *use* Synthetic Substitute, Ceramic in 0SR ◀
Cerclage *see* Restriction
Cerebral aqueduct (Sylvius) *use* Cerebral Ventricle
Cerebral Embolic Filtration, Dual Filter X2A5312 ◀
Cerebrum *use* Brain
Cervical esophagus *use* Esophagus, Upper
Cervical facet joint
 use Cervical Vertebral Joint
 use Cervical Vertebral Joint, 2 or more
Cervical ganglion *use* Head and Neck Sympathetic Nerve
Cervical interspinous ligament *use* Head and Neck Bursa and Ligament
Cervical intertransverse ligament *use* Head and Neck Bursa and Ligament
Cervical ligamentum flavum *use* Head and Neck Bursa and Ligament
Cervical lymph node
 use Lymphatic, Right Neck
 use Lymphatic, Left Neck
Cervicectomy
 see Excision, Cervix 0UBC
 see Resection, Cervix 0UTC
Cervicothoracic facet joint *use* Cervicothoracic Vertebral Joint
Cesarean section *see* Extraction, Products of Conception 10D0
Change device in
 Abdominal Wall 0W2FX
 Back
  Lower 0W2LX
  Upper 0W2KX
 Bladder 0T2BX
 Bone
  Facial 0N2WX
  Lower 0Q2YX
  Nasal 0N2BX
  Upper 0P2YX
 Bone Marrow 072TX
 Brain 0020X
 Breast
  Left 0H2UX
  Right 0H2TX
 Bursa and Ligament
  Lower 0M2YX
  Upper 0M2XX
 Cavity, Cranial 0W21X
 Chest Wall 0W28X
 Cisterna Chyli 072LX
 Diaphragm 0B2TX
 Duct
  Hepatobiliary 0F2BX
  Pancreatic 0F2DX
 Ear
  Left 092JX
  Right 092HX
 Epididymis and Spermatic Cord 0V2MX
 Extremity
  Lower
   Left 0Y2BX
   Right 0Y29X
  Upper
   Left 0X27X
   Right 0X26X
 Eye
  Left 0821X
  Right 0820X

◀ New ◀⊪ Revised ~~deleted~~ Deleted

Change device in *(Continued)*
  Face 0W22X
  Fallopian Tube 0U28X
  Gallbladder 0F24X
  Gland
    Adrenal 0G25X
    Endocrine 0G2SX
    Pituitary 0G20X
    Salivary 0C2AX
  Head 0W20X
  Intestinal Tract
    Lower 0D2DXUZ
    Upper 0D20XUZ
  Jaw
    Lower 0W25X
    Upper 0W24X
  Joint
    Lower 0S2YX
    Upper 0R2YX
  Kidney 0T25X
  Larynx 0C2SX
  Liver 0F20X
  Lung
    Left 0B2LX
    Right 0B2KX
  Lymphatic 072NX
    Thoracic Duct 072KX
  Mediastinum 0W2CX
  Mesentery 0D2VX
  Mouth and Throat 0C2YX
  Muscle
    Lower 0K2YX
    Upper 0K2XX
  Neck 0W26X
  Nerve
    Cranial 002EX
    Peripheral 012YX
  Nose 092KX
  Omentum 0D2UX
  Ovary 0U23X
  Pancreas 0F2GX
  Parathyroid Gland 0G2RX
  Pelvic Cavity 0W2JX
  Penis 0V2SX
  Pericardial Cavity 0W2DX
  Perineum
    Female 0W2NX
    Male 0W2MX
  Peritoneal Cavity 0W2GX
  Peritoneum 0D2WX
  Pineal Body 0G21X
  Pleura 0B2QX
  Pleural Cavity
    Left 0W2BX
    Right 0W29X
  Products of Conception 10207
  Prostate and Seminal Vesicles 0V24X
  Retroperitoneum 0W2HX
  Scrotum and Tunica Vaginalis 0V28X
  Sinus 092YX
  Skin 0H2PX
  Skull 0N20X
  Spinal Canal 002UX
  Spleen 072PX
  Subcutaneous Tissue and Fascia
    Head and Neck 0J2SX
    Lower Extremity 0J2WX
    Trunk 0J2TX
    Upper Extremity 0J2VX
  Tendon
    Lower 0L2YX
    Upper 0L2XX
  Testis 0V2DX
  Thymus 072MX
  Thyroid Gland 0G2KX
  Trachea 0B21
  Tracheobronchial Tree 0B20X
  Ureter 0T29X
  Urethra 0T2DX
  Uterus and Cervix 0U2DXHZ
  Vagina and Cul-de-sac 0U2HXGZ

Change device in *(Continued)*
  Vas Deferens 0V2RX
  Vulva 0U2MX
Change device in or on
  Abdominal Wall 2W03X
  Anorectal 2Y03X5Z
  Arm
    Lower
      Left 2W0DX
      Right 2W0CX
    Upper
      Left 2W0BX
      Right 2W0AX
  Back 2W05X
  Chest Wall 2W04X
  Ear 2Y02X5Z
  Extremity
    Lower
      Left 2W0MX
      Right 2W0LX
    Upper
      Left 2W09X
      Right 2W08X
  Face 2W01X
  Finger
    Left 2W0KX
    Right 2W0JX
  Foot
    Left 2W0TX
    Right 2W0SX
  Genital Tract, Female 2Y04X5Z
  Hand
    Left 2W0FX
    Right 2W0EX
  Head 2W00X
  Inguinal Region
    Left 2W07X
    Right 2W06X
  Leg
    Lower
      Left 2W0RX
      Right 2W0QX
    Upper
      Left 2W0PX
      Right 2W0NX
  Mouth and Pharynx 2Y00X5Z
  Nasal 2Y01X5Z
  Neck 2W02X
  Thumb
    Left 2W0HX
    Right 2W0GX
  Toe
    Left 2W0VX
    Right 2W0UX
  Urethra 2Y05X5Z
Chemoembolization *see* Introduction of
    substance in or on
Chemosurgery, Skin 3E00XTZ
Chemothalamectomy *see* Destruction,
    Thalamus 0059
Chemotherapy, Infusion for cancer *see*
    Introduction of substance in or on
Chest x-ray *see* Plain Radiography, Chest BW03
Chiropractic Manipulation
  Abdomen 9WB9X
  Cervical 9WB1X
  Extremities
    Lower 9WB6X
    Upper 9WB7X
  Head 9WB0X
  Lumbar 9WB3X
  Pelvis 9WB5X
  Rib Cage 9WB8X
  Sacrum 9WB4X
  Thoracic 9WB2X
Choana *use* Nasopharynx
Cholangiogram
  see Plain Radiography, Hepatobiliary System
    and Pancreas BF0
  see Fluoroscopy, Hepatobiliary System and
    Pancreas BF1

Cholecystectomy
  see Excision, Gallbladder 0FB4
  see Resection, Gallbladder 0FT4
Cholecystojejunostomy
  see Bypass, Hepatobiliary System and
    Pancreas 0F1
  see Drainage, Hepatobiliary System and
    Pancreas 0F9
Cholecystopexy
  see Repair, Gallbladder 0FQ4
  see Reposition, Gallbladder 0FS4
Cholecystoscopy 0FJ44ZZ
Cholecystostomy
  see Bypass, Gallbladder 0F14
  see Drainage, Gallbladder 0F94
Cholecystotomy *see* Drainage, Gallbladder 0F94
Choledochectomy
  see Excision, Hepatobiliary System and
    Pancreas 0FB
  see Resection, Hepatobiliary System and
    Pancreas 0FT
Choledocholithotomy *see* Extirpation, Duct,
    Common Bile 0FC9
Choledochoplasty
  see Repair, Hepatobiliary System and
    Pancreas 0FQ
  see Replacement, Hepatobiliary System and
    Pancreas 0FR
  see Supplement, Hepatobiliary System and
    Pancreas 0FU
Choledochoscopy 0FJB8ZZ
Choledochotomy *see* Drainage, Hepatobiliary
    System and Pancreas 0F9
Cholelithotomy *see* Extirpation, Hepatobiliary
    System and Pancreas 0FC
Chondrectomy
  see Excision, Upper Joints 0RB
  see Excision, Lower Joints 0SB
  Knee *see* Excision, Lower Joints 0SB
  Semilunar cartilage *see* Excision, Lower Joints
    0SB
Chondroglossus muscle *use* Tongue, Palate,
    Pharynx Muscle
Chorda tympani *use* Facial Nerve
Chordotomy *see* Division, Central Nervous
    System 008
Choroid plexus *use* Cerebral Ventricle
Choroidectomy
  see Excision, Eye 08B
  see Resection, Eye 08T
Ciliary body
  use Eye, Right
  use Eye, Left
Ciliary ganglion *use* Head and Neck
    Sympathetic Nerve
Circle of Willis *use* Intracranial Artery
Circumcision 0VTTXZZ
Circumflex iliac artery
  use Femoral Artery, Right
  use Femoral Artery, Left
Clamp and rod internal fixation system (CRIF)
  use Internal Fixation Device in Upper Bones
  use Internal Fixation Device in Lower Bones
Clamping *see* Occlusion
Claustrum *use* Basal Ganglia
Claviculectomy
  see Excision, Upper Bones 0PB
  see Resection, Upper Bones 0PT
Claviculotomy
  see Division, Upper Bones 0P8
  see Drainage, Upper Bones 0P9
Clipping, aneurysm *see* Restriction using
    Extraluminal Device
Clitorectomy, clitoridectomy
  see Excision, Clitoris 0UBJ
  see Resection, Clitoris 0UTJ
Clolar *use* Clofarabine
Closure
  see Occlusion
  see Repair
Clysis *see* Introduction of substance in or on

Coagulation *see* Destruction
CoAxia NeuroFlo catheter *use* Intraluminal Device
Cobalt/chromium head and polyethylene socket *use* Synthetic Substitute, Metal on Polyethylene in ØSR
Cobalt/chromium head and socket *use* Synthetic Substitute, Metal in ØSR
Coccygeal body *use* Coccygeal Glomus
Coccygeus muscle
　use Trunk Muscle, Right
　use Trunk Muscle, Left
Cochlea
　use Inner Ear, Right
　use Inner Ear, Left
Cochlear implant (CI), multiple channel (electrode) *use* Hearing Device, Multiple Channel Cochlear Prosthesis in 09H
Cochlear implant (CI), single channel (electrode) *use* Hearing Device, Single Channel Cochlear Prosthesis in 09H
Cochlear Implant Treatment FØBZØ
Cochlear nerve *use* Acoustic Nerve
COGNIS® CRT-D *use* Cardiac Resynchronization Defibrillator Pulse Generator in ØJH
Colectomy
　see Excision, Gastrointestinal System ØDB
　see Resection, Gastrointestinal System ØDT
Collapse *see* Occlusion
Collection from
　Breast, Breast Milk 8EØHX62
　Indwelling Device
　　Circulatory System
　　　Blood 8CØ2X6K
　　　Other Fluid 8CØ2X6L
　　Nervous System
　　　Cerebrospinal Fluid 8CØ1X6J
　　　Other Fluid 8CØ1X6L
　Integumentary System, Breast Milk 8EØHX62
　Reproductive System, Male, Sperm 8EØVX63
Colocentesis *see* Drainage, Gastrointestinal System ØD9
Colofixation
　see Repair, Gastrointestinal System ØDQ
　see Reposition, Gastrointestinal System ØDS
Cololysis *see* Release, Gastrointestinal System ØDN
Colonic Z-Stent® *use* Intraluminal Device
Colonoscopy ØDJD8ZZ
Colopexy
　see Repair, Gastrointestinal System ØDQ
　see Reposition, Gastrointestinal System ØDS
Coloplication *see* Restriction, Gastrointestinal System ØDV
Coloproctectomy
　see Excision, Gastrointestinal System ØDB
　see Resection, Gastrointestinal System ØDT
Coloproctostomy
　see Bypass, Gastrointestinal System ØD1
　see Drainage, Gastrointestinal System ØD9
Colopuncture *see* Drainage, Gastrointestinal System ØD9
Colorrhaphy *see* Repair, Gastrointestinal System ØDQ
Colostomy
　see Bypass, Gastrointestinal System ØD1
　see Drainage, Gastrointestinal System ØD9
Colpectomy
　see Excision, Vagina ØUBG
　see Resection, Vagina ØUTG
Colpocentesis *see* Drainage, Vagina ØU9G
Colpopexy
　see Repair, Vagina ØUQG
　see Reposition, Vagina ØUSG
Colpoplasty
　see Repair, Vagina ØUQG
　see Supplement, Vagina ØUUG
Colporrhaphy *see* Repair, Vagina ØUQG
Colposcopy ØUJH8ZZ
Columella *use* Nose

Common digital vein
　use Foot Vein, Right
　use Foot Vein, Left
Common facial vein
　use Face Vein, Right
　use Face Vein, Left
Common fibular nerve *use* Peroneal Nerve
Common hepatic artery *use* Hepatic Artery
Common iliac (subaortic) lymph node *use* Lymphatic, Pelvis
Common interosseous artery
　use Ulnar Artery, Right
　use Ulnar Artery, Left
Common peroneal nerve *use* Peroneal Nerve
Complete (SE) stent *use* Intraluminal Device
Compression *see* Restriction
　Abdominal Wall 2W13X
　Arm
　　Lower
　　　Left 2W1DX
　　　Right 2W1CX
　　Upper
　　　Left 2W1BX
　　　Right 2W1AX
　Back 2W15X
　Chest Wall 2W14X
　Extremity
　　Lower
　　　Left 2W1MX
　　　Right 2W1LX
　　Upper
　　　Left 2W19X
　　　Right 2W18X
　Face 2W11X
　Finger
　　Left 2W1KX
　　Right 2W1JX
　Foot
　　Left 2W1TX
　　Right 2W1SX
　Hand
　　Left 2W1FX
　　Right 2W1EX
　Head 2W10X
　Inguinal Region
　　Left 2W17X
　　Right 2W16X
　Leg
　　Lower
　　　Left 2W1RX
　　　Right 2W1QX
　　Upper
　　　Left 2W1PX
　　　Right 2W1NX
　Neck 2W12X
　Thumb
　　Left 2W1HX
　　Right 2W1GX
　Toe
　　Left 2W1VX
　　Right 2W1UX
Computer Assisted Procedure
　Extremity
　　Lower
　　　No Qualifier 8EØYXBZ
　　　With Computerized Tomography 8EØYXBG
　　　With Fluoroscopy 8EØYXBF
　　　With Magnetic Resonance Imaging 8EØYXBH
　　Upper
　　　No Qualifier 8EØXXBZ
　　　With Computerized Tomography 8EØXXBG
　　　With Fluoroscopy 8EØXXBF
　　　With Magnetic Resonance Imaging 8EØXXBH
　Head and Neck Region
　　No Qualifier 8EØ9XBZ
　　With Computerized Tomography 8EØ9XBG
　　With Fluoroscopy 8EØ9XBF
　　With Magnetic Resonance Imaging 8EØ9XBH

Computer Assisted Procedure
　(Continued)
　Trunk Region
　　No Qualifier 8EØWXBZ
　　With Computerized Tomography 8EØWXBG
　　With Fluoroscopy 8EØWXBF
　　With Magnetic Resonance Imaging 8EØWXBH
Computerized Tomography (CT Scan)
　Abdomen BW20
　　Chest and Pelvis BW25
　Abdomen and Chest BW24
　Abdomen and Pelvis BW21
　Airway, Trachea BB2F
　Ankle
　　Left BQ2H
　　Right BQ2G
　Aorta
　　Abdominal B420
　　　Intravascular Optical Coherence B420Z2Z
　　Thoracic B320
　　　Intravascular Optical Coherence B320Z2Z
　Arm
　　Left BP2F
　　Right BP2E
　Artery
　　Celiac B421
　　　Intravascular Optical Coherence B421Z2Z
　　Common Carotid
　　　Bilateral B325
　　　Intravascular Optical Coherence B325Z2Z
　　Coronary
　　　Bypass Graft
　　　　Multiple B223
　　　　　Intravascular Optical Coherence B223Z2Z
　　　Multiple B221
　　　　Intravascular Optical Coherence B221Z2Z
　　Internal Carotid
　　　Bilateral B328
　　　Intravascular Optical Coherence B328Z2Z
　　Intracranial B32R
　　　Intravascular Optical Coherence B32RZ2Z
　　Lower Extremity
　　　Bilateral B42H
　　　　Intravascular Optical Coherence B42HZ2Z
　　　Left B42G
　　　　Intravascular Optical Coherence B42GZ2Z
　　　Right B42F
　　　　Intravascular Optical Coherence B42FZ2Z
　　Pelvic B42C
　　　Intravascular Optical Coherence B42CZ2Z
　　Pulmonary
　　　Left B32T
　　　　Intravascular Optical Coherence B32TZ2Z
　　　Right B32S
　　　　Intravascular Optical Coherence B32SZ2Z
　　Renal
　　　Bilateral B428
　　　　Intravascular Optical Coherence B428Z2Z
　　　Transplant B42M
　　　　Intravascular Optical Coherence B42MZ2Z
　　Superior Mesenteric B424
　　　Intravascular Optical Coherence B424Z2Z

◀ New　◀▥ Revised　~~deleted~~ Deleted

◀ New   ◀≡ Revised   ~~deleted~~ Deleted

Control bleeding in (Continued)
Arm ◄
  Lower ◄
    Left ØX3F ◄
    Right ØX3D ◄
  Upper ◄
    Left ØX39 ◄
    Right ØX38 ◄
Axilla ◄
  Left ØX35 ◄
  Right ØX34 ◄
Back ◄
  Lower ØW3L ◄
  Upper ØW3K ◄
Buttock ◄
  Left ØY31 ◄
  Right ØY30 ◄
Cavity, Cranial ØW31 ◄
Chest Wall ØW38 ◄
Elbow Region ◄
  Left ØX3C ◄
  Right ØX3B ◄
Extremity ◄
  Lower ◄
    Left ØY3B ◄
    Right ØY39 ◄
  Upper ◄
    Left ØX37 ◄
    Right ØX36 ◄
Face ØW32 ◄
Femoral Region ◄
  Left ØY38 ◄
  Right ØY37 ◄
Foot ◄
  Left ØY3N ◄
  Right ØY3M ◄
Gastrointestinal Tract ØW3P ◄
Genitourinary Tract ØW3R ◄
Hand ◄
  Left ØX3K ◄
  Right ØX3J ◄
Head ØW30 ◄
Inguinal Region ◄
  Left ØY36 ◄
  Right ØY35 ◄
Jaw ◄
  Lower ØW35 ◄
  Upper ØW34 ◄
Knee Region ◄
  Left ØY3G ◄
  Right ØY3F ◄
Leg ◄
  Lower ◄
    Left ØY3J ◄
    Right ØY3H ◄
  Upper ◄
    Left ØY3D ◄
    Right ØY3C ◄
Mediastinum ØW3C ◄
Neck ØW36 ◄
Oral Cavity and Throat ØW33 ◄
Pelvic Cavity ØW3J ◄
Pericardial Cavity ØW3D ◄
Perineum ◄
  Female ØW3N ◄
  Male ØW3M ◄
Peritoneal Cavity ØW3G ◄
Pleural Cavity ◄
  Left ØW3B ◄
  Right ØW39 ◄
Respiratory Tract ØW3Q ◄
Retroperitoneum ØW3H ◄
Shoulder Region ◄
  Left ØX33 ◄
  Right ØX32 ◄
Wrist Region ◄
  Left ØX3H ◄
  Right ØX3G ◄
Conus arteriosus use Ventricle, Right
Conus medullaris use Spinal Cord, Lumbar

Conversion
  Cardiac rhythm 5A2204Z
  Gastrostomy to jejunostomy feeding device
    see Insertion of device in, Jejunum ØDHA
Cook Biodesign® Fistula Plug(s) use
  Nonautologous Tissue Substitute ◄
Cook Biodesign® Hernia Graft(s) use
  Nonautologous Tissue Substitute ◄
Cook Biodesign® Layered Graft(s) use
  Nonautologous Tissue Substitute ◄
Cook Zenapro™ Layered Graft(s) use
  Nonautologous Tissue Substitute ◄
Cook Zenith AAA Endovascular Graft ◄
  use Intraluminal Device, Branched or
    Fenestrated, One or Two Arteries in
    04V ◄
  use Intraluminal Device, Branched or
    Fenestrated, Three or More Arteries in
    04V ◄
  use Intraluminal Device ◄
Coracoacromial ligament
  use Shoulder Bursa and Ligament, Right
  use Shoulder Bursa and Ligament, Left
Coracobrachialis muscle
  use Upper Arm Muscle, Right
  use Upper Arm Muscle, Left
Coracoclavicular ligament
  use Shoulder Bursa and Ligament, Right
  use Shoulder Bursa and Ligament, Left
Coracohumeral ligament
  use Shoulder Bursa and Ligament, Right
  use Shoulder Bursa and Ligament, Left
Coracoid process
  use Scapula, Right
  use Scapula, Left
Cordotomy see Division, Central Nervous
  System 008
Core needle biopsy see Excision with qualifier
  Diagnostic
CoreValve transcatheter aortic valve use
  Zooplastic Tissue in Heart and Great
  Vessels
Cormet Hip Resurfacing System use
  Resurfacing Device in Lower Joints
Corniculate cartilage use Larynx
CoRoent® XL use Interbody Fusion Device in
  Lower Joints
Coronary arteriography
  see Plain Radiography, Heart B20
  see Fluoroscopy, Heart B21
Corox (OTW) Bipolar Lead
  use Cardiac Lead, Pacemaker in 02H
  use Cardiac Lead, Defibrillator in 02H
Corpus callosum use Brain
Corpus cavernosum use Penis
Corpus spongiosum use Penis
Corpus striatum use Basal Ganglia
Corrugator supercilii muscle use Facial
  Muscle
Cortical strip neurostimulator lead use
  Neurostimulator Lead in Central Nervous
  System
Costatectomy
  see Excision, Upper Bones ØPB
  see Resection, Upper Bones ØPT
Costectomy
  see Excision, Upper Bones ØPB
  see Resection, Upper Bones ØPT
Costocervical trunk
  use Subclavian Artery, Right
  use Subclavian Artery, Left
Costochondrectomy
  see Excision, Upper Bones ØPB
  see Resection, Upper Bones ØPT
Costoclavicular ligament
  use Shoulder Bursa and Ligament, Right
  use Shoulder Bursa and Ligament, Left
Costosternoplasty
  see Repair, Upper Bones ØPQ
  see Replacement, Upper Bones ØPR
  see Supplement, Upper Bones ØPU

Costotomy
  see Division, Upper Bones ØP8
  see Drainage, Upper Bones ØP9
Costotransverse joint use Thoracic Vertebral
  Joint
Costotransverse ligament
  use Thorax Bursa and Ligament, Right
  use Thorax Bursa and Ligament, Left
Costovertebral joint use Thoracic Vertebral
  Joint
Costoxiphoid ligament
  use Thorax Bursa and Ligament, Right
  use Thorax Bursa and Ligament, Left
Counseling
  Family, for substance abuse, Other Family
    Counseling HZ63ZZZ
  Group
    12-Step HZ43ZZZ
    Behavioral HZ41ZZZ
    Cognitive HZ40ZZZ
    Cognitive-Behavioral HZ42ZZZ
    Confrontational HZ48ZZZ
    Continuing Care HZ49ZZZ
    Infectious Disease
      Post-Test HZ4CZZZ
      Pre-Test HZ4CZZZ
    Interpersonal HZ44ZZZ
    Motivational Enhancement HZ47ZZZ
    Psychoeducation HZ46ZZZ
    Spiritual HZ4BZZZ
    Vocational HZ45ZZZ
  Individual
    12-Step HZ33ZZZ
    Behavioral HZ31ZZZ
    Cognitive HZ30ZZZ
    Cognitive-Behavioral HZ32ZZZ
    Confrontational HZ38ZZZ
    Continuing Care HZ39ZZZ
    Infectious Disease
      Post-Test HZ3CZZZ
      Pre-Test HZ3CZZZ
    Interpersonal HZ34ZZZ
    Motivational Enhancement HZ37ZZZ
    Psychoeducation HZ36ZZZ
    Spiritual HZ3BZZZ
    Vocational HZ35ZZZ
  Mental Health Services
    Educational GZ60ZZZ
    Other Counseling GZ63ZZZ
    Vocational GZ61ZZZ
Countershock, cardiac 5A2204Z
Cowper's (bulbourethral) gland use Urethra
CPAP (continuous positive airway pressure)
  see Assistance, Respiratory 5A09
Craniectomy
  see Excision, Head and Facial Bones ØNB
  see Resection, Head and Facial Bones ØNT
Cranioplasty
  see Repair, Head and Facial Bones ØNQ
  see Replacement, Head and Facial Bones
    ØNR
  see Supplement, Head and Facial Bones ØNU
Craniotomy
  see Drainage, Central Nervous System 009
  see Division, Head and Facial Bones ØN8
  see Drainage, Head and Facial Bones ØN9
Creation
  ~~Female ØW4NØ~~
  ~~Male ØW4MØ~~
  Perineum ◄
    Female ØW4N0 ◄
    Male ØW4M0 ◄
  Valve ◄
    Aortic 024F0 ◄
    Mitral 024G0 ◄
    Tricuspid 024J0 ◄
Cremaster muscle use Perineum Muscle
Cribriform plate
  use Ethmoid Bone, Right
  use Ethmoid Bone, Left
Cricoid cartilage use Trachea

Cricoidectomy *see* Excision, Larynx 0CBS
Cricothyroid artery
  use Thyroid Artery, Right
  use Thyroid Artery, Left
Cricothyroid muscle
  use Neck Muscle, Right
  use Neck Muscle, Left
Crisis Intervention GZ2ZZZZ
Crural fascia
  use Subcutaneous Tissue and Fascia, Right
    Upper Leg
  use Subcutaneous Tissue and Fascia, Left
    Upper Leg
Crushing, nerve
  Cranial *see* Destruction, Central Nervous
    System 005
  Peripheral *see* Destruction, Peripheral
    Nervous System 015
Cryoablation *see* Destruction
Cryotherapy *see* Destruction
Cryptorchidectomy
  see Excision, Male Reproductive System 0VB
  see Resection, Male Reproductive System 0VT
Cryptorchiectomy
  see Excision, Male Reproductive System 0VB
  see Resection, Male Reproductive System 0VT
Cryptotomy
  see Division, Gastrointestinal System 0D8
  see Drainage, Gastrointestinal System 0D9
CT scan *see* Computerized Tomography (CT
    Scan)
CT sialogram *see* Computerized Tomography
    (CT Scan), Ear, Nose, Mouth and Throat
    B92

Cubital lymph node
  use Lymphatic, Right Upper Extremity
  use Lymphatic, Left Upper Extremity
Cubital nerve *use* Ulnar Nerve
Cuboid bone
  use Tarsal, Right
  use Tarsal, Left
Cuboideonavicular joint
  use Tarsal Joint, Right
  use Tarsal Joint, Left
Culdocentesis *see* Drainage, Cul-de-sac 0U9F
Culdoplasty
  see Repair, Cul-de-sac 0UQF
  see Supplement, Cul-de-sac 0UUF
Culdoscopy 0UJH8ZZ
Culdotomy *see* Drainage, Cul-de-sac 0U9F
Culmen *use* Cerebellum
Cultured epidermal cell autograft *use*
    Autologous Tissue Substitute
Cuneiform cartilage *use* Larynx
Cuneonavicular joint
  use Tarsal Joint, Right
  use Tarsal Joint, Left
Cuneonavicular ligament
  use Foot Bursa and Ligament, Right
  use Foot Bursa and Ligament, Left
Curettage
  see Excision
  see Extraction
Cutaneous (transverse) cervical nerve *use*
    Nerve, Cervical Plexus
CVP (central venous pressure) *see*
    Measurement, Venous 4A04

Cyclodiathermy *see* Destruction, Eye 085
Cyclophotocoagulation *see* Destruction, Eye 085
CYPHER® Stent *use* Intraluminal Device, Drug-
    eluting in Heart and Great Vessels
Cystectomy
  see Excision, Bladder 0TBB
  see Resection, Bladder 0TTB
Cystocele repair *see* Repair, Subcutaneous
    Tissue and Fascia, Pelvic Region 0JQC
Cystography
  see Plain Radiography, Urinary System BT0
  see Fluoroscopy, Urinary System BT1
Cystolithotomy *see* Extirpation, Bladder 0TCB
Cystopexy
  see Repair, Bladder 0TQB
  see Reposition, Bladder 0TSB
Cystoplasty
  see Repair, Bladder 0TQB
  see Replacement, Bladder 0TRB
  see Supplement, Bladder 0TUB
Cystorrhaphy *see* Repair, Bladder 0TQB
Cystoscopy 0TJB8ZZ
Cystostomy *see* Bypass, Bladder 0T1B
Cystostomy tube *use* Drainage Device
Cystotomy *see* Drainage, Bladder 0T9B
Cystourethrography
  see Plain Radiography, Urinary System BT0
  see Fluoroscopy, Urinary System BT1
Cystourethroplasty
  see Repair, Urinary System 0TQ
  see Replacement, Urinary System 0TR
  see Supplement, Urinary System 0TU

◀ New   ◀▥ Revised   ~~deleted~~ Deleted

D

DBS lead *use* Neurostimulator Lead in Central Nervous System
DeBakey Left Ventricular Assist Device *use* Implantable Heart Assist System in Heart and Great Vessels
Debridement
Excisional *see* Excision
Non-excisional *see* Extraction
Decompression, Circulatory 6A15
Decortication, lung *see* Excision, Respiratory System 0BD
Deep brain neurostimulator lead *use* Neurostimulator Lead in Central Nervous System
Deep cervical fascia *see* Subcutaneous Tissue and Fascia, Anterior Neck
Deep cervical vein
use Vertebral Vein, Right
use Vertebral Vein, Left
Deep circumflex iliac artery
use External Iliac Artery, Right
use External Iliac Artery, Left
Deep facial vein
use Face Vein, Right
use Face Vein, Left
Deep femoral (profunda femoris) vein
use Femoral Vein, Right
use Femoral Vein, Left
Deep femoral artery
use Femoral Artery, Right
use Femoral Artery, Left
Deep Inferior Epigastric Artery Perforator Flap
Bilateral 0HRV077
Left 0HRU077
Right 0HRT077
Deep palmar arch
use Hand Artery, Right
use Hand Artery, Left
Deep transverse perineal muscle *use* Perineum Muscle
Deferential artery
use Internal Iliac Artery, Right
use Internal Iliac Artery, Left
Defibrillator Generator
Abdomen 0JH8
Chest 0JH6
Defibrotide Sodium Anticoagulant XW0 ◄
Defitelio *use* Defibrotide Sodium Anticoagulant ◄
Delivery
Cesarean *see* Extraction, Products of Conception 10D0
Forceps *see* Extraction, Products of Conception 10D0
Manually assisted 10E0XZZ
Products of Conception 10E0XZZ
Vacuum assisted *see* Extraction, Products of Conception 10D0
Delta frame external fixator
use External Fixation Device, Hybrid in 0PH
use External Fixation Device, Hybrid in 0PS
use External Fixation Device, Hybrid in 0QH
use External Fixation Device, Hybrid in 0QS
Delta III Reverse shoulder prosthesis *use* Synthetic Substitute, Reverse Ball and Socket in 0RR
Deltoid fascia
use Subcutaneous Tissue and Fascia, Right Upper Arm
use Subcutaneous Tissue and Fascia, Left Upper Arm
Deltoid ligament
use Ankle Bursa and Ligament, Right
use Ankle Bursa and Ligament, Left
Deltoid muscle
use Shoulder Muscle, Right
use Shoulder Muscle, Left

Deltopectoral (infraclavicular) lymph node
use Lymphatic, Right Upper Extremity
use Lymphatic, Left Upper Extremity
Denervation
Cranial nerve *see* Destruction, Central Nervous System 005
Peripheral nerve *see* Destruction, Peripheral Nervous System 015
Densitometry
Plain Radiography
Femur
Left BQ04ZZ1
Right BQ03ZZ1
Hip
Left BQ01ZZ1
Right BQ00ZZ1
Spine
Cervical BR00ZZ1
Lumbar BR09ZZ1
Thoracic BR07ZZ1
Whole BR0GZZ1
Ultrasonography
Elbow
Left BP4HZZ1
Right BP4GZZ1
Hand
Left BP4PZZ1
Right BP4NZZ1
Shoulder
Left BP49ZZ1
Right BP48ZZ1
Wrist
Left BP4MZZ1
Right BP4LZZ1
Denticulate (dentate) ligament *use* Spinal Meninges
Depressor anguli oris muscle *use* Facial Muscle
Depressor labii inferioris muscle *use* Facial Muscle
Depressor septi nasi muscle *use* Facial Muscle
Depressor supercilii muscle *use* Facial Muscle
Dermabrasion *see* Extraction, Skin and Breast 0HD
Dermis *see* Skin
Descending genicular artery
use Femoral Artery, Right
use Femoral Artery, Left
Destruction
Acetabulum
Left 0Q55
Right 0Q54
Adenoids 0C5Q
Ampulla of Vater 0F5C
Anal Sphincter 0D5R
Anterior Chamber
Left 08533ZZ
Right 08523ZZ
Anus 0D5Q
Aorta
Abdominal 0450
Thoracic ◄║║
Ascending/Arch 025X ◄
Descending 025W ◄
Aortic Body 0G5D
Appendix 0D5J
Artery
Anterior Tibial
Left 045Q
Right 045P
Axillary
Left 0356
Right 0355
Brachial
Left 0358
Right 0357
Celiac 0451

Destruction *(Continued)*
Artery *(Continued)*
Colic
Left 0457
Middle 0458
Right 0456
Common Carotid
Left 035J
Right 035H
Common Iliac
Left 045D
Right 045C
External Carotid
Left 035N
Right 035M
External Iliac
Left 045J
Right 045H
Face 035R
Femoral
Left 045L
Right 045K
Foot
Left 045W
Right 045V
Gastric 0452
Hand
Left 035F
Right 035D
Hepatic 0453
Inferior Mesenteric 045B
Innominate 0352
Internal Carotid
Left 035L
Right 035K
Internal Iliac
Left 045F
Right 045E
Internal Mammary
Left 0351
Right 0350
Intracranial 035G
Lower 045Y
Peroneal
Left 045U
Right 045T
Popliteal
Left 045N
Right 045M
Posterior Tibial
Left 045S
Right 045R
Pulmonary
Left 025R
Right 025Q
Pulmonary Trunk 025P
Radial
Left 035C
Right 035B
Renal
Left 045A
Right 0459
Splenic 0454
Subclavian
Left 0354
Right 0353
Superior Mesenteric 0455
Temporal
Left 035T
Right 035S
Thyroid
Left 035V
Right 035U
Ulnar
Left 035A
Right 0359
Upper 035Y
Vertebral
Left 035Q
Right 035P

Destruction *(Continued)*
 Gland *(Continued)*
  Parotid
   Left 0C59
   Right 0C58
  Pituitary 0G50
  Sublingual
   Left 0C5F
   Right 0C5D
  Submaxillary
   Left 0C5H
   Right 0C5G
  Vestibular 0U5L
 Glenoid Cavity
  Left 0P58
  Right 0P57
 Glomus Jugulare 0G5C
 Humeral Head
  Left 0P5D
  Right 0P5C
 Humeral Shaft
  Left 0P5G
  Right 0P5F
 Hymen 0U5K
 Hypothalamus 005A
 Ileocecal Valve 0D5C
 Ileum 0D5B
 Intestine
  Large 0D5E
   Left 0D5G
   Right 0D5F
  Small 0D58
 Iris
  Left 085D3ZZ
  Right 085C3ZZ
 Jejunum 0D5A
 Joint
  Acromioclavicular
   Left 0R5H
   Right 0R5G
  Ankle
   Left 0S5G
   Right 0S5F
  Carpal
   Left 0R5R
   Right 0R5Q
  Cervical Vertebral 0R51
  Cervicothoracic Vertebral 0R54
  Coccygeal 0S56
  Elbow
   Left 0R5M
   Right 0R5L
  Finger Phalangeal
   Left 0R5X
   Right 0R5W
  Hip
   Left 0S5B
   Right 0S59
  Knee
   Left 0S5D
   Right 0S5C
  Lumbar Vertebral 0S50
  Lumbosacral 0S53
  Metacarpocarpal
   Left 0R5T
   Right 0R5S
  Metacarpophalangeal
   Left 0R5V
   Right 0R5U
  Metatarsal-Phalangeal
   Left 0S5N
   Right 0S5M
  Metatarsal-Tarsal
   Left 0S5L
   Right 0S5K
  Occipital-cervical 0R50
  Sacrococcygeal 0S55
  Sacroiliac
   Left 0S58
   Right 0S57

Destruction *(Continued)*
 Joint *(Continued)*
  Shoulder
   Left 0R5K
   Right 0R5J
  Sternoclavicular
   Left 0R5F
   Right 0R5E
  Tarsal
   Left 0S5J
   Right 0S5H
  Temporomandibular
   Left 0R5D
   Right 0R5C
  Thoracic Vertebral 0R56
  Thoracolumbar Vertebral 0R5A
  Toe Phalangeal
   Left 0S5Q
   Right 0S5P
  Wrist
   Left 0R5P
   Right 0R5N
 Kidney
  Left 0T51
  Right 0T50
 Kidney Pelvis
  Left 0T54
  Right 0T53
 Larynx 0C5S
 Lens
  Left 085K3ZZ
  Right 085J3ZZ
 Lip
  Lower 0C51
  Upper 0C50
 Liver 0F50
  Left Lobe 0F52
  Right Lobe 0F51
 Lung
  Bilateral 0B5M
  Left 0B5L
  Lower Lobe
   Left 0B5J
   Right 0B5F
  Middle Lobe, Right 0B5D
  Right 0B5K
  Upper Lobe
   Left 0B5G
   Right 0B5C
 Lung Lingula 0B5H
 Lymphatic
  Aortic 075D
  Axillary
   Left 0756
   Right 0755
  Head 0750
  Inguinal
   Left 075J
   Right 075H
  Internal Mammary
   Left 0759
   Right 0758
  Lower Extremity
   Left 075G
   Right 075F
  Mesenteric 075B
  Neck
   Left 0752
   Right 0751
  Pelvis 075C
  Thorax 0757
  Upper Extremity
   Left 0754
   Right 0753
 Mandible
  Left 0N5V
  Right 0N5T
 Maxilla
  Left 0N5S
  Right 0N5R
 Medulla Oblongata 005D

Destruction *(Continued)*
 Mesentery 0D5V
 Metacarpal
  Left 0P5Q
  Right 0P5P
 Metatarsal
  Left 0Q5P
  Right 0Q5N
 Muscle
  Abdomen
   Left 0K5L
   Right 0K5K
  Extraocular
   Left 085M
   Right 085L
  Facial 0K51
  Foot
   Left 0K5W
   Right 0K5V
  Hand
   Left 0K5D
   Right 0K5C
  Head 0K50
  Hip
   Left 0K5P
   Right 0K5N
  Lower Arm and Wrist
   Left 0K5B
   Right 0K59
  Lower Leg
   Left 0K5T
   Right 0K5S
  Neck
   Left 0K53
   Right 0K52
  Papillary 025D
  Perineum 0K5M
  Shoulder
   Left 0K56
   Right 0K55
  Thorax
   Left 0K5J
   Right 0K5H
  Tongue, Palate, Pharynx 0K54
  Trunk
   Left 0K5G
   Right 0K5F
  Upper Arm
   Left 0K58
   Right 0K57
  Upper Leg
   Left 0K5R
   Right 0K5Q
 Nasopharynx 095N
 Nerve
  Abdominal Sympathetic 015M
  Abducens 005L
  Accessory 005R
  Acoustic 005N
  Brachial Plexus 0153
  Cervical 0151
  Cervical Plexus 0153
  Facial 005M
  Femoral 015D
  Glossopharyngeal 005P
  Head and Neck Sympathetic 015K
  Hypoglossal 005S
  Lumbar 015B
  Lumbar Plexus 0159
  Lumbar Sympathetic 015N
  Lumbosacral Plexus 015A
  Median 0155
  Oculomotor 005H
  Olfactory 005F
  Optic 005G
  Peroneal 015H
  Phrenic 0152
  Pudendal 015C
  Radial 0156
  Sacral 015R
  Sacral Plexus 015Q

◀ New   ◀▥ Revised   ~~deleted~~ Deleted

Dilation *(Continued)*
　Artery *(Continued)*
　　Axillary
　　　Left 0376
　　　Right 0375
　　Brachial
　　　Left 0378
　　　Right 0377
　　Celiac 0471
　　Colic
　　　Left 0477
　　　Middle 0478
　　　Right 0476
　　Common Carotid
　　　Left 037J
　　　Right 037H
　　Common Iliac
　　　Left 047D
　　　Right 047C
　　Coronary
　　　~~Four or More Sites 0273~~
　　　~~One Site 0270~~
　　　~~Three Sites 0272~~
　　　~~Two Sites 0271~~
　　　Four or More Arteries 0273 ◀
　　　One Artery 0270 ◀
　　　Three Arteries 0272 ◀
　　　Two Arteries 0271 ◀
　　External Carotid
　　　Left 037N
　　　Right 037M
　　External Iliac
　　　Left 047J
　　　Right 047H
　　Face 037R
　　Femoral
　　　Left 047L
　　　Right 047K
　　Foot
　　　Left 047W
　　　Right 047V
　　Gastric 0472
　　Hand
　　　Left 037F
　　　Right 037D
　　Hepatic 0473
　　Inferior Mesenteric 047B
　　Innominate 0372
　　Internal Carotid
　　　Left 037L
　　　Right 037K
　　Internal Iliac
　　　Left 047F
　　　Right 047E
　　Internal Mammary
　　　Left 0371
　　　Right 0370
　　Intracranial 037G
　　Lower 047Y
　　Peroneal
　　　Left 047U
　　　Right 047T
　　Popliteal
　　　Left 047N
　　　Right 047M
　　Posterior Tibial
　　　Left 047S
　　　Right 047R
　　Pulmonary
　　　Left 027R
　　　Right 027Q
　　Pulmonary Trunk 027P
　　Radial
　　　Left 037C
　　　Right 037B
　　Renal
　　　Left 047A
　　　Right 0479
　　Splenic 0474
　　Subclavian
　　　Left 0374
　　　Right 0373

Dilation *(Continued)*
　Artery *(Continued)*
　　Superior Mesenteric 0475
　　Temporal
　　　Left 037T
　　　Right 037S
　　Thyroid
　　　Left 037V
　　　Right 037U
　　Ulnar
　　　Left 037A
　　　Right 0379
　　Upper 037Y
　　Vertebral
　　　Left 037Q
　　　Right 037P
　Bladder 0T7B
　Bladder Neck 0T7C
　Bronchus
　　Lingula 0B79
　　Lower Lobe
　　　Left 0B7B
　　　Right 0B76
　　Main
　　　Left 0B77
　　　Right 0B73
　　Middle Lobe, Right 0B75
　　Upper Lobe
　　　Left 0B78
　　　Right 0B74
　Carina 0B72
　Cecum 0D7H
　Cervix 0U7C
　Colon
　　Ascending 0D7K
　　Descending 0D7M
　　Sigmoid 0D7N
　　Transverse 0D7L
　Duct
　　Common Bile 0F79
　　Cystic 0F78
　　Hepatic
　　　Left 0F76
　　　Right 0F75
　　Lacrimal
　　　Left 087Y
　　　Right 087X
　　Pancreatic 0F7D
　　　Accessory 0F7F
　　Parotid
　　　Left 0C7C
　　　Right 0C7B
　Duodenum 0D79
　Esophagogastric Junction 0D74
　Esophagus 0D75
　　Lower 0D73
　　Middle 0D72
　　Upper 0D71
　Eustachian Tube
　　Left 097G
　　Right 097F
　Fallopian Tube
　　Left 0U76
　　Right 0U75
　Fallopian Tubes, Bilateral 0U77
　Hymen 0U7K
　Ileocecal Valve 0D7C
　Ileum 0D7B
　Intestine
　　Large 0D7E
　　　Left 0D7G
　　　Right 0D7F
　　Small 0D78
　Jejunum 0D7A
　Kidney Pelvis
　　Left 0T74
　　Right 0T73
　Larynx 0C7S
　Pharynx 0C7M
　Rectum 0D7P
　Stomach 0D76
　　Pylorus 0D77

Dilation *(Continued)*
　Trachea 0B71
　Ureter
　　Left 0T77
　　Right 0T76
　Ureters, Bilateral 0T78
　Urethra 0T7D
　Uterus 0U79
　Vagina 0U7G
　Valve
　　Aortic 027F
　　Ileocecal 0D7C
　　Mitral 027G
　　Pulmonary 027H
　　Tricuspid 027J
　Vas Deferens
　　Bilateral 0V7Q
　　Left 0V7P
　　Right 0V7N
　Vein
　　Axillary
　　　Left 0578
　　　Right 0577
　　Azygos 0570
　　Basilic
　　　Left 057C
　　　Right 057B
　　Brachial
　　　Left 057A
　　　Right 0579
　　Cephalic
　　　Left 057F
　　　Right 057D
　　Colic 0677
　　Common Iliac
　　　Left 067D
　　　Right 067C
　　Esophageal 0673
　　External Iliac
　　　Left 067G
　　　Right 067F
　　External Jugular
　　　Left 057Q
　　　Right 057P
　　Face
　　　Left 057V
　　　Right 057T
　　Femoral
　　　Left 067N
　　　Right 067M
　　Foot
　　　Left 067V
　　　Right 067T
　　Gastric 0672
　　Greater Saphenous
　　　Left 067Q
　　　Right 067P
　　Hand
　　　Left 057H
　　　Right 057G
　　Hemiazygos 0571
　　Hepatic 0674
　　Hypogastric
　　　Left 067J
　　　Right 067H
　　Inferior Mesenteric 0676
　　Innominate
　　　Left 0574
　　　Right 0573
　　Internal Jugular
　　　Left 057N
　　　Right 057M
　　Intracranial 057L
　　Lesser Saphenous
　　　Left 067S
　　　Right 067R
　　Lower 067Y
　　Portal 0678
　　Pulmonary
　　　Left 027T
　　　Right 027S

◀ New　◀▥▥ Revised　~~deleted~~ Deleted

Dilation *(Continued)*
  Vein *(Continued)*
    Renal
      Left 067B
      Right 0679
    Splenic 0671
    Subclavian
      Left 0576
      Right 0575
    Superior Mesenteric
      0675
    Upper 057Y
    Vertebral
      Left 057S
      Right 057R
    Vena Cava
      Inferior 0670
      Superior 027V
    Ventricle, Right 027K
Direct Lateral Interbody Fusion (DLIF) device
  use Interbody Fusion Device in Lower
    Joints
Disarticulation *see* Detachment
Discectomy, diskectomy
  see Excision, Upper Joints 0RB
  see Resection, Upper Joints 0RT
  see Excision, Lower Joints 0SB
  see Resection, Lower Joints 0ST
Discography
  see Plain Radiography, Axial Skeleton, Except
    Skull and Facial Bones BR0
  see Fluoroscopy, Axial Skeleton, Except Skull
    and Facial Bones BR1
Distal humerus
  use Humeral Shaft, Right
  use Humeral Shaft, Left
Distal humerus, involving joint
  use Elbow Joint, Right
  use Elbow Joint, Left
Distal radioulnar joint
  use Wrist Joint, Right
  use Wrist Joint, Left
Diversion *see* Bypass
Diverticulectomy *see* Excision, Gastrointestinal
  System 0DB
Division
  Acetabulum
    Left 0Q85
    Right 0Q84
  Anal Sphincter 0D8R
  Basal Ganglia 0088
  Bladder Neck 0T8C
  Bone
    Ethmoid
      Left 0N8G
      Right 0N8F
    Frontal
      Left 0N82
      Right 0N81
    Hyoid 0N8X
    Lacrimal
      Left 0N8J
      Right 0N8H
    Nasal 0N8B
    Occipital
      Left 0N88
      Right 0N87
    Palatine
      Left 0N8L
      Right 0N8K
    Parietal
      Left 0N84
      Right 0N83
    Pelvic
      Left 0Q83
      Right 0Q82
    Sphenoid
      Left 0N8D
      Right 0N8C
    Temporal
      Left 0N86
      Right 0N85

Division *(Continued)*
  Bone *(Continued)*
    Zygomatic
      Left 0N8N
      Right 0N8M
  Brain 0080
  Bursa and Ligament
    Abdomen
      Left 0M8J
      Right 0M8H
    Ankle
      Left 0M8R
      Right 0M8Q
    Elbow
      Left 0M84
      Right 0M83
    Foot
      Left 0M8T
      Right 0M8S
    Hand
      Left 0M88
      Right 0M87
    Head and Neck 0M80
    Hip
      Left 0M8M
      Right 0M8L
    Knee
      Left 0M8P
      Right 0M8N
    Lower Extremity
      Left 0M8W
      Right 0M8V
    Perineum 0M8K
    Shoulder
      Left 0M82
      Right 0M81
    Thorax
      Left 0M8G
      Right 0M8F
    Trunk
      Left 0M8D
      Right 0M8C
    Upper Extremity
      Left 0M8B
      Right 0M89
    Wrist
      Left 0M86
      Right 0M85
  Carpal
    Left 0P8N
    Right 0P8M
  Cerebral Hemisphere 0087
  Chordae Tendineae 0289
  Clavicle
    Left 0P8B
    Right 0P89
  Coccyx 0Q8S
  Conduction Mechanism
    0288
  Esophagogastric Junction
    0D84
  Femoral Shaft
    Left 0Q89
    Right 0Q88
  Femur
    Lower
      Left 0Q8C
      Right 0Q8B
    Upper
      Left 0Q87
      Right 0Q86
  Fibula
    Left 0Q8K
    Right 0Q8J
  Gland, Pituitary 0G80
  Glenoid Cavity
    Left 0P88
    Right 0P87
  Humeral Head
    Left 0P8D
    Right 0P8C

Division *(Continued)*
  Humeral Shaft
    Left 0P8G
    Right 0P8F
  Hymen 0U8K
  Kidneys, Bilateral 0T82
  Mandible
    Left 0N8V
    Right 0N8T
  Maxilla
    Left 0N8S
    Right 0N8R
  Metacarpal
    Left 0P8Q
    Right 0P8P
  Metatarsal
    Left 0Q8P
    Right 0Q8N
  Muscle
    Abdomen
      Left 0K8L
      Right 0K8K
    Facial 0K81
    Foot
      Left 0K8W
      Right 0K8V
    Hand
      Left 0K8D
      Right 0K8C
    Head 0K80
    Hip
      Left 0K8P
      Right 0K8N
    Lower Arm and Wrist
      Left 0K8B
      Right 0K89
    Lower Leg
      Left 0K8T
      Right 0K8S
    Neck
      Left 0K83
      Right 0K82
    Papillary 028D
    Perineum 0K8M
    Shoulder
      Left 0K86
      Right 0K85
    Thorax
      Left 0K8J
      Right 0K8H
    Tongue, Palate, Pharynx 0K84
    Trunk
      Left 0K8G
      Right 0K8F
    Upper Arm
      Left 0K88
      Right 0K87
    Upper Leg
      Left 0K8R
      Right 0K8Q
  Nerve
    Abdominal Sympathetic 018M
    Abducens 008L
    Accessory 008R
    Acoustic 008N
    Brachial Plexus 0183
    Cervical 0181
    Cervical Plexus 0180
    Facial 008M
    Femoral 018D
    Glossopharyngeal 008P
    Head and Neck Sympathetic
      018K
    Hypoglossal 008S
    Lumbar 018B
    Lumbar Plexus 0189
    Lumbar Sympathetic 018N
    Lumbosacral Plexus 018A
    Median 0185
    Oculomotor 008H
    Olfactory 008F

◀ New   ◀▦ Revised   ~~deleted~~ Deleted

◀ New   ◀ Revised   ~~deleted~~ Deleted

Drainage *(Continued)*
  Artery *(Continued)*
    Common Carotid
      Left 039J
      Right 039H
    Common Iliac
      Left 049D
      Right 049C
    External Carotid
      Left 039N
      Right 039M
    External Iliac
      Left 049J
      Right 049H
    Face 039R
    Femoral
      Left 049L
      Right 049K
    Foot
      Left 049W
      Right 049V
    Gastric 0492
    Hand
      Left 039F
      Right 039D
    Hepatic 0493
    Inferior Mesenteric 049B
    Innominate 0392
    Internal Carotid
      Left 039L
      Right 039K
    Internal Iliac
      Left 049F
      Right 049E
    Internal Mammary
      Left 0391
      Right 0390
    Intracranial 039G
    Lower 049Y
    Peroneal
      Left 049U
      Right 049T
    Popliteal
      Left 049N
      Right 049M
    Posterior Tibial
      Left 049S
      Right 049R
    Radial
      Left 039C
      Right 039B
    Renal
      Left 049A
      Right 0499
    Splenic 0494
    Subclavian
      Left 0394
      Right 0393
    Superior Mesenteric 0495
    Temporal
      Left 039T
      Right 039S
    Thyroid
      Left 039V
      Right 039U
    Ulnar
      Left 039A
      Right 0399
    Upper 039Y
    Vertebral
      Left 039Q
      Right 039P
  Auditory Ossicle
    Left 099A
    Right 0999
  Axilla
    Left 0X95
    Right 0X94
  Back
    Lower 0W9L
    Upper 0W9K

Drainage *(Continued)*
  Basal Ganglia 0098
  Bladder 0T9B
  Bladder Neck 0T9C
  Bone
    Ethmoid
      Left 0N9G
      Right 0N9F
    Frontal
      Left 0N92
      Right 0N91
    Hyoid 0N9X
    Lacrimal
      Left 0N9J
      Right 0N9H
    Nasal 0N9B
    Occipital
      Left 0N98
      Right 0N97
    Palatine
      Left 0N9L
      Right 0N9K
    Parietal
      Left 0N94
      Right 0N93
    Pelvic
      Left 0Q93
      Right 0Q92
    Sphenoid
      Left 0N9D
      Right 0N9C
    Temporal
      Left 0N96
      Right 0N95
    Zygomatic
      Left 0N9N
      Right 0N9M
  Bone Marrow 079T
  Brain 0090
  Breast
    Bilateral 0H9V
    Left 0H9U
    Right 0H9T
  Bronchus
    Lingula 0B99
    Lower Lobe
      Left 0B9B
      Right 0B96
    Main
      Left 0B97
      Right 0B93
    Middle Lobe, Right 0B95
    Upper Lobe
      Left 0B98
      Right 0B94
  Buccal Mucosa 0C94
  Bursa and Ligament
    Abdomen
      Left 0M9J
      Right 0M9H
    Ankle
      Left 0M9R
      Right 0M9Q
    Elbow
      Left 0M94
      Right 0M93
    Foot
      Left 0M9T
      Right 0M9S
    Hand
      Left 0M98
      Right 0M97
    Head and Neck 0M90
    Hip
      Left 0M9M
      Right 0M9L
    Knee
      Left 0M9P
      Right 0M9N
    Lower Extremity
      Left 0M9W
      Right 0M9V

Drainage *(Continued)*
  Bursa and Ligament *(Continued)*
    Perineum 0M9K
    Shoulder
      Left 0M92
      Right 0M91
    Thorax
      Left 0M9G
      Right 0M9F
    Trunk
      Left 0M9D
      Right 0M9C
    Upper Extremity
      Left 0M9B
      Right 0M99
    Wrist
      Left 0M96
      Right 0M95
  Buttock
    Left 0Y91
    Right 0Y90
  Carina 0B92
  Carotid Bodies, Bilateral 0G98
  Carotid Body
    Left 0G96
    Right 0G97
  Carpal
    Left 0P9N
    Right 0P9M
  Cavity, Cranial 0W91
  Cecum 0D9H
  Cerebellum 009C
  Cerebral Hemisphere 0097
  Cerebral Meninges 0091
  Cerebral Ventricle 0096
  Cervix 0U9C
  Chest Wall 0W98
  Choroid
    Left 089B
    Right 089A
  Cisterna Chyli 079L
  Clavicle
    Left 0P9B
    Right 0P99
  Clitoris 0U9J
  Coccygeal Glomus 0G9B
  Coccyx 0Q9S
  Colon
    Ascending 0D9K
    Descending 0D9M
    Sigmoid 0D9N
    Transverse 0D9L
  Conjunctiva
    Left 089T
    Right 089S
  Cord
    Bilateral 0V9H
    Left 0V9G
    Right 0V9F
  Cornea
    Left 0899
    Right 0898
  Cul-de-sac 0U9F
  Diaphragm
    Left 0B9S
    Right 0B9R
  Disc
    Cervical Vertebral 0R93
    Cervicothoracic Vertebral
      0R95
    Lumbar Vertebral 0S92
    Lumbosacral 0S94
    Thoracic Vertebral 0R99
    Thoracolumbar Vertebral
      0R9B
  Duct
    Common Bile 0F99
    Cystic 0F98
    Hepatic
      Left 0F96
      Right 0F95

◀ New   ◀▦ Revised   ~~deleted~~ Deleted

Drainage *(Continued)*
  Lung *(Continued)*
    Middle Lobe, Right ØB9D
    Right ØB9K
    Upper Lobe
      Left ØB9G
      Right ØB9C
  Lung Lingula ØB9H
  Lymphatic
    Aortic 079D
    Axillary
      Left 0796
      Right 0795
    Head 0790
    Inguinal
      Left 079J
      Right 079H
    Internal Mammary
      Left 0799
      Right 0798
    Lower Extremity
      Left 079G
      Right 079F
    Mesenteric 079B
    Neck
      Left 0792
      Right 0791
    Pelvis 079C
    Thoracic Duct 079K
    Thorax 0797
    Upper Extremity
      Left 0794
      Right 0793
  Mandible
    Left ØN9V
    Right ØN9T
  Maxilla
    Left ØN9S
    Right ØN9R
  Mediastinum ØW9C
  Medulla Oblongata 009D
  Mesentery ØD9V
  Metacarpal
    Left ØP9Q
    Right ØP9P
  Metatarsal
    Left ØQ9P
    Right ØQ9N
  Muscle
    Abdomen
      Left ØK9L
      Right ØK9K
    Extraocular
      Left 089M
      Right 089L
    Facial ØK91
    Foot
      Left ØK9W
      Right ØK9V
    Hand
      Left ØK9D
      Right ØK9C
    Head ØK90
    Hip
      Left ØK9P
      Right ØK9N
    Lower Arm and Wrist
      Left ØK9B
      Right ØK99
    Lower Leg
      Left ØK9T
      Right ØK9S
    Neck
      Left ØK93
      Right ØK92
    Perineum ØK9M
    Shoulder
      Left ØK96
      Right ØK95
    Thorax
      Left ØK9J
      Right ØK9H

Drainage *(Continued)*
  Muscle *(Continued)*
    Tongue, Palate, Pharynx ØK94
    Trunk
      Left ØK9G
      Right ØK9F
    Upper Arm
      Left ØK98
      Right ØK97
    Upper Leg
      Left ØK9R
      Right ØK9Q
  Nasopharynx 099N
  Neck ØW96
  Nerve
    Abdominal Sympathetic 019M
    Abducens 009L
    Accessory 009R
    Acoustic 009N
    Brachial Plexus 0193
    Cervical 0191
    Cervical Plexus 0190
    Facial 009M
    Femoral 019D
    Glossopharyngeal 009P
    Head and Neck Sympathetic 019K
    Hypoglossal 009S
    Lumbar 019B
    Lumbar Plexus 0199
    Lumbar Sympathetic 019N
    Lumbosacral Plexus 019A
    Median 0195
    Oculomotor 009H
    Olfactory 009F
    Optic 009G
    Peroneal 019H
    Phrenic 0192
    Pudendal 019C
    Radial 0196
    Sacral 019R
    Sacral Sympathetic 019P
    Sciatic 019F
    Thoracic 0198
    Thoracic Sympathetic 019L
    Tibial 019G
    Trigeminal 009K
    Trochlear 009J
    Ulnar 0194
    Vagus 009Q
  Nipple
    Left ØH9X
    Right ØH9W
  Nose 099K
  Omentum
    Greater ØD9S
    Lesser ØD9T
  Oral Cavity and Throat ØW93
  Orbit
    Left ØN9Q
    Right ØN9P
  Ovary
    Bilateral ØU92
    Left ØU91
    Right ØU90
  Palate
    Hard ØC92
    Soft ØC93
  Pancreas ØF9G
  Para-aortic Body ØG99
  Paraganglion Extremity ØG9F
  Parathyroid Gland ØG9R
    Inferior
      Left ØG9P
      Right ØG9N
    Multiple ØG9Q
    Superior
      Left ØG9P
      Right ØG9L
  Patella
    Left ØQ9F
    Right ØQ9D

Drainage *(Continued)*
  Pelvic Cavity ØW9J
  Penis ØV9S
  Pericardial Cavity ØW9D
  Perineum
    Female ØW9N
    Male ØW9M
  Peritoneal Cavity ØW9G
  Peritoneum ØD9W
  Phalanx
    Finger
      Left ØP9V
      Right ØP9T
    Thumb
      Left ØP9S
      Right ØP9R
    Toe
      Left ØQ9R
      Right ØQ9Q
  Pharynx ØC9M
  Pineal Body ØG91
  Pleura
    Left ØB9P
    Right ØB9N
  Pleural Cavity
    Left ØW9B
    Right ØW99
  Pons 009B
  Prepuce ØV9T
  Products of Conception
    Amniotic Fluid
      Diagnostic 1090
      Therapeutic 1090
    Fetal Blood 1090
    Fetal Cerebrospinal Fluid 1090
    Fetal Fluid, Other 1090
    Fluid, Other 1090
  Prostate ØV90
  Radius
    Left ØP9J
    Right ØP9H
  Rectum ØD9P
  Retina
    Left 089F
    Right 089E
  Retinal Vessel
    Left 089H
    Right 089G
  Retroperitoneum ØW9H
  Rib
    Left ØP92
    Right ØP91
  Sacrum ØQ91
  Scapula
    Left ØP96
    Right ØP95
  Sclera
    Left 0897
    Right 0896
  Scrotum ØV95
  Septum, Nasal 099M
  Shoulder Region
    Left ØX93
    Right ØX92
  Sinus
    Accessory 099P
    Ethmoid
      Left 099V
      Right 099U
    Frontal
      Left 099T
      Right 099S
    Mastoid
      Left 099C
      Right 099B
    Maxillary
      Left 099R
      Right 099Q
    Sphenoid
      Left 099X
      Right 099W

◀ New   ◀▦ Revised   ~~deleted~~ Deleted

Drainage *(Continued)*
  Skin
    Abdomen 0H97
    Back 0H96
    Buttock 0H98
    Chest 0H95
    Ear
      Left 0H93
      Right 0H92
    Face 0H91
    Foot
      Left 0H9N
      Right 0H9M
    Genitalia 0H9A
    Hand
      Left 0H9G
      Right 0H9F
    Lower Arm
      Left 0H9E
      Right 0H9D
    Lower Leg
      Left 0H9L
      Right 0H9K
    Neck 0H94
    Perineum 0H99
    Scalp 0H90
    Upper Arm
      Left 0H9C
      Right 0H9B
    Upper Leg
      Left 0H9J
      Right 0H9H
  Skull 0N90
  Spinal Canal 009U
  Spinal Cord
    Cervical 009W
    Lumbar 009Y
    Thoracic 009X
  Spinal Meninges 009T
  Spleen 079P
  Sternum 0P90
  Stomach 0D96
    Pylorus 0D97
  Subarachnoid Space 0095
  Subcutaneous Tissue and Fascia
    Abdomen 0J98
    Back 0J97
    Buttock 0J99
    Chest 0J96
    Face 0J91
    Foot
      Left 0J9R
      Right 0J9Q
    Hand
      Left 0J9K
      Right 0J9J
    Lower Arm
      Left 0J9H
      Right 0J9G
    Lower Leg
      Left 0J9P
      Right 0J9N
    Neck
      Anterior 0J94
      Posterior 0J95
    Pelvic Region 0J9C
    Perineum 0J9B
    Scalp 0J90
    Upper Arm
      Left 0J9F
      Right 0J9D
    Upper Leg
      Left 0J9M
      Right 0J9L
  Subdural Space 0094
  Tarsal
    Left 0Q9M
    Right 0Q9L
  Tendon
    Abdomen
      Left 0L9G
      Right 0L9F

Drainage *(Continued)*
  Tendon *(Continued)*
    Ankle
      Left 0L9T
      Right 0L9S
    Foot
      Left 0L9W
      Right 0L9V
    Hand
      Left 0L98
      Right 0L97
    Head and Neck 0L90
    Hip
      Left 0L9K
      Right 0L9J
    Knee
      Left 0L9R
      Right 0L9Q
    Lower Arm and Wrist
      Left 0L96
      Right 0L95
    Lower Leg
      Left 0L9P
      Right 0L9N
    Perineum 0L9H
    Shoulder
      Left 0L92
      Right 0L91
    Thorax
      Left 0L9D
      Right 0L9C
    Trunk
      Left 0L9B
      Right 0L99
    Upper Arm
      Left 0L94
      Right 0L93
    Upper Leg
      Left 0L9M
      Right 0L9L
  Testis
    Bilateral 0V9C
    Left 0V9B
    Right 0V99
  Thalamus 0099
  Thymus 079M
  Thyroid Gland 0G9K
    Left Lobe 0G9G
    Right Lobe 0G9H
  Tibia
    Left 0Q9H
    Right 0Q9G
  Toe Nail 0H9R
  Tongue 0C97
  Tonsils 0C9P
  Tooth
    Lower 0C9X
    Upper 0C9W
  Trachea 0B91
  Tunica Vaginalis
    Left 0V97
    Right 0V96
  Turbinate, Nasal 099L
  Tympanic Membrane
    Left 0998
    Right 0997
  Ulna
    Left 0P9L
    Right 0P9K
  Ureter
    Left 0T97
    Right 0T96
  Ureters, Bilateral 0T98
  Urethra 0T9D
  Uterine Supporting Structure 0U94
  Uterus 0U99
  Uvula 0C9N
  Vagina 0U9G
  Vas Deferens
    Bilateral 0V9Q
    Left 0V9P
    Right 0V9N

Drainage *(Continued)*
  Vein
    Axillary
      Left 0598
      Right 0597
    Azygos 0590
    Basilic
      Left 059C
      Right 059B
    Brachial
      Left 059A
      Right 0599
    Cephalic
      Left 059F
      Right 059D
    Colic 0697
    Common Iliac
      Left 069D
      Right 069C
    Esophageal 0693
    External Iliac
      Left 069G
      Right 069F
    External Jugular
      Left 059Q
      Right 059P
    Face
      Left 059V
      Right 059T
    Femoral
      Left 069N
      Right 069M
    Foot
      Left 069V
      Right 069T
    Gastric 0692
    Greater Saphenous
      Left 069Q
      Right 069P
    Hand
      Left 059H
      Right 059G
    Hemiazygos 0591
    Hepatic 0694
    Hypogastric
      Left 069J
      Right 069H
    Inferior Mesenteric 0696
    Innominate
      Left 0594
      Right 0593
    Internal Jugular
      Left 059N
      Right 059M
    Intracranial 059L
    Lesser Saphenous
      Left 069S
      Right 069R
    Lower 069Y
    Portal 0698
    Renal
      Left 069B
      Right 0699
    Splenic 0691
    Subclavian
      Left 0596
      Right 0595
    Superior Mesenteric 0695
    Upper 059Y
    Vertebral
      Left 059S
      Right 059R
  Vena Cava, Inferior 0690
  Vertebra
    Cervical 0P93
    Lumbar 0Q90
    Thoracic 0P94
  Vesicle
    Bilateral 0V93
    Left 0V92
    Right 0V91

◄ New   ◄▥▥ Revised   ~~deleted~~ Deleted

Drainage *(Continued)*
　Vitreous
　　Left 0895
　　Right 0894
　Vocal Cord
　　Left 0C9V
　　Right 0C9T
　Vulva 0U9M
　Wrist Region
　　Left 0X9H
　　Right 0X9G
Dressing
　Abdominal Wall 2W23X4Z
　Arm
　　Lower
　　　Left 2W2DX4Z
　　　Right 2W2CX4Z
　　Upper
　　　Left 2W2BX4Z
　　　Right 2W2AX4Z
　Back 2W25X4Z
　Chest Wall 2W24X4Z
　Extremity
　　Lower
　　　Left 2W2MX4Z
　　　Right 2W2LX4Z
　　Upper
　　　Left 2W29X4Z
　　　Right 2W28X4Z
　Face 2W21X4Z
　Finger
　　Left 2W2KX4Z
　　Right 2W2JX4Z
　Foot
　　Left 2W2TX4Z
　　Right 2W2SX4Z

Dressing *(Continued)*
　Hand
　　Left 2W2FX4Z
　　Right 2W2EX4Z
　Head 2W20X4Z
　Inguinal Region
　　Left 2W27X4Z
　　Right 2W26X4Z
　Leg
　　Lower
　　　Left 2W2RX4Z
　　　Right 2W2QX4Z
　　Upper
　　　Left 2W2PX4Z
　　　Right 2W2NX4Z
　Neck 2W22X4Z
　Thumb
　　Left 2W2HX4Z
　　Right 2W2GX4Z
　Toe
　　Left 2W2VX4Z
　　Right 2W2UX4Z
Driver stent (RX) (OTW) *use* Intraluminal
　Device
Drotrecogin alfa *see* Introduction of
　Recombinant Human-activated Protein C
Duct of Santorini *use* Duct, Pancreatic,
　Accessory
Duct of Wirsung *use* Duct, Pancreatic
Ductogram, mammary *see* Plain Radiography,
　Skin, Subcutaneous Tissue and Breast BH0
Ductography, mammary *see* Plain Radiography,
　Skin, Subcutaneous Tissue and Breast BH0
Ductus deferens
　use Vas Deferens, Right
　use Vas Deferens, Left

Ductus deferens *(Continued)*
　use Vas Deferens, Bilateral
　use Vas Deferens
Duodenal ampulla *use* Ampulla of Vater
Duodenectomy
　see Excision, Duodenum 0DB9
　see Resection, Duodenum 0DT9
Duodenocholedochotomy *see* Drainage,
　Gallbladder 0F94
Duodenocystostomy
　see Bypass, Gallbladder 0F14
　see Drainage, Gallbladder 0F94
Duodenoenterostomy
　see Bypass, Gastrointestinal System 0D1
　see Drainage, Gastrointestinal System 0D9
Duodenojejunal flexure *use* Jejunum
Duodenolysis *see* Release, Duodenum 0DN9
Duodenorrhaphy *see* Repair, Duodenum
　0DQ9
Duodenostomy
　see Bypass, Duodenum 0D19
　see Drainage, Duodenum 0D99
Duodenotomy *see* Drainage, Duodenum 0D99
DuraHeart Left Ventricular Assist System *use*
　Implantable Heart Assist System in Heart
　and Great Vessels
Dural venous sinus *use* Vein, Intracranial
Dura mater, intracranial *use* Dura Mater
Dura mater, spinal *use* Spinal Meninges
Durata® Defibrillation Lead *use* Cardiac Lead,
　Defibrillator in 02H
Dynesys® Dynamic Stabilization System
　use Spinal Stabilization Device, Pedicle-Based
　in 0RH
　use Spinal Stabilization Device, Pedicle-Based
　in 0SH

E

E-Luminexx™ (Biliary) (Vascular) Stent *use*
  Intraluminal Device
Earlobe
  use External Ear, Right
  use External Ear, Left
  use External Ear, Bilateral
Echocardiogram *see* Ultrasonography, Heart B24
Echography *see* Ultrasonography
ECMO *see* Performance, Circulatory 5A15
EDWARDS INTUITY Elite valve system *use*
  Zooplastic Tissue, Rapid Deployment
  Technique in New Technology ◄
EEG (electroencephalogram) *see* Measurement,
  Central Nervous 4A00
EGD (esophagogastroduodenoscopy)
  0DJ08ZZ ◄
~~EGD (esophagogastroduodenscopy) 0DJ08ZZ~~
Eighth cranial nerve *use* Acoustic Nerve
Ejaculatory duct
  use Vas Deferens, Right
  use Vas Deferens, Left
  use Vas Deferens, Bilateral
  use Vas Deferens
EKG (electrocardiogram) *see* Measurement,
  Cardiac 4A02
Electrical bone growth stimulator (EBGS)
  use Bone Growth Stimulator in Head and
    Facial Bones
  use Bone Growth Stimulator in Upper Bones
  use Bone Growth Stimulator in Lower Bones
Electrical muscle stimulation (EMS) lead *use*
  Stimulator Lead in Muscles
Electrocautery
  Destruction *see* Destruction
  Repair *see* Repair
Electroconvulsive Therapy
  Bilateral-Multiple Seizure GZB3ZZZ
  Bilateral-Single Seizure GZB2ZZZ
  Electroconvulsive Therapy, Other GZB4ZZZ
  Unilateral-Multiple Seizure GZB1ZZZ
  Unilateral-Single Seizure GZB0ZZZ
Electroencephalogram (EEG) *see* Measurement,
  Central Nervous 4A00
Electromagnetic Therapy
  Central Nervous 6A22
  Urinary 6A21
Electronic muscle stimulator lead *use*
  Stimulator Lead in Muscles
Electrophysiologic stimulation (EPS) *see*
  Measurement, Cardiac 4A02
Electroshock therapy *see* Electroconvulsive
  Therapy
Elevation, bone fragments, skull *see*
  Reposition, Head and Facial Bones 0NS
Eleventh cranial nerve *use* Accessory Nerve
Embolectomy *see* Extirpation
Embolization
  see Occlusion
  see Restriction
Embolization coil(s) *use* Intraluminal Device
EMG (electromyogram) *see* Measurement,
  Musculoskeletal 4A0F
Encephalon *use* Brain
Endarterectomy
  see Extirpation, Upper Arteries 03C
  see Extirpation, Lower Arteries 04C
Endeavor® (III) (IV) (Sprint) Zotarolimus-
  eluting Coronary Stent System *use*
  Intraluminal Device, Drug-eluting in Heart
  and Great Vessels
Endologix AFX® Endovascular AAA System
  use Intraluminal Device ◄
EndoSure® sensor *use* Monitoring Device,
  Pressure Sensor in 02H
ENDOTAK RELIANCE® (G) Defibrillation
  Lead *use* Cardiac Lead, Defibrillator in 02H
Endotracheal tube (cuffed) (double-lumen)
  use Intraluminal Device, Endotracheal
  Airway in Respiratory System

Endurant® Endovascular Stent Graft *use*
  Intraluminal Device
Endurant® II AAA stent graft system *use*
  Intraluminal Device ◄
Enlargement
  see Dilation
  see Repair
EnRhythm *use* Pacemaker, Dual Chamber in 0JH
Enterorrhaphy *see* Repair, Gastrointestinal
  System 0DQ
Enterra gastric neurostimulator *use* Stimulator
  Generator, Multiple Array in 0JH
Enucleation
  Eyeball *see* Resection, Eye 08T
  Eyeball with prosthetic implant *see*
    Replacement, Eye 08R
Ependyma *use* Cerebral Ventricle
Epic™ Stented Tissue Valve (aortic) *use*
  Zooplastic Tissue in Heart and Great Vessels
Epicel® cultured epidermal autograft *use*
  Autologous Tissue Substitute
Epidermis *use* Skin
Epididymectomy
  see Excision, Male Reproductive System
    0VB
  see Resection, Male Reproductive System
    0VT
Epididymoplasty
  see Repair, Male Reproductive System 0VQ
  see Supplement, Male Reproductive System
    0VU
Epididymorrhaphy *see* Repair, Male
  Reproductive System 0VQ
Epididymotomy *see* Drainage, Male
  Reproductive System 0V9
Epidural space, intracranial *use* Epidural Space
Epidural space, spinal *use* Spinal Canal
Epiphysiodesis
  see Fusion, Upper Joints 0RG
  see Fusion, Lower Joints 0SG
Epiploic foramen *use* Peritoneum
Epiretinal Visual Prosthesis
  Left 08H105Z
  Right 08H005Z
Episiorrhaphy *see* Repair, Perineum, Female
  0WQN
Episiotomy *see* Division, Perineum, Female
  0W8N
Epithalamus *use* Thalamus
Epitroclear lymph node
  use Lymphatic, Right Upper Extremity
  use Lymphatic, Left Upper Extremity
EPS (electrophysiologic stimulation) *see*
  Measurement, Cardiac 4A02
Eptifibatide, infusion *see* Introduction of
  Platelet Inhibitor
ERCP (endoscopic retrograde
  cholangiopancreatography) *see* Fluoroscopy,
  Hepatobiliary System and Pancreas BF1
Erector spinae muscle
  use Trunk Muscle, Right
  use Trunk Muscle, Left
Esophageal artery *use* Upper Artery ◄║║║
Esophageal obturator airway (EOA)
  use Intraluminal Device, Airway in
  Gastrointestinal System
Esophageal plexus *use* Thoracic Sympathetic
  Nerve
Esophagectomy
  see Excision, Gastrointestinal System 0DB
  see Resection, Gastrointestinal System 0DT
Esophagocoloplasty
  see Repair, Gastrointestinal System 0DQ
  see Supplement, Gastrointestinal System
    0DU
Esophagoenterostomy
  see Bypass, Gastrointestinal System 0D1
  see Drainage, Gastrointestinal System 0D9
Esophagoesophagostomy
  see Bypass, Gastrointestinal System 0D1
  see Drainage, Gastrointestinal System 0D9

Esophagogastrectomy
  see Excision, Gastrointestinal System 0DB
  see Resection, Gastrointestinal System 0DT
~~Esophagogastroduodenscopy (EGD) 0DJ08ZZ~~
Esophagogastroduodenoscopy (EGD)
  0DJ08ZZ ◄
Esophagogastroplasty
  see Repair, Gastrointestinal System 0DQ
  see Supplement, Gastrointestinal System
    0DU
Esophagogastroscopy 0DJ68ZZ
Esophagogastrostomy
  see Bypass, Gastrointestinal System 0D1
  see Drainage, Gastrointestinal System 0D9
Esophagojejunoplasty *see* Supplement,
  Gastrointestinal System 0DU
Esophagojejunostomy
  see Bypass, Gastrointestinal System 0D1
  see Drainage, Gastrointestinal System 0D9
Esophagomyotomy *see* Division,
  Esophagogastric Junction 0D84
Esophagoplasty
  see Repair, Gastrointestinal System 0DQ
  see Replacement, Esophagus 0DR5
  see Supplement, Gastrointestinal System
    0DU
Esophagoplication *see* Restriction,
  Gastrointestinal System 0DV
Esophagorrhaphy *see* Repair, Gastrointestinal
  System 0DQ
Esophagoscopy 0DJ08ZZ
Esophagotomy *see* Drainage, Gastrointestinal
  System 0D9
Esteem® implantable hearing system *use*
  Hearing Device in Ear, Nose, Sinus
ESWL (extracorporeal shock wave lithotripsy)
  see Fragmentation
Ethmoidal air cell
  use Ethmoid Sinus, Right
  use Ethmoid Sinus, Left
Ethmoidectomy
  see Excision, Ear, Nose, Sinus 09B
  see Resection, Ear, Nose, Sinus 09T
  see Excision, Head and Facial Bones 0NB
  see Resection, Head and Facial Bones 0NT
Ethmoidotomy *see* Drainage, Ear, Nose, Sinus
  099
Evacuation
  Hematoma *see* Extirpation
  Other Fluid *see* Drainage
Evera (XT)(S)(DR/VR) *use* Defibrillator
  Generator in 0JH
Everolimus-eluting coronary stent *use*
  Intraluminal Device, Drug-eluting in Heart
  and Great Vessels
Evisceration
  Eyeball *see* Resection, Eye 08T
  Eyeball with prosthetic implant *see*
    Replacement, Eye 08R
Ex-PRESS™ mini glaucoma shunt *use* Synthetic
  Substitute
Examination *see* Inspection
Exchange *see* Change device in
Excision
  Abdominal Wall 0WBF
  Acetabulum
    Left 0QB5
    Right 0QB4
  Adenoids 0CBQ
  Ampulla of Vater 0FBC
  Anal Sphincter 0DBR
  Ankle Region
    Left 0YBL
    Right 0YBK
  Anus 0DBQ
  Aorta
    Abdominal 04B0
    Thoracic ◄║║║
      Ascending/Arch 02BX ◄
      Descending 02BW ◄
  Aortic Body 0GBD
  Appendix 0DBJ

◄ New ◄║║║ Revised ~~deleted~~ Deleted

Excision *(Continued)*
  Arm
    Lower
      Left 0XBF
      Right 0XBD
    Upper
      Left 0XB9
      Right 0XB8
  Artery
    Anterior Tibial
      Left 04BQ
      Right 04BP
    Axillary
      Left 03B6
      Right 03B5
    Brachial
      Left 03B8
      Right 03B7
    Celiac 04B1
    Colic
      Left 04B7
      Middle 04B8
      Right 04B6
    Common Carotid
      Left 03BJ
      Right 03BH
    Common Iliac
      Left 04BD
      Right 04BC
    External Carotid
      Left 03BN
      Right 03BM
    External Iliac
      Left 04BJ
      Right 04BH
    Face 03BR
    Femoral
      Left 04BL
      Right 04BK
    Foot
      Left 04BW
      Right 04BV
    Gastric 04B2
    Hand
      Left 03BF
      Right 03BD
    Hepatic 04B3
    Inferior Mesenteric 04BB
    Innominate 03B2
    Internal Carotid
      Left 03BL
      Right 03BK
    Internal Iliac
      Left 04BF
      Right 04BE
    Internal Mammary
      Left 03B1
      Right 03B0
    Intracranial 03BG
    Lower 04BY
    Peroneal
      Left 04BU
      Right 04BT
    Popliteal
      Left 04BN
      Right 04BM
    Posterior Tibial
      Left 04BS
      Right 04BR
    Pulmonary
      Left 02BR
      Right 02BQ
    Pulmonary Trunk 02BP
    Radial
      Left 03BC
      Right 03BB
    Renal
      Left 04BA
      Right 04B9
    Splenic 04B4

Excision *(Continued)*
  Artery *(Continued)*
    Subclavian
      Left 03B4
      Right 03B3
    Superior Mesenteric 04B5
    Temporal
      Left 03BT
      Right 03BS
    Thyroid
      Left 03BV
      Right 03BU
    Ulnar
      Left 03BA
      Right 03B9
    Upper 03BY
    Vertebral
      Left 03BQ
      Right 03BP
  Atrium
    Left 02B7
    Right 02B6
  Auditory Ossicle
    Left 09BA0Z
    Right 09B90Z
  Axilla
    Left 0XB5
    Right 0XB4
  Back
    Lower 0WBL
    Upper 0WBK
  Basal Ganglia 00B8
  Bladder 0TBB
  Bladder Neck 0TBC
  Bone
    Ethmoid
      Left 0NBG
      Right 0NBF
    Frontal
      Left 0NB2
      Right 0NB1
    Hyoid 0NBX
    Lacrimal
      Left 0NBJ
      Right 0NBH
    Nasal 0NBB
    Occipital
      Left 0NB8
      Right 0NB7
    Palatine
      Left 0NBL
      Right 0NBK
    Parietal
      Left 0NB4
      Right 0NB3
    Pelvic
      Left 0QB3
      Right 0QB2
    Sphenoid
      Left 0NBD
      Right 0NBC
    Temporal
      Left 0NB6
      Right 0NB5
    Zygomatic
      Left 0NBN
      Right 0NBM
  Brain 00B0
  Breast
    Bilateral 0HBV
    Left 0HBU
    Right 0HBT
    Supernumerary 0HBY
  Bronchus
    Lingula 0BB9
    Lower Lobe
      Left 0BBB
      Right 0BB6
    Main
      Left 0BB7
      Right 0BB3

Excision *(Continued)*
  Bronchus *(Continued)*
    Middle Lobe, Right 0BB5
    Upper Lobe
      Left 0BB8
      Right 0BB4
  Buccal Mucosa 0CB4
  Bursa and Ligament
    Abdomen
      Left 0MBJ
      Right 0MBH
    Ankle
      Left 0MBR
      Right 0MBQ
    Elbow
      Left 0MB4
      Right 0MB3
    Foot
      Left 0MBT
      Right 0MBS
    Hand
      Left 0MB8
      Right 0MB7
    Head and Neck 0MB0
    Hip
      Left 0MBM
      Right 0MBL
    Knee
      Left 0MBP
      Right 0MBN
    Lower Extremity
      Left 0MBW
      Right 0MBV
    Perineum 0MBK
    Shoulder
      Left 0MB2
      Right 0MB1
    Thorax
      Left 0MBG
      Right 0MBF
    Trunk
      Left 0MBD
      Right 0MBC
    Upper Extremity
      Left 0MBB
      Right 0MB9
    Wrist
      Left 0MB6
      Right 0MB5
  Buttock
    Left 0YB1
    Right 0YB0
  Carina 0BB2
  Carotid Bodies, Bilateral 0GB8
  Carotid Body
    Left 0GB6
    Right 0GB7
  Carpal
    Left 0PBN
    Right 0PBM
  Cecum 0DBH
  Cerebellum 00BC
  Cerebral Hemisphere 00B7
  Cerebral Meninges 00B1
  Cerebral Ventricle 00B6
  Cervix 0UBC
  Chest Wall 0WB8
  Chordae Tendineae 02B9
  Choroid
    Left 08BB
    Right 08BA
  Cisterna Chyli 07BL
  Clavicle
    Left 0PBB
    Right 0PB9
  Clitoris 0UBJ
  Coccygeal Glomus 0GBB
  Coccyx 0QBS
  Colon
    Ascending 0DBK
    Descending 0DBM

◀ New ◀ Revised ~~deleted~~ Deleted

Excision *(Continued)*
  Kidney Pelvis
    Left 0TB4
    Right 0TB3
  Knee Region
    Left 0YBG
    Right 0YBF
  Larynx 0CBS
  Leg
    Lower
      Left 0YBJ
      Right 0YBH
    Upper
      Left 0YBD
      Right 0YBC
  Lens
    Left 08BK3Z
    Right 08BJ3Z
  Lip
    Lower 0CB1
    Upper 0CB0
  Liver 0FB0
    Left Lobe 0FB2
    Right Lobe 0FB1
  Lung
    Bilateral 0BBM
    Left 0BBL
    Lower Lobe
      Left 0BBJ
      Right 0BBF
    Middle Lobe, Right 0BBD
    Right 0BBK
    Upper Lobe
      Left 0BBG
      Right 0BBC
  Lung Lingula 0BBH
  Lymphatic
    Aortic 07BD
    Axillary
      Left 07B6
      Right 07B5
    Head 07B0
    Inguinal
      Left 07BJ
      Right 07BH
    Internal Mammary
      Left 07B9
      Right 07B8
    Lower Extremity
      Left 07BG
      Right 07BF
    Mesenteric 07BB
    Neck
      Left 07B2
      Right 07B1
    Pelvis 07BC
    Thoracic Duct 07BK
    Thorax 07B7
    Upper Extremity
      Left 07B4
      Right 07B3
  Mandible
    Left 0NBV
    Right 0NBT
  Maxilla
    Left 0NBS
    Right 0NBR
  Mediastinum 0WBC
  Medulla Oblongata 00BD
  Mesentery 0DBV
  Metacarpal
    Left 0PBQ
    Right 0PBP
  Metatarsal
    Left 0QBP
    Right 0QBN
  Muscle
    Abdomen
      Left 0KBL
      Right 0KBK

Excision *(Continued)*
  Muscle *(Continued)*
    Extraocular
      Left 08BM
      Right 08BL
    Facial 0KB1
    Foot
      Left 0KBW
      Right 0KBV
    Hand
      Left 0KBD
      Right 0KBC
    Head 0KB0
    Hip
      Left 0KBP
      Right 0KBN
    Lower Arm and Wrist
      Left 0KBB
      Right 0KB9
    Lower Leg
      Left 0KBT
      Right 0KBS
    Neck
      Left 0KB3
      Right 0KB2
    Papillary 02BD
    Perineum 0KBM
    Shoulder
      Left 0KB6
      Right 0KB5
    Thorax
      Left 0KBJ
      Right 0KBH
    Tongue, Palate, Pharynx 0KB4
    Trunk
      Left 0KBG
      Right 0KBF
    Upper Arm
      Left 0KB8
      Right 0KB7
    Upper Leg
      Left 0KBR
      Right 0KBQ
  Nasopharynx 09BN
  Neck 0WB6
  Nerve
    Abdominal Sympathetic 01BM
    Abducens 00BL
    Accessory 00BR
    Acoustic 00BN
    Brachial Plexus 01B3
    Cervical 01B1
    Cervical Plexus 01B0
    Facial 00BM
    Femoral 01BD
    Glossopharyngeal 00BP
    Head and Neck Sympathetic 01BK
    Hypoglossal 00BS
    Lumbar 01BB
    Lumbar Plexus 01B9
    Lumbar Sympathetic 01BN
    Lumbosacral Plexus 01BA
    Median 01B5
    Oculomotor 00BH
    Olfactory 00BF
    Optic 00BG
    Peroneal 01BH
    Phrenic 01B2
    Pudendal 01BC
    Radial 01B6
    Sacral 01BR
    Sacral Plexus 01BQ
    Sacral Sympathetic 01BP
    Sciatic 01BF
    Thoracic 01B8
    Thoracic Sympathetic 01BL
    Tibial 01BG
    Trigeminal 00BK
    Trochlear 00BJ
    Ulnar 01B4
    Vagus 00BQ

Excision *(Continued)*
  Nipple
    Left 0HBX
    Right 0HBW
  Nose 09BK
  Omentum
    Greater 0DBS
    Lesser 0DBT
  Orbit
    Left 0NBQ
    Right 0NBP
  Ovary
    Bilateral 0UB2
    Left 0UB1
    Right 0UB0
  Palate
    Hard 0CB2
    Soft 0CB3
  Pancreas 0FBG
  Para-aortic Body 0GB9
  Paraganglion Extremity 0GBF
  Parathyroid Gland 0GBR
    Inferior
      Left 0GBP
      Right 0GBN
    Multiple 0GBQ
    Superior
      Left 0GBM
      Right 0GBL
  Patella
    Left 0QBF
    Right 0QBD
  Penis 0VBS
  Pericardium 02BN
  Perineum
    Female 0WBN
    Male 0WBM
  Peritoneum 0DBW
  Phalanx
    Finger
      Left 0PBV
      Right 0PBT
    Thumb
      Left 0PBS
      Right 0PBR
    Toe
      Left 0QBR
      Right 0QBQ
  Pharynx 0CBM
  Pineal Body 0GB1
  Pleura
    Left 0BBP
    Right 0BBN
  Pons 00BB
  Prepuce 0VBT
  Prostate 0VB0
  Radius
    Left 0PBJ
    Right 0PBH
  Rectum 0DBP
  Retina
    Left 08BF3Z
    Right 08BE3Z
  Retroperitoneum 0WBH
  Rib
    Left 0PB2
    Right 0PB1
  Sacrum 0QB1
  Scapula
    Left 0PB6
    Right 0PB5
  Sclera
    Left 08B7XZ
    Right 08B6XZ
  Scrotum 0VB5
  Septum
    Atrial 02B5
    Nasal 09BM
    Ventricular 02BM
  Shoulder Region
    Left 0XB3
    Right 0XB2

Excision (Continued)
Sinus
  Accessory 09BP
  Ethmoid
    Left 09BV
    Right 09BU
  Frontal
    Left 09BT
    Right 09BS
  Mastoid
    Left 09BC
    Right 09BB
  Maxillary
    Left 09BR
    Right 09BQ
  Sphenoid
    Left 09BX
    Right 09BW
Skin
  Abdomen 0HB7XZ
  Back 0HB6XZ
  Buttock 0HB8XZ
  Chest 0HB5XZ
  Ear
    Left 0HB3XZ
    Right 0HB2XZ
  Face 0HB1XZ
  Foot
    Left 0HBNXZ
    Right 0HBMXZ
  Genitalia 0HBAXZ
  Hand
    Left 0HBGXZ
    Right 0HBFXZ
  Lower Arm
    Left 0HBEXZ
    Right 0HBDXZ
  Lower Leg
    Left 0HBLXZ
    Right 0HBKXZ
  Neck 0HB4XZ
  Perineum 0HB9XZ
  Scalp 0HB0XZ
  Upper Arm
    Left 0HBCXZ
    Right 0HBBXZ
  Upper Leg
    Left 0HBJXZ
    Right 0HBHXZ
Skull 0NB0
Spinal Cord
  Cervical 00BW
  Lumbar 00BY
  Thoracic 00BX
Spinal Meninges 00BT
Spleen 07BP
Sternum 0PB0
Stomach 0DB6
  Pylorus 0DB7
Subcutaneous Tissue and Fascia
  Abdomen 0JB8
  Back 0JB7
  Buttock 0JB9
  Chest 0JB6
  Face 0JB1
  Foot
    Left 0JBR
    Right 0JBQ
  Hand
    Left 0JBK
    Right 0JBJ
  Lower Arm
    Left 0JBH
    Right 0JBG
  Lower Leg
    Left 0JBP
    Right 0JBN
  Neck
    Anterior 0JB4
    Posterior 0JB5
  Pelvic Region 0JBC

Excision (Continued)
Subcutaneous Tissue and Fascia (Continued)
  Perineum 0JBB
  Scalp 0JB0
  Upper Arm
    Left 0JBF
    Right 0JBD
  Upper Leg
    Left 0JBM
    Right 0JBL
Tarsal
  Left 0QBM
  Right 0QBL
Tendon
  Abdomen
    Left 0LBG
    Right 0LBF
  Ankle
    Left 0LBT
    Right 0LBS
  Foot
    Left 0LBW
    Right 0LBV
  Hand
    Left 0LB8
    Right 0LB7
  Head and Neck 0LB0
  Hip
    Left 0LBK
    Right 0LBJ
  Knee
    Left 0LBR
    Right 0LBQ
  Lower Arm and Wrist
    Left 0LB6
    Right 0LB5
  Lower Leg
    Left 0LBP
    Right 0LBN
  Perineum 0LBH
  Shoulder
    Left 0LB2
    Right 0LB1
  Thorax
    Left 0LBD
    Right 0LBC
  Trunk
    Left 0LBB
    Right 0LB9
  Upper Arm
    Left 0LB4
    Right 0LB3
  Upper Leg
    Left 0LBM
    Right 0LBL
Testis
  Bilateral 0VBC
  Left 0VBB
  Right 0VB9
Thalamus 00B9
Thymus 07BM
Thyroid Gland
  Left Lobe 0GBG
  Right Lobe 0GBH
Tibia
  Left 0QBH
  Right 0QBG
Toe Nail 0HBRXZ
Tongue 0CB7
Tonsils 0CBP
Tooth
  Lower 0CBX
  Upper 0CBW
Trachea 0BB1
Tunica Vaginalis
  Left 0VB7
  Right 0VB6
Turbinate, Nasal 09BL
Tympanic Membrane
  Left 09B8
  Right 09B7

Excision (Continued)
Ulna
  Left 0PBL
  Right 0PBK
Ureter
  Left 0TB7
  Right 0TB6
Urethra 0TBD
Uterine Supporting Structure
  0UB4
Uterus 0UB9
Uvula 0CBN
Vagina 0UBG
Valve
  Aortic 02BF
  Mitral 02BG
  Pulmonary 02BH
  Tricuspid 02BJ
Vas Deferens
  Bilateral 0VBQ
  Left 0VBP
  Right 0VBN
Vein
  Axillary
    Left 05B8
    Right 05B7
  Azygos 05B0
  Basilic
    Left 05BC
    Right 05BB
  Brachial
    Left 05BA
    Right 05B9
  Cephalic
    Left 05BF
    Right 05BD
  Colic 06B7
  Common Iliac
    Left 06BD
    Right 06BC
  Coronary 02B4
  Esophageal 06B3
  External Iliac
    Left 06BG
    Right 06BF
  External Jugular
    Left 05BQ
    Right 05BP
  Face
    Left 05BV
    Right 05BT
  Femoral
    Left 06BN
    Right 06BM
  Foot
    Left 06BV
    Right 06BT
  Gastric 06B2
  Greater Saphenous
    Left 06BQ
    Right 06BP
  Hand
    Left 05BH
    Right 05BG
  Hemiazygos 05B1
  Hepatic 06B4
  Hypogastric
    Left 06BJ
    Right 06BH
  Inferior Mesenteric 06B6
  Innominate
    Left 05B4
    Right 05B3
  Internal Jugular
    Left 05BN
    Right 05BM
  Intracranial 05BL
  Lesser Saphenous
    Left 06BS
    Right 06BR
  Lower 06BY

◀ New   ◀||||| Revised   ~~deleted~~ Deleted

Excision (Continued)
Vein (Continued)
Portal 06B8
Pulmonary
Left 02BT
Right 02BS
Renal
Left 06BB
Right 06B9
Splenic 06B1
Subclavian
Left 05B6
Right 05B5
Superior Mesenteric 06B5
Upper 05BY
Vertebral
Left 05BS
Right 05BR
Vena Cava
Inferior 06B0
Superior 02BV
Ventricle
Left 02BL
Right 02BK
Vertebra
Cervical 0PB3
Lumbar 0QB0
Thoracic 0PB4
Vesicle
Bilateral 0VB3
Left 0VB2
Right 0VB1
Vitreous
Left 08B53Z
Right 08B43Z
Vocal Cord
Left 0CBV
Right 0CBT
Vulva 0UBM
Wrist Region
Left 0XBH
Right 0XBG
EXCLUDER® AAA Endoprosthesis ◄
use Intraluminal Device, Branched or
Fenestrated, One or Two Arteries in
04V ◄
use Intraluminal Device, Branched or
Fenestrated, Three or More Arteries in
04V ◄
use Intraluminal Device ◄
EXCLUDER® IBE Endoprosthesis use
Intraluminal Device, Branched or
Fenestrated, One or Two Arteries in
04V ◄
Exclusion, Left atrial appendage (LAA) *see*
Occlusion, Atrium, Left 02L7
Exercise, rehabilitation *see* Motor Treatment,
Rehabilitation F07
Exploration *see* Inspection
Express® (LD) Premounted Stent System *use*
Intraluminal Device
Express® Biliary SD Monorail® Premounted
Stent System *use* Intraluminal Device
Express® SD Renal Monorail® Premounted
Stent System *use* Intraluminal Device
Extensor carpi radialis muscle
use Lower Arm and Wrist Muscle, Right
use Lower Arm and Wrist Muscle, Left
Extensor carpi ulnaris muscle
use Lower Arm and Wrist Muscle, Right
use Lower Arm and Wrist Muscle, Left
Extensor digitorum brevis muscle
use Foot Muscle, Right
use Foot Muscle, Left
Extensor digitorum longus muscle
use Lower Leg Muscle, Right
use Lower Leg Muscle, Left
Extensor hallucis brevis muscle
use Foot Muscle, Right
use Foot Muscle, Left

Extensor hallucis longus muscle
use Lower Leg Muscle, Right
use Lower Leg Muscle, Left
External anal sphincter *use* Anal Sphincter
External auditory meatus
use External Auditory Canal, Right
use External Auditory Canal, Left
External fixator
use External Fixation Device in Head and
Facial Bones
use External Fixation Device in Upper Bones
use External Fixation Device in Lower Bones
use External Fixation Device in Upper Joints
use External Fixation Device in Lower Joints
External maxillary artery *use* Face Artery
External naris *use* Nose
External oblique aponeurosis *use*
Subcutaneous Tissue and Fascia, Trunk
External oblique muscle
use Abdomen Muscle, Right
use Abdomen Muscle, Left
External popliteal nerve *use* Peroneal Nerve
External pudendal artery
use Femoral Artery, Right
use Femoral Artery, Left
External pudendal vein
use Greater Saphenous Vein, Right
use Greater Saphenous Vein, Left
External urethral sphincter *use* Urethra
Extirpation
Acetabulum
Left 0QC5
Right 0QC4
Adenoids 0CCQ
Ampulla of Vater 0FCC
Anal Sphincter 0DCR
Anterior Chamber
Left 08C3
Right 08C2
Anus 0DCQ
Aorta
Abdominal 04C0
Thoracic ◄▥▥
Ascending/Arch 02CX ◄
Descending 02CW ◄
Aortic Body 0GCD
Appendix 0DCJ
Artery
Anterior Tibial
Left 04CQ
Right 04CP
Axillary
Left 03C6
Right 03C5
Brachial
Left 03C8
Right 03C7
Celiac 04C1
Colic
Left 04C7
Middle 04C8
Right 04C6
Common Carotid
Left 03CJ
Right 03CH
Common Iliac
Left 04CD
Right 04CC
Coronary
~~Four or More Sites~~
~~02C3~~
~~One Site 02C0~~
~~Three Sites 02C2~~
~~Two Sites 02C1~~
Four or More Arteries 02C3 ◄
One Artery 02C0 ◄
Three Arteries 02C2 ◄
Two Arteries 02C1 ◄
External Carotid
Left 03CN
Right 03CM

Extirpation (Continued)
Artery (Continued)
External Iliac
Left 04CJ
Right 04CH
Face 03CR
Femoral
Left 04CL
Right 04CK
Foot
Left 04CW
Right 04CV
Gastric 04C2
Hand
Left 03CF
Right 03CD
Hepatic 04C3
Inferior Mesenteric 04CB
Innominate 03C2
Internal Carotid
Left 03CL
Right 03CK
Internal Iliac
Left 04CF
Right 04CE
Internal Mammary
Left 03C1
Right 03C0
Intracranial 03CG
Lower 04CY
Peroneal
Left 04CU
Right 04CT
Popliteal
Left 04CN
Right 04CM
Posterior Tibial
Left 04CS
Right 04CR
Pulmonary
Left 02CR
Right 02CQ
Pulmonary Trunk 02CP
Radial
Left 03CC
Right 03CB
Renal
Left 04CA
Right 04C9
Splenic 04C4
Subclavian
Left 03C4
Right 03C3
Superior Mesenteric
04C5
Temporal
Left 03CT
Right 03CS
Thyroid
Left 03CV
Right 03CU
Ulnar
Left 03CA
Right 03C9
Upper 03CY
Vertebral
Left 03CQ
Right 03CP
Atrium
Left 02C7
Right 02C6
Auditory Ossicle
Left 09CA0ZZ
Right 09C90ZZ
Basal Ganglia 00C8
Bladder 0TCB
Bladder Neck 0TCC
Bone
Ethmoid
Left 0NCG
Right 0NCF

Extirpation (Continued)
Bone (Continued)
Frontal
Left 0NC2
Right 0NC1
Hyoid 0NCX
Lacrimal
Left 0NCJ
Right 0NCH
Nasal 0NCB
Occipital
Left 0NC8
Right 0NC7
Palatine
Left 0NCL
Right 0NCK
Parietal
Left 0NC4
Right 0NC3
Pelvic
Left 0QC3
Right 0QC2
Sphenoid
Left 0NCD
Right 0NCC
Temporal
Left 0NC6
Right 0NC5
Zygomatic
Left 0NCN
Right 0NCM
Brain 00C0
Breast
Bilateral 0HCV
Left 0HCU
Right 0HCT
Bronchus
Lingula 0BC9
Lower Lobe
Left 0BCB
Right 0BC6
Main
Left 0BC7
Right 0BC3
Middle Lobe, Right 0BC5
Upper Lobe
Left 0BC8
Right 0BC4
Buccal Mucosa 0CC4
Bursa and Ligament
Abdomen
Left 0MCJ
Right 0MCH
Ankle
Left 0MCR
Right 0MCQ
Elbow
Left 0MC4
Right 0MC3
Foot
Left 0MCT
Right 0MCS
Hand
Left 0MC8
Right 0MC7
Head and Neck 0MC0
Hip
Left 0MCM
Right 0MCL
Knee
Left 0MCP
Right 0MCN
Lower Extremity
Left 0MCW
Right 0MCV
Perineum 0MCK
Shoulder
Left 0MC2
Right 0MC1
Thorax
Left 0MCG
Right 0MCF

Extirpation (Continued)
Bursa and Ligament (Continued)
Trunk
Left 0MCD
Right 0MCC
Upper Extremity
Left 0MCB
Right 0MC9
Wrist
Left 0MC6
Right 0MC5
Carina 0BC2
Carotid Bodies, Bilateral 0GC8
Carotid Body
Left 0GC6
Right 0GC7
Carpal
Left 0PCN
Right 0PCM
Cavity, Cranial 0WC1
Cecum 0DCH
Cerebellum 00CC
Cerebral Hemisphere 00C7
Cerebral Meninges 00C1
Cerebral Ventricle 00C6
Cervix 0UCC
Chordae Tendineae 02C9
Choroid
Left 08CB
Right 08CA
Cisterna Chyli 07CL
Clavicle
Left 0PCB
Right 0PC9
Clitoris 0UCJ
Coccygeal Glomus 0GCB
Coccyx 0QCS
Colon
Ascending 0DCK
Descending 0DCM
Sigmoid 0DCN
Transverse 0DCL
Conduction Mechanism 02C8
Conjunctiva
Left 08CTXZZ
Right 08CSXZZ
Cord
Bilateral 0VCH
Left 0VCG
Right 0VCF
Cornea
Left 08C9XZZ
Right 08C8XZZ
Cul-de-sac 0UCF
Diaphragm
Left 0BCS
Right 0BCR
Disc
Cervical Vertebral 0RC3
Cervicothoracic Vertebral 0RC5
Lumbar Vertebral 0SC2
Lumbosacral 0SC4
Thoracic Vertebral 0RC9
Thoracolumbar Vertebral 0RCB
Duct
Common Bile 0FC9
Cystic 0FC8
Hepatic
Left 0FC6
Right 0FC5
Lacrimal
Left 08CY
Right 08CX
Pancreatic 0FCD
Accessory 0FCF
Parotid
Left 0CCC
Right 0CCB
Duodenum 0DC9
Dura Mater 00C2

Extirpation (Continued)
Ear
External
Left 09C1
Right 09C0
External Auditory Canal
Left 09C4
Right 09C3
Inner
Left 09CE0ZZ
Right 09CD0ZZ
Middle
Left 09C60ZZ
Right 09C50ZZ
Endometrium 0UCB
Epididymis
Bilateral 0VCL
Left 0VCK
Right 0VCJ
Epidural Space 00C3
Epiglottis 0CCR
Esophagogastric Junction
0DC4
Esophagus 0DC5
Lower 0DC3
Middle 0DC2
Upper 0DC1
Eustachian Tube
Left 09CG
Right 09CF
Eye
Left 08C1XZZ
Right 08C0XZZ
Eyelid
Lower
Left 08CR
Right 08CQ
Upper
Left 08CP
Right 08CN
Fallopian Tube
Left 0UC6
Right 0UC5
Fallopian Tubes, Bilateral
0UC7
Femoral Shaft
Left 0QC9
Right 0QC8
Femur
Lower
Left 0QCC
Right 0QCB
Upper
Left 0QC7
Right 0QC6
Fibula
Left 0QCK
Right 0QCJ
Finger Nail 0HCQXZZ
Gallbladder 0FC4
Gastrointestinal Tract 0WCP
Genitourinary Tract 0WCR
Gingiva
Lower 0CC6
Upper 0CC5
Gland
Adrenal
Bilateral 0GC4
Left 0GC2
Right 0GC3
Lacrimal
Left 08CW
Right 08CV
Minor Salivary 0CCJ
Parotid
Left 0CC9
Right 0CC8
Pituitary 0GC0
Sublingual
Left 0CCF
Right 0CCD

◀ New   ◀‖‖ Revised   ~~deleted~~ Deleted

Extirpation *(Continued)*
  Gland *(Continued)*
    Submaxillary
      Left 0CCH
      Right 0CCG
    Vestibular 0UCL
  Glenoid Cavity
    Left 0PC8
    Right 0PC7
  Glomus Jugulare 0GCC
  Humeral Head
    Left 0PCD
    Right 0PCC
  Humeral Shaft
    Left 0PCG
    Right 0PCF
  Hymen 0UCK
  Hypothalamus 00CA
  Ileocecal Valve 0DCC
  Ileum 0DCB
  Intestine
    Large 0DCE
      Left 0DCG
      Right 0DCF
    Small 0DC8
  Iris
    Left 08CD
    Right 08CC
  Jejunum 0DCA
  Joint
    Acromioclavicular
      Left 0RCH
      Right 0RCG
    Ankle
      Left 0SCG
      Right 0SCF
    Carpal
      Left 0RCR
      Right 0RCQ
    Cervical Vertebral 0RC1
    Cervicothoracic Vertebral
      0RC4
    Coccygeal 0SC6
    Elbow
      Left 0RCM
      Right 0RCL
    Finger Phalangeal
      Left 0RCX
      Right 0RCW
    Hip
      Left 0SCB
      Right 0SC9
    Knee
      Left 0SCD
      Right 0SCC
    Lumbar Vertebral 0SC0
    Lumbosacral 0SC3
    Metacarpocarpal
      Left 0RCT
      Right 0RCS
    Metacarpophalangeal
      Left 0RCV
      Right 0RCU
    Metatarsal-Phalangeal
      Left 0SCN
      Right 0SCM
    Metatarsal-Tarsal
      Left 0SCL
      Right 0SCK
    Occipital-cervical 0RC0
    Sacrococcygeal 0SC5
    Sacroiliac
      Left 0SC8
      Right 0SC7
    Shoulder
      Left 0RCK
      Right 0RCJ
    Sternoclavicular
      Left 0RCF
      Right 0RCE

Extirpation *(Continued)*
  Joint *(Continued)*
    Tarsal
      Left 0SCJ
      Right 0SCH
    Temporomandibular
      Left 0RCD
      Right 0RCC
    Thoracic Vertebral 0RC6
    Thoracolumbar Vertebral 0RCA
    Toe Phalangeal
      Left 0SCQ
      Right 0SCP
    Wrist
      Left 0RCP
      Right 0RCN
  Kidney
    Left 0TC1
    Right 0TC0
  Kidney Pelvis
    Left 0TC4
    Right 0TC3
  Larynx 0CCS
  Lens
    Left 08CK
    Right 08CJ
  Lip
    Lower 0CC1
    Upper 0CC0
  Liver 0FC0
    Left Lobe 0FC2
    Right Lobe 0FC1
  Lung
    Bilateral 0BCM
    Left 0BCL
    Lower Lobe
      Left 0BCJ
      Right 0BCF
    Middle Lobe, Right 0BCD
    Right 0BCK
    Upper Lobe
      Left 0BCG
      Right 0BCC
  Lung Lingula 0BCH
  Lymphatic
    Aortic 07CD
    Axillary
      Left 07C6
      Right 07C5
    Head 07C0
    Inguinal
      Left 07CJ
      Right 07CH
    Internal Mammary
      Left 07C9
      Right 07C8
    Lower Extremity
      Left 07CG
      Right 07CF
    Mesenteric 07CB
    Neck
      Left 07C2
      Right 07C1
    Pelvis 07CC
    Thoracic Duct 07CK
    Thorax 07C7
    Upper Extremity
      Left 07C4
      Right 07C3
  Mandible
    Left 0NCV
    Right 0NCT
  Maxilla
    Left 0NCS
    Right 0NCR
  Mediastinum 0WCC
  Medulla Oblongata 00CD
  Mesentery 0DCV
  Metacarpal
    Left 0PCQ
    Right 0PCP

Extirpation *(Continued)*
  Metatarsal
    Left 0QCP
    Right 0QCN
  Muscle
    Abdomen
      Left 0KCL
      Right 0KCK
    Extraocular
      Left 08CM
      Right 08CL
    Facial 0KC1
    Foot
      Left 0KCW
      Right 0KCV
    Hand
      Left 0KCD
      Right 0KCC
    Head 0KC0
    Hip
      Left 0KCP
      Right 0KCN
    Lower Arm and Wrist
      Left 0KCB
      Right 0KC9
    Lower Leg
      Left 0KCT
      Right 0KCS
    Neck
      Left 0KC3
      Right 0KC2
    Papillary 02CD
    Perineum 0KCM
    Shoulder
      Left 0KC6
      Right 0KC5
    Thorax
      Left 0KCJ
      Right 0KCH
    Tongue, Palate, Pharynx 0KC4
    Trunk
      Left 0KCG
      Right 0KCF
    Upper Arm
      Left 0KC8
      Right 0KC7
    Upper Leg
      Left 0KCR
      Right 0KCQ
  Nasopharynx 09CN
  Nerve
    Abdominal Sympathetic 01CM
    Abducens 00CL
    Accessory 00CR
    Acoustic 00CN
    Brachial Plexus 01C3
    Cervical 01C1
    Cervical Plexus 01C0
    Facial 00CM
    Femoral 01CD
    Glossopharyngeal 00CP
    Head and Neck Sympathetic 01CK
    Hypoglossal 00CS
    Lumbar 01CB
    Lumbar Plexus 01C9
    Lumbar Sympathetic 01CN
    Lumbosacral Plexus 01CA
    Median 01C5
    Oculomotor 00CH
    Olfactory 00CF
    Optic 00CG
    Peroneal 01CH
    Phrenic 01C2
    Pudendal 01CC
    Radial 01C6
    Sacral 01CR
    Sacral Plexus 01CQ
    Sacral Sympathetic 01CP
    Sciatic 01CF
    Thoracic 01C8
    Thoracic Sympathetic 01CL

Extirpation *(Continued)*
Toe Nail 0HCRXZZ
Tongue 0CC7
Tonsils 0CCP
Tooth
  Lower 0CCX
  Upper 0CCW
Trachea 0BC1
Tunica Vaginalis
  Left 0VC7
  Right 0VC6
Turbinate, Nasal 09CL
Tympanic Membrane
  Left 09C8
  Right 09C7
Ulna
  Left 0PCL
  Right 0PCK
Ureter
  Left 0TC7
  Right 0TC6
Urethra 0TCD
Uterine Supporting Structure 0UC4
Uterus 0UC9
Uvula 0CCN
Vagina 0UCG
Valve
  Aortic 02CF
  Mitral 02CG
  Pulmonary 02CH
  Tricuspid 02CJ
Vas Deferens
  Bilateral 0VCQ
  Left 0VCP
  Right 0VCN
Vein
  Axillary
    Left 05C8
    Right 05C7
  Azygos 05C0
  Basilic
    Left 05CC
    Right 05CB
  Brachial
    Left 05CA
    Right 05C9
  Cephalic
    Left 05CF
    Right 05CD
  Colic 06C7
  Common Iliac
    Left 06CD
    Right 06CC
  Coronary 02C4
  Esophageal 06C3
  External Iliac
    Left 06CG
    Right 06CF
  External Jugular
    Left 05CQ
    Right 05CP
  Face
    Left 05CV
    Right 05CT
  Femoral
    Left 06CN
    Right 06CM
  Foot
    Left 06CV
    Right 06CT
  Gastric 06C2
  Greater Saphenous
    Left 06CQ
    Right 06CP
  Hand
    Left 05CH
    Right 05CG
  Hemiazygos 05C1
  Hepatic 06C4
  Hypogastric
    Left 06CJ
    Right 06CH

Extirpation *(Continued)*
Vein *(Continued)*
  Inferior Mesenteric 06C6
  Innominate
    Left 05C4
    Right 05C3
  Internal Jugular
    Left 05CN
    Right 05CM
  Intracranial 05CL
  Lesser Saphenous
    Left 06CS
    Right 06CR
  Lower 06CY
  Portal 06C8
  Pulmonary
    Left 02CT
    Right 02CS
  Renal
    Left 06CB
    Right 06C9
  Splenic 06C1
  Subclavian
    Left 05C6
    Right 05C5
  Superior Mesenteric
    06C5
  Upper 05CY
  Vertebral
    Left 05CS
    Right 05CR
Vena Cava
  Inferior 06C0
  Superior 02CV
Ventricle
  Left 02CL
  Right 02CK
Vertebra
  Cervical 0PC3
  Lumbar 0QC0
  Thoracic 0PC4
Vesicle
  Bilateral 0VC3
  Left 0VC2
  Right 0VC1
Vitreous
  Left 08C5
  Right 08C4
Vocal Cord
  Left 0CCV
  Right 0CCT
Vulva 0UCM
Extracorporeal shock wave lithotripsy *see*
  Fragmentation
Extracranial-intracranial bypass (EC-IC) *see*
  Bypass, Upper Arteries 031
Extraction
  Auditory Ossicle
    Left 09DA0ZZ
    Right 09D90ZZ
  Bone Marrow
    Iliac 07DR
    Sternum 07DQ
    Vertebral 07DS
  Bursa and Ligament
    Abdomen
      Left 0MDJ
      Right 0MDH
    Ankle
      Left 0MDR
      Right 0MDQ
    Elbow
      Left 0MD4
      Right 0MD3
    Foot
      Left 0MDT
      Right 0MDS
    Hand
      Left 0MD8
      Right 0MD7
    Head and Neck 0MD0

Extraction *(Continued)*
  Bursa and Ligament *(Continued)*
    Hip
      Left 0MDM
      Right 0MDL
    Knee
      Left 0MDP
      Right 0MDN
    Lower Extremity
      Left 0MDW
      Right 0MDV
    Perineum 0MDK
    Shoulder
      Left 0MD2
      Right 0MD1
    Thorax
      Left 0MDG
      Right 0MDF
    Trunk
      Left 0MDD
      Right 0MDC
    Upper Extremity
      Left 0MDB
      Right 0MD9
    Wrist
      Left 0MD6
      Right 0MD5
  Cerebral Meninges 00D1
  Cornea
    Left 08D9XZ
    Right 08D8XZ
  Dura Mater 00D2
  Endometrium 0UDB
  Finger Nail 0HDQXZZ
  Hair 0HDSXZZ
  Kidney
    Left 0TD1
    Right 0TD0
  Lens
    Left 08DK3ZZ
    Right 08DJ3ZZ
  Nerve
    Abdominal Sympathetic 01DM
    Abducens 00DL
    Accessory 00DR
    Acoustic 00DN
    Brachial Plexus 01D3
    Cervical 01D1
    Cervical Plexus 01D0
    Facial 00DM
    Femoral 01DD
    Glossopharyngeal 00DP
    Head and Neck Sympathetic 01DK
    Hypoglossal 00DS
    Lumbar 01DB
    Lumbar Plexus 01D9
    Lumbar Sympathetic 01DN
    Lumbosacral Plexus 01DA
    Median 01D5
    Oculomotor 00DH
    Olfactory 00DF
    Optic 00DG
    Peroneal 01DH
    Phrenic 01D2
    Pudendal 01DC
    Radial 01D6
    Sacral 01DR
    Sacral Plexus 01DQ
    Sacral Sympathetic 01DP
    Sciatic 01DF
    Thoracic 01D8
    Thoracic Sympathetic 01DL
    Tibial 01DG
    Trigeminal 00DK
    Trochlear 00DJ
    Ulnar 01D4
    Vagus 00DQ
  Ova 0UDN
  Pleura
    Left 0BDP
    Right 0BDN

◀ New   ⬅ Revised   ~~deleted~~ Deleted

F

Face lift *see* Alteration, Face ØWØ2
Facet replacement spinal stabilization device
  use Spinal Stabilization Device, Facet
    Replacement in ØRH
  use Spinal Stabilization Device, Facet
    Replacement in ØSH
Facial artery *use* Face Artery
Factor Xa Inhibitor Reversal Agent, Andexanet
  Alfa *use* Andexanet Alfa, Factor Xa
  Inhibitor Reversal Agent ◀
False vocal cord *use* Larynx
Falx cerebri *use* Dura Mater
Fascia lata
  use Subcutaneous Tissue and Fascia, Right
    Upper Leg
  use Subcutaneous Tissue and Fascia, Left
    Upper Leg
Fasciaplasty, fascioplasty
  see Repair, Subcutaneous Tissue and Fascia ØJQ
  see Replacement, Subcutaneous Tissue and
    Fascia ØJR
Fasciectomy
  see Excision, Subcutaneous Tissue and Fascia
    ØJB
Fasciorrhaphy *see* Repair, Subcutaneous Tissue
  and Fascia ØJQ
Fasciotomy
  see Division, Subcutaneous Tissue and Fascia
    ØJ8
  see Drainage, Subcutaneous Tissue and Fascia
    ØJ9
  see Release ◀
Feeding Device
  Change device in
    Lower ØD2DXUZ
    Upper ØD2ØXUZ
  Insertion of device in
    Duodenum ØDH9
    Esophagus ØDH5
    Ileum ØDHB
    Intestine, Small ØDH8
    Jejunum ØDHA
    Stomach ØDH6
  Removal of device from
    Esophagus ØDP5
    Intestinal Tract
      Lower ØDPD
      Upper ØDPØ
    Stomach ØDP6
  Revision of device in
    Intestinal Tract
      Lower ØDWD
      Upper ØDWØ
    Stomach ØDW6
Femoral head
  use Upper Femur, Right
  use Upper Femur, Left
Femoral lymph node
  use Lymphatic, Right Lower Extremity
  use Lymphatic, Left Lower Extremity
Femoropatellar joint
  use Knee Joint, Right
  use Knee Joint, Left
  use Knee Joint, Femoral Surface, Right
  use Knee Joint, Femoral Surface, Left
Femorotibial joint
  use Knee Joint, Right
  use Knee Joint, Left
  use Knee Joint, Tibial Surface, Right
  use Knee Joint, Tibial Surface, Left
Fibular artery
  use Peroneal Artery, Right
  use Peroneal Artery, Left
Fibularis brevis muscle
  use Lower Leg Muscle, Right
  use Lower Leg Muscle, Left
Fibularis longus muscle
  use Lower Leg Muscle, Right
  use Lower Leg Muscle, Left

Fifth cranial nerve *use* Trigeminal Nerve
Filum terminale *use* Spinal Meninges ◀
Fimbriectomy
  see Excision, Female Reproductive System
    ØUB
  see Resection, Female Reproductive System
    ØUT
Fine needle aspiration
  fluid or gas *see* Drainage
  tissue *see* Excision
First cranial nerve *use* Olfactory Nerve
First intercostal nerve *use* Brachial
  Plexus
Fistulization
  see Bypass
  see Drainage
  see Repair
Fitting
  Arch bars, for fracture reduction *see*
    Reposition, Mouth and Throat ØCS
  Arch bars, for immobilization *see*
    Immobilization, Face 2W31
  Artificial limb *see* Device Fitting,
    Rehabilitation FØD
  Hearing aid *see* Device Fitting, Rehabilitation
    FØD
  Ocular prosthesis FØDZ8UZ
  Prosthesis, limb *see* Device Fitting,
    Rehabilitation FØD
  Prosthesis, ocular FØDZ8UZ
Fixation, bone
  External, with fracture reduction *see* Reposition
  External, without fracture reduction *see*
    Insertion
  Internal, with fracture reduction *see* Reposition
  Internal, without fracture reduction *see*
    Insertion
FLAIR® Endovascular Stent Graft *use*
  Intraluminal Device
Flexible Composite Mesh *use* Synthetic
  Substitute
Flexor carpi radialis muscle
  use Lower Arm and Wrist Muscle, Right
  use Lower Arm and Wrist Muscle, Left
Flexor carpi ulnaris muscle
  use Lower Arm and Wrist Muscle, Right
  use Lower Arm and Wrist Muscle, Left
Flexor digitorum brevis muscle
  use Foot Muscle, Right
  use Foot Muscle, Left
Flexor digitorum longus muscle
  use Lower Leg Muscle, Right
  use Lower Leg Muscle, Left
Flexor hallucis brevis muscle
  use Foot Muscle, Right
  use Foot Muscle, Left
Flexor hallucis longus muscle
  use Lower Leg Muscle, Right
  use Lower Leg Muscle, Left
Flexor pollicis longus muscle
  use Lower Arm and Wrist Muscle, Right
  use Lower Arm and Wrist Muscle, Left
Fluoroscopy
  Abdomen and Pelvis BW11
  Airway, Upper BB1DZZZ
  Ankle
    Left BQ1H
    Right BQ1G
  Aorta
    Abdominal B41Ø
      Laser, Intraoperative B41Ø
    Thoracic B31Ø
      Laser, Intraoperative B31Ø
    Thoraco-Abdominal B31P
      Laser, Intraoperative B31P
  Aorta and Bilateral Lower Extremity Arteries
    B41D
    Laser, Intraoperative B41D
  Arm
    Left BP1FZZZ
    Right BP1EZZZ

Fluoroscopy *(Continued)*
  Artery
    Brachiocephalic-Subclavian
      Right B311
      Laser, Intraoperative B311
    Bronchial B31L
      Laser, Intraoperative B31L
    Bypass Graft, Other B21F
    Cervico-Cerebral Arch B31Q
      Laser, Intraoperative B31Q
    Common Carotid
      Bilateral B315
        Laser, Intraoperative B315
      Left B314
        Laser, Intraoperative B314
      Right B313
        Laser, Intraoperative B313
    Coronary
      Bypass Graft
        Multiple B213
          Laser, Intraoperative B213
        Single B212
          Laser, Intraoperative B212
      Multiple B211
        Laser, Intraoperative B211
      Single B21Ø
        Laser, Intraoperative B21Ø
    External Carotid
      Bilateral B31C
        Laser, Intraoperative B31C
      Left B31B
        Laser, Intraoperative B31B
      Right B319
        Laser, Intraoperative B319
    Hepatic B412
      Laser, Intraoperative B412
    Inferior Mesenteric B415
      Laser, Intraoperative B415
    Intercostal B31L
      Laser, Intraoperative B31L
    Internal Carotid
      Bilateral B318
        Laser, Intraoperative B318
      Left B317
        Laser, Intraoperative B317
      Right B316
        Laser, Intraoperative B316
    Internal Mammary Bypass Graft
      Left B218
      Right B217
    Intra-Abdominal
      Other B41B
      Laser, Intraoperative B41B
    Intracranial B31R
      Laser, Intraoperative B31R
    Lower
      Other B41J
      Laser, Intraoperative B41J
    Lower Extremity
      Bilateral and Aorta B41D
        Laser, Intraoperative B41D
      Left B41G
        Laser, Intraoperative B41G
      Right B41F
        Laser, Intraoperative B41F
    Lumbar B419
      Laser, Intraoperative B419
    Pelvic B41C
      Laser, Intraoperative B41C
    Pulmonary
      Left B31T
        Laser, Intraoperative B31T
      Right B31S
        Laser, Intraoperative B31S
    Renal
      Bilateral B418
        Laser, Intraoperative B418
      Left B417
        Laser, Intraoperative B417
      Right B416
        Laser, Intraoperative B416

◀ New   ◀||| Revised   ~~deleted~~ Deleted

◀ New ⬅️ Revised ~~deleted~~ Deleted

Fluoroscopy, laser intraoperative
   see Fluoroscopy, Heart B21
   see Fluoroscopy, Upper Arteries
     B31
   see Fluoroscopy, Lower Arteries
     B41
Flushing *see* Irrigation
Foley catheter *use* Drainage Device
Foramen magnum
   use Bone, Occipital, Right
   use Bone, Occipital, Left
Foramen of Monro (intraventricular) *use*
   Cerebral Ventricle
Foreskin *use* Prepuce
Formula™ Balloon-Expandable Renal Stent
   System *use* Intraluminal Device
Fossa of Rosenmuller *use* Nasopharynx
Fourth cranial nerve *use* Nerve, Trochlear
Fourth ventricle *use* Cerebral Ventricle
Fovea
   use Retina, Right
   use Retina, Left
Fragmentation
   Ampulla of Vater ØFFC
   Anus ØDFQ
   Appendix ØDFJ
   Bladder ØTFB
   Bladder Neck ØTFC
   Bronchus
     Lingula ØBF9
     Lower Lobe
       Left ØBFB
       Right ØBF6
     Main
       Left ØBF7
       Right ØBF3
     Middle Lobe, Right ØBF5
     Upper Lobe
       Left ØBF8
       Right ØBF4
   Carina ØBF2
   Cavity, Cranial ØWF1
   Cecum ØDFH
   Cerebral Ventricle ØØF6
   Colon
     Ascending ØDFK
     Descending ØDFM
     Sigmoid ØDFN
     Transverse ØDFL
   Duct
     Common Bile ØFF9
     Cystic ØFF8
     Hepatic
       Left ØFF6
       Right ØFF5
     Pancreatic ØFFD
       Accessory ØFFF
     Parotid
       Left ØCFC
       Right ØCFB
   Duodenum ØDF9
   Epidural Space ØØF3
   Esophagus ØDF5
   Fallopian Tube
     Left ØUF6
     Right ØUF5
   Fallopian Tubes, Bilateral ØUF7
   Gallbladder ØFF4
   Gastrointestinal Tract ØWFP
   Genitourinary Tract ØWFR
   Ileum ØDFB
   Intestine
     Large ØDFE
       Left ØDFG
       Right ØDFF
     Small ØDF8
   Jejunum ØDFA

Fragmentation *(Continued)*
   Kidney Pelvis
     Left ØTF4
     Right ØTF3
   Mediastinum ØWFC
   Oral Cavity and Throat ØWF3
   Pelvic Cavity ØWFJ
   Pericardial Cavity ØWFD
   Pericardium Ø2FN
   Peritoneal Cavity ØWFG
   Pleural Cavity
     Left ØWFB
     Right ØWF9
   Rectum ØDFP
   Respiratory Tract ØWFQ
   Spinal Canal ØØFU
   Stomach ØDF6
   Subarachnoid Space ØØF5
   Subdural Space ØØF4
   Trachea ØBF1
   Ureter
     Left ØTF7
     Right ØTF6
   Urethra ØTFD
   Uterus ØUF9
   Vitreous
     Left Ø8F5
     Right Ø8F4
Freestyle (Stentless) Aortic Root Bioprosthesis
   use Zooplastic Tissue in Heart and Great
     Vessels
Frenectomy
   see Excision, Mouth and Throat ØCB
   see Resection, Mouth and Throat ØCT
Frenoplasty, frenuloplasty
   see Repair, Mouth and Throat ØCQ
   see Replacement, Mouth and Throat ØCR
   see Supplement, Mouth and Throat ØCU
Frenotomy
   see Drainage, Mouth and Throat ØC9
   see Release, Mouth and Throat ØCN
Frenulotomy
   see Drainage, Mouth and Throat ØC9
   see Release, Mouth and Throat ØCN
Frenulum labii inferioris *use* Lower Lip
Frenulum labii superioris *use* Upper Lip
Frenulum linguae *use* Tongue
Frenulumectomy
   see Excision, Mouth and Throat ØCB
   see Resection, Mouth and Throat ØCT
Frontal lobe *use* Cerebral Hemisphere
Frontal vein
   use Face Vein, Right
   use Face Vein, Left
Fulguration *see* Destruction
Fundoplication, gastroesophageal *see* Restriction,
   Esophagogastric Junction ØDV4
Fundus uteri *use* Uterus
Fusion
   Acromioclavicular
     Left ØRGH
     Right ØRGG
   Ankle
     Left ØSGG
     Right ØSGF
   Carpal
     Left ØRGR
     Right ØRGQ
   Cervical Vertebral ØRG1
     2 or more ØRG2
       Interbody Fusion Device, Nanotextured
         Surface XRG2Ø92 ◄
     Interbody Fusion Device, Nanotextured
       Surface XRG1Ø92 ◄
   Cervicothoracic Vertebral ØRG4
     Interbody Fusion Device, Nanotextured
       Surface XRG4Ø92 ◄

Fusion *(Continued)*
   Coccygeal ØSG6
   Elbow
     Left ØRGM
     Right ØRGL
   Finger Phalangeal
     Left ØRGX
     Right ØRGW
   Hip
     Left ØSGB
     Right ØSG9
   Knee
     Left ØSGD
     Right ØSGC
   Lumbar Vertebral ØSGØ
     2 or more ØSG1
       Interbody Fusion Device, Nanotextured
         Surface XRGCØ92 ◄
       Interbody Fusion Device, Nanotextured
         Surface XRGBØ92 ◄
   Lumbosacral ØSG3
     Interbody Fusion Device, Nanotextured
       Surface XRGDØ92 ◄
   Metacarpocarpal
     Left ØRGT
     Right ØRGS
   Metacarpophalangeal
     Left ØRGV
     Right ØRGU
   Metatarsal-Phalangeal
     Left ØSGN
     Right ØSGM
   Metatarsal-Tarsal
     Left ØSGL
     Right ØSGK
   Occipital-cervical ØRGØ
     Interbody Fusion Device, Nanotextured
       Surface XRGØØ92 ◄
   Sacrococcygeal ØSG5
   Sacroiliac
     Left ØSG8
     Right ØSG7
   Shoulder
     Left ØRGK
     Right ØRGJ
   Sternoclavicular
     Left ØRGF
     Right ØRGE
   Tarsal
     Left ØSGJ
     Right ØSGH
   Temporomandibular
     Left ØRGD
     Right ØRGC
   Thoracic Vertebral ØRG6
     2 to 7 ØRG7
       Interbody Fusion Device, Nanotextured
         Surface XRG7Ø92 ◄
     8 or more ØRG8
       Interbody Fusion Device, Nanotextured
         Surface XRG8Ø92 ◄
     Interbody Fusion Device, Nanotextured
       Surface XRG6Ø92 ◄
   Thoracolumbar Vertebral ØRGA
     Interbody Fusion Device, Nanotextured
       Surface XRGAØ92 ◄
   Toe Phalangeal
     Left ØSGQ
     Right ØSGP
   Wrist
     Left ØRGP
     Right ØRGN
Fusion screw (compression) (lag) (locking)
   use Internal Fixation Device in Upper Joints
   use Internal Fixation Device in Lower Joints

F

G

Gait training *see* Motor Treatment, Rehabilitation F07
Galea aponeurotica *use* Subcutaneous Tissue and Fascia, Scalp
Ganglion impar (ganglion of Walther) *use* Sacral Sympathetic Nerve
Ganglionectomy
  Destruction of lesion *see* Destruction
  Excision of lesion *see* Excision
Gasserian ganglion *use* Trigeminal Nerve
Gastrectomy
  Partial *see* Excision, Stomach 0DB6
  Total *see* Resection, Stomach 0DT6
  Vertical (sleeve) *see* Excision, Stomach 0DB6
Gastric electrical stimulation (GES) lead *use* Stimulator Lead in Gastrointestinal System
Gastric lymph node *use* Lymphatic, Aortic
Gastric pacemaker lead *use* Stimulator Lead in Gastrointestinal System
Gastric plexus *see* Abdominal Sympathetic Nerve
Gastrocnemius muscle
  use Lower Leg Muscle, Right
  use Lower Leg Muscle, Left
Gastrocolic ligament *use* Greater Omentum
Gastrocolic omentum *use* Greater Omentum
Gastrocolostomy
  see Bypass, Gastrointestinal System 0D1
  see Drainage, Gastrointestinal System 0D9
Gastroduodenal artery *use* Hepatic Artery
Gastroduodenectomy
  see Excision, Gastrointestinal System 0DB
  see Resection, Gastrointestinal System 0DT
Gastroduodenoscopy 0DJ08ZZ
Gastroenteroplasty
  see Repair, Gastrointestinal System 0DQ
  see Supplement, Gastrointestinal System 0DU
Gastroenterostomy
  see Bypass, Gastrointestinal System 0D1
  see Drainage, Gastrointestinal System 0D9
Gastroesophageal (GE) junction *use* Esophagogastric Junction
Gastrogastrostomy
  see Bypass, Stomach 0D16
  see Drainage, Stomach 0D96
Gastrohepatic omentum *use* Lesser Omentum
Gastrojejunostomy
  see Bypass, Stomach 0D16
  see Drainage, Stomach 0D96
Gastrolysis *see* Release, Stomach 0DN6
Gastropexy
  see Repair, Stomach 0DQ6
  see Reposition, Stomach 0DS6
Gastrophrenic ligament *use* Greater Omentum
Gastroplasty
  see Repair, Stomach 0DQ6
  see Supplement, Stomach 0DU6
Gastroplication *see* Restriction, Stomach 0DV6

Gastropylorectomy *see* Excision, Gastrointestinal System 0DB
Gastrorrhaphy *see* Repair, Stomach 0DQ6
Gastroscopy 0DJ68ZZ
Gastrosplenic ligament *use* Greater Omentum
Gastrostomy
  see Bypass, Stomach 0D16
  see Drainage, Stomach 0D96
Gastrotomy *see* Drainage, Stomach 0D96
Gemellus muscle
  use Hip Muscle, Right
  use Hip Muscle, Left
Geniculate ganglion *use* Facial Nerve
Geniculate nucleus *use* Thalamus
Genioglossus muscle *use* Tongue, Palate, Pharynx Muscle
Genioplasty *see* Alteration, Jaw, Lower 0W05
Genitofemoral nerve *use* Lumbar Plexus
Gingivectomy *see* Excision, Mouth and Throat 0CB
Gingivoplasty
  see Repair, Mouth and Throat 0CQ
  see Replacement, Mouth and Throat 0CR
  see Supplement, Mouth and Throat 0CU
Glans penis *use* Prepuce
Glenohumeral joint
  use Shoulder Joint, Right
  use Shoulder Joint, Left
Glenohumeral ligament
  use Shoulder Bursa and Ligament, Right
  use Shoulder Bursa and Ligament, Left
Glenoid fossa (of scapula)
  use Glenoid Cavity, Right
  use Glenoid Cavity, Left
Glenoid ligament (labrum)
  use Shoulder Joint, Right
  use Shoulder Joint, Left
Globus pallidus *use* Basal Ganglia
Glomectomy
  see Excision, Endocrine System 0GB
  see Resection, Endocrine System 0GT
Glossectomy
  see Excision, Tongue 0CB7
  see Resection, Tongue 0CT7
Glossoepiglottic fold *use* Epiglottis
Glossopexy
  see Repair, Tongue 0CQ7
  see Reposition, Tongue 0CS7
Glossoplasty
  see Repair, Tongue 0CQ7
  see Replacement, Tongue 0CR7
  see Supplement, Tongue 0CU7
Glossorrhaphy *see* Repair, Tongue 0CQ7
Glossotomy *see* Drainage, Tongue 0C97
Glottis *use* Larynx
Gluteal Artery Perforator Flap
  Bilateral 0HRV079
  Left 0HRU079
  Right 0HRT079
Gluteal lymph node *use* Lymphatic, Pelvis

Gluteal vein
  use Hypogastric Vein, Right
  use Hypogastric Vein, Left
Gluteus maximus muscle
  use Hip Muscle, Right
  use Hip Muscle, Left
Gluteus medius muscle
  use Hip Muscle, Right
  use Hip Muscle, Left
Gluteus minimus muscle
  use Hip Muscle, Right
  use Hip Muscle, Left
GORE EXCLUDER® AAA Endoprosthesis ◄
  use Intraluminal Device, Branched or Fenestrated, One or Two Arteries in 04V ◄
  use Intraluminal Device, Branched or Fenestrated, Three or More Arteries in 04V ◄
  use Intraluminal Device ◄
GORE EXCLUDER® IBE Endoprosthesis *use* Intraluminal Device, Branched or Fenestrated, One or Two Arteries in 04V ◄
GORE TAG® Thoracic Endoprosthesis *use* Intraluminal Device ◄
GORE® DUALMESH® *use* Synthetic Substitute
Gracilis muscle
  use Upper Leg Muscle, Right
  use Upper Leg Muscle, Left
Graft
  see Replacement
  see Supplement
Great auricular nerve *use* Lumbar Plexus
Great cerebral vein *use* Intracranial Vein
Great saphenous vein
  use Greater Saphenous Vein, Right
  use Greater Saphenous Vein, Left
Greater alar cartilage *use* Nose
Greater occipital nerve *use* Cervical Nerve
Greater splanchnic nerve *use* Thoracic Sympathetic Nerve
Greater superficial petrosal nerve *use* Facial Nerve
Greater trochanter
  use Upper Femur, Right
  use Upper Femur, Left
Greater tuberosity
  use Humeral Head, Right
  use Humeral Head, Left
Greater vestibular (Bartholin's) gland *use* Vestibular Gland
Greater wing
  use Sphenoid Bone, Right
  use Sphenoid Bone, Left
Guedel airway *use* Intraluminal Device, Airway in Mouth and Throat
Guidance, catheter placement
  EKG *see* Measurement, Physiological Systems 4A0
  Fluoroscopy *see* Fluoroscopy, Veins B51
  Ultrasound *see* Ultrasonography, Veins B54

◄ New   ◄▦ Revised   ~~deleted~~ Deleted

H

Hallux
  use Toe, 1st, Right
  use Toe, 1st, Left
Hamate bone
  use Carpal, Right
  use Carpal, Left
Hancock Bioprosthesis (aortic) (mitral) valve
  use Zooplastic Tissue in Heart and Great Vessels
Hancock Bioprosthetic Valved Conduit *use* Zooplastic Tissue in Heart and Great Vessels
Harvesting, stem cells *see* Pheresis, Circulatory 6A55
Head of fibula
  use Fibula, Right
  use Fibula, Left
Hearing Aid Assessment F14Z
Hearing Assessment F13Z
Hearing Device
  Bone Conduction
    Left 09HE
    Right 09HD
  Insertion of device in
    Left 0NH6[034]SZ
    Right 0NH5[034]SZ
  Multiple Channel Cochlear Prosthesis
    Left 09HE
    Right 09HD
  Removal of device from, Skull 0NP0
  Revision of device in, Skull 0NW0
  Single Channel Cochlear Prosthesis
    Left 09HE
    Right 09HD
Hearing Treatment F09Z
Heart Assist System
  External
    Insertion of device in, Heart 02HA
    Removal of device from, Heart 02PA
    Revision of device in, Heart 02WA
  Implantable
    Insertion of device in, Heart 02HA
    Removal of device from, Heart 02PA
    Revision of device in, Heart 02WA
HeartMate II® Left Ventricular Assist Device (LVAD) *use* Implantable Heart Assist System in Heart and Great Vessels
HeartMate XVE® Left Ventricular Assist Device (LVAD) *use* Implantable Heart Assist System in Heart and Great Vessels
HeartMate® implantable heart assist system *see* Insertion of device in, Heart 02HA
Helix
  use External Ear, Right
  use External Ear, Left
  use External Ear, Bilateral
Hematopoietic cell transplant (HCT) *see* Transfusion, Circulatory 302 ◀
Hemicolectomy *see* Resection, Gastrointestinal System 0DT
Hemicystectomy *see* Excision, Urinary System 0TB
Hemigastrectomy *see* Excision, Gastrointestinal System 0DB
Hemiglossectomy *see* Excision, Mouth and Throat 0CB
Hemilaminectomy
  see Release, Central Nervous System 00N
  see Release, Peripheral Nervous System 01N
  see Drainage, Upper Bones 0P9
  see Excision, Upper Bones 0PB
  see Release, Upper Bones 0PN

Hemilaminectomy *(Continued)*
  see Drainage, Lower Bones 0Q9
  see Excision, Lower Bones 0QB
  see Release, Lower Bones 0QN
Hemilaryngectomy *see* Excision, Larynx 0CBS
Hemimandibulectomy *see* Excision, Head and Facial Bones 0NB
Hemimaxillectomy *see* Excision, Head and Facial Bones 0NB
Hemipylorectomy *see* Excision, Gastrointestinal System 0DB
Hemispherectomy
  see Excision, Central Nervous System 00B
  see Resection, Central Nervous System 00T
Hemithyroidectomy
  see Excision, Endocrine System 0GB
  see Resection, Endocrine System 0GT
Hemodialysis 5A1D00Z
Hepatectomy
  see Excision, Hepatobiliary System and Pancreas 0FB
  see Resection, Hepatobiliary System and Pancreas 0FT
Hepatic artery proper *use* Hepatic Artery
Hepatic flexure *use* Ascending Colon
Hepatic lymph node *use* Aortic Lymphatic
Hepatic plexus *use* Abdominal Sympathetic Nerve
Hepatic portal vein *use* Portal Vein
Hepaticoduodenostomy
  see Bypass, Hepatobiliary System and Pancreas 0F1
  see Drainage, Hepatobiliary System and Pancreas 0F9
Hepaticotomy *see* Drainage, Hepatobiliary System and Pancreas 0F9
Hepatocholedochostomy *see* Drainage, Duct, Common Bile 0F99
Hepatogastric ligament *use* Lesser Omentum
Hepatopancreatic ampulla *use* Ampulla of Vater
Hepatopexy
  see Repair, Hepatobiliary System and Pancreas 0FQ
  see Reposition, Hepatobiliary System and Pancreas 0FS
Hepatorrhaphy *see* Repair, Hepatobiliary System and Pancreas 0FQ
Hepatotomy *see* Drainage, Hepatobiliary System and Pancreas 0F9
Herculink (RX) Elite Renal Stent System *use* Intraluminal Device
Herniorrhaphy
  see Repair, Anatomical Regions, General 0WQ
  see Repair, Anatomical Regions, Lower Extremities 0YQ
  with synthetic substitute
    see Supplement, Anatomical Regions, General 0WU
    see Supplement, Anatomical Regions, Lower Extremities 0YU
Hip (joint) liner *use* Liner in Lower Joints
Holter monitoring 4A12X45
Holter valve ventricular shunt *use* Synthetic Substitute
Humeroradial joint
  use Elbow Joint, Right
  use Elbow Joint, Left
Humeroulnar joint
  use Elbow Joint, Right
  use Elbow Joint, Left
Humerus, distal
  use Humeral Shaft, Right
  use Humeral Shaft, Left

Hydrocelectomy *see* Excision, Male Reproductive System 0VB
Hydrotherapy
  Assisted exercise in pool *see* Motor Treatment, Rehabilitation F07
  Whirlpool *see* Activities of Daily Living Treatment, Rehabilitation F08
Hymenectomy
  see Excision, Hymen 0UBK
  see Resection, Hymen 0UTK
Hymenoplasty
  see Repair, Hymen 0UQK
  see Supplement, Hymen 0UUK
Hymenorrhaphy *see* Repair, Hymen 0UQK
Hymenotomy
  see Division, Hymen 0U8K
  see Drainage, Hymen 0U9K
Hyoglossus muscle *use* Tongue, Palate, Pharynx Muscle
Hyoid artery
  use Thyroid Artery, Right
  use Thyroid Artery, Left
Hyperalimentation *see* Introduction of substance in or on
Hyperbaric oxygenation
  Decompression sickness treatment *see* Decompression, Circulatory 6A15
  Wound treatment *see* Assistance, Circulatory 5A05
Hyperthermia
  Radiation Therapy
    Abdomen DWY38ZZ
    Adrenal Gland DGY28ZZ
    Bile Ducts DFY28ZZ
    Bladder DTY28ZZ
    Bone, Other DPYC8ZZ
    Bone Marrow D7Y08ZZ
    Brain D0Y08ZZ
    Brain Stem D0Y18ZZ
    Breast
      Left DMY08ZZ
      Right DMY18ZZ
    Bronchus DBY18ZZ
    Cervix DUY18ZZ
    Chest DWY28ZZ
    Chest Wall DBY78ZZ
    Colon DDY58ZZ
    Diaphragm DBY88ZZ
    Duodenum DDY28ZZ
    Ear D9Y08ZZ
    Esophagus DDY08ZZ
    Eye D8Y08ZZ
    Femur DPY98ZZ
    Fibula DPYB8ZZ
    Gallbladder DFY18ZZ
    Gland
      Adrenal DGY28ZZ
      Parathyroid DGY48ZZ
      Pituitary DGY08ZZ
      Thyroid DGY58ZZ
    Glands, Salivary D9Y68ZZ
    Head and Neck DWY18ZZ
    Hemibody DWY48ZZ
    Humerus DPY68ZZ
    Hypopharynx D9Y38ZZ
    Ileum DDY48ZZ
    Jejunum DDY38ZZ
    Kidney DTY08ZZ
    Larynx D9YB8ZZ
    Liver DFY08ZZ
    Lung DBY28ZZ
    Lymphatics
      Abdomen D7Y68ZZ
      Axillary D7Y48ZZ
      Inguinal D7Y88ZZ
      Neck D7Y38ZZ
      Pelvis D7Y78ZZ
      Thorax D7Y58ZZ
    Mandible DPY38ZZ
    Maxilla DPY28ZZ
    Mediastinum DBY68ZZ

Hyperthermia *(Continued)*
  Radiation Therapy *(Continued)*
    Mouth D9Y48ZZ
    Nasopharynx D9YD8ZZ
    Neck and Head DWY18ZZ
    Nerve, Peripheral D0Y78ZZ
    Nose D9Y18ZZ
    Oropharynx D9YF8ZZ
    Ovary DUY08ZZ
    Palate
      Hard D9Y88ZZ
      Soft D9Y98ZZ
    Pancreas DFY38ZZ
    Parathyroid Gland DGY48ZZ
    Pelvic Bones DPY88ZZ
    Pelvic Region DWY68ZZ
    Pineal Body DGY18ZZ
    Pituitary Gland DGY08ZZ
    Pleura DBY58ZZ
    Prostate DVY08ZZ
    Radius DPY78ZZ
    Rectum DDY78ZZ
    Rib DPY58ZZ
    Sinuses D9Y78ZZ
    Skin
      Abdomen DHY88ZZ
      Arm DHY48ZZ
      Back DHY78ZZ
      Buttock DHY98ZZ
      Chest DHY68ZZ
      Face DHY28ZZ

Hyperthermia *(Continued)*
  Radiation Therapy *(Continued)*
    Skin *(Continued)*
      Leg DHYB8ZZ
      Neck DHY38ZZ
    Skull DPY08ZZ
    Spinal Cord D0Y68ZZ
    Spleen D7Y28ZZ
    Sternum DPY48ZZ
    Stomach DDY18ZZ
    Testis DVY18ZZ
    Thymus D7Y18ZZ
    Thyroid Gland DGY58ZZ
    Tibia DPYB8ZZ
    Tongue D9Y58ZZ
    Trachea DBY08ZZ
    Ulna DPY78ZZ
    Ureter DTY18ZZ
    Urethra DTY38ZZ
    Uterus DUY28ZZ
    Whole Body DWY58ZZ
  Whole Body 6A3Z
Hypnosis GZFZZZZ
Hypogastric artery
  use Internal Iliac Artery, Right
  use Internal Iliac Artery, Left
Hypopharynx *use* Pharynx
Hypophysectomy
  see Excision, Gland, Pituitary 0GB0
  see Resection, Gland, Pituitary 0GT0

Hypophysis *use* Gland, Pituitary
Hypothalamotomy *see* Destruction, Thalamus 0059
Hypothenar muscle
  use Hand Muscle, Right
  use Hand Muscle, Left
Hypothermia, Whole Body 6A4Z
Hysterectomy
  supracervical *see* Resection, Uterus 0UT9
  total
    see Resection, Uterus 0UT9
    see Resection, Cervix 0UTC
Hysterolysis *see* Release, Uterus 0UN9
Hysteropexy
  see Repair, Uterus 0UQ9
  see Reposition, Uterus 0US9
Hysteroplasty
  see Repair, Uterus 0UQ9
Hysterorrhaphy *see* Repair, Uterus 0UQ9
Hysteroscopy 0UJD8ZZ
Hysterotomy
  see Drainage, Uterus 0U99
Hysterotrachelectomy
  see Resection, Uterus 0UT9
  see Resection, Cervix 0UTC
Hysterotracheloplasty
  see Repair, Uterus 0UQ9
Hysterotrachelorrhaphy *see* Repair, Uterus 0UQ9

◀ New   ◀▦ Revised   ~~deleted~~ Deleted

I

IABP (Intra-aortic balloon pump) *see*
    Assistance, Cardiac 5A02
IAEMT (Intraoperative anesthetic effect
    monitoring and titration) *see* Monitoring,
    Central Nervous 4A10
Idarucizumab, Dabigatran Reversal Agent
    XW0
Ileal artery *use* Superior Mesenteric Artery
Ileectomy
    see Excision, Ileum 0DBB
    see Resection, Ileum 0DTB
Ileocolic artery *use* Superior Mesenteric Artery
Ileocolic vein *use* Colic Vein
Ileopexy
    see Repair, Ileum 0DQB
    see Reposition, Ileum 0DSB
Ileorrhaphy *see* Repair, Ileum 0DQB
Ileoscopy 0DJD8ZZ
Ileostomy
    see Bypass, Ileum 0D1B
    see Drainage, Ileum 0D9B
Ileotomy *see* Drainage, Ileum 0D9B
Ileoureterostomy *see* Bypass, Bladder 0T1B
Iliac crest
    use Pelvic Bone, Right
    use Pelvic Bone, Left
Iliac fascia
    use Subcutaneous Tissue and Fascia, Right
        Upper Leg
    use Subcutaneous Tissue and Fascia, Left
        Upper Leg
Iliac lymph node *use* Lymphatic, Pelvis
Iliacus muscle
    use Hip Muscle, Right
    use Hip Muscle, Left
Iliofemoral ligament
    use Hip Bursa and Ligament, Right
    use Hip Bursa and Ligament, Left
Iliohypogastric nerve *use* Lumbar Plexus
Ilioinguinal nerve *use* Lumbar Plexus
Iliolumbar artery
    use Internal Iliac Artery, Right
    use Internal Iliac Artery, Left
Iliolumbar ligament
    use Trunk Bursa and Ligament, Right
    use Trunk Bursa and Ligament, Left
Iliotibial tract (band)
    use Subcutaneous Tissue and Fascia, Right
        Upper Leg
    use Subcutaneous Tissue and Fascia, Left
        Upper Leg
Ilium
    use Pelvic Bone, Right
    use Pelvic Bone, Left
Ilizarov external fixator
    use External Fixation Device, Ring in 0PH
    use External Fixation Device, Ring in 0PS
    use External Fixation Device, Ring in 0QH
    use External Fixation Device, Ring in 0QS
Ilizarov-Vecklich device
    use External Fixation Device, Limb
        Lengthening in 0PH
    use External Fixation Device, Limb
        Lengthening in 0QH
Imaging, diagnostic
    see Plain Radiography
    see Fluoroscopy
    see Computerized Tomography (CT Scan)
    see Magnetic Resonance Imaging (MRI)
    see Ultrasonography
Immobilization
    Abdominal Wall 2W33X
    Arm
        Lower
            Left 2W3DX
            Right 2W3CX
        Upper
            Left 2W3BX
            Right 2W3AX
    Back 2W35X

Immobilization *(Continued)*
    Chest Wall 2W34X
    Extremity
        Lower
            Left 2W3MX
            Right 2W3LX
        Upper
            Left 2W39X
            Right 2W38X
    Face 2W31X
    Finger
        Left 2W3KX
        Right 2W3JX
    Foot
        Left 2W3TX
        Right 2W3SX
    Hand
        Left 2W3FX
        Right 2W3EX
    Head 2W30X
    Inguinal Region
        Left 2W37X
        Right 2W36X
    Leg
        Lower
            Left 2W3RX
            Right 2W3QX
        Upper
            Left 2W3PX
            Right 2W3NX
    Neck 2W32X
    Thumb
        Left 2W3HX
        Right 2W3GX
    Toe
        Left 2W3VX
        Right 2W3UX
Immunization *see* Introduction of Serum,
    Toxoid, and Vaccine
Immunotherapy *see* Introduction of
    Immunotherapeutic Substance
Immunotherapy, antineoplastic
    Interferon *see* Introduction of Low-dose
        Interleukin-2
    Interleukin-2 of high-dose *see* Introduction,
        High-dose Interleukin-2
    Interleukin-2, low-dose *see* Introduction of
        Low-dose Interleukin-2
    Monoclonal antibody *see* Introduction of
        Monoclonal Antibody
    Proleukin, high-dose *see* Introduction of
        High-dose Interleukin-2
    Proleukin, low-dose *see* Introduction of Low-
        dose Interleukin-2
Impeller Pump
    Continuous, Output 5A0221D
    Intermittent, Output 5A0211D
Implantable cardioverter-defibrillator (ICD)
    use Defibrillator Generator in 0JH
Implantable drug infusion pump (anti-
    spasmodic) (chemotherapy) (pain) *use*
    Infusion Device, Pump in Subcutaneous
    Tissue and Fascia
Implantable glucose monitoring device *use*
    Monitoring Device
Implantable hemodynamic monitor (IHM) *use*
    Monitoring Device, Hemodynamic in 0JH
Implantable hemodynamic monitoring
    system (IHMS) *use* Monitoring Device,
    Hemodynamic in 0JH
Implantable Miniature Telescope™ (IMT) use
    Synthetic Substitute, Intraocular Telescope
    in 08R
Implantation
    see Replacement
    see Insertion
Implanted (venous) (access) port *use* Vascular
    Access Device, Reservoir in Subcutaneous
    Tissue and Fascia
IMV (intermittent mandatory ventilation) *see*
    Assistance, Respiratory 5A09

In Vitro Fertilization 8E0ZXY1
Incision, abscess *see* Drainage
Incudectomy
    see Excision, Ear, Nose, Sinus 09B
    see Resection, Ear, Nose, Sinus 09T
Incudopexy
    see Repair, Ear, Nose, Sinus 09Q
    see Reposition, Ear, Nose, Sinus 09S
Incus
    use Ossicle, Auditory, Right
    use Ossicle, Auditory, Left
Induction of labor
    Artificial rupture of membranes *see* Drainage,
        Pregnancy 109
    Oxytocin *see* Introduction of Hormone
InDura, intrathecal catheter (1P) (spinal) *use*
    Infusion Device
Inferior cardiac nerve *use* Thoracic Sympathetic
    Nerve
Inferior cerebellar vein *use* Intracranial Vein
Inferior cerebral vein *use* Intracranial Vein
Inferior epigastric artery
    use External Iliac Artery, Right
    use External Iliac Artery, Left
Inferior epigastric lymph node *use* Lymphatic,
    Pelvis
Inferior genicular artery
    use Popliteal Artery, Right
    use Popliteal Artery, Left
Inferior gluteal artery
    use Internal Iliac Artery, Right
    use Internal Iliac Artery, Left
Inferior gluteal nerve *use* Sacral Plexus
    Nerve
Inferior hypogastric plexus *use* Abdominal
    Sympathetic Nerve
Inferior labial artery *use* Face Artery
Inferior longitudinal muscle *use* Tongue,
    Palate, Pharynx Muscle
Inferior mesenteric ganglion *use* Abdominal
    Sympathetic Nerve
Inferior mesenteric lymph node *use* Mesenteric
    Lymphatic
Inferior mesenteric plexus *use* Abdominal
    Sympathetic Nerve
Inferior oblique muscle
    use Extraocular Muscle, Right
    use Extraocular Muscle, Left
Inferior pancreaticoduodenal artery *use*
    Superior Mesenteric Artery
Inferior phrenic artery *use* Abdominal Aorta
Inferior rectus muscle
    use Extraocular Muscle, Right
    use Extraocular Muscle, Left
Inferior suprarenal artery
    use Renal Artery, Right
    use Renal Artery, Left
Inferior tarsal plate
    use Lower Eyelid, Right
    use Lower Eyelid, Left
Inferior thyroid vein
    use Innominate Vein, Right
    use Innominate Vein, Left
Inferior tibiofibular joint
    use Ankle Joint, Right
    use Ankle Joint, Left
Inferior turbinate *use* Nasal Turbinate
Inferior ulnar collateral artery
    use Brachial Artery, Right
    use Brachial Artery, Left
Inferior vesical artery
    use Internal Iliac Artery, Right
    use Internal Iliac Artery, Left
Infraauricular lymph node *use* Lymphatic,
    Head
Infraclavicular (deltopectoral) lymph node
    use Lymphatic, Right Upper Extremity
    use Lymphatic, Left Upper Extremity
Infrahyoid muscle
    use Neck Muscle, Right
    use Neck Muscle, Left

◀ New   ◀▥ Revised   ~~deleted~~ Deleted

Infraparotid lymph node *use* Lymphatic, Head
Infraspinatus fascia
   use Subcutaneous Tissue and Fascia, Right
      Upper Arm
   use Subcutaneous Tissue and Fascia, Left
      Upper Arm
Infraspinatus muscle
   use Shoulder Muscle, Right
   use Shoulder Muscle, Left
Infundibulopelvic ligament *use* Uterine
   Supporting Structure
Infusion *see* Introduction of substance in
   or on
Infusion Device, Pump
   Insertion of device in
      Abdomen 0JH8
      Back 0JH7
      Chest 0JH6
      Lower Arm
         Left 0JHH
         Right 0JHG
      Lower Leg
         Left 0JHP
         Right 0JHN
      Trunk 0JHT
      Upper Arm
         Left 0JHF
         Right 0JHD
      Upper Leg
         Left 0JHM
         Right 0JHL
   Removal of device from
      Lower Extremity 0JPW
      Trunk 0JPT
      Upper Extremity 0JPV
   Revision of device in
      Lower Extremity 0JWW
      Trunk 0JWT
      Upper Extremity 0JWV
Infusion, glucarpidase
   Central vein 3E043GQ
   Peripheral vein 3E033GQ
Inguinal canal
   use Inguinal Region, Right
   use Inguinal Region, Left
   use Inguinal Region, Bilateral
Inguinal triangle
   see Inguinal Region, Right
   see Inguinal Region, Left
   see Inguinal Region, Bilateral
Injection *see* Introduction of substance in
   or on
Injection reservoir, port *use* Vascular Access
   Device, Reservoir in Subcutaneous Tissue
   and Fascia
Injection reservoir, pump *use* Infusion
   Device, Pump in Subcutaneous Tissue and
   Fascia
Insemination, artificial 3E0P7LZ
Insertion
   Antimicrobial envelope *see* Introduction of
      Anti-infective
   Aqueous drainage shunt
      see Bypass, Eye 081
      see Drainage, Eye 089
   Products of Conception 10H0
   Spinal Stabilization Device
      see Insertion of device in, Upper
         Joints 0RH
      see Insertion of device in, Lower
         Joints 0SH
Insertion of device in
   Abdominal Wall 0WHF
   Acetabulum
      Left 0QH5
      Right 0QH4
   Anal Sphincter 0DHR
   Ankle Region
      Left 0YHL
      Right 0YHK
   Anus 0DHQ

Insertion of device in *(Continued)*
   Aorta
      Abdominal 04H0
      Thoracic ◄▥
         Ascending/Arch 02HX ◄
         Descending 02HW ◄
   Arm
      Lower
         Left 0XHF
         Right 0XHD
      Upper
         Left 0XH9
         Right 0XH8
   Artery
      Anterior Tibial
         Left 04HQ
         Right 04HP
      Axillary
         Left 03H6
         Right 03H5
      Brachial
         Left 03H8
         Right 03H7
      Celiac 04H1
      Colic
         Left 04H7
         Middle 04H8
         Right 04H6
      Common Carotid
         Left 03HJ
         Right 03HH
      Common Iliac
         Left 04HD
         Right 04HC
      External Carotid
         Left 03HN
         Right 03HM
      External Iliac
         Left 04HJ
         Right 04HH
      Face 03HR
      Femoral
         Left 04HL
         Right 04HK
      Foot
         Left 04HW
         Right 04HV
      Gastric 04H2
      Hand
         Left 03HF
         Right 03HD
      Hepatic 04H3
      Inferior Mesenteric 04HB
      Innominate 03H2
      Internal Carotid
         Left 03HL
         Right 03HK
      Internal Iliac
         Left 04HF
         Right 04HE
      Internal Mammary
         Left 03H1
         Right 03H0
      Intracranial 03HG
      Lower 04HY
      Peroneal
         Left 04HU
         Right 04HT
      Popliteal
         Left 04HN
         Right 04HM
      Posterior Tibial
         Left 04HS
         Right 04HR
      Pulmonary
         Left 02HR
         Right 02HQ
      Pulmonary Trunk 02HP
      Radial
         Left 03HC
         Right 03HB

Insertion of device in *(Continued)*
   Artery *(Continued)*
      Renal
         Left 04HA
         Right 04H9
      Splenic 04H4
      Subclavian
         Left 03H4
         Right 03H3
      Superior Mesenteric 04H5
      Temporal
         Left 03HT
         Right 03HS
      Thyroid
         Left 03HV
         Right 03HU
      Ulnar
         Left 03HA
         Right 03H9
      Upper 03HY
      Vertebral
         Left 03HQ
         Right 03HP
   Atrium
      Left 02H7
      Right 02H6
   Axilla
      Left 0XH5
      Right 0XH4
   Back
      Lower 0WHL
      Upper 0WHK
   Bladder 0THB
   Bladder Neck 0THC
   Bone
      Ethmoid
         Left 0NHG
         Right 0NHF
      Facial 0NHW
      Frontal
         Left 0NH2
         Right 0NH1
      Hyoid 0NHX
      Lacrimal
         Left 0NHJ
         Right 0NHH
      Lower 0QHY
      Nasal 0NHB
      Occipital
         Left 0NH8
         Right 0NH7
      Palatine
         Left 0NHL
         Right 0NHK
      Parietal
         Left 0NH4
         Right 0NH3
      Pelvic
         Left 0QH3
         Right 0QH2
      Sphenoid
         Left 0NHD
         Right 0NHC
      Temporal
         Left 0NH6
         Right 0NH5
      Upper 0PHY
      Zygomatic
         Left 0NHN
         Right 0NHM
   Brain 00H0
   Breast
      Bilateral 0HHV
      Left 0HHU
      Right 0HHT
   Bronchus
      Lingula 0BH9
      Lower Lobe
         Left 0BHB
         Right 0BH6

◄ New   ◄▥ Revised   ~~deleted~~ Deleted

Insertion of device in *(Continued)*
  Bronchus *(Continued)*
    Main
      Left 0BH7
      Right 0BH3
    Middle Lobe, Right 0BH5
    Upper Lobe
      Left 0BH8
      Right 0BH4
  Buttock
    Left 0YH1
    Right 0YH0
  Carpal
    Left 0PHN
    Right 0PHM
  Cavity, Cranial 0WH1
  Cerebral Ventricle 00H6
  Cervix 0UHC
  Chest Wall 0WH8
  Cisterna Chyli 07HL
  Clavicle
    Left 0PHB
    Right 0PH9
  Coccyx 0QHS
  Cul-de-sac 0UHF
  Diaphragm
    Left 0BHS
    Right 0BHR
  Disc
    Cervical Vertebral 0RH3
    Cervicothoracic Vertebral 0RH5
    Lumbar Vertebral 0SH2
    Lumbosacral 0SH4
    Thoracic Vertebral 0RH9
    Thoracolumbar Vertebral 0RHB
  Duct
    Hepatobiliary 0FHB
    Pancreatic 0FHD
  Duodenum 0DH9
  Ear
    Left 09HE
    Right 09HD
  Elbow Region
    Left 0XHC
    Right 0XHB
  Epididymis and Spermatic Cord
    0VHM
  Esophagus 0DH5
  Extremity
    Lower
      Left 0YHB
      Right 0YH9
    Upper
      Left 0XH7
      Right 0XH6
  Eye
    Left 08H1
    Right 08H0
  Face 0WH2
  Fallopian Tube 0UH8
  Femoral Region
    Left 0YH8
    Right 0YH7
  Femoral Shaft
    Left 0QH9
    Right 0QH8
  Femur
    Lower
      Left 0QHC
      Right 0QHB
    Upper
      Left 0QH7
      Right 0QH6
  Fibula
    Left 0QHK
    Right 0QHJ
  Foot
    Left 0YHN
    Right 0YHM
  Gallbladder 0FH4
  Gastrointestinal Tract 0WHP

Insertion of device in *(Continued)*
  Genitourinary Tract 0WHR
  Gland, Endocrine 0GHS
  Glenoid Cavity
    Left 0PH8
    Right 0PH7
  Hand
    Left 0XHK
    Right 0XHJ
  Head 0WH0
  Heart 02HA
  Humeral Head
    Left 0PHD
    Right 0PHC
  Humeral Shaft
    Left 0PHG
    Right 0PHF
  Ileum 0DHB
  Inguinal Region
    Left 0YH6
    Right 0YH5
  Intestine
    Large 0DHE
    Small 0DH8
  Jaw
    Lower 0WH5
    Upper 0WH4
  Jejunum 0DHA
  Joint
    Acromioclavicular
      Left 0RHH
      Right 0RHG
    Ankle
      Left 0SHG
      Right 0SHF
    Carpal
      Left 0RHR
      Right 0RHQ
    Cervical Vertebral 0RH1
    Cervicothoracic Vertebral 0RH4
    Coccygeal 0SH6
    Elbow
      Left 0RHM
      Right 0RHL
    Finger Phalangeal
      Left 0RHX
      Right 0RHW
    Hip
      Left 0SHB
      Right 0SH9
    Knee
      Left 0SHD
      Right 0SHC
    Lumbar Vertebral 0SH0
    Lumbosacral 0SH3
    Metacarpocarpal
      Left 0RHT
      Right 0RHS
    Metacarpophalangeal
      Left 0RHV
      Right 0RHU
    Metatarsal-Phalangeal
      Left 0SHN
      Right 0SHM
    Metatarsal-Tarsal
      Left 0SHL
      Right 0SHK
    Occipital-cervical 0RH0
    Sacrococcygeal 0SH5
    Sacroiliac
      Left 0SH8
      Right 0SH7
    Shoulder
      Left 0RHK
      Right 0RHJ
    Sternoclavicular
      Left 0RHF
      Right 0RHE
    Tarsal
      Left 0SHJ
      Right 0SHH

Insertion of device in *(Continued)*
  Joint *(Continued)*
    Temporomandibular
      Left 0RHD
      Right 0RHC
    Thoracic Vertebral 0RH6
    Thoracolumbar Vertebral 0RHA
    Toe Phalangeal
      Left 0SHQ
      Right 0SHP
    Wrist
      Left 0RHP
      Right 0RHN
  Kidney 0TH5
  Knee Region
    Left 0YHG
    Right 0YHF
  Leg
    Lower
      Left 0YHJ
      Right 0YHH
    Upper
      Left 0YHD
      Right 0YHC
  Liver 0FH0
    Left Lobe 0FH2
    Right Lobe 0FH1
  Lung
    Left 0BHL
    Right 0BHK
  Lymphatic 07HN
    Thoracic Duct 07HK
  Mandible
    Left 0NHV
    Right 0NHT
  Maxilla
    Left 0NHS
    Right 0NHR
  Mediastinum 0WHC
  Metacarpal
    Left 0PHQ
    Right 0PHP
  Metatarsal
    Left 0QHP
    Right 0QHN
  Mouth and Throat 0CHY
  Muscle
    Lower 0KHY
    Upper 0KHX
  Nasopharynx 09HN
  Neck 0WH6
  Nerve
    Cranial 00HE
    Peripheral 01HY
  Nipple
    Left 0HHX
    Right 0HHW
  Oral Cavity and Throat 0WH3
  Orbit
    Left 0NHQ
    Right 0NHP
  Ovary 0UH3
  Pancreas 0FHG
  Patella
    Left 0QHF
    Right 0QHD
  Pelvic Cavity 0WHJ
  Penis 0VHS
  Pericardial Cavity 0WHD
  Pericardium 02HN
  Perineum
    Female 0WHN
    Male 0WHM
  Peritoneal Cavity 0WHG
  Phalanx
    Finger
      Left 0PHV
      Right 0PHT
    Thumb
      Left 0PHS
      Right 0PHR

◀ New   ◀▥ Revised   ~~deleted~~ Deleted

Inspection *(Continued)*
  Extremity
    Lower
      Left ØYJB
      Right ØYJ9
    Upper
      Left ØXJ7
      Right ØXJ6
  Eye
    Left Ø8J1XZZ
    Right Ø8JØXZZ
  Face ØWJ2
  Fallopian Tube ØUJ8
  Femoral Region
    Bilateral ØYJE
    Left ØYJ8
    Right ØYJ7
  Finger Nail ØHJQXZZ
  Foot
    Left ØYJN
    Right ØYJM
  Gallbladder ØFJ4
  Gastrointestinal Tract ØWJP
  Genitourinary Tract ØWJR
  Gland
    Adrenal ØGJ5
    Endocrine ØGJS
    Pituitary ØGJØ
    Salivary ØCJA
  Great Vessel Ø2JY
  Hand
    Left ØXJK
    Right ØXJJ
  Head ØWJØ
  Heart Ø2JA
  Inguinal Region
    Bilateral ØYJA
    Left ØYJ6
    Right ØYJ5
  Intestinal Tract
    Lower ØDJD
    Upper ØDJØ
  Jaw
    Lower ØWJ5
    Upper ØWJ4
  Joint
    Acromioclavicular
      Left ØRJH
      Right ØRJG
    Ankle
      Left ØSJG
      Right ØSJF
    Carpal
      Left ØRJR
      Right ØRJQ
    Cervical Vertebral ØRJ1
    Cervicothoracic Vertebral ØRJ4
    Coccygeal ØSJ6
    Elbow
      Left ØRJM
      Right ØRJL
    Finger Phalangeal
      Left ØRJX
      Right ØRJW
    Hip
      Left ØSJB
      Right ØSJ9
    Knee
      Left ØSJD
      Right ØSJC
    Lumbar Vertebral ØSJØ
    Lumbosacral ØSJ3
    Metacarpocarpal
      Left ØRJT
      Right ØRJS
    Metacarpophalangeal
      Left ØRJV
      Right ØRJU
    Metatarsal-Phalangeal
      Left ØSJN
      Right ØSJM

Inspection *(Continued)*
  Joint *(Continued)*
    Metatarsal-Tarsal
      Left ØSJL
      Right ØSJK
    Occipital-cervical ØRJØ
    Sacrococcygeal ØSJ5
    Sacroiliac
      Left ØSJ8
      Right ØSJ7
    Shoulder
      Left ØRJK
      Right ØRJJ
    Sternoclavicular
      Left ØRJF
      Right ØRJE
    Tarsal
      Left ØSJJ
      Right ØSJH
    Temporomandibular
      Left ØRJD
      Right ØRJC
    Thoracic Vertebral ØRJ6
    Thoracolumbar Vertebral
      ØRJA
    Toe Phalangeal
      Left ØSJQ
      Right ØSJP
    Wrist
      Left ØRJP
      Right ØRJN
  Kidney ØTJ5
  Knee Region
    Left ØYJG
    Right ØYJF
  Larynx ØCJS
  Leg
    Lower
      Left ØYJJ
      Right ØYJH
    Upper
      Left ØYJD
      Right ØYJC
  Lens
    Left Ø8JKXZZ
    Right Ø8JJXZZ
  Liver ØFJØ
  Lung
    Left ØBJL
    Right ØBJK
  Lymphatic Ø7JN
    Thoracic Duct Ø7JK
  Mediastinum ØWJC
  Mesentery ØDJV
  Mouth and Throat ØCJY
  Muscle
    Extraocular
      Left Ø8JM
      Right Ø8JL
    Lower ØKJY
    Upper ØKJX
  Neck ØWJ6
  Nerve
    Cranial ØØJE
    Peripheral Ø1JY
  Nose Ø9JK
  Omentum ØDJU
  Oral Cavity and Throat ØWJ3
  Ovary ØUJ3
  Pancreas ØFJG
  Parathyroid Gland ØGJR
  Pelvic Cavity ØWJD
  Penis ØVJS
  Pericardial Cavity ØWJD
  Perineum
    Female ØWJN
    Male ØWJM
  Peritoneal Cavity ØWJG
  Peritoneum ØDJW
  Pineal Body ØGJ1
  Pleura ØBJQ

Inspection *(Continued)*
  Pleural Cavity
    Left ØWJB
    Right ØWJ9
  Products of Conception 1ØJØ
    Ectopic 1ØJ2
    Retained 1ØJ1
  Prostate and Seminal Vesicles ØVJ4
  Respiratory Tract ØWJQ
  Retroperitoneum ØWJH
  Scrotum and Tunica Vaginalis ØVJ8
  Shoulder Region
    Left ØXJ3
    Right ØXJ2
  Sinus Ø9JY
  Skin ØHJPXZZ
  Skull ØNJØ
  Spinal Canal ØØJU
  Spinal Cord ØØJV
  Spleen Ø7JP
  Stomach ØDJ6
  Subcutaneous Tissue and Fascia
    Head and Neck ØJJS
    Lower Extremity ØJJW
    Trunk ØJJT
    Upper Extremity ØJJV
  Tendon
    Lower ØLJY
    Upper ØLJX
  Testis ØVJD
  Thymus Ø7JM
  Thyroid Gland ØGJK
  Toe Nail ØHJRXZZ
  Trachea ØBJ1
  Tracheobronchial Tree ØBJØ
  Tympanic Membrane
    Left Ø9J8
    Right Ø9J7
  Ureter ØTJ9
  Urethra ØTJD
  Uterus and Cervix ØUJD
  Vagina and Cul-de-sac ØUJH
  Vas Deferens ØVJR
  Vein
    Lower Ø6JY
    Upper Ø5JY
  Vulva ØUJM
  Wall
    Abdominal ØWJF
    Chest ØWJ8
  Wrist Region
    Left ØXJH
    Right ØXJG
Instillation *see* Introduction of substance in
    or on
Insufflation *see* Introduction of substance in
    or on
Interatrial septum *use* Atrial Septum
Interbody fusion (spine) cage
    use Interbody Fusion Device in Upper Joints
    use Interbody Fusion Device in Lower Joints
Interbody Fusion Device, Nanotextured
      Surface ◀
    Cervical Vertebral XRG1092 ◀
      2 or more XRG2092 ◀
    Cervicothoracic Vertebral XRG4092 ◀
    Lumbar Vertebral XRGB092 ◀
      2 or more XRGC092 ◀
    Lumbosacral XRGD092 ◀
    Occipital-cervical XRG0092 ◀
    Thoracic Vertebral XRG6092 ◀
      2 to 7 XRG7092 ◀
      8 or more XRG8092 ◀
    Thoracolumbar Vertebral XRGA092 ◀
Intercarpal joint
    use Carpal Joint, Right
    use Carpal Joint, Left
Intercarpal ligament
    use Hand Bursa and Ligament, Right
    use Hand Bursa and Ligament, Left

◀ New   ◀IIII Revised   ~~deleted~~ Deleted

◀ New   ◀▭ Revised   ~~deleted~~ Deleted

Introduction of substance in or on *(Continued)*
  Mucous Membrane *(Continued)*
    Antineoplastic 3E00X0
    Destructive Agent 3E00XTZ
    Diagnostic Substance, Other 3E00XKZ
    Hypnotics 3E00XNZ
    Pigment 3E00XMZ
    Sedatives 3E00XNZ
    Serum 3E00X4Z
    Toxoid 3E00X4Z
    Vaccine 3E00X4Z
  Muscle 3E023GC
    Analgesics 3E023NZ
    Anesthetic, Local 3E023BZ
    Anti-infective 3E0232
    Anti-inflammatory 3E0233Z
    Antineoplastic 3E0230
    Destructive Agent 3E023TZ
    Diagnostic Substance, Other 3E023KZ
    Electrolytic Substance 3E0237Z
    Hypnotics 3E023NZ
    Nutritional Substance 3E0236Z
    Radioactive Substance 3E023HZ
    Sedatives 3E023NZ
    Serum 3E0234Z
    Toxoid 3E0234Z
    Vaccine 3E0234Z
    Water Balance Substance 3E0237Z
  Nerve
    Cranial 3E0X3GC
      Anesthetic
        Local 3E0X3BZ
        Regional 3E0X3CZ
      Anti-inflammatory 3E0X33Z
      Destructive Agent 3E0X3TZ
    Peripheral 3E0T3GC
      Anesthetic
        Local 3E0T3BZ
        Regional 3E0T3CZ
      Anti-inflammatory 3E0T33Z
      Destructive Agent 3E0T3TZ
    Plexus 3E0T3GC
      Anesthetic
        Local 3E0T3BZ
        Regional 3E0T3CZ
      Anti-inflammatory 3E0T33Z
      Destructive Agent 3E0T3TZ
  Nose 3E09
    Analgesics 3E09
    Anesthetic, Local 3E09
    Anti-infective 3E09
    Anti-inflammatory 3E09
    Antineoplastic 3E09
    Destructive Agent 3E09
    Diagnostic Substance, Other 3E09
    Hypnotics 3E09
    Radioactive Substance 3E09
    Sedatives 3E09
    Serum 3E09
    Toxoid 3E09
    Vaccine 3E09
  Pancreatic Tract 3E0J
    Analgesics 3E0J
    Anesthetic, Local 3E0J
    Anti-infective 3E0J
    Anti-inflammatory 3E0J
    Antineoplastic 3E0J
    Destructive Agent 3E0J
    Diagnostic Substance, Other 3E0J
    Electrolytic Substance 3E0J
    Gas 3E0J
    Hypnotics 3E0J
    Islet Cells, Pancreatic 3E0J
    Nutritional Substance 3E0J
    Radioactive Substance 3E0J
    Sedatives 3E0J
    Water Balance Substance 3E0J
  Pericardial Cavity 3E0Y3GC
    Analgesics 3E0Y3NZ
    Anesthetic, Local 3E0Y3BZ
    Anti-infective 3E0Y32

Introduction of substance in or on *(Continued)*
  Pericardial Cavity *(Continued)*
    Anti-inflammatory 3E0Y33Z
    Antineoplastic 3E0Y
    Destructive Agent 3E0Y3TZ
    Diagnostic Substance, Other
      3E0Y3KZ
    Electrolytic Substance 3E0Y37Z
    Gas 3E0Y
    Hypnotics 3E0Y3NZ
    Nutritional Substance 3E0Y36Z
    Radioactive Substance 3E0Y3HZ
    Sedatives 3E0Y3NZ
    Water Balance Substance 3E0Y37Z
  Peritoneal Cavity 3E0M3GC
    Adhesion Barrier 3E0M05Z
    Analgesics 3E0M3NZ
    Anesthetic, Local 3E0M3BZ
    Anti-infective 3E0M32
    Anti-inflammatory 3E0M33Z
    Antineoplastic 3E0M
    Destructive Agent 3E0M3TZ
    Diagnostic Substance, Other
      3E0M3KZ
    Electrolytic Substance 3E0M37Z
    Gas 3E0M
    Hypnotics 3E0M3NZ
    Nutritional Substance 3E0M36Z
    Radioactive Substance 3E0M3HZ
    Sedatives 3E0M3NZ
    Water Balance Substance 3E0M37Z
  Pharynx 3E0D
    Analgesics 3E0D
    Anesthetic, Local 3E0D
    Anti-infective 3E0D
    Anti-inflammatory 3E0D
    Antiarrhythmic 3E0D
    Antineoplastic 3E0D
    Destructive Agent 3E0D
    Diagnostic Substance, Other 3E0D
    Electrolytic Substance 3E0D
    Hypnotics 3E0D
    Nutritional Substance 3E0D
    Radioactive Substance 3E0D
    Sedatives 3E0D
    Serum 3E0D
    Toxoid 3E0D
    Vaccine 3E0D
    Water Balance Substance 3E0D
  Pleural Cavity 3E0L3GC
    Adhesion Barrier 3E0L05Z
    Analgesics 3E0L3NZ
    Anesthetic, Local 3E0L3BZ
    Anti-infective 3E0L32
    Anti-inflammatory 3E0L33Z
    Antineoplastic 3E0L
    Destructive Agent 3E0L3TZ
    Diagnostic Substance, Other
      3E0L3KZ
    Electrolytic Substance 3E0L37Z
    Gas 3E0L
    Hypnotics 3E0L3NZ
    Nutritional Substance 3E0L36Z
    Radioactive Substance 3E0L3HZ
    Sedatives 3E0L3NZ
    Water Balance Substance 3E0L37Z
  Products of Conception 3E0E
    Analgesics 3E0E
    Anesthetic, Local 3E0E
    Anti-infective 3E0E
    Anti-inflammatory 3E0E
    Antineoplastic 3E0E
    Destructive Agent 3E0E
    Diagnostic Substance, Other 3E0E
    Electrolytic Substance 3E0E
    Gas 3E0E
    Hypnotics 3E0E
    Nutritional Substance 3E0E
    Radioactive Substance 3E0E
    Sedatives 3E0E
    Water Balance Substance 3E0E

Introduction of substance in or on *(Continued)*
  Reproductive
    Female 3E0P
      Adhesion Barrier 3E0P05Z
      Analgesics 3E0P
      Anesthetic, Local 3E0P
      Anti-infective 3E0P
      Anti-inflammatory 3E0P
      Antineoplastic 3E0P
      Destructive Agent 3E0P
      Diagnostic Substance, Other 3E0P
      Electrolytic Substance 3E0P
      Gas 3E0P
      Hypnotics 3E0P
      Nutritional Substance 3E0P
      Ovum, Fertilized 3E0P
      Radioactive Substance 3E0P
      Sedatives 3E0P
      Sperm 3E0P
      Water Balance Substance 3E0P
    Male 3E0N
      Analgesics 3E0N
      Anesthetic, Local 3E0N
      Anti-infective 3E0N
      Anti-inflammatory 3E0N
      Antineoplastic 3E0N
      Destructive Agent 3E0N
      Diagnostic Substance, Other 3E0N
      Electrolytic Substance 3E0N
      Gas 3E0N
      Hypnotics 3E0N
      Nutritional Substance 3E0N
      Radioactive Substance 3E0N
      Sedatives 3E0N
      Water Balance Substance 3E0N
  Respiratory Tract 3E0F
    Analgesics 3E0F
    Anesthetic
      Inhalation 3E0F
      Local 3E0F
    Anti-infective 3E0F
    Anti-inflammatory 3E0F
    Antineoplastic 3E0F
    Destructive Agent 3E0F
    Diagnostic Substance, Other 3E0F
    Electrolytic Substance 3E0F
    Gas 3E0F
    Hypnotics 3E0F
    Nutritional Substance 3E0F
    Radioactive Substance 3E0F
    Sedatives 3E0F
    Water Balance Substance 3E0F
  Skin 3E00XGC
    Analgesics 3E00XNZ
    Anesthetic, Local 3E00XBZ
    Anti-infective 3E00X2
    Anti-inflammatory 3E00X3Z
    Antineoplastic 3E00X0
    Destructive Agent 3E00XTZ
    Diagnostic Substance, Other 3E00XKZ
    Hypnotics 3E00XNZ
    Pigment 3E00XMZ
    Sedatives 3E00XNZ
    Serum 3E00X4Z
    Toxoid 3E00X4Z
    Vaccine 3E00X4Z
  Spinal Canal 3E0R3GC
    Analgesics 3E0R3NZ
    Anesthetic
      Local 3E0R3BZ
      Regional 3E0R3CZ
    Anti-infective 3E0R32
    Anti-inflammatory 3E0R33Z
    Antineoplastic 3E0R30
    Destructive Agent 3E0R3TZ
    Diagnostic Substance, Other 3E0R3KZ
    Electrolytic Substance 3E0R37Z
    Gas 3E0R
    Hypnotics 3E0R3NZ
    Nutritional Substance 3E0R36Z
    Radioactive Substance 3E0R3HZ

Introduction of substance in or on *(Continued)*
  Spinal Canal *(Continued)*
    Sedatives 3E0R3NZ
    Stem Cells
      Embryonic 3E0R
      Somatic 3E0R
    Water Balance Substance 3E0R37Z
  Subcutaneous Tissue 3E013GC
    Analgesics 3E013NZ
    Anesthetic, Local 3E013BZ
    Anti-infective 3E01
    Anti-inflammatory 3E0133Z
    Antineoplastic 3E0130
    Destructive Agent 3E013TZ
    Diagnostic Substance, Other 3E013KZ
    Electrolytic Substance 3E0137Z
    Hormone 3E013V
    Hypnotics 3E013NZ
    Nutritional Substance 3E0136Z
    Radioactive Substance 3E013HZ
    Sedatives 3E013NZ
    Serum 3E0134Z
    Toxoid 3E0134Z
    Vaccine 3E0134Z
    Water Balance Substance 3E0137Z
  Vein
    Central 3E04
      Analgesics 3E04
      Anesthetic, Intracirculatory 3E04
      Anti-infective 3E04
      Anti-inflammatory 3E04
      Antiarrhythmic 3E04
      Antineoplastic 3E04
      Destructive Agent 3E04
      Diagnostic Substance, Other 3E04
      Electrolytic Substance 3E04
      Hormone 3E04
      Hypnotics 3E04
      Immunotherapeutic 3E04
      Nutritional Substance 3E04
      Platelet Inhibitor 3E04
      Radioactive Substance 3E04
      Sedatives 3E04
      Serum 3E04
      Thrombolytic 3E04
      Toxoid 3E04
      Vaccine 3E04
      Vasopressor 3E04
      Water Balance Substance 3E04
    Peripheral 3E03
      Analgesics 3E03
      Anesthetic, Intracirculatory 3E03
      Anti-infective 3E03
      Anti-inflammatory 3E03
      Antiarrhythmic 3E03
      Antineoplastic 3E03
      Destructive Agent 3E03
      Diagnostic Substance, Other 3E03
      Electrolytic Substance 3E03
      Hormone 3E03
      Hypnotics 3E03
      Immunotherapeutic 3E03
      Islet Cells, Pancreatic 3E03
      Nutritional Substance 3E03
      Platelet Inhibitor 3E03
      Radioactive Substance 3E03
      Sedatives 3E03
      Serum 3E03
      Thrombolytic 3E03
      Toxoid 3E03
      Vaccine 3E03

Introduction of substance in or on *(Continued)*
  Vein *(Continued)*
    Peripheral *(Continued)*
      Vasopressor 3E03
      Water Balance Substance 3E03
Intubation
  Airway
    see Insertion of device in, Trachea 0BH1
    see Insertion of device in, Mouth and Throat 0CHY
    see Insertion of device in, Esophagus 0DH5
  Drainage device *see* Drainage
  Feeding Device *see* Insertion of device in, Gastrointestinal System 0DH
INTUITY Elite valve system, EDWARDS *use* Zooplastic Tissue, Rapid Deployment Technique in New Technology ◀
IPPB (intermittent positive pressure breathing) *see* Assistance, Respiratory 5A09
Iridectomy
  see Excision, Eye 08B
  see Resection, Eye 08T
Iridoplasty
  see Repair, Eye 08Q
  see Replacement, Eye 08R
  see Supplement, Eye 08U
Iridotomy *see* Drainage, Eye 089
Irrigation
  Biliary Tract, Irrigating Substance 3E1J
  Brain, Irrigating Substance 3E1Q38Z
  Cranial Cavity, Irrigating Substance 3E1Q38Z
  Ear, Irrigating Substance 3E1B
  Epidural Space, Irrigating Substance 3E1S38Z
  Eye, Irrigating Substance 3E1C
  Gastrointestinal Tract
    Lower, Irrigating Substance 3E1H
    Upper, Irrigating Substance 3E1G
  Genitourinary Tract, Irrigating Substance 3E1K
  Irrigating Substance 3C1ZX8Z
  Joint, Irrigating Substance 3E1U38Z
  Mucous Membrane, Irrigating Substance 3E10
  Nose, Irrigating Substance 3E19
  Pancreatic Tract, Irrigating Substance 3E1J
  Pericardial Cavity, Irrigating Substance 3E1Y38Z
  Peritoneal Cavity
    Dialysate 3E1M39Z
    Irrigating Substance 3E1M38Z
  Pleural Cavity, Irrigating Substance 3E1L38Z
  Reproductive
    Female, Irrigating Substance 3E1P
    Male, Irrigating Substance 3E1N
  Respiratory Tract, Irrigating Substance 3E1F
  Skin, Irrigating Substance 3E10
  Spinal Canal, Irrigating Substance 3E1R38Z
Isavuconazole Anti-infective XW0
Ischiatic nerve *use* Sciatic Nerve
Ischiocavernosus muscle *use* Perineum Muscle
Ischiofemoral ligament
  use Hip Bursa and Ligament, Right
  use Hip Bursa and Ligament, Left
Ischium
  use Pelvic Bone, Right
  use Pelvic Bone, Left
Isolation 8E0ZXY6
Isotope Administration, Whole Body DWY5G
Itrel (3) (4) neurostimulator *use* Stimulator Generator, Single Array in 0JH

J

Jejunal artery *use* Superior Mesenteric Artery
Jejunectomy
  see Excision, Jejunum 0DBA
  see Resection, Jejunum 0DTA
Jejunocolostomy
  see Bypass, Gastrointestinal System 0D1
  see Drainage, Gastrointestinal System 0D9
Jejunopexy
  see Repair, Jejunum 0DQA
  see Reposition, Jejunum 0DSA
Jejunostomy
  see Bypass, Jejunum 0D1A
  see Drainage, Jejunum 0D9A
Jejunotomy *see* Drainage, Jejunum 0D9A
Joint fixation plate
  use Internal Fixation Device in Upper Joints
  use Internal Fixation Device in Lower Joints
Joint liner (insert) *use* Liner in Lower Joints
Joint spacer (antibiotic)
  use Spacer in Upper Joints
  use Spacer in Lower Joints
Jugular body *use* Glomus Jugulare
Jugular lymph node
  use Lymphatic, Right Neck
  use Lymphatic, Left Neck

K

Kappa *use* Pacemaker, Dual Chamber in 0JH
Kcentra *use* 4-Factor Prothrombin Complex Concentrate
Keratectomy, kerectomy
  see Excision, Eye 08B
  see Resection, Eye 08T
Keratocentesis *see* Drainage, Eye 089
Keratoplasty
  see Repair, Eye 08Q
  see Replacement, Eye 08R
  see Supplement, Eye 08U
Keratotomy
  see Drainage, Eye 089
  see Repair, Eye 08Q
Kirschner wire (K-wire)
  use Internal Fixation Device in Head and Facial Bones
  use Internal Fixation Device in Upper Bones
  use Internal Fixation Device in Lower Bones
  use Internal Fixation Device in Upper Joints
  use Internal Fixation Device in Lower Joints
Knee (implant) insert *use* Liner in Lower Joints
KUB x-ray *see* Plain Radiography, Kidney, Ureter and Bladder BT04
Kuntscher nail
  use Internal Fixation Device, Intramedullary in Upper Bones
  use Internal Fixation Device, Intramedullary in Lower Bones

L

Labia majora *use* Vulva
Labia minora *use* Vulva
Labial gland
  use Upper Lip
  use Lower Lip
Labiectomy
  see Excision, Female Reproductive System ØUB
  see Resection, Female Reproductive System ØUT
Lacrimal canaliculus
  use Lacrimal Duct, Right
  use Lacrimal Duct, Left
Lacrimal punctum
  use Lacrimal Duct, Right
  use Lacrimal Duct, Left
Lacrimal sac
  use Lacrimal Duct, Right
  use Lacrimal Duct, Left
Laminectomy
  see Release, Central Nervous System ØØN ◀
  see Release, Peripheral Nervous System Ø1N ◀
  see Excision, Upper Bones ØPB
  see Excision, Lower Bones ØQB
Laminotomy
  see Release, Central Nervous System ØØN
  see Release, Peripheral Nervous System Ø1N
  see Drainage, Upper Bones ØP9
  see Excision, Upper Bones ØPB
  see Release, Upper Bones ØPN
  see Drainage, Lower Bones ØQ9
  see Excision, Lower Bones ØQB
  see Release, Lower Bones ØQN
LAP-BAND® adjustable gastric banding system *use* Extraluminal Device
Laparoscopy *see* Inspection
Laparotomy
  Drainage *see* Drainage, Peritoneal Cavity ØW9G
  Exploratory *see* Inspection, Peritoneal *use* Nerve, Lumbar Plexus ØWJG
Laryngectomy
  see Excision, Larynx ØCBS
  see Resection, Larynx ØCTS
Laryngocentesis *see* Drainage, Larynx ØC9S
Laryngogram *see* Fluoroscopy, Larynx B91J
Laryngopexy
  see Repair, Larynx ØCQS
Laryngopharynx *use* Pharynx
Laryngoplasty
  see Repair, Larynx ØCQS
  see Replacement, Larynx ØCRS
  see Supplement, Larynx ØCUS
Laryngorrhaphy *see* Repair, Larynx ØCQS
Laryngoscopy ØCJS8ZZ
Laryngotomy *see* Drainage, Larynx ØC9S
Laser Interstitial Thermal Therapy
  Adrenal Gland DGY2KZZ
  Anus DDY8KZZ
  Bile Ducts DFY2KZZ
  Brain DØYØKZZ
  Brain Stem DØY1KZZ
  Breast
    Left DMYØKZZ
    Right DMY1KZZ
  Bronchus DBY1KZZ
  Chest Wall DBY7KZZ
  Colon DDY5KZZ
  Diaphragm DBY8KZZ
  Duodenum DDY2KZZ
  Esophagus DDYØKZZ
  Gallbladder DFY1KZZ
  Gland
    Adrenal DGY2KZZ
    Parathyroid DGY4KZZ
    Pituitary DGYØKZZ
    Thyroid DGY5KZZ
  Ileum DDY4KZZ
  Jejunum DDY3KZZ

Laser Interstitial Thermal Therapy
  (Continued)
  Liver DFYØKZZ
  Lung DBY2KZZ
  Mediastinum DBY6KZZ
  Nerve, Peripheral DØY7KZZ
  Pancreas DFY3KZZ
  Parathyroid Gland DGY4KZZ
  Pineal Body DGY1KZZ
  Pituitary Gland DGYØKZZ
  Pleura DBY5KZZ
  Prostate DVYØKZZ
  Rectum DDY7KZZ
  Spinal Cord DØY6KZZ
  Stomach DDY1KZZ
  Thyroid Gland DGY5KZZ
  Trachea DBYØKZZ
Lateral (brachial) lymph node
  use Lymphatic, Right Axillary
  use Lymphatic, Left Axillary
Lateral canthus
  use Upper Eyelid, Right
  use Upper Eyelid, Left
Lateral collateral ligament (LCL)
  use Knee Bursa and Ligament, Right
  use Knee Bursa and Ligament, Left
Lateral condyle of femur
  use Lower Femur, Right
  use Lower Femur, Left
Lateral condyle of tibia
  use Tibia, Right
  use Tibia, Left
Lateral cuneiform bone
  use Tarsal, Right
  use Tarsal, Left
Lateral epicondyle of femur
  use Lower Femur, Right
  use Lower Femur, Left
Lateral epicondyle of humerus
  use Humeral Shaft, Right
  use Humeral Shaft, Left
Lateral femoral cutaneous nerve *use* Lumbar Plexus
Lateral malleolus
  use Fibula, Right
  use Fibula, Left
Lateral meniscus
  use Knee Joint, Right
  use Knee Joint, Left
Lateral nasal cartilage *use* Nose
Lateral plantar artery
  use Foot Artery, Right
  use Foot Artery, Left
Lateral plantar nerve *use* Tibial Nerve
Lateral rectus muscle
  use Extraocular Muscle, Right
  use Extraocular Muscle, Left
Lateral sacral artery
  use Internal Iliac Artery, Right
  use Internal Iliac Artery, Left
Lateral sacral vein
  use Hypogastric Vein, Right
  use Hypogastric Vein, Left
Lateral sural cutaneous nerve *use* Peroneal Nerve
Lateral tarsal artery
  use Foot Artery, Right
  use Foot Artery, Left
Lateral temporomandibular ligament
  use Head and Neck Bursa and Ligament
Lateral thoracic artery
  use Axillary Artery, Right
  use Axillary Artery, Left
Latissimus dorsi muscle
  use Trunk Muscle, Right
  use Trunk Muscle, Left
Latissimus Dorsi Myocutaneous Flap
  Bilateral ØHRVØ75
  Left ØHRUØ75
  Right ØHRTØ75

Lavage
  see Irrigation
  bronchial alveolar, diagnostic *see* Drainage, Respiratory System ØB9
Least splanchnic nerve *use* Thoracic Sympathetic Nerve
Left ascending lumbar vein *use* Hemiazygos Vein
Left atrioventricular valve *use* Mitral Valve
Left auricular appendix *use* Atrium, Left
Left colic vein *use* Colic Vein
Left coronary sulcus *use* Heart, Left
Left gastric artery *use* Gastric Artery
Left gastroepiploic artery *use* Splenic Artery
Left gastroepiploic vein *use* Splenic Vein
Left inferior phrenic vein *use* Renal Vein, Left
Left inferior pulmonary vein *use* Pulmonary Vein, Left
Left jugular trunk *use* Thoracic Duct
Left lateral ventricle *use* Cerebral Ventricle
Left ovarian vein *use* Renal Vein, Left
Left second lumbar vein *use* Renal Vein, Left
Left subclavian trunk *use* Thoracic Duct
Left subcostal vein *use* Hemiazygos Vein
Left superior pulmonary vein *use* Pulmonary Vein, Left
Left suprarenal vein *use* Renal Vein, Left
Left testicular vein *use* Renal Vein, Left
Lengthening
  Bone, with device *see* Insertion of Limb Lengthening Device
  Muscle, by incision *see* Division, Muscles ØK8
  Tendon, by incision *see* Division, Tendons ØL8
Leptomeninges, intracranial *use* Cerebral Meninges
Leptomeninges, spinal *use* Spinal Meninges
Lesser alar cartilage *use* Nose
Lesser occipital nerve *use* Cervical Plexus
Lesser splanchnic nerve *use* Thoracic Sympathetic Nerve
Lesser trochanter
  use Upper Femur, Right
  use Upper Femur, Left
Lesser tuberosity
  use Humeral Head, Right
  use Humeral Head, Left
Lesser wing
  use Sphenoid Bone, Right
  use Sphenoid Bone, Left
Leukopheresis, therapeutic *see* Pheresis, Circulatory 6A55
Levator anguli oris muscle *use* Facial Muscle
Levator ani muscle *use* Perineum Muscle ◀▥
  ~~use Trunk Muscle, Right~~
  ~~use Trunk Muscle, Left~~
Levator labii superioris alaeque nasi muscle *use* Facial Muscle
Levator labii superioris muscle *use* Facial Muscle
Levator palpebrae superioris muscle
  use Upper Eyelid, Right
  use Upper Eyelid, Left
Levator scapulae muscle
  use Neck Muscle, Right
  use Neck Muscle, Left
Levator veli palatini muscle *use* Tongue, Palate, Pharynx Muscle
Levatores costarum muscle
  use Thorax Muscle, Right
  use Thorax Muscle, Left
LifeStent® (Flexstar) (XL) Vascular Stent System *use* Intraluminal Device
Ligament of head of fibula
  use Knee Bursa and Ligament, Right
  use Knee Bursa and Ligament, Left
Ligament of the lateral malleolus
  use Ankle Bursa and Ligament, Right
  use Ankle Bursa and Ligament, Left
Ligamentum flavum
  use Trunk Bursa and Ligament, Right
  use Trunk Bursa and Ligament, Left

◀ New   ◀▥ Revised   ~~deleted~~ Deleted

Ligation *see* Occlusion
Ligation, hemorrhoid *see* Occlusion, Lower
　　Veins, Hemorrhoidal Plexus
Light Therapy GZJZZZZ
Liner
　Removal of device from
　　Hip
　　　Left 0SPB09Z
　　　Right 0SP909Z
　　Knee
　　　Left 0SPD09Z
　　　Right 0SPC09Z
　Revision of device in
　　Hip
　　　Left 0SWB09Z
　　　Right 0SW909Z
　　Knee
　　　Left 0SWD09Z
　　　Right 0SWC09Z
　Supplement
　　Hip
　　　Left 0SUB09Z
　　　　Acetabular Surface 0SUE09Z
　　　　Femoral Surface 0SUS09Z
　　　Right 0SU909Z
　　　　Acetabular Surface 0SUA09Z
　　　　Femoral Surface 0SUR09Z
　　Knee
　　　Left 0SUD09
　　　　Femoral Surface 0SUU09Z
　　　　Tibial Surface 0SUW09Z
　　　Right 0SUC09
　　　　Femoral Surface 0SUT09Z
　　　　Tibial Surface 0SUV09Z
Lingual artery
　use Artery, External Carotid, Right
　use Artery, External Carotid, Left

Lingual tonsil *use* Tongue
Lingulectomy, lung
　see Excision, Lung Lingula 0BBH
　see Resection, Lung Lingula 0BTH
Lithotripsy
　see Fragmentation
　with removal of fragments *see* Extirpation
LITT (laser interstitial thermal therapy) *see*
　　Laser Interstitial Thermal Therapy
LIVIAN™ CRT-D *use* Cardiac
　　Resynchronization Defibrillator Pulse
　　Generator in 0JH
Lobectomy
　see Excision, Central Nervous System 00B
　see Excision, Respiratory System 0BB
　see Resection, Respiratory System 0BT
　see Excision, Hepatobiliary System and
　　Pancreas 0FB
　see Resection, Hepatobiliary System and
　　Pancreas 0FT
　see Excision, Endocrine System 0GB
　see Resection, Endocrine System 0GT
Lobotomy *see* Division, Brain 0080
Localization
　see Map
　see Imaging
Locus ceruleus *use* Pons
Long thoracic nerve *use* Brachial Plexus
Loop ileostomy *see* Bypass, Ileum 0D1B
Loop recorder, implantable *use* Monitoring
　　Device
Lower GI series *see* Fluoroscopy, Colon BD14
Lumbar artery *use* Abdominal Aorta
Lumbar facet joint *use* Lumbar Vertebral Joint
Lumbar ganglion *use* Lumbar Sympathetic
　　Nerve
Lumbar lymph node *use* Lymphatic, Aortic

Lumbar lymphatic trunk *use* Cisterna Chyli
Lumbar splanchnic nerve *use* Lumbar
　　Sympathetic Nerve
Lumbosacral facet joint *use* Lumbosacral Joint
Lumbosacral trunk *use* Lumbar Nerve
Lumpectomy
　see Excision
Lunate bone
　use Carpal, Right
　use Carpal, Left
Lunotriquetral ligament
　use Hand Bursa and Ligament, Right
　use Hand Bursa and Ligament, Left
Lymphadenectomy
　see Excision, Lymphatic and Hemic Systems
　　07B
　see Resection, Lymphatic and Hemic Systems
　　07T
Lymphadenotomy *see* Drainage, Lymphatic and
　　Hemic Systems 079
Lymphangiectomy
　see Excision, Lymphatic and Hemic Systems
　　07B
　see Resection, Lymphatic and Hemic Systems
　　07T
Lymphangiogram *see* Plain Radiography,
　　Lymphatic System B70
Lymphangioplasty
　see Repair, Lymphatic and Hemic Systems
　　07Q
　see Supplement, Lymphatic and Hemic
　　Systems 07U
Lymphangiorrhaphy *see* Repair, Lymphatic and
　　Hemic Systems 07Q
Lymphangiotomy *see* Drainage, Lymphatic and
　　Hemic Systems 079
Lysis *see* Release

M

Macula
  use Retina, Right
  use Retina, Left
MAGEC® Spinal Bracing and Distraction
    System *use* Magnetically Controlled
    Growth Rod(s) in New Technology ◀
Magnet extraction, ocular foreign body *see*
    Extirpation, Eye Ø8C
Magnetic Resonance Imaging (MRI)
  Abdomen BW3Ø
  Ankle
    Left BQ3H
    Right BQ3G
  Aorta
    Abdominal B43Ø
    Thoracic B33Ø
  Arm
    Left BP3F
    Right BP3E
  Artery
    Celiac B431
    Cervico-Cerebral Arch B33Q
    Common Carotid, Bilateral B335
    Coronary
      Bypass Graft, Multiple B233
      Multiple B231
    Internal Carotid, Bilateral B338
    Intracranial B33R
    Lower Extremity
      Bilateral B43H
      Left B43G
      Right B43F
    Pelvic B43C
    Renal, Bilateral B438
    Spinal B33M
    Superior Mesenteric B434
    Upper Extremity
      Bilateral B33K
      Left B33J
      Right B33H
    Vertebral, Bilateral B33G
  Bladder BT3Ø
  Brachial Plexus BW3P
  Brain BØ3Ø
  Breast
    Bilateral BH32
    Left BH31
    Right BH3Ø
  Calcaneus
    Left BQ3K
    Right BQ3J
  Chest BW33Y
  Coccyx BR3F
  Connective Tissue
    Lower Extremity BL31
    Upper Extremity BL3Ø
  Corpora Cavernosa BV3Ø
  Disc
    Cervical BR31
    Lumbar BR33
    Thoracic BR32
  Ear B93Ø
  Elbow
    Left BP3H
    Right BP3G
  Eye
    Bilateral B837
    Left B836
    Right B835
  Femur
    Left BQ34
    Right BQ33
  Fetal Abdomen BY33
  Fetal Extremity BY35
  Fetal Head BY3Ø
  Fetal Heart BY31
  Fetal Spine BY34
  Fetal Thorax BY32
  Fetus, Whole BY36

Magnetic Resonance Imaging (MRI)
    (Continued)
  Foot
    Left BQ3M
    Right BQ3L
  Forearm
    Left BP3K
    Right BP3J
  Gland
    Adrenal, Bilateral BG32
    Parathyroid BG33
    Parotid, Bilateral B936
    Salivary, Bilateral B93D
    Submandibular, Bilateral B939
    Thyroid BG34
  Head BW38
  Heart, Right and Left B236
  Hip
    Left BQ31
    Right BQ3Ø
  Intracranial Sinus B532
  Joint
    Finger
      Left BP3D
      Right BP3C
    Hand
      Left BP3D
      Right BP3C
    Temporomandibular, Bilateral BN39
  Kidney
    Bilateral BT33
    Left BT32
    Right BT31
    Transplant BT39
  Knee
    Left BQ38
    Right BQ37
  Larynx B93J
  Leg
    Left BQ3F
    Right BQ3D
  Liver BF35
  Liver and Spleen BF36
  Lung Apices BB3G
  Nasopharynx B93F
  Neck BW3F
  Nerve
    Acoustic BØ3C
    Brachial Plexus BW3P
  Oropharynx B93F
  Ovary
    Bilateral BU35
    Left BU34
    Right BU33
  Ovary and Uterus BU3C
  Pancreas BF37
  Patella
    Left BQ3W
    Right BQ3V
  Pelvic Region BW3G
  Pelvis BR3C
  Pituitary Gland BØ39
  Plexus, Brachial BW3P
  Prostate BV33
  Retroperitoneum BW3H
  Sacrum BR3F
  Scrotum BV34
  Sella Turcica BØ39
  Shoulder
    Left BP39
    Right BP38
  Sinus
    Intracranial B532
    Paranasal B932
  Spinal Cord BØ3B
  Spine
    Cervical BR3Ø
    Lumbar BR39
    Thoracic BR37
  Spleen and Liver BF36

Magnetic Resonance Imaging (MRI)
    (Continued)
  Subcutaneous Tissue
    Abdomen BH3H
    Extremity
      Lower BH3J
      Upper BH3F
    Head BH3D
    Neck BH3D
    Pelvis BH3H
    Thorax BH3G
  Tendon
    Lower Extremity BL33
    Upper Extremity BL32
  Testicle
    Bilateral BV37
    Left BV36
    Right BV35
  Toe
    Left BQ3Q
    Right BQ3P
  Uterus BU36
    Pregnant BU3B
  Uterus and Ovary BU3C
  Vagina BU39
  Vein
    Cerebellar B531
    Cerebral B531
    Jugular, Bilateral B535
    Lower Extremity
      Bilateral B53D
      Left B53C
      Right B53B
    Other B53V
    Pelvic (Iliac) Bilateral B53H
    Portal B53T
    Pulmonary, Bilateral B53S
    Renal, Bilateral B53L
    Spanchnic B53T
    Upper Extremity
      Bilateral B53P
      Left B53N
      Right B53M
  Vena Cava
    Inferior B539
    Superior B538
  Wrist
    Left BP3M
    Right BP3L
Magnetically Controlled Growth Rod(s) ◀
  Cervical XNS3 ◀
  Lumbar XNSØ ◀
  Thoracic XNS4 ◀
Malleotomy *see* Drainage, Ear, Nose, Sinus Ø99
Malleus
  use Auditory Ossicle, Right
  use Auditory Ossicle, Left
Mammaplasty, mammoplasty
  see Alteration, Skin and Breast ØHØ
  see Repair, Skin and Breast ØHQ
  see Replacement, Skin and Breast ØHR
  see Supplement, Skin and Breast ØHU
Mammary duct
  use Breast, Right
  use Breast, Left
  use Breast, Bilateral
Mammary gland
  use Breast, Right
  use Breast, Left
  use Breast, Bilateral
Mammectomy
  see Excision, Skin and Breast ØHB
  see Resection, Skin and Breast ØHT
Mammillary body *use* Hypothalamus
Mammography *see* Plain Radiography, Skin,
    Subcutaneous Tissue and Breast BH0
Mammotomy *see* Drainage, Skin and Breast ØH9
Mandibular nerve *use* Trigeminal Nerve
Mandibular notch
  use Mandible, Right
  use Mandible, Left

◀ New   ◀▥ Revised   ~~deleted~~ Deleted

Mandibulectomy
  see Excision, Head and Facial Bones ØNB
  see Resection, Head and Facial Bones ØNT
Manipulation
  Adhesions *see* Release
  Chiropractic *see* Chiropractic Manipulation
Manubrium *use* Sternum
Map
  Basal Ganglia 00K8
  Brain 00KØ
  Cerebellum 00KC
  Cerebral Hemisphere 00K7
  Conduction Mechanism 02K8
  Hypothalamus 00KA
  Medulla Oblongata 00KD
  Pons 00KB
  Thalamus 00K9
Mapping
  Doppler ultrasound *see* Ultrasonography
  Electrocardiogram only *see* Measurement,
    Cardiac 4A02
Mark IV Breathing Pacemaker System *use*
  Stimulator Generator in Subcutaneous
  Tissue and Fascia
Marsupialization
  see Drainage
  see Excision
Massage, cardiac
  External 5A12012
  Open 02QA0ZZ
Masseter muscle *use* Head Muscle
Masseteric fascia *use* Subcutaneous Tissue and
  Fascia, Face
Mastectomy
  see Excision, Skin and Breast ØHB
  see Resection, Skin and Breast ØHT
Mastoid (postauricular) lymph node
  use Lymphatic, Right Neck
  use Lymphatic, Left Neck
Mastoid air cells
  use Mastoid Sinus, Right
  use Mastoid Sinus, Left
Mastoid process
  use Temporal Bone, Right
  use Temporal Bone, Left
Mastoidectomy
  see Excision, Ear, Nose, Sinus 09B
  see Resection, Ear, Nose, Sinus 09T
Mastoidotomy *see* Drainage, Ear, Nose, Sinus
  099
Mastopexy
  see Reposition, Skin and Breast ØHS
  see Repair, Skin and Breast ØHQ
Mastorrhaphy *see* Repair, Skin and Breast ØHQ
Mastotomy *see* Drainage, Skin and Breast ØH9
Maxillary artery
  use External Carotid Artery, Right
  use External Carotid Artery, Left
Maxillary nerve *use* Trigeminal Nerve
Maximo II DR (VR) *use* Defibrillator Generator
  in ØJH
Maximo II DR CRT-D *use* Cardiac
  Resynchronization Defibrillator Pulse
  Generator in ØJH
Measurement
  Arterial
    Flow
      Coronary 4A03
      Peripheral 4A03
      Pulmonary 4A03
    Pressure
      Coronary 4A03
      Peripheral 4A03
      Pulmonary 4A03
      Thoracic, Other 4A03
    Pulse
      Coronary 4A03
      Peripheral 4A03
      Pulmonary 4A03
    Saturation, Peripheral 4A03
    Sound, Peripheral 4A03

Measurement (*Continued*)
  Biliary
    Flow 4A0C
    Pressure 4A0C
  Cardiac
    Action Currents 4A02
    Defibrillator 4B02XTZ
    Electrical Activity 4A02
      Guidance 4A02X4A
      No Qualifier 4A02X4Z
    Output 4A02
    Pacemaker 4B02XSZ
    Rate 4A02
    Rhythm 4A02
    Sampling and Pressure
      Bilateral 4A02
      Left Heart 4A02
      Right Heart 4A02
    Sound 4A02
    Total Activity, Stress 4A02XM4
  Central Nervous
    Conductivity 4A00
    Electrical Activity 4A00
    Pressure 4A000BZ
      Intracranial 4A00
    Saturation, Intracranial 4A00
    Stimulator 4B00XVZ
    Temperature, Intracranial
      4A00
  Circulatory, Volume 4A05XLZ
  Gastrointestinal
    Motility 4A0B
    Pressure 4A0B
    Secretion 4A0B
  Lymphatic
    Flow 4A06
    Pressure 4A06
  Metabolism 4A0Z
  Musculoskeletal
    Contractility 4A0F
    Stimulator 4B0FXVZ
  Olfactory, Acuity 4A08X0Z
  Peripheral Nervous
    Conductivity
      Motor 4A01
      Sensory 4A01
    Electrical Activity 4A01
    Stimulator 4B01XVZ
  Products of Conception
    Cardiac
      Electrical Activity 4A0H
      Rate 4A0H
      Rhythm 4A0H
      Sound 4A0H
    Nervous
      Conductivity 4A0J
      Electrical Activity 4A0J
      Pressure 4A0J
  Respiratory
    Capacity 4A09
    Flow 4A09
    Pacemaker 4B09XSZ
    Rate 4A09
    Resistance 4A09
    Total Activity 4A09
    Volume 4A09
  Sleep 4A0ZXQZ
  Temperature 4A0Z
  Urinary
    Contractility 4A0D73Z
    Flow 4A0D75Z
    Pressure 4A0D7BZ
    Resistance 4A0D7DZ
    Volume 4A0D7LZ
  Venous
    Flow
      Central 4A04
      Peripheral 4A04
      Portal 4A04
      Pulmonary 4A04

Measurement (*Continued*)
  Venous (*Continued*)
    Pressure
      Central 4A04
      Peripheral 4A04
      Portal 4A04
      Pulmonary 4A04
    Pulse
      Central 4A04
      Peripheral 4A04
      Portal 4A04
      Pulmonary 4A04
    Saturation, Peripheral 4A04
  Visual
    Acuity 4A07X0Z
    Mobility 4A07X7Z
    Pressure 4A07XBZ
Meatoplasty, urethra *see* Repair, Urethra ØTQD
Meatotomy *see* Drainage, Urinary System ØT9
Mechanical ventilation *see* Performance,
  Respiratory 5A19
Medial canthus
  use Lower Eyelid, Right
  use Lower Eyelid, Left
Medial collateral ligament (MCL)
  use Knee Bursa and Ligament, Right
  use Knee Bursa and Ligament, Left
Medial condyle of femur
  use Lower Femur, Right
  use Lower Femur, Left
Medial condyle of tibia
  use Tibia, Right
  use Tibia, Left
Medial cuneiform bone
  use Tarsal, Right
  use Tarsal, Left
Medial epicondyle of femur
  use Lower Femur, Right
  use Lower Femur, Left
Medial epicondyle of humerus
  use Humeral Shaft, Right
  use Humeral Shaft, Left
Medial malleolus
  use Tibia, Right
  use Tibia, Left
Medial meniscus
  use Knee Joint, Right
  use Knee Joint, Left
Medial plantar artery
  use Foot Artery, Right
  use Foot Artery, Left
Medial plantar nerve *use* Tibial Nerve
Medial popliteal nerve *use* Tibial Nerve
Medial rectus muscle
  use Extraocular Muscle, Right
  use Extraocular Muscle, Left
Medial sural cutaneous nerve *use* Tibial Nerve
Median antebrachial vein
  use Basilic Vein, Right
  use Basilic Vein, Left
Median cubital vein
  use Basilic Vein, Right
  use Basilic Vein, Left
Median sacral artery *use* Abdominal Aorta
Mediastinal lymph node *use* Lymphatic, Thorax
Mediastinoscopy ØWJC4ZZ
Medication Management GZ3ZZZZ
  for substance abuse
    Antabuse HZ83ZZZ
    Bupropion HZ87ZZZ
    Clonidine HZ86ZZZ
    Levo-alpha-acetyl-methadol (LAAM)
      HZ82ZZZ
    Methadone Maintenance HZ81ZZZ
    Naloxone HZ85ZZZ
    Naltrexone HZ84ZZZ
    Nicotine Replacement HZ80ZZZ
    Other Replacement Medication HZ89ZZZ
    Psychiatric Medication HZ88ZZZ
Meditation 8E0ZXY5

M

Medtronic Endurant® II AAA stent graft system *use* Intraluminal Device ◄

Meissner's (submucous) plexus *use* Abdominal Sympathetic Nerve

Melody® transcatheter pulmonary valve *use* Zooplastic Tissue in Heart and Great Vessels

Membranous urethra *use* Urethra

Meningeorrhaphy
  see Repair, Cerebral Meninges 00Q1
  see Repair, Spinal Meninges 00QT

Meniscectomy, knee ◄|||||
  see Excision, Joint, Knee, Right 0SBC ◄
  see Excision, Joint, Knee, Left 0SBD ◄

Mental foramen
  use Mandible, Right
  use Mandible, Left

Mentalis muscle *use* Facial Muscle

Mentoplasty *see* Alteration, Jaw, Lower 0W05

Mesenterectomy *see* Excision, Mesentery 0DBV

Mesenteriorrhaphy, mesenterorrhaphy *see* Repair, Mesentery 0DQV

Mesenteriplication *see* Repair, Mesentery 0DQV

Mesoappendix *use* Mesentery

Mesocolon *use* Mesentery

Metacarpal ligament
  use Hand Bursa and Ligament, Right
  use Hand Bursa and Ligament, Left

Metacarpophalangeal ligament
  use Hand Bursa and Ligament, Right
  use Hand Bursa and Ligament, Left

Metal on metal bearing surface *use* Synthetic Substitute, Metal in 0SR ◄

Metatarsal ligament
  use Foot Bursa and Ligament, Right
  use Foot Bursa and Ligament, Left

Metatarsectomy
  see Excision, Lower Bones 0QB
  see Resection, Lower Bones 0QT

Metatarsophalangeal (MTP) joint
  use Metatarsal-Phalangeal Joint, Right
  use Metatarsal-Phalangeal Joint, Left

Metatarsophalangeal ligament
  use Foot Bursa and Ligament, Right
  use Foot Bursa and Ligament, Left

Metathalamus *use* Thalamus

Micro-Driver stent (RX) (OTW) *use* Intraluminal Device

MicroMed HeartAssist *use* Implantable Heart Assist System in Heart and Great Vessels

Micrus CERECYTE microcoil *use* Intraluminal Device, Bioactive in Upper Arteries

Midcarpal joint
  use Carpal Joint, Right
  use Carpal Joint, Left

Middle cardiac nerve *use* Thoracic Sympathetic Nerve

Middle cerebral artery *use* Intracranial Artery

Middle cerebral vein *use* Intracranial Vein

Middle colic vein *use* Colic Vein

Middle genicular artery
  use Popliteal Artery, Right
  use Popliteal Artery, Left

Middle hemorrhoidal vein
  use Hypogastric Vein, Right
  use Hypogastric Vein, Left

Middle rectal artery
  use Internal Iliac Artery, Right
  use Internal Iliac Artery, Left

Middle suprarenal artery *use* Abdominal Aorta

Middle temporal artery
  use Temporal Artery, Right
  use Temporal Artery, Left

Middle turbinate *use* Nasal Turbinate

MIRODERM™ Biologic Wound Matrix *use* Skin Substitute, Porcine Liver Derived in New Technology ◄

MitraClip valve repair system *use* Synthetic Substitute

Mitral annulus *use* Mitral Valve

Mitroflow® Aortic Pericardial Heart Valve *use* Zooplastic Tissue in Heart and Great Vessels

Mobilization, adhesions *see* Release

Molar gland *use* Buccal Mucosa

Monitoring
  Arterial
    Flow
      Coronary 4A13
      Peripheral 4A13
      Pulmonary 4A13
    Pressure
      Coronary 4A13
      Peripheral 4A13
      Pulmonary 4A13
    Pulse
      Coronary 4A13
      Peripheral 4A13
      Pulmonary 4A13
    Saturation, Peripheral 4A13
    Sound, Peripheral 4A13
  Cardiac
    Electrical Activity 4A12
      Ambulatory 4A12X45
      No Qualifier 4A12X4Z
    Output 4A12
    Rate 4A12
    Rhythm 4A12
    Sound 4A12
    Total Activity, Stress 4A12XM4
    Vascular Perfusion, Indocyanine Green Dye 4A12XSH ◄
  Central Nervous
    Conductivity 4A10
    Electrical Activity
      Intraoperative 4A10
      No Qualifier 4A10
    Pressure 4A100BZ
      Intracranial 4A10
    Saturation, Intracranial 4A10
    Temperature, Intracranial 4A10
  Gastrointestinal
    Motility 4A1B
    Pressure 4A1B
    Secretion 4A1B
    Vascular Perfusion, Indocyanine Green Dye 4A1BXSH ◄
  Intraoperative Knee Replacement Sensor XR2
  Lymphatic
    Flow 4A16
    Pressure 4A16
  Peripheral Nervous
    Conductivity
      Motor 4A11
      Sensory 4A11
    Electrical Activity Intraoperative 4A11
    No Qualifier 4A11
  Products of Conception
    Cardiac
      Electrical Activity 4A1H
      Rate 4A1H
      Rhythm 4A1H
      Sound 4A1H
    Nervous
      Conductivity 4A1J
      Electrical Activity 4A1J
      Pressure 4A1J
  Respiratory
    Capacity 4A19
    Flow 4A19
    Rate 4A19
    Resistance 4A19
    Volume 4A19
  Skin and Breast, Vascular Perfusion, Indocyanine Green Dye 4A1GXSH ◄

Monitoring (Continued)
  Sleep 4A1ZXQZ
  Temperature 4A1Z
  Urinary
    Contractility 4A1D73Z
    Flow 4A1D75Z
    Pressure 4A1D7BZ
    Resistance 4A1D7DZ
    Volume 4A1D7LZ
  Venous
    Flow
      Central 4A14
      Peripheral 4A14
      Portal 4A14
      Pulmonary 4A14
    Pressure
      Central 4A14
      Peripheral 4A14
      Portal 4A14
      Pulmonary 4A14
    Pulse
      Central 4A14
      Peripheral 4A14
      Portal 4A14
      Pulmonary 4A14
    Saturation
      Central 4A14
      Portal 4A14
      Pulmonary 4A14

Monitoring Device, Hemodynamic
  Abdomen 0JH8
  Chest 0JH6

Mosaic Bioprosthesis (aortic) (mitral) valve *use* Zooplastic Tissue in Heart and Great Vessels

Motor Function Assessment F01

Motor Treatment F07

MR Angiography
  see Magnetic Resonance Imaging (MRI), Heart B23
  see Magnetic Resonance Imaging (MRI), Upper Arteries B33
  see Magnetic Resonance Imaging (MRI), Lower Arteries B43

MULTI-LINK (VISION)(MINI-VISION) (ULTRA) Coronary Stent System *use* Intraluminal Device

Multiple sleep latency test 4A0ZXQZ

Musculocutaneous nerve *use* Brachial Plexus Nerve

Musculopexy
  see Repair, Muscles 0KQ
  see Reposition, Muscles 0KS

Musculophrenic artery
  use Internal Mammary Artery, Right
  use Internal Mammary Artery, Left

Musculoplasty
  see Repair, Muscles 0KQ
  see Supplement, Muscles 0KU

Musculorrhaphy *see* Repair, Muscles 0KQ

Musculospiral nerve *use* Radial Nerve

Myectomy
  see Excision, Muscles 0KB
  see Resection, Muscles 0KT

Myelencephalon *use* Medulla Oblongata

Myelogram
  CT *see* Computerized Tomography (CT Scan), Central Nervous System B02
  MRI *see* Magnetic Resonance Imaging (MRI), Central Nervous System B03

Myenteric (Auerbach's) plexus *use* Abdominal Sympathetic Nerve

Myomectomy *see* Excision, Female Reproductive System 0UB

Myometrium *use* Uterus

Myopexy
  see Repair, Muscles 0KQ
  see Reposition, Muscles 0KS

◄ New   ◄||||| Revised   ~~deleted~~ Deleted

Myoplasty
    see Repair, Muscles ØKQ
    see Supplement, Muscles ØKU
Myorrhaphy see Repair, Muscles ØKQ
Myoscopy see Inspection, Muscles ØKJ
Myotomy
    see Division, Muscles ØK8
    see Drainage, Muscles ØK9

Myringectomy
    see Excision, Ear, Nose, Sinus Ø9B
    see Resection, Ear, Nose, Sinus Ø9T
Myringoplasty
    see Repair, Ear, Nose, Sinus Ø9Q
    see Replacement, Ear, Nose, Sinus Ø9R
    see Supplement, Ear, Nose, Sinus Ø9U

Myringostomy see Drainage, Ear, Nose, Sinus
    Ø99
Myringotomy see Drainage, Ear, Nose, Sinus
    Ø99

N

◄ New   ◄⫯⫯⫯ Revised   ~~deleted~~ Deleted

Nonimaging Nuclear Medicine Probe
    (Continued)
  Extremity
    Lower CP5PZZZ
    Upper CP5NZZZ
  Head and Neck CW5B
  Heart C25YYZZ
    Right and Left C256
  Lymphatics
    Head C75J
    Head and Neck C755
    Lower Extremity C75P
    Neck C75K
    Pelvic C75D
    Trunk C75M
    Upper Chest C75L
    Upper Extremity C75N
  Lymphatics and Hematologic System
    C75YYZZ

Nonimaging Nuclear Medicine Probe
    (Continued)
  Musculoskeletal System, Other CP5YYZZ
  Neck and Chest CW56
  Neck and Head CW5B
  Pelvic Region CW5J
  Pelvis and Abdomen CW51
  Spine CP55ZZZ
Nonimaging Nuclear Medicine Uptake
  Endocrine System CG4YYZZ
  Gland, Thyroid CG42
Nostril *use* Nose
Novacor Left Ventricular Assist Device *use*
    Implantable Heart Assist System in Heart
    and Great Vessels
Novation® Ceramic AHS® (Articulation Hip
    System) *use* Synthetic Substitute, Ceramic
    in ØSR

Nuclear medicine
  see Planar Nuclear Medicine Imaging
  see Tomographic (Tomo) Nuclear Medicine
      Imaging
  see Positron Emission Tomographic (PET)
      Imaging
  see Nonimaging Nuclear Medicine Uptake
  see Nonimaging Nuclear Medicine Probe
  see Nonimaging Nuclear Medicine Assay
  see Systemic Nuclear Medicine Therapy
Nuclear scintigraphy *see* Nuclear Medicine
Nutrition, concentrated substances
  Enteral infusion 3EØG36Z
  Parenteral (peripheral) infusion *see*
      Introduction of Nutritional Substance

O

Obliteration *see* Destruction
Obturator artery
  use Internal Iliac Artery, Right
  use Internal Iliac Artery, Left
Obturator lymph node *use* Lymphatic,
  Pelvis
Obturator muscle
  use Hip Muscle, Right
  use Hip Muscle, Left
Obturator nerve *use* Lumbar Plexus
Obturator vein
  use Hypogastric Vein, Right
  use Hypogastric Vein, Left
Obtuse margin *use* Heart, Left
Occipital artery
  use External Carotid Artery, Right
  use External Carotid Artery, Left
Occipital lobe *use* Cerebral Hemisphere
Occipital lymph node
  use Lymphatic, Right Neck
  use Lymphatic, Left Neck
Occipitofrontalis muscle *use* Facial Muscle
Occlusion
  Ampulla of Vater ØFLC
  Anus ØDLQ
  Aorta, Abdominal 04L0
  Artery
    Anterior Tibial
      Left 04LQ
      Right 04LP
    Axillary
      Left 03L6
      Right 03L5
    Brachial
      Left 03L8
      Right 03L7
    Celiac 04L1
    Colic
      Left 04L7
      Middle 04L8
      Right 04L6
    Common Carotid
      Left 03LJ
      Right 03LH
    Common Iliac
      Left 04LD
      Right 04LC
    External Carotid
      Left 03LN
      Right 03LM
    External Iliac
      Left 04LJ
      Right 04LH
    Face 03LR
    Femoral
      Left 04LL
      Right 04LK
    Foot
      Left 04LW
      Right 04LV
    Gastric 04L2
    Hand
      Left 03LF
      Right 03LD
    Hepatic 04L3
    Inferior Mesenteric 04LB
    Innominate 03L2
    Internal Carotid
      Left 03LL
      Right 03LK
    Internal Iliac
      Left 04LF
      Right 04LE
    Internal Mammary
      Left 03L1
      Right 03L0
    Intracranial 03LG
    Lower 04LY

Occlusion (*Continued*)
  Artery (*Continued*)
    Peroneal
      Left 04LU
      Right 04LT
    Popliteal
      Left 04LN
      Right 04LM
    Posterior Tibial
      Left 04LS
      Right 04LR
    Pulmonary, Left 02LR
    Radial
      Left 03LC
      Right 03LB
    Renal
      Left 04LA
      Right 04L9
    Splenic 04L4
    Subclavian
      Left 03L4
      Right 03L3
    Superior Mesenteric 04L5
    Temporal
      Left 03LT
      Right 03LS
    Thyroid
      Left 03LV
      Right 03LU
    Ulnar
      Left 03LA
      Right 03L9
    Upper 03LY
    Vertebral
      Left 03LQ
      Right 03LP
  Atrium, Left 02L7
  Bladder ØTLB
  Bladder Neck ØTLC
  Bronchus
    Lingula ØBL9
    Lower Lobe
      Left ØBLB
      Right ØBL6
    Main
      Left ØBL7
      Right ØBL3
    Middle Lobe, Right ØBL5
    Upper Lobe
      Left ØBL8
      Right ØBL4
  Carina ØBL2
  Cecum ØDLH
  Cisterna Chyli 07LL
  Colon
    Ascending ØDLK
    Descending ØDLM
    Sigmoid ØDLN
    Transverse ØDLL
  Cord
    Bilateral ØVLH
    Left ØVLG
    Right ØVLF
  Cul-de-sac ØULF
  Duct
    Common Bile ØFL9
    Cystic ØFL8
    Hepatic
      Left ØFL6
      Right ØFL5
    Lacrimal
      Left Ø8LY
      Right Ø8LX
    Pancreatic ØFLD
      Accessory ØFLF
    Parotid
      Left ØCLC
      Right ØCLB
  Duodenum ØDL9
  Esophagogastric Junction ØDL4

Occlusion (*Continued*)
  Esophagus ØDL5
    Lower ØDL3
    Middle ØDL2
    Upper ØDL1
  Fallopian Tube
    Left ØUL6
    Right ØUL5
  Fallopian Tubes, Bilateral ØUL7
  Ileocecal Valve ØDLC
  Ileum ØDLB
  Intestine
    Large ØDLE
      Left ØDLG
      Right ØDLF
    Small ØDL8
  Jejunum ØDLA
  Kidney Pelvis
    Left ØTL4
    Right ØTL3
  Left atrial appendage (LAA) *see* Occlusion,
    Atrium, Left 02L7
  Lymphatic
    Aortic 07LD
    Axillary
      Left 07L6
      Right 07L5
    Head 07L0
    Inguinal
      Left 07LJ
      Right 07LH
    Internal Mammary
      Left 07L9
      Right 07L8
    Lower Extremity
      Left 07LG
      Right 07LF
    Mesenteric 07LB
    Neck
      Left 07L2
      Right 07L1
    Pelvis 07LC
    Thoracic Duct 07LK
    Thorax 07L7
    Upper Extremity
      Left 07L4
      Right 07L3
  Rectum ØDLP
  Stomach ØDL6
    Pylorus ØDL7
  Trachea ØBL1
  Ureter
    Left ØTL7
    Right ØTL6
  Urethra ØTLD
  Vagina ØULG
  Valve, Pulmonary 02LH ◄
  Vas Deferens
    Bilateral ØVLQ
    Left ØVLP
    Right ØVLN
  Vein
    Axillary
      Left 05L8
      Right 05L7
    Azygos 05L0
    Basilic
      Left 05LC
      Right 05LB
    Brachial
      Left 05LA
      Right 05L9
    Cephalic
      Left 05LF
      Right 05LD
    Colic 06L7
    Common Iliac
      Left 06LD
      Right 06LC
    Esophageal 06L3

◄ New   ◄▌ Revised   ~~deleted~~ Deleted

Occlusion *(Continued)*
Vein *(Continued)*
External Iliac
Left 06LG
Right 06LF
External Jugular
Left 05LQ
Right 05LP
Face
Left 05LV
Right 05LT
Femoral
Left 06LN
Right 06LM
Foot
Left 06LV
Right 06LT
Gastric 06L2
Greater Saphenous
Left 06LQ
Right 06LP
Hand
Left 05LH
Right 05LG
Hemiazygos 05L1
Hepatic 06L4
Hypogastric
Left 06LJ
Right 06LH
Inferior Mesenteric 06L6
Innominate
Left 05L4
Right 05L3
Internal Jugular
Left 05LN
Right 05LM
Intracranial 05LL
Lesser Saphenous
Left 06LS
Right 06LR
Lower 06LY
Portal 06L8
Pulmonary
Left 02LT
Right 02LS
Renal
Left 06LB
Right 06L9
Splenic 06L1
Subclavian
Left 05L6
Right 05L5
Superior Mesenteric 06L5
Upper 05LY
Vertebral
Left 05LS
Right 05LR
Vena Cava
Inferior 06L0
Superior 02LV
Occupational therapy *see* Activities of Daily
Living Treatment, Rehabilitation F08
Odentectomy
see Excision, Mouth and Throat 0CB
see Resection, Mouth and Throat 0CT
Olecranon bursa
use Elbow Bursa and Ligament,
Right
use Elbow Bursa and Ligament,
Left
Olecranon process
use Ulna, Right
use Ulna, Left
Olfactory bulb *use* Olfactory Nerve
Omentectomy, omentumectomy
see Excision, Gastrointestinal System
0DB
see Resection, Gastrointestinal System
0DT
Omentofixation *see* Repair, Gastrointestinal
System 0DQ

Omentoplasty
see Repair, Gastrointestinal System 0DQ
see Replacement, Gastrointestinal System 0DR
see Supplement, Gastrointestinal System 0DU
Omentorrhaphy *see* Repair, Gastrointestinal
System 0DQ
Omentotomy *see* Drainage, Gastrointestinal
System 0D9
Omnilink Elite Vascular Balloon Expandable
Stent System *use* Intraluminal Device
Onychectomy
see Excision, Skin and Breast 0HB
see Resection, Skin and Breast 0HT
Onychoplasty
see Repair, Skin and Breast 0HQ
see Replacement, Skin and Breast 0HR
Onychotomy *see* Drainage, Skin and Breast 0H9
Oophorectomy
see Excision, Female Reproductive System
0UB
see Resection, Female Reproductive System
0UT
Oophoropexy
see Repair, Female Reproductive System 0UQ
see Reposition, Female Reproductive System
0US
Oophoroplasty
see Repair, Female Reproductive System 0UQ
see Supplement, Female Reproductive System
0UU
Oophororrhaphy *see* Repair, Female
Reproductive System 0UQ
Oophorostomy *see* Drainage, Female
Reproductive System 0U9
Oophorotomy
see Division, Female Reproductive System
0U8
see Drainage, Female Reproductive System
0U9
Oophorrhaphy *see* Repair, Female Reproductive
System 0UQ
Open Pivot (mechanical) valve *use* Synthetic
Substitute
Open Pivot Aortic Valve Graft (AVG) *use*
Synthetic Substitute
Ophthalmic artery *use* Intracranial Artery ◀▥▥
~~use Internal Carotid Artery, Right~~
~~use Internal Carotid Artery, Left~~
Ophthalmic nerve *use* Trigeminal Nerve
Ophthalmic vein *use* Intracranial Vein
Opponensplasty
Tendon replacement *see* Replacement,
Tendons 0LR
Tendon transfer *see* Transfer, Tendons 0LX
Optic chiasma *use* Optic Nerve
Optic disc
use Retina, Right
use Retina, Left
Optic foramen
use Sphenoid Bone, Right
use Sphenoid Bone, Left
Optical coherence tomography, intravascular
see Computerized Tomography (CT Scan)
Optimizer™ III implantable pulse generator
use Contractility Modulation Device in 0JH
Orbicularis oculi muscle
use Upper Eyelid, Right
use Upper Eyelid, Left
Orbicularis oris muscle *use* Facial Muscle
Orbital Atherectomy Technology X2C
Orbital fascia *use* Subcutaneous Tissue and
Fascia, Face
Orbital portion of ethmoid bone
use Orbit, Right
use Orbit, Left
Orbital portion of frontal bone
use Orbit, Right
use Orbit, Left
Orbital portion of lacrimal bone
use Orbit, Right
use Orbit, Left

Orbital portion of maxilla
use Orbit, Right
use Orbit, Left
Orbital portion of palatine bone
use Orbit, Right
use Orbit, Left
Orbital portion of sphenoid bone
use Orbit, Right
use Orbit, Left
Orbital portion of zygomatic bone
use Orbit, Right
use Orbit, Left
Orchectomy, orchidectomy, orchiectomy
see Excision, Male Reproductive System 0VB
see Resection, Male Reproductive System 0VT
Orchidoplasty, orchioplasty
see Repair, Male Reproductive System 0VQ
see Replacement, Male Reproductive System
0VR
see Supplement, Male Reproductive System
0VU
Orchidorrhaphy, orchiorrhaphy *see* Repair,
Male Reproductive System 0VQ
Orchidotomy, orchiotomy, orchotomy *see*
Drainage, Male Reproductive System
0V9
Orchiopexy
see Repair, Male Reproductive System 0VQ
see Reposition, Male Reproductive System
0VS
Oropharyngeal airway (OPA) *use* Intraluminal
Device, Airway in Mouth and Throat
Oropharynx *use* Pharynx
~~Ossicular chain~~
~~use Auditory Ossicle, Right~~
~~use Auditory Ossicle, Left~~
Ossiculectomy
see Excision, Ear, Nose, Sinus 09B
see Resection, Ear, Nose, Sinus 09T
Ossiculotomy *see* Drainage, Ear, Nose, Sinus
099
Ostectomy
see Excision, Head and Facial Bones 0NB
see Resection, Head and Facial Bones 0NT
see Excision, Upper Bones 0PB
see Resection, Upper Bones 0PT
see Excision, Lower Bones 0QB
see Resection, Lower Bones 0QT
Osteoclasis
see Division, Head and Facial Bones 0N8
see Division, Upper Bones 0P8
see Division, Lower Bones 0Q8
Osteolysis
see Release, Head and Facial Bones 0NN
see Release, Upper Bones 0PN
see Release, Lower Bones 0QN
Osteopathic Treatment
Abdomen 7W09X
Cervical 7W01X
Extremity
Lower 7W06X
Upper 7W07X
Head 7W00X
Lumbar 7W03X
Pelvis 7W05X
Rib Cage 7W08X
Sacrum 7W04X
Thoracic 7W02X
Osteopexy
see Repair, Head and Facial Bones 0NQ
see Reposition, Head and Facial Bones 0NS
see Repair, Upper Bones 0PQ
see Reposition, Upper Bones 0PS
see Repair, Lower Bones 0QQ
see Reposition, Lower Bones 0QS
Osteoplasty
see Repair, Head and Facial Bones 0NQ
see Replacement, Head and Facial Bones
0NR
see Supplement, Head and Facial Bones
0NU

Osteoplasty *(Continued)*
  see Repair, Upper Bones ØPQ
  see Replacement, Upper Bones ØPR
  see Supplement, Upper Bones ØPU
  see Repair, Lower Bones ØQQ
  see Replacement, Lower Bones ØQR
  see Supplement, Lower Bones ØQU
Osteorrhaphy
  see Repair, Head and Facial Bones ØNQ
  see Repair, Upper Bones ØPQ
  see Repair, Lower Bones ØQQ
Osteotomy, ostotomy
  see Division, Head and Facial Bones ØN8
  see Drainage, Head and Facial Bones ØN9
  see Division, Upper Bones ØP8
  see Drainage, Upper Bones ØP9
  see Division, Lower Bones ØQ8
  see Drainage, Lower Bones ØQ9
Otic ganglion *use* Head and Neck Sympathetic
  Nerve
Otoplasty
  see Repair, Ear, Nose, Sinus Ø9Q
  see Replacement, Ear, Nose, Sinus Ø9R
  see Supplement, Ear, Nose, Sinus Ø9U

Otoscopy *see* Inspection, Ear, Nose, Sinus Ø9J
Oval window
  use Middle Ear, Right
  use Middle Ear, Left
Ovarian artery *use* Abdominal Aorta
Ovarian ligament *use* Uterine Supporting
  Structure
Ovariectomy
  see Excision, Female Reproductive System
    ØUB
  see Resection, Female Reproductive System
    ØUT
Ovariocentesis *see* Drainage, Female
  Reproductive System ØU9
Ovariopexy
  see Repair, Female Reproductive System
    ØUQ
  see Reposition, Female Reproductive System
    ØUS
Ovariotomy
  see Division, Female Reproductive System
    ØU8
  see Drainage, Female Reproductive System
    ØU9

Ovatio™ CRT-D *use* Cardiac Resynchronization
  Defibrillator Pulse Generator in ØJH
Oversewing
  Gastrointestinal ulcer *see* Repair,
    Gastrointestinal System ØDQ
  Pleural bleb *see* Repair, Respiratory System
    ØBQ
Oviduct
  use Fallopian Tube, Right
  use Fallopian Tube, Left
Oxidized zirconium ceramic hip bearing
  surface *use* Synthetic Substitute, Ceramic
  on Polyethylene in ØSR
Oximetry, Fetal pulse 10H073Z
Oxygenation
  Extracorporeal membrane (ECMO) *see*
    Performance, Circulatory 5A15
  Hyperbaric *see* Assistance, Circulatory 5AØ5
  Supersaturated *see* Assistance, Circulatory
    5AØ5

◀ New   ◀▥ Revised   ~~deleted~~ Deleted

P

Pacemaker
Dual Chamber
Abdomen ØJH8
Chest ØJH6
Intracardiac ◀
Insertion of device in ◀
Atrium ◀
Left 02H7 ◀
Right 02H6 ◀
Vein, Coronary 02H4 ◀
Ventricle ◀
Left 02HL ◀
Right 02HK ◀
Removal of device from, Heart 02PA ◀
Revision of device in, Heart 02WA ◀
Single Chamber
Abdomen ØJH8
Chest ØJH6
Single Chamber Rate Responsive
Abdomen ØJH8
Chest ØJH6
Packing
Abdominal Wall 2W43X5Z
Anorectal 2Y43X5Z
Arm
Lower
Left 2W4DX5Z
Right 2W4CX5Z
Upper
Left 2W4BX5Z
Right 2W4AX5Z
Back 2W45X5Z
Chest Wall 2W44X5Z
Ear 2Y42X5Z
Extremity
Lower
Left 2W4MX5Z
Right 2W4LX5Z
Upper
Left 2W49X5Z
Right 2W48X5Z
Face 2W41X5Z
Finger
Left 2W4KX5Z
Right 2W4JX5Z
Foot
Left 2W4TX5Z
Right 2W4SX5Z
Genital Tract, Female 2Y44X5Z
Hand
Left 2W4FX5Z
Right 2W4EX5Z
Head 2W40X5Z
Inguinal Region
Left 2W47X5Z
Right 2W46X5Z
Leg
Lower
Left 2W4RX5Z
Right 2W4QX5Z
Upper
Left 2W4PX5Z
Right 2W4NX5Z
Mouth and Pharynx 2Y40X5Z
Nasal 2Y41X5Z
Neck 2W42X5Z
Thumb
Left 2W4HX5Z
Right 2W4GX5Z
Toe
Left 2W4VX5Z
Right 2W4UX5Z
Urethra 2Y45X5Z
Paclitaxel-eluting coronary stent
use Intraluminal Device, Drug-eluting in Heart and Great Vessels

Paclitaxel-eluting peripheral stent
use Intraluminal Device, Drug-eluting in Upper Arteries
use Intraluminal Device, Drug-eluting in Lower Arteries
Palatine gland *use* Buccal Mucosa
Palatine tonsil *use* Tonsils
Palatine uvula *use* Uvula
Palatoglossal muscle *use* Tongue, Palate, Pharynx Muscle
Palatopharyngeal muscle *use* Tongue, Palate, Pharynx Muscle
Palatoplasty
see Repair, Mouth and Throat ØCQ
see Replacement, Mouth and Throat ØCR
see Supplement, Mouth and Throat ØCU
Palatorrhaphy *see* Repair, Mouth and Throat ØCQ
Palmar (volar) digital vein
use Hand Vein, Right
use Hand Vein, Left
Palmar (volar) metacarpal vein
use Hand Vein, Right
use Hand Vein, Left
Palmar cutaneous nerve
use Radial Nerve
use Median Nerve
Palmar fascia (aponeurosis)
use Subcutaneous Tissue and Fascia, Right Hand
use Subcutaneous Tissue and Fascia, Left Hand
Palmar interosseous muscle
use Hand Muscle, Right
use Hand Muscle, Left
Palmar ulnocarpal ligament
use Wrist Bursa and Ligament, Right
use Wrist Bursa and Ligament, Left
Palmaris longus muscle
use Lower Arm and Wrist Muscle, Right
use Lower Arm and Wrist Muscle, Left
Pancreatectomy
see Excision, Pancreas ØFBG
see Resection, Pancreas ØFTG
Pancreatic artery *use* Splenic Artery
Pancreatic plexus *use* Abdominal Sympathetic Nerve
Pancreatic vein *use* Splenic Vein
Pancreaticoduodenostomy *see* Bypass, Hepatobiliary System and Pancreas ØF1
Pancreaticosplenic lymph node *use* Lymphatic, Aortic
Pancreatogram, endoscopic retrograde *see* Fluoroscopy, Pancreatic Duct BF18
Pancreatolithotomy *see* Extirpation, Pancreas ØFCG
Pancreatotomy
see Division, Pancreas ØF8G
see Drainage, Pancreas ØF9G
Panniculectomy
see Excision, Skin, Abdomen ØHB7
see Excision, Abdominal Wall ØWBF
Paraaortic lymph node *use* Lymphatic, Aortic
Paracentesis
Eye *see* Drainage, Eye Ø89
Peritoneal Cavity *see* Drainage, Peritoneal Cavity ØW9G
Tympanum *see* Drainage, Ear, Nose, Sinus Ø99
Pararectal lymph node *use* Lymphatic, Mesenteric
Parasternal lymph node *use* Lymphatic, Thorax
Parathyroidectomy
see Excision, Endocrine System ØGB
see Resection, Endocrine System ØGT
Paratracheal lymph node *use* Lymphatic, Thorax
Paraurethral (Skene's) gland *use* Vestibular Gland
Parenteral nutrition, total *see* Introduction of Nutritional Substance
Parietal lobe *use* Cerebral Hemisphere
Parotid lymph node *use* Lymphatic, Head
Parotid plexus *use* Facial Nerve

Parotidectomy
see Excision, Mouth and Throat ØCB
see Resection, Mouth and Throat ØCT
Pars flaccida
use Tympanic Membrane, Right
use Tympanic Membrane, Left
Partial joint replacement
Hip *see* Replacement, Lower Joints ØSR
Knee *see* Replacement, Lower Joints ØSR
Shoulder *see* Replacement, Upper Joints ØRR
Partially absorbable mesh *use* Synthetic Substitute
Patch, blood, spinal 3E0S3GC
Patellapexy
see Repair, Lower Bones ØQQ
see Reposition, Lower Bones ØQS
Patellaplasty
see Repair, Lower Bones ØQQ
see Replacement, Lower Bones ØQR
see Supplement, Lower Bones ØQU
Patellar ligament
use Knee Bursa and Ligament, Right
use Knee Bursa and Ligament, Left
Patellar tendon
use Knee Tendon, Right
use Knee Tendon, Left
Patellectomy
see Excision, Lower Bones ØQB
see Resection, Lower Bones ØQT
Patellofemoral joint
use Knee Joint, Right
use Knee Joint, Left
use Knee Joint, Femoral Surface, Right
use Knee Joint, Femoral Surface, Left
Pectineus muscle
use Upper Leg Muscle, Right
use Upper Leg Muscle, Left
Pectoral (anterior) lymph node
use Lymphatic, Right Axillary
use Lymphatic, Left Axillary
Pectoral fascia *use* Subcutaneous Tissue and Fascia, Chest
Pectoralis major muscle
use Thorax Muscle, Right
use Thorax Muscle, Left
Pectoralis minor muscle
use Thorax Muscle, Right
use Thorax Muscle, Left
Pedicle-based dynamic stabilization device
use Spinal Stabilization Device, Pedicle-Based in ØRH
use Spinal Stabilization Device, Pedicle-Based in ØSH
PEEP (positive end expiratory pressure) *see* Assistance, Respiratory 5A09
PEG (percutaneous endoscopic gastrostomy) ØDH63UZ
PEJ (percutaneous endoscopic jejunostomy) ØDHA3UZ
Pelvic splanchnic nerve
use Abdominal Sympathetic Nerve
use Sacral Sympathetic Nerve
Penectomy
see Excision, Male Reproductive System ØVB
see Resection, Male Reproductive System ØVT
Penile urethra *use* Urethra
Perceval sutureless valve *use* Zooplastic Tissue, Rapid Deployment Technique in New Technology ◀
Percutaneous endoscopic gastrojejunostomy (PEG/J) tube *use* Feeding Device in Gastrointestinal System
Percutaneous endoscopic gastrostomy (PEG) tube *use* Feeding Device in Gastrointestinal System
Percutaneous nephrostomy catheter *use* Drainage Device
Percutaneous transluminal coronary angioplasty (PTCA) *see* Dilation, Heart and Great Vessels 027

Performance
  Biliary
    Multiple, Filtration 5A1C60Z
    Single, Filtration 5A1C00Z
  Cardiac
    Continuous
      Output 5A1221Z
      Pacing 5A1223Z
    Intermittent, Pacing 5A1213Z
    Single, Output, Manual 5A12012
  Circulatory, Continuous, Oxygenation,
    Membrane 5A15223
  Respiratory
    24-96 Consecutive Hours, Ventilation
      5A1945Z
    Greater than 96 Consecutive Hours,
      Ventilation 5A1955Z
    Less than 24 Consecutive Hours,
      Ventilation 5A1935Z
    Single, Ventilation, Nonmechanical
      5A19054
  Urinary
    Multiple, Filtration 5A1D60Z
    Single, Filtration 5A1D00Z
Perfusion see Introduction of substance in
  or on
Perfusion, donor organ ◀
  Heart 6AB50BZ ◀
  Kidney(s) 6ABT0BZ ◀
  Liver 6ABF0BZ ◀
  Lung(s) 6ABB0BZ ◀
Pericardiectomy
  see Excision, Pericardium 02BN
  see Resection, Pericardium 02TN
Pericardiocentesis
  see Drainage, Cavity, Pericardial 0W9D
Pericardiolysis see Release, Pericardium
  02NN
Pericardiophrenic artery
  use Internal Mammary Artery, Right
  use Internal Mammary Artery, Left
Pericardioplasty
  see Repair, Pericardium 02QN
  see Replacement, Pericardium 02RN
  see Supplement, Pericardium 02UN
Pericardiorrhaphy see Repair, Pericardium
  02QN
Pericardiostomy see Drainage, Cavity,
  Pericardial 0W9D
Pericardiotomy see Drainage, Cavity, Pericardial
  0W9D
Perimetrium use Uterus
Peripheral parenteral nutrition see Introduction
  of Nutritional Substance
Peripherally inserted central catheter (PICC)
  use Infusion Device
Peritoneal dialysis 3E1M39Z
Peritoneocentesis
  see Drainage, Peritoneum 0D9W
  see Drainage, Cavity, Peritoneal 0W9G
Peritoneoplasty
  see Repair, Peritoneum 0DQW
  see Replacement, Peritoneum 0DRW
  see Supplement, Peritoneum 0DUW
Peritoneoscopy 0DJW4ZZ
Peritoneotomy see Drainage, Peritoneum 0D9W
Peritoneumectomy
  see Excision, Peritoneum 0DBW
Peroneus brevis muscle
  use Lower Leg Muscle, Right
  use Lower Leg Muscle, Left
Peroneus longus muscle
  use Lower Leg Muscle, Right
  use Lower Leg Muscle, Left
Pessary ring use Intraluminal Device, Pessary in
  Female Reproductive System
PET scan see Positron Emission Tomographic
  (PET) Imaging
Petrous part of temporal bone
  use Temporal Bone, Right
  use Temporal Bone, Left

Phacoemulsification, lens
  With IOL implant see Replacement, Eye
    08R
  Without IOL implant see Extraction, Eye
    08D
Phalangectomy
  see Excision, Upper Bones 0PB
  see Resection, Upper Bones 0PT
  see Excision, Lower Bones 0QB
  see Resection, Lower Bones 0QT
Phallectomy
  see Excision, Penis 0VBS
  see Resection, Penis 0VTS
Phalloplasty
  see Repair, Penis 0VQS
  see Supplement, Penis 0VUS
Phallotomy see Drainage, Penis 0V9S
Pharmacotherapy, for substance abuse
  Antabuse HZ93ZZZ
  Bupropion HZ97ZZZ
  Clonidine HZ96ZZZ
  Levo-alpha-acetyl-methadol (LAAM)
    HZ92ZZZ
  Methadone Maintenance HZ91ZZZ
  Naloxone HZ95ZZZ
  Naltrexone HZ94ZZZ
  Nicotine Replacement HZ90ZZZ
  Psychiatric Medication HZ98ZZZ
  Replacement Medication, Other
    HZ99ZZZ
Pharyngeal constrictor muscle use Tongue,
  Palate, Pharynx Muscle
Pharyngeal plexus use Vagus Nerve
Pharyngeal recess use Nasopharynx
Pharyngeal tonsil use Adenoids
Pharyngogram see Fluoroscopy, Pharynx
  B91G
Pharyngoplasty
  see Repair, Mouth and Throat 0CQ
  see Replacement, Mouth and Throat
    0CR
  see Supplement, Mouth and Throat 0CU
Pharyngorrhaphy see Repair, Mouth and Throat
  0CQ
Pharyngotomy see Drainage, Mouth and Throat
  0C9
Pharyngotympanic tube
  use Eustachian Tube, Right
  use Eustachian Tube, Left
Pheresis
  Erythrocytes 6A55
  Leukocytes 6A55
  Plasma 6A55
  Platelets 6A55
  Stem Cells
    Cord Blood 6A55
    Hematopoietic 6A55
Phlebectomy
  see Excision, Upper Veins 05B
  see Extraction, Upper Veins 05D
  see Excision, Lower Veins 06B
  see Extraction, Lower Veins 06D
Phlebography
  see Plain Radiography, Veins B50
  Impedance 4A04X51
Phleborrhaphy
  see Repair, Upper Veins 05Q
  see Repair, Lower Veins 06Q
Phlebotomy
  see Drainage, Upper Veins 059
  see Drainage, Lower Veins 069
Photocoagulation
  for Destruction see Destruction
  for Repair see Repair
Photopheresis, therapeutic see Phototherapy,
  Circulatory 6A65
Phototherapy
  Circulatory 6A65
  Skin 6A60
Phrenectomy, phrenoneurectomy see Excision,
  Nerve, Phrenic 01B2

Phrenemphraxis see Destruction, Nerve,
  Phrenic 0152
Phrenic nerve stimulator generator use
  Stimulator Generator in Subcutaneous
  Tissue and Fascia
Phrenic nerve stimulator lead use
  Diaphragmatic Pacemaker Lead in
  Respiratory System
Phreniclasis see Destruction, Nerve, Phrenic
  0152
Phrenicoexeresis see Extraction, Nerve, Phrenic
  01D2
Phrenicotomy see Division, Nerve, Phrenic
  0182
Phrenicotripsy see Destruction, Nerve, Phrenic
  0152
Phrenoplasty
  see Repair, Respiratory System 0BQ
  see Supplement, Respiratory System 0BU
Phrenotomy see Drainage, Respiratory System
  0B9
Physiatry see Motor Treatment, Rehabilitation F07
Physical medicine see Motor Treatment,
  Rehabilitation F07
Physical therapy see Motor Treatment,
  Rehabilitation F07
PHYSIOMESH™ Flexible Composite Mesh use
  Synthetic Substitute
Pia mater, intracranial use Cerebral Meninges
Pia mater, spinal use Spinal Meninges
Pinealectomy
  see Excision, Pineal Body 0GB1
  see Resection, Pineal Body 0GT1
Pinealoscopy 0GJ14ZZ
Pinealotomy see Drainage, Pineal Body 0G91
Pinna
  use External Ear, Right
  use External Ear, Left
  use External Ear, Bilateral
Pipeline™ Embolization device (PED) use
  Intraluminal Device
Piriform recess (sinus) use Pharynx
Piriformis muscle
  use Hip Muscle, Right
  use Hip Muscle, Left
Pisiform bone
  use Carpal, Right
  use Carpal, Left
Pisohamate ligament
  use Hand Bursa and Ligament, Right
  use Hand Bursa and Ligament, Left
Pisometacarpal ligament
  use Hand Bursa and Ligament, Right
  use Hand Bursa and Ligament, Left
Pituitectomy
  see Excision, Gland, Pituitary 0GB0
  see Resection, Gland, Pituitary 0GT0
Plain film radiology see Plain Radiography
Plain Radiography
  Abdomen BW00ZZZ
  Abdomen and Pelvis BW01ZZZ
  Abdominal Lymphatic
    Bilateral B701
    Unilateral B700
  Airway, Upper BB0DZZZ
  Ankle
    Left BQ0H
    Right BQ0G
  Aorta
    Abdominal B400
    Thoracic B300
    Thoraco-Abdominal B30P
  Aorta and Bilateral Lower Extremity Arteries
    B40D
  Arch
    Bilateral BN0DZZZ
    Left BN0CZZZ
    Right BN0BZZZ
  Arm
    Left BP0FZZZ
    Right BP0EZZZ

◀ New   ◀▦ Revised   ~~deleted~~ Deleted

◀ New   ◀‖‖ Revised   ~~deleted~~ Deleted

◀ New   ◀▥ Revised   ~~deleted~~ Deleted

Plaque Radiation (*Continued*)
  Lymphatics
    Abdomen D7Y6FZZ
    Axillary D7Y4FZZ
    Inguinal D7Y8FZZ
    Neck D7Y3FZZ
    Pelvis D7Y7FZZ
    Thorax D7Y5FZZ
  Mandible DPY3FZZ
  Maxilla DPY2FZZ
  Mediastinum DBY6FZZ
  Mouth D9Y4FZZ
  Nasopharynx D9YDFZZ
  Neck and Head DWY1FZZ
  Nerve, Peripheral D0Y7FZZ
  Nose D9Y1FZZ
  Ovary DUY0FZZ
  Palate
    Hard D9Y8FZZ
    Soft D9Y9FZZ
  Pancreas DFY3FZZ
  Parathyroid Gland DGY4FZZ
  Pelvic Bones DPY8FZZ
  Pelvic Region DWY6FZZ
  Pharynx D9YCFZZ
  Pineal Body DGY1FZZ
  Pituitary Gland DGY0FZZ
  Pleura DBY5FZZ
  Prostate DVY0FZZ
  Radius DPY7FZZ
  Rectum DDY7FZZ
  Rib DPY5FZZ
  Sinuses D9Y7FZZ
  Skin
    Abdomen DHY8FZZ
    Arm DHY4FZZ
    Back DHY7FZZ
    Buttock DHY9FZZ
    Chest DHY6FZZ
    Face DHY2FZZ
    Foot DHYCFZZ
    Hand DHY5FZZ
    Leg DHYBFZZ
    Neck DHY3FZZ
  Skull DPY0FZZ
  Spinal Cord D0Y6FZZ
  Spleen D7Y2FZZ
  Sternum DPY4FZZ
  Stomach DDY1FZZ
  Testis DVY1FZZ
  Thymus D7Y1FZZ
  Thyroid Gland DGY5FZZ
  Tibia DPYBFZZ
  Tongue D9Y5FZZ
  Trachea DBY0FZZ
  Ulna DPY7FZZ
  Ureter DTY1FZZ
  Urethra DTY3FZZ
  Uterus DUY2FZZ
  Whole Body DWY5FZZ
Plasmapheresis, therapeutic 6A550Z3
Plateletpheresis, therapeutic 6A550Z2
Platysma muscle
  use Neck Muscle, Right
  use Neck Muscle, Left
Pleurectomy
  see Excision, Respiratory System ØBB
  see Resection, Respiratory System ØBT
Pleurocentesis *see* Drainage, Anatomical
  Regions, General ØW9
Pleurodesis, pleurosclerosis
  Chemical Injection *see* Introduction of
    substance in or on, Pleural Cavity 3EØL
  Surgical *see* Destruction, Respiratory System
    ØB5
Pleurolysis *see* Release, Respiratory System
  ØBN
Pleuroscopy ØBJQ4ZZ
Pleurotomy *see* Drainage, Respiratory System
  ØB9

Plica semilunaris
  use Conjunctiva, Right
  use Conjunctiva, Left
Plication *see* Restriction
Pneumectomy
  see Excision, Respiratory System ØBB
  see Resection, Respiratory System ØBT
Pneumocentesis *see* Drainage, Respiratory
  System ØB9
Pneumogastric nerve *use* Vagus Nerve
Pneumolysis *see* Release, Respiratory System
  ØBN
Pneumonectomy *see* Resection, Respiratory
  System ØBT
Pneumonolysis *see* Release, Respiratory System
  ØBN
Pneumonopexy
  see Repair, Respiratory System ØBQ
  see Reposition, Respiratory System ØBS
Pneumonorrhaphy *see* Repair, Respiratory
  System ØBQ
Pneumonotomy *see* Drainage, Respiratory
  System ØB9
Pneumotaxic center *use* Pons
Pneumotomy *see* Drainage, Respiratory System
  ØB9
Pollicization *see* Transfer, Anatomical Regions,
  Upper Extremities ØXX
Polyethylene socket *use* Synthetic Substitute,
  Polyethylene in ØSR
Polymethylmethacrylate (PMMA) *use*
  Synthetic Substitute
Polypectomy, gastrointestinal *see* Excision,
  Gastrointestinal System ØDB
Polypropylene mesh *use* Synthetic Substitute
Polysomnogram 4A1ZXQZ
Pontine tegmentum *use* Pons
Popliteal ligament
  use Knee Bursa and Ligament, Right
  use Knee Bursa and Ligament, Left
Popliteal lymph node
  use Lymphatic, Right Lower Extremity
  use Lymphatic, Left Lower Extremity
Popliteal vein
  use Femoral Vein, Right
  use Femoral Vein, Left
Popliteus muscle
  use Lower Leg Muscle, Right
  use Lower Leg Muscle, Left
Porcine (bioprosthetic) valve *use* Zooplastic
  Tissue in Heart and Great Vessels
Positive end expiratory pressure *see*
  Performance, Respiratory 5A19
Positron Emission Tomographic (PET)
  Imaging
  Brain CØ3Ø
  Bronchi and Lungs CB32
  Central Nervous System CØ3YYZZ
  Heart C23YYZZ
  Lungs and Bronchi CB32
  Myocardium C23G
  Respiratory System CB3YYZZ
  Whole Body CW3NYZZ
Positron emission tomography *see* Positron
  Emission Tomographic (PET) Imaging
Postauricular (mastoid) lymph node
  use Lymphatic, Right Neck
  use Lymphatic, Left Neck
Postcava *use* Inferior Vena Cava
Posterior (subscapular) lymph node
  use Lymphatic, Right Axillary
  use Lymphatic, Left Axillary
Posterior auricular artery
  use External Carotid Artery, Right
  use External Carotid Artery, Left
Posterior auricular nerve *use* Facial
  Nerve
Posterior auricular vein
  use External Jugular Vein, Right
  use External Jugular Vein, Left

Posterior cerebral artery *use* Intracranial
  Artery
Posterior chamber
  use Eye, Right
  use Eye, Left
Posterior circumflex humeral artery
  use Axillary Artery, Right
  use Axillary Artery, Left
Posterior communicating artery *use* Intracranial
  Artery
Posterior cruciate ligament (PCL)
  use Knee Bursa and Ligament, Right
  use Knee Bursa and Ligament, Left
Posterior facial (retromandibular) vein
  use Face Vein, Right
  use Face Vein, Left
Posterior femoral cutaneous nerve *use* Sacral
  Plexus Nerve
Posterior inferior cerebellar artery (PICA) *use*
  Intracranial Artery
Posterior interosseous nerve *use* Radial Nerve
Posterior labial nerve *use* Pudendal Nerve
Posterior scrotal nerve *use* Pudendal Nerve
Posterior spinal artery
  use Vertebral Artery, Right
  use Vertebral Artery, Left
Posterior tibial recurrent artery
  use Anterior Tibial Artery, Right
  use Anterior Tibial Artery, Left
Posterior ulnar recurrent artery
  use Ulnar Artery, Right
  use Ulnar Artery, Left
Posterior vagal trunk *use* Vagus Nerve
PPN (peripheral parenteral nutrition) *see*
  Introduction of Nutritional Substance
Preauricular lymph node *use* Lymphatic, Head
Precava *use* Superior Vena Cava
Prepatellar bursa
  use Knee Bursa and Ligament, Right
  use Knee Bursa and Ligament, Left
Preputiotomy *see* Drainage, Male Reproductive
  System ØV9
Pressure support ventilation *see* Performance,
  Respiratory 5A19
PRESTIGE® Cervical Disc *use* Synthetic
  Substitute
Pretracheal fascia *use* Subcutaneous Tissue and
  Fascia, Anterior Neck
Prevertebral fascia *use* Subcutaneous Tissue
  and Fascia, Posterior Neck
PrimeAdvanced neurostimulator (SureScan)
  (MRI Safe) *use* Stimulator Generator,
  Multiple Array in ØJH
Princeps pollicis artery
  use Hand Artery, Right
  use Hand Artery, Left
Probing, duct
  Diagnostic *see* Inspection
  Dilation *see* Dilation
PROCEED™ Ventral Patch *use* Synthetic
  Substitute
Procerus muscle *use* Facial Muscle
Proctectomy
  see Excision, Rectum ØDBP
  see Resection, Rectum ØDTP
Proctoclysis *see* Introduction of substance in or
  on, Gastrointestinal Tract, Lower 3EØH
Proctocolectomy
  see Excision, Gastrointestinal System ØDB
  see Resection, Gastrointestinal System ØDT
Proctocolpoplasty
  see Repair, Gastrointestinal System ØDQ
  see Supplement, Gastrointestinal System
    ØDU
Proctoperineoplasty
  see Repair, Gastrointestinal System ØDQ
  see Supplement, Gastrointestinal System
    ØDU
Proctoperineorrhaphy *see* Repair,
  Gastrointestinal System ØDQ

Proctopexy
  see Repair, Rectum ØDQP
  see Reposition, Rectum ØDSP
Proctoplasty
  see Repair, Rectum ØDQP
  see Supplement, Rectum ØDUP
Proctorrhaphy see Repair, Rectum ØDQP
Proctoscopy ØDJD8ZZ
Proctosigmoidectomy
  see Excision, Gastrointestinal System ØDB
  see Resection, Gastrointestinal System ØDT
Proctosigmoidoscopy ØDJD8ZZ
Proctostomy see Drainage, Rectum ØD9P
Proctotomy see Drainage, Rectum ØD9P
Prodisc-C use Synthetic Substitute
Prodisc-L use Synthetic Substitute
Production, atrial septal defect see Excision,
    Septum, Atrial Ø2B5
Profunda brachii
  use Brachial Artery, Right
  use Brachial Artery, Left
Profunda femoris (deep femoral) vein
  use Femoral Vein, Right
  use Femoral Vein, Left
PROLENE Polypropylene Hernia System
    (PHS) use Synthetic Substitute
Pronator quadratus muscle
  use Lower Arm and Wrist Muscle, Right
  use Lower Arm and Wrist Muscle, Left
Pronator teres muscle
  use Lower Arm and Wrist Muscle, Right
  use Lower Arm and Wrist Muscle, Left
Prostatectomy
  see Excision, Prostate ØVBØ
  see Resection, Prostate ØVTØ
Prostatic urethra use Urethra
Prostatomy, prostatotomy see Drainage,
    Prostate ØV9Ø
Protecta XT CRT-D use Cardiac
    Resynchronization Defibrillator Pulse
    Generator in ØJH
Protecta XT DR (XT VR) use Defibrillator
    Generator in ØJH
Protégé® RX Carotid Stent System use
    Intraluminal Device
Proximal radioulnar joint
  use Elbow Joint, Right
  use Elbow Joint, Left
Psoas muscle
  use Hip Muscle, Right
  use Hip Muscle, Left
PSV (pressure support ventilation) see
    Performance, Respiratory 5A19
Psychoanalysis GZ54ZZZ
Psychological Tests
  Cognitive Status GZ14ZZZ
  Developmental GZ10ZZZ
  Intellectual and Psychoeducational GZ12ZZZ
  Neurobehavioral Status GZ14ZZZ
  Neuropsychological GZ13ZZZ
  Personality and Behavioral GZ11ZZZ
Psychotherapy
  Family, Mental Health Services GZ72ZZZ
  Group
    GZHZZZZ
    Mental Health Services GZHZZZZ

Psychotherapy (Continued)
  Individual
    see Psychotherapy, Individual, Mental
        Health Services
    for substance abuse
      12-Step HZ53ZZZ
      Behavioral HZ51ZZZ
      Cognitive HZ50ZZZ
      Cognitive-Behavioral HZ52ZZZ
      Confrontational HZ58ZZZ
      Interactive HZ55ZZZ
      Interpersonal HZ54ZZZ
      Motivational Enhancement HZ57ZZZ
      Psychoanalysis HZ5BZZZ
      Psychodynamic HZ5CZZZ
      Psychoeducation HZ56ZZZ
      Psychophysiological HZ5DZZZ
      Supportive HZ59ZZZ
    Mental Health Services
      Behavioral GZ51ZZZ
      Cognitive GZ52ZZZ
      Cognitive-Behavioral GZ58ZZZ
      Interactive GZ50ZZZ
      Interpersonal GZ53ZZZ
      Psychoanalysis GZ54ZZZ
      Psychodynamic GZ55ZZZ
      Psychophysiological GZ59ZZZ
      Supportive GZ56ZZZ
PTCA (percutaneous transluminal coronary
    angioplasty) see Dilation, Heart and Great
    Vessels Ø27
Pterygoid muscle use Head Muscle
Pterygoid process
  use Sphenoid Bone, Right
  use Sphenoid Bone, Left
Pterygopalatine (sphenopalatine) ganglion use
    Head and Neck Sympathetic Nerve
Pubic ligament
  use Trunk Bursa and Ligament, Right
  use Trunk Bursa and Ligament, Left
Pubis
  use Pelvic Bone, Right
  use Pelvic Bone, Left
Pubofemoral ligament
  use Hip Bursa and Ligament, Right
  use Hip Bursa and Ligament, Left
Pudendal nerve use Sacral Plexus
Pull-through, rectal see Resection, Rectum
    ØDTP
Pulmoaortic canal use Pulmonary Artery,
    Left
Pulmonary annulus use Pulmonary Valve
Pulmonary artery wedge monitoring see
    Monitoring, Arterial 4A13
Pulmonary plexus
  use Vagus Nerve
  use Thoracic Sympathetic Nerve
Pulmonic valve use Pulmonary Valve
Pulpectomy see Excision, Mouth and Throat
    ØCB
Pulverization see Fragmentation
Pulvinar use Thalamus
Pump reservoir use Infusion Device, Pump in
    Subcutaneous Tissue and Fascia
Punch biopsy see Excision with qualifier
    Diagnostic

Puncture see Drainage
Puncture, lumbar see Drainage, Spinal Canal
    ØØ9U
Pyelography
  see Plain Radiography, Urinary System
      BTØ
  see Fluoroscopy, Urinary System BT1
Pyeloileostomy, urinary diversion see Bypass,
    Urinary System ØT1
Pyeloplasty
  see Repair, Urinary System ØTQ
  see Replacement, Urinary System ØTR
  see Supplement, Urinary System ØTU
Pyelorrhaphy see Repair, Urinary System ØTQ
Pyeloscopy ØTJ58ZZ
Pyelostomy
  see Bypass, Urinary System ØT1
  see Drainage, Urinary System ØT9
Pyelotomy see Drainage, Urinary System ØT9
Pylorectomy
  see Excision, Stomach, Pylorus ØDB7
  see Resection, Stomach, Pylorus ØDT7
Pyloric antrum use Stomach, Pylorus
Pyloric canal use Stomach, Pylorus
Pyloric sphincter use Stomach, Pylorus
Pylorodiosis see Dilation, Stomach, Pylorus
    ØD77
Pylorogastrectomy
  see Excision, Gastrointestinal System ØDB
  see Resection, Gastrointestinal System ØDT
Pyloroplasty
  see Repair, Stomach, Pylorus ØDQ7
  see Supplement, Stomach, Pylorus ØDU7
Pyloroscopy ØDJ68ZZ
Pylorotomy see Drainage, Stomach, Pylorus
    ØD97
Pyramidalis muscle
  use Abdomen Muscle, Right
  use Abdomen Muscle, Left

Q

Quadrangular cartilage use Nasal Septum
Quadrant resection of breast see Excision, Skin
    and Breast ØHB
Quadrate lobe use Liver
Quadratus femoris muscle
  use Hip Muscle, Right
  use Hip Muscle, Left
Quadratus lumborum muscle
  use Trunk Muscle, Right
  use Trunk Muscle, Left
Quadratus plantae muscle
  use Foot Muscle, Right
  use Foot Muscle, Left
Quadriceps (femoris)
  use Upper Leg Muscle, Right
  use Upper Leg Muscle, Left
Quarantine 8EØZXY6

◄ New   ◄ Revised   ~~deleted~~ Deleted

R

Radial collateral carpal ligament
  use Wrist Bursa and Ligament, Right
  use Wrist Bursa and Ligament, Left
Radial collateral ligament
  use Elbow Bursa and Ligament, Right
  use Elbow Bursa and Ligament, Left
Radial notch
  use Ulna, Right
  use Ulna, Left
Radial recurrent artery
  use Radial Artery, Right
  use Radial Artery, Left
Radial vein
  use Brachial Vein, Right
  use Brachial Vein, Left
Radialis indicis
  use Hand Artery, Right
  use Hand Artery, Left
Radiation Therapy
  see Beam Radiation
  see Brachytherapy
  see Stereotactic Radiosurgery
Radiation treatment *see* Radiation
    Therapy
Radiocarpal joint
  use Wrist Joint, Right
  use Wrist Joint, Left
Radiocarpal ligament
  use Wrist Bursa and Ligament, Right
  use Wrist Bursa and Ligament, Left
Radiography *see* Plain Radiography
Radiology, analog *see* Plain Radiography
Radiology, diagnostic *see* Imaging,
    Diagnostic
Radioulnar ligament
  use Wrist Bursa and Ligament, Right
  use Wrist Bursa and Ligament, Left
Range of motion testing *see* Motor
    Function Assessment, Rehabilitation
    F01
REALIZE® Adjustable Gastric Band *use*
    Extraluminal Device
Reattachment
  Abdominal Wall ØWMFØZZ
  Ampulla of Vater ØFMC
  Ankle Region
    Left ØYMLØZZ
    Right ØYMKØZZ
  Arm
    Lower
      Left ØXMFØZZ
      Right ØXMDØZZ
    Upper
      Left ØXM9ØZZ
      Right ØXM8ØZZ
  Axilla
    Left ØXM5ØZZ
    Right ØXM4ØZZ
  Back
    Lower ØWMLØZZ
    Upper ØWMKØZZ
  Bladder ØTMB
  Bladder Neck ØTMC
  Breast
    Bilateral ØHMVXZZ
    Left ØHMUXZZ
    Right ØHMTXZZ
  Bronchus
    Lingula ØBM9ØZZ
    Lower Lobe
      Left ØBMBØZZ
      Right ØBM6ØZZ
    Main
      Left ØBM7ØZZ
      Right ØBM3ØZZ
    Middle Lobe, Right ØBM5ØZZ
    Upper Lobe
      Left ØBM8ØZZ
      Right ØBM4ØZZ

Reattachment *(Continued)*
  Bursa and Ligament
    Abdomen
      Left ØMMJ
      Right ØMMH
    Ankle
      Left ØMMR
      Right ØMMQ
    Elbow
      Left ØMM4
      Right ØMM3
    Foot
      Left ØMMT
      Right ØMMS
    Hand
      Left ØMM8
      Right ØMM7
    Head and Neck ØMMØ
    Hip
      Left ØMMM
      Right ØMML
    Knee
      Left ØMMP
      Right ØMMN
    Lower Extremity
      Left ØMMW
      Right ØMMV
    Perineum ØMMK
    Shoulder
      Left ØMM2
      Right ØMM1
    Thorax
      Left ØMMG
      Right ØMMF
    Trunk
      Left ØMMD
      Right ØMMC
    Upper Extremity
      Left ØMMB
      Right ØMM9
    Wrist
      Left ØMM6
      Right ØMM5
  Buttock
    Left ØYM1ØZZ
    Right ØYMØØZZ
  Carina ØBM2ØZZ
  Cecum ØDMH
  Cervix ØUMC
  Chest Wall ØWM8ØZZ
  Clitoris ØUMJXZZ
  Colon
    Ascending ØDMK
    Descending ØDMM
    Sigmoid ØDMN
    Transverse ØDML
  Cord
    Bilateral ØVMH
    Left ØVMG
    Right ØVMF
  Cul-de-sac ØUMF
  Diaphragm
    Left ØBMSØZZ
    Right ØBMRØZZ
  Duct
    Common Bile ØFM9
    Cystic ØFM8
    Hepatic
      Left ØFM6
      Right ØFM5
    Pancreatic ØFMD
      Accessory ØFMF
  Duodenum ØDM9
  Ear
    Left Ø9M1XZZ
    Right Ø9MØXZZ
  Elbow Region
    Left ØXMCØZZ
    Right ØXMBØZZ
  Esophagus ØDM5

Reattachment *(Continued)*
  Extremity
    Lower
      Left ØYMBØZZ
      Right ØYM9ØZZ
    Upper
      Left ØXM7ØZZ
      Right ØXM6ØZZ
  Eyelid
    Lower
      Left Ø8MRXZZ
      Right Ø8MQXZZ
    Upper
      Left Ø8MPXZZ
      Right Ø8MNXZZ
  Face ØWM2ØZZ
  Fallopian Tube
    Left ØUM6
    Right ØUM5
  Fallopian Tubes, Bilateral
      ØUM7
  Femoral Region
    Left ØYM8ØZZ
    Right ØYM7ØZZ
  Finger
    Index
      Left ØXMPØZZ
      Right ØXMNØZZ
    Little
      Left ØXMWØZZ
      Right ØXMVØZZ
    Middle
      Left ØXMRØZZ
      Right ØXMQØZZ
    Ring
      Left ØXMTØZZ
      Right ØXMSØZZ
  Foot
    Left ØYMNØZZ
    Right ØYMMØZZ
  Forequarter
    Left ØXM1ØZZ
    Right ØXMØØZZ
  Gallbladder ØFM4
  Gland
    Adrenal
      Left ØGM2
      Right ØGM3
  Hand
    Left ØXMKØZZ
    Right ØXMJØZZ
  Hindquarter
    Bilateral ØYM4ØZZ
    Left ØYM3ØZZ
    Right ØYM2ØZZ
  Hymen ØUMK
  Ileum ØDMB
  Inguinal Region
    Left ØYM6ØZZ
    Right ØYM5ØZZ
  Intestine
    Large ØDME
      Left ØDMG
      Right ØDMF
    Small ØDM8
  Jaw
    Lower ØWM5ØZZ
    Upper ØWM4ØZZ
  Jejunum ØDMA
  Kidney
    Left ØTM1
    Right ØTMØ
  Kidney Pelvis
    Left ØTM4
    Right ØTM3
  Kidneys, Bilateral ØTM2
  Knee Region
    Left ØYMGØZZ
    Right ØYMFØZZ

R

Reattachment *(Continued)*
Leg
Lower
Left 0YMJ0ZZ
Right 0YMH0ZZ
Upper
Left 0YMD0ZZ
Right 0YMC0ZZ
Lip
Lower 0CM10ZZ
Upper 0CM00ZZ
Liver 0FM0
Left Lobe 0FM2
Right Lobe 0FM1
Lung
Left 0BML0ZZ
Lower Lobe
Left 0BMJ0ZZ
Right 0BMF0ZZ
Middle Lobe, Right 0BMD0ZZ
Right 0BMK0ZZ
Upper Lobe
Left 0BMG0ZZ
Right 0BMC0ZZ
Lung Lingula 0BMH0ZZ
Muscle
Abdomen
Left 0KML
Right 0KMK
Facial 0KM1
Foot
Left 0KMW
Right 0KMV
Hand
Left 0KMD
Right 0KMC
Head 0KM0
Hip
Left 0KMP
Right 0KMN
Lower Arm and Wrist
Left 0KMB
Right 0KM9
Lower Leg
Left 0KMT
Right 0KMS
Neck
Left 0KM3
Right 0KM2
Perineum 0KMM
Shoulder
Left 0KM6
Right 0KM5
Thorax
Left 0KMJ
Right 0KMH
Tongue, Palate, Pharynx 0KM4
Trunk
Left 0KMG
Right 0KMF
Upper Arm
Left 0KM8
Right 0KM7
Upper Leg
Left 0KMR
Right 0KMQ
Neck 0WM60ZZ
Nipple
Left 0HMXXZZ
Right 0HMWXZZ
Nose 09MKXZZ
Ovary
Bilateral 0UM2
Left 0UM1
Right 0UM0
Palate, Soft 0CM30ZZ
Pancreas 0FMG
Parathyroid Gland 0GMR
Inferior
Left 0GMP
Right 0GMN

Reattachment *(Continued)*
Parathyroid Gland *(Continued)*
Multiple 0GMQ
Superior
Left 0GMM
Right 0GML
Penis 0VMSXZZ
Perineum
Female 0WMN0ZZ
Male 0WMM0ZZ
Rectum 0DMP
Scrotum 0VM5XZZ
Shoulder Region
Left 0XM30ZZ
Right 0XM20ZZ
Skin
Abdomen 0HM7XZZ
Back 0HM6XZZ
Buttock 0HM8XZZ
Chest 0HM5XZZ
Ear
Left 0HM3XZZ
Right 0HM2XZZ
Face 0HM1XZZ
Foot
Left 0HMNXZZ
Right 0HMMXZZ
Genitalia 0HMAXZZ
Hand
Left 0HMGXZZ
Right 0HMFXZZ
Lower Arm
Left 0HMEXZZ
Right 0HMDXZZ
Lower Leg
Left 0HMLXZZ
Right 0HMKXZZ
Neck 0HM4XZZ
Perineum 0HM9XZZ
Scalp 0HM0XZZ
Upper Arm
Left 0HMCXZZ
Right 0HMBXZZ
Upper Leg
Left 0HMJXZZ
Right 0HMHXZZ
Stomach 0DM6
Tendon
Abdomen
Left 0LMG
Right 0LMF
Ankle
Left 0LMT
Right 0LMS
Foot
Left 0LMW
Right 0LMV
Hand
Left 0LM8
Right 0LM7
Head and Neck 0LM0
Hip
Left 0LMK
Right 0LMJ
Knee
Left 0LMR
Right 0LMQ
Lower Arm and Wrist
Left 0LM6
Right 0LM5
Lower Leg
Left 0LMP
Right 0LMN
Perineum 0LMH
Shoulder
Left 0LM2
Right 0LM1
Thorax
Left 0LMD
Right 0LMC
Trunk
Left 0LMB
Right 0LM9

Reattachment *(Continued)*
Tendon *(Continued)*
Upper Arm
Left 0LM4
Right 0LM3
Upper Leg
Left 0LMM
Right 0LML
Testis
Bilateral 0VMC
Left 0VMB
Right 0VM9
Thumb
Left 0XMM0ZZ
Right 0XML0ZZ
Thyroid Gland
Left Lobe 0GMG
Right Lobe 0GMH
Toe
1st
Left 0YMQ0ZZ
Right 0YMP0ZZ
2nd
Left 0YMS0ZZ
Right 0YMR0ZZ
3rd
Left 0YMU0ZZ
Right 0YMT0ZZ
4th
Left 0YMW0ZZ
Right 0YMV0ZZ
5th
Left 0YMY0ZZ
Right 0YMX0ZZ
Tongue 0CM70ZZ
Tooth
Lower 0CMX
Upper 0CMW
Trachea 0BM10ZZ
Tunica Vaginalis
Left 0VM7
Right 0VM6
Ureter
Left 0TM7
Right 0TM6
Ureters, Bilateral 0TM8
Urethra 0TMD
Uterine Supporting Structure 0UM4
Uterus 0UM9
Uvula 0CMN0ZZ
Vagina 0UMG
Vulva 0UMMXZZ
Wrist Region
Left 0XMH0ZZ
Right 0XMG0ZZ
Rebound HRD® (Hernia Repair Device) *use*
Synthetic Substitute
Recession
see Repair
see Reposition
Reclosure, disrupted abdominal wall
0WQFXZZ
Reconstruction
see Repair
see Replacement
see Supplement
Rectectomy
see Excision, Rectum 0DBP
see Resection, Rectum 0DTP
Rectocele repair
see Repair, Subcutaneous Tissue and Fascia,
Pelvic Region 0JQC
Rectopexy
see Repair, Gastrointestinal System 0DQ
see Reposition, Gastrointestinal System 0DS
Rectoplasty
see Repair, Gastrointestinal System 0DQ
see Supplement, Gastrointestinal System 0DU
Rectorrhaphy *see* Repair, Gastrointestinal
System 0DQ
Rectoscopy 0DJD8ZZ

◀ New   ◀▥ Revised   ~~deleted~~ Deleted

Rectosigmoid junction *use* Colon, Sigmoid
Rectosigmoidectomy
  see Excision, Gastrointestinal System ØDB
  see Resection, Gastrointestinal System ØDT
Rectostomy *see* Drainage, Rectum ØD9P
Rectotomy *see* Drainage, Rectum ØD9P
Rectus abdominis muscle
  use Abdomen Muscle, Right
  use Abdomen Muscle, Left
Rectus femoris muscle
  use Upper Leg Muscle, Right
  use Upper Leg Muscle, Left
Recurrent laryngeal nerve *use* Vagus Nerve
Reduction
  Dislocation *see* Reposition
  Fracture *see* Reposition
  Intussusception, intestinal *see* Reposition, Gastrointestinal System ØDS
  Mammoplasty *see* Excision, Skin and Breast ØHB
  Prolapse *see* Reposition
  Torsion *see* Reposition
  Volvulus, gastrointestinal *see* Reposition, Gastrointestinal System ØDS
Refusion *see* Fusion
Rehabilitation
  see Speech Assessment, Rehabilitation FØØ
  see Motor Function Assessment, Rehabilitation FØ1
  see Activities of Daily Living Assessment, Rehabilitation FØ2
  see Speech Treatment, Rehabilitation FØ6
  see Motor Treatment, Rehabilitation FØ7
  see Activities of Daily Living Treatment, Rehabilitation FØ8
  see Hearing Treatment, Rehabilitation FØ9
  see Cochlear Implant Treatment, Rehabilitation FØB
  see Vestibular Treatment, Rehabilitation FØC
  see Device Fitting, Rehabilitation FØD
  see Caregiver Training, Rehabilitation FØF
Reimplantation
  see Reattachment
  see Reposition
  see Transfer
Reinforcement
  see Repair
  see Supplement
Relaxation, scar tissue *see* Release
Release
  Acetabulum
    Left ØQN5
    Right ØQN4
  Adenoids ØCNQ
  Ampulla of Vater ØFNC
  Anal Sphincter ØDNR
  Anterior Chamber
    Left Ø8N33ZZ
    Right Ø8N23ZZ
  Anus ØDNQ
  Aorta
    Abdominal Ø4NØ
    Thoracic ◀▥
      Ascending/Arch Ø2NX ◀
      Descending Ø2NW ◀
  Aortic Body ØGND
  Appendix ØDNJ
  Artery
    Anterior Tibial
      Left Ø4NQ
      Right Ø4NP
    Axillary
      Left Ø3N6
      Right Ø3N5
    Brachial
      Left Ø3N8
      Right Ø3N7
    Celiac Ø4N1
    Colic
      Left Ø4N7
      Middle Ø4N8
      Right Ø4N6

Release *(Continued)*
  Artery *(Continued)*
    Common Carotid
      Left Ø3NJ
      Right Ø3NH
    Common Iliac
      Left Ø4ND
      Right Ø4NC
    External Carotid
      Left Ø3NN
      Right Ø3NM
    External Iliac
      Left Ø4NJ
      Right Ø4NH
    Face Ø3NR
    Femoral
      Left Ø4NL
      Right Ø4NK
    Foot
      Left Ø4NW
      Right Ø4NV
    Gastric Ø4N2
    Hand
      Left Ø3NF
      Right Ø3ND
    Hepatic Ø4N3
    Inferior Mesenteric Ø4NB
    Innominate Ø3N2
    Internal Carotid
      Left Ø3NL
      Right Ø3NK
    Internal Iliac
      Left Ø4NF
      Right Ø4NE
    Internal Mammary
      Left Ø3N1
      Right Ø3NØ
    Intracranial Ø3NG
    Lower Ø4NY
    Peroneal
      Left Ø4NU
      Right Ø4NT
    Popliteal
      Left Ø4NN
      Right Ø4NM
    Posterior Tibial
      Left Ø4NS
      Right Ø4NR
    Pulmonary
      Left Ø2NR
      Right Ø2NQ
    Pulmonary Trunk Ø2NP
    Radial
      Left Ø3NC
      Right Ø3NB
    Renal
      Left Ø4NA
      Right Ø4N9
    Splenic Ø4N4
    Subclavian
      Left Ø3N4
      Right Ø3N3
    Superior Mesenteric Ø4N5
    Temporal
      Left Ø3NT
      Right Ø3NS
    Thyroid
      Left Ø3NV
      Right Ø3NU
    Ulnar
      Left Ø3NA
      Right Ø3N9
    Upper Ø3NY
    Vertebral
      Left Ø3NQ
      Right Ø3NP
  Atrium
    Left Ø2N7
    Right Ø2N6
  Auditory Ossicle
    Left Ø9NAØZZ
    Right Ø9N9ØZZ

Release *(Continued)*
  Basal Ganglia ØØN8
  Bladder ØTNB
  Bladder Neck ØTNC
  Bone
    Ethmoid
      Left ØNNG
      Right ØNNF
    Frontal
      Left ØNN2
      Right ØNN1
    Hyoid ØNNX
    Lacrimal
      Left ØNNJ
      Right ØNNH
    Nasal ØNNB
    Occipital
      Left ØNN8
      Right ØNN7
    Palatine
      Left ØNNL
      Right ØNNK
    Parietal
      Left ØNN4
      Right ØNN3
    Pelvic
      Left ØQN3
      Right ØQN2
    Sphenoid
      Left ØNND
      Right ØNNC
    Temporal
      Left ØNN6
      Right ØNN5
    Zygomatic
      Left ØNNN
      Right ØNNM
  Brain ØØNØ
  Breast
    Bilateral ØHNV
    Left ØHNU
    Right ØHNT
  Bronchus
    Lingula ØBN9
    Lower Lobe
      Left ØBNB
      Right ØBN6
    Main
      Left ØBN7
      Right ØBN3
    Middle Lobe, Right ØBN5
    Upper Lobe
      Left ØBN8
      Right ØBN4
  Buccal Mucosa ØCN4
  Bursa and Ligament
    Abdomen
      Left ØMNJ
      Right ØMNH
    Ankle
      Left ØMNR
      Right ØMNQ
    Elbow
      Left ØMN4
      Right ØMN3
    Foot
      Left ØMNT
      Right ØMNS
    Hand
      Left ØMN8
      Right ØMN7
    Head and Neck ØMNØ
    Hip
      Left ØMNM
      Right ØMNL
    Knee
      Left ØMNP
      Right ØMNN
    Lower Extremity
      Left ØMNW
      Right ØMNV

◀ New   ◀||| Revised   ~~deleted~~ Deleted

Release *(Continued)*
  Joint *(Continued)*
    Temporomandibular
      Left ØRND
      Right ØRNC
    Thoracic Vertebral ØRN6
    Thoracolumbar Vertebral
      ØRNA
    Toe Phalangeal
      Left ØSNQ
      Right ØSNP
    Wrist
      Left ØRNP
      Right ØRNN
  Kidney
    Left ØTN1
    Right ØTNØ
  Kidney Pelvis
    Left ØTN4
    Right ØTN3
  Larynx ØCNS
  Lens
    Left Ø8NK3ZZ
    Right Ø8NJ3ZZ
  Lip
    Lower ØCN1
    Upper ØCNØ
  Liver ØFNØ
    Left Lobe ØFN2
    Right Lobe ØFN1
  Lung
    Bilateral ØBNM
    Left ØBNL
    Lower Lobe
      Left ØBNJ
      Right ØBNF
    Middle Lobe, Right ØBND
    Right ØBNK
    Upper Lobe
      Left ØBNG
      Right ØBNC
  Lung Lingula ØBNH
  Lymphatic
    Aortic Ø7ND
    Axillary
      Left Ø7N6
      Right Ø7N5
    Head Ø7NØ
    Inguinal
      Left Ø7NJ
      Right Ø7NH
    Internal Mammary
      Left Ø7N9
      Right Ø7N8
    Lower Extremity
      Left Ø7NG
      Right Ø7NF
    Mesenteric Ø7NB
    Neck
      Left Ø7N2
      Right Ø7N1
    Pelvis Ø7NC
    Thoracic Duct Ø7NK
    Thorax Ø7N7
    Upper Extremity
      Left Ø7N4
      Right Ø7N3
  Mandible
    Left ØNNV
    Right ØNNT
  Maxilla
    Left ØNNS
    Right ØNNR
  Medulla Oblongata ØØND
  Mesentery ØDNV
  Metacarpal
    Left ØPNQ
    Right ØPNP
  Metatarsal
    Left ØQNP
    Right ØQNN

Release *(Continued)*
  Muscle
    Abdomen
      Left ØKNL
      Right ØKNK
    Extraocular
      Left Ø8NM
      Right Ø8NL
    Facial ØKN1
    Foot
      Left ØKNW
      Right ØKNV
    Hand
      Left ØKND
      Right ØKNC
    Head ØKNØ
    Hip
      Left ØKNP
      Right ØKNN
    Lower Arm and Wrist
      Left ØKNB
      Right ØKN9
    Lower Leg
      Left ØKNT
      Right ØKNS
    Neck
      Left ØKN3
      Right ØKN2
    Papillary Ø2ND
    Perineum ØKNM
    Shoulder
      Left ØKN6
      Right ØKN5
    Thorax
      Left ØKNJ
      Right ØKNH
    Tongue, Palate, Pharynx ØKN4
    Trunk
      Left ØKNG
      Right ØKNF
    Upper Arm
      Left ØKN8
      Right ØKN7
    Upper Leg
      Left ØKNR
      Right ØKNQ
  Nasopharynx Ø9NN
  Nerve
    Abdominal Sympathetic Ø1NM
    Abducens ØØNL
    Accessory ØØNR
    Acoustic ØØNN
    Brachial Plexus Ø1N3
    Cervical Ø1N1
    Cervical Plexus Ø1NØ
    Facial ØØNM
    Femoral Ø1ND
    Glossopharyngeal ØØNP
    Head and Neck Sympathetic Ø1NK
    Hypoglossal ØØNS
    Lumbar Ø1NB
    Lumbar Plexus Ø1N9
    Lumbar Sympathetic Ø1NN
    Lumbosacral Plexus Ø1NA
    Median Ø1N5
    Oculomotor ØØNH
    Olfactory ØØNF
    Optic ØØNG
    Peroneal Ø1NH
    Phrenic Ø1N2
    Pudendal Ø1NC
    Radial Ø1N6
    Sacral Ø1NR
    Sacral Plexus Ø1NQ
    Sacral Sympathetic Ø1NP
    Sciatic Ø1NF
    Thoracic Ø1N8
    Thoracic Sympathetic Ø1NL
    Tibial Ø1NG
    Trigeminal ØØNK
    Trochlear ØØNJ
    Ulnar Ø1N4
    Vagus ØØNQ

Release *(Continued)*
  Nipple
    Left ØHNX
    Right ØHNW
  Nose Ø9NK
  Omentum
    Greater ØDNS
    Lesser ØDNT
  Orbit
    Left ØNNQ
    Right ØNNP
  Ovary
    Bilateral ØUN2
    Left ØUN1
    Right ØUNØ
  Palate
    Hard ØCN2
    Soft ØCN3
  Pancreas ØFNG
  Para-aortic Body ØGN9
  Paraganglion Extremity ØGNF
  Parathyroid Gland ØGNR
    Inferior
      Left ØGNP
      Right ØGNN
    Multiple ØGNQ
    Superior
      Left ØGNM
      Right ØGNL
  Patella
    Left ØQNF
    Right ØQND
  Penis ØVNS
  Pericardium Ø2NN
  Peritoneum ØDNW
  Phalanx
    Finger
      Left ØPNV
      Right ØPNT
    Thumb
      Left ØPNS
      Right ØPNR
    Toe
      Left ØQNR
      Right ØQNQ
  Pharynx ØCNM
  Pineal Body ØGN1
  Pleura
    Left ØBNP
    Right ØBNN
  Pons ØØNB
  Prepuce ØVNT
  Prostate ØVNØ
  Radius
    Left ØPNJ
    Right ØPNH
  Rectum ØDNP
  Retina
    Left Ø8NF3ZZ
    Right Ø8NE3ZZ
  Retinal Vessel
    Left Ø8NH3ZZ
    Right Ø8NG3ZZ
  Rib
    Left ØPN2
    Right ØPN1
  Sacrum ØQN1
  Scapula
    Left ØPN6
    Right ØPN5
  Sclera
    Left Ø8N7XZZ
    Right Ø8N6XZZ
  Scrotum ØVN5
  Septum
    Atrial Ø2N5
    Nasal Ø9NM
    Ventricular Ø2NM
  Sinus
    Accessory Ø9NP
    Ethmoid
      Left Ø9NV
      Right Ø9NU

◀ New   ◀ Revised   ~~deleted~~ Deleted

Release *(Continued)*
  Vein *(Continued)*
    Renal
      Left 06NB
      Right 06N9
    Splenic 06N1
    Subclavian
      Left 05N6
      Right 05N5
    Superior Mesenteric 06N5
    Upper 05NY
    Vertebral
      Left 05NS
      Right 05NR
  Vena Cava
    Inferior 06N0
    Superior 02NV
  Ventricle
    Left 02NL
    Right 02NK
  Vertebra
    Cervical 0PN3
    Lumbar 0QN0
    Thoracic 0PN4
  Vesicle
    Bilateral 0VN3
    Left 0VN2
    Right 0VN1
  Vitreous
    Left 08N53ZZ
    Right 08N43ZZ
  Vocal Cord
    Left 0CNV
    Right 0CNT
  Vulva 0UNM
Relocation *see* Reposition
Removal
  Abdominal Wall 2W53X
  Anorectal 2Y53X5Z
  Arm
    Lower
      Left 2W5DX
      Right 2W5CX
    Upper
      Left 2W5BX
      Right 2W5AX
  Back 2W55X
  Chest Wall 2W54X
  Ear 2Y52X5Z
  Extremity
    Lower
      Left 2W5MX
      Right 2W5LX
    Upper
      Left 2W59X
      Right 2W58X
  Face 2W51X
  Finger
    Left 2W5KX
    Right 2W5JX
  Foot
    Left 2W5TX
    Right 2W5SX
  Genital Tract, Female 2Y54X5Z
  Hand
    Left 2W5FX
    Right 2W5EX
  Head 2W50X
  Inguinal Region
    Left 2W57X
    Right 2W56X
  Leg
    Lower
      Left 2W5RX
      Right 2W5QX
    Upper
      Left 2W5PX
      Right 2W5NX
  Mouth and Pharynx 2Y50X5Z
  Nasal 2Y51X5Z
  Neck 2W52X

Removal *(Continued)*
  Thumb
    Left 2W5HX
    Right 2W5GX
  Toe
    Left 2W5VX
    Right 2W5UX
  Urethra 2Y55X5Z
Removal of device from
  Abdominal Wall 0WPF
  Acetabulum
    Left 0QP5
    Right 0QP4
  Anal Sphincter 0DPR
  Anus 0DPQ
  Artery
    Lower 04PY
    Upper 03PY
  Back
    Lower 0WPL
    Upper 0WPK
  Bladder 0TPB
  Bone
    Facial 0NPW
    Lower 0QPY
    Nasal 0NPB
    Pelvic
      Left 0QP3
      Right 0QP2
    Upper 0PPY
  Bone Marrow 07PT
  Brain 00P0
  Breast
    Left 0HPU
    Right 0HPT
  Bursa and Ligament
    Lower 0MPY
    Upper 0MPX
  Carpal
    Left 0PPN
    Right 0PPM
  Cavity, Cranial 0WP1
  Cerebral Ventricle 00P6
  Chest Wall 0WP8
  Cisterna Chyli 07PL
  Clavicle
    Left 0PPB
    Right 0PP9
  Coccyx 0QPS
  Diaphragm 0BPT
  Disc
    Cervical Vertebral 0RP3
    Cervicothoracic Vertebral 0RP5
    Lumbar Vertebral 0SP2
    Lumbosacral 0SP4
    Thoracic Vertebral 0RP9
    Thoracolumbar Vertebral 0RPB
  Duct
    Hepatobiliary 0FPB
    Pancreatic 0FPD
  Ear
    Inner
      Left 09PE
      Right 09PD
    Left 09PJ
    Right 09PH
  Epididymis and Spermatic Cord 0VPM
  Esophagus 0DP5
  Extremity
    Lower
      Left 0YPB
      Right 0YP9
    Upper
      Left 0XP7
      Right 0XP6
  Eye
    Left 08P1
    Right 08P0
  Face 0WP2
  Fallopian Tube 0UP8

Removal of device from *(Continued)*
  Femoral Shaft
    Left 0QP9
    Right 0QP8
  Femur
    Lower
      Left 0QPC
      Right 0QPB
    Upper
      Left 0QP7
      Right 0QP6
  Fibula
    Left 0QPK
    Right 0QPJ
  Finger Nail 0HPQX
  Gallbladder 0FP4
  Gastrointestinal Tract 0WPP
  Genitourinary Tract 0WPR
  Gland
    Adrenal 0GP5
    Endocrine 0GPS
    Pituitary 0GP0
    Salivary 0CPA
  Glenoid Cavity
    Left 0PP8
    Right 0PP7
  Great Vessel 02PY
  Hair 0HPSX
  Head 0WP0
  Heart 02PA
  Humeral Head
    Left 0PPD
    Right 0PPC
  Humeral Shaft
    Left 0PPG
    Right 0PPF
  Intestinal Tract
    Lower 0DPD
    Upper 0DP0
  Jaw
    Lower 0WP5
    Upper 0WP4
  Joint
    Acromioclavicular
      Left 0RPH
      Right 0RPG
    Ankle
      Left 0SPG
      Right 0SPF
    Carpal
      Left 0RPR
      Right 0RPQ
    Cervical Vertebral 0RP1
    Cervicothoracic Vertebral 0RP4
    Coccygeal 0SP6
    Elbow
      Left 0RPM
      Right 0RPL
    Finger Phalangeal
      Left 0RPX
      Right 0RPW
    Hip
      Left 0SPB
        Acetabular Surface 0SPE ◄
        Femoral Surface 0SPS ◄
      Right 0SP9
        Acetabular Surface 0SPA ◄
        Femoral Surface 0SPR ◄
    Knee
      Left 0SPD
        Femoral Surface 0SPU ◄
        Tibial Surface 0SPW ◄
      Right 0SPC
        Femoral Surface 0SPT ◄
        Tibial Surface 0SPV ◄
    Lumbar Vertebral 0SP0
    Lumbosacral 0SP3
    Metacarpocarpal
      Left 0RPT
      Right 0RPS

Removal of device from (Continued)
  Joint (Continued)
    Metacarpophalangeal
      Left 0RPV
      Right 0RPU
    Metatarsal-Phalangeal
      Left 0SPN
      Right 0SPM
    Metatarsal-Tarsal
      Left 0SPL
      Right 0SPK
    Occipital-cervical 0RP0
    Sacrococcygeal 0SP5
    Sacroiliac
      Left 0SP8
      Right 0SP7
    Shoulder
      Left 0RPK
      Right 0RPJ
    Sternoclavicular
      Left 0RPF
      Right 0RPE
    Tarsal
      Left 0SPJ
      Right 0SPH
    Temporomandibular
      Left 0RPD
      Right 0RPC
    Thoracic Vertebral 0RP6
    Thoracolumbar Vertebral
      0RPA
    Toe Phalangeal
      Left 0SPQ
      Right 0SPP
    Wrist
      Left 0RPP
      Right 0RPN
  Kidney 0TP5
  Larynx 0CPS
  Lens
    Left 08PK3JZ
    Right 08PJ3JZ
  Liver 0FP0
  Lung
    Left 0BPL
    Right 0BPK
  Lymphatic 07PN
    Thoracic Duct 07PK
  Mediastinum 0WPC
  Mesentery 0DPV
  Metacarpal
    Left 0PPQ
    Right 0PPP
  Metatarsal
    Left 0QPP
    Right 0QPN
  Mouth and Throat 0CPY
  Muscle
    Extraocular
      Left 08PM
      Right 08PL
    Lower 0KPY
    Upper 0KPX
  Neck 0WP6
  Nerve
    Cranial 00PE
    Peripheral 01PY
  Nose 09PK
  Omentum 0DPU
  Ovary 0UP3
  Pancreas 0FPG
  Parathyroid Gland 0GPR
  Patella
    Left 0QPF
    Right 0QPD
  Pelvic Cavity 0WPJ
  Penis 0VPS
  Pericardial Cavity 0WPD
  Perineum
    Female 0WPN
    Male 0WPM

Removal of device from (Continued)
  Peritoneal Cavity 0WPG
  Peritoneum 0DPW
  Phalanx
    Finger
      Left 0PPV
      Right 0PPT
    Thumb
      Left 0PPS
      Right 0PPR
    Toe
      Left 0QPR
      Right 0QPQ
  Pineal Body 0GP1
  Pleura 0BPQ
  Pleural Cavity
    Left 0WPB
    Right 0WP9
  Products of Conception 10P0
  Prostate and Seminal Vesicles 0VP4
  Radius
    Left 0PPJ
    Right 0PPH
  Rectum 0DPP
  Respiratory Tract 0WPQ
  Retroperitoneum 0WPH
  Rib
    Left 0PP2
    Right 0PP1
  Sacrum 0QP1
  Scapula
    Left 0PP6
    Right 0PP5
  Scrotum and Tunica Vaginalis
    0VP8
  Sinus 09PY
  Skin 0HPPX
  Skull 0NP0
  Spinal Canal 00PU
  Spinal Cord 00PV
  Spleen 07PP
  Sternum 0PP0
  Stomach 0DP6
  Subcutaneous Tissue and Fascia
    Head and Neck 0JPS
    Lower Extremity 0JPW
    Trunk 0JPT
    Upper Extremity 0JPV
  Tarsal
    Left 0QPM
    Right 0QPL
  Tendon
    Lower 0LPY
    Upper 0LPX
  Testis 0VPD
  Thymus 07PM
  Thyroid Gland 0GPK
  Tibia
    Left 0QPH
    Right 0QPG
  Toe Nail 0HPRX
  Trachea 0BP1
  Tracheobronchial Tree 0BP0
  Tympanic Membrane
    Left 09P8
    Right 09P7
  Ulna
    Left 0PPL
    Right 0PPK
  Ureter 0TP9
  Urethra 0TPD
  Uterus and Cervix 0UPD
  Vagina and Cul-de-sac 0UPH
  Vas Deferens 0VPR
  Vein
    Azygos 05P0 ◄
    Innominate ◄
      Left 05P4 ◄
      Right 05P3 ◄
    Lower 06PY
    Upper 05PY

Removal of device from (Continued)
  Vertebra
    Cervical 0PP3
    Lumbar 0QP0
    Thoracic 0PP4
  Vulva 0UPM
Renal calyx
  use Kidney, Right
  use Kidney, Left
  use Kidneys, Bilateral
  use Kidney
Renal capsule
  use Kidney, Right
  use Kidney, Left
  use Kidneys, Bilateral
  use Kidney
Renal cortex
  use Kidney, Right
  use Kidney, Left
  use Kidneys, Bilateral
  use Kidney
Renal dialysis see Performance, Urinary 5A1D
Renal plexus use Abdominal Sympathetic
  Nerve
Renal segment
  use Kidney, Right
  use Kidney, Left
  use Kidneys, Bilateral
  use Kidney
Renal segmental artery
  use Renal Artery, Right
  use Renal Artery, Left
Reopening, operative site
  Control of bleeding see Control bleeding in
  Inspection only see Inspection ◄▥
Repair
  Abdominal Wall 0WQF
  Acetabulum
    Left 0QQ5
    Right 0QQ4
  Adenoids 0CQQ
  Ampulla of Vater 0FQC
  Anal Sphincter 0DQR
  Ankle Region
    Left 0YQL
    Right 0YQK
  Anterior Chamber
    Left 08Q33ZZ
    Right 08Q23ZZ
  Anus 0DQQ
  Aorta
    Abdominal 04Q0
    Thoracic ◄▥
      Ascending/Arch 02QX ◄
      Descending 02QW ◄
  Aortic Body 0GQD
  Appendix 0DQJ
  Arm
    Lower
      Left 0XQF
      Right 0XQD
    Upper
      Left 0XQ9
      Right 0XQ8
  Artery
    Anterior Tibial
      Left 04QQ
      Right 04QP
    Axillary
      Left 03Q6
      Right 03Q5
    Brachial
      Left 03Q8
      Right 03Q7
    Celiac 04Q1
    Colic
      Left 04Q7
      Middle 04Q8
      Right 04Q6
    Common Carotid
      Left 03QJ
      Right 03QH

◄ New   ◄▥ Revised   ~~deleted~~ Deleted

Repair *(Continued)*
  Artery *(Continued)*
    Common Iliac
      Left 04QD
      Right 04QC
    Coronary
      ~~Four or More Sites 02Q3~~
      ~~One Site 02Q0~~
      ~~Three Sites 02Q2~~
      ~~Two Sites 02Q1~~
      Four or More Arteries 02Q3 ◄
      One Artery 02Q0 ◄
      Three Arteries 02Q2 ◄
      Two Arteries 02Q1 ◄
    External Carotid
      Left 03QN
      Right 03QM
    External Iliac
      Left 04QJ
      Right 04QH
    Face 03QR
    Femoral
      Left 04QL
      Right 04QK
    Foot
      Left 04QW
      Right 04QV
    Gastric 04Q2
    Hand
      Left 03QF
      Right 03QD
    Hepatic 04Q3
    Inferior Mesenteric 04QB
    Innominate 03Q2
    Internal Carotid
      Left 03QL
      Right 03QK
    Internal Iliac
      Left 04QF
      Right 04QE
    Internal Mammary
      Left 03Q1
      Right 03Q0
    Intracranial 03QG
    Lower 04QY
    Peroneal
      Left 04QU
      Right 04QT
    Popliteal
      Left 04QN
      Right 04QM
    Posterior Tibial
      Left 04QS
      Right 04QR
    Pulmonary
      Left 02QR
      Right 02QQ
    Pulmonary Trunk 02QP
    Radial
      Left 03QC
      Right 03QB
    Renal
      Left 04QA
      Right 04Q9
    Splenic 04Q4
    Subclavian
      Left 03Q4
      Right 03Q3
    Superior Mesenteric 04Q5
    Temporal
      Left 03QT
      Right 03QS
    Thyroid
      Left 03QV
      Right 03QU
    Ulnar
      Left 03QA
      Right 03Q9
    Upper 03QY
    Vertebral
      Left 03QQ
      Right 03QP

Repair *(Continued)*
  Atrium
    Left 02Q7
    Right 02Q6
  Auditory Ossicle
    Left 09QA0ZZ
    Right 09Q90ZZ
  Axilla
    Left 0XQ5
    Right 0XQ4
  Back
    Lower 0WQL
    Upper 0WQK
  Basal Ganglia 00Q8
  Bladder 0TQB
  Bladder Neck 0TQC
  Bone
    Ethmoid
      Left 0NQG
      Right 0NQF
    Frontal
      Left 0NQ2
      Right 0NQ1
    Hyoid 0NQX
    Lacrimal
      Left 0NQJ
      Right 0NQH
    Nasal 0NQB
    Occipital
      Left 0NQ8
      Right 0NQ7
    Palatine
      Left 0NQL
      Right 0NQK
    Parietal
      Left 0NQ4
      Right 0NQ3
    Pelvic
      Left 0QQ3
      Right 0QQ2
    Sphenoid
      Left 0NQD
      Right 0NQC
    Temporal
      Left 0NQ6
      Right 0NQ5
    Zygomatic
      Left 0NQN
      Right 0NQM
  Brain 00Q0
  Breast
    Bilateral 0HQV
    Left 0HQU
    Right 0HQT
    Supernumerary 0HQY
  Bronchus
    Lingula 0BQ9
    Lower Lobe
      Left 0BQB
      Right 0BQ6
    Main
      Left 0BQ7
      Right 0BQ3
    Middle Lobe, Right 0BQ5
    Upper Lobe
      Left 0BQ8
      Right 0BQ4
  Buccal Mucosa 0CQ4
  Bursa and Ligament
    Abdomen
      Left 0MQJ
      Right 0MQH
    Ankle
      Left 0MQR
      Right 0MQQ
    Elbow
      Left 0MQ4
      Right 0MQ3
    Foot
      Left 0MQT
      Right 0MQS

Repair *(Continued)*
  Bursa and Ligament *(Continued)*
    Hand
      Left 0MQ8
      Right 0MQ7
    Head and Neck 0MQ0
    Hip
      Left 0MQM
      Right 0MQL
    Knee
      Left 0MQP
      Right 0MQN
    Lower Extremity
      Left 0MQW
      Right 0MQV
    Perineum 0MQK
    Shoulder
      Left 0MQ2
      Right 0MQ1
    Thorax
      Left 0MQG
      Right 0MQF
    Trunk
      Left 0MQD
      Right 0MQC
    Upper Extremity
      Left 0MQB
      Right 0MQ9
    Wrist
      Left 0MQ6
      Right 0MQ5
  Buttock
    Left 0YQ1
    Right 0YQ0
  Carina 0BQ2
  Carotid Bodies, Bilateral 0GQ8
  Carotid Body
    Left 0GQ6
    Right 0GQ7
  Carpal
    Left 0PQN
    Right 0PQM
  Cecum 0DQH
  Cerebellum 00QC
  Cerebral Hemisphere 00Q7
  Cerebral Meninges 00Q1
  Cerebral Ventricle 00Q6
  Cervix 0UQC
  Chest Wall 0WQ8
  Chordae Tendineae 02Q9
  Choroid
    Left 08QB
    Right 08QA
  Cisterna Chyli 07QL
  Clavicle
    Left 0PQB
    Right 0PQ9
  Clitoris 0UQJ
  Coccygeal Glomus 0GQB
  Coccyx 0QQS
  Colon
    Ascending 0DQK
    Descending 0DQM
    Sigmoid 0DQN
    Transverse 0DQL
  Conduction Mechanism 02Q8
  Conjunctiva
    Left 08QTXZZ
    Right 08QSXZZ
  Cord
    Bilateral 0VQH
    Left 0VQG
    Right 0VQF
  Cornea
    Left 08Q9XZZ
    Right 08Q8XZZ
  Cul-de-sac 0UQF
  Diaphragm
    Left 0BQS
    Right 0BQR

◀ New   ◀▥ Revised   ~~deleted~~ Deleted

Repair *(Continued)*
  Kidney Pelvis
    Left 0TQ4
    Right 0TQ3
  Knee Region
    Left 0YQG
    Right 0YQF
  Larynx 0CQS
  Leg
    Lower
      Left 0YQJ
      Right 0YQH
    Upper
      Left 0YQD
      Right 0YQC
  Lens
    Left 08QK3ZZ
    Right 08QJ3ZZ
  Lip
    Lower 0CQ1
    Upper 0CQ0
  Liver 0FQ0
    Left Lobe 0FQ2
    Right Lobe 0FQ1
  Lung
    Bilateral 0BQM
    Left 0BQL
    Lower Lobe
      Left 0BQJ
      Right 0BQF
    Middle Lobe, Right 0BQD
    Right 0BQK
    Upper Lobe
      Left 0BQG
      Right 0BQC
  Lung Lingula 0BQH
  Lymphatic
    Aortic 07QD
    Axillary
      Left 07Q6
      Right 07Q5
    Head 07Q0
    Inguinal
      Left 07QJ
      Right 07QH
    Internal Mammary
      Left 07Q9
      Right 07Q8
    Lower Extremity
      Left 07QG
      Right 07QF
    Mesenteric 07QB
    Neck
      Left 07Q2
      Right 07Q1
    Pelvis 07QC
    Thoracic Duct 07QK
    Thorax 07Q7
    Upper Extremity
      Left 07Q4
      Right 07Q3
  Mandible
    Left 0NQV
    Right 0NQT
  Maxilla
    Left 0NQS
    Right 0NQR
  Mediastinum 0WQC
  Medulla Oblongata 00QD
  Mesentery 0DQV
  Metacarpal
    Left 0PQQ
    Right 0PQP
  Metatarsal
    Left 0QQP
    Right 0QQN
  Muscle
    Abdomen
      Left 0KQL
      Right 0KQK

Repair *(Continued)*
  Muscle *(Continued)*
    Extraocular
      Left 08QM
      Right 08QL
    Facial 0KQ1
    Foot
      Left 0KQW
      Right 0KQV
    Hand
      Left 0KQD
      Right 0KQC
    Head 0KQ0
    Hip
      Left 0KQP
      Right 0KQN
    Lower Arm and Wrist
      Left 0KQB
      Right 0KQ9
    Lower Leg
      Left 0KQT
      Right 0KQS
    Neck
      Left 0KQ3
      Right 0KQ2
    Papillary 02QD
    Perineum 0KQM
    Shoulder
      Left 0KQ6
      Right 0KQ5
    Thorax
      Left 0KQJ
      Right 0KQH
    Tongue, Palate, Pharynx 0KQ4
    Trunk
      Left 0KQG
      Right 0KQF
    Upper Arm
      Left 0KQ8
      Right 0KQ7
    Upper Leg
      Left 0KQR
      Right 0KQQ
  Nasopharynx 09QN
  Neck 0WQ6
  Nerve
    Abdominal Sympathetic 01QM
    Abducens 00QL
    Accessory 00QR
    Acoustic 00QN
    Brachial Plexus 01Q3
    Cervical 01Q1
    Cervical Plexus 01Q0
    Facial 00QM
    Femoral 01QD
    Glossopharyngeal 00QP
    Head and Neck Sympathetic 01QK
    Hypoglossal 00QS
    Lumbar 01QB
    Lumbar Plexus 01Q9
    Lumbar Sympathetic 01QN
    Lumbosacral Plexus 01QA
    Median 01Q5
    Oculomotor 00QH
    Olfactory 00QF
    Optic 00QG
    Peroneal 01QH
    Phrenic 01Q2
    Pudendal 01QC
    Radial 01Q6
    Sacral 01QR
    Sacral Plexus 01QQ
    Sacral Sympathetic 01QP
    Sciatic 01QF
    Thoracic 01Q8
    Thoracic Sympathetic 01QL
    Tibial 01QG
    Trigeminal 00QK
    Trochlear 00QJ
    Ulnar 01Q4
    Vagus 00QQ

Repair *(Continued)*
  Nipple
    Left 0HQX
    Right 0HQW
  Nose 09QK
  Omentum
    Greater 0DQS
    Lesser 0DQT
  Orbit
    Left 0NQQ
    Right 0NQP
  Ovary
    Bilateral 0UQ2
    Left 0UQ1
    Right 0UQ0
  Palate
    Hard 0CQ2
    Soft 0CQ3
  Pancreas 0FQG
  Para-aortic Body 0GQ9
  Paraganglion Extremity 0GQF
  Parathyroid Gland 0GQR
    Inferior
      Left 0GQP
      Right 0GQN
    Multiple 0GQQ
    Superior
      Left 0GQM
      Right 0GQL
  Patella
    Left 0QQF
    Right 0QQD
  Penis 0VQS
  Pericardium 02QN
  Perineum
    Female 0WQN
    Male 0WQM
  Peritoneum 0DQW
  Phalanx
    Finger
      Left 0PQV
      Right 0PQT
    Thumb
      Left 0PQS
      Right 0PQR
    Toe
      Left 0QQR
      Right 0QQQ
  Pharynx 0CQM
  Pineal Body 0GQ1
  Pleura
    Left 0BQP
    Right 0BQN
  Pons 00QB
  Prepuce 0VQT
  Products of Conception 10Q0
  Prostate 0VQ0
  Radius
    Left 0PQJ
    Right 0PQH
  Rectum 0DQP
  Retina
    Left 08QF3ZZ
    Right 08QE3ZZ
  Retinal Vessel
    Left 08QH3ZZ
    Right 08QG3ZZ
  Rib
    Left 0PQ2
    Right 0PQ1
  Sacrum 0QQ1
  Scapula
    Left 0PQ6
    Right 0PQ5
  Sclera
    Left 08Q7XZZ
    Right 08Q6XZZ
  Scrotum 0VQ5
  Septum
    Atrial 02Q5
    Nasal 09QM
    Ventricular 02QM

◀ New ◀||| Revised ~~deleted~~ Deleted

Replacement *(Continued)*
  Disc *(Continued)*
    Thoracic Vertebral ØRR90
    Thoracolumbar Vertebral ØRRBØ
  Duct
    Common Bile ØFR9
    Cystic ØFR8
    Hepatic
      Left ØFR6
      Right ØFR5
    Lacrimal
      Left Ø8RY
      Right Ø8RX
    Pancreatic ØFRD
      Accessory ØFRF
    Parotid
      Left ØCRC
      Right ØCRB
  Ear
    External
      Bilateral Ø9R2
      Left Ø9R1
      Right Ø9RØ
    Inner
      Left Ø9REØ
      Right Ø9RDØ
    Middle
      Left Ø9R6Ø
      Right Ø9R5Ø
  Epiglottis ØCRR
  Esophagus ØDR5
  Eye
    Left Ø8R1
    Right Ø8RØ
  Eyelid
    Lower
      Left Ø8RR
      Right Ø8RQ
    Upper
      Left Ø8RP
      Right Ø8RN
  Femoral Shaft
    Left ØQR9
    Right ØQR8
  Femur
    Lower
      Left ØQRC
      Right ØQRB
    Upper
      Left ØQR7
      Right ØQR6
  Fibula
    Left ØQRK
    Right ØQRJ
  Finger Nail ØHRQX
  Gingiva
    Lower ØCR6
    Upper ØCR5
  Glenoid Cavity
    Left ØPR8
    Right ØPR7
  Hair ØHRSX
  Humeral Head
    Left ØPRD
    Right ØPRC
  Humeral Shaft
    Left ØPRG
    Right ØPRF
  Iris
    Left Ø8RD3
    Right Ø8RC3
  Joint
    Acromioclavicular
      Left ØRRHØ
      Right ØRRGØ
    Ankle
      Left ØSRG
      Right ØSRF
    Carpal
      Left ØRRRØ
      Right ØRRQØ

Replacement *(Continued)*
  Joint *(Continued)*
    Cervical Vertebral ØRR10
    Cervicothoracic Vertebral ØRR40
    Coccygeal ØSR60
    Elbow
      Left ØRRMØ
      Right ØRRLØ
    Finger Phalangeal
      Left ØRRXØ
      Right ØRRWØ
    Hip
      Left ØSRB
        Acetabular Surface ØSRE
        Femoral Surface ØSRS
      Right ØSR9
        Acetabular Surface ØSRA
        Femoral Surface ØSRR
    Knee
      Left ØSRD
        Femoral Surface ØSRU
        Tibial Surface ØSRW
      Right ØSRC
        Femoral Surface ØSRT
        Tibial Surface ØSRV
    Lumbar Vertebral ØSR00
    Lumbosacral ØSR30
    Metacarpocarpal
      Left ØRRTØ
      Right ØRRSØ
    Metacarpophalangeal
      Left ØRRVØ
      Right ØRRUØ
    Metatarsal-Phalangeal
      Left ØSRNØ
      Right ØSRMØ
    Metatarsal-Tarsal
      Left ØSRLØ
      Right ØSRKØ
    Occipital-cervical ØRR00
    Sacrococcygeal ØSR50
    Sacroiliac
      Left ØSR80
      Right ØSR70
    Shoulder
      Left ØRRK
      Right ØRRJ
    Sternoclavicular
      Left ØRRFØ
      Right ØRREØ
    Tarsal
      Left ØSRJØ
      Right ØSRHØ
    Temporomandibular
      Left ØRRDØ
      Right ØRRCØ
    Thoracic Vertebral ØRR60
    Thoracolumbar Vertebral
      ØRRAØ
    Toe Phalangeal
      Left ØSRQØ
      Right ØSRPØ
    Wrist
      Left ØRRPØ
      Right ØRRNØ
  Kidney Pelvis
    Left ØTR4
    Right ØTR3
  Larynx ØCRS
  Lens
    Left Ø8RK3ØZ
    Right Ø8RJ3ØZ
  Lip
    Lower ØCR1
    Upper ØCRØ
  Mandible
    Left ØNRV
    Right ØNRT
  Maxilla
    Left ØNRS
    Right ØNRR

Replacement *(Continued)*
  Mesentery ØDRV
  Metacarpal
    Left ØPRQ
    Right ØPRP
  Metatarsal
    Left ØQRP
    Right ØQRN
  Muscle, Papillary Ø2RD
  Nasopharynx Ø9RN
  Nipple
    Left ØHRX
    Right ØHRW
  Nose Ø9RK
  Omentum
    Greater ØDRS
    Lesser ØDRT
  Orbit
    Left ØNRQ
    Right ØNRP
  Palate
    Hard ØCR2
    Soft ØCR3
  Patella
    Left ØQRF
    Right ØQRD
  Pericardium Ø2RN
  Peritoneum ØDRW
  Phalanx
    Finger
      Left ØPRV
      Right ØPRT
    Thumb
      Left ØPRS
      Right ØPRR
    Toe
      Left ØQRR
      Right ØQRQ
  Pharynx ØCRM
  Radius
    Left ØPRJ
    Right ØPRH
  Retinal Vessel
    Left Ø8RH3
    Right Ø8RG3
  Rib
    Left ØPR2
    Right ØPR1
  Sacrum ØQR1
  Scapula
    Left ØPR6
    Right ØPR5
  Sclera
    Left Ø8R7X
    Right Ø8R6X
  Septum
    Atrial Ø2R5
    Nasal Ø9RM
    Ventricular Ø2RM
  Skin
    Abdomen ØHR7
    Back ØHR6
    Buttock ØHR8
    Chest ØHR5
    Ear
      Left ØHR3
      Right ØHR2
    Face ØHR1
    Foot
      Left ØHRN
      Right ØHRM
    Genitalia ØHRA
    Hand
      Left ØHRG
      Right ØHRF
    Lower Arm
      Left ØHRE
      Right ØHRD
    Lower Leg
      Left ØHRL
      Right ØHRK

◀ New   ◀▥ Revised   ~~deleted~~ Deleted

◄ New   ◄▥ Revised   ~~deleted~~ Deleted

Reposition *(Continued)*
  Fallopian Tube
    Left 0US6
    Right 0US5
  Fallopian Tubes, Bilateral 0US7
  Femoral Shaft
    Left 0QS9
    Right 0QS8
  Femur
    Lower
      Left 0QSC
      Right 0QSB
    Upper
      Left 0QS7
      Right 0QS6
  Fibula
    Left 0QSK
    Right 0QSJ
  Gallbladder 0FS4
  Gland
    Adrenal
      Left 0GS2
      Right 0GS3
    Lacrimal
      Left 08SW
      Right 08SV
  Glenoid Cavity
    Left 0PS8
    Right 0PS7
  Hair 0HSSXZZ
  Humeral Head
    Left 0PSD
    Right 0PSC
  Humeral Shaft
    Left 0PSG
    Right 0PSF
  Ileum 0DSB
  Iris
    Left 08SD3ZZ
    Right 08SC3ZZ
  Jejunum 0DSA
  Joint
    Acromioclavicular
      Left 0RSH
      Right 0RSG
    Ankle
      Left 0SSG
      Right 0SSF
    Carpal
      Left 0RSR
      Right 0RSQ
    Cervical Vertebral 0RS1
    Cervicothoracic Vertebral
      0RS4
    Coccygeal 0SS6
    Elbow
      Left 0RSM
      Right 0RSL
    Finger Phalangeal
      Left 0RSX
      Right 0RSW
    Hip
      Left 0SSB
      Right 0SS9
    Knee
      Left 0SSD
      Right 0SSC
    Lumbar Vertebral 0SS0
    Lumbosacral 0SS3
    Metacarpocarpal
      Left 0RST
      Right 0RSS
    Metacarpophalangeal
      Left 0RSV
      Right 0RSU
    Metatarsal-Phalangeal
      Left 0SSN
      Right 0SSM
    Metatarsal-Tarsal
      Left 0SSL
      Right 0SSK

Reposition *(Continued)*
  Joint *(Continued)*
    Occipital-cervical 0RS0
    Sacrococcygeal 0SS5
    Sacroiliac
      Left 0SS8
      Right 0SS7
    Shoulder
      Left 0RSK
      Right 0RSJ
    Sternoclavicular
      Left 0RSF
      Right 0RSE
    Tarsal
      Left 0SSJ
      Right 0SSH
    Temporomandibular
      Left 0RSD
      Right 0RSC
    Thoracic Vertebral 0RS6
    Thoracolumbar Vertebral 0RSA
    Toe Phalangeal
      Left 0SSQ
      Right 0SSP
    Wrist
      Left 0RSP
      Right 0RSN
  Kidney
    Left 0TS1
    Right 0TS0
  Kidney Pelvis
    Left 0TS4
    Right 0TS3
  Kidneys, Bilateral 0TS2
  Lens
    Left 08SK3ZZ
    Right 08SJ3ZZ
  Lip
    Lower 0CS1
    Upper 0CS0
  Liver 0FS0
  Lung
    Left 0BSL0ZZ
    Lower Lobe
      Left 0BSJ0ZZ
      Right 0BSF0ZZ
    Middle Lobe, Right 0BSD0ZZ
    Right 0BSK0ZZ
    Upper Lobe
      Left 0BSG0ZZ
      Right 0BSC0ZZ
  Lung Lingula 0BSH0ZZ
  Mandible
    Left 0NSV
    Right 0NST
  Maxilla
    Left 0NSS
    Right 0NSR
  Metacarpal
    Left 0PSQ
    Right 0PSP
  Metatarsal
    Left 0QSP
    Right 0QSN
  Muscle
    Abdomen
      Left 0KSL
      Right 0KSK
    Extraocular
      Left 08SM
      Right 08SL
    Facial 0KS1
    Foot
      Left 0KSW
      Right 0KSV
    Hand
      Left 0KSD
      Right 0KSC
    Head 0KS0
    Hip
      Left 0KSP
      Right 0KSN

Reposition *(Continued)*
  Muscle *(Continued)*
    Lower Arm and Wrist
      Left 0KSB
      Right 0KS9
    Lower Leg
      Left 0KST
      Right 0KSS
    Neck
      Left 0KS3
      Right 0KS2
    Perineum 0KSM
    Shoulder
      Left 0KS6
      Right 0KS5
    Thorax
      Left 0KSJ
      Right 0KSH
    Tongue, Palate, Pharynx 0KS4
    Trunk
      Left 0KSG
      Right 0KSF
    Upper Arm
      Left 0KS8
      Right 0KS7
    Upper Leg
      Left 0KSR
      Right 0KSQ
  Nerve
    Abducens 00SL
    Accessory 00SR
    Acoustic 00SN
    Brachial Plexus 01S3
    Cervical 01S1
    Cervical Plexus 01S0
    Facial 00SM
    Femoral 01SD
    Glossopharyngeal 00SP
    Hypoglossal 00SS
    Lumbar 01SB
    Lumbar Plexus 01S9
    Lumbosacral Plexus 01SA
    Median 01S5
    Oculomotor 00SH
    Olfactory 00SF
    Optic 00SG
    Peroneal 01SH
    Phrenic 01S2
    Pudendal 01SC
    Radial 01S6
    Sacral 01SR
    Sacral Plexus 01SQ
    Sciatic 01SF
    Thoracic 01S8
    Tibial 01SG
    Trigeminal 00SK
    Trochlear 00SJ
    Ulnar 01S4
    Vagus 00SQ
  Nipple
    Left 0HSXXZZ
    Right 0HSWXZZ
  Nose 09SK
  Orbit
    Left 0NSQ
    Right 0NSP
  Ovary
    Bilateral 0US2
    Left 0US1
    Right 0US0
  Palate
    Hard 0CS2
    Soft 0CS3
  Pancreas 0FSG
  Parathyroid Gland 0GSR
    Inferior
      Left 0GSP
      Right 0GSN
    Multiple 0GSQ
    Superior
      Left 0GSM
      Right 0GSL

◀ New   ◀▦ Revised   ~~deleted~~ Deleted

◄ New   ◄ㅔ Revised   ~~deleted~~ Deleted

Resection (*Continued*)
  Bone (*Continued*)
    Parietal
      Left 0NT40ZZ
      Right 0NT30ZZ
    Pelvic
      Left 0QT30ZZ
      Right 0QT20ZZ
    Sphenoid
      Left 0NTD0ZZ
      Right 0NTC0ZZ
    Temporal
      Left 0NT60ZZ
      Right 0NT50ZZ
    Zygomatic
      Left 0NTN0ZZ
      Right 0NTM0ZZ
  Breast
    Bilateral 0HTV0ZZ
    Left 0HTU0ZZ
    Right 0HTT0ZZ
    Supernumerary 0HTY0ZZ
  Bronchus
    Lingula 0BT9
    Lower Lobe
      Left 0BTB
      Right 0BT6
    Main
      Left 0BT7
      Right 0BT3
    Middle Lobe, Right 0BT5
    Upper Lobe
      Left 0BT8
      Right 0BT4
  Bursa and Ligament
    Abdomen
      Left 0MTJ
      Right 0MTH
    Ankle
      Left 0MTR
      Right 0MTQ
    Elbow
      Left 0MT4
      Right 0MT3
    Foot
      Left 0MTT
      Right 0MTS
    Hand
      Left 0MT8
      Right 0MT7
    Head and Neck 0MT0
    Hip
      Left 0MTM
      Right 0MTL
    Knee
      Left 0MTP
      Right 0MTN
    Lower Extremity
      Left 0MTW
      Right 0MTV
    Perineum 0MTK
    Shoulder
      Left 0MT2
      Right 0MT1
    Thorax
      Left 0MTG
      Right 0MTF
    Trunk
      Left 0MTD
      Right 0MTC
    Upper Extremity
      Left 0MTB
      Right 0MT9
    Wrist
      Left 0MT6
      Right 0MT5
  Carina 0BT2
  Carotid Bodies, Bilateral 0GT8
  Carotid Body
    Left 0GT6
    Right 0GT7

Resection (*Continued*)
  Carpal
    Left 0PTN0ZZ
    Right 0PTM0ZZ
  Cecum 0DTH
  Cerebral Hemisphere 00T7
  Cervix 0UTC
  Chordae Tendineae 02T9
  Cisterna Chyli 07TL
  Clavicle
    Left 0PTB0ZZ
    Right 0PT90ZZ
  Clitoris 0UTJ
  Coccygeal Glomus 0GTB
  Coccyx 0QTS0ZZ
  Colon
    Ascending 0DTK
    Descending 0DTM
    Sigmoid 0DTN
    Transverse 0DTL
  Conduction Mechanism
    02T8
  Cord
    Bilateral 0VTH
    Left 0VTG
    Right 0VTF
  Cornea
    Left 08T9XZZ
    Right 08T8XZZ
  Cul-de-sac 0UTF
  Diaphragm
    Left 0BTS
    Right 0BTR
  Disc
    Cervical Vertebral 0RT30ZZ
    Cervicothoracic Vertebral 0RT50ZZ
    Lumbar Vertebral 0ST20ZZ
    Lumbosacral 0ST40ZZ
    Thoracic Vertebral 0RT90ZZ
    Thoracolumbar Vertebral 0RTB0ZZ
  Duct
    Common Bile 0FT9
    Cystic 0FT8
    Hepatic
      Left 0FT6
      Right 0FT5
    Lacrimal
      Left 08TY
      Right 08TX
    Pancreatic 0FTD
      Accessory 0FTF
    Parotid
      Left 0CTC0ZZ
      Right 0CTB0ZZ
  Duodenum 0DT9
  Ear
    External
      Left 09T1
      Right 09T0
    Inner
      Left 09TE0ZZ
      Right 09TD0ZZ
    Middle
      Left 09T60ZZ
      Right 09T50ZZ
  Epididymis
    Bilateral 0VTL
    Left 0VTK
    Right 0VTJ
  Epiglottis 0CTR
  Esophagogastric Junction 0DT4
  Esophagus 0DT5
    Lower 0DT3
    Middle 0DT2
    Upper 0DT1
  Eustachian Tube
    Left 09TG
    Right 09TF
  Eye
    Left 08T1XZZ
    Right 08T0XZZ

Resection (*Continued*)
  Eyelid
    Lower
      Left 08TR
      Right 08TQ
    Upper
      Left 08TP
      Right 08TN
  Fallopian Tube
    Left 0UT6
    Right 0UT5
  Fallopian Tubes, Bilateral 0UT7
  Femoral Shaft
    Left 0QT90ZZ
    Right 0QT80ZZ
  Femur
    Lower
      Left 0QTC0ZZ
      Right 0QTB0ZZ
    Upper
      Left 0QT70ZZ
      Right 0QT60ZZ
  Fibula
    Left 0QTK0ZZ
    Right 0QTJ0ZZ
  Finger Nail 0HTQXZZ
  Gallbladder 0FT4
  Gland
    Adrenal
      Bilateral 0GT4
      Left 0GT2
      Right 0GT3
    Lacrimal
      Left 08TW
      Right 08TV
    Minor Salivary 0CTJ0ZZ
    Parotid
      Left 0CT90ZZ
      Right 0CT80ZZ
    Pituitary 0GT0
    Sublingual
      Left 0CTF0ZZ
      Right 0CTD0ZZ
    Submaxillary
      Left 0CTH0ZZ
      Right 0CTG0ZZ
    Vestibular 0UTL
  Glenoid Cavity
    Left 0PT80ZZ
    Right 0PT70ZZ
  Glomus Jugulare 0GTC
  Humeral Head
    Left 0PTD0ZZ
    Right 0PTC0ZZ
  Humeral Shaft
    Left 0PTG0ZZ
    Right 0PTF0ZZ
  Hymen 0UTK
  Ileocecal Valve 0DTC
  Ileum 0DTB
  Intestine
    Large 0DTE
      Left 0DTG
      Right 0DTF
    Small 0DT8
  Iris
    Left 08TD3ZZ
    Right 08TC3ZZ
  Jejunum 0DTA
  Joint
    Acromioclavicular
      Left 0RTH0ZZ
      Right 0RTG0ZZ
    Ankle
      Left 0STG0ZZ
      Right 0STF0ZZ
    Carpal
      Left 0RTR0ZZ
      Right 0RTQ0ZZ
    Cervicothoracic Vertebral 0RT40ZZ
    Coccygeal 0ST60ZZ

◀ New   ◀‖‖ Revised   ~~deleted~~ Deleted

◀ New   ◀◀ Revised   ~~deleted~~ Deleted

Resection *(Continued)*
Spleen 07TP
Sternum 0PT00ZZ
Stomach 0DT6
  Pylorus 0DT7
Tarsal
  Left 0QTM0ZZ
  Right 0QTL0ZZ
Tendon
  Abdomen
    Left 0LTG
    Right 0LTF
  Ankle
    Left 0LTT
    Right 0LTS
  Foot
    Left 0LTW
    Right 0LTV
  Hand
    Left 0LT8
    Right 0LT7
  Head and Neck 0LT0
  Hip
    Left 0LTK
    Right 0LTJ
  Knee
    Left 0LTR
    Right 0LTQ
  Lower Arm and Wrist
    Left 0LT6
    Right 0LT5
  Lower Leg
    Left 0LTP
    Right 0LTN
  Perineum 0LTH
  Shoulder
    Left 0LT2
    Right 0LT1
  Thorax
    Left 0LTD
    Right 0LTC
  Trunk
    Left 0LTB
    Right 0LT9
  Upper Arm
    Left 0LT4
    Right 0LT3
  Upper Leg
    Left 0LTM
    Right 0LTL
Testis
  Bilateral 0VTC
  Left 0VTB
  Right 0VT9
Thymus 07TM
Thyroid Gland 0GTK
  Left Lobe 0GTG
  Right Lobe 0GTH
Tibia
  Left 0QTH0ZZ
  Right 0QTG0ZZ
Toe Nail 0HTRXZZ
Tongue 0CT7
Tonsils 0CTP
Tooth
  Lower 0CTX0Z
  Upper 0CTW0Z
Trachea 0BT1
Tunica Vaginalis
  Left 0VT7
  Right 0VT6
Turbinate, Nasal 09TL
Tympanic Membrane
  Left 09T8
  Right 09T7
Ulna
  Left 0PTL0ZZ
  Right 0PTK0ZZ
Ureter
  Left 0TT7
  Right 0TT6

Resection *(Continued)*
Urethra 0TTD
Uterine Supporting Structure 0UT4
Uterus 0UT9
Uvula 0CTN
Vagina 0UTG
Valve, Pulmonary 02TH
Vas Deferens
  Bilateral 0VTQ
  Left 0VTP
  Right 0VTN
Vesicle
  Bilateral 0VT3
  Left 0VT2
  Right 0VT1
Vitreous
  Left 08T53ZZ
  Right 08T43ZZ
Vocal Cord
  Left 0CTV
  Right 0CTT
Vulva 0UTM
Restoration, Cardiac, Single, Rhythm
  5A2204Z
RestoreAdvanced neurostimulator (SureScan)
  (MRI Safe) *use* Stimulator Generator,
  Multiple Array Rechargeable in 0JH
RestoreSensor neurostimulator (SureScan)
  (MRI Safe) *use* Stimulator Generator,
  Multiple Array Rechargeable in 0JH
RestoreUltra neurostimulator (SureScan)
  (MRI Safe) *use* Stimulator Generator,
  Multiple Array Rechargeable in
  0JH
Restriction
Ampulla of Vater 0FVC
Anus 0DVQ
Aorta
  Abdominal 04V0
    Ascending/Arch, Intraluminal Device,
      Branched or Fenestrated 02VX ◄
    Descending, Intraluminal Device,
      Branched or Fenestrated 02VW ◄
  Thoracic ◄▥
    Intraluminal Device, Branched or
      Fenestrated 04V0 ◄
Artery
  Anterior Tibial
    Left 04VQ
    Right 04VP
  Axillary
    Left 03V6
    Right 03V5
  Brachial
    Left 03V8
    Right 03V7
  Celiac 04V1
  Colic
    Left 04V7
    Middle 04V8
    Right 04V6
  Common Carotid
    Left 03VJ
    Right 03VH
  Common Iliac
    ~~Left 04VD~~
    ~~Right 04VC~~
    Left, Intraluminal Device, Branched or
      Fenestrated 04VD ◄
    Right, Intraluminal Device, Branched or
      Fenestrated 04VC ◄
  External Carotid
    Left 03VN
    Right 03VM
  External Iliac
    Left 04VJ
    Right 04VH
  Face 03VR
  Femoral
    Left 04VL
    Right 04VK

Restriction *(Continued)*
Artery *(Continued)*
  Foot
    Left 04VW
    Right 04VV
  Gastric 04V2
  Hand
    Left 03VF
    Right 03VD
  Hepatic 04V3
  Inferior Mesenteric 04VB
  Innominate 03V2
  Internal Carotid
    Left 03VL
    Right 03VK
  Internal Iliac
    Left 04VF
    Right 04VE
  Internal Mammary
    Left 03V1
    Right 03V0
  Intracranial 03VG
  Lower 04VY
  Peroneal
    Left 04VU
    Right 04VT
  Popliteal
    Left 04VN
    Right 04VM
  Posterior Tibial
    Left 04VS
    Right 04VR
  Pulmonary
    Left 02VR
    Right 02VQ
  Pulmonary Trunk 02VP
  Radial
    Left 03VC
    Right 03VB
  Renal
    Left 04VA
    Right 04V9
  Splenic 04V4
  Subclavian
    Left 03V4
    Right 03V3
  Superior Mesenteric 04V5
  Temporal
    Left 03VT
    Right 03VS
  Thyroid
    Left 03VV
    Right 03VU
  Ulnar
    Left 03VA
    Right 03V9
  Upper 03VY
  Vertebral
    Left 03VQ
    Right 03VP
Bladder 0TVB
Bladder Neck 0TVC
Bronchus
  Lingula 0BV9
  Lower Lobe
    Left 0BVB
    Right 0BV6
  Main
    Left 0BV7
    Right 0BV3
  Middle Lobe, Right 0BV5
  Upper Lobe
    Left 0BV8
    Right 0BV4
Carina 0BV2
Cecum 0DVH
Cervix 0UVC
Cisterna Chyli 07VL
Colon
  Ascending 0DVK
  Descending 0DVM

◀ New   ◀|||| Revised   ~~deleted~~ Deleted

◀ New   ◀▥ Revised   ~~deleted~~ Deleted

Revision of device in *(Continued)*
Subcutaneous Tissue and Fascia *(Continued)*
Trunk ØJWT
Upper Extremity ØJWV
Tarsal
Left ØQWM
Right ØQWL
Tendon
Lower ØLWY
Upper ØLWX
Testis ØVWD
Thymus Ø7WM
Thyroid Gland ØGWK
Tibia
Left ØQWH
Right ØQWG
Toe Nail ØHWRX
Trachea ØBW1
Tracheobronchial Tree ØBWØ
Tympanic Membrane
Left Ø9W8
Right Ø9W7
Ulna
Left ØPWL
Right ØPWK
Ureter ØTW9
Urethra ØTWD
Uterus and Cervix ØUWD
Vagina and Cul-de-sac ØUWH
Valve
Aortic Ø2WF
Mitral Ø2WG
Pulmonary Ø2WH
Tricuspid Ø2WJ
Vas Deferens ØVWR
Vein
Azygos Ø5WØ ◄
Innominate ◄
Left Ø5W4 ◄
Right Ø5W3 ◄
Lower Ø6WY
Upper Ø5WY
Vertebra
Cervical ØPW3
Lumbar ØQWØ
Thoracic ØPW4
Vulva ØUWM

Revo MRI™ SureScan® pacemaker *use*
Pacemaker, Dual Chamber in ØJH
rhBMP-2 *use* Recombinant Bone Morphogenetic
Protein
Rheos® System device *use* Stimulator
Generator in Subcutaneous Tissue
and Fascia
Rheos® System lead *use* Stimulator Lead in
Upper Arteries
Rhinopharynx *use* Nasopharynx
Rhinoplasty
see Alteration, Nose Ø9ØK
see Repair, Nose Ø9QK
see Replacement, Nose Ø9RK
see Supplement, Nose Ø9UK
Rhinorrhaphy *see* Repair, Nose Ø9QK
Rhinoscopy Ø9JKXZZ
Rhizotomy
see Division, Central Nervous System
ØØ8
see Division, Peripheral Nervous System
Ø18
Rhomboid major muscle
use Trunk Muscle, Right
use Trunk Muscle, Left
Rhomboid minor muscle
use Trunk Muscle, Right
use Trunk Muscle, Left
Rhythm electrocardiogram *see* Measurement,
Cardiac 4AØ2
Rhytidectomy *see* Face lift
Right ascending lumbar vein *use* Azygos
Vein
Right atrioventricular valve *use* Tricuspid
Valve
Right auricular appendix *use* Atrium,
Right
Right colic vein *use* Colic Vein
Right coronary sulcus *use* Heart, Right
Right gastric artery *use* Gastric Artery
Right gastroepiploic vein *use* Superior
Mesenteric Vein
Right inferior phrenic vein *use* Inferior Vena
Cava
Right inferior pulmonary vein *use* Pulmonary
Vein, Right
Right jugular trunk *use* Lymphatic, Right
Neck

Right lateral ventricle *use* Cerebral Ventricle
Right lymphatic duct *use* Lymphatic, Right
Neck
Right ovarian vein *use* Inferior Vena Cava
Right second lumbar vein *use* Inferior Vena
Cava
Right subclavian trunk *use* Lymphatic, Right
Neck
Right subcostal vein *use* Azygos Vein
Right superior pulmonary vein *use* Pulmonary
Vein, Right
Right suprarenal vein *use* Inferior Vena Cava
Right testicular vein *use* Inferior Vena Cava
Rima glottidis *use* Larynx
Risorius muscle *use* Facial Muscle
RNS System lead *use* Neurostimulator Lead in
Central Nervous System
RNS system neurostimulator generator *use*
Neurostimulator Generator in Head and
Facial Bones
Robotic Assisted Procedure
Extremity
Lower 8EØY
Upper 8EØX
Head and Neck Region 8EØ9
Trunk Region 8EØW
Rotation of fetal head
Forceps 10SØ7ZZ
Manual 10SØXZZ
Round ligament of uterus *use* Uterine
Supporting Structure
Round window
use Inner Ear, Right
use Inner Ear, Left
Roux-en-Y operation
see Bypass, Gastrointestinal System ØD1
see Bypass, Hepatobiliary System and
Pancreas ØF1
Rupture
Adhesions *see* Release
Fluid collection *see* Drainage

◄ New   ◄IIII Revised   ~~deleted~~ Deleted

S

Sacral ganglion *use* Sacral Sympathetic Nerve
Sacral lymph node *use* Lymphatic, Pelvis
Sacral nerve modulation (SNM) lead *use* Stimulator Lead in Urinary System
Sacral neuromodulation lead *use* Stimulator Lead in Urinary System
Sacral splanchnic nerve *use* Sacral Sympathetic Nerve
Sacrectomy *see* Excision, Lower Bones ØQB
Sacrococcygeal ligament
   use Trunk Bursa and Ligament, Right
   use Trunk Bursa and Ligament, Left
Sacrococcygeal symphysis *use* Sacrococcygeal Joint
Sacroiliac ligament
   use Trunk Bursa and Ligament, Right
   use Trunk Bursa and Ligament, Left
Sacrospinous ligament
   use Trunk Bursa and Ligament, Right
   use Trunk Bursa and Ligament, Left
Sacrotuberous ligament
   use Trunk Bursa and Ligament, Right
   use Trunk Bursa and Ligament, Left
Salpingectomy
   see Excision, Female Reproductive System ØUB
   see Resection, Female Reproductive System ØUT
Salpingolysis *see* Release, Female Reproductive System ØUN
Salpingopexy
   see Repair, Female Reproductive System ØUQ
   see Reposition, Female Reproductive System ØUS
Salpingopharyngeus muscle *use* Tongue, Palate, Pharynx Muscle
Salpingoplasty
   see Repair, Female Reproductive System ØUQ
   see Supplement, Female Reproductive System ØUU
Salpingorrhaphy *see* Repair, Female Reproductive System ØUQ
Salpingoscopy ØUJ88ZZ
Salpingostomy *see* Drainage, Female Reproductive System ØU9
Salpingotomy *see* Drainage, Female Reproductive System ØU9
Salpinx
   use Fallopian Tube, Right
   use Fallopian Tube, Left
Saphenous nerve *use* Femoral Nerve
SAPIEN transcatheter aortic valve *use* Zooplastic Tissue in Heart and Great Vessels
Sartorius muscle
   use Upper Leg Muscle, Right
   use Upper Leg Muscle, Left
Scalene muscle
   use Neck Muscle, Right
   use Neck Muscle, Left
Scan
   Computerized Tomography (CT) *see* Computerized Tomography (CT Scan)
   Radioisotope *see* Planar Nuclear Medicine Imaging
Scaphoid bone
   use Carpal, Right
   use Carpal, Left
Scapholunate ligament
   use Hand Bursa and Ligament, Right
   use Hand Bursa and Ligament, Left
Scaphotrapezium ligament
   use Hand Bursa and Ligament, Right
   use Hand Bursa and Ligament, Left
Scapulectomy
   see Excision, Upper Bones ØPB
   see Resection, Upper Bones ØPT
Scapulopexy
   see Repair, Upper Bones ØPQ
   see Reposition, Upper Bones ØPS

Scarpa's (vestibular) ganglion *use* Acoustic Nerve
Sclerectomy *see* Excision, Eye Ø8B
Sclerotherapy, mechanical *see* Destruction
Sclerotomy *see* Drainage, Eye Ø89
Scrotectomy
   see Excision, Male Reproductive System ØVB
   see Resection, Male Reproductive System ØVT
Scrotoplasty
   see Repair, Male Reproductive System ØVQ
   see Supplement, Male Reproductive System ØVU
Scrotorrhaphy *see* Repair, Male Reproductive System ØVQ
Scrototomy *see* Drainage, Male Reproductive System ØV9
Sebaceous gland *use* Skin
Second cranial nerve *use* Optic Nerve
Section, cesarean *see* Extraction, Pregnancy 1ØD
Secura (DR) (VR) *use* Defibrillator Generator in ØJH
Sella turcica
   use Sphenoid Bone, Right
   use Sphenoid Bone, Left
Semicircular canal
   use Inner Ear, Right
   use Inner Ear, Left
Semimembranosus muscle
   use Upper Leg Muscle, Right
   use Upper Leg Muscle, Left
Semitendinosus muscle
   use Upper Leg Muscle, Right
   use Upper Leg Muscle, Left
Seprafilm *use* Adhesion Barrier
Septal cartilage *use* Nasal Septum
Septectomy
   see Excision, Heart and Great Vessels Ø2B
   see Resection, Heart and Great Vessels Ø2T
   see Excision, Ear, Nose, Sinus Ø9B
   see Resection, Ear, Nose, Sinus Ø9T
Septoplasty
   see Repair, Heart and Great Vessels Ø2Q
   see Replacement, Heart and Great Vessels Ø2R
   see Supplement, Heart and Great Vessels Ø2U
   see Repair, Ear, Nose, Sinus Ø9Q
   see Replacement, Ear, Nose, Sinus Ø9R
   see Reposition, Ear, Nose, Sinus Ø9S
   see Supplement, Ear, Nose, Sinus Ø9U
Septotomy *see* Drainage, Ear, Nose, Sinus Ø99
Sequestrectomy, bone *see* Extirpation
Serratus anterior muscle
   use Thorax Muscle, Right
   use Thorax Muscle, Left
Serratus posterior muscle
   use Trunk Muscle, Right
   use Trunk Muscle, Left
Seventh cranial nerve *use* Facial Nerve
Sheffield hybrid external fixator
   use External Fixation Device, Hybrid in ØPH
   use External Fixation Device, Hybrid in ØPS
   use External Fixation Device, Hybrid in ØQH
   use External Fixation Device, Hybrid in ØQS
Sheffield ring external fixator
   use External Fixation Device, Ring in ØPH
   use External Fixation Device, Ring in ØPS
   use External Fixation Device, Ring in ØQH
   use External Fixation Device, Ring in ØQS
Shirodkar cervical cerclage ØUVC7ZZ
Shock Wave Therapy, Musculoskeletal 6A93
Short gastric artery *use* Splenic Artery
Shortening
   see Excision
   see Repair
   see Reposition
Shunt creation *see* Bypass
Sialoadenectomy
   Complete *see* Resection, Mouth and Throat ØCT
   Partial *see* Excision, Mouth and Throat ØCB
Sialodochoplasty
   see Repair, Mouth and Throat ØCQ
   see Replacement, Mouth and Throat ØCR
   see Supplement, Mouth and Throat ØCU

Sialoectomy
   see Excision, Mouth and Throat ØCB
   see Resection, Mouth and Throat ØCT
Sialography *see* Plain Radiography, Ear, Nose, Mouth and Throat B9Ø
Sialolithotomy *see* Extirpation, Mouth and Throat ØCC
Sigmoid artery *use* Inferior Mesenteric Artery
Sigmoid flexure *use* Sigmoid Colon
Sigmoid vein *use* Inferior Mesenteric Vein
Sigmoidectomy
   see Excision, Gastrointestinal System ØDB
   see Resection, Gastrointestinal System ØDT
Sigmoidorrhaphy *see* Repair, Gastrointestinal System ØDQ
Sigmoidoscopy ØDJD8ZZ
Sigmoidotomy *see* Drainage, Gastrointestinal System ØD9
Single lead pacemaker (atrium) (ventricle) *use* Pacemaker, Single Chamber in ØJH
Single lead rate responsive pacemaker (atrium) (ventricle) *use* Pacemaker, Single Chamber Rate Responsive in ØJH
Sinoatrial node *use* Conduction Mechanism
Sinogram
   Abdominal Wall *see* Fluoroscopy, Abdomen and Pelvis BW11
   Chest Wall *see* Plain Radiography, Chest BWØ3
   Retroperitoneum *see* Fluoroscopy, Abdomen and Pelvis BW11
Sinus venosus *use* Atrium, Right
Sinusectomy
   see Excision, Ear, Nose, Sinus Ø9B
   see Resection, Ear, Nose, Sinus Ø9T
Sinusoscopy Ø9JY4ZZ
Sinusotomy *see* Drainage, Ear, Nose, Sinus Ø99
Sirolimus-eluting coronary stent *use* Intraluminal Device, Drug-eluting in Heart and Great Vessels
Sixth cranial nerve *use* Abducens Nerve
Size reduction, breast *see* Excision, Skin and Breast ØHB
SJM Biocor® Stented Valve System *use* Zooplastic Tissue in Heart and Great Vessels
Skene's (paraurethral) gland *use* Vestibular Gland
Skin Substitute, Porcine Liver Derived, Replacement XHRPXL2 ◄
Sling
   Fascial, orbicularis muscle (mouth) *see* Supplement, Muscle, Facial ØKU1
   Levator muscle, for urethral suspension *see* Reposition, Bladder Neck ØTSC
   Pubococcygeal, for urethral suspension *see* Reposition, Bladder Neck ØTSC
   Rectum *see* Reposition, Rectum ØDSP
Small bowel series *see* Fluoroscopy, Bowel, Small BD13
Small saphenous vein
   use Lesser Saphenous Vein, Right
   use Lesser Saphenous Vein, Left
Snaring, polyp, colon *see* Excision, Gastrointestinal System ØDB
Solar (celiac) plexus *use* Abdominal Sympathetic Nerve
Soleus muscle
   use Lower Leg Muscle, Right
   use Lower Leg Muscle, Left
Spacer
   Insertion of device in
     Disc
       Lumbar Vertebral ØSH2
       Lumbosacral ØSH4
     Joint
       Acromioclavicular
         Left ØRHH
         Right ØRHG
       Ankle
         Left ØSHG
         Right ØSHF

◄ New   ◄ᷟ Revised   ~~deleted~~ Deleted

Spacer *(Continued)*
Insertion of device in *(Continued)*
Joint *(Continued)*
Carpal
Left 0RHR
Right 0RHQ
Cervical Vertebral 0RH1
Cervicothoracic Vertebral 0RH4
Coccygeal 0SH6
Elbow
Left 0RHM
Right 0RHL
Finger Phalangeal
Left 0RHX
Right 0RHW
Hip
Left 0SHB
Right 0SH9
Knee
Left 0SHD
Right 0SHC
Lumbar Vertebral 0SH0
Lumbosacral 0SH3
Metacarpocarpal
Left 0RHT
Right 0RHS
Metacarpophalangeal
Left 0RHV
Right 0RHU
Metatarsal-Phalangeal
Left 0SHN
Right 0SHM
Metatarsal-Tarsal
Left 0SHL
Right 0SHK
Occipital-cervical 0RH0
Sacrococcygeal 0SH5
Sacroiliac
Left 0SH8
Right 0SH7
Shoulder
Left 0RHK
Right 0RHJ
Sternoclavicular
Left 0RHF
Right 0RHE
Tarsal
Left 0SHJ
Right 0SHH
Temporomandibular
Left 0RHD
Right 0RHC
Thoracic Vertebral 0RH6
Thoracolumbar Vertebral 0RHA
Toe Phalangeal
Left 0SHQ
Right 0SHP
Wrist
Left 0RHP
Right 0RHN
Removal of device from
Acromioclavicular
Left 0RPH
Right 0RPG
Ankle
Left 0SPG
Right 0SPF
Carpal
Left 0RPR
Right 0RPQ
Cervical Vertebral 0RP1
Cervicothoracic Vertebral 0RP4
Coccygeal 0SP6
Elbow
Left 0RPM
Right 0RPL
Finger Phalangeal
Left 0RPX
Right 0RPW
Hip
Left 0SPB
Right 0SP9

Spacer *(Continued)*
Removal of device from *(Continued)*
Knee
Left 0SPD
Right 0SPC
Lumbar Vertebral 0SP0
Lumbosacral 0SP3
Metacarpocarpal
Left 0RPT
Right 0RPS
Metacarpophalangeal
Left 0RPV
Right 0RPU
Metatarsal-Phalangeal
Left 0SPN
Right 0SPM
Metatarsal-Tarsal
Left 0SPL
Right 0SPK
Occipital-cervical 0RP0
Sacrococcygeal 0SP5
Sacroiliac
Left 0SP8
Right 0SP7
Shoulder
Left 0RPK
Right 0RPJ
Sternoclavicular
Left 0RPF
Right 0RPE
Tarsal
Left 0SPJ
Right 0SPH
Temporomandibular
Left 0RPD
Right 0RPC
Thoracic Vertebral 0RP6
Thoracolumbar Vertebral 0RPA
Toe Phalangeal
Left 0SPQ
Right 0SPP
Wrist
Left 0RPP
Right 0RPN
Revision of device in
Acromioclavicular
Left 0RWH
Right 0RWG
Ankle
Left 0SWG
Right 0SWF
Carpal
Left 0RWR
Right 0RWQ
Cervical Vertebral 0RW1
Cervicothoracic Vertebral 0RW4
Coccygeal 0SW6
Elbow
Left 0RWM
Right 0RWL
Finger Phalangeal
Left 0RWX
Right 0RWW
Hip
Left 0SWB
Right 0SW9
Knee
Left 0SWD
Right 0SWC
Lumbar Vertebral 0SW0
Lumbosacral 0SW3
Metacarpocarpal
Left 0RWT
Right 0RWS
Metacarpophalangeal
Left 0RWV
Right 0RWU
Metatarsal-Phalangeal
Left 0SWN
Right 0SWM

Spacer *(Continued)*
Revision of device in *(Continued)*
Metatarsal-Tarsal
Left 0SWL
Right 0SWK
Occipital-cervical 0RW0
Sacrococcygeal 0SW5
Sacroiliac
Left 0SW8
Right 0SW7
Shoulder
Left 0RWK
Right 0RWJ
Sternoclavicular
Left 0RWF
Right 0RWE
Tarsal
Left 0SWJ
Right 0SWH
Temporomandibular
Left 0RWD
Right 0RWC
Thoracic Vertebral 0RW6
Thoracolumbar Vertebral 0RWA
Toe Phalangeal
Left 0SWQ
Right 0SWP
Wrist
Left 0RWP
Right 0RWN
Spectroscopy
Intravascular 8E023DZ
Near infrared 8E023DZ
Speech Assessment F00
Speech therapy *see* Speech Treatment, Rehabilitation F06
Speech Treatment F06
Sphenoidectomy
see Excision, Ear, Nose, Sinus 09B
see Resection, Ear, Nose, Sinus 09T
see Excision, Head and Facial Bones 0NB
see Resection, Head and Facial Bones 0NT
Sphenoidotomy *see* Drainage, Ear, Nose, Sinus 099
Sphenomandibular ligament *use* Head and Neck Bursa and Ligament
Sphenopalatine (pterygopalatine) ganglion *use* Head and Neck Sympathetic Nerve
Sphincterorrhaphy, anal *see* Repair, Sphincter, Anal 0DQR
Sphincterotomy, anal
see Division, Sphincter, Anal 0D8R
see Drainage, Sphincter, Anal 0D9R
Spinal cord neurostimulator lead *use* Neurostimulator Lead in Central Nervous System
Spinal growth rods, magnetically controlled *use* Magnetically Controlled Growth Rod(s) in New Technology ◀
Spinal nerve, cervical *use* Cervical Nerve
Spinal nerve, lumbar *use* Lumbar Nerve
Spinal nerve, sacral *use* Sacral Nerve
Spinal nerve, thoracic *use* Thoracic Nerve
Spinal Stabilization Device
Facet Replacement
Cervical Vertebral 0RH1
Cervicothoracic Vertebral 0RH4
Lumbar Vertebral 0SH0
Lumbosacral 0SH3
Occipital-cervical 0RH0
Thoracic Vertebral 0RH6
Thoracolumbar Vertebral 0RHA
Interspinous Process
Cervical Vertebral 0RH1
Cervicothoracic Vertebral 0RH4
Lumbar Vertebral 0SH0
Lumbosacral 0SH3
Occipital-cervical 0RH0
Thoracic Vertebral 0RH6
Thoracolumbar Vertebral 0RHA

◀ New ◀▥▥ Revised ~~deleted~~ Deleted

Spinal Stabilization Device *(Continued)*
  Pedicle-Based
    Cervical Vertebral ØRH1
    Cervicothoracic Vertebral ØRH4
    Lumbar Vertebral ØSHØ
    Lumbosacral ØSH3
    Occipital-cervical ØRHØ
    Thoracic Vertebral ØRH6
    Thoracolumbar Vertebral ØRHA
Spinous process
  use Cervical Vertebra
  use Thoracic Vertebra
  use Lumbar Vertebra
Spiral ganglion *use* Acoustic Nerve
Spiration IBV™ Valve System *use* Intraluminal
    Device, Endobronchial Valve in
    Respiratory System
Splenectomy
  see Excision, Lymphatic and Hemic Systems
    Ø7B
  see Resection, Lymphatic and Hemic Systems
    Ø7T
Splenic flexure *use* Transverse Colon
Splenic plexus *use* Abdominal Sympathetic
    Nerve
Splenius capitis muscle *use* Head Muscle
Splenius cervicis muscle
  use Neck Muscle, Right
  use Neck Muscle, Left
Splenolysis *see* Release, Lymphatic and Hemic
    Systems Ø7N
Splenopexy
  see Repair, Lymphatic and Hemic Systems Ø7Q
  see Reposition, Lymphatic and Hemic
    Systems Ø7S
Splenoplasty *see* Repair, Lymphatic and Hemic
    Systems Ø7Q
Splenorrhaphy *see* Repair, Lymphatic and
    Hemic Systems Ø7Q
Splenotomy *see* Drainage, Lymphatic and
    Hemic Systems Ø79
Splinting, musculoskeletal *see* Immobilization,
    Anatomical Regions 2W3
SPY system intravascular fluorescence
    angiography *see* Monitoring, Physiological
    Systems 4A1 ◄
Stapedectomy
  see Excision, Ear, Nose, Sinus Ø9B
  see Resection, Ear, Nose, Sinus Ø9T
Stapediolysis *see* Release, Ear, Nose, Sinus Ø9N
Stapedioplasty
  see Repair, Ear, Nose, Sinus Ø9Q
  see Replacement, Ear, Nose, Sinus Ø9R
  see Supplement, Ear, Nose, Sinus Ø9U
Stapedotomy *see* Drainage, Ear, Nose, Sinus Ø99
Stapes
  use Auditory Ossicle, Right
  use Auditory Ossicle, Left
Stellate ganglion *use* Head and Neck
    Sympathetic Nerve
Stem cell transplant *see* Transfusion,
    Circulatory 3Ø2 ◄
Stensen's duct
  use Parotid Duct, Right
  use Parotid Duct, Left
Stent, intraluminal (cardiovascular)
    (gastrointestinal)(hepatobiliary)(urinary)
  use Intraluminal Device
Stented tissue valve *use* Zooplastic Tissue in
    Heart and Great Vessels
Stereotactic Radiosurgery
  Abdomen DW23
  Adrenal Gland DG22
  Bile Ducts DF22
  Bladder DT22
  Bone Marrow D72Ø
  Brain DØ2Ø
  Brain Stem DØ21
  Breast
    Left DM2Ø
    Right DM21
  Bronchus DB21

Stereotactic Radiosurgery *(Continued)*
  Cervix DU21
  Chest DW22
  Chest Wall DB27
  Colon DD25
  Diaphragm DB28
  Duodenum DD22
  Ear D92Ø
  Esophagus DD2Ø
  Eye D82Ø
  Gallbladder DF21
  Gamma Beam
    Abdomen DW23JZZ
    Adrenal Gland DG22JZZ
    Bile Ducts DF22JZZ
    Bladder DT22JZZ
    Bone Marrow D72ØJZZ
    Brain DØ2ØJZZ
    Brain Stem DØ21JZZ
    Breast
      Left DM2ØJZZ
      Right DM21JZZ
    Bronchus DB21JZZ
    Cervix DU21JZZ
    Chest DW22JZZ
    Chest Wall DB27JZZ
    Colon DD25JZZ
    Diaphragm DB28JZZ
    Duodenum DD22JZZ
    Ear D92ØJZZ
    Esophagus DD2ØJZZ
    Eye D82ØJZZ
    Gallbladder DF21JZZ
    Gland
      Adrenal DG22JZZ
      Parathyroid DG24JZZ
      Pituitary DG2ØJZZ
      Thyroid DG25JZZ
    Glands, Salivary D926JZZ
    Head and Neck DW21JZZ
    Ileum DD24JZZ
    Jejunum DD23JZZ
    Kidney DT2ØJZZ
    Larynx D92BJZZ
    Liver DF2ØJZZ
    Lung DB22JZZ
    Lymphatics
      Abdomen D726JZZ
      Axillary D724JZZ
      Inguinal D728JZZ
      Neck D723JZZ
      Pelvis D727JZZ
      Thorax D725JZZ
    Mediastinum DB26JZZ
    Mouth D924JZZ
    Nasopharynx D92DJZZ
    Neck and Head DW21JZZ
    Nerve, Peripheral DØ27JZZ
    Nose D921JZZ
    Ovary DU2ØJZZ
    Palate
      Hard D928JZZ
      Soft D929JZZ
    Pancreas DF23JZZ
    Parathyroid Gland DG24JZZ
    Pelvic Region DW26JZZ
    Pharynx D92CJZZ
    Pineal Body DG21JZZ
    Pituitary Gland DG2ØJZZ
    Pleura DB25JZZ
    Prostate DV2ØJZZ
    Rectum DD27JZZ
    Sinuses D927JZZ
    Spinal Cord DØ26JZZ
    Spleen D722JZZ
    Stomach DD21JZZ
    Testis DV21JZZ
    Thymus D721JZZ
    Thyroid Gland DG25JZZ
    Tongue D925JZZ
    Trachea DB2ØJZZ
    Ureter DT21JZZ

Stereotactic Radiosurgery *(Continued)*
  Gamma Beam *(Continued)*
    Urethra DT23JZZ
    Uterus DU22JZZ
  Gland
    Adrenal DG22
    Parathyroid DG24
    Pituitary DG2Ø
    Thyroid DG25
  Glands, Salivary D926
  Head and Neck DW21
  Ileum DD24
  Jejunum DD23
  Kidney DT2Ø
  Larynx D92B
  Liver DF2Ø
  Lung DB22
  Lymphatics
    Abdomen D726
    Axillary D724
    Inguinal D728
    Neck D723
    Pelvis D727
    Thorax D725
  Mediastinum DB26
  Mouth D924
  Nasopharynx D92D
  Neck and Head DW21
  Nerve, Peripheral DØ27
  Nose D921
  Other Photon
    Abdomen DW23DZZ
    Adrenal Gland DG22DZZ
    Bile Ducts DF22DZZ
    Bladder DT22DZZ
    Bone Marrow D72ØDZZ
    Brain DØ2ØDZZ
    Brain Stem DØ21DZZ
    Breast
      Left DM2ØDZZ
      Right DM21DZZ
    Bronchus DB21DZZ
    Cervix DU21DZZ
    Chest DW22DZZ
    Chest Wall DB27DZZ
    Colon DD25DZZ
    Diaphragm DB28DZZ
    Duodenum DD22DZZ
    Ear D92ØDZZ
    Esophagus DD2ØDZZ
    Eye D82ØDZZ
    Gallbladder DF21DZZ
    Gland
      Adrenal DG22DZZ
      Parathyroid DG24DZZ
      Pituitary DG2ØDZZ
      Thyroid DG25DZZ
    Glands, Salivary D926DZZ
    Head and Neck DW21DZZ
    Ileum DD24DZZ
    Jejunum DD23DZZ
    Kidney DT2ØDZZ
    Larynx D92BDZZ
    Liver DF2ØDZZ
    Lung DB22DZZ
    Lymphatics
      Abdomen D726DZZ
      Axillary D724DZZ
      Inguinal D728DZZ
      Neck D723DZZ
      Pelvis D727DZZ
      Thorax D725DZZ
    Mediastinum DB26DZZ
    Mouth D924DZZ
    Nasopharynx D92DDZZ
    Neck and Head DW21DZZ
    Nerve, Peripheral DØ27DZZ
    Nose D921DZZ
    Ovary DU2ØDZZ
    Palate
      Hard D928DZZ
      Soft D929DZZ

Stereotactic Radiosurgery (Continued)
  Other Photon (Continued)
    Pancreas DF23DZZ
    Parathyroid Gland DG24DZZ
    Pelvic Region DW26DZZ
    Pharynx D92CDZZ
    Pineal Body DG21DZZ
    Pituitary Gland DG20DZZ
    Pleura DB25DZZ
    Prostate DV20DZZ
    Rectum DD27DZZ
    Sinuses D927DZZ
    Spinal Cord D026DZZ
    Spleen D722DZZ
    Stomach DD21DZZ
    Testis DV21DZZ
    Thymus D721DZZ
    Thyroid Gland DG25DZZ
    Tongue D925DZZ
    Trachea DB20DZZ
    Ureter DT21DZZ
    Urethra DT23DZZ
    Uterus DU22DZZ
  Ovary DU20
  Palate
    Hard D928
    Soft D929
  Pancreas DF23
  Parathyroid Gland DG24
  Particulate
    Abdomen DW23HZZ
    Adrenal Gland DG22HZZ
    Bile Ducts DF22HZZ
    Bladder DT22HZZ
    Bone Marrow D720HZZ
    Brain D020HZZ
    Brain Stem D021HZZ
    Breast
      Left DM20HZZ
      Right DM21HZZ
    Bronchus DB21HZZ
    Cervix DU21HZZ
    Chest DW22HZZ
    Chest Wall DB27HZZ
    Colon DD25HZZ
    Diaphragm DB28HZZ
    Duodenum DD22HZZ
    Ear D920HZZ
    Esophagus DD20HZZ
    Eye D820HZZ
    Gallbladder DF21HZZ
    Gland
      Adrenal DG22HZZ
      Parathyroid DG24HZZ
      Pituitary DG20HZZ
      Thyroid DG25HZZ
    Glands, Salivary D926HZZ
    Head and Neck DW21HZZ
    Ileum DD24HZZ
    Jejunum DD23HZZ
    Kidney DT20HZZ
    Larynx D92BHZZ
    Liver DF20HZZ
    Lung DB22HZZ
    Lymphatics
      Abdomen D726HZZ
      Axillary D724HZZ
      Inguinal D728HZZ
      Neck D723HZZ
      Pelvis D727HZZ
      Thorax D725HZZ
    Mediastinum DB26HZZ
    Mouth D924HZZ
    Nasopharynx D92DHZZ
    Neck and Head DW21HZZ
    Nerve, Peripheral D027HZZ
    Nose D921HZZ
    Ovary DU20HZZ
    Palate
      Hard D928HZZ
      Soft D929HZZ
    Pancreas DF23HZZ

Stereotactic Radiosurgery (Continued)
  Particulate (Continued)
    Parathyroid Gland DG24HZZ
    Pelvic Region DW26HZZ
    Pharynx D92CHZZ
    Pineal Body DG21HZZ
    Pituitary Gland DG20HZZ
    Pleura DB25HZZ
    Prostate DV20HZZ
    Rectum DD27HZZ
    Sinuses D927HZZ
    Spinal Cord D026HZZ
    Spleen D722HZZ
    Stomach DD21HZZ
    Testis DV21HZZ
    Thymus D721HZZ
    Thyroid Gland DG25HZZ
    Tongue D925HZZ
    Trachea DB20HZZ
    Ureter DT21HZZ
    Urethra DT23HZZ
    Uterus DU22HZZ
  Pelvic Region DW26
  Pharynx D92C
  Pineal Body DG21
  Pituitary Gland DG20
  Pleura DB25
  Prostate DV20
  Rectum DD27
  Sinuses D927
  Spinal Cord D026
  Spleen D722
  Stomach DD21
  Testis DV21
  Thymus D721
  Thyroid Gland DG25
  Tongue D925
  Trachea DB20
  Ureter DT21
  Urethra DT23
  Uterus DU22
Sternoclavicular ligament
  use Shoulder Bursa and Ligament, Right
  use Shoulder Bursa and Ligament, Left
Sternocleidomastoid artery
  use Thyroid Artery, Right
  use Thyroid Artery, Left
Sternocleidomastoid muscle
  use Neck Muscle, Right
  use Neck Muscle, Left
Sternocostal ligament
  use Thorax Bursa and Ligament, Right
  use Thorax Bursa and Ligament, Left
Sternotomy
  see Division, Sternum 0P80
  see Drainage, Sternum 0P90
Stimulation, cardiac
  Cardioversion 5A2204Z
  Electrophysiologic testing see Measurement,
    Cardiac 4A02
Stimulator Generator
  Insertion of device in
    Abdomen 0JH8
    Back 0JH7
    Chest 0JH6
    Multiple Array
      Abdomen 0JH8
      Back 0JH7
      Chest 0JH6
    Multiple Array Rechargeable
      Abdomen 0JH8
      Back 0JH7
      Chest 0JH6
  Removal of device from, Subcutaneous Tissue
    and Fascia, Trunk 0JPT
  Revision of device in, Subcutaneous Tissue
    and Fascia, Trunk 0JWT
  Single Array
    Abdomen 0JH8
    Back 0JH7
    Chest 0JH6

Stimulator Generator (Continued)
  Single Array Rechargeable
    Abdomen 0JH8
    Back 0JH7
    Chest 0JH6
Stimulator Lead
  Insertion of device in
    Anal Sphincter 0DHR
    Artery
      Left 03HL
      Right 03HK
    Bladder 0THB
    Muscle
      Lower 0KHY
      Upper 0KHX
    Stomach 0DH6
    Ureter 0TH9
  Removal of device from
    Anal Sphincter 0DPR
    Artery, Upper 03PY
    Bladder 0TPB
    Muscle
      Lower 0KPY
      Upper 0KPX
    Stomach 0DP6
    Ureter 0TP9
  Revision of device in
    Anal Sphincter 0DWR
    Artery, Upper 03WY
    Bladder 0TWB
    Muscle
      Lower 0KWY
      Upper 0KWX
    Stomach 0DW6
    Ureter 0TW9
Stoma
  Excision
    Abdominal Wall 0WBFXZ2
    Neck 0WB6XZ2
  Repair
    Abdominal Wall 0WQFXZ2
    Neck 0WQ6XZ2
Stomatoplasty
  see Repair, Mouth and Throat 0CQ
  see Replacement, Mouth and Throat 0CR
  see Supplement, Mouth and Throat 0CU
Stomatorrhaphy see Repair, Mouth and Throat
    0CQ
Stratos LV use Cardiac Resynchronization
    Pacemaker Pulse Generator in 0JH
Stress test
  4A02XM4
  4A12XM4
Stripping see Extraction
Study
  Electrophysiologic stimulation, cardiac see
    Measurement, Cardiac 4A02
  Ocular motility 4A07X7Z
  Pulmonary airway flow measurement see
    Measurement, Respiratory 4A09
  Visual acuity 4A07X0Z
Styloglossus muscle use Tongue, Palate,
    Pharynx Muscle
Stylomandibular ligament use Head and Neck
    Bursa and Ligament
Stylopharyngeus muscle use Tongue, Palate,
    Pharynx Muscle
Subacromial bursa
  use Shoulder Bursa and Ligament, Right
  use Shoulder Bursa and Ligament, Left
Subaortic (common iliac) lymph node use
    Lymphatic, Pelvis
Subarachnoid space, intracranial use
    Subarachnoid Space
Subarachnoid space, spinal use Spinal Canal
Subclavicular (apical) lymph node
  use Lymphatic, Right Axillary
  use Lymphatic, Left Axillary
Subclavius muscle
  use Thorax Muscle, Right
  use Thorax Muscle, Left

◀ New   ◀▦ Revised   deleted Deleted

◀ New   ◀▥ Revised   ~~deleted~~ Deleted

Supplement *(Continued)*
  Disc *(Continued)*
    Thoracic Vertebral 0RU9
    Thoracolumbar Vertebral
      0RUB
  Duct
    Common Bile 0FU9
    Cystic 0FU8
    Hepatic
      Left 0FU6
      Right 0FU5
    Lacrimal
      Left 08UY
      Right 08UX
    Pancreatic 0FUD
      Accessory 0FUF
  Duodenum 0DU9
  Dura Mater 00U2
  Ear
    External
      Bilateral 09U2
      Left 09U1
      Right 09U0
    Inner
      Left 09UE0
      Right 09UD0
    Middle
      Left 09U60
      Right 09U50
  Elbow Region
    Left 0XUC
    Right 0XUB
  Epididymis
    Bilateral 0VUL
    Left 0VUK
    Right 0VUJ
  Epiglottis 0CUR
  Esophagogastric Junction 0DU4
  Esophagus 0DU5
    Lower 0DU3
    Middle 0DU2
    Upper 0DU1
  Extremity
    Lower
      Left 0YUB
      Right 0YU9
    Upper
      Left 0XU7
      Right 0XU6
  Eye
    Left 08U1
    Right 08U0
  Eyelid
    Lower
      Left 08UR
      Right 08UQ
    Upper
      Left 08UP
      Right 08UN
  Face 0WU2
  Fallopian Tube
    Left 0UU6
    Right 0UU5
  Fallopian Tubes, Bilateral 0UU7
  Femoral Region
    Bilateral 0YUE
    Left 0YU8
    Right 0YU7
  Femoral Shaft
    Left 0QU9
    Right 0QU8
  Femur
    Lower
      Left 0QUC
      Right 0QUB
    Upper
      Left 0QU7
      Right 0QU6
  Fibula
    Left 0QUK
    Right 0QUJ

Supplement *(Continued)*
  Finger
    Index
      Left 0XUP
      Right 0XUN
    Little
      Left 0XUW
      Right 0XUV
    Middle
      Left 0XUR
      Right 0XUQ
    Ring
      Left 0XUT
      Right 0XUS
  Foot
    Left 0YUN
    Right 0YUM
  Gingiva
    Lower 0CU6
    Upper 0CU5
  Glenoid Cavity
    Left 0PU8
    Right 0PU7
  Hand
    Left 0XUK
    Right 0XUJ
  Head 0WU0
  Heart 02UA
  Humeral Head
    Left 0PUD
    Right 0PUC
  Humeral Shaft
    Left 0PUG
    Right 0PUF
  Hymen 0UUK
  Ileocecal Valve 0DUC
  Ileum 0DUB
  Inguinal Region
    Bilateral 0YUA
    Left 0YU6
    Right 0YU5
  Intestine
    Large 0DUE
      Left 0DUG
      Right 0DUF
    Small 0DU8
  Iris
    Left 08UD
    Right 08UC
  Jaw
    Lower 0WU5
    Upper 0WU4
  Jejunum 0DUA
  Joint
    Acromioclavicular
      Left 0RUH
      Right 0RUG
    Ankle
      Left 0SUG
      Right 0SUF
    Carpal
      Left 0RUR
      Right 0RUQ
    Cervical Vertebral 0RU1
    Cervicothoracic Vertebral
      0RU4
    Coccygeal 0SU6
    Elbow
      Left 0RUM
      Right 0RUL
    Finger Phalangeal
      Left 0RUX
      Right 0RUW
    Hip
      Left 0SUB
        Acetabular Surface 0SUE
        Femoral Surface 0SUS
      Right 0SU9
        Acetabular Surface 0SUA
        Femoral Surface 0SUR

Supplement *(Continued)*
  Joint *(Continued)*
    Knee
      Left 0SUD
        Femoral Surface 0SUU09Z
        Tibial Surface 0SUW09Z
      Right 0SUC
        Femoral Surface 0SUT09Z
        Tibial Surface 0SUV09Z
    Lumbar Vertebral 0SU0
    Lumbosacral 0SU3
    Metacarpocarpal
      Left 0RUT
      Right 0RUS
    Metacarpophalangeal
      Left 0RUV
      Right 0RUU
    Metatarsal-Phalangeal
      Left 0SUN
      Right 0SUM
    Metatarsal-Tarsal
      Left 0SUL
      Right 0SUK
    Occipital-cervical 0RU0
    Sacrococcygeal 0SU5
    Sacroiliac
      Left 0SU8
      Right 0SU7
    Shoulder
      Left 0RUK
      Right 0RUJ
    Sternoclavicular
      Left 0RUF
      Right 0RUE
    Tarsal
      Left 0SUJ
      Right 0SUH
    Temporomandibular
      Left 0RUD
      Right 0RUC
    Thoracic Vertebral 0RU6
    Thoracolumbar Vertebral 0RUA
    Toe Phalangeal
      Left 0SUQ
      Right 0SUP
    Wrist
      Left 0RUP
      Right 0RUN
  Kidney Pelvis
    Left 0TU4
    Right 0TU3
  Knee Region
    Left 0YUG
    Right 0YUF
  Larynx 0CUS
  Leg
    Lower
      Left 0YUJ
      Right 0YUH
    Upper
      Left 0YUD
      Right 0YUC
  Lip
    Lower 0CU1
    Upper 0CU0
  Lymphatic
    Aortic 07UD
    Axillary
      Left 07U6
      Right 07U5
    Head 07U0
    Inguinal
      Left 07UJ
      Right 07UH
    Internal Mammary
      Left 07U9
      Right 07U8
    Lower Extremity
      Left 07UG
      Right 07UF
    Mesenteric 07UB

◄ New ◄⁞ Revised ~~deleted~~ Deleted

Supplement *(Continued)*
  Thumb
    Left 0XUM
    Right 0XUL
  Tibia
    Left 0QUH
    Right 0QUG
  Toe
    1st
      Left 0YUQ
      Right 0YUP
    2nd
      Left 0YUS
      Right 0YUR
    3rd
      Left 0YUU
      Right 0YUT
    4th
      Left 0YUW
      Right 0YUV
    5th
      Left 0YUY
      Right 0YUX
  Tongue 0CU7
  Trachea 0BU1
  Tunica Vaginalis
    Left 0VU7
    Right 0VU6
  Turbinate, Nasal 09UL
  Tympanic Membrane
    Left 09U8
    Right 09U7
  Ulna
    Left 0PUL
    Right 0PUK
  Ureter
    Left 0TU7
    Right 0TU6
  Urethra 0TUD
  Uterine Supporting Structure 0UU4
  Uvula 0CUN
  Vagina 0UUG
  Valve
    Aortic 02UF
    Mitral 02UG
    Pulmonary 02UH
    Tricuspid 02UJ
  Vas Deferens
    Bilateral 0VUQ
    Left 0VUP
    Right 0VUN
  Vein
    Axillary
      Left 05U8
      Right 05U7
    Azygos 05U0
    Basilic
      Left 05UC
      Right 05UB
    Brachial
      Left 05UA
      Right 05U9
    Cephalic
      Left 05UF
      Right 05UD
    Colic 06U7
    Common Iliac
      Left 06UD
      Right 06UC
    Esophageal 06U3
    External Iliac
      Left 06UG
      Right 06UF
    External Jugular
      Left 05UQ
      Right 05UP

Supplement *(Continued)*
  Vein *(Continued)*
    Face
      Left 05UV
      Right 05UT
    Femoral
      Left 06UN
      Right 06UM
    Foot
      Left 06UV
      Right 06UT
    Gastric 06U2
    Greater Saphenous
      Left 06UQ
      Right 06UP
    Hand
      Left 05UH
      Right 05UG
    Hemiazygos 05U1
    Hepatic 06U4
    Hypogastric
      Left 06UJ
      Right 06UH
    Inferior Mesenteric 06U6
    Innominate
      Left 05U4
      Right 05U3
    Internal Jugular
      Left 05UN
      Right 05UM
    Intracranial 05UL
    Lesser Saphenous
      Left 06US
      Right 06UR
    Lower 06UY
    Portal 06U8
    Pulmonary
      Left 02UT
      Right 02US
    Renal
      Left 06UB
      Right 06U9
    Splenic 06U1
    Subclavian
      Left 05U6
      Right 05U5
    Superior Mesenteric 06U5
    Upper 05UY
    Vertebral
      Left 05US
      Right 05UR
  Vena Cava
    Inferior 06U0
    Superior 02UV
  Ventricle
    Left 02UL
    Right 02UK
  Vertebra
    Cervical 0PU3
    Lumbar 0QU0
    Thoracic 0PU4
  Vesicle
    Bilateral 0VU3
    Left 0VU2
    Right 0VU1
  Vocal Cord
    Left 0CUV
    Right 0CUT
  Vulva 0UUM
  Wrist Region
    Left 0XUH
    Right 0XUG
Supraclavicular (Virchow's) lymph node
  use Lymphatic, Right Neck
  use Lymphatic, Left Neck
Supraclavicular nerve *use* Cervical Plexus

Suprahyoid lymph node *use* Lymphatic,
  Head
Suprahyoid muscle
  use Neck Muscle, Right
  use Neck Muscle, Left
Suprainguinal lymph node *use* Lymphatic,
  Pelvis
Supraorbital vein
  use Face Vein, Right
  use Face Vein, Left
Suprarenal gland
  use Adrenal Gland, Left
  use Adrenal Gland, Right
  use Adrenal Gland, Bilateral
  use Adrenal Gland
Suprarenal plexus *use* Abdominal Sympathetic
  Nerve
Suprascapular nerve *use* Brachial Plexus Nerve
Supraspinatus fascia
  use Subcutaneous Tissue and Fascia, Right
    Upper Arm
  use Subcutaneous Tissue and Fascia, Left
    Upper Arm
Supraspinatus muscle
  use Shoulder Muscle, Right
  use Shoulder Muscle, Left
Supraspinous ligament
  use Trunk Bursa and Ligament, Right
  use Trunk Bursa and Ligament, Left
Suprasternal notch *use* Sternum
Supratrochlear lymph node
  use Lymphatic, Right Upper Extremity
  use Lymphatic, Left Upper Extremity
Sural artery
  use Popliteal Artery, Right
  use Popliteal Artery, Left
Suspension
  Bladder Neck *see* Reposition, Bladder Neck
    0TSC
  Kidney *see* Reposition, Urinary System 0TS
  Urethra *see* Reposition, Urinary System 0TS
  Urethrovesical *see* Reposition, Bladder Neck
    0TSC
  Uterus *see* Reposition, Uterus 0US9
  Vagina *see* Reposition, Vagina 0USG
Suture
  Laceration repair *see* Repair
  Ligation *see* Occlusion
Suture Removal
  Extremity
    Lower 8E0YXY8
    Upper 8E0XXY8
  Head and Neck Region 8E09XY8
  Trunk Region 8E0WXY8
Sutureless valve, Perceval *use* Zooplastic
  Tissue, Rapid Deployment Technique in
  New Technology ◀
Sweat gland *use* Skin
Sympathectomy
  see Excision, Peripheral Nervous System 01B
SynCardia Total Artificial Heart *use* Synthetic
  Substitute
Synchra CRT-P *use* Cardiac Resynchronization
  Pacemaker Pulse Generator in 0JH
SynchroMed pump *use* Infusion Device, Pump
  in Subcutaneous Tissue and Fascia
Synechiotomy, iris *see* Release, Eye 08N
Synovectomy
  Lower joint *see* Excision, Lower Joints 0SB
  Upper joint *see* Excision, Upper Joints 0RB
Systemic Nuclear Medicine Therapy
  Abdomen CW70
  Anatomical Regions, Multiple CW7YYZZ
  Chest CW73
  Thyroid CW7G
  Whole Body CW7N

T

Takedown
Arteriovenous shunt *see* Removal of device from, Upper Arteries Ø3P
Arteriovenous shunt, with creation of new shunt *see* Bypass, Upper Arteries Ø31
Stoma *see* Repair
Talent® Converter *use* Intraluminal Device
Talent® Occluder *use* Intraluminal Device
Talent® Stent Graft (abdominal) (thoracic) *use* Intraluminal Device
Talocalcaneal (subtalar) joint
use Tarsal Joint, Right
use Tarsal Joint, Left
Talocalcaneal ligament
use Foot Bursa and Ligament, Right
use Foot Bursa and Ligament, Left
Talocalcaneonavicular joint
use Tarsal Joint, Right
use Tarsal Joint, Left
Talocalcaneonavicular ligament
use Foot Bursa and Ligament, Right
use Foot Bursa and Ligament, Left
Talocrural joint
use Ankle Joint, Right
use Ankle Joint, Left
Talofibular ligament
use Ankle Bursa and Ligament, Right
use Ankle Bursa and Ligament, Left
Talus bone
use Tarsal, Right
use Tarsal, Left
TandemHeart® System *use* External Heart Assist System in Heart and Great Vessels
Tarsectomy
see Excision, Lower Bones ØQB
see Resection, Lower Bones ØQT
Tarsometatarsal joint
use Metatarsal-Tarsal Joint, Right
use Metatarsal-Tarsal Joint, Left
Tarsometatarsal ligament
use Foot Bursa and Ligament, Right
use Foot Bursa and Ligament, Left
Tarsorrhaphy *see* Repair, Eye Ø8Q
Tattooing
Cornea 3EØCXMZ
Skin *see* Introduction of substance in or on Skin 3EØØ
TAXUS® Liberté® Paclitaxel-eluting Coronary Stent System *use* Intraluminal Device, Drug-eluting in Heart and Great Vessels
TBNA (transbronchial needle aspiration) *see* Drainage, Respiratory System ØB9
Telemetry
4A12X4Z
Ambulatory 4A12X45
Temperature gradient study 4AØZXKZ
Temporal lobe *use* Cerebral Hemisphere
Temporalis muscle *use* Head Muscle
Temporoparietalis muscle *use* Head Muscle
Tendolysis *see* Release, Tendons ØLN
Tendonectomy
see Excision, Tendons ØLB
see Resection, Tendons ØLT
Tendonoplasty, tenoplasty
see Repair, Tendons ØLQ
see Replacement, Tendons ØLR
see Supplement, Tendons ØLU
Tendorrhaphy *see* Repair, Tendons ØLQ
Tendototomy
see Division, Tendons ØL8
see Drainage, Tendons ØL9
Tenectomy, tenonectomy
see Excision, Tendons ØLB
see Resection, Tendons ØLT
Tenolysis *see* Release, Tendons ØLN
Tenontorrhaphy *see* Repair, Tendons ØLQ
Tenontotomy
see Division, Tendons ØL8
see Drainage, Tendons ØL9

Tenorrhaphy *see* Repair, Tendons ØLQ
Tenosynovectomy
see Excision, Tendons ØLB
see Resection, Tendons ØLT
Tenotomy
see Division, Tendons ØL8
see Drainage, Tendons ØL9
Tensor fasciae latae muscle
use Hip Muscle, Right
use Hip Muscle, Left
Tensor veli palatini muscle *use* Tongue, Palate, Pharynx Muscle
Tenth cranial nerve *use* Vagus Nerve
Tentorium cerebelli *use* Dura Mater
Teres major muscle
use Shoulder Muscle, Right
use Shoulder Muscle, Left
Teres minor muscle
use Shoulder Muscle, Right
use Shoulder Muscle, Left
Termination of pregnancy
Aspiration curettage 10A07ZZ
Dilation and curettage 10A07ZZ
Hysterotomy 10A00ZZ
Intra-amniotic injection 10A03ZZ
Laminaria 10A07ZW
Vacuum 10A07Z6
Testectomy
see Excision, Male Reproductive System ØVB
see Resection, Male Reproductive System ØVT
Testicular artery *use* Abdominal Aorta
Testing
Glaucoma 4A07XBZ
Hearing *see* Hearing Assessment, Diagnostic Audiology F13
Mental health *see* Psychological Tests
Muscle function, electromyography (EMG) *see* Measurement, Musculoskeletal 4A0F
Muscle function, manual *see* Motor Function Assessment, Rehabilitation F01
Neurophysiologic monitoring, intra-operative *see* Monitoring, Physiological Systems 4A1
Range of motion *see* Motor Function Assessment, Rehabilitation F01
Vestibular function *see* Vestibular Assessment, Diagnostic Audiology F15
Thalamectomy *see* Excision, Thalamus 00B9
Thalamotomy
see Drainage, Thalamus 0099
Thenar muscle
use Hand Muscle, Right
use Hand Muscle, Left
Therapeutic Massage
Musculoskeletal System 8E0KX1Z
Reproductive System
Prostate 8E0VX1C
Rectum 8E0VX1D
Therapeutic occlusion coil(s) *use* Intraluminal Device
Thermography 4A0ZXKZ
Thermotherapy, prostate *see* Destruction, Prostate 0V50
Third cranial nerve *use* Oculomotor Nerve
Third occipital nerve *use* Cervical Nerve
Third ventricle *use* Cerebral Ventricle
Thoracectomy *see* Excision, Anatomical Regions, General 0WB
Thoracentesis *see* Drainage, Anatomical Regions, General 0W9
Thoracic aortic plexus *use* Thoracic Sympathetic Nerve
Thoracic esophagus *use* Esophagus, Middle
Thoracic facet joint *use* Thoracic Vertebral Joint
Thoracic ganglion *use* Thoracic Sympathetic Nerve
Thoracoacromial artery
use Axillary Artery, Right
use Axillary Artery, Left

Thoracocentesis *see* Drainage, Anatomical Regions, General 0W9
Thoracolumbar facet joint *use* Thoracolumbar Vertebral Joint
Thoracoplasty
see Repair, Anatomical Regions, General 0WQ
see Supplement, Anatomical Regions, General 0WU
Thoracostomy tube *use* Drainage Device
Thoracostomy, for lung collapse *see* Drainage, Respiratory System 0B9
Thoracotomy *see* Drainage, Anatomical Regions, General 0W9
Thoratec IVAD (Implantable Ventricular Assist Device) *use* Implantable Heart Assist System in Heart and Great Vessels
Thoratec Paracorporeal Ventricular Assist Device *use* External Heart Assist System in Heart and Great Vessels
Thrombectomy *see* Extirpation
Thymectomy
see Excision, Lymphatic and Hemic Systems 07B
see Resection, Lymphatic and Hemic Systems 07T
Thymopexy
see Repair, Lymphatic and Hemic Systems 07Q
see Reposition, Lymphatic and Hemic Systems 07S
Thymus gland *use* Thymus
Thyroarytenoid muscle
use Neck Muscle, Right
use Neck Muscle, Left
Thyrocervical trunk
use Thyroid Artery, Right
use Thyroid Artery, Left
Thyroid cartilage *use* Larynx
Thyroidectomy
see Excision, Endocrine System 0GB
see Resection, Endocrine System 0GT
Thyroidorrhaphy *see* Repair, Endocrine System 0GQ
Thyroidoscopy 0GJK4ZZ
Thyroidotomy *see* Drainage, Endocrine System 0G9
Tibial insert *use* Liner in Lower Joints
Tibialis anterior muscle
use Lower Leg Muscle, Right
use Lower Leg Muscle, Left
Tibialis posterior muscle
use Lower Leg Muscle, Right
use Lower Leg Muscle, Left
Tibiofemoral joint
use Knee Joint, Right
use Knee Joint, Left
use Knee Joint, Tibial Surface, Right
use Knee Joint, Tibial Surface, Left
TigerPaw® system for closure of left atrial appendage *use* Extraluminal Device
Tissue bank graft *use* Nonautologous Tissue Substitute
Tissue Expander
Insertion of device in
Breast
Bilateral 0HHV
Left 0HHU
Right 0HHT
Nipple
Left 0HHX
Right 0HHW
Subcutaneous Tissue and Fascia
Abdomen 0JH8
Back 0JH7
Buttock 0JH9
Chest 0JH6
Face 0JH1
Foot
Left 0JHR
Right 0JHQ
Hand
Left 0JHK
Right 0JHJ

◀ New ◀‖ Revised ~~deleted~~ Deleted

Tissue Expander *(Continued)*
  Insertion of device in *(Continued)*
    Subcutaneous Tissue and Fascia
      (Continued)
      Lower Arm
        Left ØJHH
        Right ØJHG
      Lower Leg
        Left ØJHP
        Right ØJHN
      Neck
        Anterior ØJH4
        Posterior ØJH5
      Pelvic Region ØJHC
      Perineum ØJHB
      Scalp ØJHØ
      Upper Arm
        Left ØJHF
        Right ØJHD
      Upper Leg
        Left ØJHM
        Right ØJHL
  Removal of device from
    Breast
      Left ØHPU
      Right ØHPT
    Subcutaneous Tissue and Fascia
      Head and Neck ØJPS
      Lower Extremity ØJPW
      Trunk ØJPT
      Upper Extremity ØJPV
  Revision of device in
    Breast
      Left ØHWU
      Right ØHWT
    Subcutaneous Tissue and Fascia
      Head and Neck ØJWS
      Lower Extremity ØJWW
      Trunk ØJWT
      Upper Extremity ØJWV
Tissue expander (inflatable) (injectable)
  use Tissue Expander in Skin and Breast
  use Tissue Expander in Subcutaneous Tissue
    and Fascia
Tissue Plasminogen Activator (tPA)(r-tPA) *use*
  Thrombolytic, Other
Titanium Sternal Fixation System (TSFS)
  use Internal Fixation Device, Rigid Plate in ØPS
  use Internal Fixation Device, Rigid Plate in ØPH
Tomographic (Tomo) Nuclear Medicine
    Imaging
  Abdomen CW2Ø
  Abdomen and Chest CW24
  Abdomen and Pelvis CW21
  Anatomical Regions, Multiple CW2YYZZ
  Bladder, Kidneys and Ureters CT23
  Brain CØ2Ø
  Breast CH2YYZZ
    Bilateral CH22
    Left CH21
    Right CH2Ø
  Bronchi and Lungs CB22
  Central Nervous System CØ2YYZZ
  Cerebrospinal Fluid CØ25
  Chest CW23
  Chest and Abdomen CW24
  Chest and Neck CW26
  Digestive System CD2YYZZ
  Endocrine System CG2YYZZ
  Extremity
    Lower CW2D
      Bilateral CP2F
      Left CP2D
      Right CP2C
    Upper CW2M
      Bilateral CP2B
      Left CP29
      Right CP28
  Gallbladder CF24
  Gastrointestinal Tract CD27
  Gland, Parathyroid CG21
  Head and Neck CW2B

Tomographic (Tomo) Nuclear Medicine
    Imaging *(Continued)*
  Heart C22YYZZ
    Right and Left C226
  Hepatobiliary System and Pancreas CF2YYZZ
  Kidneys, Ureters and Bladder CT23
  Liver CF25
  Liver and Spleen CF26
  Lungs and Bronchi CB22
  Lymphatics and Hematologic System
    C72YYZZ
  Musculoskeletal System, Other CP2YYZZ
  Myocardium C22G
  Neck and Chest CW26
  Neck and Head CW2B
  Pancreas and Hepatobiliary System CF2YYZZ
  Pelvic Region CW2J
  Pelvis CP26
  Pelvis and Abdomen CW21
  Pelvis and Spine CP27
  Respiratory System CB2YYZZ
  Skin CH2YYZZ
  Skull CP21
  Skull and Cervical Spine CP23
  Spine
    Cervical CP22
    Cervical and Skull CP23
    Lumbar CP2H
    Thoracic CP2G
    Thoracolumbar CP2J
  Spine and Pelvis CP27
  Spleen C722
  Spleen and Liver CF26
  Subcutaneous Tissue CH2YYZZ
  Thorax CP24
  Ureters, Kidneys and Bladder CT23
  Urinary System CT2YYZZ
Tomography, computerized *see* Computerized
  Tomography (CT Scan)
Tongue, base of *use* Pharynx ◀
Tonometry 4AØ7XBZ
Tonsillectomy
  see Excision, Mouth and Throat ØCB
  see Resection, Mouth and Throat ØCT
Tonsillotomy *see* Drainage, Mouth and Throat
  ØC9
Total Anomalous Pulmonary Venous Return
  (TAPVR) repair ◀
  see Bypass, Atrium, Left Ø217 ◀
  see Bypass, Vena Cava, Superior Ø21V ◀
Total artificial (replacement) heart *use* Synthetic
  Substitute
Total parenteral nutrition (TPN) *see*
  Introduction of Nutritional Substance
Trachectomy
  see Excision, Trachea ØBB1
  see Resection, Trachea ØBT1
Trachelectomy
  see Excision, Cervix ØUBC
  see Resection, Cervix ØUTC
Trachelopexy
  see Repair, Cervix ØUQC
  see Reposition, Cervix ØUSC
Tracheloplasty
  see Repair, Cervix ØUQC
Trachelorrhaphy *see* Repair, Cervix ØUQC
Trachelotomy *see* Drainage, Cervix ØU9C
Tracheobronchial lymph node *see* Lymphatic,
  Thorax
Tracheoesophageal fistulization ØB11ØD6
Tracheolysis *see* Release, Respiratory System ØBN
Tracheoplasty
  see Repair, Respiratory System ØBQ
  see Supplement, Respiratory System ØBU
Tracheorrhaphy *see* Repair, Respiratory System
  ØBQ
Tracheoscopy ØBJ18ZZ
Tracheostomy *see* Bypass, Respiratory System
  ØB1
Tracheostomy Device
  Bypass, Trachea ØB11
  Change device in, Trachea ØB21XFZ

Tracheostomy Device *(Continued)*
  Removal of device from, Trachea ØBP1
  Revision of device in, Trachea ØBW1
Tracheostomy tube *use* Tracheostomy Device in
  Respiratory System
Tracheotomy *see* Drainage, Respiratory System
  ØB9
Traction
  Abdominal Wall 2W63X
  Arm
    Lower
      Left 2W6DX
      Right 2W6CX
    Upper
      Left 2W6BX
      Right 2W6AX
  Back 2W65X
  Chest Wall 2W64X
  Extremity
    Lower
      Left 2W6MX
      Right 2W6LX
    Upper
      Left 2W69X
      Right 2W68X
  Face 2W61X
  Finger
    Left 2W6KX
    Right 2W6JX
  Foot
    Left 2W6TX
    Right 2W6SX
  Hand
    Left 2W6FX
    Right 2W6EX
  Head 2W60X
  Inguinal Region
    Left 2W67X
    Right 2W66X
  Leg
    Lower
      Left 2W6RX
      Right 2W6QX
    Upper
      Left 2W6PX
      Right 2W6NX
  Neck 2W62X
  Thumb
    Left 2W6HX
    Right 2W6GX
  Toe
    Left 2W6VX
    Right 2W6UX
Tractotomy *see* Division, Central Nervous
  System ØØ8
Tragus
  use External Ear, Right
  use External Ear, Left
  use External Ear, Bilateral
Training, caregiver *see* Caregiver Training
TRAM (transverse rectus abdominis
  myocutaneous) flap reconstruction
  Free *see* Replacement, Skin and Breast
    ØHR
  Pedicled *see* Transfer, Muscles ØKX
Transection *see* Division
Transfer
  Buccal Mucosa ØCX4
  Bursa and Ligament
    Abdomen
      Left ØMXJ
      Right ØMXH
    Ankle
      Left ØMXR
      Right ØMXQ
    Elbow
      Left ØMX4
      Right ØMX3
    Foot
      Left ØMXT
      Right ØMXS

◀ New   ◀|||| Revised   ~~deleted~~ Deleted

Transfusion *(Continued)*
  Artery *(Continued)*
    Peripheral
      Antihemophilic Factors 3025
      Blood
        Platelets 3025
        Red Cells 3025
          Frozen 3025
        White Cells 3025
        Whole 3025
      Bone Marrow 3025
      Factor IX 3025
      Fibrinogen 3025
      Globulin 3025
      Plasma
        Fresh 3025
        Frozen 3025
      Plasma Cryoprecipitate 3025
      Serum Albumin 3025
      Stem Cells
        Cord Blood 3025
        Hematopoietic 3025
  Products of Conception
    Antihemophilic Factors 3027
    Blood
      Platelets 3027
      Red Cells 3027
        Frozen 3027
      White Cells 3027
      Whole 3027
    Factor IX 3027
    Fibrinogen 3027
    Globulin 3027
    Plasma
      Fresh 3027
      Frozen 3027
    Plasma Cryoprecipitate 3027
    Serum Albumin 3027
  Vein
    4-Factor Prothrombin Complex
      Concentrate 3028[03]B1
    Central
      Antihemophilic Factors 3024
      Blood
        Platelets 3024
        Red Cells 3024
          Frozen 3024
        White Cells 3024
        Whole 3024
      Bone Marrow 3024
      Factor IX 3024
      Fibrinogen 3024
      Globulin 3024
      Plasma
        Fresh 3024
        Frozen 3024
      Plasma Cryoprecipitate 3024
      Serum Albumin 3024
      Stem Cells
        Cord Blood 3024
        Embryonic 3024
        Hematopoietic 3024
    Peripheral
      Antihemophilic Factors 3023
      Blood
        Platelets 3023
        Red Cells 3023
          Frozen 3023
        White Cells 3023
        Whole 3023
      Bone Marrow 3023
      Factor IX 3023
      Fibrinogen 3023
      Globulin 3023
      Plasma
        Fresh 3023
        Frozen 3023

Transfusion *(Continued)*
  Vein *(Continued)*
    Peripheral *(Continued)*
      Plasma Cryoprecipitate 3023
      Serum Albumin 3023
      Stem Cells
        Cord Blood 3023
        Embryonic 3023
        Hematopoietic 3023
Transplant *see* Transplantation ◀
Transplantation
  Bone marrow *see* Transfusion, Circulatory
    302 ◀
  Esophagus 0DY50Z
  Face 0WY20Z ◀
  Hand ◀
    Left 0XYK0Z ◀
    Right 0XYJ0Z ◀
  Heart 02YA0Z
  Hematopoietic cell *see* Transfusion,
    Circulatory 302 ◀
  Intestine
    Large 0DYE0Z
    Small 0DY80Z
  Kidney
    Left 0TY10Z
    Right 0TY00Z
  Liver 0FY00Z
  Lung
    Bilateral 0BYM0Z
    Left 0BYL0Z
    Lower Lobe
      Left 0BYJ0Z
      Right 0BYF0Z
    Middle Lobe, Right 0BYD0Z
    Right 0BYK0Z
    Upper Lobe
      Left 0BYG0Z
      Right 0BYC0Z
  Lung Lingula 0BYH0Z
  Ovary
    Left 0UY10Z
    Right 0UY00Z
  Pancreas 0FYG0Z
  Products of Conception 10Y0
  Spleen 07YP0Z
  Stem cell *see* Transfusion, Circulatory 302 ◀
  Stomach 0DY60Z
  Thymus 07YM0Z
Transposition
  see Reposition
  see Transfer
Transversalis fascia *use* Subcutaneous Tissue
  and Fascia, Trunk
Transverse (cutaneous) cervical nerve *use*
  Cervical Plexus
Transverse acetabular ligament
  use Hip Bursa and Ligament, Right
  use Hip Bursa and Ligament, Left
Transverse facial artery
  use Temporal Artery, Right
  use Temporal Artery, Left
Transverse humeral ligament
  use Shoulder Bursa and Ligament,
    Right
  use Shoulder Bursa and Ligament, Left
Transverse ligament of atlas *use* Head and
  Neck Bursa and Ligament
Transverse Rectus Abdominis Myocutaneous
  Flap
  Replacement
    Bilateral 0HRV076
    Left 0HRU076
    Right 0HRT076
  Transfer
    Left 0KXL
    Right 0KXK

Transverse scapular ligament
  use Shoulder Bursa and Ligament, Right
  use Shoulder Bursa and Ligament, Left
Transverse thoracis muscle
  use Thorax Muscle, Right
  use Thorax Muscle, Left
Transversospinalis muscle
  use Trunk Muscle, Right
  use Trunk Muscle, Left
Transversus abdominis muscle
  use Abdomen Muscle, Right
  use Abdomen Muscle, Left
Trapezium bone
  use Carpal, Right
  use Carpal, Left
Trapezius muscle
  use Trunk Muscle, Right
  use Trunk Muscle, Left
Trapezoid bone
  use Carpal, Right
  use Carpal, Left
Triceps brachii muscle
  use Upper Arm Muscle, Right
  use Upper Arm Muscle, Left
Tricuspid annulus *use* Tricuspid Valve
Trifacial nerve *use* Trigeminal Nerve
Trifecta™ Valve (aortic) *use* Zooplastic Tissue in
  Heart and Great Vessels
Trigone of bladder *use* Bladder
Trimming, excisional *see* Excision
Triquetral bone
  use Carpal, Right
  use Carpal, Left
Trochanteric bursa
  use Hip Bursa and Ligament, Right
  use Hip Bursa and Ligament, Left
TUMT (Transurethral microwave
  thermotherapy of prostate) 0V507ZZ
TUNA (transurethral needle ablation of
  prostate) 0V507ZZ
Tunneled central venous catheter *use* Vascular
  Access Device in Subcutaneous Tissue and
  Fascia
Tunneled spinal (intrathecal) catheter *use*
  Infusion Device
Turbinectomy
  see Excision, Ear, Nose, Sinus 09B
  see Resection, Ear, Nose, Sinus 09T
Turbinoplasty
  see Repair, Ear, Nose, Sinus 09Q
  see Replacement, Ear, Nose, Sinus 09R
  see Supplement, Ear, Nose, Sinus 09U
Turbinotomy
  see Division, Ear, Nose, Sinus 098
  see Drainage, Ear, Nose, Sinus 099
TURP (transurethral resection of prostate)
  see Excision, Prostate 0VB0
  see Resection, Prostate 0VT0
Twelfth cranial nerve *use* Hypoglossal Nerve
Two lead pacemaker *use* Pacemaker, Dual
  Chamber in 0JH
Tympanic cavity
  use Middle Ear, Right
  use Middle Ear, Left
Tympanic nerve *use* Glossopharyngeal Nerve
Tympanic part of temporal bone
  use Temporal Bone, Right
  use Temporal Bone, Left
Tympanogram *see* Hearing Assessment,
  Diagnostic Audiology F13
Tympanoplasty
  see Repair, Ear, Nose, Sinus 09Q
  see Replacement, Ear, Nose, Sinus 09R
  see Supplement, Ear, Nose, Sinus 09U
Tympanosympathectomy *see* Excision, Nerve,
  Head and Neck Sympathetic 01BK
Tympanotomy *see* Drainage, Ear, Nose, Sinus
  099

U

Ulnar collateral carpal ligament
use Wrist Bursa and Ligament, Right
use Wrist Bursa and Ligament, Left
Ulnar collateral ligament
use Elbow Bursa and Ligament, Right
use Elbow Bursa and Ligament, Left
Ulnar notch
use Radius, Right
use Radius, Left
Ulnar vein
use Brachial Vein, Right
use Brachial Vein, Left
Ultrafiltration
Hemodialysis *see* Performance, Urinary 5A1D
Therapeutic plasmapheresis *see* Pheresis, Circulatory 6A55
Ultraflex™ Precision Colonic Stent System *use* Intraluminal Device
ULTRAPRO Hernia System (UHS) *use* Synthetic Substitute
ULTRAPRO Partially Absorbable Lightweight Mesh *use* Synthetic Substitute
ULTRAPRO Plug *use* Synthetic Substitute
Ultrasonic osteogenic stimulator
use Bone Growth Stimulator in Head and Facial Bones
use Bone Growth Stimulator in Upper Bones
use Bone Growth Stimulator in Lower Bones
Ultrasonography
Abdomen BW40ZZZ
Abdomen and Pelvis BW41ZZZ
Abdominal Wall BH49ZZZ
Aorta
Abdominal, Intravascular B440ZZ3
Thoracic, Intravascular B340ZZ3
Appendix BD48ZZZ
Artery
Brachiocephalic-Subclavian, Right, Intravascular B341ZZ3
Celiac and Mesenteric, Intravascular B44KZZ3
Common Carotid
Bilateral, Intravascular B345ZZ3
Left, Intravascular B344ZZ3
Right, Intravascular B343ZZ3
Coronary
Multiple B241YZZ
Intravascular B241ZZ3
Transesophageal B241ZZ4
Single B240YZZ
Intravascular B240ZZ3
Transesophageal B240ZZ4
Femoral, Intravascular B44LZZ3
Inferior Mesenteric, Intravascular B445ZZ3
Internal Carotid
Bilateral, Intravascular B348ZZ3
Left, Intravascular B347ZZ3
Right, Intravascular B346ZZ3
Intra-Abdominal, Other, Intravascular B44BZZ3
Intracranial, Intravascular B34RZZ3
Lower Extremity
Bilateral, Intravascular B44HZZ3
Left, Intravascular B44GZZ3
Right, Intravascular B44FZZ3
Mesenteric and Celiac, Intravascular B44KZZ3
Ophthalmic, Intravascular B34VZZ3
Penile, Intravascular B44NZZ3
Pulmonary
Left, Intravascular B34TZZ3
Right, Intravascular B34SZZ3
Renal
Bilateral, Intravascular B448ZZ3
Left, Intravascular B447ZZ3
Right, Intravascular B446ZZ3
Subclavian, Left, Intravascular B342ZZ3
Superior Mesenteric, Intravascular B444ZZ3

Ultrasonography *(Continued)*
Artery *(Continued)*
Upper Extremity
Bilateral, Intravascular B34KZZ3
Left, Intravascular B34JZZ3
Right, Intravascular B34HZZ3
Bile Duct BF40ZZZ
Bile Duct and Gallbladder BF43ZZZ
Bladder BT40ZZZ
and Kidney BT4JZZZ
Brain B040ZZZ
Breast
Bilateral BH42ZZZ
Left BH41ZZZ
Right BH40ZZZ
Chest Wall BH4BZZZ
Coccyx BR4FZZZ
Connective Tissue
Lower Extremity BL41ZZZ
Upper Extremity BL40ZZZ
Duodenum BD49ZZZ
Elbow
Left, Densitometry BP4HZZ1
Right, Densitometry BP4GZZ1
Esophagus BD41ZZZ
Extremity
Lower BH48ZZZ
Upper BH47ZZZ
Eye
Bilateral B847ZZZ
Left B846ZZZ
Right B845ZZZ
Fallopian Tube
Bilateral BU42
Left BU41
Right BU40
Fetal Umbilical Cord BY47ZZZ
Fetus
First Trimester, Multiple Gestation BY4BZZZ
Second Trimester, Multiple Gestation BY4DZZZ
Single
First Trimester BY49ZZZ
Second Trimester BY4CZZZ
Third Trimester BY4FZZZ
Third Trimester, Multiple Gestation BY4GZZZ
Gallbladder BF42ZZZ
Gallbladder and Bile Duct BF43ZZZ
Gastrointestinal Tract BD47ZZZ
Gland
Adrenal
Bilateral BG42ZZZ
Left BG41ZZZ
Right BG40ZZZ
Parathyroid BG43ZZZ
Thyroid BG44ZZZ
Hand
Left, Densitometry BP4PZZ1
Right, Densitometry BP4NZZ1
Head and Neck BH4CZZZ
Heart
Left B245YZZ
Intravascular B245ZZ3
Transesophageal B245ZZ4
Pediatric B24DYZZ
Intravascular B24DZZ3
Transesophageal B24DZZ4
Right B244YZZ
Intravascular B244ZZ3
Transesophageal B244ZZ4
Right and Left B246YZZ
Intravascular B246ZZ3
Transesophageal B246ZZ4
Heart with Aorta B24BYZZ
Intravascular B24BZZ3
Transesophageal B24BZZ4
Hepatobiliary System, All BF4CZZZ

Ultrasonography *(Continued)*
Hip
Bilateral BQ42ZZZ
Left BQ41ZZZ
Right BQ40ZZZ
Kidney
and Bladder BT4JZZZ
Bilateral BT43ZZZ
Left BT42ZZZ
Right BT41ZZZ
Transplant BT49ZZZ
Knee
Bilateral BQ49ZZZ
Left BQ48ZZZ
Right BQ47ZZZ
Liver BF45ZZZ
Liver and Spleen BF46ZZZ
Mediastinum BB4CZZZ
Neck BW4FZZZ
Ovary
Bilateral BU45
Left BU44
Right BU43
Ovary and Uterus BU4C
Pancreas BF47ZZZ
Pelvic Region BW4GZZZ
Pelvis and Abdomen BW41ZZZ
Penis BV4BZZZ
Pericardium B24CYZZ
Intravascular B24CZZ3
Transesophageal B24CZZ4
Placenta BY48ZZZ
Pleura BB4BZZZ
Prostate and Seminal Vesicle BV49ZZZ
Rectum BD4CZZZ
Sacrum BR4FZZZ
Scrotum BV44ZZZ
Seminal Vesicle and Prostate BV49ZZZ
Shoulder
Left, Densitometry BP49ZZ1
Right, Densitometry BP48ZZ1
Spinal Cord B04BZZZ
Spine
Cervical BR40ZZZ
Lumbar BR49ZZZ
Thoracic BR47ZZZ
Spleen and Liver BF46ZZZ
Stomach BD42ZZZ
Tendon
Lower Extremity BL43ZZZ
Upper Extremity BL42ZZZ
Ureter
Bilateral BT48ZZZ
Left BT47ZZZ
Right BT46ZZZ
Urethra BT45ZZZ
Uterus BU46
Uterus and Ovary BU4C
Vein
Jugular
Left, Intravascular B544ZZ3
Right, Intravascular B543ZZ3
Lower Extremity
Bilateral, Intravascular B54DZZ3
Left, Intravascular B54CZZ3
Right, Intravascular B54BZZ3
Portal, Intravascular B54TZZ3
Renal
Bilateral, Intravascular B54LZZ3
Left, Intravascular B54KZZ3
Right, Intravascular B54JZZ3
Spanchnic, Intravascular B54TZZ3
Subclavian
Left, Intravascular B547ZZ3
Right, Intravascular B546ZZ3
Upper Extremity
Bilateral, Intravascular B54PZZ3
Left, Intravascular B54NZZ3
Right, Intravascular B54MZZ3

◀ New ◀▦ Revised ~~deleted~~ Deleted

Ultrasonography *(Continued)*
  Vena Cava
    Inferior, Intravascular B549ZZ3
    Superior, Intravascular B548ZZ3
  Wrist
    Left, Densitometry BP4MZZ1
    Right, Densitometry BP4LZZ1
Ultrasound bone healing system
  use Bone Growth Stimulator in Head and
      Facial Bones
  use Bone Growth Stimulator in Upper Bones
  use Bone Growth Stimulator in Lower Bones
Ultrasound Therapy
  Heart 6A75
  No Qualifier 6A75
  Vessels
    Head and Neck 6A75
    Other 6A75
    Peripheral 6A75
Ultraviolet Light Therapy, Skin 6A80
Umbilical artery
  use Internal Iliac Artery, Right
  use Internal Iliac Artery, Left
Uniplanar external fixator
  use External Fixation Device, Monoplanar in
      0PH
  use External Fixation Device, Monoplanar
      in 0PS
  use External Fixation Device, Monoplanar in
      0QH
  use External Fixation Device, Monoplanar
      in 0QS
Upper GI series *see* Fluoroscopy,
    Gastrointestinal, Upper BD15
Ureteral orifice
  use Ureter, Left
  use Ureter
  use Ureter, Right
  use Ureters, Bilateral
Ureterectomy
  see Excision, Urinary System 0TB
  see Resection, Urinary System 0TT
Ureterocolostomy *see* Bypass, Urinary System
    0T1
Ureterocystostomy *see* Bypass, Urinary System
    0T1
Ureteroenterostomy *see* Bypass, Urinary System
    0T1
Ureteroileostomy *see* Bypass, Urinary System
    0T1
Ureterolithotomy *see* Extirpation, Urinary
    System 0TC
Ureterolysis *see* Release, Urinary System 0TN
Ureteroneocystostomy
  see Bypass, Urinary System 0T1
  see Reposition, Urinary System 0TS
Ureteropelvic junction (UPJ)
  use Kidney Pelvis, Right
  use Kidney Pelvis, Left
Ureteropexy
  see Repair, Urinary System 0TQ
  see Reposition, Urinary System 0TS
Ureteroplasty
  see Repair, Urinary System 0TQ
  see Replacement, Urinary System 0TR
  see Supplement, Urinary System 0TU
Ureteroplication *see* Restriction, Urinary
    System 0TV
Ureteropyelography *see* Fluoroscopy, Urinary
    System BT1
Ureterorrhaphy *see* Repair, Urinary System 0TQ
Ureteroscopy 0TJ98ZZ
Ureterostomy
  see Bypass, Urinary System 0T1
  see Drainage, Urinary System 0T9
Ureterotomy *see* Drainage, Urinary System 0T9
Ureteroureterostomy *see* Bypass, Urinary
    System 0T1
Ureterovesical orifice
  use Ureter, Right
  use Ureter, Left

Ureterovesical orifice *(Continued)*
  use Ureters, Bilateral
  use Ureter
Urethral catheterization, indwelling
    0T9B70Z
Urethrectomy
  see Excision, Urethra 0TBD
  see Resection, Urethra 0TTD
Urethrolithotomy *see* Extirpation, Urethra
    0TCD
Urethrolysis *see* Release, Urethra 0TND
Urethropexy
  see Repair, Urethra 0TQD
  see Reposition, Urethra 0TSD
Urethroplasty
  see Repair, Urethra 0TQD
  see Replacement, Urethra 0TRD
  see Supplement, Urethra 0TUD
Urethrorrhaphy *see* Repair, Urethra 0TQD
Urethroscopy 0TJD8ZZ
Urethrotomy *see* Drainage, Urethra 0T9D
Uridine Triacetate XW0DX82 ◄
Urinary incontinence stimulator lead *use*
    Stimulator Lead in Urinary System
Urography *see* Fluoroscopy, Urinary System
    BT1
Uterine Artery
  use Internal Iliac Artery, Right
  use Internal Iliac Artery, Left
Uterine artery embolization (UAE) *see*
    Occlusion, Lower Arteries 04L
Uterine cornu *use* Uterus
Uterine tube
  use Fallopian Tube, Right
  use Fallopian Tube, Left
Uterine vein
  use Hypogastric Vein, Right
  use Hypogastric Vein, Left
Uvulectomy
  see Excision, Uvula 0CBN
  see Resection, Uvula 0CTN
Uvulorrhaphy *see* Repair, Uvula 0CQN
Uvulotomy *see* Drainage, Uvula 0C9N

V

Vaccination *see* Introduction of Serum, Toxoid,
    and Vaccine
Vacuum extraction, obstetric 10D07Z6
Vaginal artery
  use Internal Iliac Artery, Right
  use Internal Iliac Artery, Left
Vaginal pessary *use* Intraluminal Device,
    Pessary in Female Reproductive System
Vaginal vein
  use Hypogastric Vein, Right
  use Hypogastric Vein, Left
Vaginectomy
  see Excision, Vagina 0UBG
  see Resection, Vagina 0UTG
Vaginofixation
  see Repair, Vagina 0UQG
  see Reposition, Vagina 0USG
Vaginoplasty
  see Repair, Vagina 0UQG
  see Supplement, Vagina 0UUG
Vaginorrhaphy *see* Repair, Vagina 0UQG
Vaginoscopy 0UJH8ZZ
Vaginotomy *see* Drainage, Female Reproductive
    System 0U9
Vagotomy *see* Division, Nerve, Vagus 008Q
Valiant Thoracic Stent Graft *use* Intraluminal
    Device
Valvotomy, valvulotomy
  see Division, Heart and Great Vessels
    028
  see Release, Heart and Great Vessels 02N
Valvuloplasty
  see Repair, Heart and Great Vessels 02Q
  see Replacement, Heart and Great Vessels 02R
  see Supplement, Heart and Great Vessels 02U

Vascular Access Device
  Insertion of device in
    Abdomen 0JH8
    Chest 0JH6
    Lower Arm
      Left 0JHH
      Right 0JHG
    Lower Leg
      Left 0JHP
      Right 0JHN
    Upper Arm
      Left 0JHF
      Right 0JHD
    Upper Leg
      Left 0JHM
      Right 0JHL
  Removal of device from
    Lower Extremity 0JPW
    Trunk 0JPT
    Upper Extremity 0JPV
  Reservoir
    Insertion of device in
      Abdomen 0JH8
      Chest 0JH6
      Lower Arm
        Left 0JHH
        Right 0JHG
      Lower Leg
        Left 0JHP
        Right 0JHN
      Upper Arm
        Left 0JHF
        Right 0JHD
      Upper Leg
        Left 0JHM
        Right 0JHL
    Removal of device from
      Lower Extremity 0JPW
      Trunk 0JPT
      Upper Extremity 0JPV
    Revision of device in
      Lower Extremity 0JWW
      Trunk 0JWT
      Upper Extremity 0JWV
  Revision of device in
    Lower Extremity 0JWW
    Trunk 0JWT
    Upper Extremity 0JWV
Vasectomy *see* Excision, Male Reproductive
    System 0VB
Vasography
  see Plain Radiography, Male Reproductive
      System BV0
  see Fluoroscopy, Male Reproductive System
      BV1
Vasoligation *see* Occlusion, Male Reproductive
    System 0VL
Vasorrhaphy *see* Repair, Male Reproductive
    System 0VQ
Vasostomy *see* Bypass, Male Reproductive
    System 0V1
Vasotomy
  Drainage *see* Drainage, Male Reproductive
      System 0V9
  With ligation *see* Occlusion, Male
      Reproductive System 0VL
Vasovasostomy *see* Repair, Male Reproductive
    System 0VQ
Vastus intermedius muscle
  use Upper Leg Muscle, Right
  use Upper Leg Muscle, Left
Vastus lateralis muscle
  use Upper Leg Muscle, Right
  use Upper Leg Muscle, Left
Vastus medialis muscle
  use Upper Leg Muscle, Right
  use Upper Leg Muscle, Left
VCG (vectorcardiogram) *see* Measurement,
    Cardiac 4A02
Vectra® Vascular Access Graft *use* Vascular
    Access Device in Subcutaneous Tissue and
    Fascia

Venectomy
see Excision, Upper Veins 05B
see Excision, Lower Veins 06B
Venography
see Plain Radiography, Veins B50
see Fluoroscopy, Veins B51
Venorrhaphy
see Repair, Upper Veins 05Q
see Repair, Lower Veins 06Q
Venotripsy
see Occlusion, Upper Veins 05L
see Occlusion, Lower Veins 06L
Ventricular fold use Larynx
Ventriculoatriostomy see Bypass, Central
Nervous System 001
Ventriculocisternostomy see Bypass, Central
Nervous System 001
Ventriculogram, cardiac
Combined left and right heart see
Fluoroscopy, Heart, Right and Left
B216
Left ventricle see Fluoroscopy, Heart, Left
B215
Right ventricle see Fluoroscopy, Heart, Right
B214
Ventriculopuncture, through previously
implanted catheter 8C01X6J
Ventriculoscopy 00J04ZZ
Ventriculostomy
External drainage see Drainage, Cerebral
Ventricle 0096
Internal shunt see Bypass, Cerebral Ventricle
0016
Ventriculovenostomy see Bypass, Cerebral
Ventricle 0016
Ventrio™ Hernia Patch use Synthetic Substitute
VEP (visual evoked potential) 4A07X0Z
Vermiform appendix use Appendix
Vermilion border
use Upper Lip
use Lower Lip
Versa use Pacemaker, Dual Chamber in 0JH
Version, obstetric
External 10S0XZZ
Internal 10S07ZZ
Vertebral arch
use Cervical Vertebra
use Thoracic Vertebra
use Lumbar Vertebra
Vertebral canal use Spinal Canal
Vertebral foramen
use Cervical Vertebra
use Thoracic Vertebra
use Lumbar Vertebra
Vertebral lamina
use Cervical Vertebra
use Thoracic Vertebra
use Lumbar Vertebra
Vertebral pedicle
use Cervical Vertebra
use Thoracic Vertebra
use Lumbar Vertebra
Vesical vein
use Hypogastric Vein, Right
use Hypogastric Vein, Left

Vesicotomy see Drainage, Urinary System 0T9
Vesiculectomy
see Excision, Male Reproductive System 0VB
see Resection, Male Reproductive System
0VT
Vesiculogram, seminal see Plain Radiography,
Male Reproductive System BV0
Vesiculotomy see Drainage, Male Reproductive
System 0V9
Vestibular (Scarpa's) ganglion use Acoustic
Nerve
Vestibular Assessment F15Z
Vestibular nerve use Acoustic Nerve
Vestibular Treatment F0C
Vestibulocochlear nerve use Acoustic Nerve
VH-IVUS (virtual histology intravascular
ultrasound) see Ultrasonography, Heart
B24
Virchow's (supraclavicular) lymph node
use Lymphatic, Right Neck
use Lymphatic, Left Neck
Virtuoso (II) (DR) (VR) use Defibrillator
Generator in 0JH
Vistogard® use Uridine Triacetate ◄
Vitrectomy
see Excision, Eye 08B
see Resection, Eye 08T
Vitreous body
use Vitreous, Right
use Vitreous, Left
Viva (XT)(S) use Cardiac Resynchronization
Defibrillator Pulse Generator in 0JH
Vocal fold
use Vocal Cord, Right
use Vocal Cord, Left
Vocational
Assessment see Activities of Daily Living
Assessment, Rehabilitation F02
Retraining see Activities of Daily Living
Treatment, Rehabilitation F08
Volar (palmar) digital vein
use Hand Vein, Right
use Hand Vein, Left
Volar (palmar) metacarpal vein
use Hand Vein, Right
use Hand Vein, Left
Vomer bone use Nasal Septum
Vomer of nasal septum use Nasal Bone
Voraxaze use Glucarpidase
Vulvectomy
see Excision, Female Reproductive System
0UB
see Resection, Female Reproductive System
0UT

W

WALLSTENT® Endoprosthesis use
Intraluminal Device
Washing see Irrigation
Wedge resection, pulmonary see Excision,
Respiratory System 0BB
Window see Drainage
Wiring, dental 2W31X9Z

X

Xact Carotid Stent System use Intraluminal
Device
X-ray see Plain Radiography
X-STOP® Spacer
use Spinal Stabilization Device, Interspinous
Process in 0RH
use Spinal Stabilization Device, Interspinous
Process in 0SH
Xenograft use Zooplastic Tissue in Heart and
Great Vessels
XIENCE Everolimus Eluting Coronary Stent
System use Intraluminal Device, Drug-
eluting in Heart and Great Vessels
Xiphoid process use Sternum
XLIF® System use Interbody Fusion Device in
Lower Joints

Y

Yoga Therapy 8E0ZXY4

Z

Z-plasty, skin for scar contracture see Release,
Skin and Breast 0HN
Zenith AAA Endovascular Graft ◄
use Intraluminal Device, Branched or
Fenestrated, One or Two Arteries in
04V ◄
use Intraluminal Device, Branched or
Fenestrated, Three or More Arteries in
04V ◄
use Intraluminal Device ◄
Zenith Flex® AAA Endovascular Graft use
Intraluminal Device
Zenith TX2® TAA Endovascular Graft use
Intraluminal Device
Zenith® Renu™ AAA Ancillary Graft use
Intraluminal Device
Zilver® PTX® (paclitaxel) Drug-Eluting
Peripheral Stent
use Intraluminal Device, Drug-eluting in
Upper Arteries
use Intraluminal Device, Drug-eluting in
Lower Arteries
Zimmer® NexGen® LPS Mobile Bearing Knee
use Synthetic Substitute
Zimmer® NexGen® LPS-Flex Mobile Knee use
Synthetic Substitute
Zonule of Zinn
use Lens, Right
use Lens, Left
Zooplastic Tissue, Rapid Deployment
Technique, Replacement X2RF ◄
Zotarolimus-eluting coronary stent use
Intraluminal Device, Drug-eluting in Heart
and Great Vessels
Zygomatic process of frontal bone
use Frontal Bone, Right
use Frontal Bone, Left
Zygomatic process of temporal bone
use Temporal Bone, Right
use Temporal Bone, Left
Zygomaticus muscle use Facial Muscle
Zyvox use Oxazolidinones

◄ New   ◄IIII Revised   deleted Deleted

Appendices

DEFINITIONS
SECTION-CHARACTER

SECTION Ø - MEDICAL AND SURGICAL
CHARACTER 3 - OPERATION

Alteration	**Definition:** Modifying the anatomic structure of a body part without affecting the function of the body part **Explanation:** Principal purpose is to improve appearance **Includes/Examples:** Face lift, breast augmentation
Bypass	**Definition:** Altering the route of passage of the contents of a tubular body part **Explanation:** Rerouting contents of a body part to a downstream area of the normal route, to a similar route and body part, or to an abnormal route and dissimilar body part. Includes one or more anastomoses, with or without the use of a device **Includes/Examples:** Coronary artery bypass, colostomy formation
Change	**Definition:** Taking out or off a device from a body part and putting back an identical or similar device in or on the same body part without cutting or puncturing the skin or a mucous membrane **Explanation:** All CHANGE procedures are coded using the approach EXTERNAL **Includes/Examples:** Urinary catheter change, gastrostomy tube change
Control	**Definition:** Stopping, or attempting to stop, postprocedural or other acute bleeding **Explanation:** The site of the bleeding is coded as an anatomical region and not to a specific body part **Includes/Examples:** Control of post-prostatectomy hemorrhage, control of intracranial subdural hemorrhage, control of bleeding duodenal ulcer, control of retroperitoneal hemorrhage
Creation	**Definition:** Putting in or on biological or synthetic material to form a new body part that to the extent possible replicates the anatomic structure or function of an absent body part **Explanation:** Used for gender reassignment surgery and corrective procedures in individuals with congenital anomalies **Includes/Examples:** Creation of vagina in a male, creation of right and left atrioventricular valve from common atrioventricular valve
Destruction	**Definition:** Physical eradication of all or a portion of a body part by the direct use of energy, force, or a destructive agent **Explanation:** None of the body part is physically taken out **Includes/Examples:** Fulguration of rectal polyp, cautery of skin lesion

Detachment	**Definition:** Cutting off all or a portion of the upper or lower extremities **Explanation:** The body part value is the site of the detachment, with a qualifier if applicable to further specify the level where the extremity was detached **Includes/Examples:** Below knee amputation, disarticulation of shoulder
Dilation	**Definition:** Expanding an orifice or the lumen of a tubular body part **Explanation:** The orifice can be a natural orifice or an artificially created orifice. Accomplished by stretching a tubular body part using intraluminal pressure or by cutting part of the orifice or wall of the tubular body part **Includes/Examples:** Percutaneous transluminal angioplasty, pyloromyotomy
Division	**Definition:** Cutting into a body part, without draining fluids and/or gases from the body part, in order to separate or transect a body part **Explanation:** All or a portion of the body part is separated into two or more portions **Includes/Examples:** Spinal cordotomy, osteotomy
Drainage	**Definition:** Taking or letting out fluids and/or gases from a body part **Explanation:** The qualifier DIAGNOSTIC is used to identify drainage procedures that are biopsies **Includes/Examples:** Thoracentesis, incision and drainage
Excision	**Definition:** Cutting out or off, without replacement, a portion of a body part **Explanation:** The qualifier DIAGNOSTIC is used to identify excision procedures that are biopsies **Includes/Examples:** Partial nephrectomy, liver biopsy
Extirpation	**Definition:** Taking or cutting out solid matter from a body part **Explanation:** The solid matter may be an abnormal byproduct of a biological function or a foreign body; it may be imbedded in a body part or in the lumen of a tubular body part. The solid matter may or may not have been previously broken into pieces **Includes/Examples:** Thrombectomy, choledocholithotomy
Extraction	**Definition:** Pulling or stripping out or off all or a portion of a body part by the use of force **Explanation:** The qualifier DIAGNOSTIC is used to identify extraction procedures that are biopsies **Includes/Examples:** Dilation and curettage, vein stripping

SECTION Ø - MEDICAL AND SURGICAL
CHARACTER 3 - OPERATION

Fragmentation	**Definition:** Breaking solid matter in a body part into pieces **Explanation:** Physical force (e.g., manual, ultrasonic) applied directly or indirectly is used to break the solid matter into pieces. The solid matter may be an abnormal byproduct of a biological function or a foreign body. The pieces of solid matter are not taken out **Includes/Examples:** Extracorporeal shockwave lithotripsy, transurethral lithotripsy	**Release**	**Definition:** Freeing a body part from an abnormal physical constraint by cutting or by the use of force **Explanation:** Some of the restraining tissue may be taken out but none of the body part is taken out **Includes/Examples:** Adhesiolysis, carpal tunnel release
Fusion	**Definition:** Joining together portions of an articular body part rendering the articular body part immobile **Explanation:** The body part is joined together by fixation device, bone graft, or other means **Includes/Examples:** Spinal fusion, ankle arthrodesis	**Removal**	**Definition:** Taking out or off a device from a body part **Explanation:** If a device is taken out and a similar device put in without cutting or puncturing the skin or mucous membrane, the procedure is coded to the root operation CHANGE. Otherwise, the procedure for taking out a device is coded to the root operation REMOVAL **Includes/Examples:** Drainage tube removal, cardiac pacemaker removal
Insertion	**Definition:** Putting in a nonbiological appliance that monitors, assists, performs, or prevents a physiological function but does not physically take the place of a body part **Includes/Examples:** Insertion of radioactive implant, insertion of central venous catheter	**Repair**	**Definition:** Restoring, to the extent possible, a body part to its normal anatomic structure and function **Explanation:** Used only when the method to accomplish the repair is not one of the other root operations **Includes/Examples:** Colostomy takedown, suture of laceration
Inspection	**Definition:** Visually and/or manually exploring a body part **Explanation:** Visual exploration may be performed with or without optical instrumentation. Manual exploration may be performed directly or through intervening body layers **Includes/Examples:** Diagnostic arthroscopy, exploratory laparotomy	**Replacement**	**Definition:** Putting in or on biological or synthetic material that physically takes the place and/or function of all or a portion of a body part **Explanation:** The body part may have been taken out or replaced, or may be taken out, physically eradicated, or rendered nonfunctional during the Replacement procedure. A Removal procedure is coded for taking out the device used in a previous replacement procedure **Includes/Examples:** Total hip replacement, bone graft, free skin graft
Map	**Definition:** Locating the route of passage of electrical impulses and/or locating functional areas in a body part **Explanation:** Applicable only to the cardiac conduction mechanism and the central nervous system **Includes/Examples:** Cardiac mapping, cortical mapping	**Reposition**	**Definition:** Moving to its normal location, or other suitable location, all or a portion of a body part **Explanation:** The body part is moved to a new location from an abnormal location, or from a normal location where it is not functioning correctly. The body part may or may not be cut out or off to be moved to the new location **Includes/Examples:** Reposition of undescended testicle, fracture reduction
Occlusion	**Definition:** Completely closing an orifice or the lumen of a tubular body part **Explanation:** The orifice can be a natural orifice or an artificially created orifice **Includes/Examples:** Fallopian tube ligation, ligation of inferior vena cava	**Resection**	**Definition:** Cutting out or off, without replacement, all of a body part **Includes/Examples:** Total nephrectomy, total lobectomy of lung
Reattachment	**Definition:** Putting back in or on all or a portion of a separated body part to its normal location or other suitable location **Explanation:** Vascular circulation and nervous pathways may or may not be reestablished **Includes/Examples:** Reattachment of hand, reattachment of avulsed kidney		

SECTION Ø - MEDICAL AND SURGICAL
CHARACTER 3 - OPERATION

Restriction	**Definition:** Partially closing an orifice or the lumen of a tubular body part **Explanation:** The orifice can be a natural orifice or an artificially created orifice **Includes/Examples:** Esophagogastric fundoplication, cervical cerclage
Revision	**Definition:** Correcting, to the extent possible, a portion of a malfunctioning device or the position of a displaced device **Explanation:** Revision can include correcting a malfunctioning or displaced device by taking out or putting in components of the device such as a screw or pin **Includes/Examples:** Adjustment of position of pacemaker lead, recementing of hip prosthesis
Supplement	**Definition:** Putting in or on biological or synthetic material that physically reinforces and/or augments the function of a portion of a body part **Explanation:** The biological material is non-living, or is living and from the same individual. The body part may have been previously replaced, and the Supplement procedure is performed to physically reinforce and/or augment the function of the replaced body part **Includes/Examples:** Herniorrhaphy using mesh, free nerve graft, mitral valve ring annuloplasty, put a new acetabular liner in a previous hip replacement
Transfer	**Definition:** Moving, without taking out, all or a portion of a body part to another location to take over the function of all or a portion of a body part **Explanation:** The body part transferred remains connected to its vascular and nervous supply **Includes/Examples:** Tendon transfer, skin pedicle flap transfer
Transplantation	**Definition:** Putting in or on all or a portion of a living body part taken from another individual or animal to physically take the place and/or function of all or a portion of a similar body part **Explanation:** The native body part may or may not be taken out, and the transplanted body part may take over all or a portion of its function **Includes/Examples:** Kidney transplant, heart transplant

SECTION Ø - MEDICAL AND SURGICAL
CHARACTER 4 - BODY PART

1st Toe, Left 1st Toe, Right	**Includes:** Hallux
Abdomen Muscle, Left Abdomen Muscle, Right	**Includes:** External oblique muscle Internal oblique muscle Pyramidalis muscle Rectus abdominis muscle Transversus abdominis muscle
Abdominal Aorta	**Includes:** Inferior phrenic artery Lumbar artery Median sacral artery Middle suprarenal artery Ovarian artery Testicular artery
Abdominal Sympathetic Nerve	**Includes:** Abdominal aortic plexus Auerbach's (myenteric) plexus Celiac (solar) plexus Celiac ganglion Gastric plexus Hepatic plexus Inferior hypogastric plexus Inferior mesenteric ganglion Inferior mesenteric plexus Meissner's (submucous) plexus Myenteric (Auerbach's) plexus Pancreatic plexus Pelvic splanchnic nerve Renal plexus Solar (celiac) plexus Splenic plexus Submucous (Meissner's) plexus Superior hypogastric plexus Superior mesenteric ganglion Superior mesenteric plexus Suprarenal plexus

SECTION Ø - MEDICAL AND SURGICAL
CHARACTER 4 - BODY PART

Abducens Nerve	**Includes:** Sixth cranial nerve
Accessory Nerve	**Includes:** Eleventh cranial nerve
Acoustic Nerve	**Includes:** Cochlear nerve Eighth cranial nerve Scarpa's (vestibular) ganglion Spiral ganglion Vestibular (Scarpa's) ganglion Vestibular nerve Vestibulocochlear nerve
Adenoids	**Includes:** Pharyngeal tonsil
Adrenal Gland Adrenal Gland, Left Adrenal Gland, Right Adrenal Glands, Bilateral	**Includes:** Suprarenal gland
Ampulla of Vater	**Includes:** Duodenal ampulla Hepatopancreatic ampulla
Anal Sphincter	**Includes:** External anal sphincter Internal anal sphincter
Ankle Bursa and Ligament, Left Ankle Bursa and Ligament, Right	**Includes:** Calcaneofibular ligament Deltoid ligament Ligament of the lateral malleolus Talofibular ligament
Ankle Joint, Left Ankle Joint, Right	**Includes:** Inferior tibiofibular joint Talocrural joint
Anterior Chamber, Left Anterior Chamber, Right	**Includes:** Aqueous humour
Anterior Tibial Artery, Left Anterior Tibial Artery, Right	**Includes:** Anterior lateral malleolar artery Anterior medial malleolar artery Anterior tibial recurrent artery Dorsalis pedis artery Posterior tibial recurrent artery
Anus	**Includes:** Anal orifice
Aortic Valve	**Includes:** Aortic annulus

Appendix	**Includes:** Vermiform appendix
Ascending Colon	**Includes:** Hepatic flexure
Atrial Septum	**Includes:** Interatrial septum
Atrium, Left	**Includes:** Atrium pulmonale Left auricular appendix
Atrium, Right	**Includes:** Atrium dextrum cordis Right auricular appendix Sinus venosus
Auditory Ossicle, Left Auditory Ossicle, Right	**Includes:** Incus Malleus Stapes
Axillary Artery, Left Axillary Artery, Right	**Includes:** Anterior circumflex humeral artery Lateral thoracic artery Posterior circumflex humeral artery Subscapular artery Superior thoracic artery Thoracoacromial artery
Azygos Vein	**Includes:** Right ascending lumbar vein Right subcostal vein
Basal Ganglia	**Includes:** Basal nuclei Claustrum Corpus striatum Globus pallidus Substantia nigra Subthalamic nucleus
Basilic Vein, Left Basilic Vein, Right	**Includes:** Median antebrachial vein Median cubital vein
Bladder	**Includes:** Trigone of bladder
Brachial Artery, Left Brachial Artery, Right	**Includes:** Inferior ulnar collateral artery Profunda brachii Superior ulnar collateral artery

SECTION Ø - MEDICAL AND SURGICAL
CHARACTER 4 - BODY PART

Body Part	
Brachial Plexus	**Includes:** Axillary nerve Dorsal scapular nerve First intercostal nerve Long thoracic nerve Musculocutaneous nerve Subclavius nerve Suprascapular nerve
Brachial Vein, Left Brachial Vein, Right	**Includes:** Radial vein Ulnar vein
Brain	**Includes:** Cerebrum Corpus callosum Encephalon
Breast, Bilateral Breast, Left Breast, Right	**Includes:** Mammary duct Mammary gland
Buccal Mucosa	**Includes:** Buccal gland Molar gland Palatine gland
Carotid Bodies, Bilateral Carotid Body, Left Carotid Body, Right	**Includes:** Carotid glomus
Carpal Joint, Left Carpal Joint, Right	**Includes:** Intercarpal joint Midcarpal joint
Carpal, Left Carpal, Right	**Includes:** Capitate bone Hamate bone Lunate bone Pisiform bone Scaphoid bone Trapezium bone Trapezoid bone Triquetral bone
Celiac Artery	**Includes:** Celiac trunk
Cephalic Vein, Left Cephalic Vein, Right	**Includes:** Accessory cephalic vein
Cerebellum	**Includes:** Culmen
Cerebral Hemisphere	**Includes:** Frontal lobe Occipital lobe Parietal lobe Temporal lobe
Cerebral Meninges	**Includes:** Arachnoid mater, intracranial Leptomeninges, intracranial Pia mater, intracranial
Cerebral Ventricle	**Includes:** Aqueduct of Sylvius Cerebral aqueduct (Sylvius) Choroid plexus Ependyma Foramen of Monro (intraventricular) Fourth ventricle Interventricular foramen (Monro) Left lateral ventricle Right lateral ventricle Third ventricle
Cervical Nerve	**Includes:** Greater occipital nerve Spinal nerve, cervical Suboccipital nerve Third occipital nerve
Cervical Plexus	**Includes:** Ansa cervicalis Cutaneous (transverse) cervical nerve Great auricular nerve Lesser occipital nerve Supraclavicular nerve Transverse (cutaneous) cervical nerve
Cervical Vertebra	**Includes:** Spinous process Vertebral arch Vertebral foramen Vertebral lamina Vertebral pedicle
Cervical Vertebral Joint	**Includes:** Atlantoaxial joint Cervical facet joint

Cervical Vertebral
   Joints, 2 or
   more
	Includes:
	Cervical facet joint

Cervicothoracic Vertebral Joint	**Includes:** Cervicothoracic facet joint
Cisterna Chyli	**Includes:** Intestinal lymphatic trunk Lumbar lymphatic trunk
Coccygeal Glomus	**Includes:** Coccygeal body

SECTION Ø - MEDICAL AND SURGICAL
CHARACTER 4 - BODY PART

Colic Vein	**Includes:** Ileocolic vein Left colic vein Middle colic vein Right colic vein	Ethmoid Bone, Left Ethmoid Bone, Right	**Includes:** Cribriform plate
Conduction Mechanism	**Includes:** Atrioventricular node Bundle of His Bundle of Kent Sinoatrial node	Ethmoid Sinus, Left Ethmoid Sinus, Right	**Includes:** Ethmoidal air cell
Conjunctiva, Left Conjunctiva, Right	**Includes:** Plica semilunaris	Eustachian Tube, Left Eustachian Tube, Right	**Includes:** Auditory tube Pharyngotympanic tube
Dura Mater	**Includes:** Diaphragma sellae Dura mater, intracranial Falx cerebri Tentorium cerebelli	External Auditory Canal, Left External Auditory Canal, Right	**Includes:** External auditory meatus
Elbow Bursa and Ligament, Left Elbow Bursa and Ligament, Right	**Includes:** Annular ligament Olecranon bursa Radial collateral ligament Ulnar collateral ligament	External Carotid Artery, Left External Carotid Artery, Right	**Includes:** Ascending pharyngeal artery Internal maxillary artery Lingual artery Maxillary artery Occipital artery Posterior auricular artery Superior thyroid artery
Elbow Joint, Left Elbow Joint, Right	**Includes:** Distal humerus, involving joint Humeroradial joint Humeroulnar joint Proximal radioulnar joint	External Ear, Bilateral External Ear, Left External Ear, Right	**Includes:** Antihelix Antitragus Auricle Earlobe Helix Pinna Tragus
Epidural Space	**Includes:** Epidural space, intracranial Extradural space, intracranial	External Iliac Artery, Left External Iliac Artery, Right	**Includes:** Deep circumflex iliac artery Inferior epigastric artery
Epiglottis	**Includes:** Glossoepiglottic fold	External Jugular Vein, Left External Jugular Vein, Right	**Includes:** Posterior auricular vein
Esophagogastric Junction	**Includes:** Cardia Cardioesophageal junction Gastroesophageal (GE) junction	Extraocular Muscle, Left Extraocular Muscle, Right	**Includes:** Inferior oblique muscle Inferior rectus muscle Lateral rectus muscle Medial rectus muscle Superior oblique muscle Superior rectus muscle
Esophagus, Lower	**Includes:** Abdominal esophagus		
Esophagus, Middle	**Includes:** Thoracic esophagus	Eye, Left Eye, Right	**Includes:** Ciliary body Posterior chamber
Esophagus, Upper	**Includes:** Cervical esophagus		

SECTION Ø - MEDICAL AND SURGICAL
CHARACTER 4 - BODY PART

Face Artery	**Includes:** Angular artery Ascending palatine artery External maxillary artery Facial artery Inferior labial artery Submental artery Superior labial artery
Face Vein, Left Face Vein, Right	**Includes:** Angular vein Anterior facial vein Common facial vein Deep facial vein Frontal vein Posterior facial (retromandibular) vein Supraorbital vein
Facial Muscle	**Includes:** Buccinator muscle Corrugator supercilii muscle Depressor anguli oris muscle Depressor labii inferioris muscle Depressor septi nasi muscle Depressor supercilii muscle Levator anguli oris muscle Levator labii superioris alaeque nasi muscle Levator labii superioris muscle Mentalis muscle Nasalis muscle Occipitofrontalis muscle Orbicularis oris muscle Procerus muscle Risorius muscle Zygomaticus muscle
Facial Nerve	**Includes:** Chorda tympani Geniculate ganglion Greater superficial petrosal nerve Nerve to the stapedius Parotid plexus Posterior auricular nerve Seventh cranial nerve Submandibular ganglion
Fallopian Tube, Left Fallopian Tube, Right	**Includes:** Oviduct Salpinx Uterine tube
Femoral Artery, Left Femoral Artery, Right	**Includes:** Circumflex iliac artery Deep femoral artery Descending genicular artery External pudendal artery Superficial epigastric artery

Femoral Nerve	**Includes:** Anterior crural nerve Saphenous nerve
Femoral Shaft, Left Femoral Shaft, Right	**Includes:** Body of femur
Femoral Vein, Left Femoral Vein, Right	**Includes:** Deep femoral (profunda femoris) vein Popliteal vein Profunda femoris (deep femoral) vein
Fibula, Left Fibula, Right	**Includes:** Body of fibula Head of fibula Lateral malleolus
Finger Nail	**Includes:** Nail bed Nail plate
Finger Phalangeal Joint, Left Finger Phalangeal Joint, Right	**Includes:** Interphalangeal (IP) joint
Foot Artery, Left Foot Artery, Right	**Includes:** Arcuate artery Dorsal metatarsal artery Lateral plantar artery Lateral tarsal artery Medial plantar artery
Foot Bursa and Ligament, Left Foot Bursa and Ligament, Right	**Includes:** Calcaneocuboid ligament Cuneonavicular ligament Intercuneiform ligament Interphalangeal ligament Metatarsal ligament Metatarsophalangeal ligament Subtalar ligament Talocalcaneal ligament Talocalcaneonavicular ligament Tarsometatarsal ligament
Foot Muscle, Left Foot Muscle, Right	**Includes:** Abductor hallucis muscle Adductor hallucis muscle Extensor digitorum brevis muscle Extensor hallucis brevis muscle Flexor digitorum brevis muscle Flexor hallucis brevis muscle Quadratus plantae muscle

SECTION Ø - MEDICAL AND SURGICAL
CHARACTER 4 - BODY PART

Foot Vein, Left Foot Vein, Right	**Includes:** Common digital vein Dorsal metatarsal vein Dorsal venous arch Plantar digital vein Plantar metatarsal vein Plantar venous arch
Frontal Bone, Left Frontal Bone, Right	**Includes:** Zygomatic process of frontal bone
Gastric Artery	**Includes:** Left gastric artery Right gastric artery
Glenoid Cavity, Left Glenoid Cavity, Right	**Includes:** Glenoid fossa (of scapula)
Glomus Jugulare	**Includes:** Jugular body
Glossopharyngeal Nerve	**Includes:** Carotid sinus nerve Ninth cranial nerve Tympanic nerve
Greater Omentum	**Includes:** Gastrocolic ligament Gastrocolic omentum Gastrophrenic ligament Gastrosplenic ligament
Greater Saphenous Vein, Left Greater Saphenous Vein, Right	**Includes:** External pudendal vein Great saphenous vein Superficial circumflex iliac vein Superficial epigastric vein
Hand Artery, Left Hand Artery, Right	**Includes:** Deep palmar arch Princeps pollicis artery Radialis indicis Superficial palmar arch
Hand Bursa and Ligament, Left Hand Bursa and Ligament, Right	**Includes:** Carpometacarpal ligament Intercarpal ligament Interphalangeal ligament Lunotriquetral ligament Metacarpal ligament Metacarpophalangeal ligament Pisohamate ligament Pisometacarpal ligament Scapholunate ligament Scaphotrapezium ligament

Hand Muscle, Left Hand Muscle, Right	**Includes:** Hypothenar muscle Palmar interosseous muscle Thenar muscle
Hand Vein, Left Hand Vein, Right	**Includes:** Dorsal metacarpal vein Palmar (volar) digital vein Palmar (volar) metacarpal vein Superficial palmar venous arch Volar (palmar) digital vein Volar (palmar) metacarpal vein
Head and Neck Bursa and Ligament	**Includes:** Alar ligament of axis Cervical interspinous ligament Cervical intertransverse ligament Cervical ligamentum flavum Interspinous ligament Lateral temporomandibular ligament Sphenomandibular ligament Stylomandibular ligament Transverse ligament of atlas
Head and Neck Sympathetic Nerve	**Includes:** Cavernous plexus Cervical ganglion Ciliary ganglion Internal carotid plexus Otic ganglion Pterygopalatine (sphenopalatine) ganglion Sphenopalatine (pterygopalatine) ganglion Stellate ganglion Submandibular ganglion Submaxillary ganglion
Head Muscle	**Includes:** Auricularis muscle Masseter muscle Pterygoid muscle Splenius capitis muscle Temporalis muscle Temporoparietalis muscle
Heart, Left	**Includes:** Left coronary sulcus Obtuse margin
Heart, Right	**Includes:** Right coronary sulcus
Hemiazygos Vein	**Includes** Left ascending lumbar vein Left subcostal vein
Hepatic Artery	**Includes:** Common hepatic artery Gastroduodenal artery Hepatic artery proper

SECTION Ø - MEDICAL AND SURGICAL
CHARACTER 4 - BODY PART

Hip Bursa and Ligament, Left Hip Bursa and Ligament, Right	**Includes:** Iliofemoral ligament Ischiofemoral ligament Pubofemoral ligament Transverse acetabular ligament Trochanteric bursa
Hip Joint, Left Hip Joint, Right	**Includes:** Acetabulofemoral joint
Hip Muscle, Left Hip Muscle, Right	**Includes:** Gemellus muscle Gluteus maximus muscle Gluteus medius muscle Gluteus minimus muscle Iliacus muscle Obturator muscle Piriformis muscle Psoas muscle Quadratus femoris muscle Tensor fasciae latae muscle
Humeral Head, Left Humeral Head, Right	**Includes:** Greater tuberosity Lesser tuberosity Neck of humerus (anatomical) (surgical)
Humeral Shaft, Left Humeral Shaft, Right	**Includes:** Distal humerus Humerus, distal Lateral epicondyle of humerus Medial epicondyle of humerus
Hypogastric Vein, Left Hypogastric Vein, Right	**Includes:** Gluteal vein Internal iliac vein Internal pudendal vein Lateral sacral vein Middle hemorrhoidal vein Obturator vein Uterine vein Vaginal vein Vesical vein
Hypoglossal Nerve	**Includes:** Twelfth cranial nerve
Hypothalamus	**Includes:** Mammillary body
Inferior Mesenteric Artery	**Includes:** Sigmoid artery Superior rectal artery
Inferior Mesenteric Vein	**Includes:** Sigmoid vein Superior rectal vein

Inferior Vena Cava	**Includes:** Postcava Right inferior phrenic vein Right ovarian vein Right second lumbar vein Right suprarenal vein Right testicular vein
Inguinal Region, Bilateral Inguinal Region, Left Inguinal Region, Right	**Includes:** Inguinal canal Inguinal triangle
Inner Ear, Left Inner Ear, Right	**Includes:** Bony labyrinth Bony vestibule Cochlea Round window Semicircular canal
Innominate Artery	**Includes:** Brachiocephalic artery Brachiocephalic trunk
Innominate Vein, Left Innominate Vein, Right	**Includes:** Brachiocephalic vein Inferior thyroid vein
Internal Carotid Artery, Left Internal Carotid Artery, Right	**Includes:** Caroticotympanic artery Carotid sinus
Internal Iliac Artery, Left Internal Iliac Artery, Right	**Includes:** Deferential artery Hypogastric artery Iliolumbar artery Inferior gluteal artery Inferior vesical artery Internal pudendal artery Lateral sacral artery Middle rectal artery Obturator artery Superior gluteal artery Umbilical artery Uterine Artery Vaginal artery
Internal Mammary Artery, Left Internal Mammary Artery, Right	**Includes:** Anterior intercostal artery Internal thoracic artery Musculophrenic artery Pericardiophrenic artery Superior epigastric artery

SECTION Ø - MEDICAL AND SURGICAL
CHARACTER 4 - BODY PART

Intracranial Artery	**Includes:** Anterior cerebral artery Anterior choroidal artery Anterior communicating artery Basilar artery Circle of Willis Internal carotid artery, intracranial portion Middle cerebral artery Ophthalmic artery Posterior cerebral artery Posterior communicating artery Posterior inferior cerebellar artery (PICA)
Intracranial Vein	**Includes:** Anterior cerebral vein Basal (internal) cerebral vein Dural venous sinus Great cerebral vein Inferior cerebellar vein Inferior cerebral vein Internal (basal) cerebral vein Middle cerebral vein Ophthalmic vein Superior cerebellar vein Superior cerebral vein
Jejunum	**Includes:** Duodenojejunal flexure
Kidney	**Includes:** Renal calyx Renal capsule Renal cortex Renal segment
Kidney Pelvis, Left Kidney Pelvis, Right	**Includes:** Ureteropelvic junction (UPJ)
Kidney, Left Kidney, Right Kidneys, Bilateral	**Includes:** Renal calyx Renal capsule Renal cortex Renal segment
Knee Bursa and Ligament, Left Knee Bursa and Ligament, Right	**Includes:** Anterior cruciate ligament (ACL) Lateral collateral ligament (LCL) Ligament of head of fibula Medial collateral ligament (MCL) Patellar ligament Popliteal ligament Posterior cruciate ligament (PCL) Prepatellar bursa
Knee Joint, Femoral Surface, Left Knee Joint, Femoral Surface, Right	**Includes:** Femoropatellar joint Patellofemoral joint

Knee Joint, Left Knee Joint, Right	**Includes:** Femoropatellar joint Femorotibial joint Lateral meniscus Medial meniscus Patellofemoral joint Tibiofemoral joint
Knee Joint, Tibial Surface, Left Knee Joint, Tibial Surface, Right	**Includes:** Femorotibial joint Tibiofemoral joint
Knee Tendon, Left Knee Tendon, Right	**Includes:** Patellar tendon
Lacrimal Duct, Left Lacrimal Duct, Right	**Includes:** Lacrimal canaliculus Lacrimal punctum Lacrimal sac Nasolacrimal duct
Larynx	**Includes:** Aryepiglottic fold Arytenoid cartilage Corniculate cartilage ~~Cricoid cartilage~~ Cuneiform cartilage False vocal cord Glottis Rima glottidis Thyroid cartilage Ventricular fold
Lens, Left Lens, Right	**Includes:** Zonule of Zinn
Lesser Omentum	**Includes:** Gastrohepatic omentum Hepatogastric ligament
Lesser Saphenous Vein, Left Lesser Saphenous Vein, Right	**Includes:** Small saphenous vein
Liver	**Includes:** Quadrate lobe
Lower Arm and Wrist Muscle, Left Lower Arm and Wrist Muscle, Right	**Includes:** Anatomical snuffbox Brachioradialis muscle Extensor carpi radialis muscle Extensor carpi ulnaris muscle Flexor carpi radialis muscle Flexor carpi ulnaris muscle Flexor pollicis longus muscle Palmaris longus muscle Pronator quadratus muscle Pronator teres muscle

SECTION Ø - MEDICAL AND SURGICAL
CHARACTER 4 - BODY PART

Body Part	
Lower Eyelid, Left Lower Eyelid, Right	**Includes:** Inferior tarsal plate Medial canthus
Lower Femur, Left Lower Femur, Right	**Includes:** Lateral condyle of femur Lateral epicondyle of femur Medial condyle of femur Medial epicondyle of femur
Lower Leg Muscle, Left Lower Leg Muscle, Right	**Includes:** Extensor digitorum longus muscle Extensor hallucis longus muscle Fibularis brevis muscle Fibularis longus muscle Flexor digitorum longus muscle Flexor hallucis longus muscle Gastrocnemius muscle Peroneus brevis muscle Peroneus longus muscle Popliteus muscle Soleus muscle Tibialis anterior muscle Tibialis posterior muscle
Lower Leg Tendon, Left Lower Leg Tendon, Right	**Includes:** Achilles tendon
Lower Lip	**Includes:** Frenulum labii inferioris Labial gland Vermilion border
Lumbar Nerve	**Includes:** Lumbosacral trunk Spinal nerve, lumbar Superior clunic (cluneal) nerve
Lumbar Plexus	**Includes:** Accessory obturator nerve Genitofemoral nerve Iliohypogastric nerve Ilioinguinal nerve Lateral femoral cutaneous nerve Obturator nerve Superior gluteal nerve
Lumbar Spinal Cord	**Includes:** Cauda equina Conus medullaris
Lumbar Sympathetic Nerve	**Includes:** Lumbar ganglion Lumbar splanchnic nerve

Body Part	
Lumbar Vertebra	**Includes:** Spinous process Vertebral arch Vertebral foramen Vertebral lamina Vertebral pedicle
Lumbar Vertebral Joint	**Includes:** Lumbar facet joint
Lumbosacral Joint	**Includes:** Lumbosacral facet joint
Lymphatic, Aortic	**Includes:** Celiac lymph node Gastric lymph node Hepatic lymph node Lumbar lymph node Pancreaticosplenic lymph node Paraaortic lymph node Retroperitoneal lymph node
Lymphatic, Head	**Includes:** Buccinator lymph node Infraauricular lymph node Infraparotid lymph node Parotid lymph node Preauricular lymph node Submandibular lymph node Submaxillary lymph node Submental lymph node Subparotid lymph node Suprahyoid lymph node
Lymphatic, Left Axillary	**Includes:** Anterior (pectoral) lymph node Apical (subclavicular) lymph node Brachial (lateral) lymph node Central axillary lymph node Lateral (brachial) lymph node Pectoral (anterior) lymph node Posterior (subscapular) lymph node Subclavicular (apical) lymph node Subscapular (posterior) lymph node
Lymphatic, Left Lower Extremity	**Includes:** Femoral lymph node Popliteal lymph node
Lymphatic, Left Neck	**Includes:** Cervical lymph node Jugular lymph node Mastoid (postauricular) lymph node Occipital lymph node Postauricular (mastoid) lymph node Retropharyngeal lymph node Supraclavicular (Virchow's) lymph node Virchow's (supraclavicular) lymph node

APPENDIX A

SECTION 0 - MEDICAL AND SURGICAL
CHARACTER 4 - BODY PART

Lymphatic, Left Upper Extremity	**Includes:** Cubital lymph node Deltopectoral (infraclavicular) lymph node Epitrochlear lymph node Infraclavicular (deltopectoral) lymph node Supratrochlear lymph node
Lymphatic, Mesenteric	**Includes:** Inferior mesenteric lymph node Pararectal lymph node Superior mesenteric lymph node
Lymphatic, Pelvis	**Includes:** Common iliac (subaortic) lymph node Gluteal lymph node Iliac lymph node Inferior epigastric lymph node Obturator lymph node Sacral lymph node Subaortic (common iliac) lymph node Suprainguinal lymph node
Lymphatic, Right Axillary	**Includes:** Anterior (pectoral) lymph node Apical (subclavicular) lymph node Brachial (lateral) lymph node Central axillary lymph node Lateral (brachial) lymph node Pectoral (anterior) lymph node Posterior (subscapular) lymph node Subclavicular (apical) lymph node Subscapular (posterior) lymph node
Lymphatic, Right Lower Extremity	**Includes:** Femoral lymph node Popliteal lymph node
Lymphatic, Right Neck	**Includes:** Cervical lymph node Jugular lymph node Mastoid (postauricular) lymph node Occipital lymph node Postauricular (mastoid) lymph node Retropharyngeal lymph node Right jugular trunk Right lymphatic duct Right subclavian trunk Supraclavicular (Virchow's) lymph node Virchow's (supraclavicular) lymph node
Lymphatic, Right Upper Extremity	**Includes:** Cubital lymph node Deltopectoral (infraclavicular) lymph node Epitrochlear lymph node Infraclavicular (deltopectoral) lymph node Supratrochlear lymph node

Lymphatic, Thorax	**Includes:** Intercostal lymph node Mediastinal lymph node Parasternal lymph node Paratracheal lymph node Tracheobronchial lymph node
Main Bronchus, Right	**Includes:** Bronchus Intermedius Intermediate bronchus
Mandible, Left Mandible, Right	**Includes:** Alveolar process of mandible Condyloid process Mandibular notch Mental foramen
Mastoid Sinus, Left Mastoid Sinus, Right	**Includes:** Mastoid air cells
Maxilla, Left Maxilla, Right	**Includes:** Alveolar process of maxilla
Maxillary Sinus, Left Maxillary Sinus, Right	**Includes:** Antrum of Highmore
Median Nerve	**Includes:** Anterior interosseous nerve Palmar cutaneous nerve
Medulla Oblongata	**Includes:** Myelencephalon
Mesentery	**Includes:** Mesoappendix Mesocolon
Metacarpocarpal Joint, Left Metacarpocarpal Joint, Right	**Includes:** Carpometacarpal (CMC) joint
Metatarsal-Phalangeal Joint, Left Metatarsal-Phalangeal Joint, Right	**Includes:** Metatarsophalangeal (MTP) joint
Metatarsal-Tarsal Joint, Left Metatarsal-Tarsal Joint, Right	**Includes:** Tarsometatarsal joint
Middle Ear, Left Middle Ear, Right	**Includes:** Oval window Tympanic cavity
Minor Salivary Gland	**Includes:** Anterior lingual gland

SECTION Ø - MEDICAL AND SURGICAL
CHARACTER 4 - BODY PART

Mitral Valve	**Includes:** Bicuspid valve Left atrioventricular valve Mitral annulus
Nasal Bone	**Includes:** Vomer of nasal septum
Nasal Septum	**Includes:** Quadrangular cartilage Septal cartilage Vomer bone
Nasal Turbinate	**Includes:** Inferior turbinate Middle turbinate Nasal concha Superior turbinate
Nasopharynx	**Includes:** Choana Fossa of Rosenmuller Pharyngeal recess Rhinopharynx
Neck Muscle, Left Neck Muscle, Right	**Includes:** Anterior vertebral muscle Arytenoid muscle Cricothyroid muscle Infrahyoid muscle Levator scapulae muscle Platysma muscle Scalene muscle Splenius cervicis muscle Sternocleidomastoid muscle Suprahyoid muscle Thyroarytenoid muscle
Nipple, Left Nipple, Right	**Includes:** Areola
Nose	**Includes:** Columella External naris Greater alar cartilage Internal naris Lateral nasal cartilage Lesser alar cartilage Nasal cavity Nostril
Occipital Bone, Left Occipital Bone, Right	**Includes:** Foramen magnum
Oculomotor Nerve	**Includes:** Third cranial nerve
Olfactory Nerve	**Includes:** First cranial nerve Olfactory bulb
Optic Nerve	**Includes:** Optic chiasma Second cranial nerve
Orbit, Left Orbit, Right	**Includes:** Bony orbit Orbital portion of ethmoid bone Orbital portion of frontal bone Orbital portion of lacrimal bone Orbital portion of maxilla Orbital portion of palatine bone Orbital portion of sphenoid bone Orbital portion of zygomatic bone
Pancreatic Duct	**Includes:** Duct of Wirsung
Pancreatic Duct, Accessory	**Includes:** Duct of Santorini
Parotid Duct, Left Parotid Duct, Right	**Includes:** Stensen's duct
Pelvic Bone, Left Pelvic Bone, Right	**Includes:** Iliac crest Ilium Ischium Pubis
Pelvic Cavity	**Includes:** Retropubic space
Penis	**Includes:** Corpus cavernosum Corpus spongiosum
Perineum Muscle	**Includes:** Bulbospongiosus muscle Cremaster muscle Deep transverse perineal muscle Ischiocavernosus muscle Levator ani muscle Superficial transverse perineal muscle
Peritoneum	**Includes:** Epiploic foramen
Peroneal Artery, Left Peroneal Artery, Right	**Includes:** Fibular artery
Peroneal Nerve	**Includes:** Common fibular nerve Common peroneal nerve External popliteal nerve Lateral sural cutaneous nerve

APPENDIX A

SECTION Ø - MEDICAL AND SURGICAL
CHARACTER 4 - BODY PART

Pharynx	**Includes:** Base of Tongue Hypopharynx Laryngopharynx Oropharynx Piriform recess (sinus) Tongue, base of
Phrenic Nerve	**Includes:** Accessory phrenic nerve
Pituitary Gland	**Includes:** Adenohypophysis Hypophysis Neurohypophysis
Pons	**Includes:** Apneustic center Basis pontis Locus ceruleus Pneumotaxic center Pontine tegmentum Superior olivary nucleus
Popliteal Artery, Left Popliteal Artery, Right	**Includes:** Inferior genicular artery Middle genicular artery Superior genicular artery Sural artery
Portal Vein	**Includes:** Hepatic portal vein
Prepuce	**Includes:** Foreskin Glans penis
Pudendal Nerve	**Includes:** Posterior labial nerve Posterior scrotal nerve
Pulmonary Artery, Left	**Includes:** Arterial canal (duct) Botallo's duct Pulmoaortic canal
Pulmonary Valve	**Includes:** Pulmonary annulus Pulmonic valve
Pulmonary Vein, Left	**Includes:** Left inferior pulmonary vein Left superior pulmonary vein
Pulmonary Vein, Right	**Includes:** Right inferior pulmonary vein Right superior pulmonary vein
Radial Artery, Left Radial Artery, Right	**Includes:** Radial recurrent artery

Radial Nerve	**Includes:** Dorsal digital nerve Musculospiral nerve Palmar cutaneous nerve Posterior interosseous nerve
Radius, Left Radius, Right	**Includes:** Ulnar notch
Rectum	**Includes:** Anorectal junction
Renal Artery, Left Renal Artery, Right	**Includes:** Inferior suprarenal artery Renal segmental artery
Renal Vein, Left	**Includes:** Left inferior phrenic vein Left ovarian vein Left second lumbar vein Left suprarenal vein Left testicular vein
Retina, Left Retina, Right	**Includes:** Fovea Macula Optic disc
Retroperitoneum	**Includes:** Retroperitoneal space
Sacral Nerve	**Includes:** Spinal nerve, sacral
Sacral Plexus	**Includes:** Inferior gluteal nerve Posterior femoral cutaneous nerve Pudendal nerve
Sacral Sympathetic Nerve	**Includes:** Ganglion impar (ganglion of Walther) Pelvic splanchnic nerve Sacral ganglion Sacral splanchnic nerve
Sacrococcygeal Joint	**Includes:** Sacrococcygeal symphysis
Scapula, Left Scapula, Right	**Includes:** Acromion (process) Coracoid process
Sciatic Nerve	**Includes:** Ischiatic nerve

SECTION Ø - MEDICAL AND SURGICAL
CHARACTER 4 - BODY PART

Shoulder Bursa and Ligament, Left Shoulder Bursa and Ligament, Right	**Includes:** Acromioclavicular ligament Coracoacromial ligament Coracoclavicular ligament Coracohumeral ligament Costoclavicular ligament Glenohumeral ligament Interclavicular ligament Sternoclavicular ligament Subacromial bursa Transverse humeral ligament Transverse scapular ligament	Spleen	**Includes:** Accessory spleen
Shoulder Joint, Left Shoulder Joint, Right	**Includes:** Glenohumeral joint Glenoid ligament (labrum)	Splenic Artery	**Includes:** Left gastroepiploic artery Pancreatic artery Short gastric artery
Shoulder Muscle, Left Shoulder Muscle, Right	**Includes:** Deltoid muscle Infraspinatus muscle Subscapularis muscle Supraspinatus muscle Teres major muscle Teres minor muscle	Splenic Vein	**Includes:** Left gastroepiploic vein Pancreatic vein
		Sternum	**Includes:** Manubrium Suprasternal notch Xiphoid process
Sigmoid Colon	**Includes:** Rectosigmoid junction Sigmoid flexure	Stomach, Pylorus	**Includes:** Pyloric antrum Pyloric canal Pyloric sphincter
Skin	**Includes:** Dermis Epidermis Sebaceous gland Sweat gland	Subarachnoid Space	**Includes:** Subarachnoid space, intracranial
Sphenoid Bone, Left Sphenoid Bone, Right	**Includes:** Greater wing Lesser wing Optic foramen Pterygoid process Sella turcica	Subclavian Artery, Left Subclavian Artery, Right	**Includes:** Costocervical trunk Dorsal scapular artery Internal thoracic artery
		Subcutaneous Tissue and Fascia, Anterior Neck	**Includes:** Deep cervical fascia Pretracheal fascia
Spinal Canal	**Includes:** Epidural space, spinal Extradural space, spinal Subarachnoid space, spinal Subdural space, spinal Vertebral canal	Subcutaneous Tissue and Fascia, Chest	**Includes:** Pectoral fascia
		Subcutaneous Tissue and Fascia, Face	**Includes:** Masseteric fascia Orbital fascia
		Subcutaneous Tissue and Fascia, Left Foot	**Includes:** Plantar fascia (aponeurosis)
Spinal Meninges	**Includes:** Arachnoid mater, spinal Denticulate (dentate) ligament Dura mater, spinal Filum terminale Leptomeninges, spinal Pia mater, spinal	Subcutaneous Tissue and Fascia, Left Hand	**Includes:** Palmar fascia (aponeurosis)
		Subcutaneous Tissue and Fascia, Left Lower Arm	**Includes:** Antebrachial fascia Bicipital aponeurosis
		Subcutaneous Tissue and Fascia, Left Upper Arm	**Includes:** Axillary fascia Deltoid fascia Infraspinatus fascia Subscapular aponeurosis Supraspinatus fascia

SECTION Ø - MEDICAL AND SURGICAL
CHARACTER 4 - BODY PART

Body Part	Includes
Subcutaneous Tissue and Fascia, Left Upper Leg	**Includes:** Crural fascia Fascia lata Iliac fascia Iliotibial tract (band)
Subcutaneous Tissue and Fascia, Posterior Neck	**Includes:** Prevertebral fascia
Subcutaneous Tissue and Fascia, Right Foot	**Includes:** Plantar fascia (aponeurosis)
Subcutaneous Tissue and Fascia, Right Hand	**Includes:** Palmar fascia (aponeurosis)
Subcutaneous Tissue and Fascia, Right Lower Arm	**Includes:** Antebrachial fascia Bicipital aponeurosis
Subcutaneous Tissue and Fascia, Right Upper Arm	**Includes:** Axillary fascia Deltoid fascia Infraspinatus fascia Subscapular aponeurosis Supraspinatus fascia
Subcutaneous Tissue and Fascia, Right Upper Leg	**Includes:** Crural fascia Fascia lata Iliac fascia Iliotibial tract (band)
Subcutaneous Tissue and Fascia, Scalp	**Includes:** Galea aponeurotica
Subcutaneous Tissue and Fascia, Trunk	**Includes:** External oblique aponeurosis Transversalis fascia
Subdural Space	**Includes:** Subdural space, intracranial
Submaxillary Gland, Left Submaxillary Gland, Right	**Includes:** Submandibular gland
Superior Mesenteric Artery	**Includes:** Ileal artery Ileocolic artery Inferior pancreaticoduodenal artery Jejunal artery
Superior Mesenteric Vein	**Includes:** Right gastroepiploic vein

Body Part	Includes
Superior Vena Cava	**Includes:** Precava
Tarsal Joint, Left Tarsal Joint, Right	**Includes:** Calcaneocuboid joint Cuboideonavicular joint Cuneonavicular joint Intercuneiform joint Subtalar (talocalcaneal) joint Talocalcaneal (subtalar) joint Talocalcaneonavicular joint
Tarsal, Left Tarsal, Right	**Includes:** Calcaneus Cuboid bone Intermediate cuneiform bone Lateral cuneiform bone Medial cuneiform bone Navicular bone Talus bone
Temporal Artery, Left Temporal Artery, Right	**Includes:** Middle temporal artery Superficial temporal artery Transverse facial artery
Temporal Bone, Left Temporal Bone, Right	**Includes:** Mastoid process Petrous part of temporal bone Tympanic part of temporal bone Zygomatic process of temporal bone
Thalamus	**Includes:** Epithalamus Geniculate nucleus Metathalamus Pulvinar
Thoracic Aorta, Ascending/Arch	**Includes:** Aortic arch Ascending aorta
Thoracic Duct	**Includes:** Left jugular trunk Left subclavian trunk
Thoracic Nerve	**Includes:** Intercostal nerve Intercostobrachial nerve Spinal nerve, thoracic Subcostal nerve

SECTION Ø - MEDICAL AND SURGICAL
CHARACTER 4 - BODY PART

Thoracic Sympathetic Nerve	**Includes:** Cardiac plexus Esophageal plexus Greater splanchnic nerve Inferior cardiac nerve Least splanchnic nerve Lesser splanchnic nerve Middle cardiac nerve Pulmonary plexus Superior cardiac nerve Thoracic aortic plexus Thoracic ganglion
Thoracic Vertebra	**Includes:** Spinous process Vertebral arch Vertebral foramen Vertebral lamina Vertebral pedicle
Thoracic Vertebral Joint	**Includes:** Costotransverse joint Costovertebral joint Thoracic facet joint
Thoracolumbar Vertebral Joint	**Includes:** Thoracolumbar facet joint
Thorax Bursa and Ligament, Left Thorax Bursa and Ligament, Right	**Includes:** Costotransverse ligament Costoxiphoid ligament Sternocostal ligament
Thorax Muscle, Left Thorax Muscle, Right	**Includes:** Intercostal muscle Levatores costarum muscle Pectoralis major muscle Pectoralis minor muscle Serratus anterior muscle Subclavius muscle Subcostal muscle Transverse thoracis muscle
Thymus	**Includes:** Thymus gland
Thyroid Artery, Left Thyroid Artery, Right	**Includes:** Cricothyroid artery Hyoid artery Sternocleidomastoid artery Superior laryngeal artery Superior thyroid artery Thyrocervical trunk

Tibia, Left Tibia, Right	**Includes:** Lateral condyle of tibia Medial condyle of tibia Medial malleolus
Tibial Nerve	**Includes:** Lateral plantar nerve Medial plantar nerve Medial popliteal nerve Medial sural cutaneous nerve
Toe Nail	**Includes:** Nail bed Nail plate
Toe Phalangeal Joint, Left Toe Phalangeal Joint, Right	**Includes:** Interphalangeal (IP) joint
Tongue	**Includes:** Frenulum linguae Lingual tonsil
Tongue, Palate, Pharynx Muscle	**Includes:** Chrondroglossus muscle Genioglossus muscle Hyoglossus muscle Inferior longitudinal muscle Levator veli palatini muscle Palatoglossal muscle Palatopharyngeal muscle Pharyngeal constrictor muscle Salpingopharyngeus muscle Styloglossus muscle Stylopharyngeus muscle Superior longitudinal muscle Tensor veli palatini muscle
Tonsils	**Includes:** Palatine tonsil
Trachea	**Includes:** Cricoid cartilage
Transverse Colon	**Includes:** Splenic flexure
Tricuspid Valve	**Includes:** Right atrioventricular valve Tricuspid annulus
Trigeminal Nerve	**Includes:** Fifth cranial nerve Gasserian ganglion Mandibular nerve Maxillary nerve Ophthalmic nerve Trifacial nerve

SECTION Ø - MEDICAL AND SURGICAL
CHARACTER 4 - BODY PART

Trochlear Nerve	**Includes:** Fourth cranial nerve
Trunk Bursa and Ligament, Left Trunk Bursa and Ligament, Right	**Includes:** Iliolumbar ligament Interspinous ligament Intertransverse ligament Ligamentum flavum Pubic ligament Sacrococcygeal ligament Sacroiliac ligament Sacrospinous ligament Sacrotuberous ligament Supraspinous ligament
Trunk Muscle, Left Trunk Muscle, Right	**Includes:** Coccygeus muscle Erector spinae muscle Interspinalis muscle Intertransversarius muscle Latissimus dorsi muscle Quadratus lumborum muscle Rhomboid major muscle Rhomboid minor muscle Serratus posterior muscle Transversospinalis muscle Trapezius muscle
Tympanic Membrane, Left Tympanic Membrane, Right	**Includes:** Pars flaccida
Ulna, Left Ulna, Right	**Includes:** Olecranon process Radial notch
Ulnar Artery, Left Ulnar Artery, Right	**Includes:** Anterior ulnar recurrent artery Common interosseous artery Posterior ulnar recurrent artery
Ulnar Nerve	**Includes:** Cubital nerve
Upper Arm Muscle, Left Upper Arm Muscle, Right	**Includes:** Biceps brachii muscle Brachialis muscle Coracobrachialis muscle Triceps brachii muscle
Upper Artery	**Includes:** Aortic intercostal artery Bronchial artery Esophageal artery Subcostal artery

Upper Eyelid, Left Upper Eyelid, Right	**Includes:** Lateral canthus Levator palpebrae superioris muscle Orbicularis oculi muscle Superior tarsal plate
Upper Femur, Left Upper Femur, Right	**Includes:** Femoral head Greater trochanter Lesser trochanter Neck of femur
Upper Leg Muscle, Left Upper Leg Muscle, Right	**Includes:** Adductor brevis muscle Adductor longus muscle Adductor magnus muscle Biceps femoris muscle Gracilis muscle Pectineus muscle Quadriceps (femoris) Rectus femoris muscle Sartorius muscle Semimembranosus muscle Semitendinosus muscle Vastus intermedius muscle Vastus lateralis muscle Vastus medialis muscle
Upper Lip	**Includes:** Frenulum labii superioris Labial gland Vermilion border
Ureter Ureter, Left Ureter, Right Ureters, Bilateral	**Includes:** Ureteral orifice Ureterovesical orifice
Urethra	**Includes:** Bulbourethral (Cowper's) gland Cowper's (bulbourethral) gland External urethral sphincter Internal urethral sphincter Membranous urethra Penile urethra Prostatic urethra
Uterine Supporting Structure	**Includes:** Broad ligament Infundibulopelvic ligament Ovarian ligament Round ligament of uterus
Uterus	**Includes:** Fundus uteri Myometrium Perimetrium Uterine cornu
Uvula	**Includes:** Palatine uvula

SECTION Ø - MEDICAL AND SURGICAL
CHARACTER 4 - BODY PART

Vagus Nerve	**Includes:** Anterior vagal trunk Pharyngeal plexus Pneumogastric nerve Posterior vagal trunk Pulmonary plexus Recurrent laryngeal nerve Superior laryngeal nerve Tenth cranial nerve
Vas Deferens Vas Deferens, Bilateral Vas Deferens, Left Vas Deferens, Right	**Includes:** Ductus deferens Ejaculatory duct
Ventricle, Right	**Includes:** Conus arteriosus
Ventricular Septum	**Includes:** Interventricular septum

Vertebral Artery,
  Left
Vertebral Artery,
  Right
	Includes:
	Anterior spinal artery
	Posterior spinal artery

Vertebral Vein, Left Vertebral Vein, Right	**Includes:** Deep cervical vein Suboccipital venous plexus

Vestibular Gland	**Includes:** Bartholin's (greater vestibular) gland Greater vestibular (Bartholin's) gland Paraurethral (Skene's) gland Skene's (paraurethral) gland
Vitreous, Left Vitreous, Right	**Includes:** Vitreous body
Vocal Cord, Left Vocal Cord, Right	**Includes:** Vocal fold
Vulva	**Includes:** Labia majora Labia minora

Wrist Bursa and
  Ligament, Left
Wrist Bursa and
  Ligament, Right
	Includes:
	Palmar ulnocarpal ligament
	Radial collateral carpal ligament
	Radiocarpal ligament
	Radioulnar ligament
	Ulnar collateral carpal ligament

Wrist Joint, Left Wrist Joint, Right	**Includes:** Distal radioulnar joint Radiocarpal joint

SECTION Ø - MEDICAL AND SURGICAL
CHARACTER 5 - APPROACH

External	**Definition:** Procedures performed directly on the skin or mucous membrane and procedures performed indirectly by the application of external force through the skin or mucous membrane
Open	**Definition:** Cutting through the skin or mucous membrane and any other body layers necessary to expose the site of the procedure
Percutaneous	**Definition:** Entry, by puncture or minor incision, of instrumentation through the skin or mucous membrane and any other body layers necessary to reach the site of the procedure
Percutaneous Endoscopic	**Definition:** Entry, by puncture or minor incision, of instrumentation through the skin or mucous membrane and any other body layers necessary to reach and visualize the site of the procedure

Via Natural or Artificial Opening	**Definition:** Entry of instrumentation through a natural or artificial external opening to reach the site of the procedure
Via Natural or Artificial Opening Endoscopic	**Definition:** Entry of instrumentation through a natural or artificial external opening to reach and visualize the site of the procedure
Via Natural or Artificial Opening With Percutaneous Endoscopic Assistance	**Definition:** Entry of instrumentation through a natural or artificial external opening and entry, by puncture or minor incision, of instrumentation through the skin or mucous membrane and any other body layers necessary to aid in the performance of the procedure

APPENDIX A

SECTION Ø - MEDICAL AND SURGICAL
CHARACTER 6 - DEVICE

Device	Includes
Artificial Sphincter in Gastrointestinal System	**Includes:** Artificial anal sphincter (AAS) Artificial bowel sphincter (neosphincter)
Artificial Sphincter in Urinary System	**Includes:** AMS 8ØØ® Urinary Control System Artificial urinary sphincter (AUS)
Autologous Arterial Tissue in Heart and Great Vessels	**Includes:** Autologous artery graft
Autologous Arterial Tissue in Lower Arteries	**Includes:** Autologous artery graft
Autologous Arterial Tissue in Lower Veins	**Includes:** Autologous artery graft
Autologous Arterial Tissue in Upper Arteries	**Includes:** Autologous artery graft
Autologous Arterial Tissue in Upper Veins	**Includes:** Autologous artery graft
Autologous Tissue Substitute	**Includes:** Autograft Cultured epidermal cell autograft Epicel® cultured epidermal autograft
Autologous Venous Tissue in Heart and Great Vessels	**Includes:** Autologous vein graft
Autologous Venous Tissue in Lower Arteries	**Includes:** Autologous vein graft
Autologous Venous Tissue in Lower Veins	**Includes:** Autologous vein graft
Autologous Venous Tissue in Upper Arteries	**Includes:** Autologous vein graft
Autologous Venous Tissue in Upper Veins	**Includes:** Autologous vein graft
Bone Growth Stimulator in Head and Facial Bones	**Includes:** Electrical bone growth stimulator (EBGS) Ultrasonic osteogenic stimulator Ultrasound bone healing system
Bone Growth Stimulator in Lower Bones	**Includes:** Electrical bone growth stimulator (EBGS) Ultrasonic osteogenic stimulator Ultrasound bone healing system
Bone Growth Stimulator in Upper Bones	**Includes:** Electrical bone growth stimulator (EBGS) Ultrasonic osteogenic stimulator Ultrasound bone healing system
Cardiac Lead in Heart and Great Vessels	**Includes:** Cardiac contractility modulation lead
Cardiac Lead, Defibrillator for Insertion in Heart and Great Vessels	**Includes:** ACUITY™ Steerable Lead Attain Ability® lead Attain StarFix® (OTW) lead Cardiac resynchronization therapy (CRT) lead Corox (OTW) Bipolar Lead Durata® Defibrillation Lead ENDOTAK RELIANCE® (G) Defibrillation Lead
Cardiac Lead, Pacemaker for Insertion in Heart and Great Vessels	**Includes:** ACUITY™ Steerable Lead Attain Ability® Lead Attain StarFix® (OTW) lead Cardiac resynchronization therapy (CRT) lead Corox (OTW) Bipolar Lead
Cardiac Resynchronization Defibrillator Pulse Generator for Insertion in Subcutaneous Tissue and Fascia	**Includes:** COGNIS® CRT-D Concerto II CRT-D Consulta CRT-D CONTAK RENEWAL® 3 RF (HE) CRT-D LIVIAN™ CRT-D Maximo II DR CRT-D Ovatio™ CRT-D Protecta XT CRT-D Viva (XT)(S)
Cardiac Resynchronization Pacemaker Pulse Generator for Insertion in Subcutaneous Tissue and Fascia	**Includes:** Consulta CRT-P Stratos LV Synchra CRT-P
Contraceptive Device in Female Reproductive System	**Includes:** Intrauterine device (IUD)
Contraceptive Device in Subcutaneous Tissue and Fascia	**Includes:** Subdermal progesterone implant
Contractility Modulation Device for Insertion in Subcutaneous Tissue and Fascia	**Includes:** Optimizer™ III implantable pulse generator

SECTION Ø - MEDICAL AND SURGICAL
CHARACTER 6 - DEVICE

Defibrillator Generator for Insertion in Subcutaneous Tissue and Fascia	**Includes:** Implantable cardioverter-defibrillator (ICD) Maximo II DR (VR) Protecta XT DR (XT VR) Secura (DR) (VR) Evera (XT)(S)(DR/VR) Virtuoso (II) (DR) (VR)
Diaphragmatic Pacemaker Lead in Respiratory System	**Includes:** Phrenic nerve stimulator lead
Drainage Device	**Includes:** Cystostomy tube Foley catheter Percutaneous nephrostomy catheter Thoracostomy tube
External Fixation Device in Head and Facial Bones	**Includes:** External fixator
External Fixation Device in Lower Bones	**Includes:** External fixator
External Fixation Device in Lower Joints	**Includes:** External fixator
External Fixation Device in Upper Bones	**Includes:** External fixator
External Fixation Device in Upper Joints	**Includes:** External fixator
External Fixation Device, Hybrid for Insertion in Upper Bones	**Includes:** Delta frame external fixator Sheffield hybrid external fixator
External Fixation Device, Hybrid for Insertion in Lower Bones	**Includes:** Delta frame external fixator Sheffield hybrid external fixator
External Fixation Device, Hybrid for Reposition in Upper Bones	**Includes:** Delta frame external fixator Sheffield hybrid external fixator
External Fixation Device, Hybrid for Reposition in Lower Bones	**Includes:** Delta frame external fixator Sheffield hybrid external fixator
External Fixation Device, Limb Lengthening for Insertion in Upper Bones	**Includes:** Ilizarov-Vecklich device
External Fixation Device, Limb Lengthening for Insertion in Lower Bones	**Includes:** Ilizarov-Vecklich device
External Fixation Device, Monoplanar for Insertion in Upper Bones	**Includes:** Uniplanar external fixator
External Fixation Device, Monoplanar for Insertion in Lower Bones	**Includes:** Uniplanar external fixator
External Fixation Device, Monoplanar for Reposition in Upper Bones	**Includes:** Uniplanar external fixator
External Fixation Device, Monoplanar for Reposition in Lower Bones	**Includes:** Uniplanar external fixator
External Fixation Device, Ring for Insertion in Upper Bones	**Includes:** Ilizarov external fixator Sheffield ring external fixator
External Fixation Device, Ring for Insertion in Lower Bones	**Includes:** Ilizarov external fixator Sheffield ring external fixator
External Fixation Device, Ring for Reposition in Upper Bones	**Includes:** Ilizarov external fixator Sheffield ring external fixator
External Fixation Device, Ring for Reposition in Lower Bones	**Includes:** Ilizarov external fixator Sheffield ring external fixator
External Heart Assist System in Heart and Great Vessels	**Includes:** Biventricular external heart assist system BVS 5ØØØ Ventricular Assist Device Centrimag® Blood Pump TandemHeart® System Thoratec Paracorporeal Ventricular Assist Device

APPENDIX A

SECTION Ø - MEDICAL AND SURGICAL
CHARACTER 6 - DEVICE

Extraluminal Device	**Includes:** LAP-BAND® adjustable gastric banding system REALIZE® Adjustable Gastric Band TigerPaw® system for closure of left atrial appendage
Feeding Device in Gastrointestinal System	**Includes:** Percutaneous endoscopic gastrojejunostomy (PEG/J) tube Percutaneous endoscopic gastrostomy (PEG) tube
Hearing Device in Ear, Nose, Sinus	**Includes:** Esteem® implantable hearing system
Hearing Device in Head and Facial Bones	**Includes:** Bone anchored hearing device
Hearing Device, Bone Conduction for Insertion in Ear, Nose, Sinus	**Includes:** Bone anchored hearing device
Hearing Device, Multiple Channel Cochlear Prosthesis for Insertion in Ear, Nose, Sinus	**Includes:** Cochlear implant (CI), multiple channel (electrode)
Hearing Device, Single Channel Cochlear Prosthesis for Insertion in Ear, Nose, Sinus	**Includes:** Cochlear implant (CI), single channel (electrode)
Implantable Heart Assist System in Heart and Great Vessels	**Includes:** Berlin Heart Ventricular Assist Device DeBakey Left Ventricular Assist Device DuraHeart Left Ventricular Assist System HeartMate II® Left Ventricular Assist Device (LVAD) HeartMate XVE® Left Ventricular Assist Device (LVAD) MicroMed HeartAssist Novacor Left Ventricular Assist Device Thoratec IVAD (Implantable Ventricular Assist Device)
Infusion Device	**Includes:** Ascenda Intrathecal Catheter InDura, intrathecal catheter (1P) (spinal) Non-tunneled central venous catheter Peripherally inserted central catheter (PICC) Tunneled spinal (intrathecal) catheter
Infusion Device, Pump in Subcutaneous Tissue and Fascia	**Includes:** Implantable drug infusion pump (anti-spasmodic) (chemotherapy) (pain) Injection reservoir, pump Pump reservoir Subcutaneous injection reservoir, pump SynchroMed pump
Interbody Fusion Device in Lower Joints	**Includes:** Axial Lumbar Interbody Fusion System AxiaLIF® System CoRoent® XL Direct Lateral Interbody Fusion (DLIF) device EXtreme Lateral Interbody Fusion (XLIF) device Interbody fusion (spine) cage XLIF® System
Interbody Fusion Device in Upper Joints	**Includes:** BAK/C® Interbody Cervical Fusion System Interbody fusion (spine) cage
Internal Fixation Device in Head and Facial Bones	**Includes:** Bone screw (interlocking) (lag) (pedicle) (recessed) Kirschner wire (K-wire) Neutralization plate
Internal Fixation Device in Lower Bones	**Includes:** Bone screw (interlocking) (lag) (pedicle) (recessed) Clamp and rod internal fixation system (CRIF) Kirschner wire (K-wire) Neutralization plate
Internal Fixation Device in Lower Joints	**Includes:** Fusion screw (compression) (lag) (locking) Joint fixation plate Kirschner wire (K-wire)
Internal Fixation Device in Upper Bones	**Includes:** Bone screw (interlocking) (lag) (pedicle) (recessed) Clamp and rod internal fixation system (CRIF) Kirschner wire (K-wire) Neutralization plate
Internal Fixation Device in Upper Joints	**Includes:** Fusion screw (compression) (lag) (locking) Joint fixation plate Kirschner wire (K-wire)
Internal Fixation Device, Intramedullary in Lower Bones	**Includes:** Intramedullary (IM) rod (nail) Intramedullary skeletal kinetic distractor (ISKD) Kuntscher nail
Internal Fixation Device, Intramedullary in Upper Bones	**Includes:** Intramedullary (IM) rod (nail) Intramedullary skeletal kinetic distractor (ISKD) Kuntscher nail
Internal Fixation Device, Rigid Plate for Insertion in Upper Bones	**Includes:** Titanium Sternal Fixation System (TSFS)

SECTION Ø - MEDICAL AND SURGICAL
CHARACTER 6 - DEVICE

Internal Fixation Device, Rigid Plate for Reposition in Upper Bones	**Includes:** Titanium Sternal Fixation System (TSFS)
Intraluminal Device	**Includes:** Absolute Pro Vascular (OTW) Self-Expanding Stent System Acculink (RX) Carotid Stent System AFX® Endovascular AAA System AneuRx® AAA Advantage® Assurant (Cobalt) stent Carotid WALLSTENT® Monorail® Endoprosthesis CoAxia NeuroFlo catheter Colonic Z-Stent® Complete (SE) stent Cook Zenith AAA Endovascular Graft Driver stent (RX) (OTW) E-Luminexx™ (Biliary) (Vascular) Stent Embolization coil(s) Endologix AFX® Endovascular AAA System Endurant® Endovascular Stent Graft Endurant® II AAA stent graft system EXCLUDER® AAA Endoprosthesis Express® (LD) Premounted Stent System Express® Biliary SD Monorail® Premounted Stent System Express® SD Renal Monorail® Premounted Stent System FLAIR® Endovascular Stent Graft Formula™ Balloon-Expandable Renal Stent System GORE EXCLUDER® AAA Endoprosthesis GORE TAG® Thoracic Endoprosthesis Herculink (RX) Elite Renal Stent System LifeStent® (Flexstar) (XL) Vascular Stent System Medtronic Endurant® II AAA stent graft system Micro-Driver stent (RX) (OTW) MULTI-LINK (VISION)(MINI-VISION)(ULTRA) Coronary Stent System Omnilink Elite Vascular Balloon Expandable Stent System Pipeline™ Embolization device (PED) Protégé® RX Carotid Stent System Stent, intraluminal (cardiovascular) (gastrointestinal)(hepatobiliary)(urinary) Talent® Converter Talent® Occluder Talent® Stent Graft (abdominal) (thoracic) Therapeutic occlusion coil(s) Ultraflex™ Precision Colonic Stent System Valiant Thoracic Stent Graft WALLSTENT® Endoprosthesis Xact Carotid Stent System Zenith AAA Endovascular Graft Zenith Flex® AAA Endovascular Graft Zenith® Renu™ AAA Ancillary Graft Zenith TX2® TAA Endovascular Graft

Intraluminal Device, Airway in Ear, Nose, Sinus	**Includes:** Nasopharyngeal airway (NPA)
Intraluminal Device, Airway in Gastrointestinal System	**Includes:** Esophageal obturator airway (EOA)
Intraluminal Device, Airway in Mouth and Throat	**Includes:** Guedel airway Oropharyngeal airway (OPA)
Intraluminal Device, Bioactive in Upper Arteries	**Includes:** Bioactive embolization coil(s) Micrus CERECYTE microcoil
Intraluminal Device, Branched or Fenestrated, One or Two Arteries for Restriction in Lower Arteries	**Includes:** Cook Zenith AAA Endovascular Graft EXCLUDER® AAA Endoprosthesis EXCLUDER® IBE Endoprosthesis GORE EXCLUDER® AAA Endoprosthesis GORE EXCLUDER® IBE Endoprosthesis Zenith AAA Endovascular Graft
Intraluminal Device, Branched or Fenestrated, Three or More Arteries for Restriction in Lower Arteries	**Includes:** Cook Zenith AAA Endovascular Graft EXCLUDER® AAA Endoprosthesis GORE EXCLUDER® AAA Endoprosthesis Zenith AAA Endovascular Graft
Intraluminal Device, Drug-eluting in Heart and Great Vessels	**Includes:** CYPHER® Stent Endeavor® (III) (IV) (Sprint) Zotarolimus-eluting Coronary Stent System Everolimus-eluting coronary stent Paclitaxel-eluting coronary stent Sirolimus-eluting coronary stent TAXUS® Liberté® Paclitaxel-eluting Coronary Stent System XIENCE Everolimus Eluting Coronary Stent System Zotarolimus-eluting coronary stent
Intraluminal Device, Drug-eluting in Lower Arteries	**Includes:** Paclitaxel-eluting peripheral stent Zilver® PTX® (paclitaxel) Drug-Eluting Peripheral Stent
Intraluminal Device, Drug-eluting in Upper Arteries	**Includes:** Paclitaxel-eluting peripheral stent Zilver® PTX® (paclitaxel) Drug-Eluting Peripheral Stent
Intraluminal Device, Endobronchial Valve in Respiratory System	**Includes:** Spiration IBV™ Valve System

SECTION Ø - MEDICAL AND SURGICAL
CHARACTER 6 - DEVICE

Intraluminal Device, Endotracheal Airway in Respiratory System	**Includes:** Endotracheal tube (cuffed) (double-lumen)
Intraluminal Device, Pessary in Female Reproductive System	**Includes:** Pessary ring Vaginal pessary
Liner in Lower Joints	**Includes:** Acetabular cup Hip (joint) liner Joint liner (insert) Knee (implant) insert Tibial insert
Monitoring Device	**Includes:** Blood glucose monitoring system Cardiac event recorder Continuous Glucose Monitoring (CGM) device Implantable glucose monitoring device Loop recorder, implantable Reveal (DX) (XT)
Monitoring Device, Hemodynamic for Insertion in Subcutaneous Tissue and Fascia	**Includes:** Implantable hemodynamic monitor (IHM) Implantable hemodynamic monitoring system (IHMS)
Monitoring Device, Pressure Sensor for Insertion in Heart and Great Vessels	**Includes:** CardioMEMS® pressure sensor EndoSure® sensor
Neurostimulator Lead in Central Nervous System	**Includes:** Cortical strip neurostimulator lead DBS lead Deep brain neurostimulator lead RNS System lead Spinal cord neurostimulator lead
Neurostimulator Lead in Peripheral Nervous System	**Includes:** InterStim® Therapy lead
Neurostimulator Generator in Head and Facial Bones	**Includes:** RNS system neurostimulator generator
Nonautologous Tissue Substitute	**Includes:** Acellular Hydrated Dermis Bone bank bone graft Cook Biodesign® Fistula Plug(s) Cook Biodesign® Hernia Graft(s) Cook Biodesign® Layered Graft(s) Cook Zenapro™ Layered Graft(s) Tissue bank graft

Pacemaker, Dual Chamber for Insertion in Subcutaneous Tissue and Fascia	**Includes:** Advisa (MRI) EnRhythm Kappa Revo MRI™ SureScan® pacemaker Two lead pacemaker Versa
Pacemaker, Single Chamber for Insertion in Subcutaneous Tissue and Fascia	**Includes:** Single lead pacemaker (atrium) (ventricle)
Pacemaker, Single Chamber Rate Responsive for Insertion in Subcutaneous Tissue and Fascia	**Includes:** Single lead rate responsive pacemaker (atrium) (ventricle)
Radioactive Element	**Includes:** Brachytherapy seeds
Resurfacing Device in Lower Joints	**Includes:** CONSERVE® PLUS Total Resurfacing Hip System Cormet Hip Resurfacing System
Spacer in Lower Joints	**Includes:** Joint spacer (antibiotic)
Spacer in Upper Joints	**Includes:** Joint spacer (antibiotic)
Spinal Stabilization Device, Facet Replacement for Insertion in Upper Joints	**Includes:** Facet replacement spinal stabilization device
Spinal Stabilization Device, Facet Replacement for Insertion in Lower Joints	**Includes:** Facet replacement spinal stabilization device
Spinal Stabilization Device, Interspinous Process for Insertion in Upper Joints	**Includes:** Interspinous process spinal stabilization device X-STOP® Spacer
Spinal Stabilization Device, Interspinous Process for Insertion in Lower Joints	**Includes:** Interspinous process spinal stabilization device X-STOP® Spacer
Spinal Stabilization Device, Pedicle-Based for Insertion in Upper Joints	**Includes:** Dynesys® Dynamic Stabilization System Pedicle-based dynamic stabilization device

SECTION Ø - MEDICAL AND SURGICAL
CHARACTER 6 - DEVICE

Spinal Stabilization Device, Pedicle-Based for Insertion in Lower Joints	**Includes:** Dynesys® Dynamic Stabilization System Pedicle-based dynamic stabilization device
Stimulator Generator in Subcutaneous Tissue and Fascia	**Includes:** Baroreflex Activation Therapy® (BAT®) Diaphragmatic pacemaker generator Mark IV Breathing Pacemaker System Phrenic nerve stimulator generator Rheos® System device
Stimulator Generator, Multiple Array for Insertion in Subcutaneous Tissue and Fascia	**Includes:** Activa PC neurostimulator Enterra gastric neurostimulator Neurostimulator generator, multiple channel PrimeAdvanced neurostimulator (SureScan) (MRI Safe)
Stimulator Generator, Multiple Array Rechargeable for Insertion in Subcutaneous Tissue and Fascia	**Includes:** Activa RC neurostimulator Neurostimulator generator, multiple channel rechargeable RestoreAdvanced neurostimulator (SureScan) (MRI Safe) RestoreSensor neurostimulator (SureScan) (MRI Safe) RestoreUltra neurostimulator (SureScan) (MRI Safe)
Stimulator Generator, Single Array for Insertion in Subcutaneous Tissue and Fascia	**Includes:** Activa SC neurostimulator InterStim® Therapy neurostimulator Itrel (3) (4) neurostimulator Neurostimulator generator, single channel
Stimulator Generator, Single Array Rechargeable for Insertion in Subcutaneous Tissue and Fascia	**Includes:** Neurostimulator generator, single channel rechargeable
Stimulator Lead in Gastrointestinal System	**Includes:** Gastric electrical stimulation (GES) lead Gastric pacemaker lead
Stimulator Lead in Muscles	**Includes:** Electrical muscle stimulation (EMS) lead Electronic muscle stimulator lead Neuromuscular electrical stimulation (NEMS) lead
Stimulator Lead in Upper Arteries	**Includes:** Baroreflex Activation Therapy® (BAT®) Carotid (artery) sinus (baroreceptor) lead Rheos® System lead

Stimulator Lead in Urinary System	**Includes:** Sacral nerve modulation (SNM) lead Sacral neuromodulation lead Urinary incontinence stimulator lead
Synthetic Substitute	**Includes:** AbioCor® Total Replacement Heart AMPLATZER® Muscular VSD Occluder Annuloplasty ring Bard® Composix® (E/X) (LP) mesh Bard® Composix® Kugel® patch Bard® Dulex™ mesh Bard® Ventralex™ hernia patch BRYAN® Cervical Disc System Ex-PRESS™ mini glaucoma shunt Flexible Composite Mesh GORE® DUALMESH® Holter valve ventricular shunt MitraClip valve repair system Nitinol framed polymer mesh Open Pivot (mechanical) valve Open Pivot Aortic Valve Graft (AVG) Partially absorbable mesh PHYSIOMESH™ Flexible Composite Mesh Polymethylmethacrylate (PMMA) Polypropylene mesh PRESTIGE® Cervical Disc PROCEED™ Ventral Patch Prodisc-C Prodisc-L PROLENE Polypropylene Hernia System (PHS) Rebound HRD® (Hernia Repair Device) SynCardia Total Artificial Heart Total artificial (replacement) heart ULTRAPRO Hernia System (UHS) ULTRAPRO Partially Absorbable Lightweight Mesh ULTRAPRO Plug Ventrio™ Hernia Patch Zimmer® NexGen® LPS Mobile Bearing Knee Zimmer® NexGen® LPS-Flex Mobile Knee
Synthetic Substitute, Ceramic for Replacement in Lower Joints	**Includes:** Ceramic on ceramic bearing surface Novation® Ceramic AHS® (Articulation Hip System)
Synthetic Substitute, Ceramic on Polyethylene for Replacement in Lower Joints	**Includes:** Oxidized zirconium ceramic hip bearing surface
Synthetic Substitute, Intraocular Telescope for Replacement in Eye	**Includes:** Implantable Miniature Telescope™ (IMT)

SECTION 0 - MEDICAL AND SURGICAL
CHARACTER 6 - DEVICE

Synthetic Substitute, Metal for Replacement in Lower Joints	**Includes:** Cobalt/chromium head and socket Metal on metal bearing surface
Synthetic Substitute, Metal on Polyethylene for Replacement in Lower Joints	**Includes:** Cobalt/chromium head and polyethylene socket
Synthetic Substitute, Polyethylene for Replacement in Lower Joints	**Includes:** Polyethylene socket
Synthetic Substitute, Reverse Ball and Socket for Replacement in Upper Joints	**Includes:** Delta III Reverse shoulder prosthesis Reverse® Shoulder Prosthesis
Tissue Expander in Skin and Breast	**Includes:** Tissue expander (inflatable) (injectable)
Tissue Expander in Subcutaneous Tissue and Fascia	**Includes:** Tissue expander (inflatable) (injectable)
Tracheostomy Device in Respiratory System	**Includes:** Tracheostomy tube

Vascular Access Device in Subcutaneous Tissue and Fascia	**Includes:** Tunneled central venous catheter Vectra® Vascular Access Graft
Vascular Access Device, Reservoir in Subcutaneous Tissue and Fascia	**Includes:** Implanted (venous) (access) port Injection reservoir, port Subcutaneous injection reservoir, port
Zooplastic Tissue in Heart and Great Vessels	**Includes:** 3f (Aortic) Bioprosthesis valve Bovine pericardial valve Bovine pericardium graft Contegra Pulmonary Valved Conduit CoreValve transcatheter aortic valve Epic™ Stented Tissue Valve (aortic) Freestyle (Stentless) Aortic Root Bioprosthesis Hancock Bioprosthesis (aortic) (mitral) valve Hancock Bioprosthetic Valved Conduit Melody® transcatheter pulmonary valve Mitroflow® Aortic Pericardial Heart Valve Mosaic Bioprosthesis (aortic) (mitral) valve Porcine (bioprosthetic) valve SAPIEN transcatheter aortic valve SJM Biocor® Stented Valve System Stented tissue valve Trifecta™ Valve (aortic) Xenograft

SECTION 1 - OBSTETRICS
CHARACTER 3 - OPERATION

Abortion	**Definition:** Artificially terminating a pregnancy
Change	**Definition:** Taking out or off a device from a body part and putting back an identical or similar device in or on the same body part without cutting or puncturing the skin or a mucous membrane **Explanation:** All CHANGE procedures are coded using the approach EXTERNAL
Delivery	**Definition:** Assisting the passage of the products of conception from the genital canal
Drainage	**Definition:** Taking or letting out fluids and/or gases from a body part by the use of force **Explanation:** The qualifier DIAGNOSTIC is used to identify drainage procedures that are biopsies

Extraction	**Definition:** Pulling or stripping out or off all or a portion of a body part **Explanation:** The qualifier DIAGNOSTIC is used to identify extraction procedures that are biopsies
Insertion	**Definition:** Putting in a nonbiological appliance that monitors, assists, performs, or prevents a physiological function but does not physically take the place of a body part
Inspection	**Definition:** Visually and/or manually exploring a body part **Explanation:** Visual exploration may be performed with or without optical instrumentation. Manual exploration may be performed directly or through intervening body layers

SECTION 1 - OBSTETRICS
CHARACTER 3 - OPERATION

Removal	**Definition:** Taking out or off a device from a body part, region or orifice **Explanation:** If a device is taken out and a similar device put in without cutting or puncturing the skin or mucous membrane, the procedure is coded to the root operation CHANGE. Otherwise, the procedure for taking out a device is coded to the root operation REMOVAL
Repair	**Definition:** Restoring, to the extent possible, a body part to its normal anatomic structure and function **Explanation:** Used only when the method to accomplish the repair is not one of the other root operations

Reposition	**Definition:** Moving to its normal location or other suitable location all or a portion of a body part **Explanation:** The body part is moved to a new location from an abnormal location, or from a normal location where it is not functioning correctly. The body part may or may not be cut out or off to be moved to the new location
Resection	**Definition:** Cutting out or off, without replacement, all of a body part
Transplantation	**Definition:** Putting in or on all or a portion of a living body part taken from another individual or animal to physically take the place and/or function of all or a portion of a similar body part **Explanation:** The native body part may or may not be taken out, and the transplanted body part may take over all or a portion of its function

SECTION 1 - OBSTETRICS
CHARACTER 5 - APPROACH

External	**Definition:** Procedures performed directly on the skin or mucous membrane and procedures performed indirectly by the application of external force through the skin or mucous membrane
Open	**Definition:** Cutting through the skin or mucous membrane and any other body layers necessary to expose the site of the procedure
Percutaneous	**Definition:** Entry, by puncture or minor incision, of instrumentation through the skin or mucous membrane and any other body layers necessary to reach the site of the procedure

Percutaneous Endoscopic	**Definition:** Entry, by puncture or minor incision, of instrumentation through the skin or mucous membrane and any other body layers necessary to reach and visualize the site of the procedure
Via Natural or Artificial Opening	**Definition:** Entry of instrumentation through a natural or artificial external opening to reach the site of the procedure
Via Natural or Artificial Opening Endoscopic	**Definition:** Entry of instrumentation through a natural or artificial external opening to reach and visualize the site of the procedure

SECTION 2 - PLACEMENT
CHARACTER 3 - OPERATION

Change	**Definition:** Taking out or off a device from a body part and putting back an identical or similar device in or on the same body part without cutting or puncturing the skin or a mucous membrane
Compression	**Definition:** Putting pressure on a body region
Dressing	**Definition:** Putting material on a body region for protection

Immobilization	**Definition:** Limiting or preventing motion of a body region
Packing	**Definition:** Putting material in a body region or orifice
Removal	**Definition:** Taking out or off a device from a body part
Traction	**Definition:** Exerting a pulling force on a body region in a distal direction

SECTION 2 - PLACEMENT
CHARACTER 5 - APPROACH

External	**Definition:** Procedures performed directly on the skin or mucous membrane and procedures performed indirectly by the application of external force through the skin or mucous membrane

SECTION 3 - ADMINISTRATION
CHARACTER 3 - OPERATION

Introduction	**Definition:** Putting in or on a therapeutic, diagnostic, nutritional, physiological, or prophylactic substance except blood or blood products

Irrigation	**Definition:** Putting in or on a cleansing substance
Transfusion	**Definition:** Putting in blood or blood products

SECTION 3 - ADMINISTRATION
CHARACTER 5 - APPROACH

External	**Definition:** Procedures performed directly on the skin or mucous membrane and procedures performed indirectly by the application of external force through the skin or mucous membrane
Open	**Definition:** Cutting through the skin or mucous membrane and any other body layers necessary to expose the site of the procedure
Percutaneous	**Definition:** Entry, by puncture or minor incision, of instrumentation through the skin or mucous membrane and any other body layers necessary to reach the site of the procedure

Via Natural or Artificial Opening	**Definition:** Entry of instrumentation through a natural or artificial external opening to reach the site of the procedure
Via Natural or Artificial Opening Endoscopic	**Definition:** Entry of instrumentation through a natural or artificial external opening to reach and visualize the site of the procedure

SECTION 3 - ADMINISTRATION
CHARACTER 6 - SUBSTANCE

4-Factor Prothrombin Complex Concentrate	**Includes:** Kcentra
Adhesion Barrier	**Includes:** Seprafilm
Anti-Infective Envelope	**Includes:** AIGISRx Antibacterial Envelope Antimicrobial envelope
Clofarabine	**Includes:** Clolar
Glucarpidase	**Includes:** Voraxaze

Human B-type Natriuretic Peptide	**Includes:** Nesiritide
Other Thrombolytic	**Includes:** Tissue Plasminogen Activator (tPA)(r-tPA)
Oxazolidinones	**Includes:** Zyvox
Recombinant Bone Morphogenetic Protein	**Includes:** Bone morphogenetic protein 2 (BMP 2) rhBMP-2

SECTION 4 - MEASUREMENT AND MONITORING
CHARACTER 3 - OPERATION

Measurement	**Definition:** Determining the level of a physiological or physical function at a point in time	Monitoring	**Definition:** Determining the level of a physiological or physical function repetitively over a period of time

SECTION 4 - MEASUREMENT AND MONITORING
CHARACTER 5 - APPROACH

External	**Definition:** Procedures performed directly on the skin or mucous membrane and procedures performed indirectly by the application of external force through the skin or mucous membrane	Percutaneous Endoscopic	**Definition:** Entry, by puncture or minor incision, of instrumentation through the skin or mucous membrane and any other body layers necessary to reach and visualize the site of the procedure
Open	**Definition:** Cutting through the skin or mucous membrane and any other body layers necessary to expose the site of the procedure	Via Natural or Artificial Opening	**Definition:** Entry of instrumentation through a natural or artificial external opening to reach the site of the procedure
Percutaneous	**Definition:** Entry, by puncture or minor incision, of instrumentation through the skin or mucous membrane and any other body layers necessary to reach the site of the procedure	Via Natural or Artificial Opening Endoscopic	**Definition:** Entry of instrumentation through a natural or artificial external opening to reach and visualize the site of the procedure

SECTION 5 - EXTRACORPOREAL ASSISTANCE AND PERFORMANCE
CHARACTER 3 - OPERATION

Assistance	**Definition:** Taking over a portion of a physiological function by extracorporeal means	Restoration	**Definition:** Returning, or attempting to return, a physiological function to its original state by extracorporeal means.
Performance	**Definition:** Completely taking over a physiological function by extracorporeal means		

APPENDIX A

SECTION 6 - EXTRACORPOREAL THERAPIES
CHARACTER 3 - OPERATION

Atmospheric Control	**Definition:** Extracorporeal control of atmospheric pressure and composition	Pheresis	**Definition:** Extracorporeal separation of blood products
Decompression	**Definition:** Extracorporeal elimination of undissolved gas from body fluids	Phototherapy	**Definition:** Extracorporeal treatment by light rays
Electromagnetic Therapy	**Definition:** Extracorporeal treatment by electromagnetic rays	Shock Wave Therapy	**Definition:** Extracorporeal treatment by shock waves
Hyperthermia	**Definition:** Extracorporeal raising of body temperature	Ultrasound Therapy	**Definition:** Extracorporeal treatment by ultrasound
Hypothermia	**Definition:** Extracorporeal lowering of body temperature	Ultraviolet Light Therapy	**Definition:** Extracorporeal treatment by ultraviolet light
Perfusion	**Definition:** Extracorporeal treatment by diffusion of therapeutic fluid		

SECTION 7 - OSTEOPATHIC
CHARACTER 3 - OPERATION

Treatment	**Definition:** Manual treatment to eliminate or alleviate somatic dysfunction and related disorders

SECTION 7 - OSTEOPATHIC
CHARACTER 5 - APPROACH

External	**Definition:** Procedures performed directly on the skin or mucous membrane and procedures performed indirectly by the application of external force through the skin or mucous membrane

SECTION 8 - OTHER PROCEDURES
CHARACTER 3 - OPERATION

Other Procedures	**Definition:** Methodologies which attempt to remediate or cure a disorder or disease

SECTION 8 - OTHER PROCEDURES
CHARACTER 5 - APPROACH

External	**Definition:** Procedures performed directly on the skin or mucous membrane and procedures performed indirectly by the application of external force through the skin or mucous membrane
Percutaneous	**Definition:** Entry, by puncture or minor incision, of instrumentation through the skin or mucous membrane and any other body layers necessary to reach the site of the procedure
Percutaneous Endoscopic	**Definition:** Entry, by puncture or minor incision, of instrumentation through the skin or mucous membrane and any other body layers necessary to reach and visualize the site of the procedure

Via Natural or Artificial Opening	**Definition:** Entry of instrumentation through a natural or artificial external opening to reach the site of the procedure
Via Natural or Artificial Opening Endoscopic	**Definition:** Entry of instrumentation through a natural or artificial external opening to reach and visualize the site of the procedure

SECTION 9 - CHIROPRACTIC
CHARACTER 3 - OPERATION

Manipulation	**Definition:** Manual procedure that involves a directed thrust to move a joint past the physiological range of motion, without exceeding the anatomical limit

SECTION 9 - CHIROPRACTIC
CHARACTER 5 - APPROACH

External	**Definition:** Procedures performed directly on the skin or mucous membrane and procedures performed indirectly by the application of external force through the skin or mucous membrane

SECTION B - IMAGING
CHARACTER 3 - TYPE

Computerized Tomography (CT Scan)	**Definition:** Computer reformatted digital display of multiplanar images developed from the capture of multiple exposures of external ionizing radiation	Plain Radiography	**Definition:** Planar display of an image developed from the capture of external ionizing radiation on photographic or photoconductive plate
Fluoroscopy	**Definition:** Single plane or bi-plane real time display of an image developed from the capture of external ionizing radiation on a fluorescent screen. The image may also be stored by either digital or analog means	Ultrasonography	**Definition:** Real time display of images of anatomy or flow information developed from the capture of reflected and attenuated high frequency sound waves
Magnetic Resonance Imaging (MRI)	**Definition:** Computer reformatted digital display of multiplanar images developed from the capture of radiofrequency signals emitted by nuclei in a body site excited within a magnetic field		

SECTION C - NUCLEAR MEDICINE
CHARACTER 3 - TYPE

Nonimaging Nuclear Medicine Assay	**Definition:** Introduction of radioactive materials into the body for the study of body fluids and blood elements, by the detection of radioactive emissions	Planar Nuclear Medicine Imaging	**Definition:** Introduction of radioactive materials into the body for single plane display of images developed from the capture of radioactive emissions
Nonimaging Nuclear Medicine Probe	**Definition:** Introduction of radioactive materials into the body for the study of distribution and fate of certain substances by the detection of radioactive emissions; or, alternatively, measurement of absorption of radioactive emissions from an external source	Positron Emission Tomographic (PET) Imaging	**Definition:** Introduction of radioactive materials into the body for three dimensional display of images developed from the simultaneous capture, 18Ø degrees apart, of radioactive emissions
		Systemic Nuclear Medicine Therapy	**Definition:** Introduction of unsealed radioactive materials into the body for treatment
Nonimaging Nuclear Medicine Uptake	**Definition:** Introduction of radioactive materials into the body for measurements of organ function, from the detection of radioactive emissions	Tomographic (Tomo) Nuclear Medicine Imaging	**Definition:** Introduction of radioactive materials into the body for three dimensional display of images developed from the capture of radioactive emissions

SECTION F - PHYSICAL REHABILITATION AND DIAGNOSTIC AUDIOLOGY
CHARACTER 3 - TYPE

Activities of Daily Living Assessment	**Definition:** Measurement of functional level for activities of daily living	Hearing Treatment	**Definition:** Application of techniques to improve, augment, or compensate for hearing and related functional impairment
Activities of Daily Living Treatment	**Definition:** Exercise or activities to facilitate functional competence for activities of daily living	Motor and/or Nerve Function Assessment	**Definition:** Measurement of motor, nerve, and related functions
Caregiver Training	**Definition:** Training in activities to support patient's optimal level of function	Motor Treatment	**Definition:** Exercise or activities to increase or facilitate motor function
Cochlear Implant Treatment	**Definition:** Application of techniques to improve the communication abilities of individuals with cochlear implant	Speech Assessment	**Definition:** Measurement of speech and related functions
Device Fitting	**Definition:** Fitting of a device designed to facilitate or support achievement of a higher level of function	Speech Treatment	**Definition:** Application of techniques to improve, augment, or compensate for speech and related functional impairment
Hearing Aid Assessment	**Definition:** Measurement of the appropriateness and/or effectiveness of a hearing device	Vestibular Assessment	**Definition:** Measurement of the vestibular system and related functions
Hearing Assessment	**Definition:** Measurement of hearing and related functions	Vestibular Treatment	**Definition:** Application of techniques to improve, augment, or compensate for vestibular and related functional impairment

SECTION F - PHYSICAL REHABILITATION AND DIAGNOSTIC AUDIOLOGY
CHARACTER 5 - TYPE QUALIFIER

Acoustic Reflex Decay	**Definition:** Measures reduction in size/strength of acoustic reflex over time **Includes/Examples:** Includes site of lesion test	Alternate Binaural or Monaural Loudness Balance	**Definition:** Determines auditory stimulus parameter that yields the same objective sensation **Includes/Examples:** Sound intensities that yield same loudness perception
Acoustic Reflex Patterns	**Definition:** Defines site of lesion based upon presence/absence of acoustic reflexes with ipsilateral vs. contralateral stimulation	Anthropometric Characteristics	**Definition:** Measures edema, body fat composition, height, weight, length and girth
Acoustic Reflex Threshold	**Definition:** Determines minimal intensity that acoustic reflex occurs with ipsilateral and/or contralateral stimulation	Aphasia (Assessment)	**Definition:** Measures expressive and receptive speech and language function including reading and writing
Aerobic Capacity and Endurance	**Definition:** Measures autonomic responses to positional changes; perceived exertion, dyspnea or angina during activity; performance during exercise protocols; standard vital signs; and blood gas analysis or oxygen consumption	Aphasia (Treatment)	**Definition:** Applying techniques to improve, augment, or compensate for receptive/expressive language impairments
		Articulation/Phonology (Assessment)	**Definition:** Measures speech production

SECTION F - PHYSICAL REHABILITATION AND DIAGNOSTIC AUDIOLOGY
CHARACTER 5 - TYPE QUALIFIER

Articulation/Phonology (Treatment)	**Definition:** Applying techniques to correct, improve, or compensate for speech productive impairment
Assistive Listening Device	**Definition:** Assists in use of effective and appropriate assistive listening device/system
Assistive Listening System/Device Selection	**Definition:** Measures the effectiveness and appropriateness of assistive listening systems/devices
Assistive, Adaptive, Supportive or Protective Devices	**Explanation:** Devices to facilitate or support achievement of a higher level of function in wheelchair mobility; bed mobility; transfer or ambulation ability; bath and showering ability; dressing; grooming; personal hygiene; play or leisure
Auditory Evoked Potentials	**Definition:** Measures electric responses produced by the VIIIth cranial nerve and brainstem following auditory stimulation
Auditory Processing (Assessment)	**Definition:** Evaluates ability to receive and process auditory information and comprehension of spoken language
Auditory Processing (Treatment)	**Definition:** Applying techniques to improve the receiving and processing of auditory information and comprehension of spoken language
Augmentative/ Alternative Communication System (Assessment)	**Definition:** Determines the appropriateness of aids, techniques, symbols, and/or strategies to augment or replace speech and enhance communication **Includes/Examples:** Includes the use of telephones, writing equipment, emergency equipment, and TDD
Augmentative/ Alternative Communication System (Treatment)	**Includes/Examples:** Includes augmentative communication devices and aids
Aural Rehabilitation	**Definition:** Applying techniques to improve the communication abilities associated with hearing loss
Aural Rehabilitation Status	**Definition:** Measures impact of a hearing loss including evaluation of receptive and expressive communication skills

Bathing/Showering	**Includes/Examples:** Includes obtaining and using supplies; soaping, rinsing, and drying body parts; maintaining bathing position; and transferring to and from bathing positions
Bathing/Showering Techniques	**Definition:** Activities to facilitate obtaining and using supplies, soaping, rinsing and drying body parts, maintaining bathing position, and transferring to and from bathing positions
Bed Mobility (Assessment)	**Definition:** Transitional movement within bed
Bed Mobility (Treatment)	**Definition:** Exercise or activities to facilitate transitional movements within bed
Bedside Swallowing and Oral Function	**Includes/Examples:** Bedside swallowing includes assessment of sucking, masticating, coughing, and swallowing. Oral function includes assessment of musculature for controlled movements, structures and functions to determine coordination and phonation
Bekesy Audiometry	**Definition:** Uses an instrument that provides a choice of discrete or continuously varying pure tones; choice of pulsed or continuous signal
Binaural Electroacoustic Hearing Aid Check	**Definition:** Determines mechanical and electroacoustic function of bilateral hearing aids using hearing aid test box
Binaural Hearing Aid (Assessment)	**Definition:** Measures the candidacy, effectiveness, and appropriateness of hearing aids **Explanation:** Measures bilateral fit
Binaural Hearing Aid (Treatment)	**Explanation:** Assists in achieving maximum understanding and performance
Bithermal, Binaural Caloric Irrigation	**Definition:** Measures the rhythmic eye movements stimulated by changing the temperature of the vestibular system
Bithermal, Monaural Caloric Irrigation	**Definition:** Measures the rhythmic eye movements stimulated by changing the temperature of the vestibular system in one ear

SECTION F - PHYSICAL REHABILITATION AND DIAGNOSTIC AUDIOLOGY

CHARACTER 5 - TYPE QUALIFIER

Brief Tone Stimuli	**Definition:** Measures specific central auditory process
Cerumen Management	**Definition:** Includes examination of external auditory canal and tympanic membrane and removal of cerumen from external ear canal
Cochlear Implant	**Definition:** Measures candidacy for cochlear implant
Cochlear Implant Rehabilitation	**Definition:** Applying techniques to improve the communication abilities of individuals with cochlear implant; includes programming the device, providing patients/families with information
Communicative/ Cognitive Integration Skills (Assessment)	**Definition:** Measures ability to use higher cortical functions **Includes/Examples:** Includes orientation, recognition, attention span, initiation and termination of activity, memory, sequencing, categorizing, concept formation, spatial operations, judgment, problem solving, generalization and pragmatic communication
Communicative/ Cognitive Integration Skills (Treatment)	**Definition:** Activities to facilitate the use of higher cortical functions **Includes/Examples:** Includes level of arousal, orientation, recognition, attention span, initiation and termination of activity, memory sequencing, judgment and problem solving, learning and generalization, and pragmatic communication
Computerized Dynamic Posturography	**Definition:** Measures the status of the peripheral and central vestibular system and the sensory/motor component of balance; evaluates the efficacy of vestibular rehabilitation
Conditioned Play Audiometry	**Definition:** Behavioral measures using nonspeech and speech stimuli to obtain frequency-specific and ear-specific information on auditory status from the patient **Explanation:** Obtains speech reception threshold by having patient point to pictures of spondaic words

Coordination/Dexterity (Assessment)	**Definition:** Measures large and small muscle groups for controlled goal-directed movements **Explanation:** Dexterity includes object manipulation
Coordination/Dexterity (Treatment)	**Definition:** Exercise or activities to facilitate gross coordination and fine coordination
Cranial Nerve Integrity	**Definition:** Measures cranial nerve sensory and motor functions, including tastes, smell and facial expression
Dichotic Stimuli	**Definition:** Measures specific central auditory process
Distorted Speech	**Definition:** Measures specific central auditory process
Dix-Hallpike Dynamic	**Definition:** Measures nystagmus following Dix-Hallpike maneuver
Dressing	**Includes/Examples:** Includes selecting clothing and accessories, obtaining clothing from storage, dressing and, fastening and adjusting clothing and shoes, and applying and removing personal devices, prosthesis or orthosis
Dressing Techniques	**Definition:** Activities to facilitate selecting clothing and accessories, dressing and undressing, adjusting clothing and shoes, applying and removing devices, prostheses or orthoses
Dynamic Orthosis	**Includes/Examples:** Includes customized and prefabricated splints, inhibitory casts, spinal and other braces, and protective devices; allows motion through transfer of movement from other body parts or by use of outside forces
Ear Canal Probe Microphone	**Definition:** Real ear measures
Ear Protector Attentuation	**Definition:** Measures ear protector fit and effectiveness
Electrocochleography	**Definition:** Measures the VIIIth cranial nerve action potential
Environmental, Home and Work Barriers	**Definition:** Measures current and potential barriers to optimal function, including safety hazards, access problems and home or office design

APPENDIX A

SECTION F - PHYSICAL REHABILITATION AND DIAGNOSTIC AUDIOLOGY
CHARACTER 5 - TYPE QUALIFIER

Ergonomics and Body Mechanics	**Definition:** Ergonomic measurement of job tasks, work hardening or work conditioning needs; functional capacity; and body mechanics
Eustachian Tube Function	**Definition:** Measures eustachian tube function and patency of eustachian tube
Evoked Otoacoustic Emissions, Diagnostic	**Definition:** Measures auditory evoked potentials in a diagnostic format
Evoked Otoacoustic Emissions, Screening	**Definition:** Measures auditory evoked potentials in a screening format
Facial Nerve Function	**Definition:** Measures electrical activity of the VIIth cranial nerve (facial nerve)
Feeding/Eating (Assessment)	**Includes/Examples:** Includes setting up food, selecting and using utensils and tableware, bringing food or drink to mouth, cleaning face, hands, and clothing, and management of alternative methods of nourishment
Feeding/Eating (Treatment)	**Definition:** Exercise or activities to facilitate setting up food, selecting and using utensils and tableware, bringing food or drink to mouth, cleaning face, hands, and clothing, and management of alternative methods of nourishment
Filtered Speech	**Definition:** Uses high or low pass filtered speech stimuli to assess central auditory processing disorders, site of lesion testing
Fluency (Assessment)	**Definition:** Measures speech fluency or stuttering
Fluency (Treatment)	**Definition:** Applying techniques to improve and augment fluent speech
Gait and/or Balance	**Definition:** Measures biomechanical, arthrokinematic and other spatial and temporal characteristics of gait and balance
Gait Training/ Functional Ambulation	**Definition:** Exercise or activities to facilitate ambulation on a variety of surfaces and in a variety of environments
Grooming/Personal Hygiene (Assessment)	**Includes/Examples:** Includes ability to obtain and use supplies in a sequential fashion, general grooming, oral hygiene, toilet hygiene, personal care devices, including care for artificial airways
Grooming/Personal Hygiene (Treatment)	**Definition:** Activities to facilitate obtaining and using supplies in a sequential fashion: general grooming, oral hygiene, toilet hygiene, cleaning body, and personal care devices, including artificial airways
Hearing and Related Disorders Counseling	**Definition:** Provides patients/families/ caregivers with information, support, referrals to facilitate recovery from a communication disorder **Includes/Examples:** Includes strategies for psychosocial adjustment to hearing loss for clients and families/caregivers
Hearing and Related Disorders Prevention	**Definition:** Provides patients/families/ caregivers with information and support to prevent communication disorders
Hearing Screening	**Definition:** Pass/refer measures designed to identify need for further audiologic assessment
Home Management (Assessment)	**Definition:** Obtaining and maintaining personal and household possessions and environment **Includes/Examples:** Includes clothing care, cleaning, meal preparation and cleanup, shopping, money management, household maintenance, safety procedures, and childcare/parenting
Home Management (Treatment)	**Definition:** Activities to facilitate obtaining and maintaining personal household possessions and environment **Includes/Examples:** Includes clothing care, cleaning, meal preparation and clean-up, shopping, money management, household maintenance, safety procedures, childcare/ parenting
Instrumental Swallowing and Oral Function	**Definition:** Measures swallowing function using instrumental diagnostic procedures **Explanation:** Methods include videofluoroscopy, ultrasound, manometry, endoscopy
Integumentary Integrity	**Includes/Examples:** Includes burns, skin conditions, ecchymosis, bleeding, blisters, scar tissue, wounds and other traumas, tissue mobility, turgor and texture

SECTION F - PHYSICAL REHABILITATION AND DIAGNOSTIC AUDIOLOGY

CHARACTER 5 - TYPE QUALIFIER

Manual Therapy Techniques	**Definition:** Techniques in which the therapist uses his/her hands to administer skilled movements **Includes/Examples:** Includes connective tissue massage, joint mobilization and manipulation, manual lymph drainage, manual traction, soft tissue mobilization and manipulation
Masking Patterns	**Definition:** Measures central auditory processing status
Monaural Electroacoustic Hearing Aid Check	**Definition:** Determines mechanical and electroacoustic function of one hearing aid using hearing aid test box
Monaural Hearing Aid (Assessment)	**Definition:** Measures the candidacy, effectiveness, and appropriateness of a hearing aid **Explanation:** Measures unilateral fit
Monaural Hearing Aid (Treatment)	**Explanation:** Assists in achieving maximum understanding and performance
Motor Function (Assessment)	**Definition:** Measures the body's functional and versatile movement patterns **Includes/Examples:** Includes motor assessment scales, analysis of head, trunk and limb movement, and assessment of motor learning
Motor Function (Treatment)	**Definition:** Exercise or activities to facilitate crossing midline, laterality, bilateral integration, praxis, neuromuscular relaxation, inhibition, facilitation, motor function and motor learning
Motor Speech (Assessment)	**Definition:** Measures neurological motor aspects of speech production
Motor Speech (Treatment)	**Definition:** Applying techniques to improve and augment the impaired neurological motor aspects of speech production
Muscle Performance (Assessment)	**Definition:** Measures muscle strength, power and endurance using manual testing, dynamometry or computer-assisted electromechanical muscle test; functional muscle strength, power and endurance; muscle pain, tone, or soreness; or pelvic-floor musculature **Explanation:** Muscle endurance refers to the ability to contract a muscle repeatedly over time
Muscle Performance (Treatment)	**Definition:** Exercise or activities to increase the capacity of a muscle to do work in terms of strength, power, and/or endurance **Explanation:** Muscle strength is the force exerted to overcome resistance in one maximal effort. Muscle power is work produced per unit of time, or the product of strength and speed. Muscle endurance is the ability to contract a muscle repeatedly over time
Neuromotor Development	**Definition:** Measures motor development, righting and equilibrium reactions, and reflex and equilibrium reactions
Neurophysiologic Intraoperative	**Definition:** Monitors neural status during surgery
Non-invasive Instrumental Status	**Definition:** Instrumental measures of oral, nasal, vocal, and velopharyngeal functions as they pertain to speech production
Nonspoken Language (Assessment)	**Definition:** Measures nonspoken language (print, sign, symbols) for communication
Nonspoken Language (Treatment)	**Definition:** Applying techniques that improve, augment, or compensate spoken communication
Oral Peripheral Mechanism	**Definition:** Structural measures of face, jaw, lips, tongue, teeth, hard and soft palate, pharynx as related to speech production
Orofacial Myofunctional (Assessment)	**Definition:** Measures orofacial myofunctional patterns for speech and related functions
Orofacial Myofunctional (Treatment)	**Definition:** Applying techniques to improve, alter, or augment impaired orofacial myofunctional patterns and related speech production errors
Oscillating Tracking	**Definition:** Measures ability to visually track
Pain	**Definition:** Measures muscle soreness, pain and soreness with joint movement, and pain perception **Includes/Examples:** Includes questionnaires, graphs, symptom magnification scales or visual analog scales

SECTION F - PHYSICAL REHABILITATION AND DIAGNOSTIC AUDIOLOGY
CHARACTER 5 - TYPE QUALIFIER

Perceptual Processing (Assessment)	**Definition:** Measures stereognosis, kinesthesia, body schema, right-left discrimination, form constancy, position in space, visual closure, figure-ground, depth perception, spatial relations and topographical orientation	Pure Tone Audiometry, Air	**Definition:** Air-conduction pure tone threshold measures with appropriate masking
Perceptual Processing (Treatment)	**Definition:** Exercise and activities to facilitate perceptual processing **Explanation:** Includes stereognosis, kinesthesia, body schema, right-left discrimination, form constancy, position in space, visual closure, figure-ground, depth perception, spatial relations, and topographical orientation **Includes/Examples:** Includes stereognosis, kinesthesia, body schema, right-left discrimination, form constancy, position in space, visual closure, figure-ground, depth perception, spatial relations, and topographical orientation	Pure Tone Audiometry, Air and Bone	**Definition:** Air-conduction and bone-conduction pure tone threshold measures with appropriate masking
		Pure Tone Stenger	**Definition:** Measures unilateral nonorganic hearing loss based on simultaneous presentation of pure tones of differing volume
		Range of Motion and Joint Integrity	**Definition:** Measures quantity, quality, grade, and classification of joint movement and/or mobility **Explanation:** Range of Motion is the space, distance or angle through which movement occurs at a joint or series of joints. Joint integrity is the conformance of joints to expected anatomic, biomechanical and kinematic norms
Performance Intensity Phonetically Balanced Speech Discrimination	**Definition:** Measures word recognition over varying intensity levels		
Postural Control	**Definition:** Exercise or activities to increase postural alignment and control	Range of Motion and Joint Mobility	**Definition:** Exercise or activities to increase muscle length and joint mobility
Prosthesis	**Explanation:** Artificial substitutes for missing body parts that augment performance or function	Receptive/Expressive Language (Assessment)	**Definition:** Measures receptive and expressive language
Psychosocial Skills (Assessment)	**Definition:** The ability to interact in society and to process emotions **Includes/Examples:** Includes psychological (values, interests, self-concept); social (role performance, social conduct, interpersonal skills, self expression); self-management (coping skills, time management, self-control)	Receptive/Expressive Language (Treatment)	**Definition:** Applying techniques tot improve and augment receptive/expressive language
		Reflex Integrity	**Definition:** Measures the presence, absence, or exaggeration of developmentally appropriate, pathologic or normal reflexes
		Select Picture Audiometry	**Definition:** Establishes hearing threshold levels for speech using pictures
		Sensorineural Acuity Level	**Definition:** Measures sensorineural acuity masking presented via bone conduction
Psychosocial Skills (Treatment)	**Definition:** The ability to interact in society and to process emotions **Includes/Examples:** Includes psychological (values, interests, self-concept); social (role performance, social conduct, interpersonal skills, self expression); self-management (coping skills, time management, self-control)	Sensory Aids	**Definition:** Determines the appropriateness of a sensory prosthetic device, other than a hearing aid or assistive listening system/device
		Sensory Awareness/ Processing/Integrity	**Includes/Examples:** Includes light touch, pressure, temperature, pain, sharp/dull, proprioception, vestibular, visual, auditory, gustatory, and olfactory

SECTION F - PHYSICAL REHABILITATION AND DIAGNOSTIC AUDIOLOGY

CHARACTER 5 - TYPE QUALIFIER

Short Increment Sensitivity Index	**Definition:** Measures the ear's ability to detect small intensity changes; site of lesion test requiring a behavioral response
Sinusoidal Vertical Axis Rotational	**Definition:** Measures nystagmus following rotation
Somatosensory Evoked Potentials	**Definition:** Measures neural activity from sites throughout the body
Speech and/or Language Screening	**Definition:** Identifies need for further speech and/or language evaluation
Speech Threshold	**Definition:** Measures minimal intensity needed to repeat spondaic words
Speech-Language Pathology and Related Disorders Counseling	**Definition:** Provides patients/families with information, support, referrals to facilitate recovery from a communication disorder
Speech-Language Pathology and Related Disorders Prevention	**Definition:** Applying techniques to avoid or minimize onset and/or development of a communication disorder
Speech/Word Recognition	**Definition:** Measures ability to repeat/ identify single syllable words; scores given as a percentage; includes word recognition/ speech discrimination
Staggered Spondaic Word	**Definition:** Measures central auditory processing site of lesion based upon dichotic presentation of spondaic words
Static Orthosis	**Includes/Examples:** Includes customized and prefabricated splints, inhibitory casts, spinal and other braces, and protective devices; has no moving parts, maintains joint(s) in desired position
Stenger	**Definition:** Measures unilateral nonorganic hearing loss based on simultaneous presentation of signals of differing volume
Swallowing Dysfunction	**Definition:** Activities to improve swallowing function in coordination with respiratory function **Includes/Examples:** Includes function and coordination of sucking, mastication, coughing, swallowing

Synthetic Sentence Identification	**Definition:** Measures central auditory dysfunction using identification of third order approximations of sentences and competing messages
Temporal Ordering of Stimuli	**Definition:** Measures specific central auditory process
Therapeutic Exercise	**Definition:** Exercise or activities to facilitate sensory awareness, sensory processing, sensory integration, balance training, conditioning, reconditioning **Includes/Examples:** Includes developmental activities, breathing exercises, aerobic endurance activities, aquatic exercises, stretching and ventilatory muscle training
Tinnitus Masker (Assessment)	**Definition:** Determines candidacy for tinnitus masker
Tinnitus Masker (Treatment)	**Explanation:** Used to verify physical fit, acoustic appropriateness, and benefit; assists in achieving maximum benefit
Tone Decay	**Definition:** Measures decrease in hearing sensitivity to a tone; site of lesion test requiring a behavioral response
Transfer	**Definition:** Transitional movement from one surface to another
Transfer Training	**Definition:** Exercise or activities to facilitate movement from one surface to another
Tympanometry	**Definition:** Measures the integrity of the middle ear; measures ease at which sound flows through the tympanic membrane while air pressure against the membrane is varied
Unithermal Binaural Screen	**Definition:** Measures the rhythmic eye movements stimulated by changing the temperature of the vestibular system in both ears using warm water, screening format

APPENDIX A

SECTION F - PHYSICAL REHABILITATION AND DIAGNOSTIC AUDIOLOGY

CHARACTER 5 - TYPE QUALIFIER

Ventilation, Respiration and Circulation	**Definition:** Measures ventilatory muscle strength, power and endurance, pulmonary function and ventilatory mechanics **Includes/Examples:** Includes ability to clear airway, activities that aggravate or relieve edema, pain, dyspnea or other symptoms, chest wall mobility, cardiopulmonary response to performance of ADL and IAD, cough and sputum, standard vital signs
Vestibular	**Definition:** Applying techniques to compensate for balance disorders; includes habituation, exercise therapy, and balance retraining
Visual Motor Integration (Assessment)	**Definition:** Coordinating the interaction of information from the eyes with body movement during activity
Visual Motor Integration (Treatment)	**Definition:** Exercise or activities to facilitate coordinating the interaction of information from eyes with body movement during activity
Visual Reinforcement Audiometry	**Definition:** Behavioral measures using nonspeech and speech stimuli to obtain frequency/ear-specific information on auditory status **Includes/Examples:** Includes a conditioned response of looking toward a visual reinforcer (e.g., lights, animated toy) every time auditory stimuli are heard
Vocational Activities and Functional Community or Work Reintegration Skills (Assessment)	**Definition:** Measures environmental, home, work (job/school/play) barriers that keep patients from functioning optimally in their environment **Includes/Examples:** Includes assessment of vocational skill and interests, environment of work (job/school/play), injury potential and injury prevention or reduction, ergonomic stressors, transportation skills, and ability to access and use community resources

Vocational Activities and Functional Community or Work Reintegration Skills (Treatment)	**Definition:** Activities to facilitate vocational exploration, body mechanics training, job acquisition, and environmental or work (job/school/play) task adaptation **Includes/Examples:** Includes injury prevention and reduction, ergonomic stressor reduction, job coaching and simulation, work hardening and conditioning, driving training, transportation skills, and use of community resources
Voice (Assessment)	**Definition:** Measures vocal structure, function and production
Voice (Treatment)	**Definition:** Applying techniques to improve voice and vocal function
Voice Prosthetic (Assessment)	**Definition:** Determines the appropriateness of voice prosthetic/adaptive device to enhance or facilitate communication
Voice Prosthetic (Treatment)	**Includes/Examples:** Includes electrolarynx, and other assistive, adaptive, supportive devices
Wheelchair Mobility (Assessment)	**Definition:** Measures fit and functional abilities within wheelchair in a variety of environments
Wheelchair Mobility (Treatment)	**Definition:** Management, maintenance and controlled operation of a wheelchair, scooter or other device, in and on a variety of surfaces and environments
Wound Management	**Includes/Examples:** Includes non-selective and selective debridement (enzymes, autolysis, sharp debridement), dressings (wound coverings, hydrogel, vacuum-assisted closure), topical agents, etc.

SECTION G - MENTAL HEALTH
CHARACTER 3 - TYPE

Biofeedback	**Definition:** Provision of information from the monitoring and regulating of physiological processes in conjunction with cognitive-behavioral techniques to improve patient functioning or well-being **Includes/Examples:** Includes EEG, blood pressure, skin temperature or peripheral blood flow, ECG, electrooculogram, EMG, respirometry or capnometry, GSR/EDR, perineometry to monitor/regulate bowel/bladder activity, electrogastrogram to monitor/regulate gastric motility
Counseling	**Definition:** The application of psychological methods to treat an individual with normal developmental issues and psychological problems in order to increase function, improve well-being, alleviate distress, maladjustment or resolve crises
Crisis Intervention	**Definition:** Treatment of a traumatized, acutely disturbed or distressed individual for the purpose of short-term stabilization **Includes/Examples:** Includes defusing, debriefing, counseling, psychotherapy and/or coordination of care with other providers or agencies
Electroconvulsive Therapy	**Definition:** The application of controlled electrical voltages to treat a mental health disorder **Includes/Examples:** Includes appropriate sedation and other preparation of the individual
Family Psychotherapy	**Definition:** Treatment that includes one or more family members of an individual with a mental health disorder by behavioral, cognitive, psychoanalytic, psychodynamic or psychophysiological means to improve functioning or well-being **Explanation:** Remediation of emotional or behavioral problems presented by one or more family members in cases where psychotherapy with more than one family member is indicated
Group Psychotherapy	**Definition:** Treatment of two or more individuals with a mental health disorder by behavioral, cognitive, psychoanalytic, psychodynamic or psychophysiological means to improve functioning or well-being
Hypnosis	**Definition:** Induction of a state of heightened suggestibility by auditory, visual and tactile techniques to elicit an emotional or behavioral response
Individual Psychotherapy	**Definition:** Treatment of an individual with a mental health disorder by behavioral, cognitive, psychoanalytic, psychodynamic or psychophysiological means to improve functioning or well-being
Light Therapy	**Definition:** Application of specialized light treatments to improve functioning or well-being
Medication Management	**Definition:** Monitoring and adjusting the use of medications for the treatment of a mental health disorder
Narcosynthesis	**Definition:** Administration of intravenous barbiturates in order to release suppressed or repressed thoughts
Psychological Tests	**Definition:** The administration and interpretation of standardized psychological tests and measurement instruments for the assessment of psychological function

APPENDIX A

833

SECTION G - MENTAL HEALTH
CHARACTER 4 - QUALIFIER

Behavioral	**Definition:** Primarily to modify behavior **Includes/Examples:** Includes modeling and role playing, positive reinforcement of target behaviors, response cost, and training of self-management skills
Cognitive	**Definition:** Primarily to correct cognitive distortions and errors
Cognitive-Behavioral	**Definition:** Combining cognitive and behavioral treatment strategies to improve functioning **Explanation:** Maladaptive responses are examined to determine how cognitions relate to behavior patterns in response to an event. Uses learning principles and information-processing models
Developmental	**Definition:** Age-normed developmental status of cognitive, social and adaptive behavior skills
Intellectual and Psychoeducational	**Definition:** Intellectual abilities, academic achievement and learning capabilities (including behaviors and emotional factors affecting learning)
Interactive	**Definition:** Uses primarily physical aids and other forms of non-oral interaction with a patient who is physically, psychologically or developmentally unable to use ordinary language for communication **Includes/Examples:** Includes the use of toys in symbolic play
Interpersonal	**Definition:** Helps an individual make changes in interpersonal behaviors to reduce psychological dysfunction **Includes/Examples:** Includes exploratory techniques, encouragement of affective expression, clarification of patient statements, analysis of communication patterns, use of therapy relationship and behavior change techniques
Neurobehavioral and Cognitive Status	**Definition:** Includes neurobehavioral status exam, interview(s), and observation for the clinical assessment of thinking, reasoning and judgment, acquired knowledge, attention, memory, visual spatial abilities, language functions, and planning
Neuropsychological	**Definition:** Thinking, reasoning and judgment, acquired knowledge, attention, memory, visual spatial abilities, language functions, planning
Personality and Behavioral	**Definition:** Mood, emotion, behavior, social functioning, psychopathological conditions, personality traits and characteristics
Psychoanalysis	**Definition:** Methods of obtaining a detailed account of past and present mental and emotional experiences to determine the source and eliminate or diminish the undesirable effects of unconscious conflicts **Explanation:** Accomplished by making the individual aware of their existence, origin, and inappropriate expression in emotions and behavior
Psychodynamic	**Definition:** Exploration of past and present emotional experiences to understand motives and drives using insight-oriented techniques to reduce the undesirable effects of internal conflicts on emotions and behavior **Explanation:** Techniques include empathetic listening, clarifying self-defeating behavior patterns, and exploring adaptive alternatives
Psychophysiological	**Definition:** Monitoring and alteration of physiological processes to help the individual associate physiological reactions combined with cognitive and behavioral strategies to gain improved control of these processes to help the individual cope more effectively
Supportive	**Definition:** Formation of therapeutic relationship primarily for providing emotional support to prevent further deterioration in functioning during periods of particular stress **Explanation:** Often used in conjunction with other therapeutic approaches
Vocational	**Definition:** Exploration of vocational interests, aptitudes and required adaptive behavior skills to develop and carry out a plan for achieving a successful vocational placement **Includes/Examples:** Includes enhancing work related adjustment and/or pursuing viable options in training education or preparation

SECTION H - SUBSTANCE ABUSE TREATMENT
CHARACTER 3 - TYPE

Detoxification Services	**Definition:** Detoxification from alcohol and/or drugs **Explanation:** Not a treatment modality, but helps the patient stabilize physically and psychologically until the body becomes free of drugs and the effects of alcohol		Individual Counseling	**Definition:** The application of psychological methods to treat an individual with addictive behavior **Explanation:** Comprised of several different techniques, which apply various strategies to address drug addiction
Family Counseling	**Definition:** The application of psychological methods that includes one or more family members to treat an individual with addictive behavior **Explanation:** Provides support and education for family members of addicted individuals. Family member participation is seen as a critical area of substance abuse treatment		Individual Psychotherapy	**Definition:** Treatment of an individual with addictive behavior by behavioral, cognitive, psychoanalytic, psychodynamic or psychophysiological means
Group Counseling	**Definition:** The application of psychological methods to treat two or more individuals with addictive behavior **Explanation:** Provides structured group counseling sessions and healing power through the connection with others		Medication Management	**Definition:** Monitoring and adjusting the use of replacement medications for the treatment of addiction
			Pharmacotherapy	**Definition:** The use of replacement medications for the treatment of addiction

SECTION X - NEW TECHNOLOGY
CHARACTER 3 - OPERATION

Assistance	**Definition:** Taking over a portion of a physiological function by extracorporeal means
Extirpation	**Definition:** Taking or cutting out solid matter from a body part **Explanation:** The solid matter may be an abnormal byproduct of a biological function or foreign body; it may be imbedded in a body part or in the lumen of a tubular body part. The solid matter may or may not have been previously broken into pieces. **Includes/Examples:** Thrombectomy, choledocholithotomy
Fusion	**Definition:** Joining together portions of an articular body part rendering the articular body part immobile **Explanation:** The body part is joined together by fixation device, bone graft, or other means **Includes/Examples:** Spinal fusion, ankle arthrodesis
Insertion	**Definition:** Putting in a nonbiological appliance that monitors, assists, performs, or prevents a physiological function but does not physically take the place of a body part **Includes/Examples:** Insertion of radioactive implant, insertion of central venous catheter
Introduction	**Definition:** Putting in or on a therapeutic, diagnostic, nutritional, physiological, or prophylactic substance except blood or blood products
Monitoring	**Definition:** Determining the level of a physiological or physical function repetitively over a period of time
Removal	**Definition:** Taking out or off a device from a body part **Explanation:** If a device is taken out and a similar device put in without cutting or puncturing the skin or mucous membrane, the procedure is coded to the root operation CHANGE. Otherwise, the procedure for taking out a device is coded to the root operation REMOVAL **Includes/Examples:** Drainage tube removal, cardiac pacemaker removal
Replacement	**Definition:** Putting in or on biological or synthetic material that physically takes the place and/or function of all or a portion of a body part **Explanation:** The body part may have been taken out or replaced, or may be taken out, physically eradicated, or rendered nonfunctional during the Replacement procedure. A Removal procedure is coded for taking out the device used in a previous replacement procedure **Includes/Examples:** Total hip replacement, bone graft, free skin graft
Reposition	**Definition:** Moving to its normal location, or other suitable location, all or a portion of a body part **Explanation:** The body part is moved to a new location from an abnormal location, or from a normal location where it is not functioning correctly. The body part may or may not be cut out or off to be moved to the new location **Includes/Examples:** Reposition of undescended testicle, fracture reduction
Revision	**Definition:** Correcting, to the extent possible, a portion of a malfunctioning device or the position of a displaced device **Explanation:** Revision can include correcting a malfunctioning or displaced device by taking out or putting in components of the device such as a screw or pin **Includes/Examples:** Adjustment of position of pacemaker lead, recementing of hip prosthesis

SECTION X - NEW TECHNOLOGY
CHARACTER 5 - APPROACH

External	**Definition:** Procedures performed directly on the skin or mucous membrane and procedures performed indirectly by the application of external force through the skin or mucous membrane
Open	**Definition:** Cutting through the skin or mucous membrane and any other body layers necessary to expose the site of the procedure
Percutaneous	**Definition:** Entry, by puncture or minor incision, of instrumentation through the skin or mucous membrane and any other body layers necessary to reach the site of the procedure

Percutaneous Endoscopic	**Definition:** Entry, by puncture or minor incision, of instrumentation through the skin or mucous membrane and any other body layers necessary to reach and visualize the site of the procedure
Via Natural or Artificial Opening	**Definition:** Entry of instrumentation through a natural or artificial external opening to reach the site of the procedure
Via Natural or Artificial Opening Endoscopic	**Definition:** Entry of instrumentation through a natural or artificial external opening to reach and visualize the site of the procedure

SECTION X - NEW TECHNOLOGY
CHARACTER 6 - DEVICE / SUBSTANCE / TECHNOLOGY

Andexanet Alfa, Factor Xa Inhibitor Reversal Agent	Factor Xa Inhibitor Reversal Agent, Andexanet Alfa
Defibrotide Sodium Anticoagulant	Defitelio
Interbody Fusion Device, Nanotextured Surface in New Technology	nanoLOCK™ interbody fusion device
Magnetically Controlled Growth Rod(s) in New Technology	MAGEC® Spinal Bracing and Distraction System Spinal growth rods, magnetically controlled

Skin Substitute, Porcine Liver Derived in New Technology	MIRODERM™ Biologic Wound Matrix
Uridine Triacetate	Vistogard®
Zooplastic Tissue, Rapid Deployment Technique in New Technology	EDWARDS INTUITY Elite valve system INTUITY Elite valve system, EDWARDS Perceval sutureless valve Sutureless valve, Perceval

BODY PART KEY

Abdominal aortic plexus	**Use:** Abdominal Sympathetic Nerve
Abdominal esophagus	**Use:** Esophagus, Lower
Abductor hallucis muscle	**Use:** Foot Muscle, Right Foot Muscle, Left
Accessory cephalic vein	**Use:** Cephalic Vein, Right Cephalic Vein, Left
Accessory obturator nerve	**Use:** Lumbar Plexus
Accessory phrenic nerve	**Use:** Phrenic Nerve
Accessory spleen	**Use:** Spleen
Acetabulofemoral joint	**Use:** Hip Joint, Right Hip Joint, Left
Achilles tendon	**Use:** Lower Leg Tendon, Right Lower Leg Tendon, Left
Acromioclavicular ligament	**Use:** Shoulder Bursa and Ligament, Right Shoulder Bursa and Ligament, Left
Acromion (process)	**Use:** Scapula, Right Scapula, Left
Adductor brevis muscle	**Use:** Upper Leg Muscle, Right Upper Leg Muscle, Left
Adductor hallucis muscle	**Use:** Foot Muscle, Right Foot Muscle, Left
Adductor longus muscle Adductor magnus muscle	**Use:** Upper Leg Muscle, Right Upper Leg Muscle, Left
Adenohypophysis	**Use:** Pituitary Gland
Alar ligament of axis	**Use:** Head and Neck Bursa and Ligament
Alveolar process of mandible	**Use:** Mandible, Right Mandible, Left

Alveolar process of maxilla	**Use:** Maxilla, Right Maxilla, Left
Anal orifice	**Use:** Anus
Anatomical snuffbox	**Use:** Lower Arm and Wrist Muscle, Right Lower Arm and Wrist Muscle, Left
Angular artery	**Use:** Face Artery
Angular vein	**Use:** Face Vein, Right Face Vein, Left
Annular ligament	**Use:** Elbow Bursa and Ligament, Right Elbow Bursa and Ligament, Left
Anorectal junction	**Use:** Rectum
Ansa cervicalis	**Use:** Cervical Plexus
Antebrachial fascia	**Use:** Subcutaneous Tissue and Fascia, Right Lower Arm Subcutaneous Tissue and Fascia, Left Lower Arm
Anterior (pectoral) lymph node	**Use:** Lymphatic, Right Axillary Lymphatic, Left Axillary
Anterior cerebral artery	**Use:** Intracranial Artery
Anterior cerebral vein	**Use:** Intracranial Vein
Anterior choroidal artery	**Use:** Intracranial Artery
Anterior circumflex humeral artery	**Use:** Axillary Artery, Right Axillary Artery, Left
Anterior communicating artery	**Use:** Intracranial Artery
Anterior cruciate ligament (ACL)	**Use:** Knee Bursa and Ligament, Right Knee Bursa and Ligament, Left
Anterior crural nerve	**Use:** Femoral Nerve

BODY PART KEY

Anterior facial vein	**Use:** Face Vein, Right Face Vein, Left
Anterior intercostal artery	**Use:** Internal Mammary Artery, Right Internal Mammary Artery, Left
Anterior interosseous nerve	**Use:** Median Nerve
Anterior lateral malleolar artery	**Use:** Anterior Tibial Artery, Right Anterior Tibial Artery, Left
Anterior lingual gland	**Use:** Minor Salivary Gland
Anterior medial malleolar artery	**Use:** Anterior Tibial Artery, Right Anterior Tibial Artery, Left
Anterior spinal artery	**Use:** Vertebral Artery, Right Vertebral Artery, Left
Anterior tibial recurrent artery	**Use:** Anterior Tibial Artery, Right Anterior Tibial Artery, Left
Anterior ulnar recurrent artery	**Use:** Ulnar Artery, Right Ulnar Artery, Left
Anterior vagal trunk	**Use:** Vagus Nerve
Anterior vertebral muscle	**Use:** Neck Muscle, Right Neck Muscle, Left
Antihelix Antitragus	**Use:** External Ear, Right External Ear, Left External Ear, Bilateral
Antrum of Highmore	**Use:** Maxillary Sinus, Right Maxillary Sinus, Left
Aortic annulus	**Use:** Aortic Valve
Aortic arch	**Use:** Thoracic Aorta, Ascending/Arch
Aortic intercostal artery	**Use:** Upper Artery
Apical (subclavicular) lymph node	**Use:** Lymphatic, Right Axillary Lymphatic, Left Axillary

Apneustic center	**Use:** Pons
Aqueduct of Sylvius	**Use:** Cerebral Ventricle
Aqueous humour	**Use:** Anterior Chamber, Right Anterior Chamber, Left
Arachnoid mater	**Use:** Cerebral Meninges Spinal Meninges
Arcuate artery	**Use:** Foot Artery, Right Foot Artery, Left
Areola	**Use:** Nipple, Right Nipple, Left
Arterial canal (duct)	**Use:** Pulmonary Artery, Left
Aryepiglottic fold Arytenoid cartilage	**Use:** Larynx
Arytenoid muscle	**Use:** Neck Muscle, Right Neck Muscle, Left
Ascending aorta	**Use:** Thoracic Aorta, Ascending/Arch
Ascending palatine artery	**Use:** Face Artery
Ascending pharyngeal artery	**Use:** External Carotid Artery, Right External Carotid Artery, Left
Atlantoaxial joint	**Use:** Cervical Vertebral Joint
Atrioventricular node	**Use:** Conduction Mechanism
Atrium dextrum cordis	**Use:** Atrium, Right
Atrium pulmonale	**Use:** Atrium, Left
Auditory tube	**Use:** Eustachian Tube, Right Eustachian Tube, Left
Auerbach's (myenteric) plexus	**Use:** Abdominal Sympathetic Nerve

BODY PART KEY

Auricle	**Use:** External Ear, Right External Ear, Left External Ear, Bilateral
Auricularis muscle	**Use:** Head Muscle

Axillary fascia	**Use:**
	Subcutaneous Tissue and Fascia,
	  Right Upper Arm
	Subcutaneous Tissue and Fascia,
	  Left Upper Arm

Axillary nerve	**Use:** Brachial Plexus
Bartholin's (greater vestibular) gland	**Use:** Vestibular Gland
Basal (internal) cerebral vein	**Use:** Intracranial Vein
Basal nuclei	**Use:** Basal Ganglia
Base of Tongue	**Use:** Pharynx
Basilar artery	**Use:** Intracranial Artery
Basis pontis	**Use:** Pons
Biceps brachii muscle	**Use:** Upper Arm Muscle, Right Upper Arm Muscle, Left
Biceps femoris muscle	**Use:** Upper Leg Muscle, Right Upper Leg Muscle, Left

Bicipital aponeurosis	**Use:**
	Subcutaneous Tissue and Fascia,
	  Right Lower Arm
	Subcutaneous Tissue and Fascia,
	  Left Lower Arm

Bicuspid valve	**Use:** Mitral Valve
Body of femur	**Use:** Femoral Shaft, Right Femoral Shaft, Left
Body of fibula	**Use:** Fibula, Right Fibula, Left
Bony labyrinth	**Use:** Inner Ear, Right Inner Ear, Left

Bony orbit	**Use:** Orbit, Right Orbit, Left
Bony vestibule	**Use:** Inner Ear, Right Inner Ear, Left
Botallo's duct	**Use:** Pulmonary Artery, Left
Brachial (lateral) lymph node	**Use:** Lymphatic, Right Axillary Lymphatic, Left Axillary
Brachialis muscle	**Use:** Upper Arm Muscle, Right Upper Arm Muscle, Left
Brachiocephalic artery Brachiocephalic trunk	**Use:** Innominate Artery
Brachiocephalic vein	**Use:** Innominate Vein, Right Innominate Vein, Left
Brachioradialis muscle	**Use:** Lower Arm and Wrist Muscle, Right Lower Arm and Wrist Muscle, Left
Broad ligament	**Use:** Uterine Supporting Structure
Bronchial artery	**Use:** Upper Artery
Bronchus Intermedius	**Use:** Main Bronchus, Right
Buccal gland	**Use:** Buccal Mucosa
Buccinator lymph node	**Use:** Lymphatic, Head
Buccinator muscle	**Use:** Facial Muscle
Bulbospongiosus muscle	**Use:** Perineum Muscle
Bulbourethral (Cowper's) gland	**Use:** Urethra
Bundle of His Bundle of Kent	**Use:** Conduction Mechanism
Calcaneocuboid joint	**Use:** Tarsal Joint, Right Tarsal Joint, Left
Calcaneocuboid ligament	**Use:** Foot Bursa and Ligament, Right Foot Bursa and Ligament, Left

BODY PART KEY

Calcaneofibular ligament	**Use:** Ankle Bursa and Ligament, Right Ankle Bursa and Ligament, Left
Calcaneus	**Use:** Tarsal, Right Tarsal, Left
Capitate bone	**Use:** Carpal, Right Carpal, Left
Cardia	**Use:** Esophagogastric Junction
Cardiac plexus	**Use:** Thoracic Sympathetic Nerve
Cardioesophageal junction	**Use:** Esophagogastric Junction
Caroticotympanic artery	**Use:** Internal Carotid Artery, Right Internal Carotid Artery, Left
Carotid glomus	**Use:** Carotid Body, Left Carotid Body, Right Carotid Bodies, Bilateral
Carotid sinus	**Use:** Internal Carotid Artery, Right Internal Carotid Artery, Left
Carotid sinus nerve	**Use:** Glossopharyngeal Nerve
Carpometacarpal (CMC) joint	**Use:** Metacarpocarpal Joint, Right Metacarpocarpal Joint, Left
Carpometacarpal ligament	**Use:** Hand Bursa and Ligament, Right Hand Bursa and Ligament, Left
Cauda equina	**Use:** Lumbar Spinal Cord
Cavernous plexus	**Use:** Head and Neck Sympathetic Nerve
Celiac (solar) plexus Celiac ganglion	**Use:** Abdominal Sympathetic Nerve
Celiac lymph node	**Use:** Lymphatic, Aortic
Celiac trunk	**Use:** Celiac Artery
Central axillary lymph node	**Use:** Lymphatic, Right Axillary Lymphatic, Left Axillary
Cerebral aqueduct (Sylvius)	**Use:** Cerebral Ventricle
Cerebrum	**Use:** Brain
Cervical esophagus	**Use:** Esophagus, Upper
Cervical facet joint	**Use:** Cervical Vertebral Joint Cervical Vertebral Joints, 2 or more
Cervical ganglion	**Use:** Head and Neck Sympathetic Nerve
Cervical interspinous ligament Cervical intertransverse ligament Cervical ligamentum flavum	**Use:** Head and Neck Bursa and Ligament
Cervical lymph node	**Use:** Lymphatic, Right Neck Lymphatic, Left Neck
Cervicothoracic facet joint	**Use:** Cervicothoracic Vertebral Joint
Choana	**Use:** Nasopharynx
Chondroglossus muscle	**Use:** Tongue, Palate, Pharynx Muscle
Chorda tympani	**Use:** Facial Nerve
Choroid plexus	**Use:** Cerebral Ventricle
Ciliary body	**Use:** Eye, Right Eye, Left
Ciliary ganglion	**Use:** Head and Neck Sympathetic Nerve
Circle of Willis	**Use:** Intracranial Artery
Circumflex iliac artery	**Use:** Femoral Artery, Right Femoral Artery, Left
Claustrum	**Use:** Basal Ganglia
Coccygeal body	**Use:** Coccygeal Glomus
Coccygeus muscle	**Use:** Trunk Muscle, Right Trunk Muscle, Left

BODY PART KEY

Cochlea	Use: Inner Ear, Right Inner Ear, Left
Cochlear nerve	Use: Acoustic Nerve
Columella	Use: Nose
Common digital vein	Use: Foot Vein, Right Foot Vein, Left
Common facial vein	Use: Face Vein, Right Face Vein, Left
Common fibular nerve	Use: Peroneal Nerve
Common hepatic artery	Use: Hepatic Artery
Common iliac (subaortic) lymph node	Use: Lymphatic, Pelvis
Common interosseous artery	Use: Ulnar Artery, Right Ulnar Artery, Left
Common peroneal nerve	Use: Peroneal Nerve
Condyloid process	Use: Mandible, Right Mandible, Left
Conus arteriosus	Use: Ventricle, Right
Conus medullaris	Use: Lumbar Spinal Cord
Coracoacromial ligament	Use: Shoulder Bursa and Ligament, Right Shoulder Bursa and Ligament, Left
Coracobrachialis muscle	Use: Upper Arm Muscle, Right Upper Arm Muscle, Left
Coracoclavicular ligament Coracohumeral ligament	Use: Shoulder Bursa and Ligament, Right Shoulder Bursa and Ligament, Left
Coracoid process	Use: Scapula, Right Scapula, Left
Corniculate cartilage	Use: Larynx

Corpus callosum	Use: Brain
Corpus cavernosum Corpus spongiosum	Use: Penis
Corpus striatum	Use: Basal Ganglia
Corrugator supercilii muscle	Use: Facial Muscle
Costocervical trunk	Use: Subclavian Artery, Right Subclavian Artery, Left
Costoclavicular ligament	Use: Shoulder Bursa and Ligament, Right Shoulder Bursa and Ligament, Left
Costotransverse joint	Use: Thoracic Vertebral Joint Thoracic Vertebral Joints, 2 to 7 Thoracic Vertebral Joints, 8 or more
Costotransverse ligament	Use: Thorax Bursa and Ligament, Right Thorax Bursa and Ligament, Left
Costovertebral joint	Use: Thoracic Vertebral Joint Thoracic Vertebral Joints, 2 to 7 Thoracic Vertebral Joints, 8 or more
Costoxiphoid ligament	Use: Thorax Bursa and Ligament, Right Thorax Bursa and Ligament, Left
Cowper's (bulbourethral) gland	Use: Urethra
Cremaster muscle	Use: Perineum Muscle
Cribriform plate	Use: Ethmoid Bone, Right Ethmoid Bone, Left
Cricoid cartilage	Use: Trachea
Cricothyroid artery	Use: Thyroid Artery, Right Thyroid Artery, Left
Cricothyroid muscle	Use: Neck Muscle, Right Neck Muscle, Left

BODY PART KEY

Crural fascia	**Use:** Subcutaneous Tissue and Fascia, Right Upper Leg Subcutaneous Tissue and Fascia, Left Upper Leg
Cubital lymph node	**Use:** Lymphatic, Right Upper Extremity Lymphatic, Left Upper Extremity
Cubital nerve	**Use:** Ulnar Nerve
Cuboid bone	**Use:** Tarsal, Right Tarsal, Left
Cuboideonavicular joint	**Use:** Tarsal Joint, Right Tarsal Joint, Left
Culmen	**Use:** Cerebellum
Cuneiform cartilage	**Use:** Larynx
Cuneonavicular joint	**Use:** Tarsal Joint, Right Tarsal Joint, Left
Cuneonavicular ligament	**Use:** Foot Bursa and Ligament, Right Foot Bursa and Ligament, Left
Cutaneous (transverse) cervical nerve	**Use:** Cervical Plexus
Deep cervical fascia	**Use:** Subcutaneous Tissue and Fascia, Anterior Neck
Deep cervical vein	**Use:** Vertebral Vein, Right Vertebral Vein, Left
Deep circumflex iliac artery	**Use:** External Iliac Artery, Right External Iliac Artery, Left
Deep facial vein	**Use:** Face Vein, Right Face Vein, Left
Deep femoral (profunda femoris) vein	**Use:** Femoral Vein, Right Femoral Vein, Left
Deep femoral artery	**Use:** Femoral Artery, Right Femoral Artery, Left

Deep palmar arch	**Use:** Hand Artery, Right Hand Artery, Left
Deep transverse perineal muscle	**Use:** Perineum Muscle
Deferential artery	**Use:** Internal Iliac Artery, Right Internal Iliac Artery, Left
Deltoid fascia	**Use:** Subcutaneous Tissue and Fascia, Right Upper Arm Subcutaneous Tissue and Fascia, Left Upper Arm
Deltoid ligament	**Use:** Ankle Bursa and Ligament, Right Ankle Bursa and Ligament, Left
Deltoid muscle	**Use:** Shoulder Muscle, Right Shoulder Muscle, Left
Deltopectoral (infraclavicular) lymph node	**Use:** Lymphatic, Right Upper Extremity Lymphatic, Left Upper Extremity
Dentate ligament	**Use:** Dura Mater
Denticulate ligament	**Use:** Spinal Cord
Depressor anguli oris muscle Depressor labii inferioris muscle Depressor septi nasi muscle Depressor supercilii muscle	**Use:** Facial Muscle
Dermis	**Use:** Skin
Descending genicular artery	**Use:** Femoral Artery, Right Femoral Artery, Left
Diaphragma sellae	**Use:** Dura Mater
Distal humerus	**Use:** Humeral Shaft, Right Humeral Shaft, Left
Distal humerus, involving joint	**Use:** Elbow Joint, Right Elbow Joint, Left
Distal radioulnar joint	**Use:** Wrist Joint, Right Wrist Joint, Left
Dorsal digital nerve	**Use:** Radial Nerve

BODY PART KEY

Dorsal metacarpal vein	**Use:** Hand Vein, Right Hand Vein, Left
Dorsal metatarsal artery	**Use:** Foot Artery, Right Foot Artery, Left
Dorsal metatarsal vein	**Use:** Foot Vein, Right Foot Vein, Left
Dorsal scapular artery	**Use:** Subclavian Artery, Right Subclavian Artery, Left
Dorsal scapular nerve	**Use:** Brachial Plexus
Dorsal venous arch	**Use:** Foot Vein, Right Foot Vein, Left
Dorsalis pedis artery	**Use:** Anterior Tibial Artery, Right Anterior Tibial Artery, Left
Duct of Santorini	**Use:** Pancreatic Duct, Accessory
Duct of Wirsung	**Use:** Pancreatic Duct
Ductus deferens	**Use:** Vas Deferens, Right Vas Deferens, Left Vas Deferens, Bilateral Vas Deferens
Duodenal ampulla	**Use:** Ampulla of Vater
Duodenojejunal flexure	**Use:** Jejunum
Dura mater, intracranial	**Use:** Dura Mater
Dura mater, spinal	**Use:** Spinal Meninges
Dural venous sinus	**Use:** Intracranial Vein
Earlobe	**Use:** External Ear, Right External Ear, Left External Ear, Bilateral
Eighth cranial nerve	**Use:** Acoustic Nerve
Ejaculatory duct	**Use:** Vas Deferens, Right Vas Deferens, Left Vas Deferens, Bilateral Vas Deferens
Eleventh cranial nerve	**Use:** Accessory Nerve
Encephalon	**Use:** Brain
Ependyma	**Use:** Cerebral Ventricle
Epidermis	**Use:** Skin
Epidural space, intracranial	**Use:** Epidural Space
Epidural space, spinal	**Use:** Spinal Canal
Epiploic foramen	**Use:** Peritoneum
Epithalamus	**Use:** Thalamus
Epitrochlear lymph node	**Use:** Lymphatic, Right Upper Extremity Lymphatic, Left Upper Extremity
Erector spinae muscle	**Use:** Trunk Muscle, Right Trunk Muscle, Left
Esophageal artery	**Use:** Upper Artery
Esophageal plexus	**Use:** Thoracic Sympathetic Nerve
Ethmoidal air cell	**Use:** Ethmoid Sinus, Right Ethmoid Sinus, Left
Extensor carpi radialis muscle Extensor carpi ulnaris muscle	**Use:** Lower Arm and Wrist Muscle, Right Lower Arm and Wrist Muscle, Left
Extensor digitorum brevis muscle	**Use:** Foot Muscle, Right Foot Muscle, Left
Extensor digitorum longus muscle	**Use:** Lower Leg Muscle, Right Lower Leg Muscle, Left
Extensor hallucis brevis muscle	**Use:** Foot Muscle, Right Foot Muscle, Left

BODY PART KEY

Extensor hallucis longus muscle	**Use:** Lower Leg Muscle, Right Lower Leg Muscle, Left
External anal sphincter	**Use:** Anal Sphincter
External auditory meatus	**Use:** External Auditory Canal, Right External Auditory Canal, Left
External maxillary artery	**Use:** Face Artery
External naris	**Use:** Nose
External oblique aponeurosis	**Use:** Subcutaneous Tissue and Fascia, Trunk
External oblique muscle	**Use:** Abdomen Muscle, Right Abdomen Muscle, Left
External popliteal nerve	**Use:** Peroneal Nerve
External pudendal artery	**Use:** Femoral Artery, Right Femoral Artery, Left
External pudendal vein	**Use:** Greater Saphenous Vein, Right Greater Saphenous Vein, Left
External urethral sphincter	**Use:** Urethra
Extradural space, intracranial	**Use:** Epidural Space
Extradural space, spinal	**Use:** Spinal Canal
Facial artery	**Use:** Face Artery
False vocal cord	**Use:** Larynx
Falx cerebri	**Use:** Dura Mater
Fascia lata	**Use:** Subcutaneous Tissue and Fascia, Right Upper Leg Subcutaneous Tissue and Fascia, Left Upper Leg
Femoral head	**Use:** Upper Femur, Right Upper Femur, Left
Femoral lymph node	**Use:** Lymphatic, Right Lower Extremity Lymphatic, Left Lower Extremity
Femoropatellar joint Femorotibial joint	**Use:** Knee Joint, Right Knee Joint, Left
Fibular artery	**Use:** Peroneal Artery, Right Peroneal Artery, Left
Fibularis brevis muscle Fibularis longus muscle	**Use:** Lower Leg Muscle, Right Lower Leg Muscle, Left
Fifth cranial nerve	**Use:** Trigeminal Nerve
Filum terminale	**Use:** Spinal Meninges
First cranial nerve	**Use:** Olfactory Nerve
First intercostal nerve	**Use:** Brachial Plexus
Flexor carpi radialis muscle Flexor carpi ulnaris muscle	**Use:** Lower Arm and Wrist Muscle, Right Lower Arm and Wrist Muscle, Left
Flexor digitorum brevis muscle	**Use:** Foot Muscle, Right Foot Muscle, Left
Flexor digitorum longus muscle	**Use:** Lower Leg Muscle, Right Lower Leg Muscle, Left
Flexor hallucis brevis muscle	**Use:** Foot Muscle, Right Foot Muscle, Left
Flexor hallucis longus muscle	**Use:** Lower Leg Muscle, Right Lower Leg Muscle, Left
Flexor pollicis longus muscle	**Use:** Lower Arm and Wrist Muscle, Right Lower Arm and Wrist Muscle, Left
Foramen magnum	**Use:** Occipital Bone, Right Occipital Bone, Left
Foramen of Monro (intraventricular)	**Use:** Cerebral Ventricle
Foreskin	**Use:** Prepuce
Fossa of Rosenmuller	**Use:** Nasopharynx

APPENDIX B

BODY PART KEY

Fourth cranial nerve	**Use:** Trochlear Nerve
Fourth ventricle	**Use:** Cerebral Ventricle
Fovea	**Use:** Retina, Right / Retina, Left
Frenulum labii inferioris	**Use:** Lower Lip
Frenulum labii superioris	**Use:** Upper Lip
Frenulum linguae	**Use:** Tongue
Frontal lobe	**Use:** Cerebral Hemisphere
Frontal vein	**Use:** Face Vein, Right / Face Vein, Left
Fundus uteri	**Use:** Uterus
Galea aponeurotica	**Use:** Subcutaneous Tissue and Fascia, Scalp
Ganglion impar (ganglion of Walther)	**Use:** Sacral Sympathetic Nerve
Gasserian ganglion	**Use:** Trigeminal Nerve
Gastric lymph node	**Use:** Lymphatic, Aortic
Gastric plexus	**Use:** Abdominal Sympathetic Nerve
Gastrocnemius muscle	**Use:** Lower Leg Muscle, Right / Lower Leg Muscle, Left
Gastrocolic ligament / Gastrocolic omentum	**Use:** Greater Omentum
Gastroduodenal artery	**Use:** Hepatic Artery
Gastroesophageal (GE) junction	**Use:** Esophagogastric Junction
Gastrohepatic omentum	**Use:** Lesser Omentum
Gastrophrenic ligament / Gastrosplenic ligament	**Use:** Greater Omentum
Gemellus muscle	**Use:** Hip Muscle, Right / Hip Muscle, Left
Geniculate ganglion	**Use:** Facial Nerve
Geniculate nucleus	**Use:** Thalamus
Genioglossus muscle	**Use:** Tongue, Palate, Pharynx Muscle
Genitofemoral nerve	**Use:** Lumbar Plexus
Glans penis	**Use:** Prepuce
Glenohumeral joint	**Use:** Shoulder Joint, Right / Shoulder Joint, Left
Glenohumeral ligament	**Use:** Shoulder Bursa and Ligament, Right / Shoulder Bursa and Ligament, Left
Glenoid fossa (of scapula)	**Use:** Glenoid Cavity, Right / Glenoid Cavity, Left
Glenoid ligament (labrum)	**Use:** Shoulder Bursa and Ligament, Right / Shoulder Bursa and Ligament, Left
Globus pallidus	**Use:** Basal Ganglia
Glossoepiglottic fold	**Use:** Epiglottis
Glottis	**Use:** Larynx
Gluteal lymph node	**Use:** Lymphatic, Pelvis
Gluteal vein	**Use:** Hypogastric Vein, Right / Hypogastric Vein, Left
Gluteus maximus muscle / Gluteus medius muscle / Gluteus minimus muscle	**Use:** Hip Muscle, Right / Hip Muscle, Left
Gracilis muscle	**Use:** Upper Leg Muscle, Right / Upper Leg Muscle, Left

BODY PART KEY

Great auricular nerve	**Use:** Cervical Plexus
Great cerebral vein	**Use:** Intracranial Vein
Great saphenous vein	**Use:** Greater Saphenous Vein, Right Greater Saphenous Vein, Left
Greater alar cartilage	**Use:** Nose
Greater occipital nerve	**Use:** Cervical Nerve
Greater splanchnic nerve	**Use:** Thoracic Sympathetic Nerve
Greater superficial petrosal nerve	**Use:** Facial Nerve
Greater trochanter	**Use:** Upper Femur, Right Upper Femur, Left
Greater tuberosity	**Use:** Humeral Head, Right Humeral Head, Left
Greater vestibular (Bartholin's) gland	**Use:** Vestibular Gland
Greater wing	**Use:** Sphenoid Bone, Right Sphenoid Bone, Left
Hallux	**Use:** 1st Toe, Right 1st Toe, Left
Hamate bone	**Use:** Carpal, Right Carpal, Left
Head of fibula	**Use:** Fibula, Right Fibula, Left
Helix	**Use:** External Ear, Right External Ear, Left External Ear, Bilateral
Hepatic artery proper	**Use:** Hepatic Artery
Hepatic flexure	**Use:** Ascending Colon
Hepatic lymph node	**Use:** Lymphatic, Aortic
Hepatic plexus	**Use:** Abdominal Sympathetic Nerve
Hepatic portal vein	**Use:** Portal Vein
Hepatogastric ligament	**Use:** Lesser Omentum
Hepatopancreatic ampulla	**Use:** Ampulla of Vater
Humeroradial joint Humeroulnar joint	**Use:** Elbow Joint, Right Elbow Joint, Left
Humerus, distal	**Use:** Humeral Shaft, Right Humeral Shaft, Left
Hyoglossus muscle	**Use:** Tongue, Palate, Pharynx Muscle
Hyoid artery	**Use:** Thyroid Artery, Right Thyroid Artery, Left
Hypogastric artery	**Use:** Internal Iliac Artery, Right Internal Iliac Artery, Left
Hypopharynx	**Use:** Pharynx
Hypophysis	**Use:** Pituitary Gland
Hypothenar muscle	**Use:** Hand Muscle, Right Hand Muscle, Left
Ileal artery Ileocolic artery	**Use:** Superior Mesenteric Artery
Ileocolic vein	**Use:** Colic Vein
Iliac crest	**Use:** Pelvic Bone, Right Pelvic Bone, Left

Iliac fascia	**Use:**
	Subcutaneous Tissue and Fascia,
	  Right Upper Leg
	Subcutaneous Tissue and Fascia,
	  Left Upper Leg

BODY PART KEY

Iliac lymph node	**Use:** Lymphatic, Pelvis
Iliacus muscle	**Use:** Hip Muscle, Right Hip Muscle, Left
Iliofemoral ligament	**Use:** Hip Bursa and Ligament, Right Hip Bursa and Ligament, Left
Iliohypogastric nerve Ilioinguinal nerve	**Use:** Lumbar Plexus
Iliolumbar artery	**Use:** Internal Iliac Artery, Right Internal Iliac Artery, Left
Iliolumbar ligament	**Use:** Trunk Bursa and Ligament, Right Trunk Bursa and Ligament, Left

Iliotibial tract (band)	**Use:**
	Subcutaneous Tissue and Fascia,
	  Right Upper Leg
	Subcutaneous Tissue and Fascia,
	  Left Upper Leg

Ilium	**Use:** Pelvic Bone, Right Pelvic Bone, Left
Incus	**Use:** Auditory Ossicle, Right Auditory Ossicle, Left
Inferior cardiac nerve	**Use:** Thoracic Sympathetic Nerve
Inferior cerebellar vein Inferior cerebral vein	**Use:** Intracranial Vein
Inferior epigastric artery	**Use:** External Iliac Artery, Right External Iliac Artery, Left
Inferior epigastric lymph node	**Use:** Lymphatic, Pelvis
Inferior genicular artery	**Use:** Popliteal Artery, Right Popliteal Artery, Left
Inferior gluteal artery	**Use:** Internal Iliac Artery, Right Internal Iliac Artery, Left
Inferior gluteal nerve	**Use:** Sacral Plexus
Inferior hypogastric plexus	**Use:** Abdominal Sympathetic Nerve
Inferior labial artery	**Use:** Face Artery
Inferior longitudinal muscle	**Use:** Tongue, Palate, Pharynx Muscle
Inferior mesenteric ganglion	**Use:** Abdominal Sympathetic Nerve
Inferior mesenteric lymph node	**Use:** Lymphatic, Mesenteric
Inferior mesenteric plexus	**Use:** Abdominal Sympathetic Nerve
Inferior oblique muscle	**Use:** Extraocular Muscle, Right Extraocular Muscle, Left
Inferior pancreaticoduodenal artery	**Use:** Superior Mesenteric Artery
Inferior phrenic artery	**Use:** Abdominal Aorta
Inferior rectus muscle	**Use:** Extraocular Muscle, Right Extraocular Muscle, Left
Inferior suprarenal artery	**Use:** Renal Artery, Right Renal Artery, Left
Inferior tarsal plate	**Use:** Lower Eyelid, Right Lower Eyelid, Left
Inferior thyroid vein	**Use:** Innominate Vein, Right Innominate Vein, Left
Inferior tibiofibular joint	**Use:** Ankle Joint, Right Ankle Joint, Left
Inferior turbinate	**Use:** Nasal Turbinate
Inferior ulnar collateral artery	**Use:** Brachial Artery, Right Brachial Artery, Left
Inferior vesical artery	**Use:** Internal Iliac Artery, Right Internal Iliac Artery, Left

BODY PART KEY

Infraauricular lymph node	**Use:** Lymphatic, Head
Infraclavicular (deltopectoral) lymph node	**Use:** Lymphatic, Right Upper Extremity Lymphatic, Left Upper Extremity
Infrahyoid muscle	**Use:** Neck Muscle, Right Neck Muscle, Left
Infraparotid lymph node	**Use:** Lymphatic, Head
Infraspinatus fascia	**Use:** Subcutaneous Tissue and Fascia, Right Upper Arm Subcutaneous Tissue and Fascia, Left Upper Arm
Infraspinatus muscle	**Use:** Shoulder Muscle, Right Shoulder Muscle, Left
Infundibulopelvic ligament	**Use:** Uterine Supporting Structure
Inguinal canal Inguinal triangle	**Use:** Inguinal Region, Right Inguinal Region, Left Inguinal Region, Bilateral
Interatrial septum	**Use:** Atrial Septum
Intercarpal joint	**Use:** Carpal Joint, Right Carpal Joint, Left
Intercarpal ligament	**Use:** Hand Bursa and Ligament, Right Hand Bursa and Ligament, Left
Interclavicular ligament	**Use:** Shoulder Bursa and Ligament, Right Shoulder Bursa and Ligament, Left
Intercostal lymph node	**Use:** Lymphatic, Thorax
Intercostal muscle	**Use:** Thorax Muscle, Right Thorax Muscle, Left
Intercostal nerve Intercostobrachial nerve	**Use:** Thoracic Nerve
Intercuneiform joint	**Use:** Tarsal Joint, Right Tarsal Joint, Left

Intercuneiform ligament	**Use:** Foot Bursa and Ligament, Right Foot Bursa and Ligament, Left
Intermediate bronchus	**Use:** Main Bronchus, Right
Intermediate cuneiform bone	**Use:** Tarsal, Right Tarsal, Left
Internal (basal) cerebral vein	**Use:** Intracranial Vein
Internal anal sphincter	**Use:** Anal Sphincter
Internal carotid artery, intracranial portion	**Use:** Intracranial Artery
Internal carotid plexus	**Use:** Head and Neck Sympathetic Nerve
Internal iliac vein	**Use:** Hypogastric Vein, Right Hypogastric Vein, Left
Internal maxillary artery	**Use:** External Carotid Artery, Right External Carotid Artery, Left
Internal naris	**Use:** Nose
Internal oblique muscle	**Use:** Abdomen Muscle, Right Abdomen Muscle, Left
Internal pudendal artery	**Use:** Internal Iliac Artery, Right Internal Iliac Artery, Left
Internal pudendal vein	**Use:** Hypogastric Vein, Right Hypogastric Vein, Left
Internal thoracic artery	**Use:** Internal Mammary Artery, Right Internal Mammary Artery, Left Subclavian Artery, Right Subclavian Artery, Left
Internal urethral sphincter	**Use:** Urethra
Interphalangeal (IP) joint	**Use:** Finger Phalangeal Joint, Right Finger Phalangeal Joint, Left Toe Phalangeal Joint, Right Toe Phalangeal Joint, Left

BODY PART KEY

Interphalangeal ligament	**Use:** Hand Bursa and Ligament, Right Hand Bursa and Ligament, Left Foot Bursa and Ligament, Right Foot Bursa and Ligament, Left
Interspinalis muscle	**Use:** Trunk Muscle, Right Trunk Muscle, Left
Interspinous ligament	**Use:** Head and Neck Bursa and Ligament Trunk Bursa and Ligament, Right Trunk Bursa and Ligament, Left
Intertransversarius muscle	**Use:** Trunk Muscle, Right Trunk Muscle, Left
Intertransverse ligament	**Use:** Trunk Bursa and Ligament, Right Trunk Bursa and Ligament, Left
Interventricular foramen (Monro)	**Use:** Cerebral Ventricle
Interventricular septum	**Use:** Ventricular Septum
Intestinal lymphatic trunk	**Use:** Cisterna Chyli
Ischiatic nerve	**Use:** Sciatic Nerve
Ischiocavernosus muscle	**Use:** Perineum Muscle
Ischiofemoral ligament	**Use:** Hip Bursa and Ligament, Right Hip Bursa and Ligament, Left
Ischium	**Use:** Pelvic Bone, Right Pelvic Bone, Left
Jejunal artery	**Use:** Superior Mesenteric Artery
Jugular body	**Use:** Glomus Jugulare
Jugular lymph node	**Use:** Lymphatic, Right Neck Lymphatic, Left Neck
Labia majora Labia minora	**Use:** Vulva
Labial gland	**Use:** Upper Lip Lower Lip

Lacrimal canaliculus Lacrimal punctum Lacrimal sac	**Use:** Lacrimal Duct, Right Lacrimal Duct, Left
Laryngopharynx	**Use:** Pharynx
Lateral (brachial) lymph node	**Use:** Lymphatic, Right Axillary Lymphatic, Left Axillary
Lateral canthus	**Use:** Upper Eyelid, Right Upper Eyelid, Left
Lateral collateral ligament (LCL)	**Use:** Knee Bursa and Ligament, Right Knee Bursa and Ligament, Left
Lateral condyle of femur	**Use:** Lower Femur, Right Lower Femur, Left
Lateral condyle of tibia	**Use:** Tibia, Right Tibia, Left
Lateral cuneiform bone	**Use:** Tarsal, Right Tarsal, Left
Lateral epicondyle of femur	**Use:** Lower Femur, Right Lower Femur, Left
Lateral epicondyle of humerus	**Use:** Humeral Shaft, Right Humeral Shaft, Left
Lateral femoral cutaneous nerve	**Use:** Lumbar Plexus
Lateral malleolus	**Use:** Fibula, Right Fibula, Left
Lateral meniscus	**Use:** Knee Joint, Right Knee Joint, Left
Lateral nasal cartilage	**Use:** Nose
Lateral plantar artery	**Use:** Foot Artery, Right Foot Artery, Left
Lateral plantar nerve	**Use:** Tibial Nerve
Lateral rectus muscle	**Use:** Extraocular Muscle, Right Extraocular Muscle, Left

BODY PART KEY

Lateral sacral artery	**Use:** Internal Iliac Artery, Right Internal Iliac Artery, Left
Lateral sacral vein	**Use:** Hypogastric Vein, Right Hypogastric Vein, Left
Lateral sural cutaneous nerve	**Use:** Peroneal Nerve
Lateral tarsal artery	**Use:** Foot Artery, Right Foot Artery, Left
Lateral temporomandibular ligament	**Use:** Head and Neck Bursa and Ligament
Lateral thoracic artery	**Use:** Axillary Artery, Right Axillary Artery, Left
Latissimus dorsi muscle	**Use:** Trunk Muscle, Right Trunk Muscle, Left
Least splanchnic nerve	**Use:** Thoracic Sympathetic Nerve
Left ascending lumbar vein	**Use:** Hemiazygos Vein
Left atrioventricular valve	**Use:** Mitral Valve
Left auricular appendix	**Use:** Atrium, Left
Left colic vein	**Use:** Colic Vein
Left coronary sulcus	**Use:** Heart, Left
Left gastric artery	**Use:** Gastric Artery
Left gastroepiploic artery	**Use:** Splenic Artery
Left gastroepiploic vein	**Use:** Splenic Vein
Left inferior phrenic vein	**Use:** Renal Vein, Left
Left inferior pulmonary vein	**Use:** Pulmonary Vein, Left
Left jugular trunk	**Use:** Thoracic Duct

Left lateral ventricle	**Use:** Cerebral Ventricle
Left ovarian vein Left second lumbar vein	**Use:** Renal Vein, Left
Left subclavian trunk	**Use:** Thoracic Duct
Left subcostal vein	**Use:** Hemiazygos Vein
Left superior pulmonary vein	**Use:** Pulmonary Vein, Left
Left suprarenal vein Left testicular vein	**Use:** Renal Vein, Left
Leptomeninges, intracranial	**Use:** Cerebral Meninges
Leptomeninges, spinal	**Use:** Spinal Meninges
Lesser alar cartilage	**Use:** Nose
Lesser occipital nerve	**Use:** Cervical Plexus
Lesser splanchnic nerve	**Use:** Thoracic Sympathetic Nerve
Lesser trochanter	**Use:** Upper Femur, Right Upper Femur, Left
Lesser tuberosity	**Use:** Humeral Head, Right Humeral Head, Left
Lesser wing	**Use:** Sphenoid Bone, Right Sphenoid Bone, Left
Levator anguli oris muscle	**Use:** Facial Muscle
Levator ani muscle	**Use:** Perineum Muscle
Levator labii superioris alaeque nasi muscle Levator labii superioris muscle	**Use:** Facial Muscle
Levator palpebrae superioris muscle	**Use:** Upper Eyelid, Right Upper Eyelid, Left
Levator scapulae muscle	**Use:** Neck Muscle, Right Neck Muscle, Left

BODY PART KEY

Levator veli palatini muscle	**Use:** Tongue, Palate, Pharynx Muscle
Levatores costarum muscle	**Use:** Thorax Muscle, Right Thorax Muscle, Left
Ligament of head of fibula	**Use:** Knee Bursa and Ligament, Right Knee Bursa and Ligament, Left
Ligament of the lateral malleolus	**Use:** Ankle Bursa and Ligament, Right Ankle Bursa and Ligament, Left
Ligamentum flavum	**Use:** Trunk Bursa and Ligament, Right Trunk Bursa and Ligament, Left
Lingual artery	**Use:** External Carotid Artery, Right External Carotid Artery, Left
Lingual tonsil	**Use:** Tongue
Locus ceruleus	**Use:** Pons
Long thoracic nerve	**Use:** Brachial Plexus
Lumbar artery	**Use:** Abdominal Aorta
Lumbar facet joint	**Use:** Lumbar Vertebral Joint Lumbar Vertebral Joints, 2 or more
Lumbar ganglion	**Use:** Lumbar Sympathetic Nerve
Lumbar lymph node	**Use:** Lymphatic, Aortic
Lumbar lymphatic trunk	**Use:** Cisterna Chyli
Lumbar splanchnic nerve	**Use:** Lumbar Sympathetic Nerve
Lumbosacral facet joint	**Use:** Lumbosacral Joint
Lumbosacral trunk	**Use:** Lumbar Nerve
Lunate bone	**Use:** Carpal, Right Carpal, Left
Lunotriquetral ligament	**Use:** Hand Bursa and Ligament, Right Hand Bursa and Ligament, Left

Macula	**Use:** Retina, Right Retina, Left
Malleus	**Use:** Auditory Ossicle, Right Auditory Ossicle, Left
Mammary duct Mammary gland	**Use:** Breast, Right Breast, Left Breast, Bilateral
Mammillary body	**Use:** Hypothalamus
Mandibular nerve	**Use:** Trigeminal Nerve
Mandibular notch	**Use:** Mandible, Right Mandible, Left
Manubrium	**Use:** Sternum
Masseter muscle	**Use:** Head Muscle
Masseteric fascia	**Use:** Subcutaneous Tissue and Fascia, Face
Mastoid (postauricular) lymph node	**Use:** Lymphatic, Right Neck Lymphatic, Left Neck
Mastoid air cells	**Use:** Mastoid Sinus, Right Mastoid Sinus, Left
Mastoid process	**Use:** Temporal Bone, Right Temporal Bone, Left
Maxillary artery	**Use:** External Carotid Artery, Right External Carotid Artery, Left
Maxillary nerve	**Use:** Trigeminal Nerve
Medial canthus	**Use:** Lower Eyelid, Right Lower Eyelid, Left
Medial collateral ligament (MCL)	**Use:** Knee Bursa and Ligament, Right Knee Bursa and Ligament, Left
Medial condyle of femur	**Use:** Lower Femur, Right Lower Femur, Left

BODY PART KEY

Medial condyle of tibia	**Use:** Tibia, Right Tibia, Left
Medial cuneiform bone	**Use:** Tarsal, Right Tarsal, Left
Medial epicondyle of femur	**Use:** Lower Femur, Right Lower Femur, Left
Medial epicondyle of humerus	**Use:** Humeral Shaft, Right Humeral Shaft, Left
Medial malleolus	**Use:** Tibia, Right Tibia, Left
Medial meniscus	**Use:** Knee Joint, Right Knee Joint, Left
Medial plantar artery	**Use:** Foot Artery, Right Foot Artery, Left
Medial plantar nerve Medial popliteal nerve	**Use:** Tibial Nerve
Medial rectus muscle	**Use:** Extraocular Muscle, Right Extraocular Muscle, Left
Medial sural cutaneous nerve	**Use:** Tibial Nerve
Median antebrachial vein Median cubital vein	**Use:** Basilic Vein, Right Basilic Vein, Left
Median sacral artery	**Use:** Abdominal Aorta
Mediastinal lymph node	**Use:** Lymphatic, Thorax
Meissner's (submucous) plexus	**Use:** Abdominal Sympathetic Nerve
Membranous urethra	**Use:** Urethra
Mental foramen	**Use:** Mandible, Right Mandible, Left
Mentalis muscle	**Use:** Facial Muscle
Mesoappendix Mesocolon	**Use:** Mesentery

Metacarpal ligament Metacarpophalangeal ligament	**Use:** Hand Bursa and Ligament, Right Hand Bursa and Ligament, Left
Metatarsal ligament	**Use:** Foot Bursa and Ligament, Right Foot Bursa and Ligament, Left
Metatarsophalangeal (MTP) joint	**Use:** Metatarsal-Phalangeal Joint, Right Metatarsal-Phalangeal Joint, Left
Metatarsophalangeal ligament	**Use:** Foot Bursa and Ligament, Right Foot Bursa and Ligament, Left
Metathalamus	**Use:** Thalamus
Midcarpal joint	**Use:** Carpal Joint, Right Carpal Joint, Left
Middle cardiac nerve	**Use:** Thoracic Sympathetic Nerve
Middle cerebral artery	**Use:** Intracranial Artery
Middle cerebral vein	**Use:** Intracranial Vein
Middle colic vein	**Use:** Colic Vein
Middle genicular artery	**Use:** Popliteal Artery, Right Popliteal Artery, Left
Middle hemorrhoidal vein	**Use:** Hypogastric Vein, Right Hypogastric Vein, Left
Middle rectal artery	**Use:** Internal Iliac Artery, Right Internal Iliac Artery, Left
Middle suprarenal artery	**Use:** Abdominal Aorta
Middle temporal artery	**Use:** Temporal Artery, Right Temporal Artery, Left
Middle turbinate	**Use:** Nasal Turbinate
Mitral annulus	**Use:** Mitral Valve
Molar gland	**Use:** Buccal Mucosa
Musculocutaneous nerve	**Use:** Brachial Plexus

BODY PART KEY

Musculophrenic artery	**Use:** Internal Mammary Artery, Right Internal Mammary Artery, Left
Musculospiral nerve	**Use:** Radial Nerve
Myelencephalon	**Use:** Medulla Oblongata
Myenteric (Auerbach's) plexus	**Use:** Abdominal Sympathetic Nerve
Myometrium	**Use:** Uterus
Nail bed Nail plate	**Use:** Finger Nail Toe Nail
Nasal cavity	**Use:** Nose
Nasal concha	**Use:** Nasal Turbinate
Nasalis muscle	**Use:** Facial Muscle
Nasolacrimal duct	**Use:** Lacrimal Duct, Right Lacrimal Duct, Left
Navicular bone	**Use:** Tarsal, Right Tarsal, Left
Neck of femur	**Use:** Upper Femur, Right Upper Femur, Left
Neck of humerus (anatomical) (surgical)	**Use:** Humeral Head, Right Humeral Head, Left
Nerve to the stapedius	**Use:** Facial Nerve
Neurohypophysis	**Use:** Pituitary Gland
Ninth cranial nerve	**Use:** Glossopharyngeal Nerve
Nostril	**Use:** Nose
Obturator artery	**Use:** Internal Iliac Artery, Right Internal Iliac Artery, Left
Obturator lymph node	**Use:** Lymphatic, Pelvis
Obturator muscle	**Use:** Hip Muscle, Right Hip Muscle, Left
Obturator nerve	**Use:** Lumbar Plexus
Obturator vein	**Use:** Hypogastric Vein, Right Hypogastric Vein, Left
Obtuse margin	**Use:** Heart, Left
Occipital artery	**Use:** External Carotid Artery, Right External Carotid Artery, Left
Occipital lobe	**Use:** Cerebral Hemisphere
Occipital lymph node	**Use:** Lymphatic, Right Neck Lymphatic, Left Neck
Occipitofrontalis muscle	**Use:** Facial Muscle
Olecranon bursa	**Use:** Elbow Bursa and Ligament, Right Elbow Bursa and Ligament, Left
Olecranon process	**Use:** Ulna, Right Ulna, Left
Olfactory bulb	**Use:** Olfactory Nerve
Ophthalmic artery	**Use:** Intracranial Artery
Ophthalmic nerve	**Use:** Trigeminal Nerve
Ophthalmic vein	**Use:** Intracranial Vein
Optic chiasma	**Use:** Optic Nerve
Optic disc	**Use:** Retina, Right Retina, Left
Optic foramen	**Use:** Sphenoid Bone, Right Sphenoid Bone, Left
Orbicularis oculi muscle	**Use:** Upper Eyelid, Right Upper Eyelid, Left

BODY PART KEY

Orbicularis oris muscle	**Use:** Facial Muscle
Orbital fascia	**Use:** Subcutaneous Tissue and Fascia, Face
Orbital portion of ethmoid bone Orbital portion of frontal bone Orbital portion of lacrimal bone Orbital portion of maxilla Orbital portion of palatine bone Orbital portion of sphenoid bone Orbital portion of zygomatic bone	**Use:** Orbit, Right Orbit, Left
Oropharynx	**Use:** Pharynx
Otic ganglion	**Use:** Head and Neck Sympathetic Nerve
Oval window	**Use:** Middle Ear, Right Middle Ear, Left
Ovarian artery	**Use:** Abdominal Aorta
Ovarian ligament	**Use:** Uterine Supporting Structure
Oviduct	**Use:** Fallopian Tube, Right Fallopian Tube, Left
Palatine gland	**Use:** Buccal Mucosa
Palatine tonsil	**Use:** Tonsils
Palatine uvula	**Use:** Uvula
Palatoglossal muscle Palatopharyngeal muscle	**Use:** Tongue, Palate, Pharynx Muscle
Palmar (volar) digital vein Palmar (volar) metacarpal vein	**Use:** Hand Vein, Right Hand Vein, Left
Palmar cutaneous nerve	**Use:** Median Nerve Radial Nerve
Palmar fascia (aponeurosis)	**Use:** Subcutaneous Tissue and Fascia, Right Hand Subcutaneous Tissue and Fascia, Left Hand

Palmar interosseous muscle	**Use:** Hand Muscle, Right Hand Muscle, Left
Palmar ulnocarpal ligament	**Use:** Wrist Bursa and Ligament, Right Wrist Bursa and Ligament, Left
Palmaris longus muscle	**Use:** Lower Arm and Wrist Muscle, Right Lower Arm and Wrist Muscle, Left
Pancreatic artery	**Use:** Splenic Artery
Pancreatic plexus	**Use:** Abdominal Sympathetic Nerve
Pancreatic vein	**Use:** Splenic Vein
Pancreaticosplenic lymph node Paraaortic lymph node	**Use:** Lymphatic, Aortic
Pararectal lymph node	**Use:** Lymphatic, Mesenteric
Parasternal lymph node Paratracheal lymph node	**Use:** Lymphatic, Thorax
Paraurethral (Skene's) gland	**Use:** Vestibular Gland
Parietal lobe	**Use:** Cerebral Hemisphere
Parotid lymph node	**Use:** Lymphatic, Head
Parotid plexus	**Use:** Facial Nerve
Pars flaccida	**Use:** Tympanic Membrane, Right Tympanic Membrane, Left
Patellar ligament	**Use:** Knee Bursa and Ligament, Right Knee Bursa and Ligament, Left
Patellar tendon	**Use:** Knee Tendon, Right Knee Tendon, Left
Pectineus muscle	**Use:** Upper Leg Muscle, Right Upper Leg Muscle, Left
Pectoral (anterior) lymph node	**Use:** Lymphatic, Right Axillary Lymphatic, Left Axillary
Pectoral fascia	**Use:** Subcutaneous Tissue and Fascia, Chest

855

BODY PART KEY

Pectoralis major muscle Pectoralis minor muscle	**Use:** Thorax Muscle, Right Thorax Muscle, Left
Pelvic splanchnic nerve	**Use:** Abdominal Sympathetic Nerve Sacral Sympathetic Nerve
Penile urethra	**Use:** Urethra
Pericardiophrenic artery	**Use:** Internal Mammary Artery, Right Internal Mammary Artery, Left
Perimetrium	**Use:** Uterus
Peroneus brevis muscle Peroneus longus muscle	**Use:** Lower Leg Muscle, Right Lower Leg Muscle, Left
Petrous part of temporal bone	**Use:** Temporal Bone, Right Temporal Bone, Left
Pharyngeal constrictor muscle	**Use:** Tongue, Palate, Pharynx Muscle
Pharyngeal plexus	**Use:** Vagus Nerve
Pharyngeal recess	**Use:** Nasopharynx
Pharyngeal tonsil	**Use:** Adenoids
Pharyngotympanic tube	**Use:** Eustachian Tube, Right Eustachian Tube, Left
Pia mater, intracranial	**Use:** Cerebral Meninges
Pia mater, spinal	**Use:** Spinal Meninges
Pinna	**Use:** External Ear, Right External Ear, Left External Ear, Bilateral
Piriform recess (sinus)	**Use:** Pharynx
Piriformis muscle	**Use:** Hip Muscle, Right Hip Muscle, Left
Pisiform bone	**Use:** Carpal, Right Carpal, Left
Pisohamate ligament Pisometacarpal ligament	**Use:** Hand Bursa and Ligament, Right Hand Bursa and Ligament, Left
Plantar digital vein	**Use:** Foot Vein, Right Foot Vein, Left
Plantar fascia (aponeurosis)	**Use:** Subcutaneous Tissue and Fascia, Right Foot Subcutaneous Tissue and Fascia, Left Foot
Plantar metatarsal vein Plantar venous arch	**Use:** Foot Vein, Right Foot Vein, Left
Platysma muscle	**Use:** Neck Muscle, Right Neck Muscle, Left
Plica semilunaris	**Use:** Conjunctiva, Right Conjunctiva, Left
Pneumogastric nerve	**Use:** Vagus Nerve
Pneumotaxic center Pontine tegmentum	**Use:** Pons
Popliteal ligament	**Use:** Knee Bursa and Ligament, Right Knee Bursa and Ligament, Left
Popliteal lymph node	**Use:** Lymphatic, Right Lower Extremity Lymphatic, Left Lower Extremity
Popliteal vein	**Use:** Femoral Vein, Right Femoral Vein, Left
Popliteus muscle	**Use:** Lower Leg Muscle, Right Lower Leg Muscle, Left
Postauricular (mastoid) lymph node	**Use:** Lymphatic, Right Neck Lymphatic, Left Neck
Postcava	**Use:** Inferior Vena Cava
Posterior (subscapular) lymph node	**Use:** Lymphatic, Right Axillary Lymphatic, Left Axillary
Posterior auricular artery	**Use:** External Carotid Artery, Right External Carotid Artery, Left

BODY PART KEY

Posterior auricular nerve	**Use:** Facial Nerve
Posterior auricular vein	**Use:** External Jugular Vein, Right External Jugular Vein, Left
Posterior cerebral artery	**Use:** Intracranial Artery
Posterior chamber	**Use:** Eye, Right Eye, Left
Posterior circumflex humeral artery	**Use:** Axillary Artery, Right Axillary Artery, Left
Posterior communicating artery	**Use:** Intracranial Artery
Posterior cruciate ligament (PCL)	**Use:** Knee Bursa and Ligament, Right Knee Bursa and Ligament, Left
Posterior facial (retromandibular) vein	**Use:** Face Vein, Right Face Vein, Left
Posterior femoral cutaneous nerve	**Use:** Sacral Plexus
Posterior inferior cerebellar artery (PICA)	**Use:** Intracranial Artery
Posterior interosseous nerve	**Use:** Radial Nerve
Posterior labial nerve Posterior scrotal nerve	**Use:** Pudendal Nerve
Posterior spinal artery	**Use:** Vertebral Artery, Right Vertebral Artery, Left
Posterior tibial recurrent artery	**Use:** Anterior Tibial Artery, Right Anterior Tibial Artery, Left
Posterior ulnar recurrent artery	**Use:** Ulnar Artery, Right Ulnar Artery, Left
Posterior vagal trunk	**Use:** Vagus Nerve
Preauricular lymph node	**Use:** Lymphatic, Head
Precava	**Use:** Superior Vena Cava

Prepatellar bursa	**Use:** Knee Bursa and Ligament, Right Knee Bursa and Ligament, Left
Pretracheal fascia	**Use:** Subcutaneous Tissue and Fascia, Anterior Neck
Prevertebral fascia	**Use:** Subcutaneous Tissue and Fascia, Posterior Neck
Princeps pollicis artery	**Use:** Hand Artery, Right Hand Artery, Left
Procerus muscle	**Use:** Facial Muscle
Profunda brachii	**Use:** Brachial Artery, Right Brachial Artery, Left
Profunda femoris (deep femoral) vein	**Use:** Femoral Vein, Right Femoral Vein, Left
Pronator quadratus muscle Pronator teres muscle	**Use:** Lower Arm and Wrist Muscle, Right Lower Arm and Wrist Muscle, Left
Prostatic urethra	**Use:** Urethra
Proximal radioulnar joint	**Use:** Elbow Joint, Right Elbow Joint, Left
Psoas muscle	**Use:** Hip Muscle, Right Hip Muscle, Left
Pterygoid muscle	**Use:** Head Muscle
Pterygoid process	**Use:** Sphenoid Bone, Right Sphenoid Bone, Left
Pterygopalatine (sphenopalatine) ganglion	**Use:** Head and Neck Sympathetic Nerve
Pubic ligament	**Use:** Trunk Bursa and Ligament, Right Trunk Bursa and Ligament, Left
Pubis	**Use:** Pelvic Bone, Right Pelvic Bone, Left
Pubofemoral ligament	**Use:** Hip Bursa and Ligament, Right Hip Bursa and Ligament, Left

BODY PART KEY

Pudendal nerve	**Use:** Sacral Plexus
Pulmoaortic canal	**Use:** Pulmonary Artery, Left
Pulmonary annulus	**Use:** Pulmonary Valve
Pulmonary plexus	**Use:** Vagus Nerve Thoracic Sympathetic Nerve
Pulmonic valve	**Use:** Pulmonary Valve
Pulvinar	**Use:** Thalamus
Pyloric antrum Pyloric canal Pyloric sphincter	**Use:** Stomach, Pylorus
Pyramidalis muscle	**Use:** Abdomen Muscle, Right Abdomen Muscle, Left
Quadrangular cartilage	**Use:** Nasal Septum
Quadrate lobe	**Use:** Liver
Quadratus femoris muscle	**Use:** Hip Muscle, Right Hip Muscle, Left
Quadratus lumborum muscle	**Use:** Trunk Muscle, Right Trunk Muscle, Left
Quadratus plantae muscle	**Use:** Foot Muscle, Right Foot Muscle, Left
Quadriceps (femoris)	**Use:** Upper Leg Muscle, Right Upper Leg Muscle, Left
Radial collateral carpal ligament	**Use:** Wrist Bursa and Ligament, Right Wrist Bursa and Ligament, Left
Radial collateral ligament	**Use:** Elbow Bursa and Ligament, Right Elbow Bursa and Ligament, Left
Radial notch	**Use:** Ulna, Right Ulna, Left
Radial recurrent artery	**Use:** Radial Artery, Right Radial Artery, Left

Radial vein	**Use:** Brachial Vein, Right Brachial Vein, Left
Radialis indicis	**Use:** Hand Artery, Right Hand Artery, Left
Radiocarpal joint	**Use:** Wrist Joint, Right Wrist Joint, Left
Radiocarpal ligament Radioulnar ligament	**Use:** Wrist Bursa and Ligament, Right Wrist Bursa and Ligament, Left
Rectosigmoid junction	**Use:** Sigmoid Colon
Rectus abdominis muscle	**Use:** Abdomen Muscle, Right Abdomen Muscle, Left
Rectus femoris muscle	**Use:** Upper Leg Muscle, Right Upper Leg Muscle, Left
Recurrent laryngeal nerve	**Use:** Vagus Nerve
Renal calyx Renal capsule Renal cortex	**Use:** Kidney, Right Kidney, Left Kidneys, Bilateral Kidney
Renal plexus	**Use:** Abdominal Sympathetic Nerve
Renal segment	**Use:** Kidney, Right Kidney, Left Kidneys, Bilateral Kidney
Renal segmental artery	**Use:** Renal Artery, Right Renal Artery, Left
Retroperitoneal lymph node	**Use:** Lymphatic, Aortic
Retroperitoneal space	**Use:** Retroperitoneum
Retropharyngeal lymph node	**Use:** Lymphatic, Right Neck Lymphatic, Left Neck
Retropubic space	**Use:** Pelvic Cavity
Rhinopharynx	**Use:** Nasopharynx

BODY PART KEY

Rhomboid major muscle Rhomboid minor muscle	**Use:** Trunk Muscle, Right Trunk Muscle, Left
Right ascending lumbar vein	**Use:** Azygos Vein
Right atrioventricular valve	**Use:** Tricuspid Valve
Right auricular appendix	**Use:** Atrium, Right
Right colic vein	**Use:** Colic Vein
Right coronary sulcus	**Use:** Heart, Right
Right gastric artery	**Use:** Gastric Artery
Right gastroepiploic vein	**Use:** Superior Mesenteric Vein
Right inferior phrenic vein	**Use:** Inferior Vena Cava
Right inferior pulmonary vein	**Use:** Pulmonary Vein, Right
Right jugular trunk	**Use:** Lymphatic, Right Neck
Right lateral ventricle	**Use:** Cerebral Ventricle
Right lymphatic duct	**Use:** Lymphatic, Right Neck
Right ovarian vein Right second lumbar vein	**Use:** Inferior Vena Cava
Right subclavian trunk	**Use:** Lymphatic, Right Neck
Right subcostal vein	**Use:** Azygos Vein
Right superior pulmonary vein	**Use:** Pulmonary Vein, Right
Right suprarenal vein Right testicular vein	**Use:** Inferior Vena Cava
Rima glottidis	**Use:** Larynx
Risorius muscle	**Use:** Facial Muscle
Round ligament of uterus	**Use:** Uterine Supporting Structure
Round window	**Use:** Inner Ear, Right Inner Ear, Left
Sacral ganglion	**Use:** Sacral Sympathetic Nerve
Sacral lymph node	**Use:** Lymphatic, Pelvis
Sacral splanchnic nerve	**Use:** Sacral Sympathetic Nerve
Sacrococcygeal ligament	**Use:** Trunk Bursa and Ligament, Right Trunk Bursa and Ligament, Left
Sacrococcygeal symphysis	**Use:** Sacrococcygeal Joint
Sacroiliac ligament Sacrospinous ligament Sacrotuberous ligament	**Use:** Trunk Bursa and Ligament, Right Trunk Bursa and Ligament, Left
Salpingopharyngeus muscle	**Use:** Tongue, Palate, Pharynx Muscle
Salpinx	**Use:** Fallopian Tube, Right Fallopian Tube, Left
Saphenous nerve	**Use:** Femoral Nerve
Sartorius muscle	**Use:** Upper Leg Muscle, Right Upper Leg Muscle, Left
Scalene muscle	**Use:** Neck Muscle, Right Neck Muscle, Left
Scaphoid bone	**Use:** Carpal, Right Carpal, Left
Scapholunate ligament Scaphotrapezium ligament	**Use:** Hand Bursa and Ligament, Right Hand Bursa and Ligament, Left
Scarpa's (vestibular) ganglion	**Use:** Acoustic Nerve
Sebaceous gland	**Use:** Skin
Second cranial nerve	**Use:** Optic Nerve
Sella turcica	**Use:** Sphenoid Bone, Right Sphenoid Bone, Left

BODY PART KEY

Semicircular canal	**Use:** Inner Ear, Right Inner Ear, Left
Semimembranosus muscle Semitendinosus muscle	**Use:** Upper Leg Muscle, Right Upper Leg Muscle, Left
Septal cartilage	**Use:** Nasal Septum
Serratus anterior muscle	**Use:** Thorax Muscle, Right Thorax Muscle, Left
Serratus posterior muscle	**Use:** Trunk Muscle, Right Trunk Muscle, Left
Seventh cranial nerve	**Use:** Facial Nerve
Short gastric artery	**Use:** Splenic Artery
Sigmoid artery	**Use:** Inferior Mesenteric Artery
Sigmoid flexure	**Use:** Sigmoid Colon
Sigmoid vein	**Use:** Inferior Mesenteric Vein
Sinoatrial node	**Use:** Conduction Mechanism
Sinus venosus	**Use:** Atrium, Right
Sixth cranial nerve	**Use:** Abducens Nerve
Skene's (paraurethral) gland	**Use:** Vestibular Gland
Small saphenous vein	**Use:** Lesser Saphenous Vein, Right Lesser Saphenous Vein, Left
Solar (celiac) plexus	**Use:** Abdominal Sympathetic Nerve
Soleus muscle	**Use:** Lower Leg Muscle, Right Lower Leg Muscle, Left
Sphenomandibular ligament	**Use:** Head and Neck Bursa and Ligament
Sphenopalatine (pterygopalatine) ganglion	**Use:** Head and Neck Sympathetic Nerve

Spinal nerve, cervical	**Use:** Cervical Nerve
Spinal nerve, lumbar	**Use:** Lumbar Nerve
Spinal nerve, sacral	**Use:** Sacral Nerve
Spinal nerve, thoracic	**Use:** Thoracic Nerve
Spinous process	**Use:** Cervical Vertebra Thoracic Vertebra Lumbar Vertebra
Spiral ganglion	**Use:** Acoustic Nerve
Splenic flexure	**Use:** Transverse Colon
Splenic plexus	**Use:** Abdominal Sympathetic Nerve
Splenius capitis muscle	**Use:** Head Muscle
Splenius cervicis muscle	**Use:** Neck Muscle, Right Neck Muscle, Left
Stapes	**Use:** Auditory Ossicle, Right Auditory Ossicle, Left
Stellate ganglion	**Use:** Head and Neck Sympathetic Nerve
Stensen's duct	**Use:** Parotid Duct, Right Parotid Duct, Left
Sternoclavicular ligament	**Use:** Shoulder Bursa and Ligament, Right Shoulder Bursa and Ligament, Left
Sternocleidomastoid artery	**Use:** Thyroid Artery, Right Thyroid Artery, Left
Sternocleidomastoid muscle	**Use:** Neck Muscle, Right Neck Muscle, Left
Sternocostal ligament	**Use:** Thorax Bursa and Ligament, Right Thorax Bursa and Ligament, Left
Styloglossus muscle	**Use:** Tongue, Palate, Pharynx Muscle

BODY PART KEY

Stylomandibular ligament	**Use:** Head and Neck Bursa and Ligament
Stylopharyngeus muscle	**Use:** Tongue, Palate, Pharynx Muscle
Subacromial bursa	**Use:** Shoulder Bursa and Ligament, Right Shoulder Bursa and Ligament, Left
Subaortic (common iliac) lymph node	**Use:** Lymphatic, Pelvis
Subarachnoid space, intracranial	**Use:** Subarachnoid Space
Subarachnoid space, spinal	**Use:** Spinal Canal
Subclavicular (apical) lymph node	**Use:** Lymphatic, Right Axillary Lymphatic, Left Axillary
Subclavius muscle	**Use:** Thorax Muscle, Right Thorax Muscle, Left
Subclavius nerve	**Use:** Brachial Plexus
Subcostal artery	**Use:** Upper Artery
Subcostal muscle	**Use:** Thorax Muscle, Right Thorax Muscle, Left
Subcostal nerve	**Use:** Thoracic Nerve
Subdural space, intracranial	**Use:** Subdural Space
Subdural space, spinal	**Use:** Spinal Canal
Submandibular ganglion	**Use:** Facial Nerve Head and Neck Sympathetic Nerve
Submandibular gland	**Use:** Submaxillary Gland, Right Submaxillary Gland, Left
Submandibular lymph node	**Use:** Lymphatic, Head
Submaxillary ganglion	**Use:** Head and Neck Sympathetic Nerve
Submaxillary lymph node	**Use:** Lymphatic, Head

Submental artery	**Use:** Face Artery
Submental lymph node	**Use:** Lymphatic, Head
Submucous (Meissner's) plexus	**Use:** Abdominal Sympathetic Nerve
Suboccipital nerve	**Use:** Cervical Nerve
Suboccipital venous plexus	**Use:** Vertebral Vein, Right Vertebral Vein, Left
Subparotid lymph node	**Use:** Lymphatic, Head
Subscapular (posterior) lymph node	**Use:** Lymphatic, Right Axillary Lymphatic, Left Axillary
Subscapular aponeurosis	**Use:** Subcutaneous Tissue and Fascia, Right Upper Arm Subcutaneous Tissue and Fascia, Left Upper Arm
Subscapular artery	**Use:** Axillary Artery, Right Axillary Artery, Left
Subscapularis muscle	**Use:** Shoulder Muscle, Right Shoulder Muscle, Left
Substantia nigra	**Use:** Basal Ganglia
Subtalar (talocalcaneal) joint	**Use:** Tarsal Joint, Right Tarsal Joint, Left
Subtalar ligament	**Use:** Foot Bursa and Ligament, Right Foot Bursa and Ligament, Left
Subthalamic nucleus	**Use:** Basal Ganglia
Superficial circumflex iliac vein	**Use:** Greater Saphenous Vein, Right Greater Saphenous Vein, Left
Superficial epigastric artery	**Use:** Femoral Artery, Right Femoral Artery, Left
Superficial epigastric vein	**Use:** Greater Saphenous Vein, Right Greater Saphenous Vein, Left

BODY PART KEY

Superficial palmar arch	**Use:** Hand Artery, Right Hand Artery, Left
Superficial palmar venous arch	**Use:** Hand Vein, Right Hand Vein, Left
Superficial temporal artery	**Use:** Temporal Artery, Right Temporal Artery, Left
Superficial transverse perineal muscle	**Use:** Perineum Muscle
Superior cardiac nerve	**Use:** Thoracic Sympathetic Nerve
Superior cerebellar vein Superior cerebral vein	**Use:** Intracranial Vein
Superior clunic (cluneal) nerve	**Use:** Lumbar Nerve
Superior epigastric artery	**Use:** Internal Mammary Artery, Right Internal Mammary Artery, Left
Superior genicular artery	**Use:** Popliteal Artery, Right Popliteal Artery, Left
Superior gluteal artery	**Use:** Internal Iliac Artery, Right Internal Iliac Artery, Left
Superior gluteal nerve	**Use:** Lumbar Plexus
Superior hypogastric plexus	**Use:** Abdominal Sympathetic Nerve
Superior labial artery	**Use:** Face Artery
Superior laryngeal artery	**Use:** Thyroid Artery, Right Thyroid Artery, Left
Superior laryngeal nerve	**Use:** Vagus Nerve
Superior longitudinal muscle	**Use:** Tongue, Palate, Pharynx Muscle
Superior mesenteric ganglion	**Use:** Abdominal Sympathetic Nerve
Superior mesenteric lymph node	**Use:** Lymphatic, Mesenteric
Superior mesenteric plexus	**Use:** Abdominal Sympathetic Nerve

Superior oblique muscle	**Use:** Extraocular Muscle, Right Extraocular Muscle, Left
Superior olivary nucleus	**Use:** Pons
Superior rectal artery	**Use:** Inferior Mesenteric Artery
Superior rectal vein	**Use:** Inferior Mesenteric Vein
Superior rectus muscle	**Use:** Extraocular Muscle, Right Extraocular Muscle, Left
Superior tarsal plate	**Use:** Upper Eyelid, Right Upper Eyelid, Left
Superior thoracic artery	**Use:** Axillary Artery, Right Axillary Artery, Left
Superior thyroid artery	**Use:** External Carotid Artery, Right External Carotid Artery, Left Thyroid Artery, Right Thyroid Artery, Left
Superior turbinate	**Use:** Nasal Turbinate
Superior ulnar collateral artery	**Use:** Brachial Artery, Right Brachial Artery, Left
Supraclavicular (Virchow's) lymph node	**Use:** Lymphatic, Right Neck Lymphatic, Left Neck
Supraclavicular nerve	**Use:** Cervical Plexus
Suprahyoid lymph node	**Use:** Lymphatic, Head
Suprahyoid muscle	**Use:** Neck Muscle, Right Neck Muscle, Left
Suprainguinal lymph node	**Use:** Lymphatic, Pelvis
Supraorbital vein	**Use:** Face Vein, Right Face Vein, Left
Suprarenal gland	**Use:** Adrenal Gland, Left Adrenal Gland, Right Adrenal Glands, Bilateral Adrenal Gland

BODY PART KEY

Suprarenal plexus	**Use:** Abdominal Sympathetic Nerve
Suprascapular nerve	**Use:** Brachial Plexus
Supraspinatus fascia	**Use:** Subcutaneous Tissue and Fascia, Right Upper Arm Subcutaneous Tissue and Fascia, Left Upper Arm
Supraspinatus muscle	**Use:** Shoulder Muscle, Right Shoulder Muscle, Left
Supraspinous ligament	**Use:** Trunk Bursa and Ligament, Right Trunk Bursa and Ligament, Left
Suprasternal notch	**Use:** Sternum
Supratrochlear lymph node	**Use:** Lymphatic, Right Upper Extremity Lymphatic, Left Upper Extremity
Sural artery	**Use:** Popliteal Artery, Right Popliteal Artery, Left
Sweat gland	**Use:** Skin
Talocalcaneal (subtalar) joint	**Use:** Tarsal Joint, Right Tarsal Joint, Left
Talocalcaneal ligament	**Use:** Foot Bursa and Ligament, Right Foot Bursa and Ligament, Left
Talocalcaneonavicular joint	**Use:** Tarsal Joint, Right Tarsal Joint, Left
Talocalcaneonavicular ligament	**Use:** Foot Bursa and Ligament, Right Foot Bursa and Ligament, Left
Talocrural joint	**Use:** Ankle Joint, Right Ankle Joint, Left
Talofibular ligament	**Use:** Ankle Bursa and Ligament, Right Ankle Bursa and Ligament, Left
Talus bone	**Use:** Tarsal, Right Tarsal, Left
Tarsometatarsal joint	**Use:** Metatarsal-Tarsal Joint, Right Metatarsal-Tarsal Joint, Left

Tarsometatarsal ligament	**Use:** Foot Bursa and Ligament, Right Foot Bursa and Ligament, Left
Temporal lobe	**Use:** Cerebral Hemisphere
Temporalis muscle Temporoparietalis muscle	**Use:** Head Muscle
Tensor fasciae latae muscle	**Use:** Hip Muscle, Right Hip Muscle, Left
Tensor veli palatini muscle	**Use:** Tongue, Palate, Pharynx Muscle
Tenth cranial nerve	**Use:** Vagus Nerve
Tentorium cerebelli	**Use:** Dura Mater
Teres major muscle Teres minor muscle	**Use:** Shoulder Muscle, Right Shoulder Muscle, Left
Testicular artery	**Use:** Abdominal Aorta
Thenar muscle	**Use:** Hand Muscle, Right Hand Muscle, Left
Third cranial nerve	**Use:** Oculomotor Nerve
Third occipital nerve	**Use:** Cervical Nerve
Third ventricle	**Use:** Cerebral Ventricle
Thoracic aortic plexus	**Use:** Thoracic Sympathetic Nerve
Thoracic esophagus	**Use:** Esophagus, Middle
Thoracic facet joint	**Use:** Thoracic Vertebral Joint Thoracic Vertebral Joints, 2 to 7 Thoracic Vertebral Joints, 8 or more
Thoracic ganglion	**Use:** Thoracic Sympathetic Nerve
Thoracoacromial artery	**Use:** Axillary Artery, Right Axillary Artery, Left
Thoracolumbar facet joint	**Use:** Thoracolumbar Vertebral Joint

BODY PART KEY

Thymus gland	**Use:** Thymus
Thyroarytenoid muscle	**Use:** Neck Muscle, Right Neck Muscle, Left
Thyrocervical trunk	**Use:** Thyroid Artery, Right Thyroid Artery, Left
Thyroid cartilage	**Use:** Larynx
Tibialis anterior muscle Tibialis posterior muscle	**Use:** Lower Leg Muscle, Right Lower Leg Muscle, Left
Tibiofemoral joint	**Use:** Knee Joint, Right Knee Joint, Left Knee Joint, Tibial Surface, Right Knee Joint, Tibial Surface, Left
Tongue, base of	**Use:** Pharynx
Tracheobronchial lymph node	**Use:** Lymphatic, Thorax
Tragus	**Use:** External Ear, Right External Ear, Left External Ear, Bilateral
Transversalis fascia	**Use:** Subcutaneous Tissue and Fascia, Trunk
Transverse (cutaneous) cervical nerve	**Use:** Cervical Plexus
Transverse acetabular ligament	**Use:** Hip Bursa and Ligament, Right Hip Bursa and Ligament, Left
Transverse facial artery	**Use:** Temporal Artery, Right Temporal Artery, Left
Transverse humeral ligament	**Use:** Shoulder Bursa and Ligament, Right Shoulder Bursa and Ligament, Left
Transverse ligament of atlas	**Use:** Head and Neck Bursa and Ligament
Transverse scapular ligament	**Use:** Shoulder Bursa and Ligament, Right Shoulder Bursa and Ligament, Left
Transverse thoracis muscle	**Use:** Thorax Muscle, Right Thorax Muscle, Left
Transversospinalis muscle	**Use:** Trunk Muscle, Right Trunk Muscle, Left
Transversus abdominis muscle	**Use:** Abdomen Muscle, Right Abdomen Muscle, Left
Trapezium bone	**Use:** Carpal, Right Carpal, Left
Trapezius muscle	**Use:** Trunk Muscle, Right Trunk Muscle, Left
Trapezoid bone	**Use:** Carpal, Right Carpal, Left
Triceps brachii muscle	**Use:** Upper Arm Muscle, Right Upper Arm Muscle, Left
Tricuspid annulus	**Use:** Tricuspid Valve
Trifacial nerve	**Use:** Trigeminal Nerve
Trigone of bladder	**Use:** Bladder
Triquetral bone	**Use:** Carpal, Right Carpal, Left
Trochanteric bursa	**Use:** Hip Bursa and Ligament, Right Hip Bursa and Ligament, Left
Twelfth cranial nerve	**Use:** Hypoglossal Nerve
Tympanic cavity	**Use:** Middle Ear, Right Middle Ear, Left
Tympanic nerve	**Use:** Glossopharyngeal Nerve
Tympanic part of temporal bone	**Use:** Temporal Bone, Right Temporal Bone, Left
Ulnar collateral carpal ligament	**Use:** Wrist Bursa and Ligament, Right Wrist Bursa and Ligament, Left
Ulnar collateral ligament	**Use:** Elbow Bursa and Ligament, Right Elbow Bursa and Ligament, Left

BODY PART KEY

Ulnar notch	**Use:** Radius, Right Radius, Left
Ulnar vein	**Use:** Brachial Vein, Right Brachial Vein, Left
Umbilical artery	**Use:** Internal Iliac Artery, Right Internal Iliac Artery, Left
Ureteral orifice	**Use:** Ureter, Right Ureter, Left Ureters, Bilateral Ureter
Ureteropelvic junction (UPJ)	**Use:** Kidney Pelvis, Right Kidney Pelvis, Left
Ureterovesical orifice	**Use:** Ureter, Right Ureter, Left Ureters, Bilateral Ureter
Uterine artery	**Use:** Internal Iliac Artery, Right Internal Iliac Artery, Left
Uterine cornu	**Use:** Uterus
Uterine tube	**Use:** Fallopian Tube, Right Fallopian Tube, Left
Uterine vein	**Use:** Hypogastric Vein, Right Hypogastric Vein, Left
Vaginal artery	**Use:** Internal Iliac Artery, Right Internal Iliac Artery, Left
Vaginal vein	**Use:** Hypogastric Vein, Right Hypogastric Vein, Left
Vastus intermedius muscle Vastus lateralis muscle Vastus medialis muscle	**Use:** Upper Leg Muscle, Right Upper Leg Muscle, Left
Ventricular fold	**Use:** Larynx
Vermiform appendix	**Use:** Appendix

Vermilion border	**Use:** Upper Lip Lower Lip
Vertebral arch	**Use:** Cervical Vertebra Thoracic Vertebra Lumbar Vertebra
Vertebral canal	**Use:** Spinal Canal
Vertebral foramen Vertebral lamina Vertebral pedicle	**Use:** Cervical Vertebra Thoracic Vertebra Lumbar Vertebra
Vesical vein	**Use:** Hypogastric Vein, Right Hypogastric Vein, Left
Vestibular (Scarpa's) ganglion Vestibular nerve Vestibulocochlear nerve	**Use:** Acoustic Nerve
Virchow's (supraclavicular) lymph node	**Use:** Lymphatic, Right Neck Lymphatic, Left Neck
Vitreous body	**Use:** Vitreous, Right Vitreous, Left
Vocal fold	**Use:** Vocal Cord, Right Vocal Cord, Left
Volar (palmar) digital vein Volar (palmar) metacarpal vein	**Use:** Hand Vein, Right Hand Vein, Left
Vomer bone	**Use:** Nasal Septum
Vomer of nasal septum	**Use:** Nasal Bone
Xiphoid process	**Use:** Sternum
Zonule of Zinn	**Use:** Lens, Right Lens, Left
Zygomatic process of frontal bone	**Use:** Frontal Bone, Right Frontal Bone, Left
Zygomatic process of temporal bone	**Use:** Temporal Bone, Right Temporal Bone, Left
Zygomaticus muscle	**Use:** Facial Muscle

DEVICE KEY

3f (Aortic) Bioprosthesis valve	**Use:** Zooplastic Tissue in Heart and Great Vessels
AbioCor® Total Replacement Heart	**Use:** Synthetic Substitute
Acellular Hydrated Dermis	**Use:** Nonautologous Tissue Substitute
Acetabular cup	**Use:** Liner in Lower Joints
Activa PC neurostimulator	**Use:** Stimulator Generator, Multiple Array for Insertion in Subcutaneous Tissue and Fascia
Activa RC neurostimulator	**Use:** Stimulator Generator, Multiple Array Rechargeable for Insertion in Subcutaneous Tissue and Fascia
Activa SC neurostimulator	**Use:** Stimulator Generator, Single Array for Insertion in Subcutaneous Tissue and Fascia
ACUITY™ Steerable Lead	**Use:** Cardiac Lead, Pacemaker for Insertion in Heart and Great Vessels; Cardiac Lead, Defibrillator for Insertion in Heart and Great Vessels
Advisa (MRI)	**Use:** Pacemaker, Dual Chamber for Insertion in Subcutaneous Tissue and Fascia
AFX® Endovascular AAA System	**Use:** Intraluminal Device
AMPLATZER® Muscular VSD Occluder	**Use:** Synthetic Substitute
AMS 800® Urinary Control System	**Use:** Artificial Sphincter in Urinary System
AneuRx® AAA Advantage®	**Use:** Intraluminal Device
Annuloplasty ring	**Use:** Synthetic Substitute
Artificial anal sphincter (AAS)	**Use:** Artificial Sphincter in Gastrointestinal System
Artificial bowel sphincter (neosphincter)	**Use:** Artificial Sphincter in Gastrointestinal System
Artificial urinary sphincter (AUS)	**Use:** Artificial Sphincter in Urinary System
Assurant (Cobalt) stent	**Use:** Intraluminal Device
Attain Ability® lead	**Use:** Cardiac Lead, Pacemaker for Insertion in Heart and Great Vessels; Cardiac Lead, Defibrillator for Insertion in Heart and Great Vessels
Attain StarFix® (OTW) lead	**Use:** Cardiac Lead, Pacemaker for Insertion in Heart and Great Vessels; Cardiac Lead, Defibrillator for Insertion in Heart and Great Vessels
Autograft	**Use:** Autologous Tissue Substitute
Autologous artery graft	**Use:** Autologous Arterial Tissue in Heart and Great Vessels; Autologous Arterial Tissue in Upper Arteries; Autologous Arterial Tissue in Lower Arteries; Autologous Arterial Tissue in Upper Veins; Autologous Arterial Tissue in Lower Veins
Autologous vein graft	**Use:** Autologous Venous Tissue in Heart and Great Vessels; Autologous Venous Tissue in Upper Arteries; Autologous Venous Tissue in Lower Arteries; Autologous Venous Tissue in Upper Veins; Autologous Venous Tissue in Lower Veins
Axial Lumbar Interbody Fusion System	**Use:** Interbody Fusion Device in Lower Joints
AxiaLIF® System	**Use:** Interbody Fusion Device in Lower Joints

DEVICE KEY

BAK/C® Interbody Cervical Fusion System	**Use:** Interbody Fusion Device in Upper Joints
Bard® Composix® (E/X) (LP) mesh	**Use:** Synthetic Substitute
Bard® Composix® Kugel® patch	**Use:** Synthetic Substitute
Bard® Dulex™ mesh	**Use:** Synthetic Substitute
Bard® Ventralex™ hernia patch	**Use:** Synthetic Substitute
Baroreflex Activation Therapy® (BAT®)	**Use:** Stimulator Lead in Upper Arteries / Cardiac Rhythm Related Device in Subcutaneous Tissue and Fascia
Berlin Heart Ventricular Assist Device	**Use:** Implantable Heart Assist System in Heart and Great Vessels
Bioactive embolization coil(s)	**Use:** Intraluminal Device, Bioactive in Upper Arteries
Biventricular external heart assist system	**Use:** External Heart Assist System in Heart and Great Vessels
Blood glucose monitoring system	**Use:** Monitoring Device
Bone anchored hearing device	**Use:** Hearing Device, Bone Conduction for Insertion in Ear, Nose, Sinus / Hearing Device in Head and Facial Bones
Bone bank bone graft	**Use:** Nonautologous Tissue Substitute
Bone screw (interlocking) (lag) (pedicle) (recessed)	**Use:** Internal Fixation Device in Head and Facial Bones / Internal Fixation Device in Upper Bones / Internal Fixation Device in Lower Bones
Bovine pericardial valve	**Use:** Zooplastic Tissue in Heart and Great Vessels
Bovine pericardium graft	**Use:** Zooplastic Tissue in Heart and Great Vessels
Brachytherapy seeds	**Use:** Radioactive Element
BRYAN® Cervical Disc System	**Use:** Synthetic Substitute
BVS 5000 Ventricular Assist Device	**Use:** External Heart Assist System in Heart and Great Vessels
Cardiac contractility modulation lead	**Use:** Cardiac Lead in Heart and Great Vessels
Cardiac event recorder	**Use:** Monitoring Device
Cardiac resynchronization therapy (CRT) lead	**Use:** Cardiac Lead, Pacemaker for Insertion in Heart and Great Vessels / Cardiac Lead, Defibrillator for Insertion in Heart and Great Vessels
CardioMEMS® pressure sensor	**Use:** Monitoring Device, Pressure Sensor for Insertion in Heart and Great Vessels
Carotid (artery) sinus (baroreceptor) lead	**Use:** Stimulator Lead in Upper Arteries
Carotid WALLSTENT® Monorail® Endoprosthesis	**Use:** Intraluminal Device
Centrimag® Blood Pump	**Use:** Intraluminal Device
Ceramic on ceramic bearing surface	**Use:** Synthetic Substitute, Ceramic for Replacement in Lower Joints
Clamp and rod internal fixation system (CRIF)	**Use:** Internal Fixation Device in Upper Bones / Internal Fixation Device in Lower Bones
CoAxia NeuroFlo catheter	**Use:** Intraluminal Device
Cobalt/chromium head and polyethylene socket	**Use:** Synthetic Substitute, Metal on Polyethylene for Replacement in Lower Joints
Cobalt/chromium head and socket	**Use:** Synthetic Substitute, Metal for Replacement in Lower Joints
Cochlear implant (CI), multiple channel (electrode)	**Use:** Hearing Device, Multiple Channel Cochlear Prosthesis for Insertion in Ear, Nose, Sinus

DEVICE KEY

Cochlear implant (CI), single channel (electrode)	**Use:** Hearing Device, Single Channel Cochlear Prosthesis for Insertion in Ear, Nose, Sinus	Cook Zenith AAA Endovascular Graft	**Use:** Intraluminal Device, Branched or Fenestrated, One or Two Arteries for Restriction in Lower Arteries Intraluminal Device, Branched or Fenestrated, Three or More Arteries for Restriction in Lower Arteries Intraluminal Device
COGNIS® CRT-D	**Use:** Cardiac Resynchronization Defibrillator Pulse Generator for Insertion in Subcutaneous Tissue and Fascia		
Colonic Z-Stent®	**Use:** Intraluminal Device	CoreValve transcatheter aortic valve	**Use:** Zooplastic Tissue in Heart and Great Vessels
Complete (SE) stent	**Use:** Intraluminal Device	Cormet Hip Resurfacing System	**Use:** Resurfacing Device in Lower Joints
Concerto II CRT-D	**Use:** Cardiac Resynchronization Defibrillator Pulse Generator for Insertion in Subcutaneous Tissue and Fascia	CoRoent® XL	**Use:** Interbody Fusion Device in Lower Joints
CONSERVE® PLUS Total Resurfacing Hip System	**Use:** Resurfacing Device in Lower Joints	Corox (OTW) Bipolar Lead	**Use:** Cardiac Lead, Pacemaker for Insertion in Heart and Great Vessels Cardiac Lead, Defibrillator for Insertion in Heart and Great Vessels
Consulta CRT-D	**Use:** Cardiac Resynchronization Defibrillator Pulse Generator for Insertion in Subcutaneous Tissue and Fascia		
Consulta CRT-P	**Use:** Cardiac Resynchronization Pacemaker Pulse Generator for Insertion in Subcutaneous Tissue and Fascia	Cortical strip neurostimulator lead	**Use:** Neurostimulator Lead in Central Nervous System
		Cultured epidermal cell autograft	**Use:** Autologous Tissue Substitute
CONTAK RENEWAL® 3 RF (HE) CRT-D	**Use:** Cardiac Resynchronization Defibrillator Pulse Generator for Insertion in Subcutaneous Tissue and Fascia	CYPHER® Stent	**Use:** Intraluminal Device, Drug-eluting in Heart and Great Vessels
		Cystostomy tube	**Use:** Drainage Device
Contegra Pulmonary Valved Conduit	**Use:** Zooplastic Tissue in Heart and Great Vessels	DBS lead	**Use:** Neurostimulator Lead in Central Nervous System
Continuous Glucose Monitoring (CGM) device	**Use:** Monitoring Device	DeBakey Left Ventricular Assist Device	**Use:** Implantable Heart Assist System in Heart and Great Vessels
Cook Biodesign® Fistula Plug(s)	**Use:** Nonautologous Tissue Substitute	Deep brain neurostimulator lead	**Use:** Neurostimulator Lead in Central Nervous System
Cook Biodesign® Hernia Graft(s)	**Use:** Nonautologous Tissue Substitute	Delta frame external fixator	**Use:** External Fixation Device, Hybrid for Insertion in Upper Bones External Fixation Device, Hybrid for Reposition in Upper Bones External Fixation Device, Hybrid for Insertion in Lower Bones External Fixation Device, Hybrid for Reposition in Lower Bones
Cook Biodesign® Layered Graft(s)	**Use:** Nonautologous Tissue Substitute		
Cook Zenapro™ Layered Graft(s)	**Use:** Nonautologous Tissue Substitute		

DEVICE KEY

Delta III Reverse shoulder prosthesis	**Use:** Synthetic Substitute, Reverse Ball and Socket for Replacement in Upper Joints
Diaphragmatic pacemaker generator	**Use:** Stimulator Generator in Subcutaneous Tissue and Fascia
Direct Lateral Interbody Fusion (DLIF) device	**Use:** Interbody Fusion Device in Lower Joints
Driver stent (RX) (OTW)	**Use:** Intraluminal Device
DuraHeart Left Ventricular Assist System	**Use:** Implantable Heart Assist System in Heart and Great Vessels
Durata® Defibrillation Lead	**Use:** Cardiac Lead, Defibrillator for Insertion in Heart and Great Vessels
Dynesys® Dynamic Stabilization System	**Use:** Spinal Stabilization Device, Pedicle-Based for Insertion in Upper Joints — Spinal Stabilization Device, Pedicle-Based for Insertion in Lower Joints
E-Luminexx™ (Biliary) (Vascular) Stent	**Use:** Intraluminal Device
EDWARDS INTUITY Elite valve system	**Use:** Zooplastic Tissue, Rapid Deployment Technique in New Technology
Electrical bone growth stimulator (EBGS)	**Use:** Bone Growth Stimulator in Head and Facial Bones — Bone Growth Stimulator in Upper Bones — Bone Growth Stimulator in Lower Bones
Electrical muscle stimulation (EMS) lead	**Use:** Stimulator Lead in Muscles
Electronic muscle stimulator lead	**Use:** Stimulator Lead in Muscles
Embolization coil(s)	**Use:** Intraluminal Device
Endeavor® (III) (IV) (Sprint) Zotarolimus-eluting Coronary Stent System	**Use:** Intraluminal Device, Drug-eluting in Heart and Great Vessels
Endologix AFX® Endovascular AAA System	**Use:** Intraluminal Device

EndoSure® sensor	**Use:** Monitoring Device, Pressure Sensor for Insertion in Heart and Great Vessels
ENDOTAK RELIANCE® (G) Defibrillation Lead	**Use:** Cardiac Lead, Defibrillator for Insertion in Heart and Great Vessels
Endotracheal tube (cuffed) (double-lumen)	**Use:** Intraluminal Device, Endotracheal Airway in Respiratory System
Endurant® Endovascular Stent Graft	**Use:** Intraluminal Device
Endurant® II AAA stent graft system	**Use:** Intraluminal Device
EnRhythm	**Use:** Pacemaker, Dual Chamber for Insertion in Subcutaneous Tissue and Fascia
Enterra gastric neurostimulator	**Use:** Stimulator Generator, Multiple Array for Insertion in Subcutaneous Tissue and Fascia
Epic™ Stented Tissue Valve (aortic)	**Use:** Zooplastic Tissue in Heart and Great Vessels
Epicel® cultured epidermal autograft	**Use:** Autologous Tissue Substitute
Esophageal obturator airway (EOA)	**Use:** Intraluminal Device, Airway in Gastrointestinal System
Esteem® implantable hearing system	**Use:** Hearing Device in Ear, Nose, Sinus
Everolimus-eluting coronary stent	**Use:** Intraluminal Device, Drug-eluting in Heart and Great Vessels
Ex-PRESS™ mini glaucoma shunt	**Use:** Synthetic Substitute
EXCLUDER® AAA Endoprosthesis	**Use:** Intraluminal Device, Branched or Fenestrated, One or Two Arteries for Restriction in Lower Arteries — Intraluminal Device, Branched or Fenestrated, Three or More Arteries for Restriction in Lower Arteries

DEVICE KEY

EXCLUDER® IBE Endoprosthesis	**Use:** Intraluminal Device, Branched or Fenestrated, One or Two Arteries for Restriction in Lower Arteries
Express® (LD) Premounted Stent System	**Use:** Intraluminal Device
Express® Biliary SD Monorail® Premounted Stent System	**Use:** Intraluminal Device
Express® SD Renal Monorail® Premounted Stent System	**Use:** Intraluminal Device
External fixator	**Use:** External Fixation Device in Head and Facial Bones; External Fixation Device in Upper Bones; External Fixation Device in Lower Bones; External Fixation Device in Upper Joints; External Fixation Device in Lower Joints
EXtreme Lateral Interbody Fusion (XLIF) device	**Use:** Interbody Fusion Device in Lower Joints
Facet replacement spinal stabilization device	**Use:** Spinal Stabilization Device, Facet Replacement for Insertion in Upper Joints; Spinal Stabilization Device, Facet Replacement for Insertion in Lower Joints
FLAIR® Endovascular Stent Graft	**Use:** Intraluminal Device
Flexible Composite Mesh	**Use:** Synthetic Substitute
Foley catheter	**Use:** Drainage Device
Formula™ Balloon-Expandable Renal Stent System	**Use:** Intraluminal Device
Freestyle (Stentless) Aortic Root Bioprosthesis	**Use:** Zooplastic Tissue in Heart and Great Vessels
Fusion screw (compression) (lag) (locking)	**Use:** Internal Fixation Device in Upper Joints; Internal Fixation Device in Lower Joints
Gastric electrical stimulation (GES) lead	**Use:** Stimulator Lead in Gastrointestinal System
Gastric pacemaker lead	**Use:** Stimulator Lead in Gastrointestinal System
GORE EXCLUDER® AAA Endoprosthesis	**Use:** Intraluminal Device, Branched or Fenestrated, One or Two Arteries for Restriction in Lower Arteries
GORE EXCLUDER® IBE Endoprosthesis	**Use:** Intraluminal Device, Branched or Fenestrated, One or Two Arteries for Restriction in Lower Arteries
GORE TAG® Thoracic Endoprosthesis	**Use:** Intraluminal Device
GORE® DUALMESH®	**Use:** Synthetic Substitute
Guedel airway	**Use:** Intraluminal Device, Airway in Mouth and Throat
Hancock Bioprosthesis (aortic) (mitral) valve	**Use:** Zooplastic Tissue in Heart and Great Vessels
Hancock Bioprosthetic Valved Conduit	**Use:** Zooplastic Tissue in Heart and Great Vessels
HeartMate II® Left Ventricular Assist Device (LVAD)	**Use:** Implantable Heart Assist System in Heart and Great Vessels
HeartMate XVE® Left Ventricular Assist Device (LVAD)	**Use:** Implantable Heart Assist System in Heart and Great Vessels
Hip (joint) liner	**Use:** Liner in Lower Joints
Holter valve ventricular shunt	**Use:** Synthetic Substitute
Ilizarov external fixator	**Use:** External Fixation Device, Ring for Insertion in Upper Bones; External Fixation Device, Ring for Reposition in Upper Bones; External Fixation Device, Ring for Insertion in Lower Bones; External Fixation Device, Ring for Reposition in Lower Bones

DEVICE KEY

Ilizarov-Vecklich device	**Use:** External Fixation Device, Limb Lengthening for Insertion in Upper Bones / External Fixation Device, Limb Lengthening for Insertion in Lower Bones
Implantable cardioverter-defibrillator (ICD)	**Use:** Defibrillator Generator for Insertion in Subcutaneous Tissue and Fascia
Implantable drug infusion pump (anti-spasmodic) (chemotherapy) (pain)	**Use:** Infusion Device, Pump in Subcutaneous Tissue and Fascia
Implantable glucose monitoring device	**Use:** Monitoring Device
Implantable hemodynamic monitor (IHM)	**Use:** Monitoring Device, Hemodynamic for Insertion in Subcutaneous Tissue and Fascia
Implantable hemodynamic monitoring system (IHMS)	**Use:** Monitoring Device, Hemodynamic for Insertion in Subcutaneous Tissue and Fascia
Implantable Miniature Telescope™ (IMT)	**Use:** Synthetic Substitute, Intraocular Telescope for Replacement in Eye
Implanted (venous) (access) port	**Use:** Vascular Access Device, Reservoir in Subcutaneous Tissue and Fascia
InDura, intrathecal catheter (1P) (spinal)	**Use:** Infusion Device
Injection reservoir, port	**Use:** Vascular Access Device, Reservoir in Subcutaneous Tissue and Fascia
Injection reservoir, pump	**Use:** Infusion Device, Pump in Subcutaneous Tissue and Fascia
Interbody fusion (spine) cage	**Use:** Interbody Fusion Device in Upper Joints / Interbody Fusion Device in Lower Joints

Interspinous process spinal stabilization device	**Use:** Spinal Stabilization Device, Interspinous Process for Insertion in Upper Joints / Spinal Stabilization Device, Interspinous Process for Insertion in Lower Joints
InterStim® Therapy lead	**Use:** Neurostimulator Lead in Peripheral Nervous System
InterStim® Therapy neurostimulator	**Use:** Stimulator Generator, Single Array for Insertion in Subcutaneous Tissue and Fascia
Intramedullary (IM) rod (nail)	**Use:** Internal Fixation Device, Intramedullary in Upper Bones / Internal Fixation Device, Intramedullary in Lower Bones
Intramedullary skeletal kinetic distractor (ISKD)	**Use:** Internal Fixation Device, Intramedullary in Upper Bones / Internal Fixation Device, Intramedullary in Lower Bones
Intrauterine device (IUD)	**Use:** Contraceptive Device in Female Reproductive System
INTUITY Elite valve system, EDWARDS	**Use:** Zooplastic Tissue, Rapid Deployment Technique in New Technology
Itrel (3) (4) neurostimulator	**Use:** Stimulator Generator, Single Array for Insertion in Subcutaneous Tissue and Fascia
Joint fixation plate	**Use:** Internal Fixation Device in Upper Joints / Internal Fixation Device in Lower Joints
Joint liner (insert)	**Use:** Liner in Lower Joints
Joint spacer (antibiotic)	**Use:** Spacer in Upper Joints / Spacer in Lower Joints
Kappa	**Use:** Pacemaker, Dual Chamber for Insertion in Subcutaneous Tissue and Fascia

DEVICE KEY

Kinetra® neurostimulator	**Use:** Stimulator Generator, Multiple Array for Insertion in Subcutaneous Tissue and Fascia
Kirschner wire (K-wire)	**Use:** Internal Fixation Device in Head and Facial Bones Internal Fixation Device in Upper Bones Internal Fixation Device in Lower Bones Internal Fixation Device in Upper Joints Internal Fixation Device in Lower Joints
Knee (implant) insert	**Use:** Liner in Lower Joints
Kuntscher nail	**Use:** Internal Fixation Device, Intramedullary in Upper Bones Internal Fixation Device, Intramedullary in Lower Bones
LAP-BAND® adjustable gastric banding system	**Use:** Extraluminal Device
LifeStent® (Flexstar) (XL) Vascular Stent System	**Use:** Intraluminal Device
LIVIAN™ CRT-D	**Use:** Cardiac Resynchronization Defibrillator Pulse Generator for Insertion in Subcutaneous Tissue and Fascia
Loop recorder, implantable	**Use:** Monitoring Device
MAGEC® Spinal Bracing and Distraction System	**Use:** Magnetically Controlled Growth Rod(s) in New Technology
Mark IV Breathing Pacemaker System	Stimulator Generator in Subcutaneous Tissue and Fascia
Maximo II DR (VR)	**Use:** Defibrillator Generator for Insertion in Subcutaneous Tissue and Fascia
Maximo II DR CRT-D	**Use:** Cardiac Resynchronization Defibrillator Pulse Generator for Insertion in Subcutaneous Tissue and Fascia
Medtronic Endurant® II AAA stent graft system	**Use:** Intraluminal Device
Melody® transcatheter pulmonary valve	**Use:** Zooplastic Tissue in Heart and Great Vessels

Metal on metal bearing surface	**Use:** Synthetic Substitute, Metal for Replacement in Lower Joints
Micro-Driver stent (RX) (OTW)	**Use:** Intraluminal Device
Micrus CERECYTE microcoil	**Use:** Intraluminal Device, Bioactive in Upper Arteries
MIRODERM™ Biologic Wound Matrix	**Use:** Skin Substitute, Porcine Liver Derived in New Technology
MitraClip valve repair system	**Use:** Synthetic Substitute
Mitroflow® Aortic Pericardial Heart Valve	**Use:** Zooplastic Tissue in Heart and Great Vessels
Mosaic Bioprosthesis (aortic) (mitral) valve	**Use:** Zooplastic Tissue in Heart and Great Vessels
MULTI-LINK (VISION)(MINIVISION) (ULTRA) Coronary Stent System	**Use:** Intraluminal Device
nanoLOCK™ interbody fusion device	**Use:** Interbody Fusion Device, Nanotextured Surface in New Technology
Nasopharyngeal airway (NPA)	**Use:** Intraluminal Device, Airway in Ear, Nose, Sinus
Neuromuscular electrical stimulation (NEMS) lead	**Use:** Stimulator Lead in Muscles
Neurostimulator generator, multiple channel	**Use:** Stimulator Generator, Multiple Array for Insertion in Subcutaneous Tissue and Fascia
Neurostimulator generator, multiple channel rechargeable	**Use:** Stimulator Generator, Multiple Array Rechargeable for Insertion in Subcutaneous Tissue and Fascia
Neurostimulator generator, single channel	**Use:** Stimulator Generator, Single Array for Insertion in Subcutaneous Tissue and Fascia
Neurostimulator generator, single channel rechargeable	**Use:** Stimulator Generator, Single Array Rechargeable for Insertion in Subcutaneous Tissue and Fascia

DEVICE KEY

DEVICE KEY

Neutralization plate	**Use:** Internal Fixation Device in Head and Facial Bones Internal Fixation Device in Upper Bones Internal Fixation Device in Lower Bones
Nitinol framed polymer mesh	**Use:** Synthetic Substitute
Non-tunneled central venous catheter	**Use:** Infusion Device
Novacor Left Ventricular Assist Device	**Use:** Implantable Heart Assist System in Heart and Great Vessels
Novation® Ceramic AHS® (Articulation Hip System)	**Use:** Synthetic Substitute, Ceramic for Replacement in Lower Joints
Optimizer™ III implantable pulse generator	**Use:** Contractility Modulation Device for Insertion in Subcutaneous Tissue and Fascia
Oropharyngeal airway (OPA)	**Use:** Intraluminal Device, Airway in Mouth and Throat
Ovatio™ CRT-D	**Use:** Cardiac Resynchronization Defibrillator Pulse Generator for Insertion in Subcutaneous Tissue and Fascia
Oxidized zirconium ceramic hip bearing surface	**Use:** Synthetic Substitute, Ceramic on Polyethylene for Replacement in Lower Joints
Paclitaxel-eluting coronary stent	**Use:** Intraluminal Device, Drug-eluting in Heart and Great Vessels
Paclitaxel-eluting peripheral stent	**Use:** Intraluminal Device, Drug-eluting in Upper Arteries Intraluminal Device, Drug-eluting in Lower Arteries
Partially absorbable mesh	**Use:** Synthetic Substitute
Pedicle-based dynamic stabilization device	**Use:** Spinal Stabilization Device, Pedicle-Based for Insertion in Upper Joints Spinal Stabilization Device, Pedicle-Based for Insertion in Lower Joints

Perceval sutureless valve	**Use:** Zooplastic Tissue, Rapid Deployment Technique in New Technology
Percutaneous endoscopic gastrojejunostomy (PEG/J) tube	**Use:** Feeding Device in Gastrointestinal System
Percutaneous endoscopic gastrostomy (PEG) tube	**Use:** Feeding Device in Gastrointestinal System
Percutaneous nephrostomy catheter	**Use:** Drainage Device
Peripherally inserted central catheter (PICC)	**Use:** Infusion Device
Pessary ring	**Use:** Intraluminal Device, Pessary in Female Reproductive System
Phrenic nerve stimulator generator	**Use:** Stimulator Generator in Subcutaneous Tissue and Fascia
Phrenic nerve stimulator lead	**Use:** Diaphragmatic Pacemaker Lead in Respiratory System
PHYSIOMESH™ Flexible Composite Mesh	**Use:** Synthetic Substitute
Pipeline™ Embolization device (PED)	**Use:** Intraluminal Device
Polyethylene socket	**Use:** Synthetic Substitute, Polyethylene for Replacement in Lower Joints
Polymethylmethacrylate (PMMA)	**Use:** Synthetic Substitute
Polypropylene mesh	**Use:** Synthetic Substitute
Porcine (bioprosthetic) valve	**Use:** Zooplastic Tissue in Heart and Great Vessels
PRESTIGE® Cervical Disc	**Use:** Synthetic Substitute
PrimeAdvanced neurostimulator	**Use:** Stimulator Generator, Multiple Array for Insertion in Subcutaneous Tissue and Fascia
PROCEED™ Ventral Patch	**Use:** Synthetic Substitute
Prodisc-C	**Use:** Synthetic Substitute

APPENDIX C

DEVICE KEY

Prodisc-L	**Use:** Synthetic Substitute
PROLENE Polypropylene Hernia System (PHS)	**Use:** Synthetic Substitute
Protecta XT CRT-D	**Use:** Cardiac Resynchronization Defibrillator Pulse Generator for Insertion in Subcutaneous Tissue and Fascia
Protecta XT DR (XT VR)	**Use:** Defibrillator Generator for Insertion in Subcutaneous Tissue and Fascia
Protégé® RX Carotid Stent System	**Use:** Intraluminal Device
Pump reservoir	**Use:** Infusion Device, Pump in Subcutaneous Tissue and Fascia
PVAD™ Ventricular Assist Device	**Use:** External Heart Assist System in Heart and Great Vessels
REALIZE® Adjustable Gastric Band	**Use:** Extraluminal Device
Rebound HRD® (Hernia Repair Device)	**Use:** Synthetic Substitute
RestoreAdvanced neurostimulator	**Use:** Stimulator Generator, Multiple Array Rechargeable for Insertion in Subcutaneous Tissue and Fascia
RestoreSensor neurostimulator	**Use:** Stimulator Generator, Multiple Array Rechargeable for Insertion in Subcutaneous Tissue and Fascia
RestoreUltra neurostimulator	**Use:** Stimulator Generator, Multiple Array Rechargeable for Insertion in Subcutaneous Tissue and Fascia
Reveal (DX) (XT)	**Use:** Monitoring Device
Reverse® Shoulder Prosthesis	**Use:** Synthetic Substitute, Reverse Ball and Socket for Replacement in Upper Joints
Revo MRI™ SureScan® pacemaker	**Use:** Pacemaker, Dual Chamber for Insertion in Subcutaneous Tissue and Fascia

Rheos® System device	**Use:** Cardiac Rhythm Related Device in Subcutaneous Tissue and Fascia
Rheos® System lead	**Use:** Stimulator Lead in Upper Arteries
RNS System lead	**Use:** Neurostimulator Lead in Central Nervous System
RNS system neurostimulator generator	**Use:** Neurostimulator Generator in Head and Facial Bones
Sacral nerve modulation (SNM) lead	**Use:** Stimulator Lead in Urinary System
Sacral neuromodulation lead	**Use:** Stimulator Lead in Urinary System
SAPIEN transcatheter aortic valve	**Use:** Zooplastic Tissue in Heart and Great Vessels
Secura (DR) (VR)	**Use:** Defibrillator Generator for Insertion in Subcutaneous Tissue and Fascia
Sheffield hybrid external fixator	**Use:** External Fixation Device, Hybrid for Insertion in Upper Bones; External Fixation Device, Hybrid for Reposition in Upper Bones; External Fixation Device, Hybrid for Insertion in Lower Bones; External Fixation Device, Hybrid for Reposition in Lower Bones
Sheffield ring external fixator	**Use:** External Fixation Device, Ring for Insertion in Upper Bones; External Fixation Device, Ring for Reposition in Upper Bones; External Fixation Device, Ring for Insertion in Lower Bones; External Fixation Device, Ring for Reposition in Lower Bones
Single lead pacemaker (atrium) (ventricle)	**Use:** Pacemaker, Single Chamber for Insertion in Subcutaneous Tissue and Fascia
Single lead rate responsive pacemaker (atrium) (ventricle)	**Use:** Pacemaker, Single Chamber Rate Responsive for Insertion in Subcutaneous Tissue and Fascia
Sirolimus-eluting coronary stent	**Use:** Intraluminal Device, Drug-eluting in Heart and Great Vessels

DEVICE KEY

SJM Biocor® Stented Valve System	**Use:** Zooplastic Tissue in Heart and Great Vessels
Soletra® neurostimulator	**Use:** Stimulator Generator, Single Array for Insertion in Subcutaneous Tissue and Fascia
Spinal cord neurostimulator lead	**Use:** Neurostimulator Lead in Central Nervous System
Spinal growth rods, magnetically controlled	**Use:** Magnetically Controlled Growth Rod(s) in New Technology
Spiration IBV™ Valve System	**Use:** Intraluminal Device, Endobronchial Valve in Respiratory System
Stent (angioplasty) (embolization)	**Use:** Intraluminal Device
Stented tissue valve	**Use:** Zooplastic Tissue in Heart and Great Vessels
Stratos LV	**Use:** Cardiac Resynchronization Pacemaker Pulse Generator for Insertion in Subcutaneous Tissue and Fascia
Subcutaneous injection reservoir, port	**Use:** Vascular Access Device, Reservoir in Subcutaneous Tissue and Fascia
Subcutaneous injection reservoir, pump	**Use:** Infusion Device, Pump in Subcutaneous Tissue and Fascia
Subdermal progesterone implant	**Use:** Contraceptive Device in Subcutaneous Tissue and Fascia
Sutureless valve, Perceval	**Use:** Zooplastic Tissue, Rapid Deployment Technique in New Technology
SynCardia Total Artificial Heart	**Use:** Synthetic Substitute
Synchra CRT-P	**Use:** Cardiac Resynchronization Pacemaker Pulse Generator for Insertion in Subcutaneous Tissue and Fascia
Talent® Converter	**Use:** Intraluminal Device

Talent® Occluder	**Use:** Intraluminal Device
Talent® Stent Graft (abdominal) (thoracic)	**Use:** Intraluminal Device
TandemHeart® System	**Use:** Intraluminal Device
TAXUS® Liberté® Paclitaxel-eluting Coronary Stent System	**Use:** Intraluminal Device, Drug-eluting in Heart and Great Vessels
Therapeutic occlusion coil(s)	**Use:** Intraluminal Device
Thoracostomy tube	**Use:** Drainage Device
Thoratec IVAD (Implantable Ventricular Assist Device)	**Use:** Implantable Heart Assist System in Heart and Great Vessels
Thoratec Paracorporeal Ventricular Assist Device	**Use:** External Heart Assist System in Heart and Great Vessels
Tibial insert	**Use:** Liner in Lower Joints
TigerPaw® system for closure of left atrial appendage	**Use:** Extraluminal Device
Tissue bank graft	**Use:** Nonautologous Tissue Substitute
Tissue expander (inflatable) (injectable)	**Use:** Tissue Expander in Skin and Breast Tissue Expander in Subcutaneous Tissue and Fascia
Titanium Sternal Fixation System (TSFS)	**Use:** Internal Fixation Device, Rigid Plate for Insertion in Upper Bones Internal Fixation Device, Rigid Plate for Reposition in Upper Bones
Total artificial (replacement) heart	**Use:** Synthetic Substitute
Tracheostomy tube	**Use:** Tracheostomy Device in Respiratory System
Trifecta™ Valve (aortic)	**Use:** Zooplastic Tissue in Heart and Great Vessels
Tunneled central venous catheter	**Use:** Vascular Access Device in Subcutaneous Tissue and Fascia

APPENDIX C

DEVICE KEY

Tunneled spinal (intrathecal) catheter	**Use:** Infusion Device
Two lead pacemaker	**Use:** Pacemaker, Dual Chamber for Insertion in Subcutaneous Tissue and Fascia
Ultraflex™ Precision Colonic Stent System	**Use:** Intraluminal Device
ULTRAPRO Hernia System (UHS)	**Use:** Synthetic Substitute
ULTRAPRO Partially Absorbable Lightweight Mesh	**Use:** Synthetic Substitute
ULTRAPRO Plug	**Use:** Synthetic Substitute
Ultrasonic osteogenic stimulator	**Use:** Bone Growth Stimulator in Head and Facial Bones Bone Growth Stimulator in Upper Bones Bone Growth Stimulator in Lower Bones
Ultrasound bone healing system	**Use:** Bone Growth Stimulator in Head and Facial Bones Bone Growth Stimulator in Upper Bones Bone Growth Stimulator in Lower Bones
Uniplanar external fixator	**Use:** External Fixation Device, Monoplanar for Insertion in Upper Bones External Fixation Device, Monoplanar for Reposition in Upper Bones External Fixation Device, Monoplanar for Insertion in Lower Bones External Fixation Device, Monoplanar for Reposition in Lower Bones
Urinary incontinence stimulator lead	**Use:** Stimulator Lead in Urinary System
Vaginal pessary	**Use:** Intraluminal Device, Pessary in Female Reproductive System
Valiant Thoracic Stent Graft	**Use:** Intraluminal Device
Vectra® Vascular Access Graft	**Use:** Vascular Access Device in Subcutaneous Tissue and Fascia

Ventrio™ Hernia Patch	**Use:** Synthetic Substitute
Versa	**Use:** Pacemaker, Dual Chamber for Insertion in Subcutaneous Tissue and Fascia
Virtuoso (II) (DR) (VR)	**Use:** Defibrillator Generator for Insertion in Subcutaneous Tissue and Fascia
WALLSTENT® Endoprosthesis	**Use:** Intraluminal Device
X-STOP® Spacer	**Use:** Spinal Stabilization Device, Interspinous Process for Insertion in Upper Joints Spinal Stabilization Device, Interspinous Process for Insertion in Lower Joints
Xenograft	**Use:** Zooplastic Tissue in Heart and Great Vessels
XIENCE V Everolimus Eluting Coronary Stent System	**Use:** Intraluminal Device, Drug-eluting in Heart and Great Vessels
XLIF® System	**Use:** Interbody Fusion Device in Lower Joints
Zenith Flex® AAA Endovascular Graft	**Use:** Intraluminal Device
Zenith TX2® TAA Endovascular Graft	**Use:** Intraluminal Device
Zenith® Renu™ AAA Ancillary Graft	**Use:** Intraluminal Device
Zilver® PTX® (paclitaxel) Drug-Eluting Peripheral Stent	**Use:** Intraluminal Device, Drug-eluting in Upper Arteries Intraluminal Device, Drug-eluting in Lower Arteries
Zimmer® NexGen® LPS Mobile Bearing Knee	**Use:** Synthetic Substitute
Zimmer® NexGen® LPS-Flex Mobile Knee	**Use:** Synthetic Substitute
Zotarolimus-eluting coronary stent	**Use:** Intraluminal Device, Drug-eluting in Heart and Great Vessels

SUBSTANCE KEY

Term	ICD-10-PCS Value
AIGISRx Antibacterial Envelope Antimicrobial envelope	**Use:** Anti-Infective Envelope
Bone morphogenetic protein 2 (BMP 2)	**Use:** Recombinant Bone Morphogenetic Protein
Clolar	**Use:** Clofarabine
Defitelio	**Use:** Defibrotide Sodium Anticoagulant
Factor Xa Inhibitor Reversal Agent, Andexanet Alfa	**Use:** Andexanet Alfa, Factor Xa Inhibitor Reversal Agent
Kcentra	**Use:** 4-Factor Prothrombin Complex Concentrate

Term	ICD-10-PCS Value
Nesiritide	**Use:** Human B-type Natriuretic Peptide
rhBMP-2	**Use:** Recombinant Bone Morphogenetic Protein
Seprafilm	**Use:** Adhesion Barrier
Tissue Plasminogen Activator (tPA) (rtPA)	**Use:** Other Thrombolytic
Vistogard®	**Use:** Uridine Triacetate
Voraxaze	**Use:** Glucarpidase
Zyvox	**Use:** Oxazolidinones

DEVICE AGGREGATION TABLE

Specific Device	for Operation	in Body System	General Device
Autologous Arterial Tissue	All applicable	Heart and Great Vessels Lower Arteries Lower Veins Upper Arteries Upper Veins	**7** Autologous Tissue Substitute
Autologous Venous Tissue	All applicable	Heart and Great Vessels Lower Arteries Lower Veins Upper Arteries Upper Veins	**7** Autologous Tissue Substitute
Cardiac Lead, Defibrillator	Insertion	Heart and Great Vessels	**M** Cardiac Lead
Cardiac Lead, Pacemaker	Insertion	Heart and Great Vessels	**M** Cardiac Lead
Cardiac Resynchronization Defibrillator Pulse Generator	Insertion	Subcutaneous Tissue and Fascia	**P** Cardiac Rhythm Related Device
Cardiac Resynchronization Pacemaker Pulse Generator	Insertion	Subcutaneous Tissue and Fascia	**P** Cardiac Rhythm Related Device
Contractility Modulation Device	Insertion	Subcutaneous Tissue and Fascia	**P** Cardiac Rhythm Related Device
Defibrillator Generator	Insertion	Subcutaneous Tissue and Fascia	**P** Cardiac Rhythm Related Device
Epiretinal Visual Prosthesis	All applicable	Eye	**J** Synthetic Substitute
External Fixation Device, Hybrid	Insertion	Lower Bones Upper Bones	**5** External Fixation Device
External Fixation Device, Hybrid	Reposition	Lower Bones Upper Bones	**5** External Fixation Device
External Fixation Device, Limb Lengthening	Insertion	Lower Bones Upper Bones	**5** External Fixation Device
External Fixation Device, Monoplanar	Insertion	Lower Bones Upper Bones	**5** External Fixation Device
External Fixation Device, Monoplanar	Reposition	Lower Bones Upper Bones	**5** External Fixation Device
External Fixation Device, Ring	Insertion	Lower Bones Upper Bones	**5** External Fixation Device
External Fixation Device, Ring	Reposition	Lower Bones Upper Bones	**5** External Fixation Device
Hearing Device, Bone Conduction	Insertion	Ear, Nose, Sinus	**S** Hearing Device
Hearing Device, Multiple Channel Cochlear Prosthesis	Insertion	Ear, Nose, Sinus	**S** Hearing Device
Hearing Device, Single Channel Cochlear Prosthesis	Insertion	Ear, Nose, Sinus	**S** Hearing Device
Internal Fixation Device, Intramedullary	All applicable	Lower Bones Upper Bones	**4** Internal Fixation Device
Internal Fixation Device, Rigid Plate	Insertion	Upper Bones	**4** Internal Fixation Device
Internal Fixation Device, Rigid Plate	Reposition	Upper Bones	**4** Internal Fixation Device
Intraluminal Device, Pessary	All applicable	Female Reproductive System	**D** Intraluminal Device

DEVICE AGGREGATION TABLE

Specific Device	for Operation	in Body System	General Device
Intraluminal Device, Airway	All applicable	Ear, Nose, Sinus Gastrointestinal System Mouth and Throat	**D** Intraluminal Device
Intraluminal Device, Bioactive	All applicable	Upper Arteries	**D** Intraluminal Device
Intraluminal Device, Branched or Fenestrated, One or Two Arteries	Restriction	Heart and Great Vessels Lower Arteries	**D** Intraluminal Device
Intraluminal Device, Branched or Fenestrated, Three or More Arteries	Restriction	Heart and Great Vessels Lower Arteries	**D** Intraluminal Device
Intraluminal Device, Drug-eluting	All applicable	Heart and Great Vessels Lower Arteries Upper Arteries	**D** Intraluminal Device
Intraluminal Device, Drug-eluting, Four or More	All applicable	Heart and Great Vessels Lower Arteries Upper Arteries	**D** Intraluminal Device
Intraluminal Device, Drug-eluting, Three	All applicable	Heart and Great Vessels Lower Arteries Upper Arteries	**D** Intraluminal Device
Intraluminal Device, Drug-eluting, Two	All applicable	Heart and Great Vessels Lower Arteries Upper Arteries	**D** Intraluminal Device
Intraluminal Device, Endobronchial Valve	All applicable	Respiratory System	**D** Intraluminal Device
Intraluminal Device, Endotracheal Airway	All applicable	Respiratory System	**D** Intraluminal Device
Intraluminal Device, Four or More	All applicable	Heart and Great Vessels Lower Arteries Upper Arteries	**D** Intraluminal Device
Intraluminal Device, Radioactive	All applicable	Heart and Great Vessels	**D** Intraluminal Device
Intraluminal Device, Three	All applicable	Heart and Great Vessels Lower Arteries Upper Arteries	**D** Intraluminal Device
Intraluminal Device, Two	All applicable	Heart and Great Vessels Lower Arteries Upper Arteries	**D** Intraluminal Device
Monitoring Device, Hemodynamic	Insertion	Subcutaneous Tissue and Fascia	**2** Monitoring Device
Monitoring Device, Pressure Sensor	Insertion	Heart and Great Vessels	**2** Monitoring Device
Pacemaker, Dual Chamber	Insertion	Subcutaneous Tissue and Fascia	**P** Cardiac Rhythm Related Device
Pacemaker, Single Chamber	Insertion	Subcutaneous Tissue and Fascia	**P** Cardiac Rhythm Related Device
Pacemaker, Single Chamber Rate Responsive	Insertion	Subcutaneous Tissue and Fascia	**P** Cardiac Rhythm Related Device
Spinal Stabilization Device, Facet Replacement	Insertion	Lower Joints Upper Joints	**4** Internal Fixation Device
Spinal Stabilization Device, Interspinous Process	Insertion	Lower Joints Upper Joints	**4** Internal Fixation Device
Spinal Stabilization Device, Pedicle-Based	Insertion	Lower Joints Upper Joints	**4** Internal Fixation Device

DEVICE AGGREGATION TABLE

Specific Device	for Operation	in Body System	General Device
Stimulator Generator, Multiple Array	Insertion	Subcutaneous Tissue and Fascia	**M** Stimulator Generator
Stimulator Generator, Multiple Array Rechargeable	Insertion	Subcutaneous Tissue and Fascia	**M** Stimulator Generator
Stimulator Generator, Single Array	Insertion	Subcutaneous Tissue and Fascia	**M** Stimulator Generator
Stimulator Generator, Single Array Rechargeable	Insertion	Subcutaneous Tissue and Fascia	**M** Stimulator Generator
Synthetic Substitute, Ceramic	Replacement	Lower Joints	**J** Synthetic Substitute
Synthetic Substitute, Ceramic on Polyethylene	Replacement	Lower Joints	**J** Synthetic Substitute
Synthetic Substitute, Intraocular Telescope	Replacement	Eye	**J** Synthetic Substitute
Synthetic Substitute, Metal	Replacement	Lower Joints	**J** Synthetic Substitute
Synthetic Substitute, Metal on Polyethylene	Replacement	Lower Joints	**J** Synthetic Substitute
Synthetic Substitute, Polyethylene	Replacement	Lower Joints	**J** Synthetic Substitute
Synthetic Substitute, Reverse Ball and Socket	Replacement	Upper Joints	**J** Synthetic Substitute
Synthetic Substitute, Unicondylar	Replacement	Lower Joints	**J** Synthetic Substitute